Baran and Dawber's
**Diseases of the Nails
and their Management**

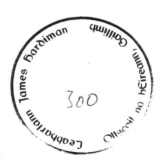

# Baran and Dawber's
# Diseases of the Nails and their Management

EDITED BY

## R. Baran
MD
Le Grand Palais, Nail Disease Centre, Cannes, France

## R.P.R. Dawber
MA, MB, ChB, FRCP
Consultant Dermatologist and Clinical Senior Lecturer,
Department of Dermatology, The Churchill Hospital, Oxford, UK

## D.A.R. de Berker
MB, BS, MRCP
Consultant Dermatologist and Honorary Senior Lecturer,
Department of Dermatology, Bristol Royal Infirmary, Bristol, UK

## E. Haneke
Prof Dr Med
Klinikk Bunas, Sandvika, Oslo, Norway

## A. Tosti
MD
Professor of Dermatology, Istituto di Clinica Dermatologica,
dell' Universita di Bologna, Bologna, Italy

THIRD EDITION

*b*

**Blackwell
Science**

© 1984, 1994, 2001 by
Blackwell Science Ltd
Editorial Offices:
Osney Mead, Oxford OX2 0EL
25 John Street, London WC1N 2BS
23 Ainslie Place, Edinburgh EH3 6AJ
350 Main Street, Malden
  MA 02148-5018, USA
54 University Street, Carlton
  Victoria 3053, Australia
10, rue Casimir Delavigne
  75006 Paris, France

Other Editorial Offices:
Blackwell Wissenschafts-Verlag GmbH
Kurfürstendamm 57
10707 Berlin, Germany

Blackwell Science KK
MG Kodenmacho Building
7–10 Kodenmacho Nihombashi
Chuo-ku, Tokyo 104, Japan

Iowa State University Press
A Blackwell Science Company
2121 S. State Avenue
Ames, Iowa 50014-8300, USA

First published 1984
Second edition 1994
Reprinted 1995, 1997
Third edition 2001

Set by Graphicraft Limited, Hong Kong
Printed and bound in Italy by
Rotolito Lombarda SpA, Milan

The Blackwell Science logo is a
trade mark of Blackwell Science Ltd,
registered at the United Kingdom
Trade Marks Registry

DISTRIBUTORS

Marston Book Services Ltd
PO Box 269
Abingdon, Oxon OX14 4YN
(*Orders*: Tel: 01235 465500
        Fax: 01235 465555)

The Americas
Blackwell Publishing
c/o AIDC
PO Box 20
50 Winter Sport Lane
Williston, VT 05495-0020
(*Orders*: Tel: 800 216 2522
        Fax: 802 864 7626)

Australia
Blackwell Science Pty Ltd
54 University Street
Carlton, Victoria 3053
(*Orders*: Tel: 3 9347 0300
        Fax: 3 9347 5001)

A catalogue record for this title
is available from the British Library

ISBN 0-632-05358-5

Library of Congress
Cataloging-in-publication Data

Baran and Dawber's diseases of the nails and their management /
edited by R. Baran . . . [et al.].—3rd ed.
    p. ; cm.
    Includes bibliographical references and index.
    ISBN 0-632-05358-5
    1. Nails (Anatomy)—Diseases.
    2. Nail manifestations of general diseases.
    I. Title: Diseases of the nails and their management.
    II. Baran, R. (Robert)
    III. Dawber, R. P. R. (Rodney P. R.)
    IV. Diseases of the nails and their management.
    [DNLM: 1. Nail Diseases.
    2. Nails—abnormalities. WR 475 B2251 2001]
    RL165 .D57 2001
    616.5′47—dc21
                                    00-058490

For further information on
Blackwell Science, visit our website:
www.blackwell-science.com

# Contents

# Contributors

**R. Baran** MD
Nail Disease Centre, Le Grand Palais,
42 rue des Serbes,
06400 Cannes, France

**D.A.R. de Berker** MB, BS, MRCP
Consultant Dermatologist and Honorary Senior Lecturer,
Department of Dermatology,
Bristol Royal Infirmary,
Bristol, UK

**E. Brauer** MD (*Deceased*)
Formerly Associate Professor of Clinical Dermatology,
New York University School of Medicine,
New York,
NY, USA

**G.J. Brauner** MD
Associate Clinical Professor of Dermatology,
New York Medical College,
Valhalla,
NY, USA

**R.P.R. Dawber** MA, MB, ChB, FRCP
Consultant Dermatologist and Clinical Senior Lecturer,
Department of Dermatology,
The Churchill Hospital,
Oxford, UK

**J.-L. Drapé** MD, PhD
C.I.E.R.M.,
Hôpital de Bicêtre,
Université Paris Sud,
Le Kremlin-Bicêtre, France

**E. Haneke** Prof Dr Med
Klinikk Bunas, 1337
Sandvika, Oslo, Norway

**R.J. Hay** MA, DM, FRCP, MRCPath
Mary Dunhill Professor of Cutaneous Medicine,
St John's Institute of Dermatology,
St Thomas's Hospital,
London, UK

**L. Juhlin** MD
Professor and Head, Department of Dermatology,
University Hospital,
S-751 85 Uppsala, Sweden

**J.F. Kreusch** PhD, MD
Dermatological Clinic,
University of Luebeck,
23538 Luebeck, Germany

**B. Richert** MD
Department of Dermatology,
Polyclinique Lucien Brull,
4200 Liege, Belgium

**R.J.G. Rycroft** MA, MB, BChir, MD, FRCP
Consultant Dermatologist,
St John's Institute of Dermatology,
St Thomas's Hospital,
London, UK

**A. Tosti** MD
Professor of Dermatology,
Istituto di Clinica Dermatologica
dell' Universita di Bologna,
40138 Bologna, Italy

**E.G. Zook** MD
Professor of Surgery and Chairman,
Southern Illinois School of Medicine,
Institute of Plastic Surgery,
Springfield,
IL 62708, USA

# Preface to the Third Edition

It is now over 20 years since we first conceived the idea of a detailed reference book on all aspects of nail science, nail disorders and their treatment. By that time in our lecturing and teaching commitments around the world we had been privileged to work with a vast array of great experts in the field, all beginning to move across traditional specialty boundaries—one saw podiatrists with great operating skills working with dermatological and plastic surgeons; beauticians showing doctors that aesthetic and 'functional' remedies may at times be more relevant than formal medical therapeutics; geneticists seeing that the nail apparatus may give more specific insight into mechanisms of hereditary diseases than other sites . . . and so on. Blackwell Science accepted the project and the first edition appeared in 1984.

The 'cross-fertilization' between specialists has continued apace during the last 17 years to the extent that expanding knowledge and better medical and surgical treatments have led to the Third Edition being 50% larger than the First Edition. This expansion has been controlled and enhanced by the editorial team increasing to five—David de Berker, Antonella Tosti and Eckart Haneke have great breadth of experience in the scientific and clinical aspects of the nail apparatus and those used to the Second Edition will recognize this input well beyond their specific contributions to many chapters. There has been considerable enlargement of the sections on nail apparatus tumours and nail surgery; this is due almost entirely to the new contributions by Elvin Zook and Jean-Luc Drapé. Last but not least we welcome Bernard Richert; his clinical experience has been carefully applied to the physical signs section. Significant changes have occurred in the understanding and treatment of onychomycosis since the Second Edition and this is reflected in the fungal diseases section.

Many clinical figures included in this edition have been contributed by colleagues from all over the world and we offer them our most grateful thanks; we hope that all their contributions have been acknowledged in the text and apologise if inadvertently we have failed to do so at any point. After three editions of this book it is time for a very particular acknowledgement to be made to Nicole Baran. Those directly involved will know of her immense administrative commitment far beyond the call of duty! One can truly say that she is the great catalyst that has made the book gel.

Robert Baran
Rodney Dawber

# Preface to the First Edition

Since the earliest publication by Heller there have been several books written on diseases of the nail: in particular the works of Alkiewicz and Pfister; Pardo-Castello and Pardo; Samman, Sertoli and Zaïas must be mentioned as they are of high quality and extremely useful, mainly to dermatologists.

For many years we have felt that there is a need for a comprehensive reference book on all aspects of the nail in health and disease. It is evident that in different cultures nail abnormalities are often seen by a variety of specialists, e.g. traumatic and genetic dystrophies are rarely seen initially by dermatologists whilst cosmetic and industrial problems may be handled by dermatologists, industrial health experts, cosmetologists or chiropodists. These are a few examples of the need for a reference book to 'cross' speciality, and even more important, parochial, national medical barriers. We believe that a satisfactory book on the nail must do this. The world is small! We have both travelled widely in recent years and do hope that the content and style of the book succeeds in this aim.

Some people may be surprised to find a Frenchman and Englishman apparently having agreed with each other for long enough to produce a book of this nature—not all French and English are enemies! We have worked diligently to benefit from our language differences and to combine the differences in training and interests and hope that this first truly international book, including authors from France, Germany, Sweden, UK and USA, will be of use world-wide.

Though the chapters have been contributed by specific authors, we must point out that the book is very much a group activity; in particular, the editors have contributed much from their own files to every section. This applies to the script, references and figures, and therefore any errors of fact, emphasis or quality of picture may be the fault of the editors rather than the named chapter writers!

The inclusion of colour pictures has obviously made the book more expensive than with black and white pictures alone. We gave considerable thought to this and decided to include them as important diagnostic aids because of the photogenic nature of the nail; and the fact that between the ten authors we had a unique opportunity to pool material collected over many years.

## Acknowledgements

An undertaking of this kind is quite impossible without the help of a vast number of colleagues the world over who have encouraged, cajoled and constructively disagreed with us over the many years that we have been interested in nails; and more specifically we must thank those who have provided details and pictures of their patients—these are acknowledged in the script.

We are deeply indebted to Georges Achten, Peter Samman and Nardo Zaïas who at various times have stimulated our interest in this field; without their help in our careers this book would not have materialized in any shape or form.

We are very grateful to Dr Gerald Godfrey and Chris Gummer who gave great assistance in formulating the final text.

Robert Baran
Rodney Dawber

# CHAPTER 1

# Science of the nail apparatus

**R.P.R. Dawber, D.A.R. de Berker & R. Baran**

## Gross anatomy and terminology

The nail is an opalescent window through to the vascular nail bed. It is held in place by the nail folds, origin at the matrix and attachment to the nail bed. It ends at a free edge distally, overlying the hyponychium. These structures are illustrated in Figs 1.1 and 1.2. The definition of the components of the nail unit are as follows:

**Nail plate (nail):** Durable keratinized structure which continues growing throughout life.

**Lateral nail folds:** The cutaneous folded structures providing the lateral borders to the nail.

**Proximal nail fold (posterior nail fold):** Cutaneous folded structure providing the visible proximal border of the nail, continuous with the cuticle. On the undersurface this becomes the dorsal matrix.

**Cuticle (eponychium):** The layer of epidermis extending from the proximal nail fold and adhering to the dorsal aspect of the nail plate.

**Nail matrix (nail root):** Traditionally, this can be split into three parts (Lewis 1954). The dorsal matrix is synonymous with the ventral aspect of the proximal nail fold. Intermediate matrix (germinative matrix) is the epithelial structure starting at the point that the dorsal matrix folds back on itself to underlie the proximal nail. The ventral matrix is synonymous with the nail bed and starts at the border of the lunula, where the intermediate matrix stops. It is limited distally by the hyponychium.

**Lunula (half moon):** The convex margin of the intermediate matrix seen through the nail. It is more pale than adjacent nail bed. It is most commonly visible on the thumbs and great toes. It may be concealed by the proximal nail fold.

**Nail bed (ventral matrix, sterile matrix):** The vascular bed upon which the nail rests extending from the lunula to the hyponychium. This is the major territory seen through the nail plate.

**Onychodermal band:** The distal margin of the nail bed has a contrasting hue in comparison with the rest of the nail bed (Terry 1955). Normally, this is a transverse band of 1–1.5 mm of a deeper pink (Caucasian) or brown (Afro-Carribean). Its colour, or presence, may vary with disease or compression which influences the vascular supply (Fig. 1.3). Sonnex *et al.* (1991) examined 1000 nails from thumbs and fingers in 100 subjects, alive and dead. In addition to clinical observation they obtained histology from cadavers. Their findings can be summarized in Table 1.1. The onychocorneal band represents the first barrier to penetration of materials to beneath the nail plate. Disruption of this barrier by disease or trauma precipitates a range of further events affecting the nail bed. The white appearance of the central band represents the transmission of light from the digit tip through the stratum corneum and up through the nail. If the digit is placed against a black surface, the band appears dark.

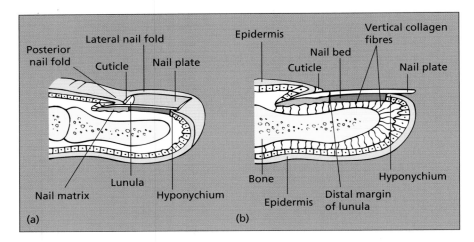

Fig. 1.1 Longitudinal section of a digit showing the dorsal nail apparatus.

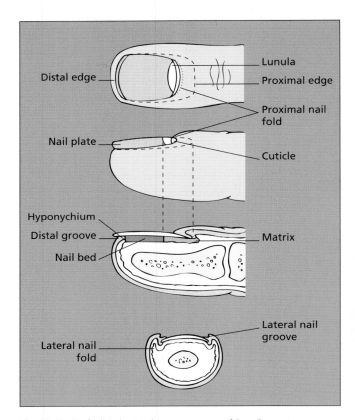

Fig. 1.2 The tip of a digit showing the component parts of the nail apparatus.

**Hyponychium (contains the Solenhorn):** The cutaneous margin underlying free nail, bordered distally by the distal groove.

**Distal groove (limiting furrow):** A cutaneous ridge demarcating the border between subungual structures and the finger pulp.

## References

Lewis, B.L. (1954) Microscopic studies of fetal and mature nail and surrounding soft tissue. *Archives of Dermatology and Syphilis* 70, 732–744.

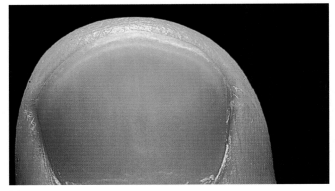

(a)

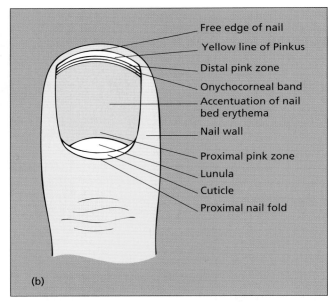

(b)

Fig. 1.3 (a) Onychodermal band. (b) Diagrammatic representation of the morphological features of the normal nail; detail of the distal physiological colour bands are shown. (Courtesy of T.S. Sonnex and W.A.D. Griffiths, St John's Institute of Dermatology.)

**Table 1.1** Clinical appearance of distal zones of the nail bed.

| Zone | Sub-zone | Appearance |
|---|---|---|
| Free edge | | Clear grey |
| Onychocorneal band | | |
| I | Distal pink zone | 0.5–2 mm distal pink margin, may merge with free edge |
| II | Central white band | 0.1–1 mm distal white band representing the point of attachment of the stratum corneum arising from the digit pulp |
| III | Proximal pink gradient | Merging with nail bed |

Sonnex, T.S., Griffiths, W.A.D. & Nicol, W.J. (1991) The nature and significance of the transverse white band of human nails. *Seminars in Dermatology* **10**, 12–16.

Terry, R.B. (1955) The onychodermal band in health and disease. *Lancet* **i**, 179–181.

## Embryology

### Morphogenesis

#### 8–12 weeks

Individual digits are discernible from the 8th week of gestation (Lewis 1954). The first embryonic element of the nail unit is the nail anlage present from 9 weeks as the epidermis overlying the dorsal tip of the digit. At 10 weeks a distinct region can be seen and is described as the primary nail field. This almost overlies the tip of the terminal phalanx, with clear proximal and lateral grooves in addition to a well-defined distal groove. The prominence of this groove is partly due to the distal ridge, thrown up proximally, accentuating the contour. The primary nail field grows proximally by a wedge of germinative matrix cells extending back from the tip of the digit. These cells are proximal to both the distal groove and ridge. The spatial relationship of these two latter structures remains relatively constant as the former becomes the vestigial distal groove and the latter the hyponychium (Fig. 1.4).

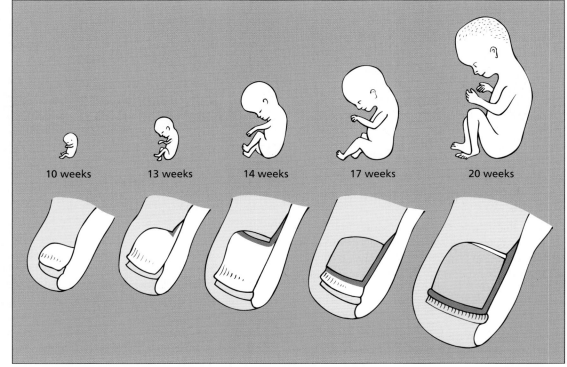

**Fig. 1.4** Embryogenesis of the nail apparatus. 10 weeks: the primary nail field can be seen with proximal, lateral and distal grooves. The latter is accentuated by a distal ridge. 13 weeks: a wedge of matrix primordium moves proximally, with the invagination of the proximal nail fold above. 14 weeks: the nail plate emerges. 17 weeks: the nail plate covers most of the nail bed and the distal ridge starts to flatten. 20 weeks: the nail plate extends to the distal ridge, now termed hyponychium. Finger and nail grow roughly in tandem from now on. Fetuses are one-fifth of the actual size.

10 weeks    13 weeks    14 weeks    17 weeks    20 weeks

### 13–14 weeks

Differential growth of the slowly developing primary nail field and surrounding tissue results in the emergence of overhanging proximal and lateral nail folds. Depending on the point of reference, the nail folds may be interpreted as overhanging (Warwick & Williams 1973) or the matrix as invaginating. By 13 weeks the nail field is well defined in the finger, with the matrix primordium underlying a proximal nail fold. By 14 weeks the nail plate is seen emerging from beneath the proximal nail fold, with elements arising from the lunula as well as more proximal matrix.

### 17 weeks to birth

At 17 weeks, the nail plate covers most of the nail bed and the distal ridge has flattened. From 20 weeks, the nail unit and finger grow in tandem, with the nail plate abutting the distal ridge. This now becomes termed the hyponychium. The nail bed epithelium no longer produces keratohyalin, with a more parakeratotic appearance. By birth the nail plate extends to the distal groove, which becomes progressively less prominent. The nail may curve over the volar surface of the finger. It may also demonstrate koilonychia. This deformity is normal in the very young and a function of the thinness of the nail plate. It reverses with age.

## Tissue differentiation

Keratin synthesis can be identified in the nail unit from the earliest stages of its differentiation (Moll *et al.* 1988). In 12- and 13-week embryos, the nail-matrix anlage is a thin epithelial wedge penetrating from the dorsal epidermis into the dermis. This wedge is thought to represent the 'ventral matrix primordium'. Keratin represents about 80% of the intracellular structural protein of epithelial cells. It belongs to the family of intermediate filaments. There are many different keratins with varied structural properties and localization within animals. They are divided into two groups, the first of which are 'soft', epithelial keratins commonly found in the skin. The second is 'hard', trichocyte or hair/nail keratins found in hair, nail, thymus, tooth primordia and tongue. Unfortunately, the funding for research and the access of researchers to scalp rather than nail matrix as a substrate for study means that these keratins are most commonly referred to in the literature as hair keratins. We feel that it is more precise to refer to them by their physical characteristics as 'hard' keratins rather than by a misleading epithet defining only one of their origins.

By week 15, hard keratins are seen throughout the nail bed and matrix. This could have significance concerning theories of nail embryogenesis and growth, where debate exists as to the contribution made by the nail bed to nail growth (Lewis 1954; Zaias 1963; Hashimoto *et al.* 1966; Zaias & Alvarez 1968;

Johnson *et al.* 1991). However, at 22 weeks, the layer of hard keratin positive cells remains very thin in the nail bed, whereas it is considerably thickened in the matrix. In the adult nail, there have been reports of both the presence (Baden & Kubilus 1984) and absence (Heid *et al.* 1988; Moll *et al.* 1988; de Berker *et al.* 1992; Westgate *et al.* 1997) of hard keratins in the nail bed.

Histological observation at 13 and 14 weeks reveals parakeratotic cells just distal to this nail plate primordium staining for disulphydryl groups. This contrasts to adjacent epithelium, suggesting the start of nail plate differentiation. This early differentiation represents matrix formation and Merkel cells have been detected in the matrix primordium of human fetuses between weeks 9 and 15 (Moll & Moll 1993). Merkel cells may play a role in the development of epidermal appendages and are detectable using monoclonal antibodies specific to keratin 20. Their role in ontogenesis would explain their disappearance from the nail matrix after week 22 (Moll & Moll 1993). However, this is not a universal finding, with an abundance of Merkel cells identified in the matrix of young adult and cadaver nail specimens in one study (Cameli *et al.* 1998).

At the 13–22-week stage there is coincident increase in the expression of hard keratins and the development of keratohyalin granules.

By 25 weeks, most features of nail unit differentiation are complete. Changes may still occur in the chemical constitution of the nail plate after this date. A decrease in sulphur and aluminium and a rise in chlorine has been noted as a feature of full-term newborns in comparison with the nail plate of premature babies (Sirota *et al.* 1988). An elevated aluminium level may correspond to bone abnormalities which lead to osteopenia.

## Factors in embryogenesis

The nail plate grows from the 15th week of gestation until death. Many factors act upon it in this time and influence its appearance. Because it is a rugged structure, growing over a cycle of 4–18 months, it provides a record of the effects of these influences. To consider the different formative mechanisms, it is important to distinguish:

1 embryogenesis;
2 regrowth;
3 growth.

There is overlap in all these processes, with the main clues concerning embryogenesis deriving from fetal studies and analysis of congenital abnormalities. Regrowth is the growth of the nail plate following its removal. This may be for therapeutic reasons or following accidental trauma with associated damage. Observations of this process add to our understanding of both growth and embryogenesis. Growth is the continuous process of nail plate generation over a fully differentiated nail bed and hyponychium. Embryogenesis is the subject of this section.

In the chick limb bud formation there is a complex interaction between mesoderm and ectoderm. Initially, the mesoderm induces the development of the apical ectodermal ridge (AER). The mesoderm then becomes dependent upon the AER for the creation of the limb. Removal of the AER results in a halt of mesodermal differentiation. Replacing the underlying mesoderm with mesoderm from another part of the limb primordium still results in normal differentiation (Zwilling 1968). However, the AER continues to be dependent upon the mesoderm, which must be of limb type. Replacement of limb mesoderm with somite mesoderm causes flattening of the AER. These morphogenetic interactions occur prior to cytodifferentiation (Grant 1978). In the human, cases of anonychia secondary to phenytoin (Hanson & Smith 1975) might implicate the drug at this stage, prior to 8 weeks. Drugs have been argued as being contributory to congenital nail dystrophies mainly affecting the index finger (Higashi *et al.* 1975).

Dermal–epidermal interactions in appendage formation have been closely examined using the hair follicle, where the role of the dermal papilla is central in the induction of epidermal differentiation, both *in vivo* and *in vitro* (Jahoda 1984; Reynolds *et al.* 1993).

Other congenital abnormalities highlight the debate that spans embryogenesis, growth and regrowth. Congenital onychodysplasia of the index fingers (COIF) is frequently associated with abnormalities of the terminal phalanges and interphalangeal joints (Baran 1980). The nail may be absent, small or composed of several small nails on the dorsal tip of the affected finger. The bony abnormality varies, with the most marked change being bifurcation of the terminal phalanx on lateral X-ray (Millman & Strier 1982). However, a bony abnormality is not mandatory in this condition or other conditions with ectopic nail (Aoki & Suzuki 1984). A normal nail may overly an abnormal bone on other than the index finger (Kinoshita & Nagano 1976). COIF appears to demonstrate an association between abnormalities of bone and nail, rather than the presence of a strict relationship. It may represent a fault of mesoderm/ectoderm interaction at the stage when these layers are mutually dependent. It has been suggested that a vascular abnormality may provide the common factor between pathology in the two embryonic layers (Kitayama & Tsukada 1983). If this is the case, it appears likely that any vascular abnormality arises due to a defect of patterned embryogenesis rather than a random event, given that a form of COIF can occur in the big toe of individuals with involved fingers (Koizumi *et al.* 1998).

An interpretation based upon a mutual mesodermal and ectodermal fault would fit with the observation of two cases of congenital anonychia and hypoplastic nails combined with hypoplastic phalanges (Baran & Juhlin 1986). These cases were used as a foil for the suggestion of a mechanism of 'bone dependent nail formation'. It might also be argued in reverse that the bone was dependent upon the nail.

## References

Aoki, K. & Suzuki, H. (1984) The morphology and hardness of the nail in two cases of congenital onychoheterotopia. *British Journal of Dermatology* **110**, 717–723.

Baden, H.P. & Kubilus, J. (1984) A comparative study of the immunologic properties of hoof and nail fibrous proteins. *Journal of Investigative Dermatology* **83**, 327–331.

Baran, R. (1980) Syndrome d'Iso et Kikuchi (COIF syndrome); 2 cas avec revue de la littérature (44 cas). *Annales de Dermatologie et de Vénéréologie* **107**, 431–435.

Baran, R. & Juhlin, L. (1986) Bone dependent nail formation. *British Journal of Dermatology* **114**, 371–375.

de Berker, D., Leigh, I. & Wojnarowska, F. (1992) Patterns of keratin expression in the nail unit—an indicator of regional matrix differentiation. *British Journal of Dermatology* **127**, 423.

Cameli, N., Ortonne, J.P., Picardo, M., Peluso, A.M. & Tosti, A. (1998) Distribution of Merkel cells in adult human nail matrix (letter). *British Journal of Dermatology* **139**, 541.

Grant, P. (ed.) (1978) Limb morphogenesis: a dialog between an ectodermal sheet and mesoderm. In: *Biology of Developing Systems*, pp. 414–421. Holt, Rinehart and Winston, New York.

Hanson, J.W. & Smith, D.W. (1975) The fetal hydantoin syndrome. *Journal of Pediatrics* **87**, 285–290.

Hashimoto, K., Gross, B.G., Nelson, R. & Lever, W.F. (1966) The ultrastructure of the skin of human embryos. III. The formation of the nail in 16–18 week old embryos. *Journal of Investigative Dermatology* **47**, 205–207.

Heid, H.W., Moll, I. & Franke, W.W. (1988) Patterns of trichocytic and epithelial cytokeratins in mammalian tissues. II. Concomitant and mutually exclusive synthesis of trichocytic and epithelial cytokeratins in diverse human and bovine tissues. *Differentiation* **37**, 215–230.

Higashi, N., Ikegami, T. & Asada, Y. (1975) Congenital nail defects of the index finger. *Japanese Journal of Clinical Dermatology* **29**, 699–701.

Jahoda, C.A.B. (1984) Induction of hair growth by implantation of cultured dermal papilla cells. *Nature* **311**, 560–562.

Johnson, M., Comaish, J.S. & Shuster, S. (1991) Nail is produced by the normal nail bed: a controversy resolved. *British Journal of Dermatology* **125**, 27–29.

Kinoshita, Y. & Nagano, T. (1976) Congenital defects of the index finger. *Japanese Journal of Plastic and Reconstructive Surgery* **19**, 23.

Kitayama, Y. & Tsukada, S. (1983) Congenital onychodysplasia. Report of 11 cases. *Archives of Dermatology* **119**, 8–12.

Koizumi, H., Tomoyori, T. & Ohkawara, A. (1998) Congenital onychodysplasia of the index fingers with anomaly of the great toe. *Acta Dermato-Venereologica* **78**, 478–479.

Lewis, B.L. (1954) Microscopic studies of fetal and mature nail and surounding soft tissue. *Archives of Dermatology and Syphilis* **70**, 732–744.

Millman, A.J. & Strier, R.P. (1982) Congenital onychodysplasia of the index fingers. *Journal of the American Academy of Dermatology* **7**, 57–65.

Moll, I., Heid, H.W., Franke, W.W. & Moll, R. (1988) Patterns of expression of trichocytic and epithelial cytokeratins in mammalian tissues. *Differentiation* **39**, 167–184.

Moll, I. & Moll, R. (1993) Merkel cells in ontogenesis of human nails. *Archives of Dermatological Research* **285**, 366–371.

Reynolds, A.J., Lawrence, C.M. & Jahoda, C.A. (1993) Human hair follicle germinative epidermal cell culture. *Journal of Investigative Dermatology* **101**, 634–638.

Sirota, L., Straussberg, R., Fishman, P. *et al.* (1988) X-ray microanalysis of the fingernails in term and preterm infants. *Pediatric Dermatology* **5**, 184–186.

Warwick, R. & Williams, P.L. (eds) (1973) *Gray's Anatomy*, 35th edn. Longman, Harlow, Essex.

Westgate, G.E., Tidman, N., de Berker, D., Blount, M.A., Philpott, M.P. & Leigh, I.M. (1997) Characterisation of LH Tric 1, a new monospecific monoclonal antibody to the hair keratin Ha 1 Br. *Journal of Dermatology* **137**, 24–31.

Zaias, N. (1963) Embryology of the human nail. *Archives of Dermatology* **87**, 37–53.

Zaias, N. & Alvarez, J. (1968) The formation of the primate nail plate. An autoradiographic study in the squirrel monkey. *Journal of Investigative Dermatology* **51**, 120–136.

Zwilling, E. (1968) Morphogenetic phases in development. In: *The Emergence of Order in Developing Systems.* (eds M. Locke), pp. 184–207. Academic Press, New York.

# Regional anatomy

## Histological preparation

High quality sections of the nail unit are difficult to obtain. Nails are very hard and tend to split or tear. In biopsies containing nail plate and soft subungual and periungual tissue, the nail plate is often torn from the matrix and other adjacent structures by the microtome. This effect can be diminished by softening the nail, which may be less practical if there are soft tissue attachments requiring histological examination.

### Nail softening techniques

#### Nail alone

There are several different techniques to soften the nail plate. Lewis (1954) recommended routine fixation in 10% formalin and processing as usual. Earlier methods employed used fixation with potassium bichromate, sodium sulphate and water. The section is then decalcified with nitric acid and embedded in collodion. Alkiewicz and Pfister (1976) recommended softening the nail with thioglycollate or hydrogen peroxide. Nail fragments are kept in 10% potassium thioglycollate at 37°C for 5 days or in 20–30% hydrogen peroxide for 5–6 days. The nail is then fixed by boiling in formalin for 1 min before cutting 10–15 μm sections.

Although softening of nail clippings for histology is not mandatory, it is possible and may be helpful. Suarez *et al.* (1991) suggest soaking the clipping for 2 days in a mix of mercuric chloride, chromic acid, nitric acid and 95% alcohol.

The specimen is then transferred to absolute alcohol, xylene, successive paraffin mixtures, sectioned at 4 μm and placed on gelatinized slides. An alternative method, described for preserving histological detail in the nail plate, entails fixation in a mix of 5% trichloracetic acid and 10% formalin for the initial 24 h (Alvarez & Zaias 1967). This is followed by a modified polyethylene glycol-pyroxylin embedding method.

#### Nail and soft tissue

In nail biopsies containing soft tissue, more gentle methods of preparation are necessary. The specimen can be soaked in distilled water for a few hours before placing in formalin (Bennett 1976). Good results are obtained with routine fixation and embedding if permanent wave solution, thioglycollate or 10% potassium hydroxide solution, is applied with a cotton swab to the surface of the paraffin block every two or three sections. Lewin *et al.* (1973) suggests applying 1% aqueous polysorbate 40 to the cut surface of the block for 1 h at 4°C.

Sections will sometimes adhere to normal slides, but when there is nail alone, the material tends to curl as it dries and may fall off. This means that it may be necessary to use gelatinized or 3-aminopropyltriethoxysilane (APES) slides. Given the difficulty in obtaining high quality sections it is worth cutting many at different levels to maximize the chance of getting what you need.

Routine staining with haematoxylin and eosin is sufficient for most cases. Periodic acid Schiff (PAS) and Grocott's silver stain can be used to demonstrate fungi; a blancophore fluorochromation selectively delineates fungal walls (Haneke 1991). Toluidine blue at pH 5 allows better visualization of the details of the nail plate (Achten 1963; Achten *et al.* 1991). Fontana's argentaffin reaction demonstrates melanin. Haemoglobin is identified using a peroxidase reaction. Prussian Blue and Perl stains are not helpful in the identification of blood in the nail. They are specific to the haemosiderin product of haemoglobin breakdown caused by macrophages. This does not occur in the nail (Achten & Wanet 1973; Alkiewicz & Pfister 1976; Baran & Haneke 1984).

Masson-Goldner's trichrome stain is very useful to study the keratinization process and Giemsa stain reveals slight changes in the nail keratin.

Polarization microscopy shows the regular arrangement of keratin filaments and birefringence is said to be absent in disorders of nail formation such as leuconychia.

## Nail matrix and lunula

For simplicity, the nail matrix (syn. intermediate matrix) will be defined as the most proximal region of the nail bed extending to the lunula. This is commonly considered to be the source of the bulk of the nail plate, although further contributions may come from other parts of the nail unit (qv. nail growth). Contrast with these other regions helps characterize the matrix.

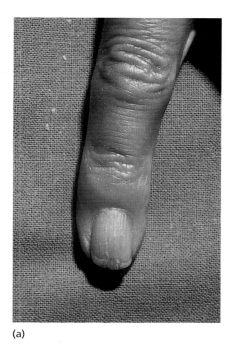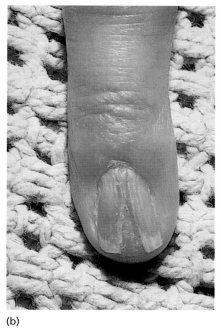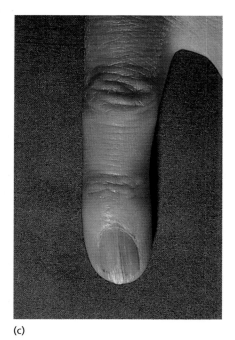

(a)             (b)             (c)

**Fig. 1.5** Longitudinal nail biopsy of Zaias: (a) before biopsy; (b) 5 weeks after; (c) 3 months later.

The matrix is vulnerable to surgical and accidental trauma; a longitudinal biopsy of greater than 3 mm width is likely to leave a permanent dystrophy (Zaias 1967) (Fig. 1.5). Once matrix damage has occurred, it is difficult to effectively repair it (Nakayama *et al.* 1990; Pessa *et al.* 1990). This accounts for the relatively small amount of histological information on normal nail matrix.

It is possible to make distinctions between distal and proximal matrix on functional grounds, given that 81% of cell numbers in the nail plate are provided by the proximal 50% of the nail matrix (de Berker *et al.* 1996b) and surgery to distal matrix is less likely to cause scarring than more proximal surgery.

Clinically, the matrix is synonymous with the lunula, or half moon, which can be seen through the nail emerging from beneath the proximal nail fold as a pale convex structure. This is most prominent on the thumb, becoming less prominent in a gradient towards the little finger. It is rarely seen on the toes. The absence of a clinically identifiable lunula may mean that the vascular tone of the nail bed and matrix have obscured it or that the proximal nail fold extends so far along the nail plate that it lies over the entire matrix.

High resolution magnetic resonance imaging idenitifies the matrix and dermal zones beneath. Drapé *et al.* (1996) described a zone beneath the distal matrix where there is loose connective tissue and a dense microvascular network. It may be the presence of this network that accounts for the variable sign of red lunulae in some systemic conditions (Wilkerson & Wilkin 1989; Cohen 1996). However, the histological observations of Lewin suggested that there is diminished vascularity and increased dermal collagen beneath the matrix contributing to

the pallor which helps identify the area (Lewin 1965). This has been confirmed in a more recent study utilizing injection of gelatinized Indian ink into amputation specimens (Wolfram-Gabel & Sick 1995).

The thinner epidermis of the nail bed may account for the contrast between white and pink appearance of the lunula and bed, respectively (Burrows 1917). Many suggestions have been made to account for the appearance of the lunula (Burrows 1917, 1919; Ham & Leeson 1961; Achten 1963; Lewin 1965; Baran & Gioanni 1969):
1 The matrix epithelium in the lunula has more nuclei than the nail bed, making it appear parakeratotic with an altered colour.
2 The surface of the nail is smoother and more shiny proximally.
3 The thicker epidermis of the lunula obscures the underlying vasculature.
4 The nail attachment at the lunula is less firm, allowing greater refraction and reflection at the nail/soft tissue interface.
5 The underlying dermis has less capillaries in it.
6 The underlying dermis is of looser texture.

Macroscopically, the distal margin of the matrix is convex and is easily distinguished from the contiguous nail bed once the nail is removed, even if the difference is not clear prior to avulsion. The nail bed is a more deep red and has surface corrugations absent from the matrix. At the proximal margin of the matrix, the contour of the lunula is repeated. At the lateral apices, a subtle ligamentous attachment has been described, arising as a dorsal expansion of the lateral ligament of the distal interphalangeal joint (Guero *et al.* 1994). Lack of balance between the symmetrical tension on these attachments may

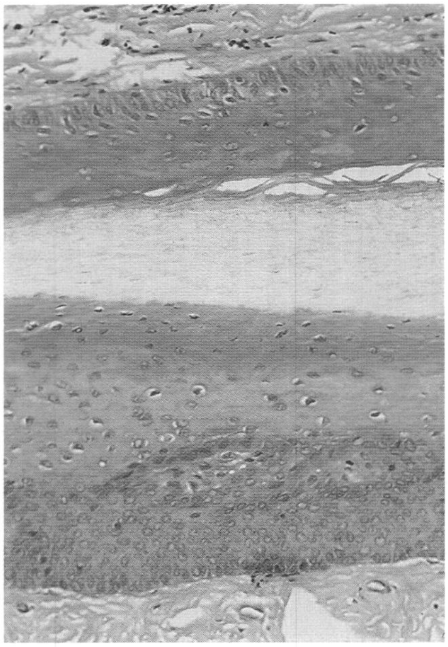

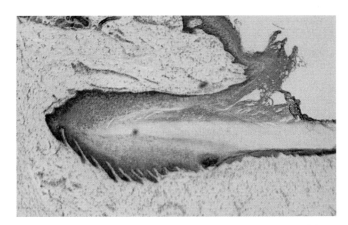

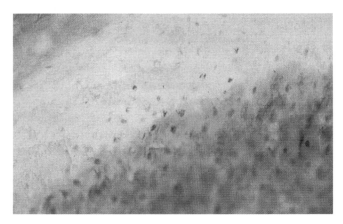

**Fig. 1.7** Keratin stain of the nail apparatus delineating the epithelial structures of the matrix and proximal nail fold.

**Fig. 1.6** A granular layer is absent from the germinal matrix (lower part) and the ventral aspect of the proximal nail fold (upper part).

explain some forms of acquired and congenital malalignment (de Berker & Baran 1998).

### Routine histology

The cells of the nail matrix are distinct from the adjacent nail bed distally and the ventral surface of the nail fold, lying at an angle above. The nail matrix is the thickest area of stratified squamous epithelium in the midline of the nail unit, comparable with the hyponychium. There are long rete ridges characteristically descending at a slightly oblique angle, their tips pointing distally. Laterally, the matrix rete ridges are less marked, whereas those of the nail bed nail folds become prominent.

Unlike the overlying nail fold, but like the nail bed, the matrix has no granular layer (Fig. 1.6). The demarcation between overlying nail fold and matrix is enhanced by the altered morphology of the rete ridges. At their junction at the apex of the matrix and origin of the nail, the first matrix epithelial ridge may have a bobbed appearance like a lopped sheep's tail. Periodic acid Schiff staining is marked at both the distal and proximal margins of the intermediate matrix (Fig. 1.7).

Distally, there is often a step reduction in the epithelial thickness at the transition of the matrix with the nail bed. This represents the edge of the lunula.

Nail is formed from the matrix as cells become larger and more pale and eventually the nucleus disintegrates. There is progression with flattening, elongation and further pallor. Occasionally retained shrunken or fragmented nuclei persist to be included into the nail plate. Lewis (1954) called these 'pertinax bodies'. They can give an impression of the longitudinal progression of growth in the nail plate (Fig. 1.8).

**Fig. 1.8** Pertinax bodies can be seen as the nuclear remnants within the nail plate.

Melanocytes are present in the matrix where they reach a density of up to $300/mm^2$ (Higashi 1968; Higashi & Saito 1969; Tosti *et al.* 1994; de Berker *et al.* 1996a; Perrin *et al.* 1997). They are dendritic cells found in the epibasal layers and most prominent in the distal matrix (Tosti *et al.* 1994; de Berker *et al.* 1996a; Perrin *et al.* 1997). This point can be refined in terms of the functional status of the melanocytes. Ortonne described melanocytes of the proximal matrix as being in a single compartment of largely dormant cells. Those in the distal matrix are in two compartments, with both a dormant and functionally differentiated population. Longitudinal melanonychia most commonly arises from pigment contributed to the nail plate by these differentiated distal melanocytes. Ortonne also defined a smaller population of nail bed melanocytes, with approximately 25% of the number found in the matrix and none of these were differentiated in terms of DOPA staining. This differs from the observations of de Berker *et al.* (1996a) where the nail bed was noted to lack melanocyte markers.

The suprabasal location of nail matrix melanocytes can lead to difficulties in the interpretation of histological specimens obtained to exclude dysplasia in instances of melanonychia, given that ascending melanocytes is a sign of dysplasia in normal epidermis. This complication may be related to the fact that the differentiation of melanocytes in the matrix is different from that found elsewhere given that they typically do not produce pigment in Caucasians and they are detected by the antibody HMB-45, which recognizes melanoma cells and fetal melanocytes but not mature melanocytes (Tosti *et al.* 1994). In spite of these difficulties of interpretation, melanoma is a relatively rare cause of subungual pigmentation, although it is usually considered necessary to exclude it histologically, particularly in white adults (Tosti *et al.* 1994; Molina & Sanchez 1995).

Melanin in the nail plate is composed of granules derived from matrix melanocytes (Zaias 1963). Longitudinal melanonychia may be a benign phenomenon, particularly in Afro-Caribbeans—77% of black people will have a melanonychia by the age of 20 and almost 100% by 50 (Monash 1932; Leyden *et al.* 1972). The Japanese also have a high prevalence of longitudinal melanonychia, being present in 10–20% of adults (Kopf & Waldo 1980). In a study of 15 benign melanonychia in Japanese patients, they were found to arise from an increase in activity and number of DOPA-positive melanocytes in the matrix, not a melanocytic naevus (Higashi 1968). Longitudinal melanonychia in Caucasians is more sinister. Oropeza (1986) stated that a subungual pigmented lesion in this group has a higher chance of being malignant than of being benign.

There is only a thin layer of dermis dividing the matrix from the terminal phalanx. This has a rich vascular supply (see below) and an elastin and collagen infrastructure giving attachment to periosteum.

### Electron microscopy

Transmission electron microscopy confirms that in many respects, matrix epithelium is similar to normal cutaneous epithelium. (Hashimoto 1971a,b,c,d). The basal cells contain desmosomes and hemidesmosomes and interdigitate freely. Differentiating cells are rich in ribosomes and polysomes and contain more RNA than equivalent cutaneous epidermal cells. As cell differentiation proceeds towards the nail plate, there is an accumulation of cytoplasmic microfibrils (7.5–10 nm). These fibrils are haphazardly arranged within the cells up to the transitional zone. Beyond this, they become aligned with the axis of nail plate growth.

Membrane-coating granules (Odland bodies) are formed within the differentiating cells. They are discharged onto the cell surface in the transitional zone and have been thought to contribute to the thickness of the plasma membrane. They may also have a role in the firm adherence of the squamous cells within the nail plate, which is a notable characteristic (Parent *et al.* 1985). The glycoprotein characteristics of cell membrane complexes isolated from nail plate may reflect the constituents of these granules (Allen *et al.* 1991).

Mitochondria are degraded during the transitional phase, whilst RNA-containing ribosomes are evident up to the stage of plasma membrane thickening. Vacuoles containing lipid and other products of cytolysis are seen at the transitional stage. Dorsal matrix cells start to show nuclear shrinkage at this point, whereas the nuclei in the matrix remain intact to a higher level.

## References

Achten, G. (1963) L'ongle normal et pathologique. *Dermatologica* **126**, 229–245.

Achten, G. & Wanet, J. (1973) Pathologie der nagel. In: *Spezielle Pathologische Anatomie*, Vol. 7 (eds W. Doerr, G. Seifert & E. Uehlinger), pp. 487–528. Springer Verlag, New York.

Achten, G., Andre, J. & Laporte, M. (1991) Nails in light and electron microscopy. *Seminars in Dermatology* **10**, 54–64.

Alkiewicz, J. & Pfister, R. (1976) *Atlas der Nagelkrankheiten*, p. 8. Schattauer-Verlag, Stuttgart.

Allen, A.K., Ellis, J. & Rivett, D.E. (1991) The presence of glycoproteins in the cell membrane complex of variety of keratin fibres. *Biochimica et Biophysica Acta* **1074**, 331–333.

Alvarez, R. & Zaias, N. (1967) A modified polyethylene glycol-pyroxylin embedding method specially suited for nails. *Journal of Investigative Dermatology* **49**, 409–410.

Baran, R. & Gioanni, T. (1969) Les dyschromies ungueales. *Hospital (Paris)* **57**, 101–107.

Baran, R. & Haneke, E. (1984) Diagnostik und Therapie der streifenformigen nagelpigmentierung. *Hautarzt* **35**, 359–365.

Bennett, J. (1976) Technique of biopsy of nails. *Dermatologic Surgery and Oncology* **2**, 325–326.

de Berker, D.A.R. & Baran, R. (1998) Acquired malalignment: a complication of lateral longitudinal biopsy. *Acta Dermato-Venereologica* **78**, 468–470.

de Berker, D., Dawber, R.P.R., Thody, A. & Graham, A. (1996a) Melanocytes are absent from normal nail bed; the basis of a clinical dictum. *British Journal of Dermatology* **134**, 564.

de Berker, D.A.R., MaWhinney, B. & Sviland, L. (1996b) Quantification of regional matrix nail production. *British Journal of Dermatology* **134**, 1083–1086.

Burrows, M.T. (1917) The significance of the lunula of the nail. *Anatomical Record* **12**, 161–166.

Burrows, M.T. (1919) The significance of the lunula of the nail. *Johns Hopkins Medical Journal* **18**, 357–361.

Cohen, P.R. (1996) The lunula. *Journal of the American Academy of Dermatology* **34**, 943–953.

Drapé, J.L., Wolfram-Gabel, R., Idy-Peretti, I. *et al.* (1996) The lunula: a magnetic resonance imaging approach to the subnail matrix area. *Journal of Investigative Dermatology* **106**, 1081–1085.

Guero, S., Guichard, S. & Fraitag, S.R. (1994) Ligamentary structure at the base of the nail. *Surgical and Radiological Anatomy* **16**, 47–52.

Ham, A.W. & Leeson, T.S. (eds) (1961) *Histology*, 4th edn. Pitman Medical, London.

Haneke, E. (1991) Fungal infections of the nail. *Seminars in Dermatology* **10**, 41–53.

Hashimoto, K. (1971a) The marginal band: a demonstration of the thickened cellular envelope of the human nail. *Archives of Dermatology* **103**, 387–393.

Hashimoto, K. (1971b) Ultrastructure of the human toenail. II. *Journal of Ultrastructural Research* **36**, 391–410.

Hashimoto, K. (1971c) Ultrastructure of the human toenail: I proximal nail matrix. *Journal of Investigative Dermatology* **56**, 235–246.

Hashimoto, K. (1971d) Ultrastructure of the human toenail. Cell migration, keratinization and formation of the intercellular cement. *Archiv für Dermatologische Forschung* **240**, 1–22.

Higashi, N. (1968) Melanocytes of nail matrix and nail pigmentation. *Archives of Dermatology* **97**, 570–574.

Higashi, N. & Saito, T. (1969) Horizontal distribution of the DOPA-positive melanocytes in the nail matrix. *Journal of Investigative Dermatology* **53**, 163–165.

Kopf, A.W. & Waldo, F. (1980) Melanonychia striata. *Australasian Journal of Dermatology* **21**, 59–70.

Lewin, K. (1965) The normal finger nail. *British Journal of Dermatology* **77**, 421–430.

Lewin, K., Dewitt, S. & Lawson, R. (1973) Softening techniques for nail biopsy. *Archives of Dermatology* **107**, 223–224.

Lewis, B.L. (1954) Microscopic studies of fetal and mature nail and the surrounding soft tissue. *Archives of Dermatological Syphilology* **70**, 732–744.

Leyden, J.J., Spot, D.A. & Goldsmith, H. (1972) Diffuse banded melanin pigmentation in nails. *Archives of Dermatology* **105**, 548–550.

Molina, D. & Sanchez, J.L. (1995) Pigmented longitudinal bands of the nail. A clinicopathologic study. *American Journal of Dermatopathology* **17**, 539–541.

Monash, S. (1932) Normal pigmentation in the nails of negroes. *Archives of Dermatology* **25**, 876–881.

Nakayama, Y., Iino, T., Uchida, A. *et al.* (1990) Vascularised free nail grafts nourished by arterial inflow from the venous system. *Plastic and Reconstructive Surgery* **85**, 239–245.

Oropeza, R. (1986) Melanomas of special sites. In: *Cancer of the Skin: Biology, Diagnosis, Management*, Vol. 2. pp. 974–987. Blackwell Scientific Publications, Oxford.

Parent, D., Achten, G. & Stouffs-Vanhoof, F. (1985) Ultrastructure of the normal human nail. *American Journal of Dermatopathology* **7**, 529–535.

Perrin, C., Michiels, J.F., Pisani, A. & Ortonne, J.P. (1997) Anatomic distribution of melanocytes in normal nail unit: an immunohistochemical investigation. *American Journal of Dermatopathology* **19**, 462–467.

Pessa, J.E., Tsai, T.M., Li, Y. & Kleinert, H.E. (1990) The repair of nail deformities with the non-vascularised nail bed graft. Indications and results. *Journal of Hand Surgery* **15A**, 466–470.

Suarez, S.M., Silvers, D.N. & Scher, R.K. (1991) Histologic evaluation of nail clippings for diagnosing onychomycosis. *Archives of Dermatology* **127**, 1517–1519.

Tosti, A., Cameli, N., Piraccini, B.M. *et al.* (1994) Characterization of nail matrix melanocytes with anti-PEP1, anti-PEP8, TMH-1, and HMB-45 antibodies. *Journal of the American Academy of Dermatology* **31** (2 Part 1), 193–196.

Wilkerson, M.G. & Wilkin, J.K. (1989) Red lunulae revisited: a clinical and histopathologic examination. *Journal of the American Academy of Dermatology* **20**, 453–457.

Wolfram-Gabel, R. & Sick, H. (1995) Vascular networks of the periphery of the fingernail. *Journal of Hand Surgery [Br]* **20B**, 488–492.

Zaias, N. (1963) Embryology of the human nail. *Archives of Dermatology* **87**, 37–53.

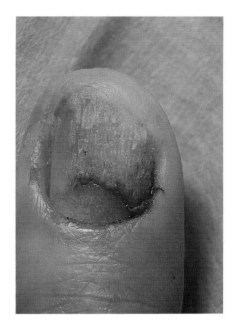

**Fig. 1.9** The epidermis of the nail bed has longitudinal ridges visible after nail avulsion.

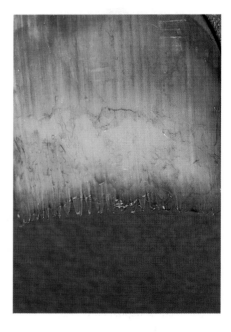

**Fig. 1.10** The undersurface of the nail plate shows longitudinal ridging which matches that seen on the nail bed. This pattern is lost at the margin of the lunula, where the nail is in continuity with the matrix from which it arises.

Zaias, N. (1967) The longitudinal nail biopsy. *Journal of Investigative Dermatology* **49**, 406–408.

## Nail bed and hyponychium

The nail bed extends from the distal margin of the lunula to the hyponychium. It is also called the ventral matrix depending on whether or not you believe that it contributes to the substance of the nail plate (see 'Nail growth' below). Avulsion of the nail plate reveals a pattern of longitudinal epidermal ridges stretching to the lunula (Fig. 1.9). On the underside of the nail plate is a complementary set of ridges, which has led to the description of the nail being led up the nail bed as if on rails (Fig. 1.10). The

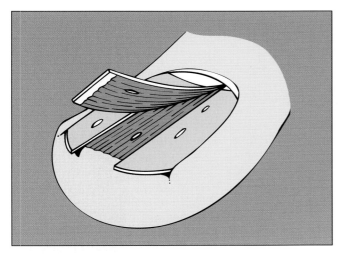

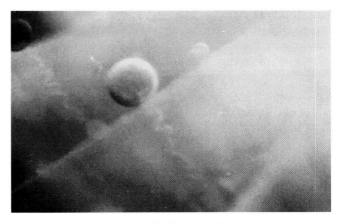

**Fig. 1.13** Sweat pores in the distal nail bed (Maricq 1967).

**Fig. 1.11** The appearance of splinter haemorrhages. Haem from longitudinal nail bed vessels is deposited on the underside of the nail plate. This grows out in the shape of a splinter.

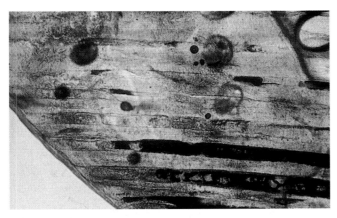

**Fig. 1.12** The undersurface of the nail has dark-stained blood in the longitudinal grooves corresponding to splinter haemorrhages.

small vessels of the nail bed are orientated in the same axis. This is demonstrated by splinter haemorrhages (Figs 1.11 & 1.12), where haem is deposited on the undersurface of the nail plate and grows out with it. The free edge of a nail loses the ridges, suggesting that they are softer than the main nail plate structure. The nail bed also loses these ridges shortly after loss of the overlying nail. It is likely that the ridges are generated at the margin of the lunula on the ventral surface of the nail to be imprinted upon the nail bed.

The epidermis of the nail bed is thin over the bulk of its territory. It becomes thicker at the nail folds where it develops rete ridges. It has no granular layer except in disease states. The dermis is sparse, with little fat, firm collagenous adherence to the underlying periosteum and no sebaceous or follicular appendages (Lewin 1965). Sweat ducts can be seen at the distal margin of the nail bed using *in vivo* magnification (Fig. 1.13) (Maricq 1967).

The hyponychium lies between the distal ridge and the nail plate and represents a space as much as a surface. The distal ridge (see 'Factors in embryogenesis' above) is seen from the 10th week of gestation onwards. The hyponychium and onychocorneal band may be the focus or origin of subungual hyperkeratosis in some diseases such as pityriasis rubra pilaris (see below) or pachyonychia congenita (see below). In these instances, and in some elderly people, it can be thought of as the solenhorn described by Pinkus (1927).

Pterygium inversum unguis is a further condition characterized by changes in the distal nail bed and hyponychium (Caputo & Prandi 1973). There is tough, fibrotic tissue tethering the free edge of the nail plate to the underlying soft structures. It is found in both congenital (Odom *et al.* 1974) and acquired forms (Patterson 1977). The aetiology is not clear. Patterson proposed that it was a combination of a genetic predisposition and microvascular ischaemia.

The hyponychium and overhanging free nail provide a crevice. This is a reservoir for microbes, relevant in surgery and the dissemination of infection. After 10 min of scrubbing the fingers with povidone iodine, nail clippings were cultured for bacteria, yeasts and moulds (Rayan & Flournoy 1987). In 19 out of 20 patients *Staphylococcus epidermidis* was isolated, seven patients had an additional bacteria, eight had moulds and three had yeasts. These findings could have significance to both surgeons and patients.

The hand to mouth transfer of bacteria is suggested by the high incidence of *Helicobacter pylori* beneath the nails of those who are seropositive for antibodies and have oral carriage. Dowsett *et al.* (1999) found that 58% of those with tongue *H. pylori* had it beneath the index fingernail, representing a significant ($P = 0.002$) association.

## Nail folds

The proximal and lateral nail folds give purchase to the nail plate by enclosing more than 75% of its periphery. They also provide a physical seal against the penetration of materials to vulnerable subungual and proximal regions.

The epidermal structure of the lateral nail folds is unremarkable, and comparable with normal skin. There is a tendency to hyperkeratosis, sometimes associated with trauma. When the trauma arises from the ingrowth of the nail, considerable soft tissue hypertrophy can result, with repeated infection (qv. ingrowing nails).

The proximal nail fold has three parts. Its upper aspect is normal glabrous skin, providing no direct influence upon the nail plate. At the point where its distal margin meets the nail plate it forms the cuticle (eponychium). In health, the cuticle adheres firmly to the dorsal aspect of the nail plate, achieving a seal. Its disruption may be associated with systemic disorders (collagen vascular) or local dermatoses. In the latter it may be the avenue of contact allergens or microbes. The ventral aspect of the proximal nail fold is apposed to the dorsal aspect of the nail. It contrasts with the adjacent matrix by being thinner, with shorter rete ridges and having a granular layer. Keratins expressed in the proximal nail fold may differ on its dorsal and ventral aspects and can contrast with expression elsewhere in the nail unit (de Berker *et al.* 2000; see 'Nail growth' below).

The proximal nail fold has significance in four main areas:
**1** It may contribute to the generation of nail plate through a putative dorsal matrix on its ventral aspect.
**2** It may influence the direction of growth of the nail plate by directing it obliquely over the nail bed.
**3** Nail fold microvasculature can provide useful information in some pathological conditions.
**4** When inflamed it can influence nail plate morphology as seen in eczema, psoriasis, habit tic deformity and paronychia.

The first two issues are dealt with in the section on nail growth (see 'Nail growth' below), the latter under vasculature (see 'Vasculature' below) and dermatological diseases and the nail (see Chapter 5).

## References

de Berker, D., Wojnarowska, F., Sviland, L. *et al.* (2000) Keratin expression in the normal nail unit: markers of regional differentiation. *British Journal of Dermatology* 142, 89–96.

Caputo, R. & Prandi, G. (1973) Pterygium inversum unguis. *Archives of Dermatology* 108, 817–818.

Dowsett, S.A., Archila, L., Segreto, V.A. *et al.* (1999) *Helicobacter pylori* infection in indigenous families of Central America: serostatus and oral and fingernail carriage. *Journal of Clinical Microbiology* 37, 2456–2460.

Lewin, K. (1965) The normal finger nail. *British Journal of Dermatology* 77, 421–430.

Maricq, H.R. (1967) Observation and photography of sweat ducts of the fingers *in vivo*. *Journal of Investigative Dermatology* 48, 399–401.

Odom, R.B., Stein, K.M. & Maibach, H.I. (1974) Congenital, painful aberrant hyponychium. *Archives of Dermatology* 110, 89–90.

Patterson, J.W. (1977) Pterygium inversum unguis-like changes in scleroderma. *Archives of Dermatology* 113, 1429–1430.

Pinkus, F. (1927) In: *Handbuch der Haut und Geschlechtskrankeiten* (eds J.J. Jadassohn), pp. 267–289. Springer, Berlin.

Rayan, G.M. & Flournoy, D.J. (1987) Microbiologic flora of human fingernails. *Journal of Hand Surgery* 12A, 605–607.

## Immunohistochemistry of periungual tissues

### Keratins

The most extensive immunohistological investigations of the nail unit have utilized keratin antibodies. The nail plate (Lynch *et al.* 1986; Heid *et al.* 1988), human embryonic nail unit (Heid *et al.* 1988; Moll *et al.* 1988; Lacour *et al.* 1991), accessory digit nail unit (de Berker *et al.* 1992, 1999; Sinclair *et al.* 1994) and adult nail unit (Haneke 1990; Lacour *et al.* 1991; de Berker *et al.* 2000) have all been examined.

Using the antibody 34βE12, Haneke (1990) demonstrated positivity of the basal two-thirds of the matrix. This antibody detects keratins 5, 10 and 11, indicating the presence of one or more of these at this location. Using monospecific antibodies, de Berker *et al.* (1992, 2000) detected keratins 1 and 10 in a suprabasal location in the matrix and noted their absence from the nail bed (Fig. 1.14) (see 'Nail growth' above and 'Nail plate' below). Keratins 1 and 10 are 'soft' epithelial keratins found suprabasally in normal skin (Purkis *et al.* 1990) and characteristic of cornification with terminal keratinocyte differentiation. Their absence from normal nail bed is reversed in disease where nail bed cornificaton is often seen, alongside development of a granular layer and expression of keratins 1 and 10 (de Berker *et al.* 1995). The development of a granular layer in subungual tissues can be interpreted as a pathological sign in nail histology, seen in a range of diseases and probably associated with changes in keratin expression (Fanti *et al.* 1994).

Ha-1 is found in the matrix. Ha-1 is a 'hard' keratin. Keratin 7 has been found at other sites in the nail unit and hair follicle, whereas Ha-1, detected by the monoclonal anti-keratin antibody LH TRIC 1, is limited to the matrix of the nail (Fig. 1.15) and the germinal matrix of the hair follicle (de Berker *et al.* 1992; Westgate *et al.* 1997). Keratin 19 is probably not found in the adult matrix (Moll *et al.* 1988; Haneke 1990; de Berker *et al.* 2000). However, Moll *et al.* (1988) did detect keratin 19 at this site in 15-week embryo nail units. Keratin 19 is also

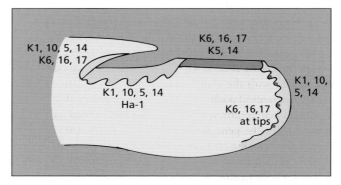

**Fig. 1.14** Distribution of keratins in the human periungual and subungual tissues.

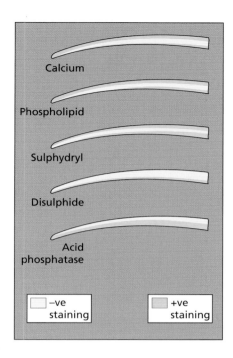

**Fig. 1.15** The histochemistry of the human nail plate (after Jarrett & Spearman 1966). Nail plates were sectioned and stained. Index, calcium; middle, phospholipid; ring, sulphydryl; little, disulphide; thumb, acid phosphatase.

found in the outer root sheath of the hair follicle and lingual papilla (Heid *et al.* 1988).

The co-localization of hard and soft keratins within single cells of the matrix has been observed by several workers in bovine hoof (Kitahara & Ogawa 1993) and human nail (Kitahara & Ogawa 1994, 1997; de Berker *et al.* 2000), suggesting that these cells are contributing both forms of keratin to the nail plate. This dual differentiation continues into *in vitro* culture of bovine hoof matrix cells (Kitahara & Ogawa 1994). Culture of human nail matrix confirms the persistence of hard keratin expression (Picardo *et al.* 1994; Nagae *et al.* 1995).

Markers for keratins 8 and 20 are thought to be specific to Merkel cells in the epidermis. Positive immunostaining for these keratins has been noted by Lacour *et al.* (1991) in adult nail matrix and de Berker *et al.* (2000) in infant accessory digits. Some workers have failed to detect Merkel cells and whilst it seems likely that they are present in fetal and young adult matrix, it may be that the cells are less common or absent as people age (Boot *et al.* 1992).

The nail bed appears to have a distinct identity with respect to keratin expression. Keratins 6, 16 and, to a lesser degree, 17 are all found in the nail bed and are largely absent from the matrix (de Berker *et al.* 2000). This finding has gained clinical significance with the characterization of the underlying fault in some variants of pachyonychia congenita where abnormalities of nail bed keratin lead to a grossly thicknened nail plate. Mutations in the gene for keratin 17 have been reported in a large Scottish kindred with the PC-2, or Jackson–Lawlor, phenotype (Munro *et al.* 1994; McLean *et al.* 1995). There is a cross-over with steatocystoma multiplex where the same mutation of keratin 17 may cause this phenotype which appears

to be independent of the specific keratin 17 mutation (Corden & McLean 1996; Hohl 1997; Covello *et al.* 1998). Mutations in the gene coding for K6b produce a phenotype seen with K17 gene mutations (Smith *et al.* 1998). Mutations in the K6a (Bowden *et al.* 1995) and K16 (McLean *et al.* 1995) genes have been reported in PC-1, originally described as the Jadassohn–Lewandsky variant of pachyonychia congenita.

Expression of keratins 6, 16 and 17 extend beyond the nail bed onto the digit pulp and are thought to match the physical characteristics of this skin which is adapted to high degrees of physical stress (Swensson *et al.* 1998). In particular, expression of keratin 17 is found at the base of epidermal ridges, which might also support the idea that this keratin is associated with stem cell function.

### Non-keratin immunohistochemistry

Haneke (1990) has provided a review of other important immunohistochemically detectable antigens. Involucrin is a protein necessary for the formation of the cellular envelope in keratinizing epithelia. It is strongly positive in the upper two thirds of the matrix and elsewhere in the nail unit (Baden 1994) and weakly detected in the suprabasal layers. Pancornulin and sciellin are also detected in the matrix (Baden 1994) The antibody HHF35 is considered specific to actin. It has been found to show a strong membranous staining and weak cytoplasmic staining of matrix cells (Haneke 1990).

In the dermis, vimentin was strongly positive in fibroblasts and vascular endothelial cells. Vimentin and desmin were expressed in the smooth muscle wall of some vessels. S100 stain, for cells of neural crest origin, revealed perivascular nerves, glomus bodies and Meissner's corpuscles distally.

Filaggrin could not be demonstrated in the matrix in Haneke's work or by electron microscopy (Heid *et al.* 1988). However, Manabe and O'Guin (1994) have detected the coexistence of trichohyalin and filaggrin in monkey nail, located in the area they term the 'dorsal matrix' which is likely to correspond to the most proximal aspect of the human nail matrix as it merges with the undersurface of the proximal nail fold. Kitahara and Ogawa (1997) have identified filaggrin in the human nail in the same location and O'Keefe *et al.* (1993) have found trichohyalin in the 'ventral matrix' of human nail, which is synonymous with the nail bed. Manabe noted that these two proteins coexist with keratins 6 and 16, which are more characteristic of nail bed than matrix. It is argued that filaggrin and trichohyalin may act to stabilize the intermediate filament network of K6 and K16, which are normally associated with unstable or hyperproliferative states.

The plasminogen activator inhibitor, PAI-Type 2, has been detected in the nail bed and matrix where it has been argued that it may have a role in protecting against programmed cell death (Lavker *et al.* 1998).

The basement membrane zone of the entire nail unit has been examined, employing a wide range of monoclonal and

**Table 1.2** Analysis of nail unit basement membrane zone using monoclonal and polyclonal antibodies.

| | Digit 1 | | | | | Digit 2 | | | | Digit 3 | |
| | Nail apparatus | | | | Proximal phalangeal skin | Nail apparatus | | | | | |
| | Fold | Matrix | Bed | HN | | Fold | Matrix | Bed | HN | Split skin | Intact skin |
|---|---|---|---|---|---|---|---|---|---|---|---|
| *Mono. Ab* | | | | | | | | | | | |
| LH7:2 | + | + | + | + | + | + | + | + | + | epi | + |
| L3d | + | + | + | + | + | + | + | + | + | epi | + |
| Co1 IV | + | + | + | + | + | + | + | + | + | epi | + |
| GB3 | + | + | + | + | + | + | + | + | + | epi | + |
| LH24 | + | + | + | + | + | + | + | + | + | epi | + |
| LH39 | + | + | + | + | + | + | + | + | + | epi | + |
| GDA | + | + | + | + | + | + | + | + | + | epi | + |
| Tenascin | + | + | + | + | + | + | + | + | + | epi | + |
| a6 | + | + | + | + | + | + | + | + | + | epi | + |
| G71 | + | + | + | + | + | + | + | + | + | epi | + |
| *Poly. Ab* | | | | | | | | | | | |
| Fibronectin | − | − | − | − | − | − | − | − | − | − | − |
| Laminin | + | + | + | + | + | + | + | + | + | derm | + |
| BP 220 kDa | + | + | + | + | + | + | + | + | + | epi | + |
| EBA 250 kDa | + | + | + | + | + | + | + | + | + | derm | + |
| LAD 285 kDa | + | + | + | + | + | + | + | + | + | epi | + |
| LAD ? kDa | + | + | + | + | + | + | + | + | + | derm | + |

HN, Hyponychium.

polyclonal antibodies (Sinclair *et al.* 1994). Collagen VII, fibronectin, chondroitin sulphate and tenascin were among the antigens detected. All except tenascin were present in a quantity and pattern indistinguishable from normal skin. Tenascin was absent from the nail bed, which was attributed to the fact that the dermal papillae are altered or considered absent (Table 1.2).

## References

Baden, H. (1994) Common transglutaminase substrates shared by hair, epidermis and nail and their function. *Journal of Dermatologic Science* 7 (Suppl.), S20–S26.

de Berker, D., Leigh, I. & Wojnarowska, F. (1992) Patterns of keratin expression in the nail unit—an indicator of regional matrix differentiation. *British Journal of Dermatology* 127, 423.

de Berker, D., Sviland, L. & Angus, B.A. (1995) Suprabasal keratin expression in the nail bed: a marker of dystrophic nail differentiation. *British Journal of Dermatology* 133 (Suppl. 45), 16.

de Berker, D., Wojnarowska, F., Sviland, L. *et al.* (2000) Keratin expression in the normal nail unit: markers of regional differentiation. *British Journal of Dermatology* 142, 89–96.

Boot, P.M., Rowden, G. & Walsh, N. (1992) The distribution of Merkel cells in human fetal and adult skin. *American Journal of Dermatopathology* 14, 391–396.

Bowden, P.E., Haley, J.L., Kansky, A. *et al.* (1995) Mutation of a type II keratin gene (K6a) in pachyonychia congenita. *Nature Genetics* 10, 363–365.

Corden, L.D. & McLean, W.H. (1996) Human keratin disease: hereditary fragility of specific epithelial tissues. *Experimental Dermatology* 5, 297–307.

Covello, S.P., Smith, F.J.D., Sillevis Smitt, J.H. *et al.* (1998) Keratin 17 mutations cause either steatocystoma multiplex or pachyonychia congenita type 2. *British Journal of Dermatology* 139, 475–480.

Fanti, P.A., Tosti, A., Cameli, N. & Varotti, C. (1994) Nail matrix hypergranulosis. *American Journal of Dermatopathology* 16, 607–610.

Haneke, E. (1990) The human nail matrix—flow cytometric and immunohistochemical studies. In: *Clinical Dermatology in the Year 2000*. Book of Abstracts, May.

Heid, W.H., Moll, I. & Franke, W.W. (1988) Patterns of expression of trichocytic and epithelial cytokeratins in mammalian tissues. II. Concomitant and mutually exclusive synthesis of trichocytic and epithelial cytokeratins in diverse human and bovine tissues. *Differentiation* 37, 215–230.

Hohl, D. (1997) Steatocystoma multiplex and oligosymptomatic pachyonychia congenita of the Jackson–Lawler type. *Dermatology* 195, 86–88.

Kitahara, T. & Ogawa, H. (1993) Coexpression of keratins characteristic of skin and nail differentiation in nail cells. *Journal of Investigative Dermatology* 100, 171–175.

Kitahara, T. & Ogawa, H. (1994) Variation of differentiation in nail and bovine hoof cells. *Journal of Investigative Dermatology* 102, 725–729.

Kitahara, T. & Ogawa, H. (1997) Cellular features of differentiation in the nail. *Microscopic Research Techniques* 38, 436–442.

Lacour, J.P., Dubois, D., Pisani, A. & Ortonne, J.P. (1991) Anatomical mapping of Merkel cells in normal human adult epidermis. *British Journal of Dermatology* **125**, 535–542.

Lavker, R.M., Risse, B., Brown, H. *et al.* (1998) Localisation of plasminogen activator inhibitor Type 2 (PAI-2) in hair and nail: implications for terminal differentiation. *Journal of Investigative Dermatology* **110**, 917–922.

Lynch, M.H., O'Guin, W.M., Hardy, C. *et al.* (1986) Acid and basic hair/nail ('hard') keratins: their co-localisation in upper corticle and cuticle cells of the human hair folicle and their relationship to 'soft' keratins. *Journal of Cell Biology* **103**, 2593–2606.

McLean, W.H.I., Rugg, E.L., Luny, D.P. *et al.* (1995) Keratin 16 and 17 mutations cause pachyonychia congenita. *Nature Genetics* **9**, 273–278.

Manabe, M. & O'Guin, W.M. (1994) Existence of trichohyalin-keratohyalin hybrid granules: co-localisation of 2 major intermediate filament-associated proteins in non-follicular epithelia. *Differentiation* **58**, 65–75.

Moll, I., Heid, H.W., Franke, W.W. & Moll, R. (1988) Patterns of expression of trichocytic and epithelial cytokeratins in mammalian tissues. *Differentiation* **39**, 167–184.

Munro, C.S., Carter, S., Bryce, S. *et al.* (1994) A gene for pachyonychia congenita is closely linked with the gene cluster on 17q12-q21. *Journal of Medical Genetics* **31**, 675–678.

Nagae, H., Nakanishi, H., Urano, Y. & Arase, S. (1995) Serial cultivation of human nail matrix cells under serum-free conditions. *Journal of Dermatology* **22**, 560–566.

O'Keefe, E.J., Hamilton, E.H., Lee, S.C. & Steiner, P. (1993) Trichohyalin: a structural protein of hair, tongue, nail and epidermis. *Journal of Investigative Dermatology* **101**, 65s–71s.

Picardo, M., Tosti, A., Marchese, C. *et al.* (1994) Characterisation of cultured nail matrix cells. *Journal of the American Academy of Dermatology* **30**, 434–440.

Purkis, P.E., Steel, J.B., Mackenzie, I.C. *et al.* (1990) Antibody markers of basal cells in complex epithelia. *Journal of Cellular Science* **97**, 39–50.

Sinclair, R.D., Wojnarowska, F. & Dawber, R.P.R. (1994) The basement membrane zone of the nail. *British Journal of Dermatology* **131**, 499–505.

Smith, F.J., Corden, L.D., Rugg, E.L. *et al.* (1997) Missense mutations in keratin 17 cause either pachyonychia congenita type 2 or a phenotype resembling steatocystoma multiplex. *Journal of Investigative Dermatology* **108**, 220–223.

Smith, F.J., Jonkman, M.F., van Goor, H. *et al.* (1998) A mutation in human keratin K6b produces a phenocopy of the K17 disorder pachyonychia congenita type 2. *Human Molecular Genetics* **7**, 1143–1148.

Swensson, O., Langbein, L., McMillan, J.R. *et al.* (1998) Specialised keratin expression pattern in human ridged skin as an adaptation to high physical stress. *British Journal of Dermatology* **139**, 767–775.

Westgate, G.E., Tidman, N., de Berker, D. *et al.* (1997) Characterization of LH Tric-1, a new monospecific monoclonal antibody to the trichocyte keratin Ha1. *British Journal of Dermatology* **137**, 24–30.

## Nail plate

The nail plate is composed of compacted keratinized epithelial cells. It covers the nail bed and intermediate matrix. It is curved in both the longitudinal and transverse axes. This allows it to be embedded in nail folds at its proximal and lateral margins, which provide strong attachment and make the free edge a useful tool. This feature is more marked in the toes than the fingers. In the great toe, the lateral margins of the matrix and nail extend almost half way around the terminal phalanx. This provides strength appropriate to the foot (Fig. 1.16).

The upper surface of the nail plate is smooth and may have a variable number of longitudinal ridges that change with age. These ridges are sufficiently specific to allow forensic identification and the distinction between identical twins (Diaz *et al.* 1990). The ventral surface also has longitudinal ridges that correspond to complementary ridges on the upper aspect of the nail bed (see 'Nail bed' above) to which it is bonded (Fig. 1.17). These nail ridges may be best examined using polarized light. They can also be used for forensic identification (Apolinar & Rowe 1980), as may blood groups from fragments of nail plate (Garg 1983).

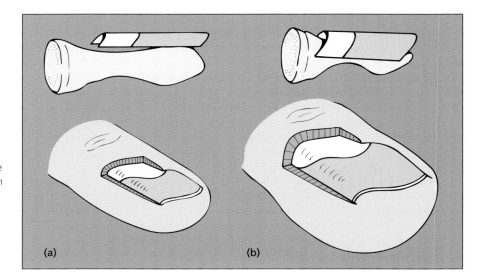

**Fig. 1.16** Nail plate association with soft tissue and bone in the finger and toe. (a) In the finger, the nail plate has modest transverse curvature and shallow association with soft tissues. (b) In the great toe, the nail plate has more marked transverse curvature and deep soft tissue association. This makes it strong—appropriate to the foot—but also accounts for the tendency to ingrow and the need for deep lateral extirpation at lateral matricectomy.

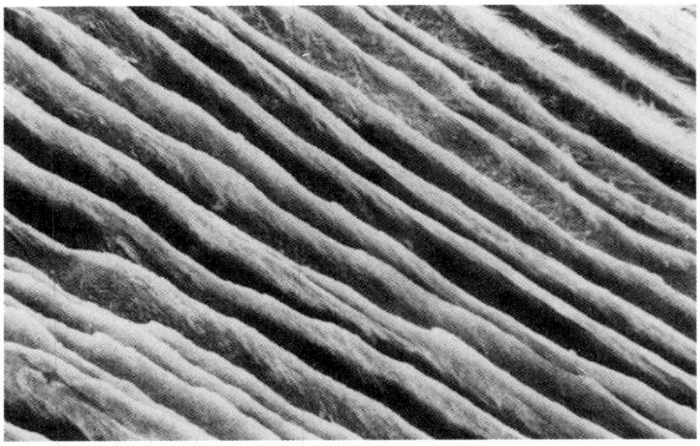

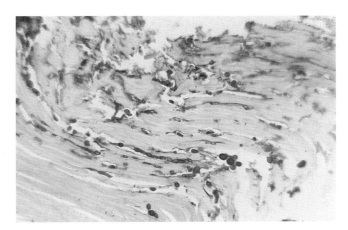

**Fig. 1.17** Scanning electron micrograph of the nail bed demonstrating longitudinal ridges.

**Fig. 1.19** Fungal spores and hyphae can be seen in the stained section of a nail clipping taken from a nail with onychomycosis.

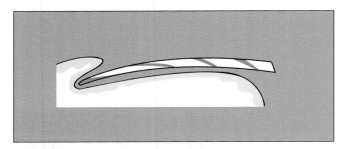

**Fig. 1.18** Shaded areas represent 7-day periods of nail growth, separated by 1 month with transition of nail from horizontal to oblique axis over 4 months.

The nail plate gains thickness and density as it grows distally (Johnson *et al.* 1991) according to analysis of surgical specimens. *In vivo* ultrasound suggests that there may be an 8.8% reduction in thickness distally (Finlay *et al.* 1987). A thick nail plate may imply a long intermediate matrix. This stems from the process whereby the longitudinal axis of the intermediate matrix becomes the vertical axis of the nail plate (Fig. 1.18). Other factors, like linear rate of nail growth (Samman & White 1964), vascular supply, subungual hyperkeratosis and drugs also influence thickness.

The tendency to describe a dorsal, intermediate and ventral matrix, has generated description of corresponding layers of the nail plate deriving from the different matrix zones. Whether or not the three demarcations of the nail matrix exist, it is important to recognize the basic principle that proximal regions of matrix produce dorsal nail plate and distal matrix produces ventral nail plate.

### Light microscopy

Lewis (1954) described a silver stain that delineates the nail plate zones. Three regions of nail plate have been histochemically defined (Jarrett & Spearman 1966) (Fig. 1.15). The dorsal plate has a relatively high calcium, phospholipid and sulphydryl group content. It has little acid phosphatase activity and is physically hard. The phospholipid content may provide some water resistance. The intermediate nail plate has a high acid phosphatase activity, probably corresponding to the number of retained nuclear remnants. There is a high number of disulphide bonds, low content of bound sulphydryl groups, phospholipid and calcium. Controversy allows that the ventral nail plate may be a variable entity (Samman 1961). Jarrett and Spearman (1966) described it as a layer only one or two cells thick. These cells are eosinophilic and move both upwards and forward with nail growth. With respect to calcium, phospholipid and sulphydryl groups it is the same as the dorsal nail plate. It shares a high acid phosphatase and frequency of disulphide bonds with the intermediate nail plate.

Ultrasound examination of *in vivo* and avulsed nail plates suggests that it has the physical characteristics of a bilamellar structure (Jemec & Serup 1989). There is a superficial dry compartment and a deep humid one. This has been given as evidence against the existence of a ventral matrix contribution to the nail plate.

In clinical practice, histology of the nail plate may be useful in the identification of fungal infections in culture-negative specimens (Haneke 1991; Suarez *et al.* 1991) (Fig. 1.19). It may also be used to identify the dorso-ventral location of melanin in the nail clipping of a longitudinal melanonychia and hence allow prediction of the site of melanocyte activity in the intermediate matrix (Baran & Kechijian 1989; Dawber & Colver 1991).

Germann *et al.* (1980) utilized a form of tape-stripping in conjunction with light microscopy to examine dorsal nail plate corneocyte morphology in disease and health. She found that conditions of rapid nail growth (psoriasis and infancy) resulted in smaller cell size. Sonnex *et al.* (1991) describes the histology of transverse white lines in the nail.

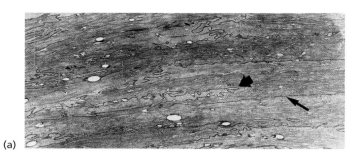

(a)

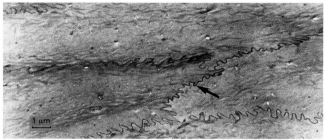

(b)

**Fig. 1.20** (a) Transmission electron micrograph of the upper part of the nail plate. The corneocytes are flattened and joined laterally by infrequent deep interdigitations (broad arrow). (b) The cell membranes between adjacent cell layers are discretely indented and in parts without invaginations—Thiery's technique. (Courtesy of Professor G. Achten.)

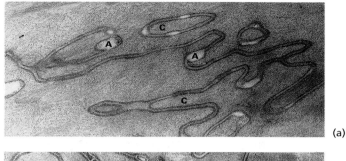

(a)

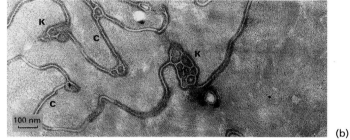

(b)

**Fig. 1.21** (a) Upper part of the nail plate showing ampullar dilatations (A). (b) Lower part of the nail plate showing anchoring knots (K). The only cell-to-cell coupling observed (C) is a desmosome. (Courtesy of Professor G. Achten.)

### Electron microscopy

Scanning electron microscopy has added to our understanding of onychoschizia (Shelley & Shelley 1984; Wallis *et al.* 1991) as well as basic nail plate structure (Forslind & Thyresson 1975; Dawber 1980). In the normal nail corneocytes can be seen adherent to the dorsal aspect of the nail plate. In cross-section, the compaction of the lamellar structure is visible. Both these features can be seen to be disrupted in onychoschizia following repeated immersion and drying of the nail plates.

Transmission electron microscopy has been used to identify the relationship between the corneocytes of the nail plate (Parent *et al.* 1985). Using Thierry's tissue processing techniques, material for the following description has been provided. Cell membranes and intercellular junctions are easily discernible (Fig. 1.20). Even though at low magnification one can differentiate the dorsal and intermediate layers of the nail plate, the exact boundary is unclear using transmission electron microscopy. Cells on the dorsal ($34 \times 60 \times 2.2\ \mu m$) aspect are half as thick as ventral cells ($40 \times 50 \times 5.5\ \mu m$), with a gradation of sizes in between. In the dorsal nail plate, large intercellular spaces are present corresponding to ampullar dilatations (Figs 1.21 & 1.22). These gradually diminish in the deeper layers and are absent in the ventral region. At this site, cells are joined by complete folds, membranes of adjacent cells appearing to penetrate each other to form 'anchoring knots'.

Corneocytes of the dorsal nail plate are joined laterally by infrequent deep interdigitations. The plasma membranes between adjacent cell layers are more discretely indented, often with no

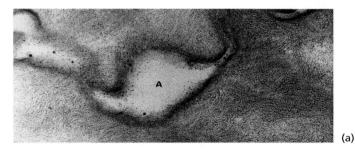

(a)

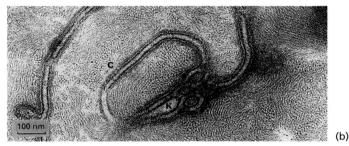

(b)

**Fig. 1.22** Upper part of the nail plate as in Fig. 1.20, in greater detail. (Courtesy of Professor G. Achten.)

invaginations (Fig. 1.20). In the deeper parts of the nail plate the interdigitations are more numerous, but more shallow (Fig. 1.20). No tight gap junctions are seen in either of the major nail layers in this series (Parent *et al.* 1985), although they were identified previously by Forslind and Thyresson (1975). The intercellular material is homogeneous and separated from

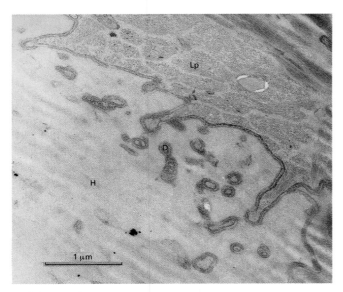

**Fig. 1.23** Corneocytes of the lowest part of the nail plate (Lp) sending out numerous digitations (D) penetrating the hyponychial nail bed cells (H). (Courtesy of Professor G. Achten.)

the cell membrane by two thin electron-dense lines. The space between the cell membranes varies from 25 nm to 35 nm (Figs 1.20 & 1.22). No complete desmosomal structures are seen.

Nail bed cells show considerable infolding and inter-digitation at their junction with the nail plate cells (Fig. 1.23).

They are polygonal and show no specific alignment. They are between 6 and 20 μm across and show neither tight nor gap junctions. They do, however, have desmosomal connections of the type seen in normal epidermis. (Fig. 1.24).

Cells of the hyponychium are distinguished from the nail plate on the basis of morphology, staining affinities and size.

Using different preparation techniques, other workers have demonstrated other anatomical details. On the cytoplasmic side of the cell membranes of nail plate cells lies a layer of protein particles (Hashimoto 1971a,b; Caputo *et al.* 1982). Other staining techniques suggest that the single type of intercellular bond described by Parent *et al.* (1985) may be a spot desmo-some (Arnn & Stoehelin 1981).

## References

Apolinar, E. & Rowe, W.F. (1980) Examination of human fingernail ridges by means of polarized light. *Journal of Forensic Science CA* **25**, 154–161.

Arnn, Y. & Stoehelin, L.A. (1981) The structure and function of spot desmosomes. *International Journal of Dermatology* **20**, 331–339.

Baran, R. & Kechijian, P. (1989) Longitudinal melanonychia diagnosis and management. *Journal of the American Academy of Dermatology* **21**, 1165–1175.

Caputo, R., Gasparini, G. & Contini, D. (1982) A freeze-fracture study of the human nail plate. *Archives of Dermatological Research* **272**, 117–125.

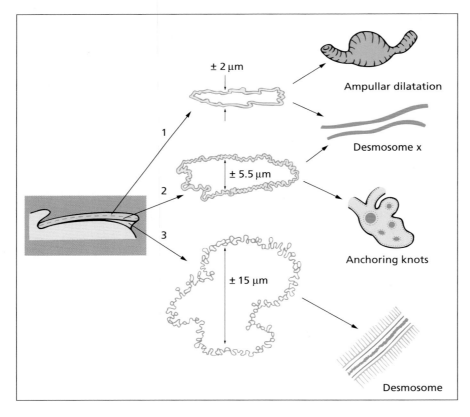

**Fig. 1.24** Intercellular junctions of the three parts of the nail: 1, upper plate; 2, lower plate; 3, hyponychial ventral nail with desmosome as seen by Thiery's technique. (Courtesy of Professor G. Achten.)

Dawber, R.P.R. (1980) The ultrastructure and growth of human nails. *Archives of Dermatological Research* **269**, 197–204.

Dawber, R.P.R. & Colver, G.B. (1991) The spectrum of malignant melanoma of the nail apparatus. *Seminars in Dermatology* **10**, 82–87.

Diaz, A.A., Boehm, A.F. & Rowe, W.F. (1990) Comparison of finger-nail ridge patterns of monozygotic twins. *Journal of Forensic Science CA* **35**, 97–102.

Finlay, A.Y., Moseley, H. & Duggan, T.C. (1987) Ultrasound transmission time: an *in vivo* guide to nail thickness. *British Journal of Dermatology* **117**, 765–770.

Forslind, B. & Thyresson, N. (1975) On the structures of the normal nail. *Archiv für Dermatologische Forschung* **251**, 199–204.

Garg, R.K. (1983) Determination of ABO (H) blood group substances from finger and toenails. *Zeitschrift für Rechtsmedizin* **91**, 17–19.

Germann, H., Barran, W. & Plewig, G. (1980) Morphology of corneocytes from human nail plates. *Journal of Investigative Dermatology* **74**, 115–118.

Haneke, E. (1991) Fungal infections of the nail. *Seminars in Dermatology* **10**, 41–53.

Hashimoto, K. (1971a) The marginal band: a demonstration of the thickened cellular envelope of the human nail. *Archives of Dermatology* **103**, 387–393.

Hashimoto, K. (1971b) Ultrastructure of the human toenail. II. *Journal of Ultrastructural Research* **36**, 391–410.

Jarrett, A. & Spearman, R.I.C. (1966) The histochemistry of the human nail. *Archives of Dermatology* **94**, 652–657.

Jemec, G.B.E. & Serup, J. (1989) Ultrasound structure of the human nail plate. *Archives of Dermatology* **125**, 643–646.

Johnson, M., Comaish, J.S. & Shuster, S. (1991) Nail is produced by the normal nail bed: a controversy resolved. *British Journal of Dermatology* **125**, 27–29.

Lewis, B.L. (1954) Microscopic studies of fetal and mature nail and surrounding soft tissue. *Archives of Dermatology and Syphilis* **70**, 732–744.

Parent, D., Achten, G. & Stouffs-Vamhoof, F. (1985) Ultrastructure of the normal human nail. *American Journal of Dermatopathology* **7**, 529–535.

Samman, P.D. (1961) The ventral nail. *Archives of Dermatology* **84**, 1030–1033.

Samman, P.D. & White, W.F. (1964) The 'yellow nail' syndrome. *British Journal of Dermatology* **76**, 153–157.

Shelley, W.B. & Shelley, D. (1984) Onychschizia: scanning electron microscopy. *Journal of the American Academy of Dermatology* **10**, 623–627.

Sonnex, T.S., Griffiths, W.A.D. & Nicol, W.J. (1991) The nature and significance of the transverse white band of human nails. *Seminars in Dermatology* **10**, 12–16.

Suarez, S.M., Silvers, D.N., Scher, R.K. *et al.* (1991) Histologic evaluation of nail clippings for diagnosing onychomycosis. *Archives of Dermatology* **127**, 1517–1519.

Wallis, M.S., Bowen, W.R. & Guin, J.D. (1991) Pathogenesis of onychoschizia (lamellar dystrophy). *Journal of the American Academy of Dermatology* **24**, 44–48.

## Vascular supply

### Arterial supply

The vascular supply of the finger is considered in detail here. Many of the anatomical principles may be extended to the anatomy of the foot and toe, whilst details can be sought elsewhere (Warwick & Williams 1973).

The radial and ulnar arteries supply deep and superficial palmar arcades that act as large anastomoses between the two vessels. From these arcades extend branches aligned with the phalanges. Four arteries supply each digit, two on either side. The dorsal digital arteries are small and arise as branches of the radial artery. They undertake anastomoses with the superficial and deep palmar arches and the palmar digital vessels before passing distally into the finger. The palmar digital arteries provide the main blood supply to the fingers. They receive contributions from the deep and superficial palmar arcades. Although paired, one is normally dominant (Smith *et al.* 1991a). They anastomose via dorsal and palmar arches around the distal phalanx. The palmar arch is located in a protected position, beneath the maximal padding of the finger pulp and tucked into a recess behind the protruberant phalangeal boss (Fig. 1.25). This is of functional value as it protects against occlusion of the blood supply when the fingers exert maintained grip.

The dorsal nail fold arch (superficial arcade) lies just distal to the distal interphalangeal joint. It supplies the nail fold and extensor tendon insertion. It is tortuous, with numerous branches to the intermediate nail matrix. Its transverse passage across the finger can be roughly located by pushing proximally on the free edge of the nail plate. This produces a faint crease about 5 mm proximal to the cuticle and is both the cul de sac of the proximal nail fold and the line of the dorsal nail fold arch.

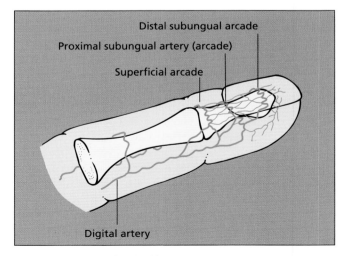

**Fig. 1.25** Arterial supply of the distal finger.

The subungual region is supplied by distal and proximal subungual arcades, arising in turn from an anastomosis of the palmar arch and the dorsal nail fold arch. A helpful study on adults and fetuses was performed by Flint (1955) and more recently by Wolfram-Gabel and Sick (1995).

The tortuosity of the main vessels in the finger is a notable feature. Vessels may turn through 270° and resemble a coiled spring (Smith *et al.* 1991a). Functionally, this can be interpreted as protection against occlusion by kinking in an articulated longitudinal structure.

### Venous drainage

Venous drainage of the finger is by deep and superficial systems. The deep system corresponds to the arterial supply. Superficially, there exist the dorsal and palmar digital veins. These are in a prominent branching network, particularly on the dorsal aspect. However, in the microsurgical techniques needed to restore amputations, it appears that distally, the palmar superficial veins are largest (Smith *et al.* 1991b).

Although the arterial supply to the nail unit is substantial, the matrix will tolerate only limited trauma before scarring (Zaias 1967). A longitudinal biopsy of greater than 3 mm is likely to leave a permanent dystrophy. Equally, it appears to need a precise, not just abundant, blood supply. Non-vascularized split thickness nail bed grafting is moderately successful for the nail bed, but not for intermediate matrix (Pessa *et al.* 1990). This is in the presence of otherwise adequate local blood supply at sites of previous trauma. Toenail matrix grafts can be made successful if they are transplanted with associated soft tissue and a venous pedicle (Nakayama *et al.* 1990). The local arterial supply is then anastomosed through this pedicle.

### Effects of altered vascular supply

Impaired arterial supply can have a considerable effect upon the finger pulp and nail unit. Lynn *et al.* (1955) claimed that there was almost complete correlation between occluded arteriographic findings and the presence of paronychial infection or ulceration, ridged brittle fingernails or phlyctenular gangrene. Samman and Strickland (1962) reviewed the nail dystrophies of 41 patients with features of peripheral vascular disease. In this uncontrolled study, he observed that onycholysis, Beau's lines, thin brittle nails and yellow discoloration were all attributable to ischaemia in the absence of other causes. It has also been suggested that congenital onychodysplasias may result from digital ischaemia *in utero* (Kitayama & Tsukada 1983). Immobilization might be associated with diminished local blood supply and has been noted to reduce nail growth (Dawber 1981). Conversely, the increased growth associated with arteriovenous shunts may reflect the role of greater blood flow (Orentreich *et al.* 1979). Clubbing constitutes a change in both the nail and nail bed. It is believed that it arises secondary to neurovascular pathology. Post-mortem studies suggest that it is due to increased blood flow with vasodilatation rather than vessel hyperplasia (Currie & Gallagher 1988).

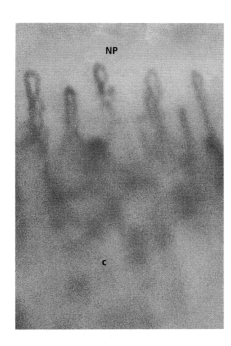

**Fig. 1.26** Capillary loops visible in the proximal nail fold. NP, nail plate; c, cuticle.

### Nail fold vessels

The nail fold capillary network (Gilje *et al.* 1974) is seen easily with a ×4 magnifying lens, dermatoscope or an ophthalmoscope. With the latter it should be set at +40 and the lens held very close to a drop of oil on the nail fold. It is similar to the normal cutaneous plexus in health, except that the capillary loops are more horizontal and visible throughout their length. The loops are in tiers of uniform size, with peaks equidistant from the base of the cuticle (Fig. 1.26) (Ryan 1973). The venous arm is more dilated and tortuous than the arterial arm. There is a wide range of morphologies within the normal population (Davies & Landau 1966). Features in some disorders may be sufficiently gross to be useful without magnification; erythema and haemorrhages being the most obvious.

In the first 10 years of life, the pattern of nail fold vessels is immature (Basserga *et al.* 1996). Microscopy of small vessels in adulthood can be of diagnostic value in some connective tissue diseases (Buchanan & Humpston 1968; Granier *et al.* 1986). Pathological features include venous plexus visibility, density of capillary population, avascular fields, haemorrhages, giant capillaries and cessation of blood flow following cooling. When determined quantitatively, using television microscopy, Studer found it possible to distinguish between systemic and disseminated cutaneous lupus erythematosus, and between localized and systemic sclerosis (Studer *et al.* 1991). In patients with undifferentiated connective tissue disease, it may be possible to predict which will progress to systemic sclerosis by undertaking quantitative analysis of nail fold vessel dimensions.

The larger the vessels the more likely that the condition is going to progress (Ohtsuka *et al*. 1998). The mechanism of dilated vessel evolution may in part arise from impaired fibrinolysis, macroglobulinaemia and cryoglobulinaemia (Ryan 1973).

Fibrinogen may increase in subjects in renal failure on continuous ambulatory peritoneal dialysis. This has been proposed as a cause for the changes seen in nail fold vessels of such patients in proportion to abnormalities of urea and uric acid clearances (Schumann *et al*. 1996). Nail fold vessel changes may also occur in psoriasis and appear to correlate with nail pitting, onycholyis and periungual psoriatic plaques (Ohtsuka *et al*. 1994). However, it can be imagined that clinical or subclinical elements of cutaneous psoriasis may represent the underlying change in vessel pattern.

The capillary networks in the normal nail fold of toes and fingers have been compared using video-microscopy. It has revealed a greater density of capillaries in the toe nail fold, but with a reduced rate of flow (Richardson & Schwartz 1984). The exact pattern of an individual's nail fold vessels can be used as an identifying characteristic (Krylova & Soboleva 1995).

Intravenous bolus doses of Na-fluorescein dye have been followed through nail fold microscopy (Bollinger *et al*. 1979). There is rapid and uniform leakage from the capillaries in normal subjects to within 10 μm of the capillaries. It is suggested that a sheath of collagen may prevent diffusion beyond this point. The same procedure has been followed in patients with rheumatoid arthritis demonstrating decreased flow rates and abnormal flow patterns, but no change in vessel leakage (Grassi *et al*. 1989).

Nail fold microscopy has been used for the investigation of Raynaud's phenomenon (Mahler *et al*. 1987). It is possible to assess vascular toxicity affecting nail fold vessels following chemotherapy, using the same method (Hansen *et al*. 1990).

Ultimately, histological information on the vessels and tissue of the nail folds may be helpful. The technique and benefits of nail fold biopsy have been described (Schnitzler *et al*. 1976). Amyloid deposits, subintimal hyalinosis and severe dermal fibrosis are cited as useful supplementary information yielded by biopsy.

## Glomus bodies

The term glomus is defined as a ball, tuft or cluster, a small conglomeration or plexus of cavernous blood vessels. In the skin it is an end organ apparatus in which there is an arteriovenous anastomosis bypassing the intermediary capillary bed. This anastomosis includes the afferent artery and the Sucquet–Hoyer canal. The latter is surrounded by structures including cuboidal epithelioid cells and cells possibly of smooth muscle or pericyte origin (Zimmerman type). These are surrounded by a rich nerve supply and then the efferent vein which connects with the venous system outside the glomus capsule.

The nail bed is richly supplied with glomus bodies and their presence in histological specimens should be interpreted in this context, rather than assuming that their abundance has some pathological significance. These are neurovascular bodies which act as arteriovenous anastomoses (AVA). AVAs are connections between the arterial and venous side of the circulation with no intervening capillaries. Each glomus body is an encapsulated oval organ 300 μm long composed of a tortuous vessel uniting an artery and venule, a nerve supply and a capsule. It contains many modified large muscle cells, resembling epithelioid cells and cholinergic nerves. Digital nail beds contain 93–501 glomus bodies per cm$^3$. They lie parallel to the capillary resevoirs which they bypass. They are able to contract asynchronously with their associated arterioles such that in the cold, arterioles constrict and glomus bodies dilate. They can thus serve as regulators of capillary circulation, acquiring the name 'the peripheral heart of Masson' (Masson 1937). They are particularly important in the preservation of blood supply to the peripheries in cold conditions.

Nail bed infarcts and splinter haemorrhage can be seen in a range of systemic disorders and local mechanical and dermatological abnormalities (see below).

## Nerve supply (Fig. 1.27)

The periungual soft tissues are innervated by dorsal branches of paired digital nerves. Wilgis and Maxwell (1979) stated that the digital nerve is composed of three major fascicles supplying the digit tip, with the main branch passing under the nail bed and innervating both nail bed and matrix (Zook 1988). Winkelmann (1960) showed many nerve endings adjacent to the epithelial surface, mainly in the nail folds.

## References

Basserga, M., Bonacci, E., Cammarota, M.G. & d'Amico, N. (1996) La cappilaroscopia periungueale nello studio del microcircolo in età pediatrica. *Minerva Pediatrics* **48**, 297–301.

Bollinger, A., Jäger, K., Roten, A., Timeus, C. & Mahler, F. (1979) Diffusion, pericapillary distribution and clearance of Na-fluorescein in the human nail fold. *Pflügers Archives* **382**, 137–143.

Buchanan, I. & Humpston, D.J. (1968) Nail fold capillaries in connective tissue disorders. *Lancet* **41**, 845–847.

Currie, A.E. & Gallagher, P.J. (1988) The pathology of clubbing: vascular changes in the nail bed. *British Journal of the Chest* **82**, 382–385.

Davies, E. & Landau, J. (eds) (1966) *Clinical Capillary Microscopy.* C.C. Thomas, Springfield, IL.

Dawber, R.P.R. (1981) The effect of immobilization upon finger nail growth. *Clinical and Experimental Dermatology* **6**, 533–535.

Flint, M.H. (1955) Some observations on the vascular supply of the nail bed and terminal segments of the finger. *British Journal of Plastic Surgery* **8**, 186–195.

Gilje, O., Kierland, R. & Baldes, E.J. (1974) Capillary microscopy in the diagnosis of dermatologic diseases. *Journal of Investigative Dermatology* **22**, 199–206.

Granier, F., Vayssairat, M., Priollet, P. *et al.* (1986) Nail fold capillary microsopy in mixed connective tissue disease. *Arthritis and Rheumatism* **29**, 189–195.

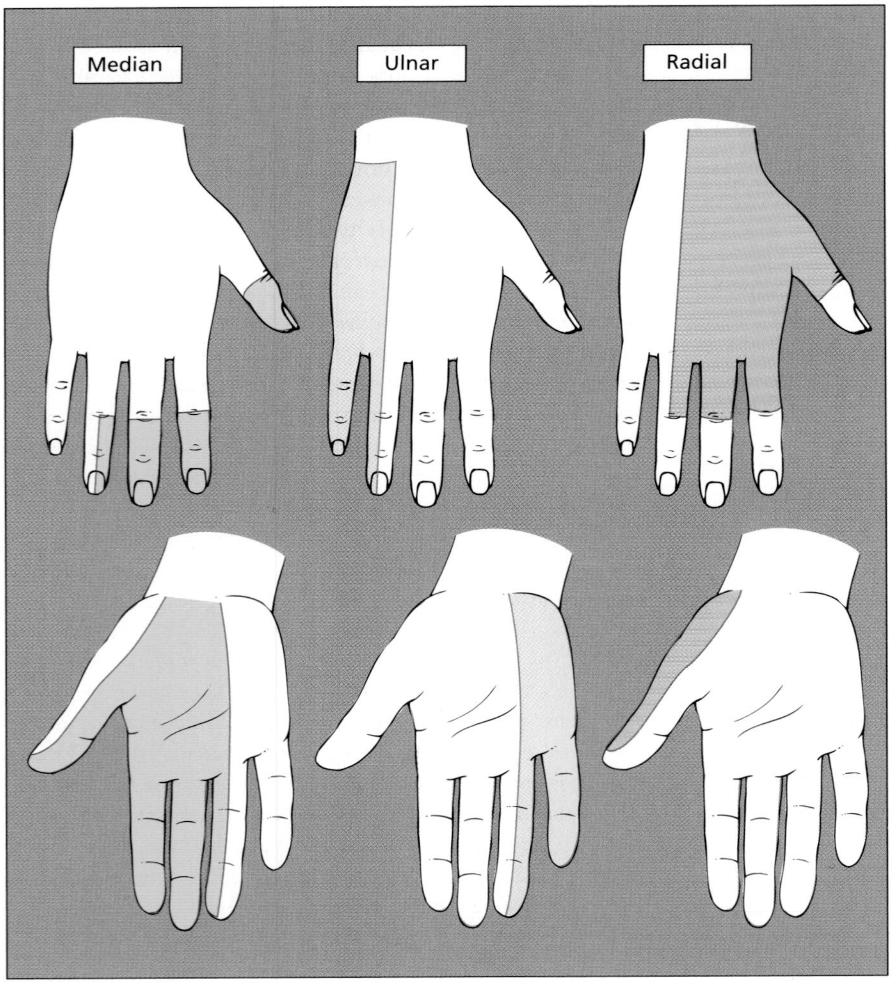

**Fig. 1.27** Sensory supply of the hand.

Grassi, W., Felder, M., Thüring-Vollenweider, U. & Bollinger, A. (1989) Microvascular dynamics at the nail fold in rheumatoid arthritis. *Clinical and Experimental Rheumatology* **7**, 47–53.

Hansen, S.W., Olsen, N., Rossing, N. & Rorth, M. (1990) Vascular toxicity and the mechanism underlying Raynaud's phenomenon in patients treated with cisplatin, vinblastine and bleomycin. *Annals of Oncology* **1**, 289–292.

Kitayama, Y. & Tsukada, S. (1983) Congenital onychodysplasia. Report of 11 cases. *Archives of Dermatology* **119**, 8–12.

Krylova, N.V. & Soboleva, T.M. (1995) The use of capillaroscopy of the skin of the nail wall in personal identification. *Sudebno-Meditsinnskaia Ekspertiza* **38**, 16–19.

Lynn, R.B., Steiner, R.E. & Van Wyck, F.A.F. (1955) Arteriographic appearances of the digital arteries of the hands in Raynaud's disease. *Lancet* i, 471–474.

Mahler, F., Saner, H., Boss, C. *et al.* (1987) Local cold exposure test for capillaroscopic examination of patients with Raynaud's syndrome. *Microvascular Research* **33**, 422–427.

Masson, P. (ed.) (1937) *Les Glomus neurovasculaires*. Hermann et Cie, Paris.

Nakayama, Y., Iino, T., Uchida, A., Kiyosawa, T. & Soeda, S. (1990) Vascularised free nail grafts nourished by arterial inflow from the venous system. *Plastic and Reconstructive Surgery* **85**, 239–245.

Ohtsuka, T., Tamura, T., Yamakage, A. & Yamazaki, S. (1998) The predictive value of quantitative nail fold capillary microscopy in patients with undifferentiated connective tissue disease. *British Journal of Dermatology* **139**, 622–629.

Ohtsuka, T., Yamakage, A. & Miyachi, Y. (1994) Statistical definition of nail fold capillary pattern in patients with psoriasis. *International Journal of Dermatology* **33**, 779–782.

Orentreich, N., Markofsky, J. & Vogelman, J.H. (1979) The effect of ageing on linear nail growth. *Journal of Investigative Dermatology* **73**, 126–130.

Pessa, J.E., Tsai, T.M., Li, Y. & Kleinert, H.E. (1990) The repair of nail deformities with the non-vascularised nail bed graft: indications and results. *Journal of Hand Surgery* **15A**, 466–470.

Richardson, D. & Schwartz, R. (1984) Comparison of resting capillary flow dynamics in the finger and toe nail folds. *Microcirculation, Endothelium and Lymphatics* **1**, 645–656.

Ryan, T.J. (1973) Direct observations of blood vessels in the superficial vasculature system of the skin. In: *The Physiology and Pathophysiology of the Skin*, Vol. 2 (ed. A. Jarrett), pp. 658–659. Academic Press, London.

Samman, P. & Strickland, B. (1962) Abnormalities of the finger nails associated with impaired peripheral blood supply. *British Journal of Dermatology* **74**, 165–173.

Schumann, L., Korten, G., Holdt, B. & Holtz, M. (1996) Microcirculation of the fingernail fold in CAPD patients: preliminary observations. *Peritoneal Dialysis International* **16**, 412–416.

Schnitzler, L., Baran, R., Civatte, J., Schubert, B., Verret, J.L. & Hurez, D. (1976) Biopsy of the proximal nail fold in collagen diseases. *Journal of Dermatologic Surgery* **2**, 313–315.

Smith, D.O., Oura, C., Kimura, C. & Toshimori, K. (1991a) Artery anatomy and tortuosity in the distal finger. *Journal of Hand Surgery* **16A**, 297–302.

Smith, D.O., Oura, C., Kimura, C. & Toshimori, K. (1991b) The distal venous anatomy of the finger. *Journal of Hand Surgery* **16A**, 303–307.

Studer, A., Hunziker, T., Lutolf, O. *et al.* (1991) Quantitative nail fold capillary microscopy in cutaneous and systemic lupus erythematosus and localised and systemic scleroderma. *Journal of the American Academy of Dermatology* **24**, 941–945.

Warwick, R. & Williams, P.L. (1973) *Gray's Anatomy*, 35th edn. Longman, Harlow, Essex.

Wilgis, E.F.S. & Maxwell, G.P. (1979) Distal digital nerve graft. *Journal of Hand Surgery* **4**, 439–443.

Winkelmann, R.K. (1960) Similarities in cutaneous nerve end-organs. In: *Advances in Biology of Skin: Cutaneous Innervation* (ed. W. Montagna), pp. 48–62. Pergamon, New York.

Wolfram-Gabel, R. & Sick, H. (1995) Vascular networks of the periphery of the fingernail. *Journal of Hand Surgery [Br]* **20**, 488–492.

Zaias, N. (1967) The longitudinal nail biopsy. *Journal of Investigative Dermatology* **49**, 406–408.

Zook, E.G. (1988) Injuries of the fingernail. In: *Operative Hand Surgery* (ed. D.P. Green), 2nd edn. Churchill Livingstone, New York.

## Comparative anatomy and function

The comparative anatomy of the nail unit can be considered from two aspects. There is the comparison of the nail with other ectodermal structures and most particularly hair and its follicle. The nail can also be viewed in an evolutionary setting alongside the hoof and claw. In this respect the functional qualities of the nail or its equivalent are exemplified by the morphological differences in different species. The human nail can be considered to have many mechanical and social functions, the most prominent of which are:
- fine manipulation;
- scratching;
- physical protection of the extremity;
- a vehicle for cosmetics and aesthetic manipulation.

In comparison with other species, the first three functions have evolved with detailed physical modifications in the form of the hoof, claw and nail.

### The nail and other appendages

An appendage is formed through the interaction of mesoderm and ectoderm, which in differentiated states usually means the interaction between dermis and epidermis. Those appendages most closely related to nail include hair and tooth. There are many shared aspects of different appendages, illustrated by diseases, morphology and analysis of the biological constituents.

Congenital abnormalities of hair, tooth and nail coexist in several conditions underlining their common ground. Ectodermal dysplasias represent a group of disorders in which these appendages as well as eccrine sweat glands, may be affected in association with skin changes.

In some conditions only two of the appendages seem to be affected, such as the hair and nail changes described by Barbareschi *et al.* (1997) or tooth and nail changes in the hypodontia and nail dysplasia syndrome (Witkop tooth and nail syndrome) (Murdoch-Kinch *et al.* 1993; Garzon & Paller 1996). Alternatively, the same genetic defect, such as a mutation in the gene for keratin 17, may underlie two separate diseases where the nail is abnormal in one phenotype and hair follicle in the other (Smith *et al.* 1997). Presumably an additional factor determines which of the possible phenotypes prevails.

Whilst diseases illustrate inter-relationships between appendages, further common ground can be defined in terms of morphology. Achten (1968) noted that the nail unit was comparable in some respects to a hair follicle, sectioned longitudinally and laid on its side (Fig. 1.28). The hair bulb was considered analogous to the intermediate nail matrix and the cortex to the nail plate. As a model to stimulate thought, this idea is helpful. It also encourages the consideration of other manipulations of the hair follicle that might fit the analogy more tightly. The nail unit could be seen as in Fig. 1.28, as an unfolded form of the hair follicle, producing a hair with no cortex, just hard cuticle. Scanning electron microscopy of the nail confirms that its structure is more similar to compacted cuticular cells than cortical fibres. A third model could represent the nail unit as a form of follicle abbreviated on one side, providing a modified form of outer root sheath to mould and direct nail growth in the manner of the proximal nail fold (Fig. 1.28). The matrix and other epithelial components of tooth can be seen in a similar comparative light and even the lingual papilla which shares some keratin expression with the nail, shows some morphological similarities with the nail and hair follicle (Manabe & O'Guin 1994). In pachyonychia congenita where alopecia is found, transverse sections of scalp follicles reveal dyskeratosis of the outer root sheath, attracting comparisons with the nail bed (Templeton & Wiegand 1997).

Constituents of some appendages, such as keratin and trichohyalin, are both specific in their physical attributes and specific to certain appendages. A considerable amount of biochemical work on hair and nail illustrates this point. In one study (Dekio & Jidoi 1989) two-dimensional electrophoresis was used to determine the presence of nine keratins in human hair and nail. Those of molecular weights 76, 73, 64, 61 and 55 kDa were common to hair and nail. One component of 61 kDa was specific to hair, and two components, both with a molecular weight of 50 kDa, were specific to nail. Further definition of these proteins was given by Heid *et al.* (1988) who employed gel electrophoresis, immunoblotting, peptide mapping and

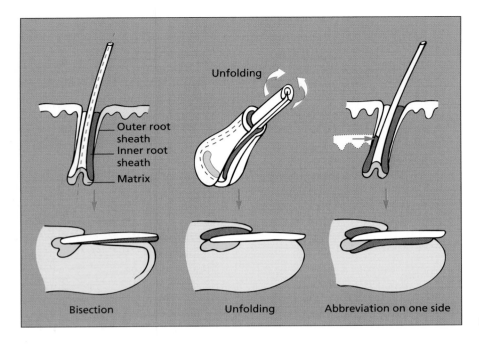

Fig. **1.28** Models of hair follicle/nail unit homology.

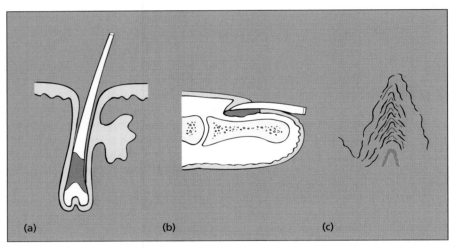

Fig. **1.29** Localization of immunoreactivity of the hard keratin Ha-1 in (a) the anagen hair follicle (×200), (b) the nail unit (×10) and (c) the human lingual papilla (×500). (After Westgate *et al.* 1997.)

complementary keratin binding analysis. Heid found that whilst nail plate contained both 'soft' epithelial and 'hard' hair/nail keratins, plucked hairs contained only the latter. By contrast, 'soft' epithelial keratins could be detected in the hair follicle and coexpressed with 'hard' keratins in a pattern also seen in the nail matrix. Although these 'hard' keratins are found in small amounts in the embryonic thymus and lingual papilla, they can generally be thought to be a feature of the hair/nail differentiation. Common ground between the lingual papilla and nail is demonstrated in the nail dystrophy of dyskeratosis congenita, where there are oral changes including changes in expression of keratins of the lingual papillae (Ogden *et al.* 1992).

The proposal that different appendages have common paths of early differentiation was pursued further by Lynch *et al.*

(1986) who suggested that the precursor cells of hair cortex and nail plate share a major pathway of epithelial differentiation. She felt that the acidic 44 kDa/46 kDa and basic 56–60 kDa 'hard' keratins represent a coexpressed keratin pair that defines hair/nail tissue.

More recently, immunohistochemistry with monospecific antibodies has facilitated mapping out the distribution of certain hard keratins such as Ha-1, found in hair follicle, nail matrix and lingual papilla (Westgate *et al.* 1997) (Fig. 1.29).

The character of the nail plate and hair has led to their use in assays of circulating metabolites. They both lend themselves to this because they are long-lasting structures that may afford historical information. Additionally, their protein constituents bind metabolites and they provide accessible specimens. This allows both hair and nail to be used in the detection of systemic

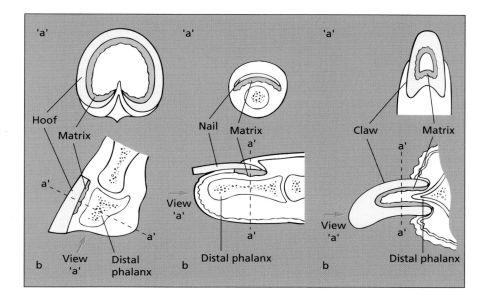

**Fig. 1.30** Comparison of hoof, nail and claw and their matrix (red) origins.

metabolites which may have disappeared from the blood many weeks previously (see 'Exogenous materials in nail analysis' below).

## Phylogenetic comparisons

The structure of claws and hooves and their evolutionary relationship to the human nail has been well reviewed (Spearman 1978). In higher primates, nails have developed with the acquisition of manual dexterity. Other mammals do not possess such flattened claws from which nails have evolved. (Fig. 1.30).

The lowest evolutionary level at which claws are seen is in the amphibia (Lucas & Strettenheim 1972). The matrix contributes the greatest mass to the nail plate in man and other primates, with a lesser contribution from the dorsal and nail bed matrices. Claws (Kato 1977) are formed from an extensive germinal matrix, which occupies the territory of the nail bed in primates. It is sometimes described as comprising a dorsal and ventral component (Mueller *et al.* 1993), where differential growth of these components is responsible for the curve. The orientation of the matrix and hence growth of nail, may be influenced by the shape of the underlying phalanx (Kato 1977). It is postulated that their sharp tip is produced by a dominant midline matrix.

Claws are significantly more three dimensional than nails and this is achieved by the coronal distribution of matrix tissue around the terminal phalanx. If this is recognized, the comparisons between other hard keratinized animal appendages such as horns and beaks becomes obvious. All these structures share physical and biochemical attributes specific to their biological character and function. In some respects the upper beak has more in common with the morphology of the nail than do claws and comparisons have been made in both structure and constituents between beak and claw (Gillespie *et al.* 1982). The dis-

orders of claws presenting to one university veterinary service demonstrated a preponderance of trauma and bacterial infection (Scott & Miller 1992) (Table 1.3). This differs from dermatological experience in humans where complaints are usually attributable to dermatoses such as psoriasis or eczema or to fungal infection.

Claws and talons are harder than nails, probably because of the content of calcium as crystalline hydroxyapatite within keratinocytes (cf. human nails; Pautard 1964). A study of onychomadesis (nail shedding) in dogs looked at mineral constituents of normal claws, human nails and the hooves of cows and pigs (Harvey & Markwell 1996). It appears that there is no particular pattern of homology between different species in this respect (Table 1.4).

Orientation of keratin microfibrils may contribute to their strength. Fourier-transform Raman spectroscopy shows that bird and reptile claws are made up mainly of β-sheeted keratin in contrast to the predominantly α-helical keratin conformation of human nail keratin (Akhtar & Edwards 1997).

**Table 1.3** Proportion of diagnoses of dogs with disorders of the claws from a study of 196 affected dogs. (Adapted from Scott & Miller 1992.)

| Diagnosis | % of cases |
| --- | --- |
| Bacterial paronychia | 35.5 |
| Trauma | 22 |
| Neoplasia | 14 |
| Fungal | 4 |
| Lupoid | 4 |
| Bullous disorder | 4 |
| Demodicosis | 1 |
| Systemic illness | 0.5 |
| Idiopathic | 15 |

**Table 1.4** Mineral content (expressed as mg/kg, standard error in parentheses). (Adapted from Harvey & Markwell 1996.)

| Mineral | Dog claw | Porcine hoof | Bovine hoof | Human nail |
|---|---|---|---|---|
| Calcium | 771 (83) | 1699 (50) | 1481 (25) | 671 (806) |
| Magnesium | 238 (21) | 220 (10) | 300 (11) | 100 (121) |
| Iron | 268 (31) | 73 (8) | 17 (1.1) | 29 (64) |
| Potassium | 430 (53) | 1050 (30) | 785 (53) | – |
| Sodium | 676 (50) | – | 523 (16) | 2400 (1800) |
| Copper | 6.3 (0.5) | 4.6 (0.13) | 8.3 (0.3) | 29 (89) |
| Zinc | 129 (5) | 160 (4) | 128 (1.7) | 106 (154) |

Claws and nails have more in common with each other than they do with hooves. However, the bovine hoof has provided a useful source of research tissue for experiments on colocalization of hard and soft keratin expression in matrix cells and the characteristics of matrix cells in tissue culture (Kitahara & Ogawa 1994). Hooves have evolved to provide a 'bulky claw' for weight bearing and locomotion over hard ground (Sisson & Grossman 1953). It is interesting that among the prosimians, tarsiers have nails on all digits apart from the 2nd and 3rd digits of the hindlimb which bear claws (Spearman 1978). In hooves the nail fold and root have been displaced backwards with a forwards extension of the nail bed. The hard 'soft plate' under hooves is produced from an area equivalent to the subungual part of the claw. In some animals, cloven hooves have only developed on the digits that touch the floor. In horses, the single large hoof is produced from the 3rd digit. The typical hoof shape is due to a deep, backwardly placed root matrix with the ventral plate formed from the subungual epidermis. The microfibrils in hooves are from 25 to 100 μm in diameter. The orientation of the fibrils is along the main axis of the hoof, similar to the hair cortex.

## References

Achten, G. (1968) Normale histologie und histochemie des nagels. In: *Handbuch der Haut- und Geschlechtskrankeiten*, Vol. 1 (ed. J. Jadassohn), pp. 339–376. Springer-Verlag, Berlin.

Akhtar, W. & Edwards, H.G. (1997) Fourier-transform Raman spectroscopy of mammalian and avian keratotic biopolymers. *Spectrochemica Acta A, Molecular and Biomolecular Spectroscopy* **53A**, 81–90.

Barbareschi, M., Cambiaghi, S., Crupi, A.C. & Tadini, G. (1997) Family with 'pure' hair-nail ectodermal dysplasia. *American Journal of Medical Genetics* **72**, 91–93.

Dekio, S. & Jidoi, J. (1989) Comparison of human hair and nail low-sulfur protein compositions on two-dimensional electrophoresis. *Journal of Dermatology* **16**, 284–288.

Garzon, M.C. & Paller, A.S. (1996) What syndrome is this? Witkop tooth and nail syndrome. *Pediatric Dermatology* **13**, 63–65.

Gillespie, J.M., Marshall, R.C. & Woods, E.F. (1982) A comparison of lizard claw keratin proteins with those of avian beak and claw. *Journal of Molecular Evolution* **18**, 121–129.

Harvey, R.G. & Markwell, P.J. (1996) The mineral composition of nails in normal dogs and comparison with shed nails in canine idiopathic onychomadesis. *Veterinary Dermatology* **7**, 29–34.

Heid, H.W., Moll, I. & Franke, W.W. (1988) Patterns of expression of trichocytic and epithelial cytokeratins in mammalian tissues. *Differentiation* **37**, 215–230.

Kato, T. (1977) A study on the development of the cat claw. *Hiroshima Journal of Medical Science* **26**, 103–126.

Kitahara, T. & Ogawa, H. (1994) Variation of differentiation in nail and bovine hoof cells. *Journal of Investigative Dermatology* **102**, 725–729.

Lucas, A.M. & Strettenheim, P.R. (1972) *Avian Anatomy Integument. Part 2. Agricultural Handbook, No. 362.* US Government Printing Office, Washington DC.

Lynch, M.H., O'Guin, W.M., Hardy, C. *et al.* (1986) Acidic and basic hair/nail ('hard') keratins: their co-localization in upper cortical and cuticle cells and the human hair follicle and their relationship to 'soft' keratins. *Journal of Cell Biology* **103**, 2593–2606.

Manabe, M. & O'Guin, W.M. (1994) Existence of trichohyalin-keratohyalin hybrid granules: co-localisation of 2 major intermediate filament-associated proteins in non-follicular epithelia. *Differentiation* **58**, 65–75.

Mueller, R.S., Sterner-Kock, A. & Stannard, A.A. (1993) Microanatomy of the canine claw. *Veterinary Dermatology* **4**, 5–11.

Murdoch-Kinch, C.A., Miles, D.A. & Poon, C.K. (1993) Hypodontia and nail dysplasia syndrome. Report of a case. *Oral Surgery, Oral Medicine and Oral Pathology* **75**, 403–406.

Ogden, G.R., Chisholm, D.M., Leigh, I.M. & Lane, E.B. (1992) Cytokeratin profiles in dyskeratosis congenita: an immunocytochemical investigation of lingual hyperkeratosis. *Journal of Oral Pathology and Medicine* **21**, 353–357.

Pautard, F.G.E. (1964) Calcification of keratin. In: *Progress in Biological Sciences in Relation to Dermatology*, Vol. 2 (eds A.J. Rook & R.E. Champion), p. 227. Cambridge University Press.

Scott, D.W. & Miller, W.H. (1992) Disorders of the claw and clawbed in dogs. *Compendium* **14**, 1448–1458.

Sisson, S. & Grossman, J.D. (eds) (1953) *The Anatomy of the Domestic Animals.* W.B. Saunders, Philadelphia.

Smith, F.J.D., Corden, L.D., Rugg, E.L. *et al.* (1997) Missense mutations in keratin 17 cause either pachyonychia congenita type 2 or a phenotype resembling steatocystoma multiplex. *Journal of Investigative Dermatology* **108**, 220–223.

Spearman, R.I.C. (1978) The physiology of the nail. In: *The Physiology and Pathophysiology of the Skin*, Vol. 5 (ed. A. Jarrett), p. 1827. Academic Press, New York.

Templeton, S.F. & Wiegand, S.E. (1997) Pachyonychia congenita-associated alopecia. A microscopic analysis using transverse section technique. *American Journal of Dermatopathology* **19**, 180–184.

Westgate, G.E., Tidman, N., de Berker, D., Blount, M.A., Philpott, M.P. & Leigh, I.M. (1997) Characterisation of LH Tric 1, a new monospecific monoclonal antibody to the hair keratin Ha 1. *British Journal of Dermatology* **137**, 24–31.

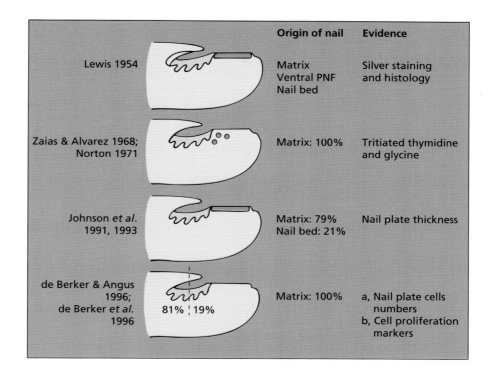

| | | Origin of nail | Evidence |
|---|---|---|---|
| Lewis 1954 | | Matrix<br>Ventral PNF<br>Nail bed | Silver staining<br>and histology |
| Zaias & Alvarez 1968;<br>Norton 1971 | | Matrix: 100% | Tritiated thymidine<br>and glycine |
| Johnson *et al.*<br>1991, 1993 | | Matrix: 79%<br>Nail bed: 21% | Nail plate thickness |
| de Berker & Angus<br>1996;<br>de Berker *et al.*<br>1996 | 81% ¦ 19% | Matrix: 100% | a, Nail plate cells<br>  numbers<br>b, Cell proliferation<br>  markers |

**Fig. 1.31** Theories of nail plate origin.

## Physiology

### Nail growth

#### Definition of the nail matrix

In the first section we have attempted to define the matrix in anatomical terms, assisted by histology and immunohistochemistry illustrating regional differentiation within the nail unit and in particular with respect to keratin expression. These measures provide indirect information on aspects of nail production and help us to address the central question of which tissues produce nail plate and which simply support and surround it. There is considerable biological and clinical relevance to this point, given that the focus of embryogenesis, damage repair and disease processes are better understood if the exact location of nail formation is established. The location or existence of nail matrix tumours is often poorly defined because there is a lack of awareness of the site and pivotal role of nail matrix disturbance in the creation of abnormal nail morphology. Equally, diagnostic biopsies or sampling can be misdirected if the likely source of nail abnormalities is not recognized at the outset; a clear prognosis following surgery or trauma cannot be given unless the clinician understands the relative contributions of the nail matrix and nail bed.

In spite of the importance of the question, controversy remains as to the relative contributions of the three putative nail matrices to the nail plate. The three contenders are the dorsal, intermediate and ventral matrix (Fig. 1.31). The first is part of the proximal nail fold, the latter is the nail bed. Lewis (1954) claimed that the nail plate demonstrated a three-layer structure on silver staining and that each layer derived from one of the possible matrices. This remains one of the indirect histological methods of defining the matrix which have been supplemented by more direct measures of nail plate productions.

#### Markers of matrix and nail bed proliferation

Zaias and Alvarez (1968) disagreed with Lewis on the basis of *in vivo* autoradiographic work on squirrel monkeys, where dynamic aspects of the process were being examined. Tritiated thymidine injected into experimental animals was only incorporated into classical matrix (or intermediate matrix to use Lewis's terminology). Norton used human subjects in further autoradiographic studies (Norton 1971). Although there was some incorporation of radiolabelled glycine in the area of the nail bed, it was in a poorly defined location, making clear statements impossible.

More recent immunohistochemical techniques have allowed us to examine proliferation markers in human tissue, without the drawbacks of autoradiography. Antibodies to proliferating cell nuclear antigen and to the antigen K1-67 associated with cell cycling, have been used on longitudinal sections of healthy and diseased nail units (de Berker & Angus 1996). Both markers demonstrated labelling indices in excess of 20% for the nail matrix in contrast with 1% or less for the nail bed in healthy tissue. In psoriatic nail and onychomycosis, the labelling index of nail bed rises to >29%. Whilst these indices do not directly measure nail plate production, a very low index for normal nail bed is consistent with other studies suggesting that the nail bed is an insignificant player in normal nail production. The situation may change in disease and the definition of nail plate becomes difficult when substantial subungual hyperkeratosis produces a ventral nail of indeterminate character (Samman 1961).

### Nail plate indicators of matrix location

Johnson *et al.* (1991, 1993) dismissed the evidence of Zaias, claiming that the methodology was flawed. She examined nail growth by the measurement of change in nail thickness along a proximal to distal longitudinal axis. She demonstrated that 21% of nail plate thickness in traumatically lost big toenails was gained as the nail grew over the nail bed. This was taken as evidence of nail bed contribution to the nail plate.

A similar study developed this observation with histology of the nail plate taken at fixed reference points along the longitudinal nail axis and comparing nail plate thickness at these sites with numbers of corneocytes in the dorso-ventral axis of the nail (de Berker *et al.* 1996). The result of this was to confirm the observation that the nail plate thickens over the nail bed but that this is not matched by an increase in nail cells. In fact, the number of cells reduces by 10%, but this was not of statistical significance. These combined studies may be reconciled if we propose that the shape of cells within the big toenail becomes altered with compaction as the nail grows. This is likely where clinical experience shows that the nail develops transverse rippling where there is habitual distal trauma.

If the loss of nail cell numbers along the nail bed is a genuine observation, it might suggest that they are being shed from the nail surface. This is compatible with the status of nail plate as a modified form of stratum corneum. Heikkilä *et al.* (1996) provides evidence in support of this where nail growth was measured by making indentations on the nail surface and measuring the change in the volume of these grooves as they reach the free edge. There was a reduction of volume by 30–35%, which was taken as evidence of a nail bed contribution to the nail plate. However, this interpretation is less believable than the possibility that the nail is losing cells from the surface, and histology of grooves in a similar study shows that this is likely to be the case (de Berker 1997).

### Flow cytometry of matrix cells

Haneke and Kiesewetter (unpublished data) have performed flow cytometry on matrix cells obtained during surgical lateral matrixectomy for ingrowing nail. This demonstrated 94% of the matrix cells were in G0/1 phase, 3.4% in S phase and 2% in G2 + M phase. The corresponding values for matrix connective tissue cells were 96.6% for G0/1, 2.3% for S and 1.1% for G2 + M phases. The differences between matrix cells and associated connective tissue were statistically significant. It suggests that the percentage of cells in the phase of DNA synthesis and mitosis (S plus G2 + M phases) in the nail matrix is much lower than that of hair matrix cells and equals that of the cells in the hair root sheath. However, the values may have been underestimated in this experiment if the matrixectomies failed to sample the most basal matrix cells as can happen in this operation. Also, this technique was not applied to distinguish nail bed from matrix and does not directly address the issue of which tissues are primarily involved in nail plate production.

### Ultrasound as a tool to define nail matrix

Ultrasound studies of the nail plate have done little to support the notion that the nail bed contributes significantly to its substance (Finlay *et al.* 1987; Jemec & Serup 1989). Jemec claimed that the nail plate had a clear two-part structure, none of which appeared to come from the nail bed. Finlay observed that the nail plate had a more rapid ultrasound transmission distally; paradoxical if one imagines a nail bed contribution. This last comment is almost diametrically opposite that of Johnson *et al.* (1991).

### Clinical markers of matrix location

The clearest demonstration of nail generation is the effect of digit amputation at different levels. Trauma within the lunula is more likely to cause irreparable nail changes than that of the nail bed (Nishi *et al.* 1996). This observation is true for adults and children alike, although the likelihood of normal regrowth is greater in children with similar trauma (Libbin & Neufeld 1988). Longitudinal biopsies of the entire nail unit within the midzone of the nail are said to cause a chronic split if the width of the biopsy exceeds 3 mm (Zaias 1967). However, there are several factors in addition to the width of the biopsy that can contribute to scarring with longitudinal biopsies and smaller biopsies in the midzone can also give long-term problems.

In some circumstances, most commonly old age, there is a pattern of subungual hyperkeratosis associated with nail thickening whch gives the impression of a nail bed contribution to the nail plate. Historically, this has been referred to as the solehorn (Fig. 1.32) and considered a germinal element of the hyponychium. Samman considered this issue in the context of a patient with pustular psoriasis (Samman 1961). He concluded that the ventral nail is a movable feast, manifesting itself in certain pathological circumstances.

## Normal nail morphology

The main issues in normal nail morphology are: why is it flat? and why is the free edge rounded and not pointed? Factors influencing nail plate thickness are dealt with earlier (see 'Nail plate' above).

### Why does nail grow out straight?

The first question was addressed in an article by Kligman

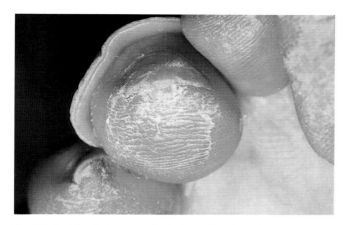

**Fig. 1.32** Vestigial solenhorn seen as focal subungual hyperkeratosis.

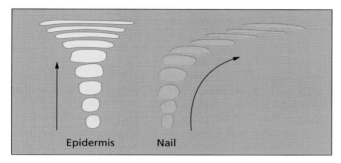

Epidermis    Nail

**Fig. 1.33** Change in shape and direction of the cells within the epidermis and the nail matrix. (After Kligman 1961.)

(1961) entitled, 'Why do nails grow out instead of up?'. His hypothesis was that the proximal nail fold acts to mould the nail as it moves away from the matrix giving an oblique growth path. From observing other keratinizing epithelia, he noted that growth is normally parallel to the axis of keratinization. From this, he considerd it anomalous that nails grow out along the nail bed and not upwards (Fig. 1.33). A patient with the nervous habit of chewing off the proximal nail fold did not provide an adequate experiment to demonstrate its function. However, when given the opportunity to autograft 5-mm matrix punch biopsies from digit to forearm, nail tissue was seen to grow upwards like a cutaneous horn. This was presented as proof of the hypothesis.

Baran was in disagreement (Baran 1981), and presented evidence from surgical experience in the removal of the proximal nail fold and the lack of subsequent change in the nail. He also challenged the validity of Kligman's experiment on the basis that the underlying terminal phalanx has a great influence upon nail growth (Baran & Juhlin 1986) and this was lost in transplanting the graft to the arm. Further examples of ectopic nail growth do not resolve the issue (Kikuchi *et al.* 1984) and the relevance of acquired bone and nail changes occurring in tandem has its own literature. Carpal tunnel syndrome can result in abnormal nails alongside acroosteolysis and ischaemic

skin lesions (Tosti *et al.* 1993). The reversal of many of the skin and nail features on treatment of the carpal tunnel compression suggests a neurovascular origin to both nail and bone changes in this pattern of acroosteolysis. Where the aetiology of the osteolysis is termed idiopathic, there are also nail changes (Todd & Saxe 1994). It seems unlikely that these cases represent a specific influence of bone upon nail formation, but rather that both structures are responding to some undefined agent. There are a wide range of primary disorders in which secondary osteolysis and altered nails are recognized complications (Todd & Saxe 1994).

All the models demonstrating the influence of the different periungual tissues and bone upon the nail are flawed. Those above do not acknowledge the adherent quality of the nail bed as an influential factor, or the the guiding influence of the lateral nail being embedded in the lateral nail folds. The role of the nail bed becomes manifest in psoriasis affecting the toes where the combination of subungual hyperkeratosis and trauma can produce upward growing nails in the presence of an apparently normal proximal nail fold. It is reasonable with our present knowledge to consider horizontal nail growth as being attributable to more than one part of the nail unit (Fig. 1.34).

### What determines the contour of the free edge?

The second issue is why are nails rounded and not pointed? This has generally been accepted as being a function of the shape of the lunula, as illustrated in Fig. 1.35. The mechanism of this is seen in Fig. 1.34. Given that nails are growing continuously throughout life, it is possible to argue that we rarely see the true free edge, but observe the eroded or manicured outline. However, there are two instances when we see the genuine free edge; at birth and with regrowth following avulsion (Fig. 1.36). These appear to follow the margin of the lunula. Finally, the nail bed may have some role in determining the shape of the free edge. Trauma to the nail bed can result in nail plate dystrophies giving the free edge a scalloped contour. This can be corrected with nail bed grafts (Pessa *et al.* 1990).

### References

Baran, R. (1981) Nail growth direction revisited. *Journal of the American Academy of Dermatology* **4**, 78–83.

Baran, R. & Juhlin, L. (1986) Bone dependent nail formation. *British Journal of Dermatology* **114**, 371–375.

de Berker, D. (1997) Nail growth measurement by indentation. *Clinical and Experimental Dermatology* **22**, 109.

de Berker, D. & Angus, B. (1996) Proliferative compartments in the normal nail unit. *British Journal of Dermatology* **135**, 555–559.

de Berker, D.A.R., MaWhinney, B. & Sviland, L. (1996) Quantification of regional matrix nail production. *British Journal of Dermatology* **134**, 1083–1086.

Finlay, A.Y., Moseley, H. & Duggan, T.C. (1987) Ultrasound transmission time: an *in vivo* guide to nail thickness. *British Journal of Dermatology* **117**, 765–770.

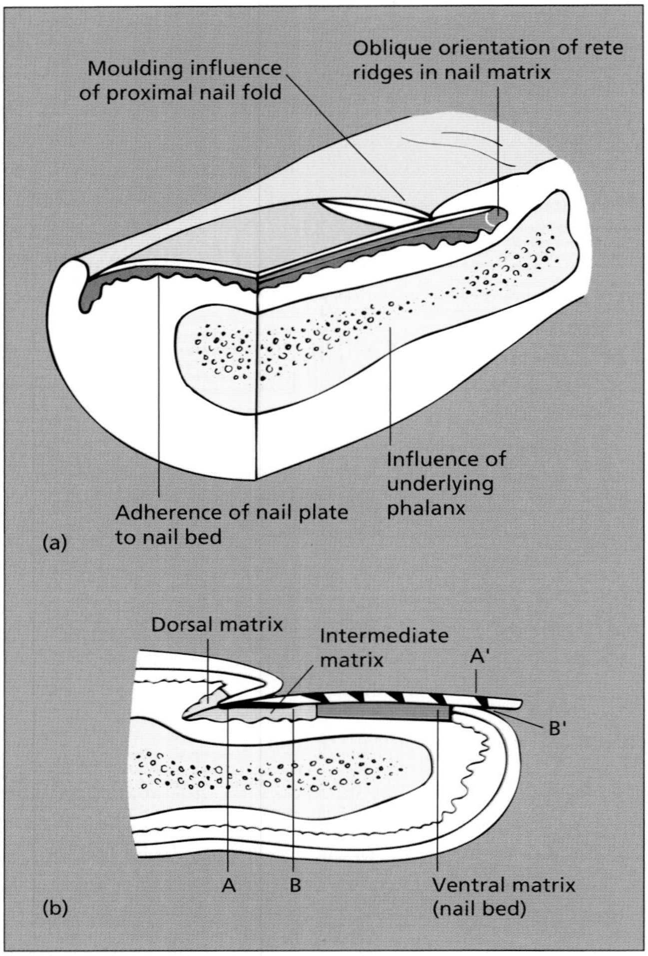

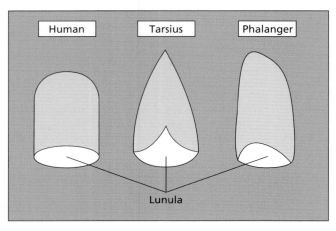

**Fig. 1.34**  Why do nails grow out instead of up? (i) Guiding restraint of proximal nail fold; (ii) inductive influence of underlying phalanx; (iii) containment by lateral nail folds; (iv) adherence to nail bed. (b) Generation of nail plate marked at monthly intervals. The horizontal axis of the intermediate axis is transformed into an oblique axis. Proximal matrix, A, generates dorsal nail A'. Distal intermediate matrix, B, generates ventral nail B'.

**Fig. 1.35**  Relationship of lunula to nail tip shape.

Heikkilä, H., Stubb, S. & Kiistala, U. (1996) Nail growth measurement employing nail indentation—an experimental follow-up study of nail growth *in situ*. *Clinical and Experimental Dermatology* **21**, 96–99.

Jemec, G.B.E. & Serup, J. (1989) Ultrasound structure of the human nail plate. *Archives of Dermatology* **125**, 643–646.

Johnson, M. & Schuster, S. (1993) Continuous formation of nail along the nail bed. *British Journal of Dermatology* **128**, 277–280.

Johnson, M., Comaish, J.S. & Shuster, S. (1991) Nail is produced by the normal nail bed: a controversy resolved. *British Journal of Dermatology* **125**, 27–28.

Kikuchi, I., Ogata, K. & Idemori, M. (1984) Vertically growing ectopic nail. *Journal of the American Academy of Dermatology* **10**, 114–116.

Kligman, A. (1961) Why do nails grow out instead of up? *Archives of Dermatology* **84**, 181–183.

Lewis, B.L. (1954) Microscopic studies of fetal and mature nail and the surrounding soft tissue. *Archives of Dermatology and Syphilis* **70**, 732–744.

Libbin, R.M. & Neufeld, D.A. (1988) Regeneration of the nail bed. *Plastic and Reconstructive Surgery* **81**, 1001–1002.

Nishi, G., Shibata, Y., Tago, K. *et al.* (1996) Nail regeneration in digits replanted after amputation through the distal phalanx. *Journal of Hand Surgery* **21A**, 229–233.

Norton, L.A. (1971) Incorporation of thymidine-methyl-$H^3$ and glycine-2-$H^3$ in the nail matrix and bed of humans. *Journal of Investigative Dermatology* **56**, 61–68.

Pessa, J.E., Tsai, T.M., Li, Y. & Kleinert, H.E. (1990) The repair of nail bed deformities with the nonvascularised nail bed graft. Indications and results. *Journal of Hand Surgery* **15A**, 466–470.

Samman, P. (1961) The ventral nail. *Archives of Dermatology* **84**, 192–195.

Todd, G. & Saxe, N. (1994) Idiopathic phalangeal osteolysis. *Archives of Dermatology* **130**, 759–762.

Tosti, A., Morelli, R., D'Alessandro, R. & Bassi, F. (1993) Carpal tunnel syndrome presenting with ischemic skin lesions, acroosteolysis and nail changes. *Journal of the American Academy of Dermatology* **29**, 287–290.

Zaias, N. (1967) The longitudinal nail biopsy. *Journal of Investigative Dermatology* **49**, 406–408.

Zaias, N. & Alvarez, J. (1968) The formation of the primate nail plate. An autoradiographic study in the squirrel monkey. *Journal of Investigative Dermatology* **51**, 120–136.

## Nail growth measurement

The literature on nail growth has relied on quantification. A range of methods have been employed, mostly requiring the imprint of a fixed reference mark on the nail and measuring its change in location relative to a fixed structure separate from the nail after a study period. Gilchrist and Dudley Buxton (1938) made a transverse scratch about 2 mm from the most distal margin of the lunula. This distance was then measured using a rule and magnifier. Changes in the distance with time provided a record of growth rate. There have been variants of this, with the scratch being made at the convex apogee of the lunula and subsequent measurements made with reference to the lunula (Hillman 1955), or alternatively making a scratch a fixed 3 mm from the cuticle and noting the change with time (Dawber

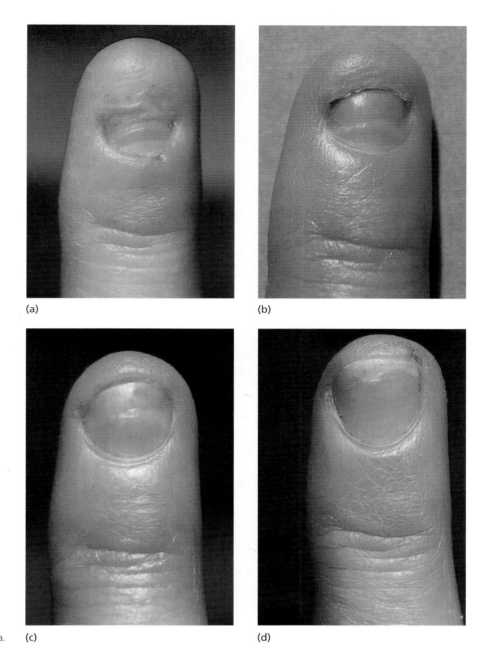

**Fig. 1.36** (a–d) Regrowth of the fingernail following traumatic avulsion. The free edge is parallel to the lunula.

(a)  (b)  (c)  (d)

1970a) (Fig. 1.37). The precision of these methods was increased by the introduction of magnified photographs before and after, and comparison of the photographs (Babcock 1955). This was modified further by Sibinga (1959) who increased the photographic magnification from a factor of 6 to 35. This made it possible to conduct studies of nail growth over a period as short as 1 month.

Babcock (1955) understood the problems in the methods involving the lunula and cuticle as reference points, as they both might conceivably change during the study. The method suggested for overcoming this was inventive, but unacceptable these days for ethical reasons. The nail was marked with a deep scratch which was then filled with bismuth amalgam. This made it radio-opaque and allowed comparison with the underlying bony reference points on X-ray. A follow up X-ray, after re-filling the scratch with amalgam, allowed growth estimation. The concern over variation in the-non-nail plate reference point can be partly surmounted by using two reference points and possibly halving the error. This can be done by making a scratch at the tip of the lunula and measuring the distance to the distal limit of the nail plate attachment, visible through the nail plate. Subsequent measurements are made from both the lunula and the edge of nail plate attachment. Their sum should always be equal as a way of verifying the method (Fig. 1.38).

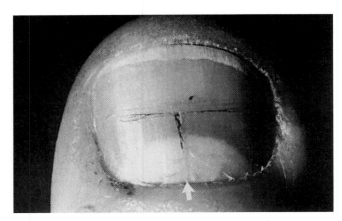

**Fig. 1.37** T-shaped mark etched on nail for nail growth measurement (Dawber 1970a). Arrow points to posterior nail fold reference point. Note the absence of a cuticle.

Surface imaging of the nail, exploiting natural irregularities, can be used in lieu of marks placed by the observer. This has been reported by de Doncker and Piérard (1994) in a study of nail growth during itraconazole therapy. The technique was not pushed to its full potential, as only clippings and not the entire *in vivo* nail plate were assessed. It was thought that longitudinal nail growth increased during therapy because surface beading became more spaced apart.

All these methods involve estimation of linear growth. As a measure of total matrix activity this could be misleading. Hamilton sought to measure volume by the following equation (Hamilton *et al.* 1955):

Thickness (mm) × breadth (mm) × length grown per day
= volume

Johnson also tried to measure volumetric growth with respect to linear growth, ignoring time (Johnson *et al.* 1991). This entailed the measurement of thickness and mass at different points in the avulsed nail plate. The method presumed that linear measurements in the longitudinal axis of the nail plate were proportional to time and that no element of compaction complicated the issue.

Attempts to measure volume take on particular significance in disease states provoking Beau's lines. In a condition where

the bulk of the nail is manifestly affected, measurement of linear growth alone may give misleading results (Fig. 1.39).

Van Noord measured the length and weight of clippings (P.A.H. Van Noord, personal communication).

## Physiological factors and nail growth

Most studies concern fingernails. Their rate of growth can vary between 1.9 and 4.4 mm/month (Sibinga 1959). A reasonable guide is 3 mm/month or 0.1 mm/day. Toenails are estimated to grow around 1 mm/month. Population studies on nail growth have given the general findings that there is little marked seasonal change and nails are unaffected by mild intercurrent illnesses (Hillman 1955; Sibinga 1959). The height or weight of the individual made no sigificant difference (Hillman 1955; Hewitt & Hillman 1966). Sex makes a small difference in early adulthood, with men having significantly ($P < 0.001$) faster linear nail growth up to the age of 19 (Hamilton *et al.* 1955). They continue to do so with gradually diminishing significance levels, up to the age of 69, when there is a crossover and women's nails grow faster than males. There is rough agreement from Hillman in an earlier study, although he found that the crossover age was around 40 (Hillman 1955). However, males continued to have a greater rate of nail growth throughout life if volume was measured, and not length (Hamilton *et al.* 1955). Children under 14 have faster growth than adults.

Pregnancy may increase the rate of nail growth (Hewitt & Hillman 1966) and poor nutrition may retard it (Gilchrist & Dudley Buxton 1938).

Temperature is an influence with unclear effects. Bean (1980) kept a slightly idiosyncratic record of his own fingernail growth by making a scratch at the free edge of his cuticle on the first day of each month for 35 years. His record showed a gradual slowing with age. It initially showed a seasonal variation with heightened growth in the warm months. This variation became less marked with age, combining with a move from Iowa to Texas where seasonal contrasts are reduced. Other studies to determine the influence of temperature have compared nail growth rates for people in temperate and polar conditions. An original study in 1958

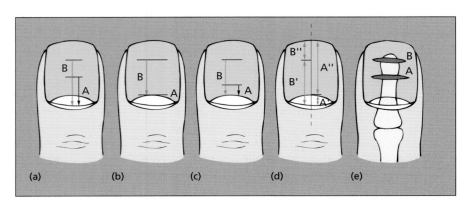

**Fig. 1.38** Methods of nail growth measurement. (a) Reference, cuticle; growth B − A; c magnifier, Dawber (1970a). (b) Reference, lunula; growth, B; Hillman (1955); c × 6 reference photo, Babcock (1955), c × 35 reference photo, Sibinga (1959). (c) Reference, lunula; growth, B − A; c magnifier, Gilchrist & Dudley Buxton (1938). (d) Reference, cuticle and nail attachment margin; growth, (B′ − A′) + (A″ − B″)/2; verification by A′ + A″ = B′ + B″. (e) Reference, bone feature on X-ray, bismuth amalgam in nail scratch; growth, depends on landmark.

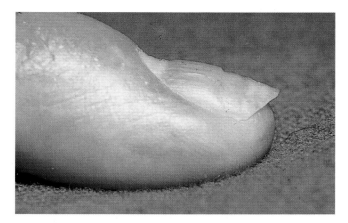

**Fig. 1.39** Side view of a nail with Beau's line, indicating the change in nail bulk.

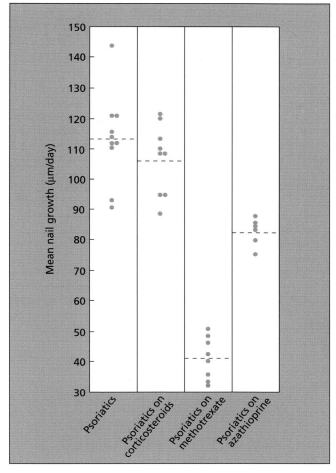

**Fig. 1.40** Effect of therapy on nail growth in psoriasis (Dawber 1970b).

(Geoghegan *et al.* 1958) found that nail growth was significantly retarded by living in the Arctic. Subsequent studies from the Antarctic found that there was no change in nail growth (Donovan 1977; Gormly & Ledingham 1983). These studies are not scientific, and it is unclear whether they are commenting on the improvement in thermal insulation since 1958 or nail physiology.

## Nail growth in disease

### Systemic disease

Insufficient numbers of seriously ill people have been followed as part of a larger study to give good statistical evidence concerning the influence of disease on nail growth. There is plenty of evidence from small numbers that some severe systemic upsets disturb nail formation. The observations of Justin Honoré Simon Beau in 1836 (Weismann 1977) detailed the development of transverse depressions upon the nails of people surviving typhoid. The form of nail growth interference represented by Beau's lines is seen in many conditions (see Beau's lines in Chapter 2). Severe illness in the form of mumps has been noted to bring linear growth to a standstill (Sibinga 1959). Other acute infections are quite variable, with 10 cases of acute febrile tuberculosis failing to have significant effect (Sibinga 1959). In the same study, chronic nephrosis produced exceptionally slow nail growth. Paradoxically, they also found that cadavers appeared to continue the growth of their nails in the 10 days post mortem during which they were assessed. The effect of death was less marked than mumps; something adults with mumps might agree with.

### Local disease

Local diseases can influence nail growth. Dawber *et al.* (1971) noted that onycholysis was associated with increased nail growth. This was true whether it was related to psoriasis or idiopathic. It is interesting that psoriasis may also produce Beau's lines and so reduce the bulk of the nail. It is not even clear whether Beau's lines represent a reduction in linear growth. They have been noted after retinoid therapy, and yet this group of drugs has been noted to increase nail growth in psoriasis (Galosi *et al.* 1985). The surface morphology of the nail in a Beau's line reflects a change in rate of nail plate production in different zones in the matrix and a loss of co-ordination with longitudinal growth; it is a product of pathology in space and time. Perhaps a nail that is growing faster is unable to accumulate bulk. Other systemic psoriasis treatments may reduce the rate of nail growth (Dawber 1970b) (Fig. 1.40).

Trauma may also influence nail growth, where wrist fractures are the most common example. Details of nail and local hair growth have been recorded in instances of reflex sympathetic dystrophy where Beau's lines and hypertrichosis on the dorsum of wrist, arm and hand may coincide. It is not clear whether the nail changes represent increased or decreased growth in these circumstances. Hypertrichosis indicates an extension of anagen, such that hairs that might normally fall

**Table 1.5** Influences on nail growth.

| Faster | Slower |
|---|---|
| Daytime | Night |
| Pregnancy (Hewitt & Hillman 1966) | 1st day of life (Schnick 1908) |
| Minor trauma/nail biting (Gilchrist & Dudley Buxton 1938; Hamilton *et al.* 1955) | |
| Right hand/dominant | Left hand/non-dominant |
| Youth | Old age (Hamilton *et al.* 1955) |
| Fingers | Toes (Pfister & Heneka 1969) |
| Summer (Bean 1980) | Winter/cold (Roberts & Sandford 1958) |
| Middle finger | Thumb and little finger (LeGros Clark & Buxton 1938; Orentreich *et al.* 1979) |
| Men | Women (LeGros Clark & Buxton 1938; Hamilton *et al.* 1955) |
| Psoriasis (Landherr *et al.* 1982) | Finger immobilization (Dawber 1981) |
| pitting (Dawber 1970a) | Fever (Sibinga 1959) |
| normal nails (Dawber 1970a) | Beau's lines (Weismann 1977) |
| onycholysis (Dawber *et al.* 1971) | |
| Pityriasis rubra pilaris (Dawber 1980) | Methotrexate, azathioprine (Dawber 1970b) |
| Etretinate (Baran 1982) | Etretinate (Baran 1982) |
| Idiopathic onycholysis of women (Dawber *et al.* 1971) | Denervation (Head & Sherrin 1905) |
| | Poor nutrition (Gilchrist & Dudley Buxton 1938) |
| Hyperthyroidism (Orentreich *et al.* 1979) | |
| L-DOPA (Miller 1973) | |
| AV shunts (Orentreich *et al.* 1979) | Yellow nail syndrome (Samman 1978) |
| Calcium/vitamin D (Hogan *et al.* 1984) | Relapsing polychondritis (Estes 1983) |
| Benoxaprofen (Fenton & Wilkinson 1983) | |

out at 5 mm or less, become longer and may gain a greater diameter. It does not necessarily mean that the hairs are growing *faster* and so in common with Beau's lines it represents a change in the pattern of appendage growth rather than a simple alteration of rate.

Immobility alone may result in a reduction in rate of nail growth and whilst this factor prevails after wrist fracture, reflex sympathetic dystrophy entails significant changes in blood supply that may have their own effects.

Table 1.5 includes influences upon nail growth that are reported, but not always of statistical significance.

## References

Babcock, M.J. (1955) Methods for measuring fingernail growth rates in nutritional studies. *Journal of Nutrition* **55**, 323–336.

Baran, R. (1982) Action therapeutique et complications due retinoide aromatique sur l'appareil ungueal. *Annales de Dermatologie et de Vénéréologie* **109**, 367–371.

Bean, W.B. (1980) Nail growth. Thirty five years of observation. *Archives of Internal Medicine* **140**, 73–76.

Dawber, R. (1970a) Fingernail growth in normal and psoriatic subjects. *British Journal of Dermatology* **82**, 454–457.

Dawber, R.P.R. (1970b) The effect of methotrexate, corticosteroids and azathioprine on fingernail growth in psoriasis. *British Journal of Dermatology* **83**, 680–683.

Dawber, R.P.R. (1980) Ultrastructure and growth of human nails. *Archives of Dermatological Research* **269**, 197–204.

Dawber, R.P.R. (1981) Effects of immobilization on nail growth. *Clinical and Experimental Dermatology* **6**, 1–4.

Dawber, R.P.R., Samman, P. & Bottoms, E. (1971) Fingernail growth in idiopathic and psoriatic onycholysis. *British Journal of Dermatology* **85**, 558–560.

de Doncker, P. & Piérard, G.E. (1994) Acquired nail beading in patients receiving itraconazole—an indicator of faster nail growth? A study using optical profilometry. *Clinical and Experimental Dermatology* **19**, 404–406.

Donovan, K.M. (1977) Antarctic environment and nail growth. *British Journal of Dermatology* **96**, 507–510.

Estes, S.A. (1983) Relapsing polychondritis. *Cutis* **32**, 471–476.

Fenton, D.A. & Wilkinson, J.D. (1983) Milia, increased nail growth and hypertrichosis following treatment with Benoxaprofen. *Journal of the Royal Society of Medicine* **76**, 525–527.

Galosi, A., Plewig, G. & Braun-Falco, O. (1985) The effect of aromatic retinoid RO 10–9359 on fingernail growth. *Archives of Dermatological Research* **277**, 138–140.

Geoghegan, B., Roberts, D.F. & Sampford, M.R. (1958) A possible climatic effect on nail growth. *Journal of Applied Physiology* **13**, 135–138.

Gilchrist, M. & Dudley Buxton, L.H. (1938) The relation of fingernail growth to nutritional status. *Journal of Anatomy* **9**, 575–582.

Gormly, P.J. & Ledingham, J.E. (1983) Nail growth in antarctic conditions. *Australian Journal of Dermatology* **24**, 86–89.

Hamilton, J.B., Terada, H. & Mestler, G.E. (1955) Studies of growth throughout the lifespan in Japanese: growth and size of nails and

**Table 1.6** Different methods of nail constituent analysis.

| Method | Element | Reference |
|---|---|---|
| I. *Structural and mineral constituents* | | |
| Raman spectroscopy | Water, proteins and lipid | Gniadecka *et al.* 1998 |
| Immunohistochemistry | Keratin | Heid *et al.* 1988 |
| Polymerase chain reaction | Deoxyribonucleic acid | Kaneshige *et al.* 1992; Tahir & Watson 1995 |
| Electron microscopy | Cystine | Salamon *et al.* 1988 |
| X-ray diffraction | Mg, Cl, Na, Ca, S, Cu | Sirota *et al.* 1988; Forslind 1970 |
| Colorimetry | Fe | Jacobs & Jenkins 1960 |
| II. *Exogenous materials* | | |
| Atomic absorption spectometry | Cd, Pb, Zn, Ca, Cr, Fe, Cu, Mn, Ni, Co, Na, K | Wilhelm *et al.* 1991; Forslind 1970; Nowak 1996 |
| Mass fragmentography | Metamphetamine | Suzuki *et al.* 1989 |
| Gas chromatography | Amphetamine, cocaine | Suzuki *et al.* 1984; Cirimele *et al.* 1995; Miller *et al.* 1994 |
| Flow injection hydride generation atomic absorption spectrometry | Arsenic | Das *et al.* 1995 |
| III. *Biological markers* | | |
| High performance liquid chromatography | Furosine (glycosylated keratin), terbinafine | Sueki *et al.* 1989; Dykes *et al.* 1990 |
| Microscopy | Lipid: triglyceride | Salamon *et al.* 1988 |
| Adsorption differential pulse voltametry | Ni | Gamelgaard & Anderson 1985 |
| Enzymic assay | Steroid sulphatase | Matsumoto *et al.* 1990 |
| Neutron activation analysis | Zinc, selenium | Rogers *et al.* 1991; Van Noord *et al.* 1987; Yoshizawa *et al.* 1998 |

their relationship to age, sex heredity and other factors. *Journal of Gerontology* 10, 401–415.

Head, H. & Sherrin, J. (1905) The consequence of injury to peripheral nerves in man. *Brain* 28, 116.

Hewitt, D. & Hillman, R.W. (1966) Relation between rate of nail growth in pregnant women and estimated previous general growth rate. *American Journal of Clinical Nutrition* 19, 436–439.

Hillman, R. (1955) Fingernail growth in the human subject. *Human Biology* 27, 274–283.

Hogan, D.B., McNair, S., Young, J. & Crilly, R. (1984) Nail growth, calcium and vitamin D. *Annals of Internal Medicine* 101, 283.

Johnson, M., Comaish, J.S. & Shuster, S. (1991) Nail is produced by the normal nail bed: a controversy resolved. *British Journal of Dermatology* 125, 27–28.

Landherr, G., Braun-Falco, O., Hofmann, C. *et al.* (1982) Fingernagelwaschtum bei psoriatikern unter puva-therapie. *Hautarzt* 33, 210–213.

LeGros Clark, W.E. & Buxton, L.H.D. (1938) Studies in nail growth. *British Journal of Dermatology* 50, 221–229.

Miller, E. (1973) Levodopa and nail growth. *New England Journal of Medicine* 288, 916.

Orentreich, N., Markofsky, J. & Vogelman, J.H. (1979) The effect of ageing on the rate of linear nail growth. *Journal of Investigative Dermatology* 73, 126–130.

Roberts, D.F. & Sandford, M.R. (1958) A possible climactic effect on nail growth. *Applied Physiology* 13, 135–137.

Pfister, R. & Heneka, J. (1969) Wachstum und Gestaltung der Zahnnagel bei Gesunden. *Archiv der Klinische und experimentale Dermatologie* 223, 263–274.

Sibinga, M.S. (1959) Observations on growth of fingernails in health and disease. *Pediatrics* 24, 225–233.

Weismann, K. (1977) J.H.S. Beau and his descriptions of transverse depressions on nails. *British Journal of Dermatology* 97, 571–572.

## Nail plate biochemical analysis

### Methods of analysis

A great range of methods have been used to analyse the organic and inorganic content of nails. Table 1.6 gives a guide, indicating how particular methods are appropriate for different constituents.

### Nail proteins

From Table 1.6 on analytical methods it is clear that a considerable number of endogenous and exogenous materials can be sought in the nail plate. The protein mesh into which the elements fit is made primarily of the intracellular protein keratin. The highly ordered structure of the proteins in the nail plate helps explain the degree of chemical and physical resistance in contrast to the characteristics of skin. The proteins of hair and nail alike have extensive folding maintained by extremely stable disulphide bonds. Although these bonds can also be found to a lesser extent in the stratum corneum of normal skin, they have a different geometry in the two sites as demonstrated by Raman spectroscopy. This is expressed as *gauche–gauche–gauche* for hair and nail and *gauche–gauche–trans* for stratum corneum (Gniadecka *et al.* 1998). The latter is less stable. The altered geometry of disulphide bonds and the extreme folding of protein molecules in hair and nail results in a different degree of hydration. The looser structure of skin allows more free water, whereas the structure of hair and nail allows very little. This contrasting degree of hydration means that skin is capable of sustaining metabolic processes not seen in nail (Gniadecka *et al.* 1998). Keratins and the associated proteins fall into the following categories:

- low sulphur proteins (40–60 kDa);
- high sulphur proteins (10–25 kDa);
- high glycine/tyrosine proteins (6–9 kDa).

It is believed that the low sulphur keratins form 10-nm filaments and the latter two groups of proteins form an interfilamentous matrix. The diversity of keratins within humans and between different species lies in the permutations of these three proteins (Gillespie & Frenkel 1974) and the diversity of the keratins themselves. Over 30 high sulphur proteins have been identified in human nail by polyacrylamide gel electrophoresis (Marshall 1980).

Nail plate keratin fibrils appear orientated in a plane parallel to the surface and in the transverse axis (Forslind 1970). They fall roughly into an 80 : 20 split between 'hard' hair type (trichocyte) keratin and 'soft', epithelial keratin (Lynch *et al.* 1986). These two variants are similar in many respects and share an X-ray diffraction pattern of α-helices in a coiled conformation, also confirmed using Raman spectroscopy (Gniadecka *et al.* 1998). Hard keratins split into the classical association of acidic and basic pairs, with extensive amino acid homologies with the epithelial forms (Hanukoglu & Fuchs 1983). In spite of regions of homology, the 'hard' and 'soft' keratins are distinguishable by immunohistochemistry (Lynch *et al.* 1986; Heid *et al.* 1988; Westgate *et al.* 1997). The relative resilience of the two groups of keratins is also reflected in their solubility in 2-mercaptoethanol. At 50 mmol/L concentrations, only epithelial 'soft' keratins are extracted from nail clippings. The concentration needs to be raised to 200 mmol/L before significant quantities of 'hard' keratin dissolve (Kitahara & Ogawa 1991).

The main lipid of nail is cholesterol. The total fat content is 0.1–1%, contrasting with the 10% found in the stratum corneum. The water content is less than that of skin, being 7–12% compared with 15–25%.

## Mineral constituents of nail

X-ray diffraction is one of the best tried methods of elemental nail analysis. Much of the initial work was done by Forslind (1970). He observed that the hardness of the nail plate is unlikely to be due to calcium, which the analogy with bone has suggested. Detailed resumés of normal nail mineral content have been made (Zaias 1990).

Much interest has been demonstrated in the analysis of nails as a source of information concerning health. A significant increase in the nail content of Na, Mg and P was noted in a survey of 50 patients with cirrhosis (Djaldetti *et al.* 1987). In a comparison of term and preterm infants, a decrease in aluminium and sulphur was found in term deliveries. The high aluminium content in preterm infants was considered of possible relevance to the osteopenia observed in this group (Sirota *et al.* 1988). Copper and iron have been observed at higher levels in the nails of male 6–11 year olds in comparison with females (Alexiou *et al.* 1980). Iron levels in the general population were found to be equal in men and women, but higher in children and highest in the neonate (Jacobs & Jenkins 1960).

## Biological markers in nail plate

In some respects, nail analysis can be compared with a blood test, but involving the examination of a less labile source of information. Analysis of chloride in nail clippings of a juvenile control population and those suffering cystic fibrosis, revealed a significant increase of chloride, by a factor of 5, in the latter. This has led to the suggestion of 'screening nail by mail' for inaccessible regions, where sending nails would be relatively easy.

The glycosylated globin molecule, used for estimation of long-term diabetic control, has been used as a model in studies measuring nail furosine in diabetes mellitus. The nail fructose-lysine content is raised in this disease and has shown a correlation with the severity of diabetic retinopathy and neuropathy (Oimomi *et al.* 1985). Nail furosine levels have also shown a good correlation with fasting glucose and may even compete with glycosylated haemoglobin as an indicator of long-term diabetic control (Sueki *et al.* 1989).

Steroid sulphatase and its substrate, cholesterol sulphate, have been assayed in the nails of children being screened for X-linked ichthyosis and found to have adequate sensitivity and accuracy to be useful (Djaldetti *et al.* 1987; Matsumoto *et al.* 1990; Serizawa *et al.* 1990). Sudan IV-positive material in nails has been measured as a guide to serum triglycerides (Salamon *et al.* 1988).

Selenium is a trace element critical for the activity of glutathione peroxidase, which may protect DNA and other cellular molecules against oxidative damage. High concentrations are seen to protect against the action of certain carcinogens in some animal models and consequently its role in human cancers has been explored. Analysis of the selenium levels of different rat tissues suggest that blood selenium may be the best indirect measure of liver selenium and nail selenium may best reflect whole body levels and the level in skeletal and heart muscle (Behne *et al.* 1996). Nail selenium levels in those being screened for oral cancer (Rogers *et al.* 1991) and carcinoma of the breast (Djaldetti *et al.* 1987; van den Brandt *et al.* 1994) showed no significant differences between affected and control patients. However, in a prospective study, toenail selenium levels had a weak predictive value for the development of advanced prostate cancer, where low levels of selenium predisposed to this malignancy (Yoshizawa *et al.* 1998). Examination of a wide range of trace elements in the nails of women with breast cancer failed to show any difference from normal controls (Garland *et al.* 1996) and analysis of nail for zinc showed no significant difference between pellagra patients with low serum zinc and normal controls (Vannucchi *et al.* 1995).

Nail clippings can be used as a source of DNA which, after amplification by the polymerase chain reaction, is of forensic use. Early work required 20–30 mg of nail (Kaneshige *et al.* 1992) and this figure has decreased to 9 mg, where the DNA for the HLA-DQa alleles are used to assess homology with blood samples (Tahir & Watson 1995).

### Exogenous materials in nail analysis

Exogenous materials can be considered in two groups: environmental and ingested substances. In the first category, cadmium, copper, lead and zinc were examined in the hair and nails of young children (Wilhelm *et al.* 1991). This was done to gauge the exposure to these substances sustained in rural and industrialized areas of Germany. Both hair and nail reflected the different environments, although the multiple correlation coefficient was higher for hair than nails.

Water taken from wells in arsenic-rich rock has resulted in arsenic poisoning on a major scale in West Bengal, India over the last 10 years. About 50% of ingested arsenic is excreted in the urine, smaller amounts in the faeces, hair and nails. Nail analysis has been used in the Bengal population as well as in other populations suffering arsenic poisoning. Levels were estimated using flow injection hydride generation atomic absorption spectroscopy which allows analysis using very small samples and enables comparisons between different tissues. The Bengal experience suggests that there are similar concentrations in hair and nail, with a trend towards higher concentrations in the latter (Das *et al.* 1995). During an episode of arsenic posioning in Alaska, the level of arsenic in nail was four times that found in hair (Harrington *et al.* 1978). A study in New Hampshire, USA, found that in subjects drinking from arsenic-rich wells, there was a doubling of toenail arsenic for a 10-fold rise in water arsenic content (Karagas *et al.* 1996).

The features of arsenic poisoning were different in Alaska and Bengal, with far more cutaneous and systemic signs of toxicity in the Bengal population in spite of similar levels in body tissues. This was attributed to coexistent dietary deficiencies and ill health in the Bengalis.

In addition to hair and nail, teeth can also act as indicators of long-term unwanted substances and, in particular, heavy metals. One account suggests that hair reflects a period of 2–5 months, nails 12–18 months and teeth a far longer period measured in years (Nowak 1996). These figures are likely to be subject to the length of the hair, the site of nail sampling (toe vs. finger) and the age of the subject.

Nickel analysis has been performed to establish occupational exposure (Gamelgaard & Anderson 1985).

The use of forensic nail drug analysis has been reported by the Japanese where over 20 000 people were arrested for the abuse of methamphetamine in 1987 (Suzuki *et al.* 1984, 1989). It was found that the drug entered the nail via both the matrix and nail bed. Chronic drug abusers could be distinguished from those with a single recent ingestion by scraping the undersur-face of the nail before analysis. This would remove the nail bed contribution and the drug it contained in the 'one-off' abuser.

Simultaneous hair and nail analysis has been performed to compare the capacity of the tissues to reflect chronic drug abuse in those taking cocaine (Miller *et al.* 1994) and amphetamines (Cirimele *et al.* 1995). Miller *et al.* (1994) found that concentrations of cocaine and its derivatives were higher in hair than in nail, whereas Cirimele *et al.* (1995) found that the concentrations of amphetamines and its metabolites were similar in both tissues. Analysis of nail clippings from the newborn by gas chromatography–mass spectroscopy can provide evidence of exposure to cocaine during embryogenesis. Given the point of nail formation, it is likely that the levels will reflect exposure after the 14th week (Skopp & Pötsch 1997). Inclusion of the antifungal, terbinafine, via the nail bed has also been observed (Dykes *et al.* 1990). Access of the drug to the nail plate via the nail bed may be one of the important factors allowing effective therapy to be delivered in less time than it takes to grow a nail (Matthieu *et al.* 1991; Munro & Shuster 1992). *In vitro* models for the uptake and delivery of terbinafine by nail plate have been employed to examine aspects of this process (Rashid *et al.* 1995).

Following single large doses of methamphetamine, it can be detected by mass fragmentography in saliva up to 2 days later, hair up to 18 days and in nail for the next 45 days (Suzuki *et al.* 1989). Chloroquine (Ofori-Adjei & Ericsson 1985) has also been measured in nail clippings for research purposes up to a year after ingestion.

### References

Alexiou, D., Koutsclinis, A., Manolidis, C. *et al.* (1980) The content of trace elements in fingernails of children. *Dermatology* **160**, 380–382.

Behne, D., Gessner, H. & Kyriakopoulos, A. (1996) Information on the selenium status of several body compartments of rats from the selenium concentrations in blood fractions, hair and nails. *Journal of Trace Elements in Medicine and Biology* **10**, 174–179.

van den Brandt, P.A., Goldbohm, R.A., vant Veer, P. *et al.* (1994) Toenail selenium levels and the risk of breast cancer. *American Journal of Epidemiology* **140**, 20–26.

Cirimele, V., Kintz, P. & Mangin, P. (1995) Detection of amphetamines in fingernails: an alternative to hair analysis. *Archives of Toxicology* **70**, 68–69.

Das, D., Chatterjee, A., Badal, K. *et al.* (1995) Arsenic in ground water in six districts of West Bengal, India: the biggest arsenic calamity in the world. *Analyst* **120**, 917–924.

Djaldetti, M., Fishman, P., Harpaz, D. & Lurie, B. (1987) X-ray microanalysis of the fingernails in cirrhotic patients. *Dermatologica* **174**, 114–116.

Dykes, P.J., Thomas, R. & Finlay, A.Y. (1990) Determination of terbinafine in nail samples during treatment for onychomycoses. *British Journal of Dermatology* **123**, 481–486.

Forslind, B. (1970) Biophysical studies of the normal nail. *Acta Dermato-Venereologica* **50**, 161–168.

Gamelgaard, B. & Anderson, J.R. (1985) Determination of nickel in human nails by adsorption differential-pulse voltametry. *Analyst* **110**, 1197–1199.

Garland, M., Morris, J.S., Colditz, G.A. et al. (1996) Toenail trace element levels and breast cancer: a prospective study. American Journal of Epidemiology 144, 653–660.

Gillespie, J.M. & Frenkel, M.J. (1974) The diversity of keratins. Comparative Biochemistry and Physiology 47B, 339–346.

Gniadecka, M., Nielsen, O. & Christensen, D. et al. (1998) Structure of water, proteins and lipids in intact human skin, hair and nail. Journal of Investigative Dermatology 110, 393–398.

Hanukoglu, I. & Fuchs, E. (1983) The cDNA sequence of a human epidermal keratin: divergence of sequence but conservation of structure among intermediate filaments. Cell 31, 243–251.

Harrington, J., Middaugh, J., Morse, D. & Housworth, J. (1978) A survey of a population exposed to high concentrations of arsenic in well water in Fairbanks, Alaska. American Journal of Epidemiology 108, 377–385.

Heid, H.W., Moll, I. & Franke, W.W. (1988) Patterns of expression of trichocytic and epithelial cytokeratins in mammalian tissues. Differentiation 37, 215–230.

Jacobs, A. & Jenkins, D.J. (1960) The iron content of finger nails. British Journal of Dermatology 72, 145–148.

Kaneshige, T., Takagi, K., Nakamura, S. et al. (1992) Genetic analysis using fingernail DNA. Nucleic Acid Research 20, 5489–5490.

Karagas, M.R., Morris, J.S. & Weiss, J.E. (1996) Toenail samples as an indicator of drinking water arsenic exposure. Cancer Epidemiology, Biomarkers and Prevention 5, 849–852.

Kitahara, T. & Ogawa, H. (1991) The extraction and characterisation of human nail keratin. Journal of Dermatological Science 2, 402–406.

Lynch, M.H., O'Guin, W.M., Hardy, C. et al. (1986) Acidic and basic hair/nail 'hard' keratins: their co-localisation in upper cortical and cuticle cells of the human hair follicle and their relationship to 'soft' keratins. Journal of Cell Biology 103, 2593–2606.

Marshall, R.C. (1980) Genetic variation in the proteins of the human nail. Journal of Investigative Dermatology 75, 264–269.

Matsumoto, T., Sakura, N. & Ueda, K. (1990) Steroid sulphatase activity in nails: screening for X-linked ichthyosis. Pediatric Dermatology 7, 266–269.

Matthieu, L., de Doncker, P., Cauwenburgh, G. et al. (1991) Itraconazole penetrates the nail via the nail matrix and the nail bed—an investigation in onychomycosis. Clinical and Experimental Dermatology 16, 374–376.

Miller, M., Martz, R. & Donnelly, B. (1994) Drugs in keratin samples from hair, fingernails and toenails. In: Second International Meeting on Clinical and Forensic Aspect of Hair Analysis (Abstract), Genoa, Italy, June 6–8, p. 39.

Munro, C.S. & Shuster, S. (1992) The route of rapid access of drugs to the distal nail plate. Acta Dermatolo-Venereologica 72, 387–388.

Nowak, B. (1996) Occurrence of heavy metals, sodium, calcium and potassium in human hair, teeth and nails. Biological Trace Element Research 52, 11–22.

Ofori-Adjei, D. & Ericsson, O. (1985) Chloroquine in nail clippings. Lancet 2 (8450), 331.

Oimomi, M., Maeda, Y., Hata, F. et al. (1985) Glycosylation levels of nail proteins in diabetic patients with retinopathy and neuropathy. Kobe Journal of Medical Science 31, 183–188.

Rashid, A., Scott, E.M. & Richardson, M.D. (1995) Inhibitory effect of terbinafine on the invasion of nails by Trichophyton mentagrophytes. Journal of the American Academy of Dermatology 33, 718–723.

Rogers, M., Thomas, D.B., Davis, S. et al. (1991) A case control study of oral cancer and pre-diagnostic concentrations of selenium and zinc in nail tissue. International Journal of Cancer 48, 182–188.

Salamon, T., Lazovic-Tepavac, O., Nikulin, A. et al. (1988) Sudan IV positive material of the nail plate related to plasma triglycerides. Dermatologica 176, 52–54.

Serizawa, S., Nagai, T., Ito, M. & Sato, Y. (1990) Cholesterol sulphate levels in the hair and nails of patients with recessive X-linked ichthyosis. Clinical and Experimental Dermatology 15, 13–15.

Sirota, L., Straussberg, R., Fishman, P., Dulitzky, F. & Djaldetti, M. (1988) X-ray microanalysis of the fingernails in term and preterm infants. Pediatric Dermatology 5, 184–186.

Skopp, G. & Pötsch, L. (1997) A case report on drug screening of nail clippings to detect prenatal drug exposure. Therapeutic Drug Monitoring 19, 386–389.

Sueki, H., Nozaki, S., Fujisawa, R. et al. (1989) Glycosylated proteins of skin, nail and hair: application as an index for long-term control of diabetes mellitus. Journal of Dermatology 16, 103–110.

Suzuki, O., Hattori, H. & Asano, M. (1984) Nails as useful materials for detection of metamphetamine or amphetamine abuse. Forensic Science International 24, 9–16.

Suzuki, S., Inoue, T., Hori, H. & Inayama, S. (1989) Analysis of methamphetamine in hair, nail, sweat and saliva by mass fragmentography. Journal of Analytical Toxicology 13, 176–178.

Tahir, M. & Watson, N. (1995) Typing of DNA HLA-DQa alleles extracted from human nail material using polymerase chain reaction. Journal of Forensic Sciences CA 40, 634–636.

Van Noord, P.A.H., Collette, H.J.A. Maas, M.J. & de Waard, F. (1987) Selenium levels in nails of premenopausal breast cancer patients assessed prediagnostically in a cohort-nested case-referent study among women screened in the DOM project. International Journal of Epidemiology 16 (Suppl.), 318–322.

Vannucchi, H.F., Varo, R.M., Cunha, D.F. & Marchini, J.S. (1995) Assessment of zinc nutritional status of pellagra patients. Alcohol and Alcoholism 30, 297–302.

Westgate, G.E., Tidman, N., de Berker, D., Blount, M.A., Philpott, M.P. & Leigh, I.M. (1997) Characterisation of LH Tric 1, a new monospecific monoclonal antibody to the hair keratin Ha 1. British Journal of Dermatology 137, 24–31.

Wilhelm, M., Hafner, D., Lombeck, I. & Ohnesorge, F.K. (1991) Monitoring of cadmium, copper, lead and zinc status in young children using toenails: comparison with scalp hair. Science of the Total Environment 103, 199–207.

Yoshizawa, K., Willett, W.C., Morris, S.J. et al. (1998) Study of the prediagnostic selenium levels in toenails and the risk of advanced prostate cancer. Journal of the National Cancer Institute 90, 1219–1224.

Zaias, N. (ed.) (1989) The Nail in Health and Disease, 2nd edn, pp. 12–13. Appleton-Lange, Norwalk, CT.

## Physical properties of nails

### Strength

The strength and physical character of the nail plate is attributable to both its constituents and design. The features of design worthy of note are the double curvature, in transverse and longitudinal axes, and the flexibility of the ventral plate compared with the dorsal aspect. The first provides rigidity, whereas the latter allows moderate flexion deformity and slightly less extension. The most proximal component of the matrix provides the corneocytes of the dorsal nail surface. These usually provide a shiny surface. When the matrix is altered by disease or the nail surface subject to trauma, this shine is lost.

## Measuring nail strength

Several techniques have been developed to study the physical properties of nails (Baden 1970; Maloney & Paquette 1977; Finlay *et al.* 1980). Maloney's studies showed changes of tensile, flexural and tearing strength with age, sex and the digit from which the nail derived. Finlay devised a 'nail flexometer' able to repeatedly flex longitudinal nail sections through 90°, recording the number it took to fracture the nail. In this way, the strength could be quantified. He noted that the immersion of nails in water for an hour increased their weight by 21%. It also made them significantly more flexible. After 2 h, the flexibility was still increasing, whilst the water content reached a plateau. Analysis of *in vivo* nail by Raman spectroscopy suggests that after soaking in water for 10 min, the α-helical protein conformation is made more loose, with greater spacing between proteins as water occupies the interstices. However, this change is seen only in distal nail, with proximal nail already manifesting a high degree of hydration before immersion (Wessel *et al.* 1999).

Mineral oil has no effect on flexibility, although it can act to maintain some of the flexibility imbued by water. This principle is applied in the treatment of onychoschizia, where repeated hydration and drying of the nail plate results in splitting at the free edge (Wallis *et al.* 1991). Zaun (1997) has used a method of assessment of brittleness that relies on the swelling properties of nail, employing the technique before and after therapy for brittle nails. Splitting can be partially overcome by applications of emollient after soaking the nails in water. The use of nail varnish can also decrease water loss (Spruit 1972).

## Permeability

The degree of nail plate swelling in alkali has been suggested as an index of disease (Zaun & Becker 1976). Normal, onychomycotic and psoriatic nails differ in the time it takes them to stop swelling, and what percentage volume increase they sustain.

Nail permeability is relevant to topical drugs on the dorsal surface and systemic drugs from the ventral surface. Trans-onychial water loss can be measured *in vivo* (Jemec *et al.* 1989), but drug penetration assay is more complicated. The simplest method is to use cadaver nails. Doing this, the permeability coefficient for water has been estimated at $16.5 \times 10^{-3}$ cm/h and that for ethanol at $5.8 \times 10^{-3}$ cm/h (Walters *et al.* 1983).

This demonstrates that the hydrated nail is more permeable to water than to alcohol and behaves like a hydrogel of high ionic strength to polar and semipolar alcohols. Combining alcohols with water may increase the permeation by the alcohol. The addition of N-acetyl-L-cysteine or mercaptoethanol to an aqueous solvent has been found to enhance the penetration of nail samples by the antifungal, tolnaftate (Kobayashi *et al.* 1998). Human nail can be substituted in such studies using an *in vitro* model for the assessment of drug penetration employing a keratin membrane prepared from bovine (Mertin & Lippold 1997a), sheep (Yang *et al.* 1997) and porcine hooves (Pittrof *et al.* 1992).

The nail is 1000 times more permeable to water than is skin (Spruit 1971; Walters *et al.* 1981) and consequently drugs required to diffuse through the nail should normally have a high degree of water solubility (Mertin & Lippold 1997b). In spite of this, there is possibly a parallel lipid pathway that allows permeation of hydrophobic molecules (Walters *et al.* 1985a) and lipid vehicles are of value because they stick better to the nail surface (Mertin & Lippold 1997a,b).

Molecular size, expressed as weight, is a further factor determining the penetration of nail by a drug. Larger molecules penetrate less well. In the field of topical antimycotics, this allows prediction of efficacy when the combined characteristics of water solubility, molecular size and minimum inhibitory concentration for antifungal activity are allowed for in a complex calculation (Mertin & Lippold 1997c). In this manner, drugs such as ciclopirox and amorolfine can be predicted to be of some value. However, more hydrophobic molecules, such as the imidazoles, itraconazole and ketoconazole, are barely able to diffuse into nail, even when it is pretreated with topical keratolytics such as papain, urea and salicylic acid (Quintanar-Guerrero *et al.* 1998).

The dense matrix of keratin and associated proteins is considered an obstacle to DMSO penetration in the nail plate, contrasting with its easier access through skin (Walters 1985a). However, it appears to facilitate the penetration of some topical antimycotics (Stüttgen & Bauer 1982). When amorolfine is applied to nail, its penetration is enhanced by pretreatment with DMSO and the penetration is further enhanced if methylene chloride is used as a vehicle for the antifungal in preference to ethanol (Franz 1992). Some medicated lacquers are also able to penetrate sufficiently to be of clinical use, particularly if their access is increased by abrading the dorsal surface of the nail plate (Ceschin-Roques *et al.* 1991; Mensing & Splanemann 1991). The concentration gradient, and hence diffusion, can be increased further by facilitating solution of the reagents, such as miconazole, by lowering the pH (Walters *et al.* 1985b). Using a solvent that evaporates will have the same effect (Marty & Dervault 1991).

There is also exchange of chemicals between nail and the internal environment and it is likely that the nail has different characteristics of drug penetration on the dorsal and ventral surfaces (Kobayashi *et al.* 1999). The significance of this is mainly with respect to inclusion of circulating materials into the nail rather than the other way around, although in a study of topical application of sodium pyrithone, Mayer *et al.* (1992) found microscopic amounts in the systemic circulation. Munro and Shuster (1992) and Matthieu *et al.* (1991) have shown that drugs can penetrate rapidly into the distal nail via the nail bed. Other drugs may be found in the nail, which makes the nail a useful source of information concerning the ingestion of some illicit drugs or environmental pollutants (see below).

Nail has been compared with other keratinous tissues, such as hair, hoof and skin, to determine how well it provides a model of *in vitro* infection by fungi (Rai & Qureshi 1994). This reveals that nail is relatively resistant to such infection and hair, feathers and horn were more easily penerated.

## Radiation penetration

The permeability of the nail plate to radiation has both advantages and drawbacks. It is the basis for treating twenty-nail dystrophy with topical PUVA (Halkier-Sørenson *et al.* 1990) and also the cause of photoonycholysis. This may be in association with photosensitizing drugs (Baran & Juhlin 1987). Benign longitudinal melanonychia can complicate phototherapy for psoriasis (Beltrani & Scher 1991).

Chronic X-irradiation is associated with carcinoma-in-situ and invasive squamous cell carcinoma (Onukak 1980). The polydactylous form of Bowen's disease is commonly related to some source of radiation (Baran & Gormley 1987). Parker and Diffey (1983) have investigated the transmission of light through the toenails of cadavers. Examining wavelengths between 300 and 600 nm, it appears that transmission at the shorter wavelength is minimal. This corresponds to UVB. If the nail plate is acting as a sunscreen it is fortuitous, but the character of the toenails studied may not be the same as fingernails, which are more commonly exposed.

A double-blind study of superficial radiotherapy in psoriatic nail dystrophy has demonstrated a definite albeit temporary benefit (Yu & King 1992). A similar temporary benefit has been demonstrated with electron beam therapy (Kwang *et al.* 1994). Both of these studies might suggest that the different forms of radiation are penetrating nail, although treatment of periungual psoriasis can have a secondary beneficial effect on subungual tissues.

## References

Baden, H.P. (1970) The physical properties of nail. *Journal of Investigative Dermatology* 55, 115.

Baran, R. & Gormley, D.E. (1987) Polydactylous Bowen's disease of the nail. *Journal of the American Academy of Dermatology* 17, 201–204.

Baran, R. & Juhlin, L. (1987) Drug induced photo onycholysis. *Journal of the American Academy of Dermatology* 17, 1012–1016.

Beltrani, V. & Scher, R. (1991) Evaluation and management of melanonychia striata in a patient receiving phototherapy. *Archives of Dermatology* 127, 319–320.

Ceschin-Roques, C.G., Hanel, H., Pruja-Bougaret, S.M., Luc, J., Vandermander, J. & Michel, G. (1991) Ciclopirox nail lacquer 8%: *in vivo* penetration into and through nails. *Skin Pharmacology* 4, 89–94.

Finlay, A.F., Frost, P., Keith, A.C. & Snipes, W. (1980) An assessment of factors influencing flexibility of human fingernails. *British Journal of Dermatology* 103, 357–365.

Franz, T.J. (1992) Absorption of amorolfine through human nail. *Dermatology* 184 (Suppl. 1), 18–20.

Halkier-Sørenson, L., Cramers, M. & Kragballe, K. (1990) Twenty nail dystrophy treated with topical PUVA. *Acta Dermato-Venereologica* 70, 510–511.

Jemec, G.B.E., Agner, T. & Serup, J. (1989) Transonychial water loss: relation to sex, age and nail plate thickness. *British Journal of Dermatology* 121, 443–446.

Kobayashi, Y., Miyamoto, M., Sugibayashi, K. & Morimoto, Y. (1998) Enhancing effect of N-acetyl-l-cysteine or 2-mercaptoethanol on the *in vitro* permeation of 5-fluorouracil or tolnaftate through the human nail plate. *Chemical and Pharmaceutical Bulletin (Tokyo)* 46, 1797–1802.

Kobayashi, Y., Miyamoto, M., Sugibayashi, K. & Morimoto, Y. (1999) Drug permeation through the three layers of the human nail plate. *Journal of Pharmacy and Pharmacology* 51, 271–278.

Kwang, T.Y., Nee, T.S. & Seng, K.T.H. (1994) A therapeutic study of nail psoriasis using electron beams (letter). *Acta Dermato-Venereologica* 75, 90.

Maloney, M.J. & Paquette, E.G. (1977) The physical properties of fingernails. I. Apparatus for physical measurements. *Journal of the Society of Comparative Chemistry* 28, 415.

Marty, J.P. & Dervault, A.M. (1991) Voie percutanée. In: *Therapeutique Dermatologique* (ed. L. Dubertret), pp. 649–663. Medecine Sciences Flammarion, Paris.

Matthieu, L., de Doncker, P., Cauwenburgh, G. *et al.* (1991) Itraconazole penetrates the nail via the nail matrix and the nail bed—an investigation in onychomycosis. *Clinical and Experimental Dermatology* 16, 374–376.

Mayer, P.R., Couch, R.C., Erickson, M.K., Woodbridge, C.B. & Brazzell, R.K. (1992) Topical and systemic absorption of sodium pyrithone following topical application to the nails of the rhesus monkey. *Skin Pharmacology* 5, 154–159.

Mensing, H. & Splanemann, V. (1991) Evaluation of the antimycotic activity of the pathological substance under the nail after treatment with RO 14–4767 nail lacquer. In: *Proceedings of the 1st EADV Congress*, pp. 21–22. Blackwell Scientific Publications, Oxford.

Mertin, D. & Lippold, B.C. (1997a) *In vitro* permeability of the human nail and of a keratin membrane from bovine hooves: penetration of chloramphenicol from lipophilic vehicles and a nail lacquer. *Journal of Pharmacy and Pharmacology* 49, 241–245.

Mertin, D. & Lippold, B.C. (1997b) *In vitro* permeability of the human nail and of a keratin membrane from bovine hooves: influence of the partition coefficient octanol/water and the water solubility of drugs on their permeability and maximum flux. *Journal of Pharmacy and Pharmacology* 49, 30–34.

Mertin, D. & Lippold, B.C. (1997c) *In vitro* permeability of the human nail and of a keratin membrane from bovine hooves: prediction of the penetration rate of antimycotics through the nail plate and their efficacy. *Journal of Pharmacy and Pharmacology* **49**, 866–872.

Munro, C.S. & Shuster, S. (1992) The route of rapid access of drugs to the distal nail plate. *Acta Dermato-Venereologica* **72**, 387–388.

Onukak, E.E. (1980) Squamous cell carcinoma of the nail bed. Diagnosis and therapeutic problems. *British Journal of Surgery* **67**, 893–895.

Parker, S.G. & Diffey, B.L. (1983) The transmission of optical radiation through human nails. *British Journal of Dermatology* **108**, 11–16.

Pittrof, F., Gerhards, J. & Erni, W. (1992) Loceryl nail lacquer—realization of a new galenical approach to onychomycosis therapy. *Clinical and Experimental Dermatology* **17** (Suppl. 1), 26–28.

Quintanar-Guerrero, D., Ganem-Quintanar, A., Tapia-Olguìn, P. *et al.* (1998) The effect of keratolytic agents on the permeability of three imidazole antimycotic drugs through the human nail. *Drug Development and Industrial Pharmacy* **24**, 685–690.

Rai, M.K. & Qureshi, S. (1994) Screening of different keratin baits for isolation of keratinophilic fungi. *Mycoses* **37**, 295–298.

Spruit, D. (1971) Measurement of water vapor loss through human nail in vivo. *Journal of Investigative Dermatology* **56**, 359–361.

Spruit, D. (1972) Effect of nail polish on hydration of the fingernail. *American Cosmetics and Perfumery* **87**, 57–58.

Stüttgen, G. & Bauer, E. (1982) Bioavailability, skin and nail penetration of topically applied antimycotics. *Mykosen* **25**, 74–80.

Wallis, M.S., Bowen, W.R. & Guin, J.D. (1991) Pathogenesis of onychoschizia (lamellar dystrophy). *Journal of the American Academy of Dermatology* **24**, 44–48.

Walters, K.A., Flynn, G.L. & Marvel, J.R. (1981) Physicochemical characterization of the human nail: 1. Pressure sealed apparatus for measuring nail plate permeability. *Journal of Investigative Dermatology* **76**, 76–79.

Walters, K.A., Flynn, G.L. & Marvel, J.R. (1983) Physicochemical characterisation of the human nail: permeation pattern for water and the homologous alcohols and differences with respect to the stratum corneum. *Journal of Pharmacy and Pharmacology* **35**, 28–33.

Walters, K.A., Flynn, G.L. & Marvel, J.R. (1985a) Physicochemical characterisation of the human nail: solvent effects on the permeation of homologous alcohols. *Journal of Pharmacy and Pharmacology* **37**, 771–775.

Walters, K.A., Flynn, G.L. & Marvel, J.R. (1985b) Penetration of the human nail plate: the effects of vehicule pH on the permeation of miconazole. *Journal of Pharmacy and Pharmacology* **37**, 418–419.

Wessel, S., Gniadecka, M., Jemec, G.B. & Wulf, H.C. (1999) Hydration of human nails investigated by NIR-FT-Raman spectroscopy. *Biochimica et Biophysica Acta* **17**, 210–216.

Yang, D., Chaumont, J.P., Makki, S. & Millet-Clerc, J. (1997) Un nouveau modéle de simulation pour étudier la pénétration topique díantifongiques en kératine dure in vitro. *Journal of Mycological Medicine* **7**, 195–198.

Yu, R.C.H. & King, C.M. (1992) A double blind study of superficial radiotherapy in psoriatic nail dystrophy. *Acta Dermato-Venereologica* **72**, 134–136.

Zaun, H. (1997) Brittle nails. Objective assessment and therapy follow-up. *Hautarzt* **48**, 455–461.

Zaun, H. & Becker, H. (1976) Die quelleigenschaften von nagelmaterial in natronlauge bei bestimmug mit einer standardisierten methode. *Arztliche Kosmetologie* **6**, 115–119.

# Imaging of the nail apparatus

## Radiology

X-ray reveals little of the soft structures of the nail unit under normal circumstances. Most isolated nail dystrophies should be X-rayed prior to surgical exploration. Clues to an exostosis, bone cyst, acroosteolysis or psoriatic arthropathy might be found. In invasive subungual squamous cell carcinoma up to 55% of patients will have radiological evidence of involvement of the underlying phalanx (Lumpkin *et al.* 1984).

Glomus tumours may provide particular radiological features. Mathis and Schulz (1948) reviewed 15 such tumours on the digit and found that nine had characteristic changes of bony erosion. This was smooth and concave in most cases, but occasionally with a punched out appearance on the phalangeal tuft. Supplementation of routine X-rays with arteriography may reveal a star-shaped telangiectatic zone (Camirand & Giroux 1970).

## Magnetic resonance imaging

Magnetic resonance imaging (MRI) (Chapter 11) is an effective method of locating tumours, particularly where there is diagnostic difficulty (Jablon *et al.* 1990; Holzberg 1992; Goettman *et al.* 1994). It can be used in a range of periungual neoplasms (Drapé *et al.* 1996a), although it is most useful when the tumour contrasts with surrounding tissues with respect to density, fluid or fat content. The most marked example of this is with mucoid cysts (Drapé *et al.* 1996b), but even normal soft tissues can be differentiated and an *in vivo* anatomical assessment made using MRI (Drapé *et al.* 1996c).

## Ultrasound

Ultrasound has been used in the nail unit both as a research tool and to aid clinical diagnosis. Finlay *et al.* (1987) used a 20-MHz pulse echo ultrasound to measure nail thickness *in vivo*, proximally and distally. The latter measurement correlated well with a micrometer gauge measurement of the free edge. Pulse transmission time was reduced by 8.8% distally, in comparison to the proximal measurement. This implies that the nail becomes thinner as it emerges, which is contrary to findings on avulsed nails (see 'Nail growth' above). He also found that the nails ranked in thickness sequentially around the hand, with the thumb being top and the little finger bottom.

Jemec's study of cadaver nails, *in situ* and avulsed, showed that nail dessication destroyed the correlation between ultrasound thickness measurements and screwgauge (Jemec & Serup 1989). This could have significance in quantification when the water content of nails can vary by 10%.

Clinically, high frequency ultrasound has been used in the diagnosis of glomus tumours. Fornage examined 12 patients and could depict the tumour in nine. The resolution of his transducer meant that lesions smaller than 3 mm could not be seen (Fornage 1988). Hirai and Fumiiri (1995) have used a 30-MHz high resolution B-mode ultrasound probe to examine nail dystrophies. The conclusion was that if the echogram detected any abnormality beneath the nail fold, the dystrophy was likely to be due to matrix pathology. The converse was true for nail bed pathology. The authors claimed that even in poorly defined tumours such as subungual malignant melanoma, the technique provided guidance as to the tumour margin.

## Profilometry

Profilometry is the technique of measuring the profile of a surface. This has been used in skin for nearly 20 years and can give a measure of wrinkling with actinic damage (Corcuff *et al.* 1983; Grove *et al.* 1989). More recently it has been used on nail surfaces to assess dystrophies where characteristic profiles are reported for the clinical features of pitting, grooves and trachyonychia (Nikkels-Tassoudji *et al.* 1995). Having established the method, it is then possible to use it as a measure of disease activity and nail growth as attempted with a study of psoriatic trachyonychia during low-dose cyclosporin therapy (Piérard & Piérard-Franchimont 1996) and the rate of nail growth during itraconazole treatment (de Doncker & Piérard 1994).

## Epiluminescence

Epiluminescence is a method of microscopic examination using reflected light. In the clinical setting this is conveniently provided by a hand-held dermatoscope. A dissection microscope is a laboratory alternative. The dermatoscope affords only low magnification, usually in the order of 10–20×. Illumination is provided from a light source within the instrument with an incident angle of 20°. Mineral oil is used at the skin surface to reduce the fraction of incident light reflected from the stratum corneum and increase the component that reveals intraepidermal detail in addition to some features of the papillary dermis. Reflection of the incident light by the stratum corneum is suppressed by immersion of the lesion in a drop of oil (Kopf *et al.* 1994; Argenyi 1997). Dermatoscopy is an established method for the examination of pigmented lesions of the skin (Binder *et al.* 1995; Delfino *et al.* 1997; Feldmann *et al.* 1998), but its use for nail pathology has not been widely considered (Stolz *et al.* 1994).

**Examples of dermatoscopy findings in a range of pigmented nail unit lesions** (courtesy of Luc Thomas, MD, Dermatology Unit, Hôtel Dieu, Lyon 69288, France)

*Ungual melanoma* (Figs 1.41–1.44)

*Ungual nevus* (Fig. 1.45)

*Ungual lentigo* (Figs 1.46–1.48)

*Drug-induced nail pigmentation* (Fig. 1.49)

## Photography

Many sophisticated systems are available for taking good photographs of the nail unit. Whilst their function might be sophisticated, their operation should be simple. It is not possible to deal with complicated equipment and tend to patients at the same time. The essentials involve a 1 : 1 macrolens, with a further magnifying filter if great detail within the nail unit is desired. This can be part of a zoom or supplemented by a further 50-mm lens. If you have a mobile system, a hand-held flash is necessary and superior to a ring flash. It gives greater flexibility than the ring flash and allows oblique lighting if needed. However, in general, the light should be directed from the tip of the finger up the limb to avoid shadows.

As with all medical photography, it is necessary to run off

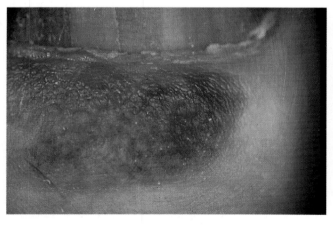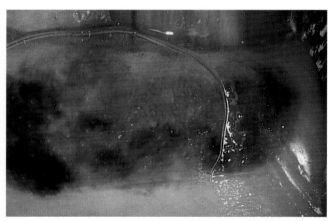

(a)          (b)

**Fig. 1.41** (a,b) Melanoma of the proximal nail fold: polymorphic pigment with asymmetric disposition of a dark ink spot, irregular network, blue-grey areas.

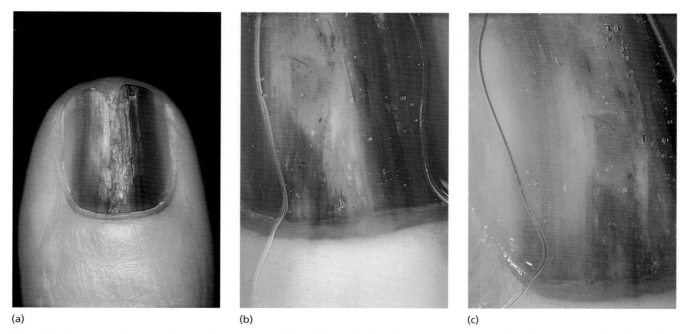

(a)                                              (b)                                              (c)

**Fig. 1.42** (a) Uneven pigment in the nail plate forming heterochrome parallel lines. (b) Pseudo-Hutchinson's sign through translucent cuticle. In the lateral portion of the nail plate (c), heterochrome linear disposition of pigmentation is more visible.

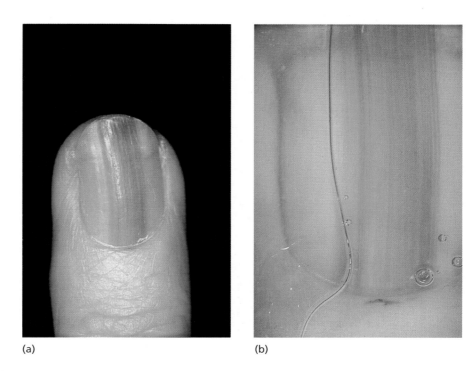

**Fig. 1.43** Hutchinson's sign (a) may be more clearly revealed when using dermatoscopy (b).

(a)                                              (b)

several films with practise shots at different settings and on different coloured skins. A dark, matt background cloth is preferable.

Video systems have been used as a research tool for nail morphometry (Goyal & Griffiths 1998). End-on and lateral views can be transfered to a computer for calculation of dimensions and provide reference measurements.

## Light

A good pocket torch is useful in the diagnostic transillumination of a myxoid cyst. Transillumination should also be used to distinguish between intrinsic nail plate chromonychia and surface changes. Wood's light may enhance the colour changes induced by tetracycline and give a yellow fluorescence. Des-

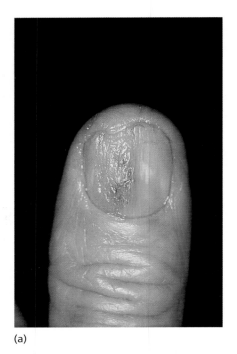

(a)

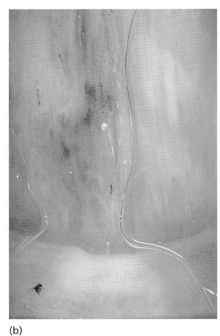

(b)

**Fig. 1.44** A destructive neoplasm of the nail bed and matrix appears initially to be without pigment (a), but this is demonstrated (b) using epiluminescence.

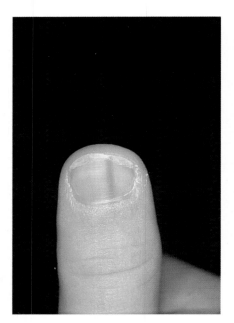

**Fig. 1.45** Acquired longitudinal melanonychia in an 8-year-old male child, has relatively homogeneous pigment using dermatoscopy, with a clinical diagnosis of a benign naevus.

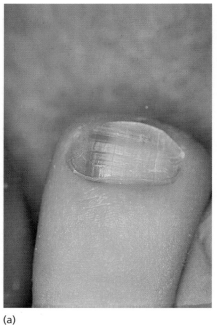

(a)

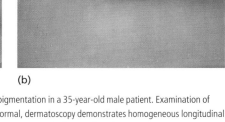

(b)

**Fig. 1.46** (a,b) Recently discovered toenail longitudinal pigmentation in a 35-year-old male patient. Examination of other nails, mucous membranes and skin was otherwise normal, dermatoscopy demonstrates homogeneous longitudinal greyish pigmentation of the nail plate. No clear parallel lines are seen. Histology confirms lentigo.

methylchlortetracycline appears reddish, and pseudomonas, yellowish-green.

Polarized light can be helpful in the examination of the underside of nails. This is done with the aid of a light microscope to identify the longitudinal ridge pattern (Apolinar & Rowe 1980).

## Other techniques

Laser Doppler can be used to assess the blood flow in the nail unit. Optical coherence tomography produces a series of cross-sectional images down to a depth of 1 mm, separated by 15 μm. It has some potential for examining periungual tissues, but has been little explored as a technique (Welzel *et al.* 1997). Confocal microscopy is in a similar category, where light penetrates the un-sectioned tissue to give three-dimensional information and has been used to examine the normal nail plate (Kaufman *et al.* 1995).

Older techniques for the assessment of shape, and clubbing in particular, include brass templates (Stavem 1959), shadowgraphs (Bentley *et al.* 1976), plaster casts and planimetry (Regan *et al.* 1967) and plethysmography (Cudowicz & Wraith 1957).

## References

Apolinar, E. & Rowe, W.F. (1980) Examination of human fingernail ridges by means of polarized light. *Journal of Forensic Science CA* **25**, 156–161.

Argenyi, Z.B. (1997) Dermoscopy (epiluminescence microscopy) of pigmented skin lesions: current status and evolving trends. *Dermatologic Clinics* **15**, 79–95.

Bentley, D., Moore, A. & Schwachman, H. (1976) Finger clubbing: a quantitative survey by analysis of the shadowgraph. *Lancet* **2**, 164–167.

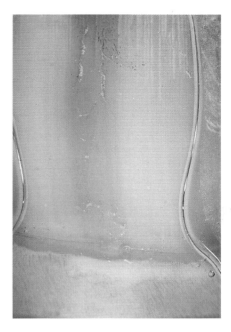

**Fig. 1.47** Lentigo.

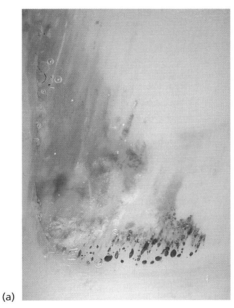

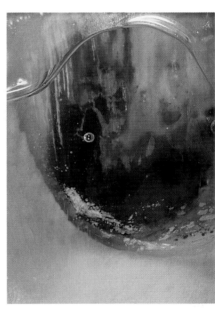

**Fig. 1.48** (a–d) Subungual haemorrhage has some longitudinal orientation because of the pattern of nail bed vessels and the longitudinal ridging of the underside of the nail plate. However, there are additional irregular elements that appear as 'lakes' of haem, which is not seen with melanocytic pathology.

(a)

(b)

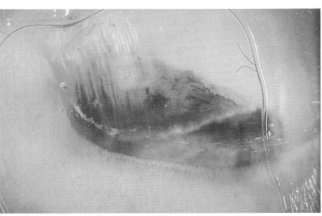

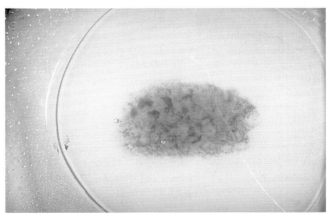

(c)

(d)

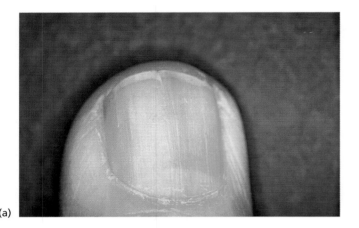

(a)

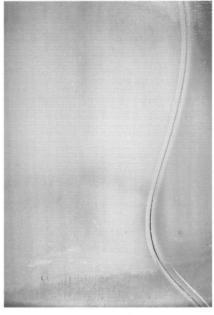

(b)

**Fig. 1.49** (a) Acquired longitudinal melanonychia involving several finger and toenails in a 72-year old male patient treated for 4 years with hydroxyurea for chronic lymphocytic leukaemia. (b) The band is homogeneous and grey.

Binder, M., Schwarz, M., Winkler, A. *et al.* (1995) Epiluminescence microscopy: a useful tool for the diagnosis of pigmented skin lesions for formally trained dermatologists. *Archives of Dermatology* **131**, 286–291.

Camirand, P. & Giroux, J.M. (1970) Subungual glomus tumour. Radiological manifestations. *Archives of Dermatology* **102**, 677–679.

Corcuff, P., de Rigal, Lévêque, J.L., Makki, S. & Agache, P. (1983) Skin relief and ageing. *Journal of the Society of Cosmetic Chemistry* **34**, 177–190.

Cudowicz, P. & Wraith, D.G. (1957) An evaluation of the clinical significance of clubbing in common lung disorders. *British Journal of Tuberculous Disease of the Chest* **51**, 14–31.

Delfino, M., Fabbrocini, G., Argenziano, G., Magliocchetti, N. & Nofroni, I. (1997) A statistical analysis of the characteristics of pigmented skin lesions using epiluminescence microscopy. *Journal of the European Academy of Dermatology and Venereology* **9**, 243–248.

de Doncker, P. & Piérard, G.E. (1994) Acquired nail beading in patients receiving itraconazole—an indicator of faster nail growth? A study using optical profilometry. *Clinical and Experimental Dermatology* **19**, 404–406.

Drapé, J.L., Idy-Peretti, I., Goettmann, S. *et al.* (1996a) Standard and high resolution MRI in glomus tumours of toes and fingertips. *Journal of the American Academy of Dermatology* **35**, 550–555.

Drapé, J.L., Idy-Peretti, I., Goettmann, S. *et al.* (1996b) MR imaging of digital mucoid cysts. *Radiology* **200**, 531–536.

Drapé, J.L., Wolfram-Gabel, R., Idy-Peretti, I. *et al.* (1996c) The lunula: a magnetic resonance imaging approach to the subnail matrix area. *Journal of Investigative Dermatology* **106**, 1081–1085.

Feldmann, R., Fellenz, C. & Gschnait, F. (1998) The ABCD rule in dermatoscopy: analysis of 500 melanocytic lesions. *Hautarzt* **49**, 473–476.

Finlay, A.Y., Moseley, H. & Duggan, T.C. (1987) Ultrasound transmission time: an *in vivo* guide to nail thickness. *British Journal of Dermatology* **117**, 765–770.

Fornage, B.D. (1988) Glomus tumours in the fingers: diagnosis with US. *Radiology* **167**, 183–185.

Goettmann, S., Drape, J.L., Idy-Peretti, I. *et al.* (1994) Magnetic resonance imaging: a new tool in the diagnosis of tumours of the nail apparatus. *British Journal of Dermatology* **130**, 701–710.

Goyal, S. & Griffiths, W.A.D. (1998) An improved methods of studying fingernail morphometry: application to the early detection of fingernail clubbing. *Journal of the American Academy of Dermatology* **39**, 640–642.

Grove, G.L., Grove, M.J. & Leyden, J.J. (1989) Optical profilometry: an objective method for quantification of facial wrinkles. *Journal of the American Academy of Dermatology* **21**, 631–637.

Hirai, T. & Fumiiri, M. (1995) Ultrasonic observation of the nail matrix. *Dermatological Surgery* **21**, 158–161.

Holzberg, M. (1992) Glomus tumour of the nail. *Archives of Dermatology* **128**, 160–162.

Jablon, M., Horowitz, A. & Bernstein, D.A. (1990) Magnetic resonance imaging of a glomus tumour of the finger tip. *Journal of Hand Surgery* **15A**, 507–509.

Jemec, G.B.E. & Serup, J. (1989) Ultrasound of the human nail plate. *Archives of Dermatology* **125**, 643–646.

Kaufman, S.C., Beuerman, R.W. & Greer, D.L. (1995) Confocal microscopy: a new tool for the study of the nail unit *Journal of the American Academy of Dermatology* **32**, 668–670.

Kopf, A.W., Salopek, T.G., Slade, J., Marghoob, A.A. & Bart, R.S. (1994) Techniques of cutaneous examination for the detection of skin cancer. *Cancer* **75**, 684–690.

Lumpkin, L.R., Rosen, T. & Tschen, J.A. (1984) Subungual squamous cell carcinoma. *Journal of the American Academy of Dermatology* **11**, 735–738.

Mathis, W.H. & Schulz, M.D. (1948) Roentgen diagnosis of glomus tumours. *Radiology* **51**, 71–76.

Nikkels-Tassoudji, N., Piérard-Franchimont, C., de Doncker, P. & Piérard, G.E. (1995) Optical profilometry of nail dystrophies. *Dermatology* **190**, 301–304.

Piérard, G.E. & Piérard-Franchimont, C. (1996) Dynamics of psoriatic trachyonychia during low dose cyclosporin A treatment: a pilot study on onychochronobiology using optical profilometry. *Dermatology* **192**, 116–119.

Regan, G.M., Tagg, B. & Thomson, M.L. (1967) Subjective measurement and objective measurement of finger clubbing. *Lancet* **1**, 530–532.

Stavem, P. (1959) Instrument for estimation of clubbing. *Lancet* **2**, 7–8.

Stolz, W., Braun-Falco, O., Bilek, P., Landthaler, M. & Cognetta, A.B. (1994) Pigmented lesions on hands and feet. In: *Color Atlas of Dermatoscopy* (ed. W. Stolz), pp. 101–107. Blackwell Scientific Publications, Oxford.

Welzel, J., Lankenau, E., Birngruber, R. & Engelhardt, R. (1997) Optical coherence tomography of the human skin. *Journal of the American Academy of Dermatology* **37**, 958–963.

# CHAPTER 2

# Physical signs

**R. Baran, R.P.R. Dawber & B. Richert**

**Modification in the configuration of the nail**
  Clubbing or hippocratic fingers
  Koilonychia
  Transverse overcurvature of the nail
  Dolichonychia
  Brachyonychia/short nails/racquet nails
  Parrot beak nails
  Curved nail of the 4th toe
  Circumferential fingernail
  Claw-like nail
  Macronychia and micronychia
  Worn-down nails
  Onychatrophy
  Anonychia
  Hypertrophy of the nail
**Modification of the nail surface**
  Longitudinal lines
  Oblique lines/chevron nail/herring-bone nail
  Transverse grooves and Beau's lines

  Pitting (pits, onychia punctata, erosions, Rosenau's depressions)
  Trachyonychia (rough nails)
  Pseudomycotic nail dystrophy (pseudomycotic onychia)
  Lamellar nail splitting (onychoschizia lamellina)
  Elkonyxis
**Modification of the nail plate and soft tissue attachments**
  Pterygium
  Onychomadesis/nail shedding—retronychia
  Onycholysis
  Subungual hyperkeratosis
**Modifications in perionychial tissues**
**Modification in the consistency of the nail**
  Causes of nail fragility
  Treatment of brittle nails
**Modification in colour: chromonychia or dyschromia**
  Causes of colour modification
  Leuconychia
  Erythronychia

## Modification in the configuration of the nail

### Clubbing or hippocratic fingers

Clubbed fingers have been known since the first century BC, when Hippocrates first described the sign in patients suffering from empyema. The morphological changes combine: (a) increased transverse and longitudinal curvature of the nails; and (b) enlargement of the soft tissue structures, strictly confined to the fingertips (Coury 1960). The increased nail curvature is most prominent in the radial three digits.

The curvature is variable; the deformity may be fusiform, shaped like a bird's beak, and clubbed, resembling a watch glass.

These shape types can be found in all of the four main forms of clubbing.

### Simple clubbing

This is the most common category. It has several elements.
1 Increased nail curvature with a transverse furrow which separates it from the rest of the nail both in the early stage and on

resolution. The onset is usually gradual and painless, except in some cases of carcinoma of the lung where clubbing may develop abruptly and may be associated with severe pain.
2 Hypertrophy of the soft tissues with elastic, oedematous infiltration of the pulp, which may spread on to the dorsal surface causing periungual swelling.
3 Hyperplasia of the dermal fibrovascular tissue, which readily extends to involve the adjacent matrix. This accounts for one of the earliest signs of clubbing, i.e. an abnormal mobility of the base of the nail, which can be rocked back and forth giving the impression that it is floating on a soft oedematous pad (Lovibond 1938). The increased vascularity is responsible for the slow return of colour when the nail is slightly pressed and released.
4 Local cyanosis described by Coury (1960), present in 60% of the cases.

In the early stages clubbing may be unilateral, though eventually both hands become affected symmetrically. Several stages of clubbing or acropachy may be distinguished: suspected, slight, average and severe. In practice the degree of the deformity may be determined by Lovibond's 'profile sign', which measures the angle between the curved nail plate and the prox-

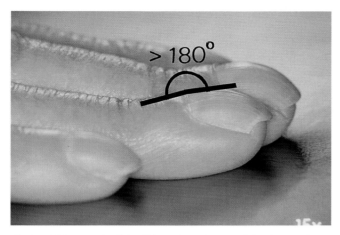

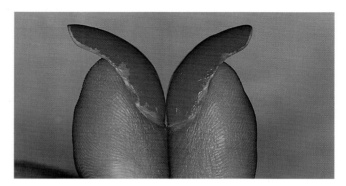

**Fig. 2.3** Clubbing—Schamroth's sign. 'Window' lost in clubbing, with prominent distal angle between the ends of the nail.

**Fig. 2.1** Clubbing—Lovibond's 'profile' sign: the angle is normally less than 160° but exceeds 180° in clubbing.

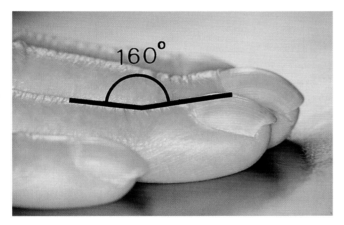

**Fig. 2.2** Clubbing—Curth's modified profile sign.

imal nail fold when the finger is viewed from the side. This is normally 160° but exceeds 180° in clubbing (Fig. 2.1). By contrast, pseudoclubbing is defined as an overcurvature of the nails in both the longitudinal and transverse axes, with preservation of a normal Lovibond's angle (Goyal *et al.* 1998). With a modified profile sign, the angle between the middle and the terminal phalanx at the interphalangeal joint is measured (Curth *et al.* 1961). In normal fingers the distal phalanx forms an almost straight (180°) extension of the middle phalanx, whereas in severe clubbing this angle may be reduced to 160° or even 140° (Fig. 2.2). However, the best indicator may well be the measurement of the hyponychial angle (Regan *et al.* 1967). This can be assessed either clinically or with the aid of a clubbing shadowgraph (Bentley *et al.* 1976), which may allow serial measurements of the angles to record any progression of finger clubbing. Other methods are described by Blumsohn (1981). In fact fixing the limits of true clubbing in minimal cases is ultimately a matter of clinical sense and habit (Coury 1960); therefore a simple clinical method was adopted by Schamroth

(1976). In the normal individual a distinct diamond-shaped aperture, or 'window', is formed at the base of the nail beds, if symmetrical fingers are placed against each other with contact on both dorsal surfaces. Early clubbing obliterates this window and demonstrates a prominent distal angle between the ends of the nails (Fig. 2.3) (Lampe & Kagan 1983). A simple and inexpensive system was recently developed to accurately visualize and quantify changes in the morphology of the nail plate by means of digital cameras and computerized analysis (Goyal *et al.* 1998). This technique allows examination of progressive changes in the nail to be correlated with therapy.

Radiological changes occur in less than one-fifth of cases. They include phalangeal demineralization and irregular thickening of the cortical diaphysis. Ungual tufts generally show considerable variations and may be prominent in advanced stages of the disease. Atrophy may be present.

Congenital clubbed fingers may be accompanied by abnormalities and deformities, such as hyperkeratosis of the palms and soles, and cortical hypertrophy of the long bones. Familial clubbing may occur in conjunction with familial hypertrophic osteoarthropathy; for some authors, simple clubbing is regarded as a mild form of the latter (Curth *et al.* 1961). Isolated watch-glass nails without their accompanying deformities are also constitutionally determined.

Very rare cases of unilateral hippocratic nails have been reported due to obstructed circulation, causalgia (Saunders & Hanna 1988), oedema of the soft tissues and dystrophies of the affected parts. Asymmetrical clubbing may be a manifestation of sarcoid bone disease (Hashmi & Kaplan 1992).

The pathological process which appears to be responsible for clubbing and its associated changes is increasing blood flow as a result of vasodilatation rather than hyperplasia of vessels in the nail bed (Currie & Gallagher 1988). In Bigler's series (Bigler 1958), nail bed thickness of the thumb was greater than 2.0 mm in clubbed digits.

Pseudoclubbing has been defined as overcurvature of the nail in both the longitudinal and transverse axes, with preservation of a normal Lovibond angle (Goyal *et al.* 1998).

## Hypertrophic osteoarthropathy

This disorder may be divided into two categories: (a) hypertrophic pulmonary osteoarthropathy; and (b) hypertrophic osteoarthropathy confined to the lower extremities.

## Hypertrophic pulmonary osteoarthropathy (Bamberger–Pierre–Marie syndrome)

This disorder is characterized by the six following signs (Coury 1960):

1 Clubbing of the nails on hands and feet.

2 Hypertrophy of the upper and lower extremities, which is similar to the deformity found in acromegaly (spade-like enlargement of the hands).

3 Joint manifestations with pseudoinflammatory, symmetrical, painful arthropathy of the large limb joints, especially those of the lower limbs. This syndrome is almost pathognomonic of malignant chest tumours, especially lung carcinoma, mesotheliomas of the pleura and less commonly bronchiectasis. Associated gynaecomastia is a further indication of malignancy.

4 There may be bone changes which consist of bilateral, proliferative periostitis with a transluscent thin line between the periosteal reaction and the thickened cortex especially over the distal ends of the long bones (Fisher *et al.* 1964). Moderate, diffuse decalcification may also be present.

5 Peripheral neurovascular disorders are common, such as local cyanosis and paraesthesia.

6 The pain and swelling often disappear with successful therapy of the underlying disease process.

A case of florid hypertrophic osteoarthropathy regressed clinically and radiologically when a celestin tube was removed (Haslock & Vasanthakumar 1988).

## Hypertrophic osteoarthropathy confined to the lower extremities

Recurrent infection of the lower extremities after an aortofemoral bypass graft is associated with pain of the legs and X-ray findings of severe hypertrophic osteoarthropathy (Gibson *et al.* 1974; Sorin *et al.* 1980; Stock 1986). This condition is restricted to the legs when the flow of blood is reversed through a patent ductus arteriosus or when sepsis occurs in the presence of an abdominal aortic prosthesis with an intestinal fistula (Stein & Little 1978).

## Pachydermoperiostosis (Touraine–Solente–Golé syndrome) (Touraine *et al.* 1935)

Pachydermoperiostosis or idiopathic hypertrophic osteoarthropathy is very rare. In most of the reported cases the digit changes usually begin at or about the time of puberty. The ends of fingers and toes are bulbous and often grotesque, with hyperhidrosis of the hands and the feet. This clubbing stops abruptly

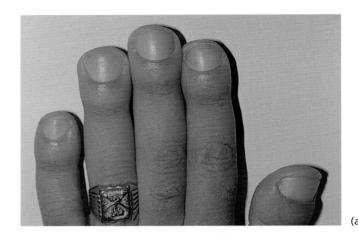

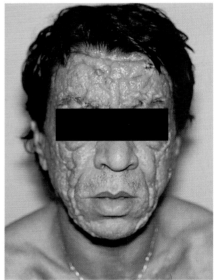

(a)

(b)

**Fig. 2.4** (a) Clubbing in pachydermoperiostosis. (Courtesy of P.Y. Venencie, Paris.) (b) Pachydermoperiostosis, severe skin changes.

at the distal interphalangeal joint (Rimoin 1965) (Fig. 2.4). In this type the lesions of the fingertips are clinically identical to those of hypertrophic pulmonary osteoarthropathy. However, in primary pachydermoperiostosis (Thappa *et al.* 2000), the thickened cortex appears radiologically homogeneous and does not encroach on the medullary space (Fisher *et al.* 1964). Acroosteolysis of the distal phalanges has been reported with increased blood flow through clubbed fingers (Fam *et al.* 1983). The pachydermal change of the extremities and face, with furrowing and oiliness of the skin, is the most characteristic feature of this disorder. Nevertheless in hypertrophic pulmonary osteoarthropathy there may be facial skin and scalp changes which are indistinguishable from those seen in primary pachydermoperiostosis; this could be explained by a common genetic factor (Vogl & Goldfischer 1962; Lindmaier *et al.* 1989). The differential diagnosis includes acromegaly, which enhances tufting of the terminal phalanges in an anchor-like shape

**Table 2.1** Classification of clubbing.

*Idiopathic forms*

Hereditary and congenital forms, sometimes associated with other anomalies
(see Table 10.5)
Familial and racial forms (black people, North Africans)
Citrullinaemia

*Acquired forms*

1 Thoracic organ disorders (involved in about 80% of cases of clubbing, often
with the common denominator of hypoxia):
(a) Bronchopulmonary diseases, especially chronic and infective
bronchiectasis, abscess and cyst of the lung, pulmonary tuberculosis
Sarcoidosis, pulmonary fibrosis, emphysema, Ayerza's syndrome, chronic
pulmonary venous congestion, asthma in infancy, mucoviscidosis
Blastomycosis, pneumonia, *Pneumocystis carinii*
(b) Thoracic tumours:
Primary or metastatic bronchopulmonary cancers, pleural tumours,
mediastinal tumours (an infrequent cause), Hodgkin's disease,
lymphoma, pseudotumour due to oesophageal dilatation
(c) Cardiovascular diseases:
Congenital heart disease associated with cyanosis (rarely non-cyanotic)
Thoracic vascular malformations—stenoses and arteriovenous aneuryms
Osler's disease (subacute bacterial endocarditis)
Congestive cardiac failure
Myxoma
Raynaud's syndrome, erythromelalgia, Maffucci's syndrome

2 Disorders of the alimentary tract (5% of cases):
(a) Oesophageal, gastric and colonic cancer; gastric leiomyosarcoma
(Rabast 1997)
(b) Diseases of the small intestine
(c) Colonic diseases with:
Amoebiasis and inflammatory states of the colon
Ulcerative colitis, Crohn's disease
Familial polyposis, Gardner's syndrome
Ascariasis
(d) Active chronic hepatitis, primary or secondary cirrhoses
(e) Purgative abuse

3 Endocrine origin:
POEMS syndrome (Myers 1991)
Diamond's syndrome (pretibial myxoedema, exophthalmos and finger
clubbing); thyroid cancer
Seip–Lawrence syndrome (Reed *et al.* 1965)

4 Haematological causes:
Primary polycythaemia or secondary polycythaemia associated with hypoxia
Methaemoglobinaemia, sulphaemoglobinaemia, haemoglobinopathies
Poisoning by phosphorus, arsenic, alcohol, mercury or beryllium

5 Miscellaneous:
AIDS (Cribier *et al.* 1998)
Hypervitaminosis A, heroin addiction (Chotkowski 1994), hashish addicts
(Barris *et al.* 1990)
Lupus erythematosus
Malnutrition, Kwashiorkor
Syringomyelia

6 Unilateral or limited to a few digits:
Aneurysm of the aorta, the subclavian artery, axillary or ulnar artery
Arteriovenous fistula (haemodialysis)
Causalgia (Saunders & Hanna 1988)
Ductus arteriosus
Hemiplegia
Juvenile hyaline fibromatosis II (Camarosa & Moreno 1987)
Pancoast–Tobias syndrome
Sarcoidosis (Hashmi & Kaplan 1992)
Subluxation of the shoulder (with paralysis of the brachial plexus), median
nerve neuritis
Tophaceous gout

7 Other unidigital forms:
Idiopathic (Stoll & Beetham 1954)
Local injury, whitlow, lymphangitis
Subungual epidermoid inclusion, osteoid osteoma, enchondroma
Takayasu's arteritis (Kaditis *et al.* 1995)
Traumatic obstruction of subclavian vein
Varices of the arm
Wart of ventral aspect proximal nail fold

8 Confined to the lower extremities: abdominal aortic graft with sepsis
Upper extremities: hashish, heroin

9 Transitory form: physiological in the newborn child (due to reversal of the
circulation at birth)

10 Occupational: acroosteolysis (exposure to vinyl chloride)

(Wendling & Guidet 1993), but does not cause acroosteolysis in contrast to pachydermoperiostosis (Guyer *et al.* 1978). Thyroid acropachy is usually associated with exophthalmos, pretibial myxoedema and disturbed thyroid function.

#### The shell nail syndrome

First reported by Cornelius and Shelley (1967), this syndrome occurs in some cases of bronchiectasis and is similar to clubbing, but there is associated atrophy of the nail bed and the underlying bone.

A comprehensive list of causes of clubbing is shown in Table 2.1.

### References

Barris, Y.I., Tan, E., Kalyoncu, F. *et al.* (1990) Digital clubbing in hashish addict. *Chest* 98, 1545–1546.
Bentley, D., Moore, A. & Schwachman, H. (1976) Finger clubbing: a quantitative survey by analysis of the shadowgraph. *Lancet* ii, 164.
Bigler, F.C. (1958) The morphology of clubbing. *American Journal of Pathology* 34, 237–241.

Blumsohn, D. (1981) Clubbing of the fingers with special reference to Schamroth's diagnostic method. *Heart and Lung* **10**, 1069–1072.

Camarosa, J.G. & Moreno, K. (1987) Juvenile hyaline fibromatosis. *Journal of the American Academy of Dermatology* **16**, 881–883.

Chotkowski, L.A. (1994) Clubbing of the fingernails in heroin addiction. *New England Journal of Medicine* **311**, 262.

Cornelius, C.E. & Shelley, W.B. (1967) Shell nail syndrome associated with bronchiectiasis. *Archives of Dermatology* **96**, 694.

Coury, C. (1960) Hippocratic fingers and hypertrophic osteoarthropathy. *British Journal of Diseases of the Chest* **54**, 202.

Cribier, B., Mena, M.L., Rey, D. *et al.* (1998) Nail changes in patients infected with HIV. *Archives of Dermatology* **134**, 1216–1220.

Currie, A.E. & Gallagher, P.J. (1988) The pathology of clubbing: vascular changes in the nail bed. *British Journal of Diseases of the Chest* **82**, 382–385.

Curth, H.O., Firschein, I.L. & Alphert, M. (1961) Familial clubbed fingers. *Archives of Dermatology* **83**, 829.

Fam, A.G., Chin-Sang, H. & Ramsay, C.A. (1983) Pachydermoperiostosis: scintigraphic, thermographic, plethysmographic, and capillaroscopic observations. *Annals of the Rheumatic Diseases* **42**, 98–102.

Fisher, D.S., Singer, D.H. & Feldman, S.M. (1964) Clubbing: a review with emphasis on hereditary acropachy. *Medicine* **43**, 459.

Gibson, T., Joye, J. & Schumauer, H.R. (1974) Localized hypertrophic osteoarthropathy with abdominal aortic prosthesis and infection. *Annals of Internal Medicine* **81**, 556–557.

Goyal, S., Griffith, W.A.D., Omarouayache, S. *et al.* (1998) An improved method of studying fingernail morphometry: application to the early detection of fingernail clubbing. *Journal of the American Academy of Dermatology* **39**, 640–642.

Guyer, P.B., Brunton, F.J. & Wren, M.W.G. (1978) Pachydermoperiostosis with acroosteolysis. A report of five cases. *Journal of Bone and Joint Surgery* **60B**, 219.

Hashmi, S. & Kaplan, D. (1992) Asymmetric clubbing as a manifestation of sarcoid bone disease. *American Journal of Medicine* **93**, 471.

Haslock, I. & Vasanthakumar, V. (1988) Disappearing hypertrophic osteoarthropathy. *British Journal of Rheumatology* **27**, 143–145.

Kaditis, A.G., Nelson, A.M. & Driscoll, D.J. (1995) Takayasu's arteritis presenting with unilateral digital clubbing. *Journal of Rheumatology* **22**, 2346–2348.

Lampe, R.M. & Kagan, A. (1983) Detection of clubbing—Schamroth's sign. *Clinical Pediatrics* **22**, 125.

Lindmaier, A., Raff, M., Seidl, G. *et al.* (1989) Pachydermoperiostose (Klinik, Klassifikation und Pathogenese). *Hautarzt* **40**, 752–757.

Lovibond, J.L. (1938) Diagnosis of clubbed fingers. *Lancet* i, 363.

Myers, B.M. (1991) POEMS syndrome with idiopathic flushing mimicking carcinoid syndrome. *American Journal of Medicine* **90**, 646–648.

Rabast, U. (1997) Trommel schlegelfinger bei eine, niedrig malignen Leiomyosarkom mit gemishter Hiatus hermie. *Deutsche Medizinische Wochenschrift* **122**, 1207–1212.

Reed, W.D., Dexter, R., Corley, C. *et al.* (1965) Congenital lipodystrophic diabetes with acanthosis nigricans. *Archives of Dermatology* **91**, 326–334.

Regan, G.M., Tagg, B. & Thomson, M.L. (1967) Subjective assessment and objective measurement of finger clubbing. *Lancet* i, 530.

Rimoin, D.L. (1965) Pachydermoperiostosis (idiopathic clubbing and periostosis). *New England Journal of Medicine* **272**, 923.

Saunders, P.R. & Hanna, M. (1988) Unilateral clubbing of fingers associated with causalgia. *British Medical Journal* **297**, 1635.

Schamroth, L. (1976) Personal experience. *South African Medical Journal* **50**, 297–300.

Sorin, S.B., Askari, A. & Rhodes, R.S. (1980) Hypertrophic osteoarthropathy of the lower extremities as a manifestation of arterial graft sepsis. *Arthritis and Rheumatism* **23**, 768–770.

Stein, H.B. & Little, H.A. (1978) Localized hypertrophic osteoarthropathy in the presence of an abdominal aortic prosthesis. *Canadian Medical Association Journal* **118**, 947–948.

Stock, C.M. (1986) Trommel schlegelfinger. Ein Symptom. *Zeitschrift für Hautkrankheiten* **61**, 1745–1748.

Stoll, B.A. & Beetham, W.R. (1954) Unidigital clubbing, with report of a case. *Medical Journal of Australia* **2**, 852–855.

Thappa, D.M., Sethuraman, G., Kumar, G.R. *et al.* (2000) Primary pachydermoperiostosis: a case report. *Journal of Dermatology* **27**, 106–109.

Touraine, A., Solente, G. & Golé, A. (1935) Un syndrome ostéodermopathique, la pachydermie plicaturée avec pachypériostose des extrémités. *Presse Médicale* **43**, 1830.

Vogl, A. & Goldfischer, S. (1962) Primary or idiopathic osteoarthropathy. *American Journal of Medicine* **33**, 166.

Wendling, D. & Guidet, M. (1993) Les dysacromélies. *Est Médecine* **7–8**, 23–25.

## Koilonychia (Table 2.2)

Koilonychia is the converse of clubbing, the nail being concave with the edges everted, the so-called 'spoon nail' (Fig. 2.5). This dystrophy, which becomes more apparent when the nail is viewed laterally, normally affects several fingers, especially the thumb. All the fingers may be involved and, less frequently, the toes. The exception is in the first few years of life when it is a common normal finding in the big toes. The underlying tissues may be healthy or affected by subungual hyperkeratosis, which is clearly visible at the margin. This would suggest psoriasis, or an occupational origin of the deformity; the first three digits are frequently involved in the latter case. The nail, which may be normal, thinned or thickened and sometimes soft, has a smooth surface when the koilonychia is idiopathic. Longitudinal splitting with koilonychia in each of the separated parts of the nail plate appears in some cases of lichen striatus, and in certain inherited conditions (Bergeron & Stone 1967). Some or all of the fingernails may, in contrast, present with a central, longitudinal ridge in place of the fissure. In the trichoonychotic hidrotic ectodermal dysplasias, for example, there is a peculiar longitudinal fold increasing distally. This divides the nail plate with separated koilonychia on each side and without abnormalities elsewhere (Fig. 2.6).

The 'serrated koilonychia' syndrome (Runne 1978) combines spoon nail and tranverse grooves involving all the digits; steroid injections in the proximal nail fold lead to a temporary improvement.

The petaloid nail is a variant of an early stage of koilonychia, in which flattening of the nail is the characteristic sign. A variety of koilonychia is the type known as 'ongle en fermoir d'épingle de nourrice', in which the deformity is shaped like the catch on

**Table 2.2** Classification of koilonychia.

*Idiopathic forms* (Rosso *et al.* 1998)
Hereditary and congenital forms, sometimes occurring with other anomalies
(Chapter 9):
    Fissured nails, in adenoma sebaceum
    Monilethrix; hyperkeratosis of the palm (Meleda type); leukonychia
    Hereditary osteo-onychodysplasia (nail–patella syndrome)
    Nezelof's syndrome (immunological defect)
    Oliver–McFerlane syndrome (Zaun *et al.* 1984)
    Normal appearance in big toes in early childhood

*Acquired forms*
Cardiovascular and haematological (Chapter 7):
    Iron deficiency anaemia (following gastrectomy; Plummer–Vinson syndrome)
    Iron malabsorption by the intestinal mucosa
    Haemoglobinopathy sickle cell
    Polycythaemia
    Haemochromatosis
    Banti's syndrome (the nails heal after splenectomy)
    Coronary disease
Infections:
    Syphilis, fungal diseases
Endocrine forms (Chapter 7):
    Acromegaly
    Diabetes (Beaven & Brooks 1984)
    Hypothyroidism
    Thyrotoxicosis
Traumatic and occupational forms (Chapter 8):
    Petrol, various solvents, engine oils
    Acids and alkalis, thioglycollate (hairdressers)
    Housewives, chimney sweeps, rickshaw boys (toes)
    Nail biting
Avitaminoses (PP, $B_2$ and especially C)
Dermatoses:
    Acanthosis nigricans, alopecia areata, connective tissue diseases,
    Cronkhite–Canada syndrome, Darier's disease, incontinentia pigmenti,
    lichen planus, porphyria cutanea tarda, psoriasis, Raynaud's disease
Kidney transplantation
Carpal tunnel syndrome

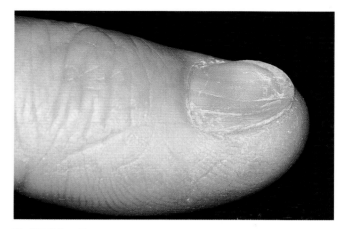

**Fig. 2.5** Koilonychia.

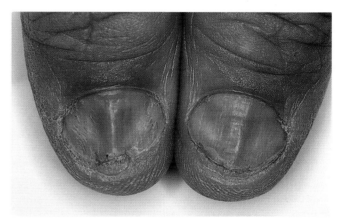

**Fig. 2.6** Koilonychia in tricho-onychotic hidrotic ectodermal dysplasia.

a safety pin. Koilonychia is commonly found in the toenails of normal children but this defect usually disappears spontaneously. In infants there is a significant correlation between koilonychia and iron deficiency; it may be noted before clinical and laboratory signs of anaemia develop (Hogan & Jones 1970). Spoon nails can be seen also in haemachromatosis, therefore iron deficiency *per se* is not the cause of the deformity. Cystine content of the nail substance is said to be lower than normal (Jalili & Al-kassab 1959). Familial cases have been reported (Almagor & Haim 1981), sometimes with associated abnormalities; these include leukonychia (Baran & Achten 1969; Crosby & Petersen 1989), onychogryphosis and monilethrix. Koilonychia may be a racial characteristic mainly in Tibetans (Anan & Harris 1988). According to Stone (1975),

nail changes in clubbing and spooning are the result of an angulation of the matrix secondary to connective tissue changes. Clubbing occurs if the distal portion of the matrix is relatively high compared with the proximal end; in spooning, the distal portion is relatively low compared with the proximal end. The lifting up of the former results from connective tissue proliferation and at times from the increase in vascular flow. The depressed distal portion of the latter may be due to distal, connective tissue anoxia and atrophy. In psoriasis or onychomycosis, the hyperkeratotic reaction in the nail bed exerts an upward pressure which is transmitted to the area of keratinization and results in a spoon nail type deformity. Minimal expansion of the dorsal aspect of the distal portion of the bony phalanx is capable of producing this effect.

As koilonychia is frequently found in the thumb, index and middle fingernails, Higashi (1985) believes that it is related to the pressure-bearing function of the fingers in handiwork. As the distal phalanx is only the heart of the distal portion of the finger, upward pressure forces cause upward deformation of the distal and lateral portions of the nail plate.

## References

Almagor, G. & Haim, S. (1981) Familial koilonychia. *Dermatologia* **162**, 400.

Anan, I.S. & Harris, P. (1988) Koilonychia in Ladakhis. *British Journal of Dermatology* **119**, 267–268.

Baran, R. & Achten, G. (1969) Les associations congénitales de Koïlonychie et de leuconychie totale. *Archives Belges de Dermatologie et Syphiligraphie* **XXV**, 13–29.

Beaven, D.W. & Brooks, S.E. (1984) *A Colour Atlas of the Nail in Clinical Diagnosis.* Wolfe Medical, London.

Bergeron, J.R. & Stone, O.J. (1967) Koilonychia. A report of familial spoon nails. *Archives of Dermatology* **95**, 351.

Crosby, D.L. & Petersen, M.J. (1989) Familial koilonychia. *Cutis* **44**, 209–210.

Higashi, N. (1985) Pathogenesis of the spooning. *Hifu* **27**, 29–34.

Hogan, G.R. & Jones, B. (1970) The relationship of koilonychia and iron deficiency in infants. *Journal of Pediatrics* **77**, 1054.

Jalili, M.A. & Al-kassab, S. (1959) Koilonychia and cystine content of nail. *Lancet* **ii**, 108–110.

Rosso, D., dos Santos Rodriguez, H., Larangeira, H. *et al.* (1998) Coiloniquia idiopatica. *Anales Brasiliera de Dermatologia* **73**, 313–315.

Runne, U. (1978) Koilonychia serrata syndrom. *Zeitschrift für Hautkrankheiten* **53**, 623.

Stone, O.J. (1975) Spoon nails and clubbing, significance and mechanisms. *Cutis* **16**, 235–241.

Zaun, H., Strenger, D., Zabransky, S. *et al.* (1984) Das syndrom der langen Wimpern (Trichomegalie syndrom, Oliver–McFerlane). *Hautarzt* **35**, 162–165.

## Transverse overcurvature of the nail

There are three main forms of overcurvature (Fig. 2.7): arched, pincer, trumpet or omega nail; tile-shaped nail; and 'plicated' nail.

Pincer nail (see Chapter 10, page 498) is a dystrophy characterized by transverse overcurvature that increases along the longitudinal axis of the nail and reaches its greatest proportion at the distal part. At this point, the lateral borders tighten around the soft tissues, which are pinched without necessarily

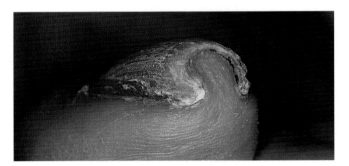

**Fig. 2.8** Pincer nail deformity.

breaking through the epidermis (Fig. 2.8). In extreme cases, they may join together, forming a tunnel, or they may roll about themselves taking the form of a cone. In certain varieties, the nails are shaped like claws, sometimes resembling pachyonychia congenita. After a while, the soft tissue may actually disappear and this may be accompanied by a resorption of the underlying bone (Cornelius & Shelley 1968).

Pincer nail is probably due to selective widening of the proximal region of the lateral matrix horns by juxta-articular osteophytes. As the shape of the distal matrix does not change the nail plate assumes a conical shape which rises above the nail bed. As the nail is tightly bound to the periosteum, it lifts a traction osteophyte from the dorsum of the underlying phalanx (Haneke 1992).

This morphological abnormality would be no more than a curiosity if the constriction were not occasionally accompanied by pain which is sometimes provoked by the lightest of touch, for example the weight of a bedsheet (Baran 1974). The origin of this dystrophy probably resides in a developmental anomaly and may be an inherited disorder (Chapman 1973). Some cases have been attributed to the wearing of ill-fitting shoes. Underlying pathology, such as subungual exostosis in the toes and inflammatory osteoarthritis, should always be looked for, especially where the fingers are involved. Higashi (1990) reported on six patients with pincer nail due to tinea unguium. The deformity resolved with oral griseofulvin. Reversible pincer nails after treatment with β-blocker is a rare aetiology (Greiner *et al.* 1998). Pincer nails as markers of gastrointestinal malignancy are exceptional (Jemec & Thomsen 1997).

The tile-shaped nail presents with an increase in the transverse curvature; the lateral edges of the nail remain parallel.

In the plicated variety of overcurvature the surface of the nail plate is almost flat, while one or both lateral margins are sharply angled forming vertical sides which are parallel (Fig. 2.9).

Although these deformities may be associated with ingrowing nails, inflammatory oedema due to the constriction of the soft tissue is unusual.

For treatment of these forms of nail overcurvature, see Chapter 10.

In terms of aetiology and pathogenesis, three different types of transverse overcurvature have to be differentiated:

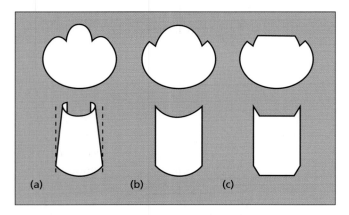

**Fig. 2.7** Transverse overcurvature showing the three subtypes: (a) pincer or trumpet nail; (b) tile-shaped nail; (c) plicated nail with sharply angled lateral margins.

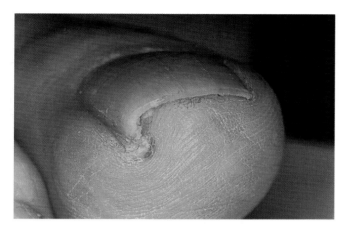

**Fig. 2.9** Unilateral variety—may have lateral pincer or plicated lateral change.

1 A symmetrical form, often hereditary and seen in several generations of a family and in several family members of the same generation; it is usually seen in toenails with both the great and the lesser nails being affected. It is usually associated with a malalignment of the nail's long axis—the great toenail is deviated laterally, the other nails medially. X-ray films show that the distal phalanx of the big toe also shows a slight lateral deviation, the base of the last phalanx is very wide and exhibits bony outgrowths pointing distally, and there is a small traction osteophyte on the dorsal tuft of the tip of the distal phalanx. Its histological examination reveals amorphous dense osseous material.

From proximal to distal, the nail bed epithelium becomes progressively more acanthotic, papillomatous and hyperkeratotic with a marked hypergranulosis and round to oval globules of inspissated serous exudate in the subungual horn. There is also a marked dilatation of some capillaries in the tip of the nail bed's papillary dermis.

2 An asymmetrical form that is acquired and may be due to trauma, surgery, some dermatoses and particularly associated with degenerative osteoarthritis of the distal interphalangeal joints of the fingers or foot deformation. This type is more frequently seen in elderly women. Radiography of the big toe also reveals a wide base of the distal phalanx with lateral and medial exostoses and sometimes also irregular subperiostal bone appositions on the processus unguicularis and a small osteophyte on the dorsal aspect of the tip of the distal phalanx. Since the matrix is intimately and firmly attached to the bone its physiological curvature is unbent, which in turn leads to a less curved nail proximally but increasing its curvature distally. This heaps up the nail plate and induces a distal dorsal traction osteophyte. Treatment is aimed at releasing the outward pressure on the matrix by selectively removing the lateral matrix horns, and at spreading the nail bed (Haneke 1999).

3 Repeated nail avulsions, injury to the distal phalanx and the nail organ as well as some dermatoses, particularly psoriasis and total dystrophic onychomycosis with secondary shrinking of the nail field, may cause transverse overcurvature of the involved nail.

## References

Baran, R. (1974) Pincer and trumpet nails. *Archives of Dermatology* 110, 639.

Chapman, R.S. (1973) Overcurvature of the nails. An inherited disorder. *British Journal of Dermatology* 89, 211–213.

Cornelius, C.E. & Shelley, W.B. (1968) Pincer nails syndrome. *Archives of Surgery* 96, 321.

Greiner, D., Schöfer, H. & Milbradt, R. (1998) Reversible transverse overcurvature of the nails (pincer nails) after treatment with a β-blocker. *Journal of the American Academy of Dermatology* 39, 486–487.

Haneke, E. (1992) Etiopathogénie et traitement de l'hypercourbure transversale de l'ongle du gros orteil. *Journal de Médecine Esthétique* 29, 123–127.

Haneke, E. (1999) Pincer nails. *Journal of the European Academy of Dermatology and Venereology* 12 (Suppl. 2), S125.

Higashi, N. (1990) Pincer nail due to tinea unguium. *Hifu* 32, 40–44.

Jemec, G. & Thomsen, K. (1997) Pincer nails and alopecia as markers of gastrointestinal malignancy. *Journal of Dermatology* 24, 479–481.

## Dolichonychia

Normally the quotient between the length and the width is 1 ± 0.1. In dolichonychia this quotient is greater (1.9) (Alkiewicz & Pfister 1976). Therefore the nails appear long and narrow. This condition may be seen in Ehlers–Danlos' syndrome, in Marfan's syndrome, in association with eunuchoidism or with hypopituitarism.

## Reference

Alkiewicz, J. & Pfister, R. (1976) *Atlas des Nagelkrankheiten*, pp. 52–53. Schattauer-Verlag, Stuttgart.

## Brachyonychia/short nails/racquet nails
(see acroosteolysis (Chapter 5) and Table 9.6)

In this condition, considered in the past as a minor sign of congenital syphilis (Ronchese 1951), the width of the nail plate (and the nail bed) is greater than the length (Fig. 2.10), which is in contrast to the normal ratio of the length to the shape. It may occur in isolation or associated with a shortening of the terminal phalanx (Basset 1962). The 'racquet thumb' is usually inherited as an autosomal dominant trait. Ronchese (1973) in a review of 113 cases of racquet thumbnail found a sex ratio of three females to one male and a higher prevalence of bilateral cases. All the fingers may be involved. The epiphyses of the terminal phalanx of the thumb are normally closing at the age of 13–14 years in girls and slightly later in boys. In individuals with hereditary defect the epiphyseal line is obliterated on the affected side at the age of 7–10 years, while it is still present

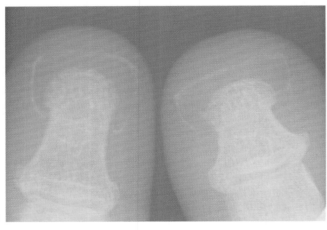

(a)

(b)

**Fig. 2.10** Brachyonychia. (a) Unilateral (right). (b) X-ray of (a) showing the shortened terminal phalanx (right).

according to age in normal thumb. Among the 31 patients with racquet nails studied by Higashi (1994), two women presented only great toenail involvement. Johnson (1966) recorded the syndrome of broad thumbs, broad great toes, facial abnormalities and mental retardation. Racquet nails have been reported in association with brachydactylia and multiple malignant Spiegler tumours (Tsambaos *et al.* 1979). Disorders associated with brachyonychia include cartilage-hair hypoplasia, acroosteolysis, Larsen syndrome, pyknodysostosis and acrodysostosis (see Table 9.6). This condition may also be acquired in bitten nail, or associated with bone resorption in hyperparathyroidism (Fairris & Rowell 1984) and psoriatic arthropathy (see Chapter 5). Thickened and large cuticle extending on the nail may mimick brachyonychia.

### References

Basset, H. (1962) Trois formes génotypiques d'ongles courts, le pouce en raquette, les doigt en raquette, les ongles courts simples. *Bulletin de la Societé Française de Dermatologie et de Syphiligraphie* **69**, 15.
Fairris, G.M. & Rowell, N.R. (1984) Acquired racket nails. *Clinical and Experimental Dermatology* **9**, 267–269.

Higashi, N. (1994) Racket nail. *Hifu* **36**, 776–779.
Johnson, C.F. (1966) Broad thumbs and broad great toes with facial abnormalities and mental retardation. *Pediatrics* **68**, 942.
Ronchese, F. (1951) Peculiar nail anomalies. *Archives of Dermatology and Syphilis* **63**, 565–580.
Ronchese, F. (1973) The racket thumbnail. *Dermatologica* **146**, 199–202.
Tsambaos, D., Greither, A. & Orfanos, C.E. (1979) Multiple malignant Spiegler tumors with brachydactyly and racket-nails. *Journal of Cutaneous Pathology* **6**, 31.

## Parrot beak nails

This peculiar, symmetrical overcurvature of the free margin of some fingernails simulates the beak of a parrot (Kandel 1971) (Fig. 2.11a,b). If the patient trims the affected nails close to the line of separation from the nail bed, no abnormality would be noted clinically.

Soaking the nails in tepid water for about 30 min causes this overcurvature to disappear temporarily. Distal hemitorsion of the nail plate observed in porphyria cutanea tarda (Baran 1981) could be clinically related to the parrot beak nail.

### References

Baran, R. (1981) *Porphyria*. In: *The Nail* (ed. M. Pierre), p. 51. Churchill Livingstone, Edinburgh.
Kandel, E. (1971) Parrot beak nails. *Lebanese Medical Journal* **24**, 433.

## Curved nail of the 4th toe (Fig. 2.11c)

The common feature of this congenital condition is a curved 4th toenail, often bilateral. Eight cases were reported by Higashi *et al.* (1999) without other anomalies of the extremities. Additional hypoplasia of the bone and soft tissue was present in the cases reported by Iwasawa *et al.* (1991). This nail deformity resembles a post-traumatic fingertip abnormality, in which the loss of the supporting tissues for the nail lead to curving of the nail. It is not clear whether the series of Iwasawa *et al.* (1991) described the same pathology as that of Egawa (1977) or Miura (1987), where the deformities of the nails in these series resembled those in that of Iwasawa *et al.* Another curved nail anomaly is Kirner's deformity, but this is usually absent before 12 years of age (David 1982). Congenital curved nail of the 4th toe is inherited as an autosomal recessive.

### References

David, P. (1982) *Green's Operative Hand Surgery*, p. 303. Churchill Livingstone, Edinburgh.
Egawa, T. (1977) Congenital clawlike fingers and toes: case report of two siblings. *Plastic and Reconstructive Surgery* **59**, 569–574.
Higashi, N., Kume, A., Tanogushi, T. *et al.* (1999) Congenital curved nail of the fourth toe. *Journal of Pediatric Dermatology (Jap)* **18**, 99–101.
Iwasawa, M., Hirose, T. & Matuso, K. (1991) Congenital curved nail of the fourth toe. *Plastic and Reconstructive Surgery* **87**, 553–554.

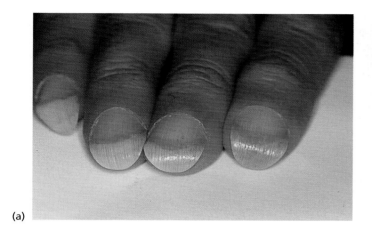

(a)

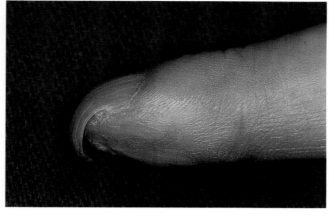

(b)

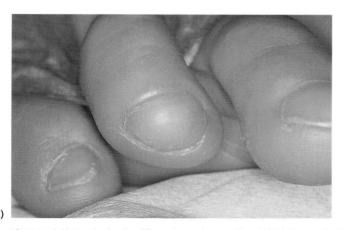

(c)

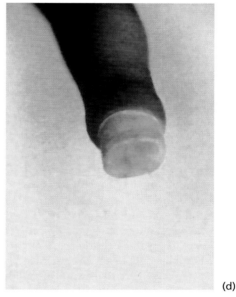

(d)

**Fig. 2.11** (a,b) Parrot beak nails—different degrees between (a) and (b). (c) Curved nail of the 4th toe. (d) Circumferential nail. (Courtesy of A. Griffiths, UK.)

Miura, T. (1987) Two families with congenital nail anomalies: nail formation in ectopic areas. *Journal of Hand Surgery* **3**, 348–351.

## Circumferential fingernail (see Chapter 9) (Fig. 2.11d)

Alves *et al.* (1999) described a tubular nail plate resembling a punch biopsy involving the left ring finger of a 7-year-old Brazilian girl. This extremely rare congenital malformation was associated with other bony and soft tissue abnormalities of the affected limb.

### Reference

Alves, G.F., Poon, E., John, J. *et al.* (1999) Circumferential fingernail. *British Journal of Dermatology* **140**, 960–962.

## Claw-like nail

One or both little toenails are often rounded like a claw. This con-

dition predominates in women wearing high heels and narrow shoes and is often associated with the development of hyperkeratosis such as calluses on the feet. Congenital claw-like fingernails and toenails have been reported (Egawa 1977). Claw nails may be curved dorsally showing a concave upper surface. This condition resembles onychogryphosis or post-traumatic hook nail.

### Reference

Egawa, T. (1977) Congenital claw-like fingers and toes: case report of two siblings. *Plastic and Reconstructive Surgery* **59**, 569–574.

## Macronychia and micronychia

The nails are larger or smaller than normal and affect one or more digits with wide or narrow nail bed areas and matrices. They may occur as an isolated defect or in association with megadactyly, as in Von Recklinghausen's disease or in epiloia. In fact macrodactyly may be the forme fruste of a wide variety

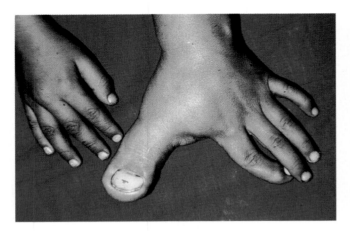

**Fig. 2.12** Macronychia associated with megadactyly.

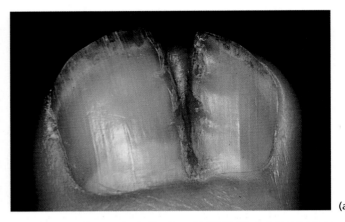

(a)

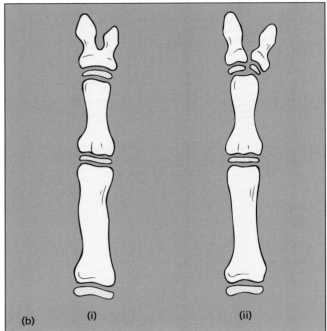

(b)  (i)  (ii)

**Fig. 2.13** (a) Duplication of the nail. (Courtesy of A. Tosti, Italy.) (b) Duplication of the nail—diagram of associated bony changes: (i) bifid distal phalanx; (ii) duplicated distal phalanx.

of connective tissue abnormalities. It has been associated with the proteus syndrome (partial gigantism, hemihypertrophy, etc.) (Fig. 2.12) (Child *et al.* 1998), Maffucci's syndrome and Klippel–Trenaunay–Weber syndrome. Greenberg *et al.* (1987) reported on a patient with epidermal naevus syndrome who also exhibited bilateral, four-finger megadactyly. Involvement of both hands and both feet of the same patient is unique (Keret *et al.* 1987).

Macrodactyly most commonly manifests in the middle and index fingers (Barsky 1967); usually corresponding to the territory supplied by the sensory branches of the median nerve, which was designated as nerve territory orientated macrodactyly or NTOM for short (Kelikian 1974). Finger incurvation may be neurological in origin (Mouly & Debeyre 1961). Macrodactyly associated with plexiform neurofibroma of the medial plantar nerve of the right foot is an unusual localization (Turra *et al.* 1986). About one-third of neural fibrolipomas are associated with overgrowth of bone and macrodactyly (Silverman & Enziger 1985; Wu 1991). Distant benign lipoblastomatosis in the axilla has been reported (Colot *et al.* 1984). As a rule, the involvement by macrodactylia fibrolipomatosis is almost always unilateral.

Pseudomegadactyly is an anecdotal presentation of chronic granulomatous paronychia resulting in hypertrophy of nail plate and bed (Mittal & Mittal 1984).

Duplication of the distal phalanx is usually accompanied by a wide digit with a bivalved nail, fissured or confluent (Fig. 2.13) (Robertson 1987; Tosti *et al.* 1992; Boutros *et al.* 1998). Nail plasty with refinements, based on a lunula, focusing on constructing a good appearance of the nail in the treatment of duplicated thumb, has been advocated by Iwasawa and Hirose (1993).

In Iso–Kikuchi's syndrome (Chapter 9) the micronychia is usually medially sited instead of a centrally placed small nail, except for a less common type termed 'rolled micronychia' (Millman & Strier 1982) where the nail is centrally sited.

Apparent micronychia may be due to overlapping of the nail surface by thickened lateral nail folds. This is sometimes seen in Turner's syndrome, in which the whole paronychium may be affected as in recalcitrant chronic paronychia (Zaias 1990). Micronychia is often observed in Zimmerman–Laband syndrome (Laband *et al.* 1964).

## References

Barsky, A.J. (1967) Macrodactyl. *Journal of Bone and Joint Surgery* **49**, 1255–1256.

Boutros, S., Weinfeld, A.B., Stafford, J. *et al.* (1998) An unusual case of polydactyly of the thumb. *Annals of Plastic Surgery* **41**, 434–435.

Child, F.J., Werring, D.J. & DuVivier, A.W.P. (1998) Proteus syndrome: diagnosis in adulthood. *British Journal of Dermatology* **139**, 132–136.

Colot, G., Castmans-Elias, S. & Philippet, G. (1984) Macrodactylie associée à une lipoblastomatose bénigne. *Annales de Chirurgie de la Main* 3, 262–265.

Greenberg, B.M., Pess, G.M. & May, J.W. (1987) Macrodactyly and the epidermal naevus syndrome. *Journal of Hand Surgery* **12A**, 730–733.

Iwasawa, M. & Hirose, T. (1993) Nail plasty in the treatment of duplicated thumb. *Annals of Plastic Surgery* **31**, 528–531.

Kelikian, H. (1974) *Congenital Deformities of the Hand and Forearm*, pp. 610–660. W.B. Saunders. Philadelphia.

Keret, D., Ger, E. & Marks, H. (1987) Macrodactyly involving both hands and both feet. *Journal of Hand Surgery* **12A**, 610–614.

Laband, P.F., Habib, G. & Humprey, G.S. (1964) Hereditary gingival fibromatosis. Report of an affected family with associated splenomegaly and skeletal and soft tissue abnormalities. *Oral Surgery* **17**, 339–351.

Millman, A.J. & Strier, R.P. (1982) Congenital onychodysplasia of the index fingers. *Journal of the American Academy of Dermatology* **7**, 57–65.

Mittal, R.L. & Mittal, R. (1984) Pseudomegadactyly. *Dermatologica* **169**, 86–87.

Mouly, R. & Debeyre, J. (1961) Le gigantisme digital: etiologie et traitement. A propos d'un cas. *Annales de Chirurgie Plastique* **6**, 187–194.

Robertson, W.W. (1987) The bifid great toe, a surgical approach. *Journal of Pediatric Orthopedics* **7**, 25–28.

Silverman, T.A. & Enziger, F.M. (1985) Fibrolipomatous hamartoma of nerve. A clinicopathologic analysis of 26 cases. *American Journal of Surgical Pathology* **9**, 7.

Tosti, A., Paoluzzi, P. & Baran, R. (1992) Doubled nail of the thumb. A rare form of polydactyly. *Dermatology* **184**, 216–218.

Turra, S., Frizziero, P., Cagnoni, G. *et al.* (1986) Macrodactyly of the foot associated with plexiform neurofibroma of the medial plantar nerve. *Journal of Pediatric Orthopedics* **6**, 489–492.

Wu, K.K. (1991) Macradactylia fibrolipomatosis of the foot. *Journal of Foot Surgery* **30**, 402–405.

Zaias, N. (1990) *The Nail in Health and Disease*. Lange and Appleton, Norwalk, CT.

## Worn-down nails

Patients with atopic dermatitis or chronic erythroderma may be 'chronic scratchers and rubbers'. The surface of the nail plate becomes glossy and shiny and the free edge is worn away. 'Usure des ongles' may also occur in many different manual occupations (Ronchese 1962) (Fig. 2.14a). This condition has been described as an occupational hazard of mushroom-pickers handling heavy, plastic bags (Schubert *et al.* 1977). A French variant of the worn-down nail syndrome, the 'bidet nail', has been reported by Baran and Moulin (1999) (Fig. 2.14b). The dystrophy of the middle three fingernails of the dominant hand involved three unrelated women. The defect was triangular with its base lying at the free edge of the nail where the thinning was maximal. All three were fastidious females in whom the desire for cleanliness verged on the obsessional. All three were traumatizing their nails against the glazed earthenware of the bidet.

## References

Baran, R. & Moulin, G. (1999) The bidet nail. A French variant of the worn down nail syndrome. *British Journal of Dermatology* **140**, 377.

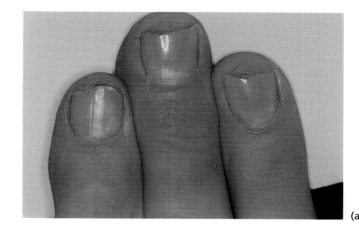

(a)

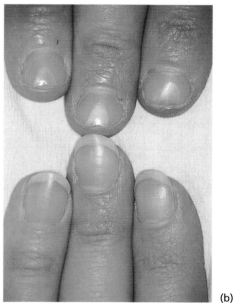

(b)

**Fig. 2.14** (a) Shiny, 'worn-down' nails. (b) Triangular defect involving the dominant hand in the 'bidet nail'.

Ronchese, F. (1962) Nails—injuries and disease. In: *Traumatic Medicine and Surgery for the Attorney*, Vol. 6, p. 626. Butterworth, Washington.

Schubert, B., Minard, J.J., Baran, R. *et al.* (1977) Onychopathie des champignonnistes. *Annales de Dermatologie et de Vénéréologie* **104**, 627.

## Onychatrophy

Acquired (e.g. lichen planus, Chapter 5) and congenital onychatrophy present as a reduction in size and thickness of the nail plate, often accompanied by fragmentation and splitting. This condition may progressively worsen, with scar tissue eventually replacing the atrophic nail plate (Fig. 2.15).

## Anonychia (see Chapter 9)

This implies absence of all or part of some or several nails

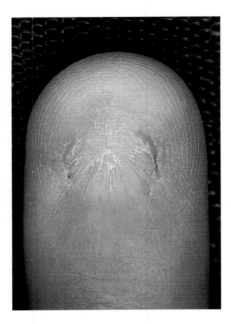

**Fig. 2.15** Scleroatrophy associated with lichen planus.

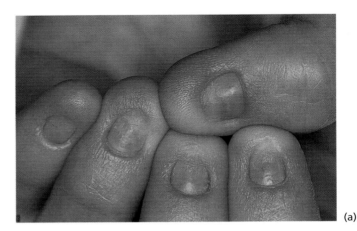

(a)

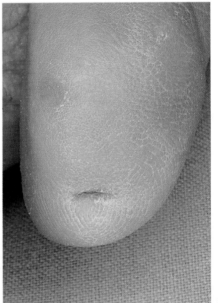

**Fig. 2.16** (a) Anonychia of all the digits. (b) Severe anonychia involving the 5th toe.

(b)

(Fig. 2.16). In aplastic anonychia, a rare congenital disorder occasionally associated with other defects such as ectrodactyly, the nail never forms (Solammadevi 1981; Aköz *et al.* 1998; Priolo *et al.* 2000). Loose horny masses are produced by the metaplastic, squamous epithelium of the matrix and the nail bed in anonychia keratodes. Kelikian (1974) states that 'one cannot conceive of a normal nail above an anomalous ungual phalanx'. It would appear that congenital anonychia and hyponychia may be 'bone territory' dependent disorders (Baran & Juhlin 1986). The development of a normal nail is not only dependent on the underlying bone but this dependence may also extend to the middle phalanx. Anonychia or hyponychia may result when the underlying phalanx is either hypoplastic or completely absent (Fig. 2.17). Congenital forms have been reported as a part of different syndromes such as the nail–patella syndrome, where hypoplasia of the nail plates is its hallmark. In the least affected cases only the ulnar half of each thumbnail is missing. Onychodystrophy-deafness and Cook syndrome are also affected by the nail anomaly (Chapter 9).

In acquired nail atrophy (anonychia atrophica), the damage to the matrix can result in a rudimentary nail reduced to a corneal layer or to progressive scar formation; it is impossible to draw a strict line between anonychia and onychatrophy. In contrast to these permanent types, a transient anonychia can be due to a local or sytemic condition, for example after etretinate therapy (Chapter 5).

## References

Aköz, T., Erdodan, B., Görgü, M. *et al.* (1998) Congenital anonychia. *Plastic and Reconstructive Surgery* **101**, 551–552.

Baran, R. & Juhlin, L. (1986) Bone dependent nail formation. *British Journal of Dermatology* **114**, 371–375.

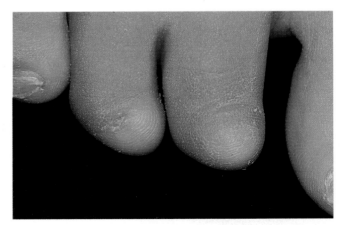

**Fig. 2.17** Severe anonychia with bone defect.

Kelikian, H. (1974) *Congenital Deformities of the Hand and Forearm.* W.B. Saunders, Philadelphia.

Priolo, M., Rosaia, L., Seri, M. *et al.* (2000) Total anonychia congenita in a woman with normal intelligence. Report of a further case. *Dermatology* 200, 84–85.

Solammadevi, S.V. (1981) Simple anonychia. *Southern Medical Journal* 74, 1555.

## Hypertrophy of the nail

Hypertrophy may be acquired, the results of dermatological or systemic conditions, including trauma, or occur as a developmental abnormality.

### Pachyonychia

Pachyonychia is characterized by thickening of the nail. When the thickening is regular and confined to the nail plate, it is due to involvement of the matrix and is sometimes called *onychauxis*. This sign has been reported in association with the eunuchoid state.

Hyperplastic subungual tissues, especially of the hyponychium, can alter the nail plate and nail consistency may be hard, as in pachyonychia congenita, or soft, as in psoriasis, pityriasis rubra pilaris, chronic eczema and onychomycosis.

In pachyonychia congenita (Jadassohn–Lewandowsky syndrome) the nails are yellow-brown in colour and extremely hard (Fig. 2.18). There is increased transverse overcurvature with a free edge shaped like a horseshoe or a barrel. All the nails are affected but the toenails are less severely involved. Recurrent paronychia results in repeated shedding of the nails.

Histology shows a normal proximal nail fold and matrix. The nail plate is normal or moderately thickened, but its structure is normal. The nail bed shows marked acanthosis, papillomatosis and huge hyperkeratosis. Groups of amorphous periodic acid–Schiff (PAS)-positive globules are arranged in vertical columns between the keratin masses of the subungual

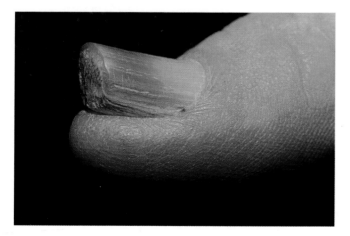

**Fig. 2.18** Pachyonychia congenita (Jadassohn–Lewandowsky syndrome).

hyperkeratosis (Alkiewicz & Lebioda 1961); they are very similar to those seen in pincer nails and probably represent serum inclusions. Electron microscopy confirms the acanthosis and shows hypergranulosis representing serum inclusions. There is no difference between classical and late-onset pachyonychia congenita (Forslind *et al.* 1973; Paller *et al.* 1991).

### Onychogryphosis (Table 2.3)

Onychogryphosis may rarely occur as a developmental abnormality but is usually acquired. It is most common in the toenail and presents as an uneven, thickened, opaque nail plate on a hyperplastic nail bed. The hallux is particularly vulnerable and the nail is often shaped like a ram's horn and is brownish in colour. Its irregular surface is marked by striations which are most frequently transverse. The matrix produces the nail plate at uneven rates; the faster growing side determines the direction of the deformity (Zaias 1990). In the case reported by Ohata *et al.* (1996), the free edge of the deformed nail plate re-entered the proximal nail fold with subsequent granulation tissue and ulcer. Onychogryphosis is obvious when the changes are marked (Fig. 2.19a). In the early stages, however, when there is just a mild hypertrophy of the nail plate, diagnosis may present some difficulty.

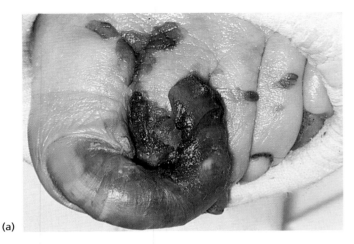

(a)

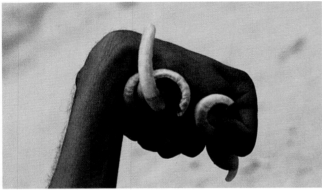

(b)

**Fig. 2.19** (a) Onychogryphosis. (b) Onychogryphosis following peripheral nervous injury.

In the elderly the dystrophy is usually caused by pressure from footwear. The bend of the nail is medially directed, accentuated by hypertrophy of the nail bed (Zaias 1990), and favoured by secondary foot anomalies such as hallux valgus.

Onychogryphosis may be related to weight-bearing function of the great toe, especially at the step-off phase. In case the free edge of the great toenail is considerably shorter than the tip of the great toe, the distal tissue bulge causes the onychogryphosis, which is due to primarily improper shorter nail cutting (Higashi & Matsumura 1988). Therefore, for these authors, surgical treatment should be that of distal ingrowing nail.

Onychogryphosis, indicating longstanding poor personal care (Möhrenschlager et al. 1999), appears in cases of self-neglect and is often seen in tramps and in senile dementia. Although this dystrophy may be a source of discomfort, or even pain when shoes are worn, it is usually accepted without complaint. In old age, fungal infection associated with onychogryphosis is not unusual (Tanaka 1986); it may be restricted to a single fingernail. Symptomatic onychogryphosis may be due to diseases such as ichthyosis and psoriasis (Fig. 2.20). Pemphigus, syphilis and variola (Heller 1927) are exceptional causes. Nail resembling cutaneous horn may occur after acral bone loss (Patki & Baran 1994).

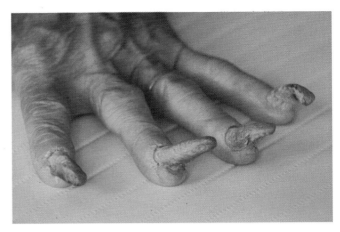

**Fig. 2.20** Onychogryphosis due to psoriasis.

Impairment of the peripheral circulation may produce onychogryphosis. Occasionally in the elderly, the pressure on the thickened onychogryphotic nail will initiate subungual gangrene (Douglas & Krull 1981). Onychogryphosis may be considered as one of the manifestions of hyperuricaemia (Horvath & Vlcek 1986).

Onychogryphosis may result from an injury to the matrix, scarring of the nail bed and pathology in the central or peripheral nervous system (Fig. 2.19b). The traumatic type is common in young people.

In hereditary onychogryphosis (Videbaek 1948; Schmidt 1965; Lubach 1982), all the nails of both hands and feet may be involved. The deformity is congenital and particularly marked during the first year of life. The disease is inherited as an autosomal dominant trait. Hemionychogryphosis may result from congenital malalignment of the big toenail and can be prevented by surgical correction of the deformity. One of the signs of the Iso–Kikuchi syndrome is hemionychogryphosis of the index finger (Chapter 9).

## References

Achten, G. & Wanet-Rouard, J. (1970) Pachyonychia. *British Journal of Dermatology* 83, 56–62.

Alkiewicz, J. & Lebioda, J. (1961) Zur Klinik und Histologie der Pachyonychia congenita. *Archiv der Klinische und experimentale Dermatologie* 112, 140–147.

Douglas, M.C. & Krull, E.A. (1981) *Diseases of the Nails. Current Therapy*, p. 712. W.B. Saunders, Philadelphia.

Forslind, B., Nylén, B., Swanbeck, G., Thyresson, M. & Thyresson, N. (1973) Pachyonychia congenita. A histologic and microradiographic study. *Acta Dermato-Venereologica* 53, 211–216.

Heller, J. (1927) Die krankheiten der Nägel. In: *Handbuch der Haut- und Geschlechtskrankheiten*, Vol. XIII/2 (ed. J.J. Jadassohn). Springer, Berlin.

Higashi, N. & Matsumura, T. (1988) The etiology of onychogryphosis of the great toenail and of ingrowing nail. *Hifu* 30, 620–623.

Horvath, G. & Vlcek, F. (1986) Uricaemia and onychogryphosis. *Ceskoslovenska Dermatologie* 81, 388–390.

Lubach, D. (1982) Erbliche onychogryphosis. *Hautarzt* 33, 331.

Ohata, C., Shirabe, H., Takagi, K. *et al.* (1996) Inychogryphosis with granulation tissue of proximal nail fold. *Skin Research* 38, 626–629.

Paller, A.S., Moore, J.A. & Scher, R. (1991) Pachyonychia congenita tarda. A late-onset form of pachyonychia congenita. *Archives of Dermatology* 127, 701–703.

Patki, A. & Baran, R. (1994) Nail resembling cutaneous horn occurring after acral bone loss. *Cutis* 54, 41–42.

Schmidt, H. (1965) Total onychogryphosis traced during 6 generations. In: *Proceedings of the Fenno-Scandinavian Association of Dermatology*, pp. 36–37.

Tanaka, T., Sohba, S. & Tanida, Y. (1986) Onychogryphosis considered to be due to tinea unguium. *Hifuka No Rinsho* 28, 1333–1337.

Videbaek, A. (1948) Hereditary onychogryphosis. *Annals of Eugenics* 14, 139.

Zaias, N. (1990) *The Nail in Health and Disease*, 2nd edn, p. 164. Lange & Appleton. Norwalk, CT.

## Modification of the nail surface

### Longitudinal lines

Longitudinal lines, or striations, may appear as indented grooves or projecting ridges.

#### Longitudinal grooves

Longitudinal grooves represent long-lasting abnormalities and can occur under the following conditions:

1 Physiological, as shallow and delicate furrows, usually parallel, and separated by low, projecting ridges. They become more prominent with age and in certain pathological states, such as lichen planus, rheumatoid arthritis, peripheral circulatory disorders, Darier's disease and other genetic anomalies.

2 Onychorrhexis is a series of narrow, longitudinal parallel furrows which have the appearance of having been scratched by an awl or by sandpaper. Sometimes dust becomes ingrained on the nail surface. Splitting of the free edge is common.

3 Tumours, such as myxoid cysts and warts, located in the proximal nail fold area, may exert pressure on the nail matrix and produce a wide, deep, longitudinal groove or canal, which will disappear if the cause is removed.

4 Median nail dystrophy. This uncommon condition consists of a longitudinal defect of the thumbnails in the midline or just off centre, starting at the cuticle and growing out of the free edge. It may be associated with an enlarged lunula (Zelger *et al.* 1974). In the cases described by Heller (1928), the base of a 2–5-mm-wide groove with steep edges showed numerous transverse defects (Fig. 2.21) Ronchese (1951) reported cases showing longitudinal fissures as 'dystrophia longitudinalis fissuriformis'. In some cases median longitudinal ridges have been observed, occasionally combined with fissures and/ or a groove, developed from the distal edge of the nail plate to the matrix. Often a few short feathery chevron-shaped cracks

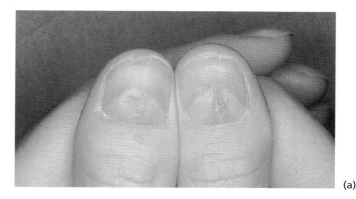

(a)

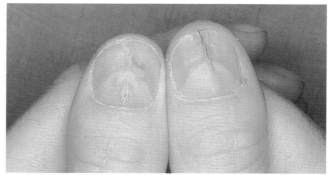

(b)

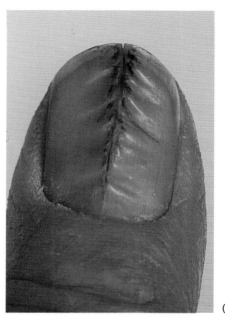

**Fig. 2.21** Median canaliform (Heller's) dystrophy: (a) early; (b) later; (c) inverted 'fir tree' appearance, reaching the distal edge.

(c)

extend laterally from the split. The so-called 'naevus striatus symmetricus of the thumbs' (Oppenheim & Cohen 1942) corresponds to this form (Leclercq 1964). Median nail dystrophy is usually symmetrical and most often affects the thumbs. Sometimes other fingers are involved, seldom the toes (usually the big toe). After several months or years, the nail returns to normal but recurrences are not exceptional. Sutton and Waisman (1975) reported a case of 'solenonychia' with a flabby filament of fleshy tissue present in the toenail canal. Familial cases have been recorded (Rehtijärvi 1971; Seller 1974). In all cases the aetiology is unknown, but Zaias (1990) suggests that the deformity is usually due to self-inflicted trauma resulting from a tic or habit. Pressure repeatedly exerted on the base of the nail probably explains the appearance of this condition as well as its enlarged reddish lunula.

It has been suggested that treatment of recalcitrant cases should be identical to that of post-traumatic nail splitting. We do not advocate this view.

### Differential diagnosis

A central longitudinal depression is found in 'washboard nail plates' (MacAulay 1966) caused by chronic, mechanical injury. Unlike Heller's dystrophy, the cuticle is pushed back and there is accompanying inflammation of the proximal nail fold. Splits due to trauma, or those occurring in the nail–patella syndrome and in pterygium, are generally obvious. Longitudinal splits may also result from Raynaud's disease, lichen striatus and trachyonychia.

### Treatment

Nail wrapping (Chapter 9) may reduce the disability produced by the fissure. Higashi et al. (1998) consider that onychorrhexis with nail splitting is caused by microtrauma to the proximal nail fold and suggest that topical steroid ointment should be applied on the fold.

### Longitudinal ridges (Fig. 2.22)

Small rectilinear projections extend from the proximal nail fold as far as the free edge of the nail; or they may stop short. They may be interrupted at regular intervals giving rise to a beaded or sausage-like appearance. Sometimes a wide, longitudinal median ridge has the appearance, in cross-section, of a circumflex accent. This condition, usually post-traumatic, may be inherited and affects mainly the thumb and fingers of both hands.

### Oblique lines/chevron nail/herring-bone nail (see Chapter 3)

In early childhood, the ridges may be oblique and converge towards the centre distally. Sometimes, in teenagers one longitudinal half of the nail may present oblique lines while the other half is covered with longitudinal ridges.

The oblique lines disappear by adult life, in contrast to the gorilla where they are life long (Pinkus 1927). The significance of chevron nail (Schuster 1996) or herring-bone nail (Parry et al. 1995) is still debatable.

### References

Heller, J. (1928) Dystrophia unguium mediana canaliformis. *Dermatologische Zeitschrift* **51**, 416–419.

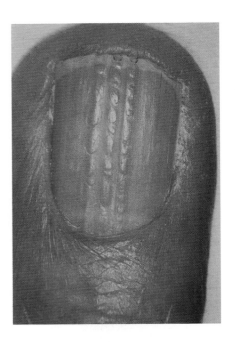

**Fig. 2.22** Longitudinal ridging with 'beaded' appearance.

Higashi, N., Kune, A., Ueda, K. *et al.* (1998) Onychorrhexis; etiology and treatment. *Hifu* **40**, 481–483.

Leclercq, R. (1964) Naevus striatus symmetricus unguis, dystrophie unguéale médiane canaliforme de Heller ou dystropie unguéale médiane en chevrons. A propos de 2 cas. *Bulletin de la Societé Française de Dermatologie et de Syphiligraphie* **71**, 655.

MacAulay, W.L. (1966) Transverse ridging of the thumbnails. *Archives of Dermatology* **93**, 421.

Oppenheim, M. & Cohen, D. (1942) Naevus striatus symmetricus unguis. *Archives of Dermatology and Syphilis* **45**, 253.

Parry, E.J., Morley, W.N. & Dawber, R.P.R. (1995) Herring bone nails: an uncommon variant of nail growth in childhood? *British Journal of Dermatology* **132**, 1021–1022.

Pinkus, F. (1927) Die normale Anatomie der Haut. In: *Handbuch der Haut- und Geschlechtskrankheiten*, Vol. 1/1 (ed. J.J. Jadassohn), p. 278. Springer, Berlin.

Rehtijärvi, K. (1971) Dystrophia unguis mediana canaliformis (Heller). *Acta Dermato-Venereologica* **51**, 315.

Ronchese, F. (1951) Peculiar nail anomalies. *Archives of Dermatology* **63**, 565.

Schuster, S. (1996) The significance of chevron nails. *British Journal of Dermatology* **135**, 151–152.

Seller, H. (1974) Dystrophic unguis mediana canaliformis. Familiäres vorkommen. *Hautarzt* **25**, 456.

Sutton, R.L. Jr & Waisman, M. (1975) *The Practitioner's Dermatology*. Yorke Medical Books, New York.

Zaias, N. (1990) *The Nail in Health and Disease*, 2nd edn. Appleton & Lange, Norwalk, CT.

Zelger, J., Wohlfarth, P. & Putz, R. (1974) Dystrophia unguium mediana canaliformis Heller. *Hautarzt* **25**, 629.

### Transverse grooves and Beau's lines
(Figs 2.23–2.25; Table 2.4)

Transverse lines in the form of sulci, limited proximally by slightly elevated ridges and affecting the surface of all nails

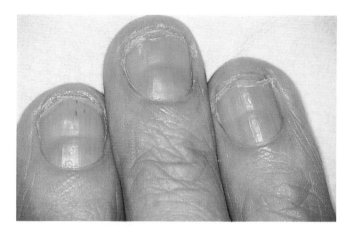

**Fig. 2.23** Beau's lines.

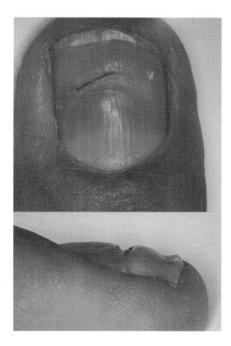

**Fig. 2.24** Beau's lines—wider depression than in Fig. 2.23.

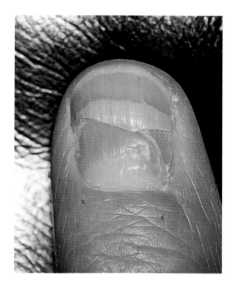

**Fig. 2.25** Latent onychomadesis.

**Table 2.4** Cause of Beau's lines. (After Requena 1991.)

| Cause | Study |
|---|---|
| Acute diseases (severe) | Beau (1846) |
| Acute hypocalcaemia | |
| Carpal tunnel syndrome | |
| Chronic paronychia | |
| Dapsone (syndrome) | Kromann et al. (1982) |
| Eczema | |
| Epileptic convulsion (severe) | |
| Fluorosis | Spira (1946) |
| Hand-foot-mouth disease | Clementz & Mancini (2000) |
| Hypopituitarism | Bieva (1973) |
| Immunobullous diseases | de Berker et al. (1995) |
| Malaria | Glew & Howard (1973) |
| Measles | |
| Menstrual cycle | Colver & Dawber (1984) |
| Metoprolol | Graber & Lapkin (1981) |
| Myelomatosis | Aberg & Graig (1966) |
| Nervous habit of repeatedly pushing back the cuticle | MacAulay (1966) |
| Overzealous manicuring | Sutton & Waisman (1975) |
| Raynaud's disease | |
| Razoxane | Tucker et al. (1984) |
| Reflex sympathetic dystrophy | O'Toole et al. (1995) |
| Retinoids | Baran (1990) |
| Transition from intrauterine to extrauterine life | Wolf et al. (1982) |
| Trauma | Ward et al. (1988) |
| Upper extremity tourniquet | Zook & Russell (1990) |
| Zinc deficiency | Weismann (1977); Higashi (1990) |

at corresponding levels, were described by Beau (1846) as 'retrospective indicators' of a number of pathological states. The condition is sometimes restricted to the thumbs and big toes. The grooves are superficial, but more marked in the middle aspect of the nail.

The transverse depression, sometimes involving the whole depth of the nail plate, appears some weeks after illness (e.g. fever). As the approximate growth rate is known (Chapters 1 and 3), it is possible to assess the approximate time of the prior causative disease which has marked the nails, the thumbnail supplies information for the previous 5–6 months, and the big toenail evidence of disease for up to 2 years. As the thumb and toes nails are most frequently affected they are the most reliable indicators of previous disease. Markings occur inconsistently on the other digits.

Beau's lines reflect a temporary reduction in matrix activity.

The length in the long axis of the furrow represents the exact duration of the disease which has affected the matrix, and the distal limit of the depression, if abrupt, indicates a sudden attack of disease, and if slopping a more protracted onset. If the activity of the entire matrix is inhibited for a period of 1–2 weeks for example, Beau's line will reach its maximum dimension causing a total division of the nail plate. Only the keratinized nail bed fills the gap between the old and new plate. This is seen in *latent* onychomadesis (Fig. 2.25) and leads to a temporary shedding of the nail (Runne & Orfanos 1981). Beau's lines are analogous to the Pohl–Pincus line found in the hair, which shows transient decreased diameter of the shaft and loss of medulla.

Physiological Beau's lines may occur in 4–5-week-old babies, marking the transition from intrauterine to extrauterine life, and monthly with each menstrual cycle. Cyclical transverse nail grooves occurring simultaneously with groups of knots in the hair have been reported (Fabry 1965). Beau's lines may be due to any severe disability and, particularly, to measles in childhood; zinc deficiency, whatever the cause, may produce transverse grooves. Antimitotic drug therapy temporarily inhibits the activity in nail matrix leading to transverse nail depression. In the interval between two series of chemotherapy, the nails are normal (Requena 1991). Transverse depressions restricted to one or two digits may indicate one of the following causes: injury, carpal tunnel syndrome, extremes of cold in Raynaud's disease. Unilateral Beau's line may develop after hand trauma involving damage to nerves and flexor tendons (Ward *et al.* 1988) or after fractured and immobilized wrist (Roberts 1993; Harford *et al.* 1995). In addition to Beau's lines, pyogenic granuloma may follow hand trauma (Price *et al.* 1994). Unilateral Beau's line has also been observed in childhood reflex sympathetic dystrophy (O'Toole *et al.* 1995). A transverse groove is the most common ischaemic deformity of the nail seen by hand surgeons following the use of the upper extremity tourniquet (Zook & Russell 1990). Fine transverse grooves, a few millimetres wide, and starting at one lateral edge of the nail plate, may appear on the whole length from its proximal part to the free margin and may occur in chronic paronychia; they may be dark or have a greenish tinge. Transverse depressions may be the consequence of a chronic condition, such as eczema. When a series of transverse grooves parallels the proximal fold rather than the distal convex curve of the lunula, the cause is likely to be repeated injury to the matrix from overzealous manicuring (Sutton & Waisman 1975). The grooves are separated by ridges of healthy nail.

A nervous habit of repeatedly pushing back the cuticle on one or several fingers can create 'washboard nails' (MacAulay 1966). Usually the proximal nail fold of the thumb on the same hand is damaged by the index finger and shows redness, swelling and scaling. This chronic, mechanical injury results in a series of transverse grooves and a large central depression running down the nail (Fig. 2.26). When the central depression does not exist, psoriasis should be suspected. Habit-tic deformity may respond to treatment with serotonin reuptake inhibitors (Vittorio & Phillips 1997), which is an antidepressant therapy for obsessive-compulsive disorders.

The 'serrated koilonychia' syndrome (Runne 1978) consists of a combination of saw-like transverse grooving of all nails with koilonychia.

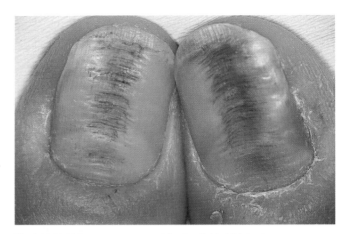

**Fig. 2.26** Multiple transverse grooves of thumbs—'habit-tic' deformity.

Total lack of nail plate synthesis may be preceded by a transverse band of leuconychia (Shelley & Shelley 1985). This indicates that initially the agent, such as a drug, caused only defective keratinization resulting in a white line. More severe disturbance results in matrix arrest and Beau's line formation. Shoreline nails are vivid evidence of their prior drug-induced erythrodermas.

To explain how transverse ridging appears, Higashi (1977) considers that the direction of nail growth is determined by three forces, that is, upward force due to nail matrix, downward force due to proximal nail fold (PNF), and outward force due to nail cul-de-sac. The former does not change because the length of matrix is fixed. Downward force fluctuates by the retraction and protrusion of the proximal nail fold, and outward force fluctuates because the length of the cul-de-sac changes by the retraction and protrusion of the latter. The decrease of downward force due to the retraction of the PNF results in thickening of the nail plate. The increase of downward force due to protrusion of the PNF results in thinning of the nail. Consequently the fluctuation of the distal end of the PNF results in ridges and furrows of the nail plate. Topical steroid ointment applied on the PNF would be the right treatment.

## References

Aberg, H. & Graig, D. (1966) Beau's lines in a case of myelomatosis. *Lancet* i, 503–504.

Baran, R. (1990) Retinoids and the nails. *Journal of Dermatological Treatment* 1, 151–154.

Beau, J.H.S. (1846) Note sur certains caractères de séméiologie rétrospective présentés par les ongles. *Archives Générales de Médecine* 11, 447.

de Berker, D., Dawber, R.P.R. & Wojnarowska, F. (1995) Beau's lines in immunobullous disease. *Clinical and Experimental Dermatology* 20, 359–360.

Bieva, L. (1973) La alteration ungueal nel morbo di Sheehan. *Chronic Dermatology* 3–4, 815.

Clementz, G.C. & Mancini, A.J. (2000) Nail matrix arrest following hand-foot-mouth disease: a report of five children. *Pediatric Dermatology* **17**, 7–11.

Colver, G.B. & Dawber, R.P.R. (1984) Multiple Beau's lines due to dysmenorrhoea. *British Journal of Dermatology* **111**, 111–113.

Fabry, H. (1965) Gleichzeitiges rhythmisches Auftreten von guerfuchen der Nägel und gruppierten Knotenbildungen der Haare. *Zeitschrift für Hautkrankheiten* **39**, 336–338.

Glew, R.H. & Howard, W.A. (1973) Transverse furrows of the nails associated with *Plasmodium vivax* malaria. *Johns Hopkins Medical Journal* **132**, 61–64.

Graber, C.W. & Lapkin, R.A. (1981) Metoprolol and alopecia. *Cutis* **28**, 633–634.

Harford, R.R., Cob, M.W. & Banner, N.T. (1995) Unilateral Beau's lines associated with a fractured and immobilized wrist. *Cutis* **56**, 263–264.

Higashi, N. (1977) How do transverse striations appear on the nail plate. *Rinsho Hifuka* **31**, 785–790.

Higashi, N. (1990) Nail changes in zinc deficiency state. *Hifu* **32**, 485–486.

Kromann, N.P., Wilhelmsen, R. & Strahl, D. (1982) The dapsone syndrome. *Archives of Dermatology* **118**, 531–532.

MacAulay, W.L. (1966) Transverse ridging of the thumbnails— 'washboard thumbnails'. *Archives of Dermatology* **93**, 421–432.

O'Toole, E.A., Gormally, S., Druim, B. *et al.* (1995) Unilateral Beau's lines in childhood. Reflex sympathetic dystrophy. *Pediatric Dermatology* **12**, 245–247.

Price, M.A., Bruce, S., Waidhofer, W. *et al.* (1994) Beau's lines and pyogenic granulomas following hand trauma. *Cutis* **54**, 248–249.

Requena, L. (1991) Chemotherapy-induced transverse ridging of the nails. *Cutis* **48**, 129–130.

Roberts, S. (1993) Post-traumatic Beau's lines. *International Journal of the Care of the Injured* **24**, 637–638.

Runne, V. & Orfanos, C.E. (1981) The human nail. *Current Problems in Dermatology* **9**, 102–149.

Shelley, W.B. & Shelley, E.D. (1985) Shoreline nails: sign of drug-induced erythroderma. *Cutis* **35**, 220–224.

Spira, L. (1946) Disturbance of pigmentation in fluorosis. *Acta Medica Scandinavica* **126**, 65–84.

Sutton, R.L. & Waisman, M. (1975) *The Practitioner's Dermatology.* Yorke Medical Books, New York.

Tucker, W.F.G., Church, R.E. & Hallam, R. (1984) Beau's lines after Razoxane therapy for psoriasis. *Archives of Dermatology* **120**, 1140.

Vittorio, C.C. & Phillips, K.A. (1997) Treatment of habit-tic deformity with fluoxetine. *Archives of Dermatology* **133**, 1203–1204.

Ward, D.J., Hudson, I. & Jeffs, J.V. (1988) Beau's lines following hand trauma. *Journal of Hand Surgery* **13B**, 411–414.

Weismann, K. (1977) Lines of Beau: possible markers of zinc deficiency. *Acta Dermato-Venereologica* **57**, 88–90.

Wolf, D., Wolf, R. & Goldberg, M.D. (1982) Beau's lines: a case report. *Cutis* **29**, 141.

Zook, E.G. & Russell, R.C. (1990) Reconstitution of a functional and esthetic nail. *Hand Clinics* **6**, 59–68.

## Pitting (pits, onychia punctata, erosions, Rosenau's depressions) (Fig. 2.27)

Pits develop as a result of defective nail formation in punctate areas located in the proximal portion of the matrix. The surface of the nail plate is covered by small punctate depressions which

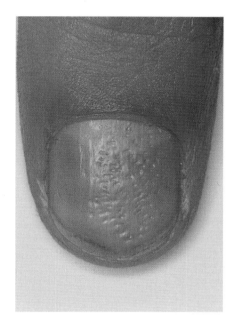

**Fig. 2.27** Pitting of the nails due to psoriasis. Irregular sized pits can be seen.

vary in number, size, depth and shape. The depth and width of the pits relates to the extent of the matrix involved; their length is determined by the duration of the matrix damage.

They are randomly distributed or uniformly arranged in series along one or several longitudinal lines, or sometimes arranged in a criss-cross pattern, they may resemble the external surface of a thimble.

Samman (1978) has shown that regular pitting could be converted to rippling or ridging (Fig. 2.28a) and these two conditions appear, at times, to be variants of uniform pitting. Nails showing pitting grow faster than the apparently normal nails.

Occasional pits occur on normal nails. Deep pits can be attributed to psoriasis. Shallow pits are usually seen in alopecia areata, eczematous dermatitis or occupational trauma. In some cases a genetic basis is possible. In secondary syphilis and pityriasis rosea, pitting occurs rarely. We have seen one case of the latter, with the pits distributed on all the fingernails at corresponding levels, in a manner analogous to that of Beau's lines.

## Reference

Samman, P.D. (1978) *The Nails in Disease*, 3rd edn., p. 180. Heinemann, London.

## Trachyonychia (rough nails)

This dystrophy was described by Alkiewicz (1950), then by Achten and Wanet-Rouard (1974), especially in relation to congenital nail atrophies, and by Samman (1979). It is characterized by a roughness of the nail surface and a grey opacity of the nail, which becomes brittle and splits at the free edge. One form may result from external chemical action (Alkiewicz 1950); other types are idiopathic, familial (Arias *et al.* 1982),

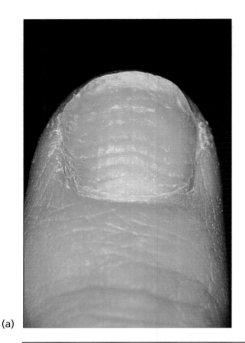

(a)

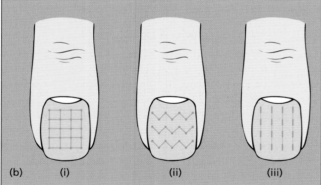

**Fig. 2.28** (a) Rippled lines of pits. (b) Pitting: (i) regular; (ii) rippled; (iii) ridged varieties.

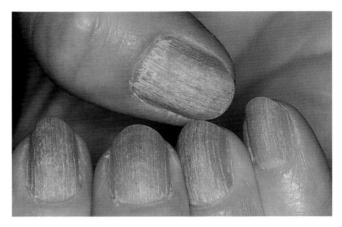

**Fig. 2.29** Trachyonychia—sandpapered appearance.

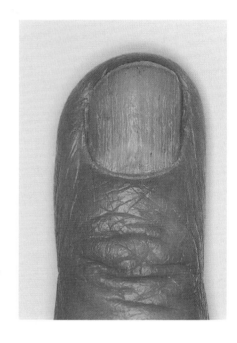

**Fig. 2.30**
Trachyonychia—nail shiny but fine stippled opalescent, longitudinal ridging.

congenital or acquired. Trachyonychia can involve one, several or all digits. The latter type, the so-called 'twenty-nail dystrophy' affecting both children and adults, may be related to a known dermatological disorder, such as lichen planus, psoriasis or alopecia areata, although these conditions may not yet be manifest. Identical nail changes have been described in ichthyosis vulgaris (James *et al.* 1981), dark red lunulae and knuckle pads (Runne 1980), selective IgA deficiency (Leong *et al.* 1982) and ectodermal dysplasia. An association with vitiligo has been reported in three cases (Peloro & Pride 1999). Tosti *et al.* (1991) have detected spongiotic inflammation of the nail apparatus in the nail biopsy specimens from 13 patients affected by severe trachyonychia involving all 20 nails. Spongiotic trachyonychia is due to a T-cell-mediated immune response. The possibility that idiopathic spongiotic trachyonychia is actually a variety of alopecia areata limited to the nails, is suggested by clinical and immunohistochemical data. In a study

of 22 cases of trachyonychia, Richert and André (1999) found spongiotic changes in 10 cases, psoriasis in six and lichen planus in six with a scarring evolution in two of them.

Some clarification of the confusion in the literature regarding this condition is indicated. It can be divided into two main types (Baran 1981):

1 The whole nail gives the appearance of having been sandpapered in a longitudinal direction. There is excessive ridging and a roughness, which deprives the nail of its natural lustre. We have designated this 'vertical striated sandpaper twenty-nail dystrophy' (Baran & Dupré 1977). It is most frequently associated with alopecia areata (Fig. 2.29), when a specific aetiology exists. It is difficult to demonstrate the condition adequately by photography.

2 In the second type of 'twenty-nail dystrophy', the nail plate is shiny, with opalescent longitudinal ridging (Fig. 2.30). The fine

stippled aspect of the nail reflects the camera flash and is clearly evident on photography. Alopecia areata may occur in association with both types.

Oral administration of biotin for 6 months resulted in a reduction of longitudinal ridging, thinning and distal notching of the nail plate in two cases of trachyonychia of childhood (Möhrenschlager *et al.* 1998).

A beneficial response following a short course of topically applied 5% 5-fluorouracil cream is anecdotal (Schissel & Elston 1998).

## References

Achten, G. & Wanet-Rouard, J.J. (1974) Atrophie unguéale et trachyonychie. *Archives Belges Dermatologique* **30**, 201.

Alkiewicz, J. (1950) Trachyonychie. *Annales de Dermatologie et de Syphiligraphie* **10**, 136.

Arias, A.M., Yung, C.W., Rendler, S. *et al.* (1982) Familial severe twenty-nail dystrophy. *Journal of the American Academy of Dermatology* **7**, 349.

Baran, R. (1981) Twenty-nail dystrophy of alopecia areata. *Archives of Dermatology* **117**, 1.

Baran, R. & Dupré, A. (1977) Vertical striated sandpaper nails. *Archives of Dermatology* **113**, 1613.

James, W.D., Odom, R.B. & Horm, R.T. (1981) Twenty-nail dystrophy and ichthyosis vulgaris. *Archives of Dermatology* **117**, 316.

Leong, A.B., Gange, R.W. & O'Connor, R.D. (1982) Twenty-nail dystrophy (trachyonychia) associated with selective IgA deficiency. *Pediatrics* **100**, 418.

Möhrenschlager, M., Schmidt, T., Ring, J. *et al.* (1998) Effects of biotin in trachyonychia of childhood. *Annales de Dermatologie et de Vénéréologie* **125** (Suppl. 1), 176.

Peloro, T.M. & Pride, H.B. (1999) Twenty-nail dystrophy and vitiligo: a rare association. *Journal of the American Academy of Dermatology* **40**, 488–490.

Richert, B. & André, J. (1999) Trachyonychia: a clinical and histological study of 22 cases. *Journal of the European Academy of Dermatology and Venereology* **12** (Suppl. 2), S126.

Runne, V. (1980) Twenty-nail dystrophy with knuckle pads. *Zeitschrift für Hautkrankheiten* **55**, 901.

Samman, P.D. (1979) Trachyonychia (rough nails). *British Journal of Dermatology* **101**, 701.

Schissel, D.J. & Elston, D.M. (1998) Topical 5-fluorouracil treatment for psoriatic trachyonychia. *Cutis* **62**, 27–28.

Tosti, A., Fanti, P.A., Morelli, R. *et al.* (1991) Spongiotic trachyonychia. *Archives of Dermatology* **127**, 584–585.

## Pseudomycotic nail dystrophy (pseudomycotic onychia)

Four cases of isolated pseudomycotic nail dystrophy were studied by Higashi *et al.* (1997). All the fingernails and toenails were simultaneously involved. Clinical features include longitudinal striations, fissuring and scaling of the surface of the nail plate with sometimes a yellow-brown discoloration.

The epithelium of the nail matrix reveals hyperplasia with a granular layer and projections similar to the crest of a wave. Inflammatory cell infiltration is present at the upper dermis of the matrix. The nail plate consists of normally keratinized layers and abnormal ones in stratiform pattern.

These findings differ histologically from that of psoriasis, lichen planus and twenty-nail dystrophy. Because of the inflammatory response of the matrix, Higashi *et al.* (1997) suggest the term 'pseudomycotic onychia'. The significance of isolated pseudomycotic nail dystrophy is not known; however it seems difficult to completely rule out alopecia areata restricted to the nail, a condition where the severe changes are sometimes 'simulating longstanding onychomycosis' (Demis & Weiner 1963). Milligan *et al.* (1988) have reported two cases involving all the digits, associated with vitiligo.

## References

Demis, D.J. & Weiner, M.A. (1963) Alopecia universalis, onychodystrophy and total vitiligo. *Archives of Dermatology* **88**, 195–201.

Higashi, N., Kume, A., Ueda, K. *et al.* (1997) Clinical and histopathological study of pseudo-mycotic onychia. *Hifu* **39**, 469–474.

Milligan, A., Barth, J.H., Graham-Brown, R.A.C. & Dawber, R.P.R. (1988) Pseudo-mycotic nail dystrophy and vitiligo. *Clinical and Experimental Dermatology* **13**, 109–110.

## Lamellar nail splitting (onychoschizia lamellina)

In this condition, found in 27–35% of normal adult women, the distal portion of the nail splits horizontally (Fig. 2.31). The nail is formed in layers analogous to the formation of scales in the skin; the thin lamellae then break off. Exogenous factors contribute to the defect. It is common in people who carry out a great deal of housework, whose nails are repeatedly soaked in water and then dried. Splitting into layers has been reported in X-linked dominant chondrodysplasia punctata (Happle

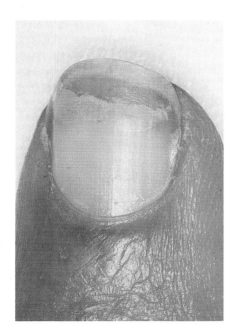

**Fig. 2.31** Onychoschizia lamellina (lamellar splitting).

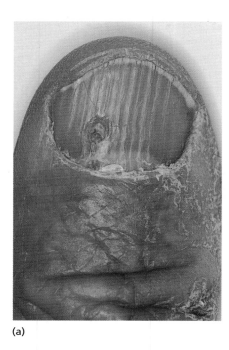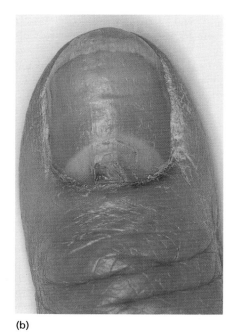

(a)        (b)        **Fig. 2.32** (a,b) Elkonyxis.

1979) and in polycythaemia vera (Graham-Brown & Homes 1980). In lichen planus, and in psoriasis treated with systemic retinoids, onychoschizia may be seen in the proximal portion of the nail (Baran 1990).

Shelley and Shelley (1984) studied with scanning electron microscopy the distal ends of nails of four women presenting with onychoschizia. The dorsal surface and tip of each nail showed horizontal lamellar separations representing single cell layers. Some cleavage lines extended proximally into the nail plate, revealing remarkable sculptured cell surfaces deep within the plate. These observations indicate that the lamellar splitting of onychoschizia occurs between cell layers. This presumably results from repeated trauma to a nail with diminished adherence between cell layers, secondary to the dissolution of intercellular cement by detergents and nail polish solvent.

Wallis *et al.* (1991) studied the *in vitro* nail changes produced by several organic solvents, detergents, other polar materials, and both acidic and basic solutions. Although other factors may influence onychoschizia, the typical changes can be produced in normal nails after a 21-day challenge of repeated exposure to water followed by dehydration. Scanning electron microscopy demonstrated unattached individual cells in empty spaces in which separation was prominent. The prominent *in vitro* changes from wetting and drying suggest that lamellar dystrophy could be managed by hydration followed by an occlusive topical agent that promotes water retention. Wallis *et al.* (1991) have successfully combined protection from exposure with hydrophilic petrolatum (Aquaphor), as a nail cream applied to the wet nails to maintain a relatively constant level of hydration. α-Hydroxy acids are more than mere moisturizers according to Leyden *et al.* (1995).

## References

Baran, R. (1990) Retinoids and the nails. *Journal of Dermatological Treatment* 1, 151–154.

Graham-Brown, R.A.C. & Homes, R. (1980) Polycythaemia rubra vera with lamellar dystrophy of the nails, a report of two cases. *Clinical and Experimental Dermatology* 5, 209.

Happle, R. (1979) X-linked dominant chondrodysplasia punctata. *Humangenitik* 53, 65.

Leyden, J.J., Lavker, R.M., Grove, G. *et al.* (1995) Alpha hydroxy acids are more than moisturizers. *Journal of Geriatric Dermatology* 3 (Suppl. A), 33A–37A.

Shelley, W.B. & Shelley, E.D. (1984) Onychoschizia, scanning electron microscopy. *Journal of the American Academy of Dermatology* 10, 623–627.

Wallis, M.S., Bowen, W.R. & Guin, J.R. (1991) Pathogenesis of onychoschizia (lamellar dystrophy). *Journal of the American Academy of Dermatology* 24, 44–48.

## Elkonyxis (Fig. 2.32)

Initially the nail appears punched out at the lunula and subsequently the disorder moves distally with the growth of the nail. It has been described in secondary syphilis, psoriasis, Reiter's syndrome and after trauma. It may be produced by etretinate (Cannata & Gambetti 1990).

## Reference

Cannata, G. & Gambetti, M. (1990) Elconyxis, une complication inconnue de l'étrétinate. *Nouvelles Dermatologiques* 9, 251.

## Modification of the nail plate and soft tissue attachments

The proximal nail fold is closely applied to the dorsal surface of the newly formed nail plate. At the free border of the proximal nail fold, the cuticle should adhere to the dorsal surface of the nail and seal the cul-de-sac. Inflammation of the proximal nail fold is called paronychia and will be described elsewhere; when this condition becomes chronic, the cuticle disappears and a 'pocket' is created between the ventral surface of the posterior nail fold and the nail.

### Pterygium

Pterygium of the nail has been described on both dorsal and ventral aspects of the nail plate. The term pterygium, which literally means 'wing', is more suitable for the dorsal pterygium ('pterygium unguis') which looks somewhat like a wing (Table 2.5). It consists of a linear forward growth of the proximal nail fold which fuses with the underlying matrix and subsequently with the nail bed dividing the nail plate in two (Fig. 2.33a). Ventral pterygium represents the same process extending from the hyponychium, anchoring to the undersurface of the nail plate with subsequent obliteration of the distal nail groove. Both conditions are non-specific abnormalities of the nail apparatus.

### Dorsal pterygium

Dorsal pterygium or pterygium unguis consists of a gradual shortening of the cul-de-sac of the proximal nail fold (PNF) with associated thinning of the nail plate until the latter

**Table 2.5** Causes of pterygium unguis (dorsal pterygium).

Burns
Cicatricial pemphigoid
Congenital
Diabetic vasculopathy
Dyskeratosis congenita
Graft-versus-host disease
Idiopathic atrophy of the nail
Lichen planus
Onychotillomania
Pemphigus foliaceus
Radiodermatitis
Raynaud's phenomenon
Sarcoidosis
Systemic lupus erythematosus
Toxic epidermal necrolysis
Trauma
Type-2 lepra reaction

becomes fissured because of the fusion of the PNF to the matrix and subsequently to the nail bed; the divided nail plate portions progressively decrease in size as the pterygium widens, resulting in two small remnants where the median part lateral segments. Complete involvement of the matrix and nail bed will produce a total loss of the plate and a permanent atrophy of the nail apparatus. It usually affects the fingers, rarely the toes (Edwards 1948). Involvement of all 20 nails has been reported in one single case only (Lembo *et al.* 1985). It is mostly acquired but exceptional congenital forms are reported. The first description was made by Friedman (1921) under the term of 'Navellierungsprozess' in a case of nail lichen planus.

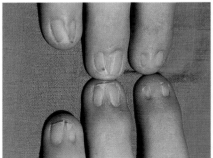
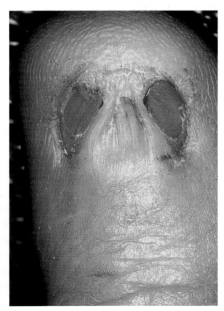

**Fig. 2.33** (a) Congenital dorsal pterygium. (Courtesy of G. Moulin, France.) (b) Dorsal pterygium in lichen planus.

(a)

(b)

Lichen planus remains its major cause (Zaias 1970) (Fig. 2.33b), but pterygium unguis has also been reported in isolated instances in various conditions. Healing of a disease involving the PNF may lead to pterygium formation as a scarring sequel. Physical factors such as trauma (Mortimer & Dawber 1985), burns, radiodermatitis (Lagrot & Gréco 1976; Richert & de la Brassine 1993) and diseases prone to develop adherence bands such as cicatricial pemphigoid (Barth *et al.* 1987), graft-versus-host disease (Liddle & Cowan 1990), toxic epidermal necrolysis (Burns & Sarkany 1978) and pemphigus foliaceus (Costa 1943) may be aetiological. There may be vascular causes such as peripheral ischaemia, which can be intermittent as in Raynaud's phenomenon (Edwards 1948) or permanent as in atherosclerosis and diabetic vasculopathy (Green & Scher 1987) and type-2 lepra reaction (Patki & Metha 1982). An idiopathic form called 'idiopathic atrophy of the nails' exists. However, this may be a variant of lichen planus and remains controversial (Tosti *et al.* 1995). There are congenital forms possibly associated with dyskeratosis congenita. Pterygium formation has also been reported in one case of sarcoidosis involving the proximal nail fold (Kalb & Grossman 1985) and in systemic lupus erythematosus (Wollina & Knopf 1992; Wollina 1995).

It seems that several coincident factors are required to produce pterygium formation. In patients suffering from dorsal pterygium (except of the traumatic or congenital type), the main characteristic is a dilatation of the nail capillary loops and the formation of a slender microvascular shunt system in the more dilatated loops (Trevisan & Tallocchi 1980). Pterygium resulting from trauma is not linked to its intensity; it may be observed in severe distal injury, it remains exceptional in repeated chronic trauma inflicted to the PNF in onychotillomania (Ameen Sait *et al.* 1985). Treatment of pterygium unguis remains very difficult and requires surgery: the nail plate is elevated from the dorsum of the nail bed and held, separated with a strip of silastic or non-adherent material. This allows the undersurface of the nail fold to epithelialize. If unsuccessful, a split-thickness graft should be placed on the undersurface of the PNF after freeing it from the nail plate (Zook 1990). If surgery is refused by the patient, injections of corticosteroids within the whole length of the pterygium may stop its progression and may even cause some flattening.

### Ventral pterygium

Ventral pterygium is a relatively recently described condition: the term pterygium inversum unguis was first coined by Caputo and Prandi (1973) to describe a condition consisting of a forward extension of the hyponychium anchoring to the undersurface of the nail plate and thus obliterating the distal nail groove (Fig. 2.34; Table 2.6). The similarity in the behaviour of the hyponychium and PNF in the two conditions led to the similarity of the name. However, the ventral pterygium does not look like a wing and does not split the nail.

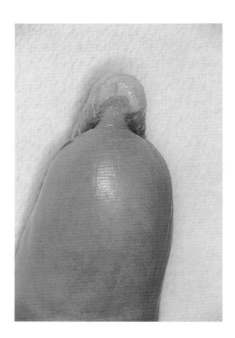

**Fig. 2.34** Ventral pterygium (pterygium inversum unguis).

**Table 2.6** Causes of pterygium inversum unguis (ventral pterygium).

Associated with lenticular atrophy of the palmar creases
Causalgia of the median nerve
Familial
Formaldehyde-containing hardeners
Lepra
Lupus erythematosus
Neurofibromatosis
Paresis
Scarring in the vicinity of the nail groove
Subungual exostosis
Systemic sclerosis

Pterygium inversum unguis (PIU) may be either congenital or acquired. The congenital form was first described by Odom *et al.* (1974) as a 'congenital, painful and aberrant hyponychium'. In some instances, the condition has been reported as familial (Christophers 1975; Dugois *et al.* 1975; Patterson 1977; Chams-Davatchi 1980; Nogita *et al.* 1991). In most reported cases the patients sought medical advice for pain or bleeding when trimming their nails (Caputo & Prandi 1973; Dugois *et al.* 1975; Drake 1976; Patterson 1977; Caputo *et al.* 1978, 1993; Daly & Johnson 1986; Morimoto & Gurevitch 1988). However, because the affection may be underestimated, especially in asymptomatic cases, Mello Filho (1985) performed a systematic digital examination on 2000 patients and found a frequency of 0.4% in the adult population. In his cases there was no familial trait and the condition was commoner in females than in males. Idiopathic forms were preponderant. Involvement of the toes remains exceptional: it may be associated with fingernails (Dugois *et al.* 1975; Morimoto & Gurevitch 1988; Caputo *et al.* 1993); restriction to the toes has been reported

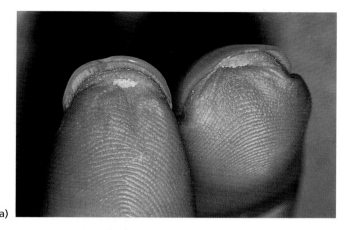

(a)

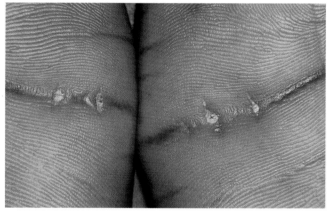

(b)

**Fig. 2.35** (a) Ventral pterygium. (b) Ventral pterygium associated with lenticular atrophy of the palmar creases. (Courtesy of A. Dupré, France.)

once only (Nogita *et al.* 1991). Women are more prone to develop this condition (Mello Filho 1985; Caputo *et al.* 1993).

By far the commonest form of PIU is the acquired form. It may sometimes be idiopathic but it is generally secondary to systemic connective tissue diseases and particularly to progressive systemic sclerosis and systemic lupus erythematosus. Its occurrence in patients suffering from such diseases has been estimated to be 16%. Furthermore, one patient with congenital PIU developed systemic lupus erythematosus at the age of 19 years.

PIU has also been described in various other conditions: it may be secondary to scarring in the vicinity of the distal nail groove (Catteral & White 1978; Caputo *et al.* 1993), it may arise from a reaction to formaldehyde-containing nail hardeners (Daly & Johnson 1986) or from a subungual exostosis (Guidetti *et al.* 1996). PIU has been reported once in neurofibromatosis (Patterson 1977), in association with lenticular atrophy of the palmar creases (Fig. 2.35) (Dupré *et al.* 1981) and causalgia of the median nerve (Runne & Orfanos 1981). Unilateral PIU of the fingers and toes has been reported 1 year after a stroke, resulting in a paresis of the same side (Morimoto & Gurevitch 1988).

The pathogenesis of PIU remains unclear. The congenital form could be related to an early defect in the developing fetal groove and ridge (Odom *et al.* 1974) or considered as a vestigial remnant of the animal claw (Caputo & Prandi 1973).

Medical treatment for PIU has not been rewarding: twice daily application of tretinoin 0.05% was useless (Odom *et al.* 1974) and electrocautery was followed by recurrence (Morimoto & Gurevitch 1988). Therapy directed towards the improvement of impaired peripheral blood flow ($\alpha$-methyldopa, Aldomet) in patients with scleroderma and Raynaud's phenomenon, while improving the latter, did not affect the nails (Patterson 1977). Surgery may be more useful and usually provides relief from pain: after avulsion of the distal 5-mm nail, a strip of nail bed and hyponychium 3–4 mm wide is resected and replaced by a split thickness graft (Zook 1990).

## References

Ameen Sait, M., Reddy, B.S.N. & Garg, B.R. (1985) Onychotillomania. *Dermatologica* **171**, 200–202.
Barth, J.H., Wojnarowska, F., Millard, P.R. & Dawber, R.P.R. (1987) Immunofluorescence of the nail bed in pemphigoid. *American Journal of Dermatopathology* **9**, 349–350.
Burns, D.A. & Sarkany, I. (1978) Junctional naevi following toxic epidermal necrolysis. *Clinical and Experimental Dermatology* **3**, 323.
Caputo, R. & Prandi, G. (1973) Pterygium inversum unguis. *Archives of Dermatology* **108**, 817–818.
Caputo, R., Crosti, C. & Menni, S. (1978) Pterigio inverso delle unghie. *Giornale Italiano di Dermatologia. Minerva Dermatologia* **113**, 559–562.
Caputo, R., Cappio, F., Rigoni, C. *et al.* (1993) Pterygium inversum unguis: report of 19 cases and review of the literature. *Archives of Dermatology* **129**, 1307–1309.
Catteral, M.D. & White, J.E. (1978) Pterygium inversum unguis. *Clinical and Experimental Dermatology* **3**, 437–438.
Chams-Davatchi, C. (1980) Pterygium inversum unguéal: à propos de trois cas. *Annales de Dermatologie et de Vénéréologie* **107**, 83–86.
Christophers, E. (1975) Familiäre subunguale Pterygien. *Hautartz* **26**, 543–544.
Costa, O.G. (1943) Lesoes ungueais no penfigo foliaceo. *Anales Brasiliera de Dermatologia* **18**, 67–73.
Daly, B.M. & Johnson, M. (1986) Pterygium inversum unguis due to nail fortifier. *Contact Dermatitis* **15**, 256–257.
Drake, L. (1976) Pterygium inversum unguis. *Archives of Dermatology* **112**, 255.
Dugois, P., Amblard, P., Martel, C. & Reymond, J.L. (1975) Pterygium inversum unguis familial. *Bulletin de la Societé Française de Dermatologie et de Syphiligraphie* **82**, 283–284.
Dupré, A., Christol, B., Bonafé, J.L. & Lasserre, J. (1981) Pterygium inversum unguis et atrophie ponctuée des plis palmaires. *Dermatologica* **162**, 209–212.
Edwards, E.A. (1948) Nail changes in functional and organic arterial disease. *New England Journal of Medicine* **239**, 362–365.
Friedman, M. (1921) Nagelveranderungen bei lichen ruber. *Archives of Dermatology and Syphilis* **135**, 174–179.
Green, R.A. & Scher, R.K. (1987) Nail changes associated with

diabetes mellitus. *Journal of the American Academy of Dermatology* **16**, 1015–1021.

Guidetti, M.S., Stinchi, C., Vezzani, C. & Tosti, A. (1996) Subungual exostosis of a finger resembling pterygium inversum unguis. *Dermatology* **193**, 354–355.

Kalb, E.R. & Grossman, M.E. (1985) Pterygium formation due to sarcoidosis. *Archives of Dermatology* **121**, 276–277.

Lagrot, F. & Gréco, J. (1976) Les lésions des ongles dans les radiodermites chroniques des mains. *Cutis (France)* **4**, 507–522.

Lembo, G., Montesano, M. & Balato, N. (1985) Complete pterygium unguis. *Cutis* **36**, 427–429.

Liddle, B.J. & Cowan, M.A. (1990) Lichen planus-like eruption and nail changes in a patient with graft-versus-host disease. *British Journal of Dermatology* **122**, 841–843.

Mello Filho, A. (1985) Ocorrencia do 'pterygium inversum unguis' em populaçao adulta. *Medicina Cutanea Ibero-Latino-Americana* **13**, 401–405.

Morimoto, S.S. & Gurevitch, A.W. (1988) Unilateral pterygium unguis. *International Journal of Dermatology* **27**, 491–494.

Mortimer, P.S. & Dawber, R.P.R. (1985) Trauma to the nail unit including occupational sports injuries. *Dermatologic Clinics* **3**, 415–420.

Nogita, T., Yamashita, H., Kawashima, M. & Hidano, A. (1991) Pterygium unguis. *Journal of the American Academy of Dermatology* **124**, 787–788.

Odom, R.B., Stein, K.M. & Maibach, H.I. (1974) Congenital, painful, aberrant hyponychium. *Archives of Dermatology* **110**, 89–90.

Patki, A.H. (1990) Pterygium inversum unguis in a patient with lepra. *Archives of Dermatology* **126**, 1110.

Patki, A.H. & Metha, J.M. (1989) Pterygium unguis in a patient with recurrent type-2 lepra reaction. *Cutis* **44**, 311–312.

Patterson, J.W. (1977) Pterygium inversum unguis-like changes in scleroderma. *Archives of Dermatology* **113**, 1429–1430.

Richert, B. & de la Brassinne, M. (1993) Subungual chronic radiodermatitis. *Dermatology* **186**, 290–293.

Runne, U. & Orfanos, C.E. (1981) The human nail. In: *Current Problems in Dermatology*, pp. 102–149. Karger, Basel.

Tosti, A., Piraccini, B.M., Fanti, P.A., Bardazzi, F. & Di Landro, A. (1995) Idiopathic atrophy of the nails: clinical and pathological study of two cases. *Dermatology* **190**, 116–118.

Trevisan, G. & Tallocchi, G. (1980) Pterygium unguis senza alterazioni acrostiffiche clinicamente rilevabili: 20 casi studiati con capillaroscopia. *Annali Italiani di Dermatological Clinical Speriment* **34**, 361–367.

Wollina, U. (1995) Symptome rheumatischer Erkrankungen am Nagelorgan. *Arthritis and Rheumatism* **15**, 22–24.

Wollina, U. & Knopf, B. (1992) Seltenere Kutane Manifestationen des Lupus erythema-todes. *Dermatologische Monatsschrift* **178**, 456–461.

Zaias, N. (1970) The nail in lichen planus. *Archives of Dermatology* **101**, 264–271.

Zook, E.G. (1990) The perionychium. In: *Operative Hand Surgery* (ed. D.P. Green), pp. 1331–1375. Churchill Livingstone, New York.

## Onychomadesis/nail shedding—retronychia
(Figs 2.36 & 2.37)

Spontaneous separation of the nail from the matrix area is called onychomadesis. At first, a cleavage appears under the proximal portion of the nail, followed by the disappearance of the juxtamatricial portion of the surface of the nail. A sort of surface ulcer is thus formed, which does not usually involve the deeper layers. This is due to a limited lesion of the proximal part of the matrix. In latent onychomadesis (Runne & Orfanos 1981) the nail plate shows a transverse split (Fig. 2.25), because of transient complete inhibition of nail growth for at least 1–2 weeks. It may be characterized by a Beau's line which has reached its maximum dimension; nevertheless the nail continues growing for some time because there is no disruption in its attachment to the nail bed. Growth ceases when it is cast off after losing this connection. In some very severe general acute diseases, such as Lyell's syndrome, the proximal edge of all the nail plates may be elevated.

Retronychia (Fig. 2.37) is the term coined by de Berker and Rendall (1999) for describing an acute onychomadesis involving patients with a 3–6-month history of inflammation in the affected digits. After ineffective conservative treatment, avulsion may reveal three generations of nail joined distally but separate proximally, with the upper and oldest generation embedded into the overlying PNF. Interestingly other nails on the hands may present Beau's line with onset synchronous with the thumb pathology in one case. All cases arose following a precipitating event altering the nail growth; bilateral in the first two and minor trauma in the third. Failure of longitudinal growth combined with a wedge-like effect of new nail beneath, directed the overlying nail upwards into the PNF. This nonrecurrent pathology resolves by loss of the nail and may be due to latent onychomadesis with nail retention favoured by posterolateral ligamentous attraction of the plate.

The terms onychoptosis defluvium, or alopecia unguium, are sometimes used to describe atraumatic nail loss. Onychomadesis usually results from serious generalized diseases, bullous dermatoses, hand, foot and mouth disease (Bernier *et al.* 1998), drug reactions, intensive X-ray therapy, acute paronychia, severe psychological stress, or it may be idiopathic. When the disease is inherited (as a dominant characteristic) the shedding may be periodic, and rarely associated with the dental condition amelogenesis imperfecta. Longitudinal fissures, recurrent onychomadesis and onychogryphosis may be associated with mild degrees of keratosis punctata. In toenails, onychomadesis may be produced by minor traumatic episodes, as in sportsman's toe. Onychomadesis and pyogenic granuloma following cast immobilization have been reported by Tosti *et al.* (2001).

Total nail loss with scarring may be due to permanent damage of the matrix following trauma, or late stages of acquired onychatrophia following lichen planus, bullous diseases or where there is defective peripheral circulation.

In texts on congenital anomalies, this defect is sometimes referred to as aplastic anonychia which does not always produce scarring.

Temporary total nail loss may also result from severe progressive onycholysis.

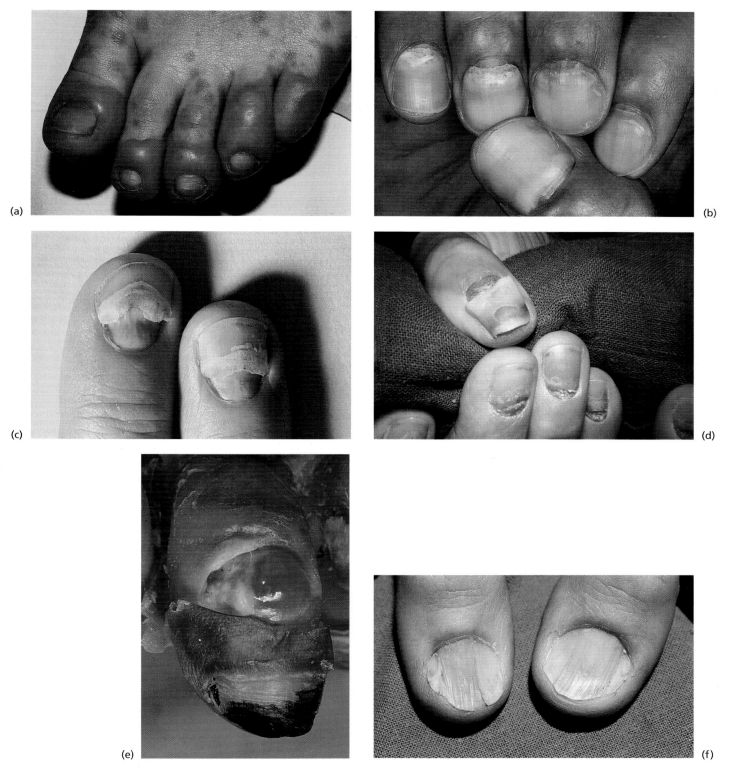

**Fig. 2.36** (a) Lyell syndrome—periungual bullae. (Courtesy of S. Goettmann-Bonvallot, France.) (b) Lyell syndrome—onychomadesis. (Courtesy of S. Goettmann-Bonvallot, France.) (c) Nail shedding—onychomadesis type. (Courtesy of A. Krebs, Switzerland.) (d) Lyell syndrome—onychomadesis with early nail shedding. (Courtesy of S. Goettmann-Bonvallot, France.) (e) Lyell syndrome—nail deglovement. (Courtesy of S. Goettmann-Bonvallot, France.) (f) Lyell syndrome—late stage.

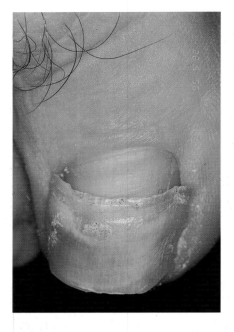

**Fig. 2.37** Onychomadesis—'retronychia' type.

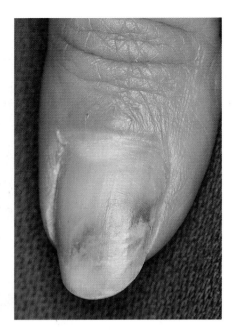

**Fig. 2.38** (a) Onycholysis —*Candida* associated with *Pseudomonas*.

## References

de Berker, D.A.R. & Rendall, J.R.S. (1999) Retronychia—proximal ingrowing nail. *Journal of the European Academy of Dermatology and Venereology* **12** (Suppl. 2), S126.

Bernier, V., Labrèze, C. & Taieb, A. (1998) Onychomadesis and hand, foot and mouth disease. *Annales de Dermatologie et de Vénéréologie* **125** (Suppl. 1), S178.

Runne, U. & Orfanos, C.E. (1981) The human nail. *Current Problems in Dermatology* **9**, 102.

Tosti, A., Piraccini, B.M. & Camacho-Martinez, F. (2001) Onychomadesis and pyogenic granuloma following cast immobilization. *Archives of Dermatology* **137**, 231–232.

## Onycholysis

Onycholysis refers to the detachment of the nail from its bed at its distal end and/or its lateral attachments (Fig. 2.38). The pattern of separation of the plate from the nail bed takes many forms. Sometimes it closely resembles the damage from a splinter under the nail, the detachment extending proximally along a convex line, giving the appearance of a half-moon. When the process reaches the matrix, onycholysis becomes complete. Involvement of the lateral edge of the nail plate alone is less common. In certain cases, the free edge rises up like a hood, or coils up on itself like a roll of paper (Fig. 2.39). Onycholysis creates a subungual space that gathers dirt and keratin debris. Water accumulates in the 'cave' beneath the nail plate and secondary infection by bacteria and yeasts ocurrs. As opposed to chronic paronychia, inflammation is rarely seen (Fleckman 1999). The greyish-white colour is due to the presence of air under the nail but the colour may vary from yellow to brown, depending on the aetiology. This area is sometimes malodorous.

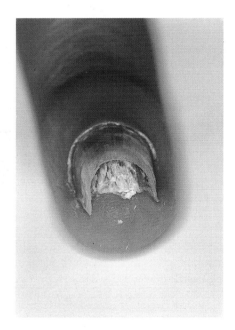

**Fig. 2.39** Onycholysis, with rolling or coiling of the nail plate (psoriasis).

In psoriasis there is usually a yellow margin visible between the pink, normal nail and the white separated area. In the 'oily spot' or 'salmon-patch' variety, the nail plate–nail bed separation may start in the middle of the nail; this is sometimes surrounded by a yellow margins. The accumulation of large amounts of serum-like exudate containing glycoprotein, in and under the affected nails (Zaias 1990), explains the colour change in this kind of onycholysis. Glycoprotein deposition is commonly found in inflammatory and eczematous diseases affecting the nail bed. Oil patches have been reported in systemic lupus erythematosus; they may be extensive in lectitis purulenta and granulomata (Runne *et al.* 1978). Onycholysis is usually symptomless and it is mainly the appearance of the nail which brings the patient to the doctor; occasionally there is slight pain associated with inflammation in the early stages. The extent of onycholysis increases progressively and can be estimated by measuring the distance separating the distal edge of the lunula from the limit of proximal detachment (Taft 1968). Transillumination of the terminal phalanx gives a good view of the area (Chapter 3).

The onset of this condition may be sudden, as in photo-onycholysis (Baran & Juhlin 1987) (Chapter 6), where there may be a triad of 'photosensitization, onycholysis and dyschromia' (Segal 1963), or when the cause is contact with chemical irritants such as hydrofluoric acid (Shewmake & Anderson 1979) or thioglycolate (Baran 1980). Sculptured onycholysis (Zaias 1990) is a self-induced nail abnormality produced by cleaning the underside of the nail plate with a sharp instrument. This results in an opaque, dead portion of the nail with a gently curved proximal 'lytic' border.

Onycholysis of the toes demonstrates some differences from the condition on the fingers. The major distinctions are governed by:
1 The lack of occupational hazards.
2 The reduced use of cosmetics on the feet.
3 The protection afforded by footwear, which reduces the risk of photoonycholysis.

The two main causes of onycholysis of the toenail, especially the great toenail are: (a) onychomycosis; and (b) repeated minor traumas.

Primary candida onycholysis is almost exclusively confined to the fingernails.

Traumatic onycholysis may have a different presentation:
1 The diagnosis is conspicuous when the nail is lifted up by a blister after strenuous exercise in new footwear, not necessarily platform shoes. The blister may have disappeared leaving an oozing nail bed. Sometimes there is only a blackish hue or thorough examination finds a distal worn-down great toenail.
2 Sometimes the diagnosis is not self-evident. A careful search must be made to look for a discrete brownish tinge, the signature of the trauma.
3 In distal and subungual onychomycosis of the toenails, the horny thickening raises their free edge with disruption of the normal nail plate–nail bed attachment; this gives rise to secondary onycholysis in this common presentation.

Baran and Badillet (1982) have questioned whether big toenail onychomycosis is ever truly primary. Its presence should always lead to a search for abnormalities of the foot, such as hyperkeratosis of the metatarsal heads, large thickening of the ball of the foot or pressure on the big toe by an overriding second toe, this being fully developed when shoes are worn. All these disorders are frequently combined with high heels, narrow and slanting shoes.

Treatment consists of a silicone rubber moulded toe cap or a silicone rubber orthodigital splint or a direct moulding splint, the device being produced *in situ*.

In summary, two entities appear clearly distinct, except when onycholysis seems the primary disease and is accompanied by both dermatophytes and plantar anomalies. In such cases, the dermatophytes may act as commensal agents and we suggest that therapy should above all remove the pressure and help to restore proper balance to the foot with fitted shoes and padding or accommodative shields.

The various conditions which can produce onycholysis are listed in Table 2.7.

## References

Angeloni, V.L., Salasche, S.J. & Ortiz, R. (1987) Nail, skin and scleral pigmentation induced by minocycline. *Cutis* 40, 229–233.

Baran, R. (1980) Acute onycholysis from rust-removing agents. *Archives of Dermatology* 116, 382–383.

Baran, R. & Badillet, G. (1982) Primary onycholysis of the big toenails. A review of 113 cases. *British Journal of Dermatology* 106, 526–534.

Baran, R. & Brun, P. (1986) Photoonycholisis induced by the fluoroquinolones pefloxacine and ofloxacine. *Dermatologica* 176, 185–188.

Baran, R. & Bureau, H. (1983) Congenital malalignment of the big toenail as a cause of ingrowing toenail in infancy. *Clinical and Experimental Dermatology* 8, 619–623.

Baran, R. & Juhlin, L. (1987) Drug-induced photo-onycholysis. Three subtypes identified in a study of 15 cases. *Journal of the American Academy of Dermatology* 17, 1012–1016.

Bazex, J., Baran, R., Monbrun, F. *et al.* (1990) Hereditary distal onycholysis. *Clinical and Experimental Dermatology* 15, 146–148.

Boss, J.M., Matthews, C.N.A., Peachey, R.D.G. *et al.* (1981) Speckled hyperpigmentation, palmo-plantar punctate keratoses and childhood blistering: a clinical triad with variable associations. *British Journal of Dermatology* 105, 579.

Brueggmeyer, C.D. & Ramirez, G. (1984) Onycholysis associated with captopril. *Lancet* i, 1352–1353.

Byrne, J.P.H., Boss, J.M. & Dawber, R.P.R. (1976) Contraceptive pill-induced porphyria cutanea tarda presenting with onycholysis of the fingernails. *Postgraduate Medical Journal* 52, 535–538.

Cliff, S. & Mortimer, P.S. (1996) Onycholysis associated with carcinoma of the lung. *Clinical and Experimental Dermatology* 21, 244.

Clouston, H.R. (1929) A hereditary ectodermal dystrophy. *Canadian Medical Association Journal* 21, 10.

Cornelius, C.E. & Shelley, W.B. (1967) Shell–nail syndrome associated with bronchiectasis. *Archives of Dermatology* 96, 694–695.

Fleckman, P. (1999) Current and future nail research. Area ripe for study. *Skin Pharmacology and Applied Skin Physiology* 12, 146–153.

Grech, V. & Vella, C. (1999) Generalized onycholysis associated with sodium valproate therapy. *European Neurology* 42, 64–65.

Guin, J.D. & Wilson, P. (1999) Onycholysis from nail lacquer: a complication of nail enhancement. *American Journal of Contact Dermatitis* 10, 34–36.

Hundeiker, M. (1969) Hereditäre Nageldysplasie der 5.Zehe. *Hautarzt* 20, 282.

Kechijian, P. (1991) Nail polish removers: are they harmful? *Seminars in Dermatology* 10, 26–28.

**Table 2.7** Classification of onycholysis: see appropriate chapters for references. (Modified from Ray 1963.)

1 *Idiopathic*
   1.1 Leukoonycholysis paradentotica (Schuppli 1963)

2 *Systemic* (Chapter 6)
   2.1 Circulatory (lupus erythematosus (Wollina 1995), Raynaud's syndrome, etc.)
   2.2 Yellow nail syndrome
   2.3 Endocrine (hypothyroidism, thyrotoxicosis, etc.)
   2.4 Pregnancy
   2.5 Syphilis (Chapter 4)
   2.6 Iron deficiency anaemia, pellagra
   2.7 Carcinoma of the lung (Cliff & Mortimer 1996)
   2.8 Shell nail syndrome (Cornelius & Shelley 1967)
   2.9 Cytotoxic drugs (bleomycin, docetraxel, doxorubicin, 5-fluorouracil, paclitaxel, mitozantrone)
      Retinoids (valproate) (Grech & Vella 1999) (Chapter 6)
      Drug-induced photoonycholysis: trypaflavine, chlorpromazine, chloramphenicol, icodextrin (Lebrun-Vignes *et al.* 1999)
      Cephaloridine (cefaloridine), cloxacillin (exceptional), clorazepate dipotassium (Torras *et al.* 1989), allopurinol (Shelley & Shelley 1985)
      Tetracylines: especially demethylchlortetracycline and doxycycline but also minocyline (Angeloni *et al.* 1987); fluoroquinolones (Baran & Brun 1986)
      Photochemotherapy with psoralens (sunlight or PUVA)
      Benoxaprofen, thiazide diuretics, flumequine (Revuz & Pouget 1983)
      Oral contraceptives (Byrne *et al.* 1976)
      Indomethacin (indometacin), captopril (Brueggmeyer & Ramirez *et al.* 1984)

3 *Congenital and/or hereditary* (Chapter 9)
   3.1 Partial hereditary onycholysis (Schulze 1966; Bazex *et al.* 1990)
   3.2 Hereditary nail dysplasia of the 5th toe (Hundeiker 1969)
   3.3 Malalignment of the big toenail (Baran & Bureau (1983)
   3.4 Speckled hyperpigmentation, palmoplantar punctate keratoses and childhood blistering (Boss *et al.* 1981)
   3.5 Hereditary ectodermal dysplasia (Clouston 1929)
   3.6 Pachyonychia congenita
   3.7 Hyperpigmentation and hypohidrosis (Sparrow *et al.* 1976)
   3.8 Hypoplastic enamel, onycholysis and hypohidrosis inherited as an autosomal dominant trait (Witkop *et al.* 1975)
   3.9 Periodic shedding, leprechaunism, Darier's disease

4 *Cutaneous diseases*
   4.1 Psoriasis, Reiter's syndrome, vesiculous or bullous disease, lichen planus, alopecia areata, multicentric reticulohistiocysis, histiocytosis-X
   4.2 Atopic dermatitis, contact dermatitis (accidental or occupational)
   4.3 Hyperhidrosis
   4.4 Tumours of the nail bed (Chapter 11)
      Pyogenic granuloma
      Bowen disease, mycosis fungoides (Mikhaël 1984)

5 *Local causes* (Chapters 7, 8 and 10)
   5.1 Traumatic (accidental, occupational, self-inflicted or mixed) (Chapters 7 and 10)
      5.1.1 As when clawing, pinching or stabbing cause trauma to the nails
      5.1.2 Foreign bodies
   5.2 Infectious (Chapter 4)
      5.2.1 Fungal (Chapter 4)
      5.2.2 Bacterial (granulomatous purulent nail bed inflammation (Chapter 10))
      5.2.3 Viral (e.g. warts, herpes simplex)
   5.3 Chemical (accidental or occupational (Chapter 7))
      5.3.1 Prolonged immersion in (hot) water with alkalies and detergents, sodium hypochlorite, etc
      5.3.2 Paint removers, rust-removing agents (Baran 1980)
      5.3.3 Sugar solution
      5.3.4 Gasoline and similar solvents
   5.4 Cosmetics (base coats, formaldehyde, false nails, depilatory products (Baran 1980); nail polish removers (Milstein 1982; Kechijian 1991; Guin & Wilson 1999))
      Nickel derived from metal pellets in nail varnish
   5.5 Physical (Chapter 7)
      Thermal injury (accidental or occupational)
      Microwaves

Lebrun-Vignes, B., Queffeulou, G., Marck, Y. *et al.* (1999) Toxidermies psoriasiformes à l'icodextrine. *Annales de Dermatologie et de Vénéréologie* **126** (2S), 18–19.

Mikhaël, G. (1984) Subungual epidermoid carcinoma. *Journal of the American Academy of Dermatology* **11**, 291–298.

Milstein, H.G. (1982) Onycholysis due to nail polish remover. *The Schoch Letter* **32**, 51.

Ray, L. (1963) Onycholysis. *Archives of Dermatology and Syphilis* **88**, 181.

Revuz, J. & Pouget, F. (1983) Photoonycholyse à l'apurone (flumequine). *Annales de Dermatologie et de Vénéréologie* **110**, 765.

Runne, U., Goerz, E. & Weese, A. (1978) Lectitis purulenta et granulomatosa. *Zeitschrift für Hautkrankheiten* **53**, 625.

Schulze, H.D. (1966) Hereditäre onycholyse partialis mit Skleronychie. *Dermatologische Wochenschrift* **30**, 766–775.

Schuppli, R. (1963) Uber eine mit Paradentose Kombinierte Veränderung der Nägel. *Zeitschrift für Hautkrankheiten* **34**, 114–117.

Segal, B.M. (1963) Photosensitivity, nail discoloration and onycholysis; side-effect of tetracycline therapy. *Archives of Internal Medicine* **112**, 165.

Shelley, W.B. & Shelley, E.D. (1985) Shoreline nails: sign of drug-induced erythroderma. *Cutis* **35**, 220–224.

Shewmake, S.W. & Anderson, B.G. (1979) Hydrofluoric acid burns. *Archives of Dermatology* **115**, 593–596.

Sparrow, G.D., Samman, P.D. & Wells, R.S. (1976) Hyperpigmentation and hypohidrosis. *Clinical and Experimental Dermatology* **1**, 527.

Taft, F.H. (1968) Onycholysis. A clinical review. *Australian Journal of Dermatology* **2**, 345.

Torras, H., Mascaro, J.M. Jr & Mascaro, J.M. (1989) Photoonycholysis caused by clorazepate dipotassium. *Journal of the Academy of Dermatology* **21**, 1304–1305.

Witkop, C.J., Brearly, L.J. & Gentry, W.D. (1975) Hypoplastic enamel, onycholysis and hypohydrosis inherited as an autosomal dominant trait. *Oral Surgery* **39**, 71–86.

Wollina, U. (1995) Symptome rheumatischer Erkrankungen am Nagelorgan. *Arthritis and Rheumatism* **15**, 22–24.

Zaias, N. (1990) *The Nail in Health and Disease*, 2nd edn. Lange & Appleton. Norwalk, CT.

## Subungual hyperkeratosis

Besides congenital nail bed hyperplasia, epithelial hyperplasia of the subungual tissues results from exudative skin diseases and may occur with any chronic inflammatory condition which involves this area (Fig. 2.40). It is especially common in psoriasis, pityriasis rubra pilaris and chronic eczema or it may be due to fungi. Histology reveals PAS-positive, homogeneous rounded- or oval-shaped amorphous masses surrounded by normal squamous cells usually separated from each other by empty spaces. These clumps, which coalesce and enlarge, have been described by Zaias (1990) in psoriasis of the nail. They are also found in some hyperkeratotic processes such as warts involving the subungual area. Subungual keratosis may also be seen in lichen planus, Reiter's disease, Sezary's syndrome, pityriasis rubra pilaris, Darier's disease and in Norwegian scabies (Achten & Wanet-Rouard 1970). The horny excres-

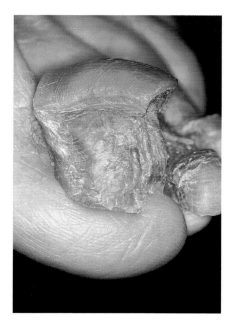

**Fig. 2.40** Huge subungual keratosis lifting up the normal nail plate.

cences of the nail bed are not very marked but the ridged structure may become apparent if the nail plate is cut shortened.

In *keratosis cristarum* (Alkiewicz & Pfister 1976) the keratinizing process is limited to the peripheral area of the nail bed (Fig. 2.41). It starts at its distal portion but may progress somewhat proximally. Acaulis (*Scopulariopsis onychomycosis*), which may present similar alterations, should be ruled out.

*Localized multinucleate distal subungual keratosis* (Baran & Perrin 1995) is a small horny lesion originating from the hyponychium or the distal nail bed. This condition is sometimes associated with erythronychia (*Onychopapilloma of the subungual tissue*) (Chapter 11).

### References

Achten, G. & Wanet-Rouard, J. (1970) Pachyonychia. *British Journal of Dermatology* **83**, 56–62.

Alkiewicz, J. & Pfister, R. (1976) *Atlas der Nagelkrankheiten*. Schattauer-Verlag, Stuttgart.

Baran, R. & Perrin, C. (1995) Localized multinucleate distal subungual keratosis. *British Journal of Dermatology* **133**, 77–82.

Zaias, N. (1990) *The Nail in Health and Disease*, 2nd edn. Lange & Appleton, Norwalk, CT.

## Modification in perionychial tissues

Paronychia, ingrowing nails, tumours of the nail folds (Baran & Tosti 1994) and periungual telangiectasia are each described in the appropriate sections. In chronic paronychia, the attachment of the proximal nail fold to the underlying nail plate by the cuticle is interrupted. Formation of a real space from a potential space results where irritants and water accumulate (Fleckman 1999).

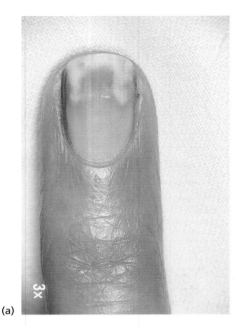

(a)

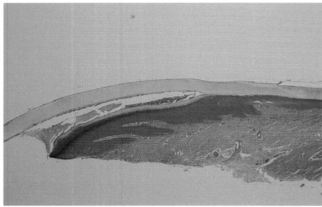

(b)

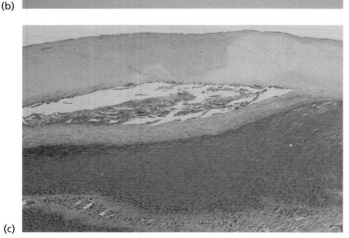

(c)

**Fig. 2.41** (a) Subungual hyperkeratosis of 'keratosis cristarum' type. (b) Histology. (Courtesy of C. Beylot & C. Perrin.) (c) Histology. (Courtesy of C. Beylot & C. Perrin.)

Thickened, hyperkeratotic, irregular ('ragged') cuticles have been reported, especially in dermatomyositis. Pushing them back is painful ('Keining-Zeichen', Kunte & Plewig 1998) but may be seen in normal careless individuals. Thickened cuticle composed of several layers and called 'polyeponychia bolboides' (onion-like) by Happle and Chang (1991) can be an unusual manifestation of factitious disorders.

Perionychial tissues are subject to trauma, such as rubbing of the proximal nail fold of the great toenail against the roof of the shoes. There may be self-inflicted erosions of the nail folds in association with neurosis. The ulnar side of the nail is most vulnerable and there may be small, triangular tags of epidermis ('hang nail') which are painful and vulnerable to secondary infection. Hang nails may also result from occupational injuries.

*Painful dorso-lateral fissures* (Fig. 2.42a) may develop distal to the lateral nail groove where there is a combination of factors such as frequent wetting, dry skin and the winter months (Dawber & Baran 1984). Sometimes these fissures converge to the tip of the finger. They also can be observed in atopic and psoriatic patients (Fig. 2.42b) and as occupational disorders in cement workers.

Chronic granulomatous paronychia is an exceptional presentation resulting in pseudomegadactyly (Mittal & Mittal 1984).

The causes of paronychias are listed in Table 2.8.

## References

Ahmed, I., Cronk, J.S., Crutchfield, C.E. *et al.* (2000) Myeloma-associated systemic amyloidosis presenting as chronic paronychia and palmodigital erythematous swelling and induration of the hands. *Journal of the American Academy of Dermatology* **42**, 339–342.

Altmeyer, H. & Merkel, K.H. (1981) Multiple systematisierte Neurome der Haut und der Schleimhaut. *Hautarzt* **32**, 240–244.

Antonio, D., Romano, F., Icône, A. *et al.* (1999) Onychomycosis caused by *Blastoschizomyces capitatus*. *Journal of Clinical Microbiology* **37**, 2927–2930.

Baran, R. & Tosti, A. (1994) Metastatic bronchogenic carcinoma to the terminal phalanx with review of 116 non-melanoma tumors to the distal digit. *Journal of the American Academy of Dermatology* **31**, 251–263.

Baran, R., Tosti, A. & Piraccini, B.M. (1997) Uncommon clinical patterns of *Fusarium* nail infection: report of three cases. *British Journal of Dermatology* **136**, 424–427.

Barton, L.L. & Anderson, L.E. (1974) Paronychia caused by HB1 organisms. *Pediatrics* **54**, 372.

Bories, A. (1998) Périonyxis révélateur d'un lupus érythémteux systémique. *Nouvelles Dermatologiques* **17**, 184–185.

Caraffini, S., Assalve, D. & Lapomarda, V. (1994) An unusual nosocomial infection. *Annali Italiani di Dermatological Clinical Speriment* **48**, 173–174.

Dawber, R.P.R. & Baran, R. (1984) Painful dorso-lateral fissure of the fingertip—an extension of the lateral nail groove. *Clinical and Experimental Dermatology* **9**, 419–420.

Derrick, E.K., Darley, C.R. & Tanner, B. (1994) Bizarre parosteal osteochondromatous proliferations of the tubular bones of the hands and feet. *Clinical and Experimental Dermatology* **19**, 53–55.

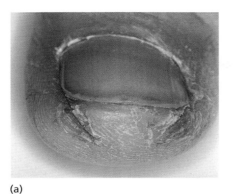

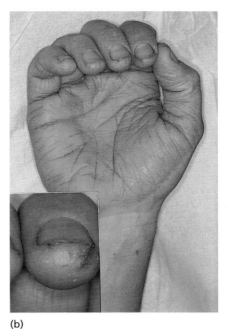

**Fig. 2.42** (a) Painful dorsolateral distal fissures.
(b) Psoriatic type.

Fleckman, P. (1999) Current and future nail research. Areas ripe for study. *Skin Pharmacology: Applied Skin Physiology* **12**, 146–153.

Fleegler, E.J. & Zeinowicz, R.J. (1990) Tumors of the perionychium. *Hand Clinics* **6**, 113–133.

Happle, R. & Chang, A. (1991) Polyeponychia bolboides: an unusual manifestation of factitious disorder. *European Journal of Dermatology* **1**, 35–37.

High, D.A., Luscombe, H.A. & Kauh, Y.C. (1985) Leukemia cutis masquerading as chronic paronychia. *International Journal of Dermatology* **24**, 595–597.

Kamalan, A., Ajithadass, K., Sentamilselvi, G. *et al.* (1992) Paronychia and black discoloration of a thumbnail caused by *Curvularia lunata*. *Mycopathology* **118**, 83–84.

Kowal-Vern, A. & Eng, A. (1993) Unusual erythema of the proximal nail fold and onychodermal band. *Cutis* **52**, 43–44.

Kunte, C. & Plewig, G. (1998) Das 'Keining-Zeich' bei Dermatomyositis. *Hautarzt* **49**, 596–597.

Mittal, R.L. & Mittal, R. (1984) Pseudomegadactyly. *Dermatologica* **169**, 86–87.

Narayani, K., Gopinathan, T. & Ipe, P.T. (1981) Pitted keratolysis. *Indian Journal of Dermatology, Venereology and Leprosy* **47**, 151–154.

Pinon, G. & Villez, J.P. (1988) Panaris à *Actinobacillus actinomycetemcomitans*. *Presse Medicale* **17**, 2138.

Raja, K.M., Khan, A.A., Hameed, A. *et al.* (1998) Unusual clinical variants of cutaneous leishmaniasis in Pakistan. *British Journal of Dermatology* **139**, 111–113.

Sagerman, S.D., Heights, A. & Lourie, G.M. (1995) *Eikenella* osteomyelititis in a chronic nail biter: a case report. *Journal of Hand Surgery (St Louis)* **20**, 71–72.

Sander, A. & Frank, B. (1997) Paronychia caused by *Bartonella henselae*. *Lancet* **350**, 1078.

Tanuma, H. (1999) Current topics in diagnosis and treatment of *Tinea unguium* in Japan. *Journal of Dermatology* **26**, 87–97.

Tosti, A. & Piraccini, B.M. (1998) Proximal subungual onychomycosis due to *Aspergillus niger*. Report of two cases. *British Journal of Dermatology* **139**, 152–169.

Tosti, A., Piraccini, B.M., Strinchi, C. *et al.* (1996) Onychomycosis due to *Scopulariopsis brevicaulis*: clinical features and response to systemic antifungals. *British Journal of Dermatology* **135**, 799–802.

## Modification in the consistency of the nail

The nail plate is a unique combination of strength and flexibility. It may be hard, soft, brittle or friable. The following definitions should be remembered (Schoon 1996).

1 Strength is the ability of the nail plate to withstand breakage.

2 Hardness measures how easily the plate is scratched or dented.

3 Flexibility determines how much the plate will bend. It is due to moisture content.

4 Brittleness shows how likely the nail is to break.

5 Toughness is a combination of strength and flexibility.

*Hard nails* are seen in pachyonychia congenita. They must be soaked for prolonged periods before they can be trimmed; large, 'professional', nail clippers are most suitable for this purpose. Jadassohn, who first described this syndrome, had to use a hammer and chisel on the hardened nails of his patient. For very soft nails the term hapalonychia is used. Such nails may be thinner than usual (less than 0.5 mm) and bend easily and break or split at the free edge. In some cases the nails, which assume a semitransparent, bluish-white hue, are referred to as 'egg-shell nails'. Hapalonychia has been noted in chronic arthritis, leprosy, myxoedema, acroasphyxia, peripheral neuritis, hemiplegia, cachexia and other states. Occupational contact with chemicals is probably the most common cause. *Soft*

**Table 2.8** Causes of paronychias.

*Bacterial*
Classical
  Erysipeloid
  Leprosy
  Milker's nodules
  *Mycobacterium marinum* infection
  Orf
  Prosector's TB verrucosa cutis
  Pseudomonas
  Staphylocci
  Streptococci
  Syphilis
  Tularaemia
Unusual
  *Actinobacillus actinomycetemcomitans* (Pinon & Villez 1988)
  *Bartonella henselae* (Sander & Frank 1997)
  *Corynebacterium* spp. (in 10% of the patients affected by pitted keratolysis)
    (Narayani *et al.* 1981)
  *Eikenella corrodens* (Barton & Anderson 1974; Sagerman *et al.* 1995)
  *Klebsiella pneumoniae* (Caraffini *et al.* 1994)
  *Serratia marcescens* (Caraffini *et al.* 1994)
  *Torulopsis maris*

*Fungal*
*Aspergillus niger* (Tosti & Piraccini 1998)
*Blastoschizomyces capitatus* (Antonio *et al.* 1999)
*Candida* spp.
*Fusarium* spp. (Baran *et al.* 1997)
*Microsporum gypseum* (Tanuma 1999)
*Scopulariopsis brevicaulis* (Tosti *et al.* 1996)
*Scytalidium* spp.
*Trichosporum beigelli* (Tanuma 1999)
*Curvularia lunata* (Kamalan *et al.* 1992)

*Parasitic*
Tungiasis
Leishmaniasis (Raja *et al.* 1998)

*Viral*
Herpetic whitlow

*Occupational*
See Table 7.4

*Dermatological disease*
Artificial nails (Chapter 9)
Atopic dermatitis
Contact dermatitis (Chapter 8)
Darier's disease
Dyskeratosis congenita
Erythema multiform
Finger sucking (children)
Frostbite
Granulomas
Hidrotic ectodermal dysplasia
Ingrowing toenails
Leukemia cutis (High *et al.* 1985)
Lichen planus
Pachyonychia congenita
Parakeratosis pustulosa
Pemphigoid, pemphigus
Pernio
Psoriasis
Radiodermatitis (chronic)

Reiter's disease
Repeated microtrauma
Rubinstein–Taybi syndrome
Stevens–Johnson Syndrome
Toxic epidermal necrolysis

*Systemic disease*
Acrodermatitis enteropathica
Acrodermatosis paraneoplastica
Chronic mucocutaneous candidiasis
Cushing's syndrome
Diabetes mellitus
Digital ischaemia
Epidermic encephalitis
Glioma
Glucagonoma syndrome
Graft-versus-host disease
Hypoparathyroidism
Immunosuppression
Job syndrome
Langerhans histiocytosis
Multiple mucosa neuroma syndrome
Myeloma-associated systemic amyloidosis (Ahmed *et al.* 2000)
Neurofibroma (Fleegler & Zeinowicz 1990)
Neuropathies (sensory or autonomic)
Primary systemic amyloidosis
Raynaud's syndrome
Sarcoidosis
Schwannoma
Systematized multiple fibrilar neuroma (Altmeyer & Merkel 1981)
Systemic lupus erythematosus (Bories 1998)
Systemic sclerosis
Tricho-oculo-vertebral syndrome
Thromboangiitis obliterans
Wiscot–Aldrich syndrome
Yellow nail syndrome
Zinc deficiency

*Drugs* (Chapter 6)
Acitretin
Docetaxel
Cephalexin
5-Fluorouracil
Cyclophosphamide/vincristine (Kowal-Vern & Eng 1993)
Etretinate
Cyclosporin
Indinavir
Isotretinoin
Lamivudine
Methotrexate
Sulphonamides
Zidovudine

*Tumours* (*primary or secondary of the nail unit*)
Bizarre parosteal osteochondromatous proliferation of the tubular bones
  (Derrick *et al.* 1994)
Bowen's disease
Enchondroma
Keratoacanthoma
Malignant melanoma
Myxoid pseudocyst
Neurofibroma
Osteoid osteoma

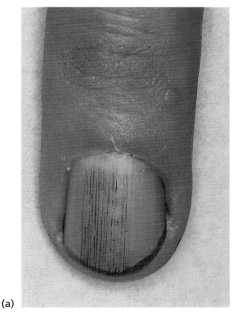

(a)

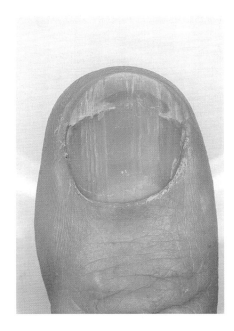

**Fig. 2.44** Transverse splitting of the lateral edges.

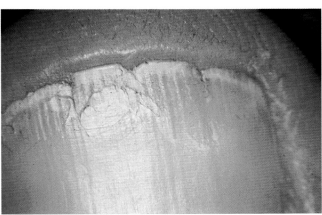

(b)

**Fig. 2.43** (a) Onychorrhexis—shallow parallel furrow in the superficial nail plate. (b) Multiple crenellated 'castle battlement' appearance.

*nail disease* (Prandi & Caccialanza 1977) is an unusual, congenital, nail dystrophy with anatomical and functional defects of the nail matrix.

*The nail fragility syndrome*, also called 'brittle nail syndrome' (Rich 1999), encompasses six main types (Baran 1978):
1 Onychorrhexis is made of shallow parallel furrows running in the superficial layer of the nail (Fig. 2.43a). It may result in an isolated split at the free edge, which sometimes extends proximally.
2 A single longitudinal split of the entire nail plate is sometimes observed. It may be produced by focal matrix lichen planus.
3 Multiple crenellated splitting, which resembles the battlements of a castle. Triangular pieces may easily be torn from the free margin (Fig. 2.43b).
4 Lamellar splitting of the free edge of the nail into fine layers (Fig. 2.31). It may occur in isolation or associated with the other types. Proximal lamellar splitting may occasionally be observed in lichen planus and during etretinate or acitretin therapy.
5 Transverse splitting and breaking of the lateral edge, usually close to the distal margin (Fig. 2.44).
6 The changes in brittle *friable* nails are often confined to the surface of the nail plate; this occurs in superficial white onychomycosis and may be seen after the application of nail polish or base coat which causes 'granulations' in the nail keratin (Fig. 2.45a) (Chapter 8). In advanced psoriasis (Fig. 2.45b) and fungal infection the friability may extend throughout the entire nail.

Changes in nail consistency may be due to impairment of one or more of the factors on which the health of the nail depends and include such elements as variations in the water content or the keratin constituent. Changes in the intercellular structures, cell membranes and intracellular changes in the arrangement of keratin fibrils have been revealed by electron microscopy (Forslind 1970). Normal nails contain approximately 15% water (Samman 1977). After prolonged immersion in water this percentage is increased and the nail becomes soft; this makes toenail trimming much easier. A low lipid content may decrease the nail's ability to retain water. If the water content is considerably reduced, the nail becomes brittle. Splitting, which results from this brittle quality, is probably partly due to repeated uptake and drying out of water.

The keratin content may be modified by chemical and physical insults, especially in occupational nail disorders (Chapter 7). Amino acid chains may be broken or distorted by alkalis, oxidizing agents and thioglycolates, such as chemicals employed in the permanent waving processes. These break or distort the multiple —S=S— bond linkages which join the

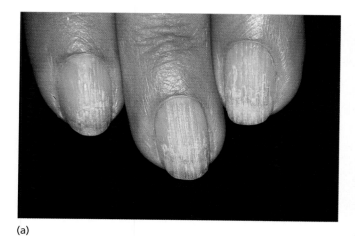

(a)

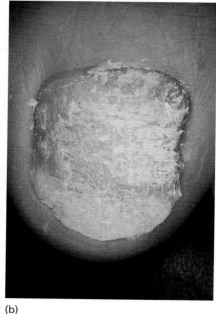

(b)

**Fig. 2.45** (a) Friability of the nail surface, here caused by nail cosmetic 'base coat'. (b) Superficial friability in psoriatic patient.

protein chains to form the keratin fibrils. Keratin structure can also be changed in genetic disorders (Price *et al.* 1980). In some congenital conditions, such as dyskeratosis congenita, the nail plate is completely absent, or reduced to thin, dystrophic remnants.

The composition of the nail plate is sometimes related to generalized disease. High sulphur contents predominate in the form of cystine, which contributes to the stability of the fibrous protein by the formation of disulphide bonds. A lack of iron can result in softening of the nail and koilonychia; conversely, the calcium content in the nail would appear to contribute little towards its hardness. Calcium is mainly in the surface of the nail, in small absorbed quantities, and X-ray diffraction shows no evidence of calcite or apatite crystals. Damage to both the central and peripheral nervous system may result in nail fragility.

## Causes of nail fragility

These may be local or, less frequently, systemic.

### Local causes

They may be due either to nail plate impairment or to matrix impairment.

The nail may be damaged by trauma or by chemical agents such as detergents, alkalis various solvents and sugar solutions and, especially, by hot water.

The nail plate requires 5–6 months in order to regenerate and therefore it is vulnerable to daily insults. Anyone carrying out a lot of household tasks is very susceptible; particularly at risk are the first three fingers of the dominant hand. Anything that slows the rate of nail growth will increase the risk. Cosmetic causes are rare. Some varnishes will damage the superficial layers of the nail. Drying may be enhanced by some nail varnish removers (Kechijian 1991), and soaking fingers in a warm soapy solution to remove the cuticle is especially dangerous—this is common practice among manicurists. It has been shown that climatic and seasonal factors may affect the hydration of the nail plate.

Fragility, due to thinning of the nail plate, may be caused by a reduction in the length of the matrix. Diminution, or even complete arrest of nail formation over a variable width, may be the result of many dermatoses such as eczema, lichen planus, psoriasis (rare) and impairment of the peripheral circulation. The frequency of nail fragility in alopecia areata lends credence to the popular belief that nail and hair disorders are often associated.

Lubach and Beckers (1992) have shown that in women the bridges between nail corneocytes are possibly weaker than in males as a constitutional characteristic. Accordingly, frequent, alternating periods of hydration and drying increase the incidence of brittle nails, particularly in women.

### General causes

Among these are included hypochromic anaemia, reduction in serum iron, arsenical intoxication, infection, diseases which produce severe generalized effects, arthritic deformities of the distal joints, deficiencies in vitamins A, C and $B_6$, osteoporosis and osteomalacia; also, there are numerous inherited defects associated with atrophy of the nail. The diverse constituents of the nail plate, especially the enzymes necessary for the formation of keratin, are subject to genetic influences and changes in them are manifested in the form of hereditary disease.

## Treatment of brittle nails

Moisture (excess hydration) and trauma must be avoided at all cost; routine household chores are particularly damaging. Protection with rubber gloves worn over light cotton glove liners should be used in order to avoid frequent direct contact with water.

A warm environment and hyperaemia may lead to faster growth. This could bring about a reduction in the time that the nail plate is exposed to repeated minor chemical and physical actions which accentuate nail fragility.

There is no efficient barrier cream able to prevent oversoftening of the nails due to water and detergents. After hydration, the nail plate should be massaged with mineral oil or a lubricating cream to prevent the nail from drying out. Under experimental conditions hydration may be further enhanced by the addition of phospholipids, which have been shown to be effective in increasing and maintaining the increased nail flexibility (Finlay *et al.* 1980). This may result from an occlusive effect of the applications, which may delay the evaporation of water. Base coat, nail polish and hard top coat act in a similar manner and also have a splint-like effect in strengthening the nail.

Some treatments claim to make the nails harder, for example by painting them daily with 5% aluminium chloride in propylene glycol and water. Such products make the nails stiff and brittle, which causes them to be less flexible and have lower strength (Schoon 1996).

Systemic treatment may be helpful. Zaun (1981, 1997) demonstrated that brittle nails tested with a standardized micrometric method, swell significantly less than normal nails: measurement of these 'swelling properties' may be the best documented and most reliable method for the treatment of brittle nails. Qualitative assessment data can also be obtained by scanning electron microscopy. Measurement of the transonychial water loss and assessment of the thickness and density of nails by ultrasound have also been used successfully.

Oral iron (given for 6 months), even in the absence of demonstrable iron deficiency, may be of some value. Campbell and McEwan (1981) suggested the following regimen: evening primrose oil (Efamol G) 2 capsules tid, pyridoxine 25–30 mg per day and ascorbic acid 2–3 g per day.

Gelatin has been abandoned and more recently biotin has been suggested for brittle nails (Colombo *et al.* 1990; Floersheim 1991; Gehring 1996).

## References

Baran, R. (1978) Fragilité des ongles. *Cutis (France)* **2**, 457.

Campbell, A.J. & McEwan, G.C. (1981) Treatment of brittle nails and dry eyes. *British Journal of Dermatology* **105**, 113.

Colombo, V.E., Gerber, F., Bronhofer, M. *et al.* (1990) Treatment of brittle fingernails and onychoschizia with biotin: scanning electron microscopy. *Journal of the American Academy of Dermatology* **23**, 1127–1132.

Finlay, A.Y., Frost, P., Keith, A.D. *et al.* (1980) An assessment of factors influencing flexibility of human fingernails. *British Journal of Dermatology* **103**, 357–365.

Floersheim, G.L. (1991) Behandlung brüchiger Fingernägel mit Biotin. *Zeitschrift für Hautkrankheiten* **64**, 31–48.

Forslind, B. (1970) Biophysical studies of the normal nail. *Acta Dermato-Venereologica* **50**, 161–180.

Gehring, W. (1996) The influence of biotin on nails of reduced quality. *Aktuelle Dermatologie* **22**, 20–24.

Kechijian, P. (1991) Nail polish removers. Are they harmful? *Seminars in Dermatology* **10**, 26–28.

Lubach, D. & Beckers, P. (1992) Wet working conditions increase brittleness of nails, but do not cause it. *Dermatology* **185**, 120–122.

Prandi, G. & Caccialanza, M. (1977) An unusual congenital nail dystrophy (soft nail diseases). *Clinical and Experimental Dermatology* **2**, 265.

Price, V.H., Odom, R.B., Ward, W.H. & Jones, F.T. (1980) Trichothiodystrophy: sulphur-deficient brittle hair as a marker for a neuroectodermal symptom complex. *Archives of Dermatology* **116**, 1375.

Rich, P. (1999) Lab reports. *Nails Magazine* July, 91.

Samman, P. (1977) Nail disorders caused by external influences. *Journal of the Society of Cosmetic Chemistry* **28**, 351–356.

Schoon, D. (1996) *Nail Structure and Product Chemistry*. Milady Publishing, Albany, NY.

Zaun, H. (1981) Der Nagel-Quellfactor als Kriteriun für Wirksamkeit und aussichtsreichen Einsatz von Nageltherapeutika bei brüchigen und splitternden Nägeln. *Arztliche Kosmetique* **11**, 242.

Zaun, H. (1997) Brüchige Nägel objektivierung und Therapie Kontrolle. *Hautarzt* **48**, 455–461.

## Modification in colour: chromonychia or dyschromia

The term chromonychia indicates an abnormality in colour of the substance or the surface of the nail plate and/or subungual tissues.

Generally, abnormalities of colour (Jeanmougin & Civatte 1983) depend on the transparency of the nail, its attachments and the character of the underlying tissues. Pigment may accumulate due to hyperproduction (melanin) or storage (copper, various drugs, exceptionally haemosiderin) or surface deposition. Subungual haematoma leads to the accumulation of blood which cannot be degraded to haemosiderin, because it is located between the nail plate on top and the newly formed deeper nail plate portion from the more distal matrix. A narrow longitudinal haemosiderin band in the nail was described by Alkiewicz and Pfister (1976). A 24-year-old patient with adult prurigo developed a brownish-red stripe in his thumbnail from the matrix slowly reaching the free edge. It grew out after about 5 months. Haemosiderin granules were demonstrated by

Prussian blue staining. Small granules were located intracellularly, large globules intercellularly.

The nails provide a long-sustained, historical record of profound temporary abnormalities of the control of skin pigment which otherwise might pass unnoticed. Colour is also affected by the state of the skin vessels, various intravascular factors such as anaemia, carbon monoxide poisoning, methaemoglobinaemia and sulfhaemoglobinaemia.

Certain important points concerning the examination of abnormal nails are worthy of mention (Daniel 1985). They should be studied with the fingers completely relaxed and not pressed against any surface. Failure to do this may alter the haemodynamics of the nail and change its appearance. The fingertip should then be blanched to see if the pigmented abnormality is grossly altered; this may help to differentiate between discoloration of the nail plate and of the vascular nail bed. If the discoloration is in the vascular bed, it will usually disappear. Further information may be gleaned by transillumination of the nail using a pentorch placed against the pulp. The nail lesions for which transillumination is especially effective include varying degrees of nail plate markings, onycholysis, subungual thickening and leuconychia. In a dark room, a single narrow strong beam of light is used underneath the flexor pad of the fingertip. The blackish lines of nail plate, pits, separations of nail plate and thicknesses are seen and differentiated readily from the diffuse homogeneous reddish glow of the normal nail plate (Goldman 1962). If the discoloration is in the matrix or soft tissue, its exact position can more easily be identified (glomus tumour, for example). To determine if the colour is within the plate, a piece of nail should be cut off and examined while immersed in water. When nail specimens are allowed to dry, their true colour may be obscured by light scattering (Baden 1987). Furthermore, if a topical agent is suspected as the cause, one can remove the discoloration by scraping or cleaning the nail plate with a solvent such as acetone. However, with the leaking out of the nail varnish responsible for nail plate staining, the dyes may penetrate the nail too deeply to be removed. If the substance is impregnated more deeply into the nail or subungually, microscopic studies of potassium hydroxide preparations or biopsy specimens, using special stains such as Fontana–Masson silver stain, may be indicated. Wood's lamp examination is sometimes useful, showing yellow lunulae with fluorescence after tetracycline therapy (Hendricks 1980), or fluorescence of the nails from quinacrine hydrochloride (Kierland *et al.* 1946). Nail composition studies might be helpful in the future.

When there is nail contact with occupationally derived agents, or topical application of therapeutic agents, the discoloration often follows the shape of the proximal nail fold (Fig. 2.46a). If the discoloration corresponds to the shape of the lunula, internal causes predominate (Zaias 1990) (Fig. 2.46b).

When examining nails, one must be aware of the occurrence of morphological changes that can be observed in apparently normal healthy individuals (Baden 1987).

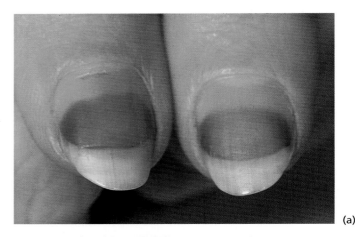

(a)

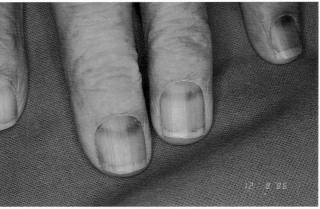

(b)

**Fig. 2.46** (a) Discoloration following the shape of the proximal nail fold—topical application. (b) Discoloration corresponding to the shape of the lunula—internal cause, in this case arsenic. (Courtesy of E. Grosshans, France.)

## Causes of colour modification

The causes are summarized in the following list; the subtypes within these broad groups are described in the chapters indicated or in the tables which accompany the list below.

**1 Exogenous causes** (see Chapters 6 and 7)

(a) Contact with occupationally derived agents (cf. Chapter 7).
(b) Topical application of therapeutic agents (Table 2.9).
(c) Tobacco, cosmetics and miscellaneous (Table 2.10).
(d) Traumatic causes (Table 2.11) (cf. Chapter 10).
(e) Physical agents (Table 2.12).

## References

Alkiewicz, J. & Pfister, R. (1976) *Atlas der Nagelkranheiten. Pathohistologie, Klinik und Differentialdiagnose*, pp. 28–29. Schattauer, Stuttgart.
Baden, H.P. (1987) *Diseases of the Hair and Nails*, p. 21. Year Book Medical Publishers, Chicago.

**Table 2.9** Causes of nail colour modification: topical application of therapeutic agents.

| Aetiology | Colour | Location | Remarks |
|---|---|---|---|
| Ammoniated mercury | Brown | Nail | |
| Amorolfine | Bluish | Nail | Rigopoulos *et al.* (1996) |
| Amphotericin B | Yellow | Nail | |
| Anthralin | Orange | Nail | |
| Arning's tincture | Orange | Nail | Cignoline |
| Chrysarobin | Orange | Nail | |
| Chlorophyll derivatives | Green | Nail | Daniel & Osment (1982) |
| Cupric sulphate | Blue | Nail | |
| Dinitrochlorobenzene | Yellow | Nail | |
| Eosin | Red | Nail | |
| Fluorescein | Yellow | Nail | |
| 5-Fluorouracil | Brown | Nail | |
| Formaldehyde | Grey | Nail | |
| Fuchsin | Purple | Nail | |
| Gentian violet | Purple | Nail | |
| Glutaraldehyde | Golden brown | Nail | |
| Hydroquinone | Grey | Nail | With light exposure |
| Iodine | Brown | Nail | |
| Iodochlorhydroxyquinolone | Orange-brown | Nail | Vioform |
| Mercurochrome | Red | Nail | |
| Mercury bichloride | Grey-blue | Nail | After sun exposure |
| Methylene blue | Blue | Nail | |
| Methyl green | Green | Nail | |
| Nitric acid and derivatives | Yellow | Nail | |
| Picric acid | Yellow | Nail | |
| Potassium permanganate | Chestnut brown | Nail | Stain may be removed from nails with 3% hydrogen peroxide, sodium propionate |
| Prophyllin | Green | Nail | |
| Pyrogallol | Brown | Nail | |
| Resorcin | Brown | Nail | |
| Rivanol | Brown | Nail | Ethacridine lactate |
| Silver nitrate | Black | Nail | |
| Sodium hypochlorite | Leukonychia | Nail | Onycholysis |
| Sublimate | Brown | Nail | |
| Tars | Black-yellow | Nail | |
| Tartrazine | Yellow | Nail | Adhesive plaster pad (Verbov 1985) |
| Tetracycline | Yellow | Nail | Treatment of acne |
| | | Lunula | Treatment of acne (Hendricks 1980) |

Baran, R. (1987) Frictional longitudinal melanonychia: a new entity. *Dermatologica* **174**, 280–284.

Baran, R. (1990) Nail biting and picking as a possible cause of longitudinal melanonychia. A study of 6 cases. *Dermatologica* **181**, 126–128.

Brodkin, R.H. & Bleiberg, J. (1973) Cutaneous microwave injury. A report of two cases. *Acta Dermato-Venereologica* **53**, 50.

Cortese, T.A. (1981) Capitrol shampoo, nail discoloration. *The Schoch Letter* **31**, item 154.

Coulson, I.H. (1993) 'Fade out' photochromonychia. *Clinical and Experimental Dermatology* **18**, 87–88.

Daniel, C.R. (1985) Nail pigmentation abnormalities. *Dermatologic Clinics* **3**, 431–443.

Daniel, C.R. & Osment, L.S. (1982) Nail pigmentation abnormalities. *Cutis* **30**, 348.

Goldman, L. (1962) Transillumination of fingertip as aid in examination of nail changes. *Archives of Dermatology* **85**, 644.

Hendricks, A.A. (1980) Yellow lunulae with fluorescence after tetracycline therapy. *Archives of Dermatology* **116**, 438–440.

Inalsingh, A. (1972) Melanonychia after treatment of malignant disease with radiation and cyclophosphamide. *Archives of Dermatology* **106**, 765.

Jeanmougin, M. & Civatte, J. (1983) Nail dyschromia. *International Journal of Dermatology* **22**, 279–290.

Jeune, R. & Ortonne, J.P. (1979) Chromonychia following thermal injury. *Acta Dermato-Venereologica* **59**, 91–92.

Kierland, R.R., Sheard, C., Mason, H.L. *et al.* (1946) Fluorescence of nails from quinacrine hydrochloride. *Journal of the American Medical Association* **131**, 809–810.

**Table 2.10** Causes of nail colour modification: tobacco, cosmetics and miscellaneous (Chapters 7 and 8).

| Aetiology | Colour | Location | Remarks |
|---|---|---|---|
| *Tobacco* | | | |
| Heavy smokers | Chestnut brown | Nail | Along the lateral nail fold and adjacent pulp of 1st, 2nd and 3rd finger |
| Quitter's nails | Tar stained | Nail | Distal tip (Verghèse 1994) |
| *Hair cosmetics* | | | |
| Chloroxine | Spectrum of colours | Nail | Active ingredient in Capitrol shampoo (Cortese 1981) |
| | | | Highly reactive to metals: |
| | | | + aluminium > bright yellow; |
| | | | + iron > green; |
| | | | + nickel > deep green; |
| | | | + stainless steel > black |
| Hair dyes | Same as dye | Nail | |
| Henna | Chestnut-brown | Nail | |
| Resorcinol | Yellow | Nail | Nail varnish (nitrocellulose) used with resorcinol-containing products (Lovemann & Fliegelman 1955) |
| *Nail cosmetics* | | | |
| False nails and formaldehyde | Bluish, reddish, then yellowish | Nail | Subungual haemorrhage and its resolution |
| Varnish | Spectrum of colours | | |
| | Orange-brown | Nail | D & C reds, especially |
| | Orange-green | Nail | Benzophenone (Schauder 1990) |
| *Bleaching agents* | | | |
| Mercury | Greyish | Nail | Mercury intoxication (Chapter 7) |
| Hydroquinone | Orange-brown | Nail | With light exposures (Mann & Hermann 1983; Coulson 1993) |
| *Miscellaneous* | | | |
| Dynap insecticide | Yellow | Nail | Daniel & Osment (1982) |
| Iron | Orange-brown | Nail | Contact exposure to elemental iron (Olsen & Jatlav 1984; Platschek & Lubach 1989) |

**Table 2.11** Traumatic causes of nail colour modification.

| Aetiology | Colour | Location | Remarks |
|---|---|---|---|
| Haematoma | Black Yellowish | Nail and bed | Depending on site of trauma Resolution of subungual haemorrhage |
| Splinter haemorrhage | Black | Bed | |
| Longitudinal melanonychia (after acute trauma) | Brown | Nail | Exceptional in Caucasians (Zehnder 1970) |
| Frictional melanonychia | Brown | Nail | Baran (1987) |
| Nail biting and picking | Brown | Nail | Baran (1990) |

Lovemann, A.B. & Fliegelman, M.T. (1955) Discoloration of the nails. *Archives of Dermatology* **72**, 153.

Mann, R.J. & Hermann, R.R.M. (1983) Nail staining due to hydroquinone skin-lightening creams. *British Journal of Dermatology* **108**, 363–365.

Olsen, T.G. & Jatlav, P. (1984) Contact exposure to elemental iron causing chromonychia. *Archives of Dermatology* **120**, 102.

Platschek, H. & Lubach, D. (1989) Braune Haar und Nagel verfärbungen. *Hautarzt* **40**, 441–442.

Rigopoulos, D., Katsambas, A., Antoniou, C. *et al.* (1996) Discoloration of the nail plate due to misuse of amorolfine 5% nail lacquer. *Acta Dermato-Venereologica* **76**, 83–84.

Schauder, S. (1990) Unvertraglichkeitsreactionen auf lichtfilter bei 58 patienten. *Zeitung Hautkranktein* **66**, 294–318.

Verbov, J. (1985) Topical tartrazine as an unusual cause of staining. *British Journal of Dermatology* **112**, 729.

Verghèse, A. (1994) Quitter's nail. *New England Journal of Medicine* **7**, 974.

**Table 2.12** Physical agents contributing to nail colour modification.

| Aetiology | Colour | Location | Remarks |
|---|---|---|---|
| Radiotherapy of digits | Brown | Nail | LM (Chapter 6) |
| Electron beam LM | | Nail | R. Baran (personal observation) |
| Radiotherapy for malignant disease elsewhere | Brown | Nail | Wide pigmented band (Inalsingh 1972) |
| Cryotherapy | Transverse | Nail | Transverse furrow |
| Thermal injury | Yellow-brown | Nail | Jeune & Ortonne (1979) |
| Microwaves | Whitish | Bed | Transverse dystrophy ridging (Brodkin & Bleiberg 1973) |

LM, Longitudinal melanonychia.

Zaias, N. (1990) *The Nail in Health and Disease*, 2nd edn. Lange & Appleton, Norwalk, CT.

Zehnder, M.A. (1970) Post traumatic nail [letter]. *New England Journal of Medicine* 282, 345.

**(f) Fungal and bacterial chromonychia** (Table 2.13) (cf. Chapter 5).

White discoloration of the nails is common with most fungal infections. The condition 'superficial white onychomycosis' (SWO) is an infection where the initial invasion occurs from the top surface of the nail plate. The disease normally presents with invasion of the superficial aspect of the nail plate together with a powdery discoloration which is chalky white. Fungal hyphae are present on the top surface of the nail. The main causes of this condition are *Trichophyton mentagrophytes*, *Microsporum persicolor*, *Fusarium*, *Aspergillus* and *Acremonium* spp. It has also been reported by Zaias (1980) that *Candida albicans* may produce this pattern of nail plate invasion in infants. Superficial black onychomycosis has been reported with *Trichophyton rubrum* (Badillet 1988) and *Scytalidium dimidiatum* (Badillet 1988; Meisel & Quadripur 1992).

The colour of the nail in dermatophyte infections may also be yellow or brown, particularly in the case of *T. mentagrophytes* which may result in streaky pigmentation of the great toenails (Soares Ribeiro *et al.* 1998). *Scopulariopsis brevicaulis* causes an infection of the toenails in which the colour is a light cinnamon brown due to the pigmentation of the fungal spores in the nail keratin.

*Acrothecium nigrum* (Young 1934) and *Fusarium oxysporum* (Ritchie & Pinkerton 1959) are said to cause a black-green discoloration of the nail. There are a large number of brown pigmented fungi and some of these cause nail disease, although it is possible that in some reported cases fungi may simply have colonized areas of onycholysis. Causes of fungal melanonychia are shown in Table 2.13.

In fungal melanonychia the nail plate appears black but the pigment is often grouped into a cluster at the distal edge. The pigmentation has irregular density and is irregularly distributed.

**Table 2.13** Fungal causes of melanonychia (some of these fungi may be only possible causative organisms).

*Acrothecium nigrum* (Young 1934)
*Aureobasidium pullulans*
*Alternaria grisea tenis*
*Candida albicans*
*Candida humicola* (Velez & Fernandez-Roldan 1996)
*Candida tropicalis*
*Chaetomium globosum* (Tanuma 1999)
*Chaetomium kunze*
*Chaetomium perpulchrum*
*Cladosporium carrionii*
*Cladosporium sphaerospermum*
*Curvularia lunata*
*Fusarium oxysporum* (Ritchie & Pinkerton 1959)
*Hormodendrum elatum* (Tanuma 1999)
*Phyllostictina sydowi*
*Pyrenochaeta unguis-hominis*
*Scopulariopsis brumptii* (Tanuma 1999)
*Scytalidium dimidiatum* (Natrassia mangifera, Hendersonula toruloidea)
*T. mentagrophytes* var. *mentagrophytes* (Soares Ribeiro *et al.* 1998)
*Trichophyton rubrum* (Badillet *et al.* 1984, 1988; Higashi 1990a; Perrin & Baran *et al.* 1994)
*Trichophyton soudanense*
*Wangiella dermatitidis* (Matsumoto *et al.* 1992)

Fungal melanonychia may have more significance than just the gross pigmentary anomaly. Black or dematiaceous fungi produce melanin which may affect virulence through enhancing resistance to phagocytosis. In addition melanin may also affect the outcome of antifungal chemotherapy. Melanin biosynthesis inhibitors such as tricyclazole may therefore contribute to the efficacy of chemotherapy.

It is likely that the production of melanin conveys an evolutionary advantage on fungi that live in the natural environment; fungi that produce melanin are more resistant to the adverse effects of ultraviolet irradiation, heat or cold than non-pigmented (hyaline) organisms. The pigment also protects against hydrolytic enzymes produced by environmental bacteria. Fungi produce different forms of melanin, although those based on DOPA or pentaketides are the most common. It is also apparent that fungi that do not appear visibly melanized may also contain melanin. The significance of fungal melanonychia is, therefore, that it represents a form of onychomycosis where the organisms are likely to be more resistant to both host or therapeutic mechanisms.

In *Candida* infections of the nail there is often a greenish discoloration at the lateral margin and near the nail fold. This is particularly prominent in paronychia or where there is extensive onycholysis. The pigment is confined to the undersurface of the nail where there is onycholysis and can be removed by scraping the area. In paronychia the pigment may involve the upper surface of the nail plate. In most cases this is due to the presence of *Pseudomonas* species, but it is not clear whether this is a result of organisms within the nail plate or whether diffusible pigment is present. It is often difficult to exclude or prove in these cases whether gram-negative bacteria are present as well (Moore & Marcus 1951).

*Pseudomonas* species can colonize any area of the nail where there is onycholysis as well as the nail fold. The pigmentation that follows this colonization varies both with the species involved and the composition of pigments produced. The colours vary correspondingly from a light green to dark green/black. *Pseudomonas* species produce a number of different diffusible pigments such as pyocyanin (dark green) and fluorescein (yellow-green). These are soluble in water, the former in chloroform as well (Bauer & Cohen 1957). This discoloration may involve the entire nail plate or simply part of it. Green striped nails may result from repeated episodes of bacterial infection with deposition of organisms and pigment during each episode (Shellow & Koplon 1968). Some help in the diagnosis can be obtained by soaking nail fragments in water or chloroform (Baran & Badillet 1978). If these turn green it is likely that *Pseudomonas* has been or is still present and this is the most likely reason for the deposition of pigment in the nail. Black discoloration of the nails due to *Proteus mirabilis* has been reported (Zuehlke & Taylor 1970; Higashi 1990b).

Pigmentation of the nail bed has been reported in pinta by Medina (1963); secondary syphilis may present with chromonychia (Chapter 5).

Nail pigmentation due to fungi and possibly also to bacteria such as *Pseudomonas* spp. and *Proteus* spp. is usually readily identified also in histological nail sections. The nail plate exhibits a diffuse yellowish to brown discoloration that stands out in haematoxylin and eosin (H&E) stain and more clearly in PAS stains.

## References

Badillet, G. (1988) Melanonychies superficielles. *Bulletin de la Societé Française de Mycologie et Médécine* **17**, 335–340.

Badillet, G., Panagiotidou, D. & Sené, S. (1984) Etude rétrospective des *Trichophyton rubrum* à pigment noir diffusible isolés à Paris de 1971 à 1980. *Bulletin de la Societé Française de Mycologie et Médécine* **13**, 117–120.

Baran, R. & Badillet, G. (1978) Les ongles verts ou syndrome chloronychique. *Cutis (France)* **2**, 469–479.

Bauer, M.F. & Cohen, B.A. (1957) The role of *Pseudomonas aeruginosa* in infection about the nails. *Archives of Dermatology* **75**, 394.

Higashi, N. (1990a) Melanonychia due to tinea unguium. *Hifu* **32**, 379–380.

Higashi, N. (1990b) *Proteus mirabilis*. *Hifu* **32**, 245–249.

Matsumoto, T., Matsudea, T., Padhye, A.A. *et al.* (1992) Fungal melanonychia: an ungual phaeohyphomycosis caused by *Wangiella dermatitis*. *Clinical and Experimental Dermatology* **17**, 83–86.

Medina, R. (1963) El Carate en Venezuela. *Dermatologique Venezuela* **3**, 160.

Meisel, C.W. & Quadripur, S.A. (1992) Onychomycosis due to *Hendersonula toruloidea*. *Hautnah Mykologie* **6**, 232–234.

Moore, M. & Marcus, M.D. (1951) Green nails: role of *Candida* and *Pseudomonas aeruginosa*. *Archives of Dermatology* **64**, 499.

Perrin, C.H. & Baran, R. (1994) Longitudinal melanonychia caused by *Trichophyton rubrum*. Histochemical and ultra structural study of two cases. *Journal of the American Academy of Dermatology* **31**, 311–316.

Ritchie, E.B. & Pinkerton, M.E. (1959) *Fusarium oxysporum* infection of the nail. *Archives of Dermatology* **79**, 705.

Shellow, W.V.R. & Koplon, B.S. (1968) Green striped nails: chromonychia due to *Pseudomonas aeruginosa*. *Archives of Dermatology* **97**, 149.

Soares Ribeiro, L.H., Maya, T.C., Piñero Macera, J. *et al.* (1998) Melanoniquia estriada: estudio de tres casos e analise comparativa da bibliografia pesquisada. *Anales Brasiliera de Dermatologia* **73**, 341–344.

Tanuma, H. (1999) Current topics in diagnosis and treatment of tinea unguium in Japan. *Journal of Dermatology* **26**, 87–90.

Velez, A. & Fernandez-Roldan, J.C. (1996) Melanonychia due to *Candida humicola*. *British Journal of Dermatology* **134**, 375–376.

Young, W.J. (1934) Pigmented micotic growth beneath the nail. *Archives of Dermatology* **30**, 186.

Zaias, N. (1980) *The Nail in Health and Disease*, 2nd edn. Lange & Appleton, Norwalk, CT.

Zuehlke, R.L. & Taylor, W.B. (1970) Black nails with *Proteus mirabilis*. *Archives of Dermatology* **102**, 154.

## 2  Effects of systemic drugs and chemicals (cf. Chapter 7)

(a) Psoralens (Table 2.14).
(b) Antimalarials (Table 2.15).

**Table 2.14** Causes of nail colour modification: psoralens (Chapter 6).

| Aetiology | Colour | Location | Remarks |
|---|---|---|---|
| 8-Methoxypsoralen | Brown | Nail and/or bed | Pigmentation may be diffuse or present as longitudinal |
| 5-Methoxypsoralen | Brown | Nail and/or bed | Bands and haemorrhages may be seen in the nail bed with |
| Trimethylpsoralen | Brown | Nail and/or bed | PUVA: photoonycholysis appears with PUVA or sunlight |

**Table 2.15** Causes of nail colour modification: antimalarials (Chapter 6).

| Aetiology | Colour | Location | Remarks |
|---|---|---|---|
| Camoquinine | Blue-grey | Bed | |
| Chloroquine | Purplish-blue | Bed | |
| Quinacrine | Blue-green, slate grey | Bed | Green-yellow or whitish |
| | White, yellow, grey | Nail and/or bed | Fluorescence under wood light |

**Table 2.16** Causes of nail colour modification: antirheumatic drugs (Chapter 6).

| Aetiology | Colour | Location | Remarks |
|---|---|---|---|
| Benoxaprofen | White | Distal bed | Onycholysis and photoonycholysis |
| D-Penicillamine | Yellow | Nail | Yellow nail syndrome |
| Gold salts | Black-brown | Nail | Latent onychomadesis |

(c) Cancer chemotherapeutic agents (cf. Chapter 6).
(d) Antirheumatic drugs (Table 2.16).
(e) Other systemic drugs and chemicals (Table 2.17).

## 3 Some essential dermatological conditions (Table 2.18; cf. Chapters 5 and 9)

## 4 Systemic infections (Table 2.19)

## 5 Non-infectious systemic conditions (cf. Chapter 6)

(a) Alimentary tract disease (Table 2.20).
(b) Cardiac failure and peripheral circulatory impairment (Table 2.21).
(c) Blood dyscrasias (Table 2.22).
(d) Renal disease (Table 2.23).
(e) Hormonal conditions (Table 2.24).
(f) Malignancies (Table 2.25).
(g) Miscellaneous (Table 2.26).

## 6 Causes of longitudinal melanonychia (Table 2.27; cf. Chapters 10 and 11)

## References

Alkiewicz, J. & Pfister, R. (1976) *Atlas der Nagelkrankheiten*, pp. 28–29. FK Schattauer-Verlag, Stuttgart.

Allenby, C.F. & Snell, P.H. (1966) Longitudinal pigmentation of the nails in Addison's disease. *British Medical Journal* 1, 1582–1583.

Aplas, V. (1957) Hyperbilirubinamische melanonychie. *Zeitschrift für Hautkrankheiten* 22, 203–207.

Aratari, E., Regesta, G. & Rebora, A. (1984) Carpal tunnel syndrome appearing with prominent skin symptoms. *Archives of Dermatology* 120, 517–519.

Azon-Masoliver, A., Mallolas, J., Gatell, J. *et al.* (1988) Zidovudine-induced nail pigmentation. *Archives of Dermatology* 124, 1570–1571.

Baran, R. (1979) Longitudinal melanotic streaks as a clue to Laugier–Hunziker syndrome. *Archives of Dermatology* 115, 1448–1449.

Baran, R. (1987) Frictional longitudinal melanonychia: a new entity. *Dermatologica* 174, 280–284.

Baran, R. (1990) Nail biting and picking as a possible cause of longitudinal melanonychia. A study of 6 cases. *Dermatologica* 181, 126–128.

Baran, R. & Barrière, H. (1986) Longitudinal melanonychia with spreading pigmentation in Laugier–Hunziker syndrome: a report of two cases. *British Journal of Dermatology* 115, 707–710.

Baran, R. & Perrin, C. (1999) Linear melanonychia due to subungual keratosis of the nail bed: a report of two cases. *British Journal of Dermatology* 140, 730–733.

Baran, R. & Simon, C. (1988) Longitudinal melanonychia: a symptom of Bowen's disease. *Journal of the American Academy of Dermatology* 18, 1359–1360.

Baran, R., Jancovici, E., Sayag, J. *et al.* (1985) Longitudinal melanonychia in lichen planus. *British Journal of Dermatology* 113, 369–370.

Bondy, P.K. & Harwick, H.J. (1969) Longitudinal banded pigmentation of nails following adrenalectomy for Cushing's syndrome. *New England Journal of Medicine* 281, 1056–1057.

Coskey, R.J., Magnell, T.D. & Bernacki, E.G. Jr (1983) Congenital subungual nevus. *Journal of the American Academy of Dermatology* 9, 747–751.

Daniel, C.R. & Scher, R.K. (1985) Nail changes caused by systemic drugs or ingestants. *Dermatologic Clinics* 3, 491–500.

Daniel, C.R. & Zaias, N. (1988) Pigmentary abnormalities of the nails with emphasis on systemic diseases. *Dermatologic Clinics* 6, 305–313.

Dawn, G., Kenwar, A.J. & Dhar, S. (1995) Nail pigmentation due to roxithromycin. *Dermatology* 191, 342–343.

De Nicola, P., Morsiani, M. & Zavagli, G. (1974) *Nail Diseases in Internal Medicine*, pp. 58–86. Charles Thomas, Springfield.

Feibleman, C.E., Stol, H. & Maize, J.C. (1980) Melanomas of the palm, sole and nailbed: a clinicopathologic study. *Cancer* 46, 2492–2504.

Fisher, B.K. & Warner, L.C. (1987) Cutaneous manifestations of the acquired immunodeficiency syndrome: update 1987. *International Journal of Dermatology* 26, 615–630.

Freyer, J.M. & Werth, V.P. (1992) Pregnancy-associated hyperpigmentation: longitudinal melanonychia. *Journal of the American Academy of Dermatology* 26, 493–494.

Granel, F., Truchetet, F. & Grandidier, M. (1997) Pigmentation diffuse associée à une infection par le virus de l'immunodéficience humain (VIH). *Annales de Dermatologie et de Vénéréologie* 124, 460–462.

Haneke, E. (1991) Laugier–Hunziker–Baran Syndrom. *Hautarzt* 42, 512–515.

Hendricks, A.A. (1980) Yellow lunulae with fluorescence after tetracycline therapy. *Archives of Dermatology* 116, 438–440.

Inalsingh, C.H.A. (1972) Melanonychia after treatment of malignant disease with radiation and cyclophosphamide. *Archives of Dermatology* 106, 765–766.

**Table 2.17** Causes of nail colour modification: other systemic drugs or chemicals (Chapter 6).

| Aetiology | Colour | Location | Remarks |
|---|---|---|---|
| Acetanilide | Cyanosis | Bed | Methaemoglobinaemia |
| Acetyl salicylic acid | Purpura | Bed | Aspirin |
| Acridine derivatives | Whitish | Distal bed | Acriflavine, trypaflavine photoonycholysis–onychoschizia |
| ACTH | Brown | Nail | Longitudinal streaks or diffuse pigmentation |
| Androgen | Half-and-half nail changes | | Bed |
| Aniline and nitrite derivatives of benzinic carbides | Purplish with cyanosis | Nail bed | Methaemoglobinaemia |
| Antimony | T. leuconychia | | Poisoning |
| Arsenic | Brownish | Nail | Sometimes longitudinal bands (arsenicism) |
| | T. leuconychia | Nail | In acute intoxication (Mees' bands) |
| Betacarotene | Yellow-brown | Bed | |
| Brome | Haemorrhage | Bed | Acute poisoning |
| Canthaxantine | Yellow | Bed | |
| Carbon monoxide | Cherry red | Bed | Cochineal pink skin |
| Caustic soda | Yellow | Nail | High doses and prolonged treatment (psychiatric) |
| Chlorpromazine | Brown | Bed | |
| Chromium salts | Yellow ochre | Nail | |
| Clomipramine | Brownish | Nail | LM (Serdaroglus et al. 1995) |
| Dinitrophenol | Yellow | Bed | |
| Fluconazole | Brown | Nail | LM |
| Fluoride (fluorosis) | White patches, T. leuconychia LM | Nail | Brittleness, Beau's line pits 'mottled nails' |
| 5-Fluorouracil | Brown | Nail | When applied directly to periungual area |
| Heparin | T. red band | Bed | Acute poisoning (Alkiewicz & Pfister 1976) |
| Iodine | Haemorrhage | Bed | |
| Ketoconazole | Brown | Nail and bed | LM; splinter haemorrhage |
| Lead | T. leuconychia | Nail | In acute poisoning; in chronic intoxication: onychomadesis, atrophy |
| Lithium carbonate | Rich golden | Distal bed | Great toenail, onychorrhexis, slow growth |
| MSH | Brown | Nail | Longitudinal streaks or diffuse pigmentation |
| Neosynephryne | Purpura | Bed | |
| Para-amino salicylic acid | Cyanosis | Bed | Methaemoglobinaemia |
| PCB (polychlorinated biphenyls) | Brown to grey line | Nail and bed | Poisoning (Yusho), deformity of the nails |
| Phenindione | Orange | Nail | External cause due to trace amounts of the drug |
| Phenolphthalein | Dark grey | Lunula | |
| Phenytoin | Ochre brown | Nail | Fetal hydantoin syndrome |
| Picric acid | Yellow | Bed | Poisoning |
| Pilocarpine | T. leuconychia | Nail | Intoxication |
| Phosphorus | Haemorrhage | Bed | Poisoning |
| Practolol | Blotchy erythema | Bed | |
| Propranolol | Psoriasis-like | Nail and bed Bed | |
| Roxithromycin | Brown | Nail | Dawn et al. (1995) |
| Santonin | Yellow | | |
| Silver | Slate blue | Lunula and bed | Fingernails (due to UVA) |
| Sulfhydrilic acid | Cyanosis | Bed | Poisoning |
| Sulphonamide | T. leuconychia | Nail | |
| Sulphone | Cyanosis | Bed | Methaemoglobinaemia |
| Thallium | Brownish T. leuconychia | Nail | Mees' bands equivalent in acute intoxication |
| Thiazide diuretics | Whitish | Distal bed | Photoonycholysis |
| Tetryl | Yellow | Bed | Nitramine; yellow staining to skin and hair |
| Timolol maleate | Brown | Nail | Eyedrops topically applied |
| TNT (absorption) | Red | Bed purpura | |
| Warfarin sodium | Purplish | Bed | |

LM, Longitudinal melanonychia; T., transverse.

**Table 2.18** Some dermatological conditions affecting nail colour.

| Aetiology | Colour | Location | Remarks |
|---|---|---|---|
| Acanthosis nigricans | Leuconychia, greyish, brownish | Nail | See Chapter 6 |
| Alopecia areata | Leuconychia yellow, brown | Nail | See Chapter 5 |
| Angioma | Reddish | Nail | See Chapter 11 |
| Coat's syndrome | Red | Bed | See Chapter 9 |
| Cronkhite–Canada syndrome | Grey or Black | Nail | See Chapter 6 |
| Dyshidrosis | T. leuconychia | Nail | |
| Enchondroma | Bluish | Bed | See Chapter 11 |
| Erythema multiforme | T. leuconychia | Nail | See Chapter 5 |
| Exostosis (subungual) | Brown | Bed | See Chapter 11 |
| Fogo selvagem | Yellowish | Nail | See Chapter 5 |
| Glomus tumour | Bluish | Bed | See Chapter 11 |
| | L. erythronychia | Bed | |
| Keratosis lichenoides chronica | Variable | Nail/Bed | See Chapter 5 |
| Laugier–Hunziker's syndrome | Brown | Nail | LM, see Chapters 10 and 11 |
| Lichen planus | Brownish | Plate/bed | LM, see Chapter 5 |
| Lupus erythematosus discoides | Reddish | Bed | See Chapter 5 |
| Melanocytic hyperplasia | Brown | Nail | LM, see Chapter 11 |
| Melanocytic naevus | Brown | Nail | LM, see Chapter 11 |
| Pityriasis rubra pilaris | Dark | Nail | See Chapter 5 |
| Post-traumatic melanonychia | Brown | Nail | LM, see Chapters 10 and 11 |
| Reiter's syndrome | Psoriasis-like | Nail/bed | See Chapter 5 |

LM, Longitudinal melanonychia; T., transverse.

**Table 2.19** Systemic infections causing modification of nail colour (Chapters 5, 6 and 7)

| Aetiology | Colour | Location | Remarks |
|---|---|---|---|
| Acute infection | T. leuconychia | Nail | |
| Jaundice | Yellow | Bed | Viral or spirochaetal |
| Leprosy | White | Bed | |
| Lymphogranuloma venereum | Red | Lunula | |
| Malaria | Grey, subungual haemorrhage, T. dark brown lines T. leuconychia | Bed | Anaemia |
| Pinta | Black | Bed | Medina (1963) |
| Pneumonia | T. leuconychia | Nail | |
| Rickettsiosis | T. leuconychia | Nail | |
| Subacute bacterial endocarditis | Splinter haemorrhages | Bed | |
| Syphilis | Brown | Bed | |
| Trichinosis | Splinter haemorrhages | Bed | |
| Visceral leishmaniasis | Diffuse grey | ? | |
| Zoster | T. leuconychia | Bed | |

T., transverse.

Jeanmougin, M. & Civatte, J. (1983) Nail dyschromia. *International Journal of Dermatology* **22**, 279–290.

Kar, H.K. (1998) Longitudinal melanonychia with fluconazole therapy. *International Journal of Dermatology* **37**, 719–720.

Kolmsee, I. & Schultka, O. (1972) Keratoma palmare et plantare dissipatum hereditarium, Pachyonychia congenita und Hypotrichosis lanuginosa, Malignes Melanom, Möller-Huntersche Glossitis, Vasculitis allergica superficialis (Bildberichte). *Hautarzt* **23**, 459–460.

Kopf, A.W. & Waldo, E. (1980) Melanonychia striata. *Australasian Journal of Dermatology* **21**, 59–70.

Krutchik, A.N., Taschina, C.K., Buzdar, A.U. *et al.* (1978) Longitudinal nail banding with breast carcinoma unrelated to chemotherapy. *Archives of Internal Medicine* **138**, 1302–1303.

Leyden, J.J., Spott, D.A. & Goldschmidt, H. (1972) Diffuse and banded melanin pigmentation in nails. *Archives of Dermatology* **105**, 548–550.

**Table 2.20** Alimentary tract disease causing nail colour modification (Chapter 6).

| Aetiology | Colour | Location | Remarks |
| --- | --- | --- | --- |
| Cirrhosis | White | Bed | Terry's nails |
| Hyperbilirubinaemia | Brown | Nail | Aplas (1957) |
| Jaundice | Yellow | Bed | |
| Ulcerative colitis | T. leuconychia | Nail | |
| | Haemorrhages | Bed | |

T., Transverse.

**Table 2.21** Causes of nail colour modification: cardiac failure and peripheral circulatory impairment (Chapter 6).

| Aetiology | Colour | Location |
| --- | --- | --- |
| Cardiac insufficiency | Red | Lunula |
| Gangrene | Black | Bed |
| Myocardial infarction | T. leuconychia | Bed |
| Lupus erythematosus (acute) | Red | Bed |
| Venous stasis | Cyanotic | Bed |
| Yellow nail syndrome | Yellow brown | Nail |

T., Transverse.

**Table 2.22** Causes of nail colour modification: blood dyscrasia (Chapter 6).

| Aetiology | Colour | Location | Remarks |
| --- | --- | --- | --- |
| Alkaline metabolic disease | Variable white | ? | De Nicola *et al.* (1974) |
| Anaemia | Pallor | Bed | |
| Carbon monoxide | Cherry red | Bed | |
| Cryoglobulinaemia | Splinter haemorrhage | Bed | |
| Gout | T. leuconychia | Nail | |
| Hyperalbuminaemia | T. leuconychia | Nail | |
| Hypoalbuminaemia | White | Bed | Muehrcke's pair bands |
| Hypocalcaemia | T. leuconychia | Nail | |
| Methaemoglobinaemia | Cyanotic | Bed | See Chapter 7 |
| Polycythaemia | Dark red | Bed | |
| Protein deficiency | T. leuconychia | Nail | |
| Sickle cell anaemia | T. leuconychia | Nail | |

T., Transverse.

**Table 2.23** Causes of nail colour modification: renal disease (Chapter 6).

| Aetiology | Colour | Location |
| --- | --- | --- |
| Kidney transplant | T. leuconychia | Nail |
| Renal failure (acute or chronic) | T. leuconychia | Nail |
| Uraemic onychopathia | | |
| Lindsay's type (Lindsay 1967) | White | Bed |
| | Pink, red or brown | Distal nail area |
| Leyden's type (Leyden *et al.* 1972) | White | Bed |
| | Brown | Distal nail area |

T., Transverse.

Lindsay, P.G. (1967) The half-and-half nail. *Archives of Internal Medicine* **119**, 583–587.

Medina, R. (1963) El carate in Venezuela. *Dermatologique Venezuela* **3**, 160.

Miura, S. & Jimbow, K. (1985) Clinical characteristics of subungual melanoma in Japan: case report and questionnaire survey of 108 cases. *Journal of Dermatology* **12**, 393–402.

Monash, S. (1932) Normal pigmentation in the nails of the Negro. *Archives of Dermatology* **25**, 876–881.

Nogaret, J.M., Andre, J., Parent, D. *et al.* (1986) Melanoma of the extremities, a little known diagnosis and difficult treatment. *Acta Chirurgie Belge* **86**, 238–244.

Pack, G.T. & Oropeza, R. (1967) Subungual melanoma. *Surgery, Gynecology and Obstetrics* **124**, 571–582.

Patterson, R. & Helwig, E.B. (1980) Subungual melanoma: a clinical pathological study. *Cancer* **46**, 2074–2087.

Positano, R.G., Lauro, T.M. & Berkowitz, B.J. (1989) Nail changes secondary to environmental influences. *Clinics in Podiatric Medicine and Surgery* **6**, 417–429.

Retsas, S. & Samman, P.D. (1983) Pigment streaks in the nail plate due to secondary malignant melanoma. *British Journal of Dermatology* **108**, 367–370.

Rudolph, R.E. (1987) Subungual basal cell carcinoma presenting as

| Aetiology | Colour | Location | Remarks |
| --- | --- | --- | --- |
| Adrenal insufficiency | Brown | Nail | LM |
| Cushing's syndrome | Brown | Nail | LM |
| Diabetes mellitus | Yellow | Nail | |
| Menstrual cycle | T. leuconychia | Nail | |
| Parathyroid insufficiency | T. leuconychia | Nail | Fingernail dystrophies |
| | Grey brown | Nail | Toenails |
| Pregnancy (Freyer & Werth 1992) | Brown | Nail | LM |

LM, Longitudinal melanonychia; T., transverse.

**Table 2.24** Causes of nail colour modification: hormonal conditions (Chapter 6).

**Table 2.25** Causes of nail colour modification: malignancies (Chapter 6).

| Aetiology | Colour | Location | Remarks |
|---|---|---|---|
| Acanthosis nigricans | Leuconychia | Nail | |
| Acrokeratosis paraneoplastica | Variable | Nail | |
| Breast carcinoma | Brown | Nail | LM |
| Carcinoid tumours of the bronchus | T. leuconychia | Nail | |
| Hodgkin's disease | T. leuconychia | Nail | |
| Intra-abdominal malignancies | T. leuconychia | Nail | |
| Lympho- or reticulosarcoma | Red | Lunula | De Nicola *et al.* (1974) |
| Malignant melanoma | Brown | Nail/bed | Surrounding soft tissues |
| Melanocytic hyperplasia (atypical) | Brown | Nail | LM |

LM, Longitudinal melanonychia; T., transverse.

**Table 2.26** Causes of nail colour modification: miscellaneous non-infectious systemic conditions (Chapter 6).

| Aetiology | Colour | Location | Remarks |
|---|---|---|---|
| Ageing | Yellow-grey | Nail | See Chapter 3 |
| Cachetic state | T. leuconychia | Nail | |
| Familial amyloidosis with polyneuropathy | Yellow | Nail | |
| Fracture | T. leuconychia | Nail | |
| Malnutrition | Brown | Nail | LM |
| Multiple system atrophy | T. reddish band | Nail bed | |
| Occupational | Variable | Nail/nail bed | See Chapter 7 |
| Pellagra | T. leuconychia | Nail | |
| Peripheral neuropathy | T. leuconychia | Nail | |
| Shock | T. leuconychia | Nail | |
| Surgery | T. leuconychia | Nail | |
| Sympathetic leuconychia | T. leuconychia | Nail | |
| Trauma | T. leuconychia | Nail | |
| Vitamin $B_{12}$ deficiency | Brown | Nail | |
| Zinc deficiency | T. leuconychia | Nail | |

LM, Longitudinal melanonychia; T., transverse.

longitudinal melanonychia. *Journal of the American Academy of Dermatology* **16**, 229–233.

Rupp, M., Khalluf, E. & Toker, C. (1987) Subungual fibrous histiocytoma mimicking melanoma. *Journal of the American Podiatric Medical Association* **77**, 141–142.

Serdaroglus, S., Kosen, V. & Ozboya, T. (1995) Band-like discoloration in nail. *Deri-Hast Frengi-Ars* **29**, 153–154.

Shelley, W.B., Rawnsley, H.M. & Pillsbury, D.M. (1964) Postirradiation melanonychia. *Archives of Dermatology* **90**, 174–176.

Stenier, C., de Beer, P., Creusy, C. *et al.* (1992) Maladie de Laugier isolée de l'ongle. *Nouvelle Dermatologie* **11**, 24–26.

Takahashi, M. & Seiji, M. (1983) Acral melanoma in Japan. *Pigment Cell Research* **6**, 150–166.

Zaias, N. (1990) *The Nail in Health and Disease*, 2nd edn. Appleton & Lange, Norwalk, CT.

Zaun, H. (1987) *Krankhafte Veränderungen des Nagels. Beiträge zur Dermatologie*, Vol. 7, No. 71. Perimed Fachbuch, Erlangen.

Zehnder, M.A. (1970) Post-traumatic nail [letter]. *New England Journal of Medicine* **282**, 345.

## 7 Congenital and inherited disease (cf. Chapter 9)

### Leuconychia (Table 2.28)

White nails are the most common chromatic abnormality of the nail and these can be divided into three main types: true leuconychia where nail plate involvement originates in the matrix; apparent leuconychia with involvement of the subungual tissue; and pseudoleuconychia.

**1** In true leuconychia resulting from a structural modification of the nail fabric itself, the nail appears opaque and white in colour owing to the diffraction of light in the parakeratotic cells; with polarized light, the nail structure appears disrupted due to disorganization of the keratin fibrils. The leuconychia may be complete, total leuconychia (rare), or incomplete, subtotal leuconychia. These forms can be temporary or permanent depending on the aetiology. Partial forms are divided into

**Table 2.27** Causes and similators of longitudinal melanonychia.

**Single band**

*Non-neoplastic*
Carpal tunnel syndrome (Aratari *et al.* 1984)
Foreign body (subungual) (N. Goldfarb, personal communication)
Haematoma (longitudinal) (Pack & Oropeza 1967)
Irradiation (local) (Shelley *et al.* 1964)
Postinflammatory (hyperpigmentation) (personal observation)
Trauma (acute) (Zehnder 1970)
Trauma (chronic) (Baran 1987, 1990)

*Neoplastic*
Melanocytic
 Acquired melanocytic naevus (Kopf & Waldo 1980)
 Congenital melanocytic naevus (Coskey *et al.* 1993)
 Proliferation of normal melanocytes (A.B. Ackerman, personal communication)
 Proliferation of atypical melanocytes (A.B. Ackerman, personal communication)
 Postoperative recurrent/persistent melanocytosis
 Melanoma *in situ* (Kopf & Waldo 1980)
 Metastatic melanoma (Kolmsee & Schultka 1972; Retsas & Samman 1983; Zaun 1987)
 Subungual melanoma (Feibleman *et al.* 1980; Kopf & Waldo 1980; Patterson & Helvig 1980; Takahashi 1983; Miura & Jimbow 1985; Nogaret *et al.* 1986)
Non-melanocytic
 Basal cell carcinoma (Rudolph 1987)
 Bowen's disease (Baran & Simon 1988)
 Mucous cyst (Daniel & Zaias 1988)
 Subungual fibrous histiocytoma (Rupp *et al.* 1987)
 Subungual linear keratotic melanonychia (Baran & Perrin 1999)
 Verruca vulgaris (A.B. Ackerman, personal communication)

**Multiple bands**

*Non-neoplastic*
Dermatologic disorders
 Laugier-Hunziker syndrome (Baran 1979; Baran & Barrière 1986; Haneke 1991; Stenier *et al.* 1992)
 Lichen planus (Baran *et al.* 1985)
 Lichen striatus (Zaias 1990)
Drugs and ingestants (Jeanmougin & Civatte 1983; Daniel & Scher 1985; Azon-Masoliver *et al.* 1988)
 Roxithromycin (Dawn *et al.* 1995)
 Antimalarials, arsenic, bleomycin
 Cytotoxic drugs (Chapter 11):
  diquat, daunorubicin, doxorubicin, fluconzole (Kar 1998), fluoride, 5-fluorouracil, gold therapy, hydroxyurea, ketoconazole (Positano *et al.* 1989), melphalan, mepracine, mercury, methotrexate, minocycline, nitrogen, mustard, nitrosourea, phenothiazine, phenytoin, psoralen, sulphonamide, tetracycline, timolol, zidovudine
Microbial immunodeficiency (Fisher & Warner 1987; Granel *et al.* 1997)
Exogenous/non-microbial
 Irradiation (systemic) (Inalsingh 1972)
Racial variation
 African-American (Monash 1932; Leyden *et al.* 1972)
 Hispanic, Indian and other dark-skinned races
 Japanese
Systemic diseases and states
 Addison's disease (Allenby & Snell 1966)
 Adrenalectomy for Cushing's disease (Bondy & Harwick 1969)
 Haemosiderosis (Alkiewicz & Pfister 1976)
 Pregnancy (Freyer & Werth 1992)

*Neoplastic*
Breast carcinoma (Krutchik *et al.* 1978)

punctate leuconychia, which is common, tranverse leuconychia, relatively common and distal leuconychia, which is very rare.

Higashi (1990) considers that the lunula presents with a white colour because the cells of the transitional zone have a high degree of hydration.

**2** Apparent leuconychia of a translucent nail plate, sometimes called leukopathia (Alkiewicz & Pfister 1976), can be further subdivided into a white appearance of the nail due to:

(i) underlying onycholysis and subungual hyperkeratosis;

(ii) modification of the matrix and/or the nail bed giving rise, for example, to an apparent macrolunula.

**3** The term pseudoleuconychia is used when the matrix is not responsible for the nail plate alteration, for example in onychomycosis, either superficial or subungual (Fig. 2.47).

A different classification of leuconychia according to the location of the defect has also been suggested by Grossman and Scher (1990), who give another meaning to some of the terms. Granulations of nail keratin resulting from nail enamel (Fig. 2.45a) look whitish as does psoriasis. A transverse strip on the left fingernail was noted 1 h following a drop of a 2-ethyl cyanoacrylate glue on it (Ena *et al.* 2000).

### True leuconychia

#### *Total leuconychia* (Fig. 2.48a)

In this rare condition the nail may be milky, chalky, bluish, ivory or porcelain white in colour. The opacity of the whiteness varies. When it is faintly opaque, it may be possible to see transverse streaks of leuconychia in a nail with total leuconychia. Involvement of the longitudinal half of the nail plate has been described in a patient presenting total leuconychia in some other digits.

Accelerated nail growth is associated with total leuconychia.

Kates *et al.* (1986) presented the pedigree of a family with 28 affected members.

#### *Subtotal leuconychia*

In this form, there is a pink arc of about 2–4 mm width distal to the white area. This can be explained by the fact that the nucleated cells in the distal area mature, lose their keratohyalin granules and then produce healthy keratin several weeks after they have been formed. Juhlin (1963) discussed the possibility that there are parakeratotic cells along the whole length of the nail; these decrease in number as they approach the distal end, thus producing the normal pink colour up to the point of separation from the nail bed. There might, however, be enough left for the nail to acquire a whitish tint when it has lost contact with the nail bed. Butterworth (1982) contends that subtotal leuconychia is a phase of total leuconychia based on the occurrence of both in different members of one family and the simultaneous occurrence in one person. In addition, either type may be found separately in some persons at different times.

**Table 2.28** Classification of leuconychia (see appropriate chapters).

*Congenital and/or hereditary*
Isolated or associated with other conditions (Table 9.9)

*Acquired*
Pseudoleuconychia
 Onychomycosis
 Keratin granulation (nail varnish, base-coat)

Apparent leuconychia
 Anaemia
 Cancer chemotherapeutic agents (Chapter 7)
 Cirrhosis
 Fly-tyer's finger (MacAulay 1990)
 Half-and-half nail (renal diseases, androgen, 5-fluorouracil) and distal crescent
  pigmentation
 Kawasaki disease
 Leprosy
 Muehrcke's lines with normal albuminaemia or hypoalbuminaemia
 Ulcerative colitis (Zaun 1980)
 Peptic ulcer disease and cholelithiasis (Ingegno & Yatto 1982)

True leuconychia
 Alkaline metabolic disease
 Acute rejection of renal allograft
 Altitude leuconychia (Botella de Maglia 1998)
 Alopecia areata
 Breast cancer
 Cachectic state
 Carcinoid tumours of the bronchus
 Cardiac insufficiency
 Crow–Fukase syndrome (POEMS) (Shelley & Shelley 1987)
 Cytotoxic and other drugs (emetine, pilocarpine, sulphonamide, cortisone,
  quinacrine, trazodone (Longstreth & Hershman 1985)
 Dysidrosis
 Endemic typhus (Alkiewicz & Pfister 1976)
 Erythema multiforme (Bryer-Ash *et al.* 1981)
 Exfoliative dermatitis
 Fasting periods in orthodox Jews
 Fracture
 Gout

Hodgkin's disease (Ronchese 1951)
Hyperalbuminaemia
Hypocalcaemia (Simpson 1954)
Immunohaemolytic anaemia
Infectious diseases and infectious fevers
Intra-abdominal malignancies
Kawazaki syndrome
Kidney transplant (Linder 1978)
Leuko-onycholysis paradentotica (Schuppli 1963)
Leprosy
Lichen plano-pilaris (Tosti *et al.* 1988)
Malaria
Malnutrition and myoedema (Conn & Smith 1965)
Menstrual cycle
Myocardial infarction (Urbach 1945)
Nitric acid, nitrite solution (Zaun 1991)
Occupational
Parasitic infections (Hepburn *et al.* 1997)
Pellagra (Donald *et al.* 1962)
Peripheral neuropathy
Pneumonia
Poisoning (antimony, arsenic, carbon monoxide, fluoride, lead, thallium)
 (Chapter 6)
Protein deficiency
Psoriasis
Psychotic episodes (acute)
Renal failure (acute or chronic) (Hudson & Dennis 1966)
*Rickettsia*
Salt plant workers (Frenk & Leu 1966)
Shock
Sickle cell anaemia
Surgery
Sympathetic leuconychia (Arnold 1979)
Systemic lupus erythematosus
Trauma
Trichinosis
Vascular impairment
Zinc deficiency
Zoster

Albright and Wheeler (1964) saw also total or partial leuconychia in a single family. In the family reported by Bettoli and Tosti (1986), in contrast, all the patients affected by total leuconychia at birth experienced a gradual improvement of the nail discoloration during the course of life.

### Transverse leuconychia

One or several nails exhibit a band, usually transverse, 1 or 2 mm wide (Thomas 1964) and often occurring at the same site in each nail resulting, for example, from acute arsenic toxicity (Mees' lines), trauma, repeated microtrauma resulting from lack of trimming and impinging on the distal part of the shoe (Baran & Perrin 1995) (Fig. 2.48b) or acute rejection of renal

allograft (Held *et al.* 1989). This condition may be inherited. Malher (1987) reported on a congenital type involving only the entire great toenail and half of the second toe of both feet.

### Punctate leuconychia

In this type, white spots of 1–3 mm in diameter occur singly or in groups; only rarely do they occur on toenails. Their appearance is usually due to repeated minor trauma to the matrix. The evolution of the spots is variable; appearing generally on contact with the cuticle, they grow distally with the nail but about half of them disappear in the course of their migration towards the free edge. This proves that parakeratotic cells are capable of maturing and losing their keratohyalin granules to produce

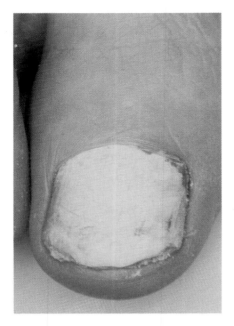

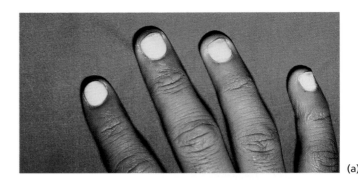

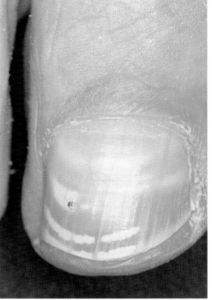

**Fig. 2.47**
Pseudoleuconychia due to
*Scopulariopsis brevicaulis.*

keratin, even though they have been without vascularization for many months. Some white spots enlarge, whilst others appear at a distance from the lunula, suggesting that the nail bed is participating by incorporating groups of nucleated cells into the nail (Mitchell 1953). A similar process could explain the exclusively distal leuconychia which is occasionally seen (Juhlin 1963). A local or general fault in normal keratinization is not the only cause of punctate leuconychia. Infiltration of air, which is known to occur in cutaneous parakeratoses, may also play a part.

**Fig. 2.48** (a) Total
leuconychia. (b)
Transverse leuconychia
due to repeated
microtrauma of the free
edge. (c) Leuconychia
variegata.

### *Leuconychia variegata* (Alkiewicz & Pfister 1976)

This consists of white irregular transverse thread-like streaks (Fig. 2.48c).

### *Longitudinal leuconychia*

Longitudinal leuconychia is a typical example of a localized metaplasia (Alkiewicz & Pfister 1976). It is characterized by a permanent greyish white longitudinal streak, 1 mm broad, below the nail plate (Fig. 2.49). Histologically there is a mound of horny cells causing the white discoloration due to a lack of transparency resulting in alteration in light diffraction.

Early stages of longitudinal splits and ridges of the nail may appear as white streaks. Two stripes in one nail may occur. Occasionally, two or three nails may be affected in the same person (Zaun 1991). Higashi *et al.* (1971) described longitudinal leuconychia resulting from parakeratotic hyperplasia of the nail bed epidermis, with or without abnormal keratinization of the deeper cells of the nail plate, due to naevoid matrix changes.

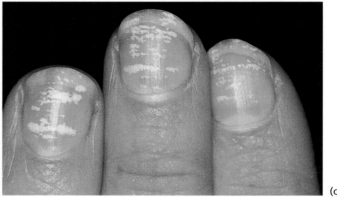

According to Zaias (1990) it represents Darier's disease, which is definitely too restrictive. Moulin *et al.* (1996) have reported epidermal hamartoma presenting as longitudinal pachyleuconychia restricted to fingernails.

When considering the aetiology of true leuconychia it is necessary to make a distinction between disorders of the nail itself and of the nail bed.

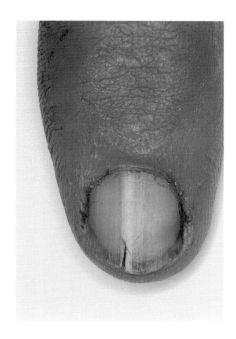

**Fig. 2.49** Isolated longitudinal leuconychia.

Congenital forms are transmitted as autosomal dominant traits. They are usually total or subtotal and are rarely punctate or striate. These congenital forms can be associated with other malformations of the nail, skin or other tissue, for example deafness (Chapter 9). The 20 digits are usually involved, but sometimes only the fingers are affected (Stevens *et al.* 1998).

Acquired forms may be exogenous or endogenous. Overzealous manicuring is the main cause of punctate leuconychia, so common in women. This can also produce transverse white striae. Traumatic transverse leuconychia lines are less homogeneous than endogenous ones in which the borders are usually smoother. In addition there are occupational causes (Chapter 7).

Endogenous leuconychia occurs after physiological phenomena, such as in neonates (Becker 1930), menstruation or severe stress, after acute diseases, such as cardiac disease (myocardial infarction), diseases of the alimentary tract (ulcerative colitis) (Wolf 1925), erythema multiforme and renal diseases, pellagra (Donald *et al.* 1962); it is also associated with shock, fractures, surgery and infectious diseases such as herpes zoster, measles, TB, syphilis and typhoid. It may be found in chronic diseases, such as autoimmune conditions (glomerulonephritis and vitiligo), neoplasia, Hodgkin's disease (Ronchese 1951), intra-abdominal malignancies, breast cancer (Hortobagyi 1983), related to chemotherapy (James & Odom 1983; Shetty 1988), metabolic disorders such as gout, immunohaemolytic anaemia (Marino 1990) and severe hyperalbuminaemia, peripheral neuropathy and also renal insufficiency. Hudson and Dennis (1966) noted that the magnitude of the bands was an indication of the severity of the illness. Transverse leuconychia has been associated with acute rejection of renal allograft (Held *et al.* 1989). Leuconychia has also been described after poisoning

with thallium, arsenic, lead, sulphonamides and pilocarpine. In acute arsenic poisoning, Mees' bands, small transverse white lines occurring at the same site in each nail, are of medicolegal interest; such bands are quite distinctive in traversing the whole nail and the proximal and distal borders are in parallel throughout their width (Krebs 1983). In chronic arsenic poisoning, white diagonal striae are said to be equally characteristic. Acquired transverse leuconychia was also described in members of an expedition who were starved of protein for 1 month, but in whom no abnormality in serum protein was demonstrated.

## Apparent leuconychia

### Terry's nail

Terry (1954) was the first to describe white opacity of the nails in patients with cirrhosis (Fig. 2.50). In the majority of cases the nails are of an opaque white colour, obscuring the lunula. This discoloration, which stops suddenly 1–2 mm from the distal edge of the nail, leaves a pink to brown area 0.5–3.0 mm wide not obscured by venous congestion and corresponding to the onychodermal band. It lies parallel to the distal part of the nail bed and may be irregular. The condition involves all nails uniformly. Revised definition and new correlations on Terry's nails have been advocated by Holzberg and Walker (1984). They found that a distal brown band was four times more frequent than the normal pink band as described by Terry. The proximal nail beds of a quarter of the patients were light pink, rather than white with a ground-glass opacity. The nail abnormality is associated with cirrhosis, and demonstrated in associations with chronic congestive heart failure, adult-onset diabetes mellitus and age. The biochemical abnormalities that were associated with Terry's nails may be related to the underlying disease and not causally related to the nail disorder. The pathological findings from all three patients who underwent biopsy demonstrated an underlying change in vascularity. Telangiectases were found in the dermis of the band.

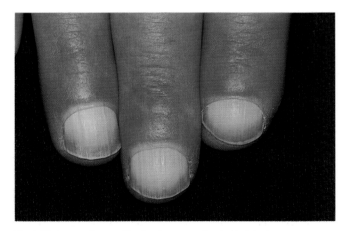

**Fig. 2.50** Apparent leuconychia—Terry's type associated with cirrhosis.

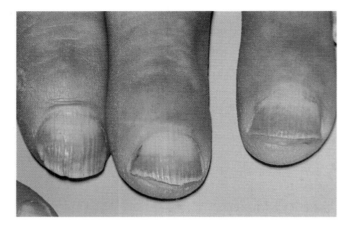

**Fig. 2.51** Uraemic 'half-and-half' nail.

### Morey and Burke's nail (1955)

This is a variation of Terry's nail (Terry 1954). The authors reported four cases in which the whitening of the nail extended to the central segment with a curved frontal edge; one of the cases had identical changes in the toes.

### Uraemic half-and-half nail (Lindsay 1967) (ongle équisegmenté hyperazotémique; Baran & Gioanni 1968)

In this disorder, the nail consists of two parts separated more or less transversely by a well-defined line; the proximal area is dull white, resembling ground glass and obscuring the lunula; the distal area is pink, reddish or brown, and occupies between 20% and 60% of the total length of the nail (average 33%) (Fig. 2.51). In typical cases diagnosis presents no difficulty, but in Terry's nail the pink distal area may occupy up to 50% of the length of the nail, in which case the two types of nail may be confused. Half-and-half nail can display a normal proximal half portion and the colour of the distal part can be due to either an increase in the number of capillaries and thickening of their walls, or melanic granules in the nail bed. Sometimes the distinctly abnormal onychodermal band extends approximately 20–25% from the distal portion of the fingernail as a distal crescent of pigmentation with pigment throughout the brown arc of the nail plate (Daniel *et al.* 1975). Half-and-half nails have occurred after chemotherapy, and in a breast cancer patient after androgen use; this patient had not required chemotherapy for her tumour (Nixon *et al.* 1981).

Nail changes similar to those reported by Terry, Lindsay and Muehrcke have been termed 'Neapolitan nail' (Horan *et al.* 1982); they are probably simply an age-related phenomenon.

### Muehrcke's paired, narrow white bands (Muehrcke 1956) (page 254)

These bands, which are parallel to the lunula, are separated

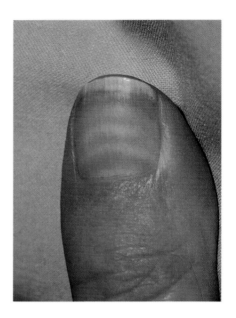

**Fig. 2.52** Apparent leuconychia—Muehrcke's paired narrow white band.

from one another, and from the lunula, by strips of pink nail (Fig. 2.52). They disappear when the serum albumin level returns to normal and reappear if it falls again. It is possible that hypoalbuminaemia produces oedema of the connective tissue in front of the lunula just below the epidermis of the nail bed, changing the compact arrangement of the collagen in this area into a looser texture, resembling the structure of the lunula; hence the whitish colour. The correlation between the presence or disappearance of the white bands, and the amount of serum albumin, seems to confirm this hypothesis. However, white fingernails preceded by multiple transverse white bands have been reported with normal serum albumin levels. Cytotoxic drugs may produce Muehrcke's bands. Unilateral Muehrcke's lines may develop after trauma (Feldman & Gammon 1989).

Apparent leuconychia may be preceded by multiple transverse white bands (Jensen 1981). They disappear when blanching the fingertips. We have observed an identical case with vascular impairment. The white bands transformed gradually into total apparent leuconychia each winter and reappeared each summer.

### Anaemia

Anaemia produces a pallor with apparent leuconychia.

### Dermatological forms of leuconychia

In psoriasis the nail may be affected by true leuconychia, due to involvement of the matrix, and apparent leuconychia, due to onycholysis, and/or to parakeratosis deposits in the nail bed. The parakeratotic cells filling the pits of the dorsum of the nail usually disappear quickly when they come from beneath the proximal nail fold. It happens that these cells adhere to each other, producing superficial white friable quality of the nail plate. One of the earliest signs of leprosy is an apparent macrolunula, which may become total in dystrophic leprosy. Leuconychia may also occur in other acquired dermatoses, such as alopecia areata, dyshidrosis or inherited conditions (Darier's disease, Hailey–Hailey's disease, etc.) (Chapter 10).

## References

Albright, S.D. & Wheeler, C.E. (1964) Leukonychia: total and partial leuconychia in a single family with review of the literature. *Archives of Dermatology* **90**, 392–399.

Alkiewicz, J. & Pfister, R. (1976) *Atlas der Nagelkrankheiten.* Schattauer-Verlag, Stuttgart.

Arnold, H.L. (1979) Sympathetic symmetric punctate leukonychia. *Archives of Dermatology* **115**, 495.

Baran, R. & Gioanni, T. (1968) Half-and-half nail (ongle équisegmenté hyperazotémique). *Bulletin de la Société Française de Dermatologie et de Syphiligraphie* **75**, 399–400.

Baran, R. & Perrin, C. (1995) Transverse leuconychia of toenail due to repeated microtrauma. *British Journal of Dermatology* **133**, 267–269.

Becker, S.W. (1930) Leukonychia striata. *Archives of Dermatology and Syphilis* **21**, 957–960.

Bettoli, V. & Tosti, A. (1986) Leukonychia totalis and partialis: a single family presenting a peculiar course of the disease. *Journal of the American Academy of Dermatology* **15**, 535.

Botella de Maglia, J. (1998) Leuconychia de la altitude. *Revista Clinica Espanola* **198**, 90–91.

Bryer-Ash, M., Kennedy, C. & Ridgway, H. (1981) A case of leuconychia striata with severe erythema multiforme. *Clinical and Experimental Dermatology* **6**, 565.

Butterworth, T. (1982) Leuconykia partialis—a phase of leukonychia totalis. *Cutis* **29**, 363–367.

Conn, R.D. & Smith, R.H. (1965) Malnutrition, myoedema and Muehrcke's lines. *Archives of Internal Medicine* **116**, 875–878.

Daniel, C.R., Bower, J.D. & Daniel, C.R. Jr (1975) The half-and-half fingernail. The most significant onychopathological indicator of chronic renal failure. *Journal of the Mississippi State Medical Association* **16**, 367–370.

Donald, G.F., Hunter, G.A. & Gillman, B.D. (1962) Transverse leuconychia due to pellagra. *Archives of Dermatology* **85** (Suppl.), 530.

Ena, P., Mazzarello, V., Fenu, G. *et al.* (2000) Leukonychia from 2-ethyl-cyanoacrylate glue. *Contact Dermatitis* **42**, 105–106.

Feldman, S.R. & Gammon, W.R. (1989) Unilateral Muehrcke's lines following trauma. *Archives of Dermatology* **125**, 133–134.

Frenk, E. & Leu, F. (1966) Leukonychie durch beruflichen Kontakt mit gesalzenen Därmen. *Hautarzt* **17**, 233–235.

Grossman, M. & Scher, R.K. (1990) Leukonychia: review and classification. *International Journal of Dermatology* **29**, 535–541.

Held, J.L., Chew, S., Grossman, M.E. *et al.* (1989) Transverse striate leukonychia associated with rejection of renal allograft. *Journal of the American Academy of Dermatology* **20**, 513–514.

Hepburn, M.J., English, J.C. & Meffert, J.J. (1997) Mee's lines in patient with multiple parasitic infections. *Cutis* **59**, 321–323.

Higashi, N. (1990) Why does the lunula shows a white colour? *Hifubyo-Shinryou* **12**, 728–729.

Higashi, N., Sugai, T. & Yamamoto, T. (1971) Leukonychia striata longitudinalis. *Archives of Dermatology* **104**, 192–196.

Holzberg, M. & Walker, H.K. (1984) Terry's nails: revised definition and new correlations. *Lancet* **i**, 896–899.

Horan, M.A., Puxty, J.A. & Fox, R.A. (1982) The white nails of old age (Neapolitan nails). *Journal of the American Geriatric Society* **30**, 734–737.

Hortobagyi, G.N. (1983) Leukonychia striata associated with breast cancer. *Journal of Surgical Oncology* **23**, 60–61.

Hudson, J.B. & Dennis, A.J. (1966) Transverse white lines in the fingernails after acute and chronic renal failure. *Archives of Internal Medicine* **117**, 276–279.

Ingegno, A.P. & Yatto, R.P. (1982) Hereditary white nails, duodenal ulcer and gallstones. *New York State Journal of Medicine* **13**, 1797.

James, W.D. & Odom, R.B. (1983) Chemotherapy induced transverse white lines in the fingernails. *Archives of Dermatology* **119**, 334.

Jensen, O. (1981) White fingernails preceded by multiple transverse white bands. *Acta Dermato-Venereologica* **61**, 261–262.

Juhlin, L. (1963) Hereditary leukonychia. *Acta Dermato-Venereologica* **43**, 136.

Kates, S.L., Harris, G.D. & Nagle, D.J. (1986) Leukonychia totalis. *Journal of Hand Surgery* **11B**, 465–466.

Krebs, A. (1983) Veränenderungen der Nägel durch Medikamente. *Aktuelle Dermatologie* **2**, 53–59.

Linder, M. (1978) Striped nails after kidney transplant. *Annals of Internal Medicine* **88**, 809.

Lindsay, P.G. (1967) The half-and-half nail. *Archives of Internal Medicine* **119**, 583.

Longstreth, G.F. & Hershman, J. (1985) Trazodone-induced hepatoxicity and leukonychia. *Journal of the American Academy of Dermatology* **13**, 149.

MacAulay, J.C. (1990) Fly tyer's finger. *Canadian Journal of Dermatology* **2**, 67.

Malher, R.H., Gerstein, W. & Watters, K. (1987) Congenital leukonychia striata. *Cutis* **39**, 453–454.

Marino, M.T. (1990) Mee's lines. *Archives of Dermatology* **126**, 827–828.

Mitchell, J.C. (1953) A clinical study of leukonychia. *British Journal of Dermatology* **65**, 121–130.

Morey, D.A. & Burke, J.O. (1955) Distinctive nail changes in advanced hepatic cirrhosis. *Gastroenterology* **29**, 258–261.

Moulin, G., Baran, R. & Perrin, C.H. (1996) Epidermal hamartoma presenting as longitudinal parchyleukonychia: a new nail genodermatosis. *Journal of the American Academy of Dermatology* **35**, 675–677.

Muehrcke, R.C. (1956) The fingernails in chronic hypoalbuminaemia. *British Medical Journal* **1**, 1327.

Nixon, D.W., Pirrozi, D., York, R.M. *et al.* (1981) Dermatologic changes after systemic cancer therapy. *Cutis* **27**, 181.

Ronchese, F. (1951) Peculiar nail anomalies. *Annales de Dermatologie et de Syphiligraphie* **63**, 565–580.

Schuppli, R. (1963) Uber eine mit Paradentose Kombinierte Veränderung der Nägel. *Zeitschrift für Hautkrankheiten* **34**, 114.

Shelley, W.B. & Shelley, E.D. (1987) The skin changes in the Crow–Fukase syndrome. *Archives of Dermatology* **123**, 85–87.

Shetty, M.R. (1988) White lines in the fingernails induced by combination chemotherapy. *British Medical Journal* **297**, 1635.

Simpson, J.A. (1954) Dermatological changes in hypocalcemia. *British Journal of Dermatology* **66**, 1.

Stevens, K.R., Leis, P.F., Perters, S. *et al.* (1998) Congenital leukonychia. *Journal of the American Academy of Dermatology* **39**, 509–512.

**Table 2.29** Causes of longitudinal erythronychia: a sign observed in different circumstances.

*Acantholytic dyskeratoses*
Acrokeratosis verruciformis (Hopf)
Acantholytic dyskeratotic epidermal naevus
Darier's disease (Zaias & Ackerman 1973)
Warty dyskeratoma (Higashi 1990; Baran & Perrin 1997)
Acantholytic epidermolysis bullosa (Hoffman *et al.* 1995)

*Dermatological condition*
Lichen planus

*Systemic disease*
Amyloidosis

*Local benign tumour*
Glomus tumour
Localized multinucleate distal subungual keratosis (Baran & Perrin 1995)
Onychopapilloma of the nail bed (Baran & Perrin 2000)

*Local malignancy*
Bowen's disease (Baran & Perrin, 2000)
Malignant melanoma (S. Goettmann-Bonvallot, unpublished data)

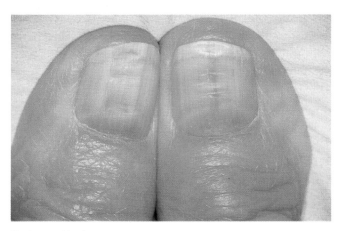

**Fig. 2.53** Red lunulae.

Terry, R.B. (1954) White nails in hepatic cirrhosis. *Lancet* i, 757.
Thomas, H.M. (1964) Transverse bands in fingernails. *Bulletin of the Johns Hopkins Hospital* 115, 238.
Tosti, A., De Padova, M.P. & Fanti, P. (1988) Nail involvement in lichen plano-pilaris. *Cutis* 42, 213–214.
Urbach, E. (1945) White cross strial of the fingernails following cardiac infarction. *Archives of Dermatology and Syphilis* 52, 106–107.
Wolf, M.S. (1925) Leukonychia striata. *Archives of Dermatology and Syphilis* 12, 520–521.
Zaias, N. (1990) *The Nail in Health and Disease*, 2nd edn. Appleton & Lange, Norwalk, CT.
Zaun, H. (1980) Milchglasnägel: Hinweis auf intestinale Erkrankungen. *Aktuelle Dermatologie* 6, 107–108.
Zaun, H. (1991) Leukonychias. *Seminars in Dermatology* 10, 17–20.

## Erythronychia

### Longitudinal erythronychia

A red longitudinal streak may be found in the nail plate in a range of disorders and patterns (Table 2.29).

## References

Baran, R. & Perrin, C.H. (1995) Localized multinucleate distal subungual keratosis. *British Journal of Dermatology* 133, 77–82.
Baran, R. & Perrin, C.H. (1997) Focal subungual warty dyskeratoma. *Dermatology* 195, 278–280.
Baran, R. & Perrin, C.H. (2000) Longitudinal erythronychia with distal subungual keratosis: onychopapilloma of the nail bed. *British Journal of Dermatology* 143, 132–135.
Higashi, N. (1990) Focal acantholytic dyskeratosis. *Hifu* 32, 507–510.

Hoffman, M.D., Fleming, M.G. & Pearson, R.W. (1995) Acantholytic epidermolysis bullosa. *Archives of Dermatology* 131, 586–589.
Zaias, N. & Ackerman, A.B. (1973) The nail in Darier–White disease. *Archives of Dermatology* 107, 193–199.

### Red lunula (Fig. 2.53; Table 2.30)

Red lunulae can be observed in patients with several cutaneous or systemic disorders (Cohen 1992) or they may be idiopathic. The sharply circumscribed erythema of the lunulae can affect all fingernails—and toenails—or only some fingernails especially the thumbs. Dark erythema may diffuse onto the proximal pink nail bed or a narrow white band may be present at the distal lunulae. The erythema of the fingernail lunulae migrated distally in a unique case of severe alopecia areata (Bergner *et al.* 1992). The erythema disappears under pressure to the nail plate. The lunular erythema usually fades slowly even without therapy. The pathogenesis of red lunulae remains undetermined. Biopsy specimens taken from the red lunula of a thumb revealed neither an increased number nor size of capillaries (Wilkerson & Wilkin 1989).

## References

Bergner, T., Donhauser, G. & Ruzicka, T. (1992) Red lunulae in severe alopecia areata. *Acta Dermato-Venereologica* 72, 203–205.
Cohen, P.R. (1992) Red lunulae: case report and literature review. *Journal of the American Academy of Dermatology* 26, 292–294.
Daniel, C.R. III (1985) Nail pigmentation abnormalities. *Dermatologic Clinics* 3, 431–443.
DeNicola, P., Morsiani, M. & Zavagli, G. (1974) *Nail Diseases in Internal Medicine*, p. 56. Charles C. Thomas, Springfield, IL.
Jorizzo, J.L., Gonzalez, E.B. & Daniels, J.C. (1983) Red lunulae in a patient with rheumatoid arthritis. *Journal of the American Academy of Dermatology* 8, 711–718.
Leider, M. (1955) I. Progression of alopecia areata through alopecia totalis to alopecia generalizata. II. Pecular nail changes (obliteration of the lunulae by erythema) while under cortisone therapy. III.

**Table 2.30**  Disorders in patients with red lunulae. (From Cohen (1992) with permission.)

| | |
|---|---|
| *Cardiovascular* (De Nicola *et al.* 1974; Jorrizo *et al.* 1983) | Carbon monoxide poisoning |
| Angina pectoris | Chronic idiopathic lymphoedema |
| Atherosclerotic disease | Corticosteroid therapy |
| Conduction abnormality |   Systemic |
| Congestive heart failure |   Topical |
| Fever-induced heart disease | Hay fever pollen desensitization |
| Hypertension | Malnutrition |
| Myocardial infarction | Senile macular degeneration |
| | Tobacco abuse |
| *Dermatological* (Leider 1955; Runne 1980; Wilkerson & Wilkin 1989) | |
| Alopecia areata | *Neoplastic* (Terry 1954; De Nicola *et al.* 1974) |
| Chronic urticaria | Hodgkin's disease |
| Lichen sclerous et atrophicus | Lymphoid follicular reticulosis |
| Psoriasis vulgaris | Lymphosarcoma |
| Twenty-nail dystrophy | Myeloid leukaemia |
| Vitiligo | Polycythaemia vera |
| | Reticulosarcoma |
| *Endocrine* (Terry 1954; Wilkerson & Wilkin 1989) | |
| Diabetes mellitus | *Neurological* (Wilkerson & Wilkin 1989) |
| Hyperthyroidism | Cerebrovascular accident |
| Not specified | |
| Thyroid disease | *Pulmonary* (Terry 1954; Wilkerson & Wilkin 1989) |
| | Chronic bronchitis |
| *Gastrointestinal* (Wilkerson & Wilkin 1989) | Chronic obstructive pulmonary disease |
| Oesophageal strictures | Emphysema |
| Irritable bowel syndrome | |
| Pyloric channel ulcer | *Renal* (Wilkerson & Wilkin 1989) |
| | Proteinuria |
| *Haematological* (Wilkerson & Wilkin 1989) | |
| Anaemia of chronic disease | *Rheumatological* (Jorizzo *et al.* 1983; Daniel 1985; Wilkerson & Wilkin 1989) |
| Idiopathic transient leucopenia | Baker's cyst |
| | Dermatomyositis |
| *Hepatic* (Terry 1954; Wilkerson & Wilkin 1989) | Lupus erythematosus (Wollina 1998) |
| Cirrhosis |   Drug-induced (procainamide) |
| |   Systemic |
| *Infectious* (De Nicola *et al.* 1974; Wilkerson & Wilkin 1989) | Osteoarthritis |
| Lymphogranuloma venereum | Polymyalgia rheumatica |
| Pneumonia | Rheumatoid arthritis |
| Tuberculosis | |
| | *Trauma* |
| *Miscellaneous* (Terry 1954; Leider 1955; Misch 1981; Daniel 1985) | Repeated microtrauma (habit tic) |
| Alcohol abuse | |

Allergic eczematous contact dermatitis from the binding of a toupee or the adhesive used to hold it in position. *Archives of Dermatology* 71, 648–649.

Misch, K.J. (1981) Red nails associated with alopecia areata. *Clinical and Experimental Dermatology* 6, 561–563.

Runne, V. (1980) Twenty-nail dystrophy mit 'knuckle pads'. *Zeitschrift für Hautkrankheiten* 55, 901–902.

Terry, R. (1954) Red half-moon in cardiac failure. *Lancet* ii, 842–844.

Wilkerson, M.G. & Wilkin, J.K. (1989) Red lunulae revisited: a clinical and histopathologic examination. *Journal of the American Academy of Dermatology* 20, 453–457.

Wollina, U. (1998) Red lunula in systemic lupus eythematosus. *Journal of the American Academy of Dermatology* 38, 1016.

CHAPTER 3

# The nail in childhood and old age

**R. Baran, R.P.R. Dawber & D.A.R. de Berker**

A classification of nail dystrophies according to age is somewhat arbitrary. Some nail diseases have a predilection for certain age groups but the relationships to age are usually not clearly defined.

Certain abnormalities may be lifelong once acquired but their presentation may be modified by the age, and underlying pathology may worsen or improve with advancing years. Habits, occupation and pastimes may have effects on the nail apparatus and are themselves influenced by the age of the patient.

Although in general nail pathology is dealt with in relation to its disease, there are some conditions which are of special significance in the very young or the very old, and these are therefore given separate attention here.

# CHILDHOOD

## Composition and morphology of the nail in childhood

### Nail constituents

Nail plate analysis may be performed using a range of techniques and usually requires only a nail clipping (Chapter 1). The normal levels of universal constituents have been examined, as have markers of disease and analysis of exogenous materials such as lead and narcotics which may provide evidence of environmental pollution.

The chloride and sodium content of nails of normal newborns is highest at birth and decreases to 50% within 3 days (Chapman *et al.* 1985). The iron content of fingernails is variable in the same individual throughout the year (Harrison & Clemena 1972). The iron status of the individual is reflected by the amount of iron present in nail samples (Sobolewski *et al.* 1978). X-ray microanalysis of the fingernails showed a decrease in sulphur and aluminium, and a higher chlorine content in term infants in comparison with preterm ones (Sirota *et al.* 1988). Elevated aluminium content in the nail of preterm infants may be a clue to the osteopenia observed in these infants (Sirota *et al.* 1988). 'Nail plate biopsies' in neonatal anabolic disorders have been advocated by Lockard *et al.* (1972). The fact that ill neonates have a significantly lower nail nitrogen content than adults suggests a pattern of nail protein accumulation which parallels that of muscle and the whole body in the developing fetus and neonate.

Steroid sulphatase and its substrate, cholesterol sulphate, have been assayed in the nails of children being screened for X-linked ichthyosis and found to have adequate sensitivity and accuracy to be useful (Matsumoto *et al.* 1990; Serizawa *et al.* 1990).

The copper content in the hair and nails of patients with hepatolenticular degeneration (Wilson's disease) is higher than normal (Martin 1964).

In cystic fibrosis, the sodium and potassium content of nail clippings has been analysed by Kopito *et al.* (1965); their concentrations in nails and hair were found to be elevated. Neutron activation analysis of sodium in nails (Roomans *et al.* 1978) has proved to be a valuable diagnostic method in children over 1 year of age, showing that there is an increased concentration of sodium and potassium in the sweat of patients with cystic fibrosis; this is compatible with the idea that these ions are of extrinsic origin (Kollberg & Landström 1974). The immediate attraction of nail sodium analysis lies in its potential as a postal screening service (Tarnoky *et al.* 1976); however, the sodium content of nail clippings can be influenced by many factors, including the subject's activities for some time before the nails are cut. A simple, unified set of instructions before obtaining samples from small children may be necessary.

Analysis of nail clippings from the newborn by gas chromatography–mass spectroscopy can provide evidence of exposure to cocaine during embryogenesis. Given the point of nail formation, it is likely that the levels will reflect exposure after the 14th week (Skopp & Pötsch 1997).

## Nail morphology

Hudson *et al.* (1988) measured index finger, nail and thumb dimensions in normal, fullterm infants within the first 3 days of life. In newborn infants the index fingernail length is $5.041 \pm 0.703$ mm and the width is $3.570 \pm 0.354$ mm. The thumb width is $9.800 \pm 0.546$ mm. These measurements are of potential value when describing syndromes in which nail shape and size are characteristically altered. One report suggests that about 75% of congenital syndromes are associated with nail abnormalities (Seaborg & Bordurtha 1989).

In infants and children with cardiopulmonary disease, measurements of the ratio of the distal phalangeal depth to the interphalangeal depth of the index finger have been performed. This measurement has been used to quantitate digital clubbing (Hudson *et al.* 1988).

The length of nails is used as a morphological criterion for the assessment of gestational age in preterm babies (Lamberti *et al.* 1981; Kolle *et al.* 1985). Premature infants may have nails which are shorter than the distal digital pulp, giving the appearance of distal ingrowing (Silverman 1990).

The five most common findings in otherwise normal children are: (a) punctate leuconychia; (b) onychophagia; (c) pitting; (d) koilonychia, especially of the big toe; and (e) lamellar splitting of the free edge.

## References

Chapman, A.L., Fegley, B. & Cho, C.T. (1985) X ray microanalysis of chloride in nails from cystic fibrosis and control patients. *European Journal of Respiratory Diseases* **66**, 218–223.

Harrison, W.W. & Clemena, G.G. (1972) Survey of the analysis of trace elements in human fingernails by spark source mass spectrometry. *Clinica Chimica Acta* **36**, 485–492.

Hudson, V.K., Flannery, D.B., Karp, W.B. *et al.* (1988) Finger and nail measurements in newborn infants. *Dysmorphic Clinical Genetics* **1**, 145–147.

Kollberg, H. & Landström, O. (1974) A methodological study of the diagnosis of cystic fibrosis by instrumental neutron activation analysis of sodium in nail clippings. *Acta Paediatrica Scandinavica* **63**, 405.

Kolle, L.A.A., Leusin, K.J. & Peer, P.G.M. (1985) Assessment of gestational age: a simplified coring system. *Journal of Perinatal Medicine* **13**, 135–138.

Kopito, L., Mahmoodian, A., Townley, R.R.W. *et al.* (1965) Studies in cystic fibrosis, analysis of nail clippings for sodium and potassium. *New England Journal of Medicine* **272**, 504.

Lamberti, G., Korner, G. & Agorastos, T. (1981) The role of skin and its appendages in the assessment of the newborn's maturity. *Journal of Perinatal Medicine* **9** (Suppl.), 147–148.

Lockard, D., Pass, R. & Cassady, G. (1972) Fingernail nitrogen content in neonates. *Pediatrics* **49**, 618.

Martin, G.M. (1984) Copper content of hair and nails of normal individual and of patients with hepatolenticular degeneration. *Nature* **202**, 903.

Matsumoto, T., Sakura, N. & Ueda, K. (1990) Steroid sulphatase activity in nails: screening for X-linked ichthyosis. *Pediatric Dermatology* **7**, 266–269.

Roomans, G.M., Afzelius, B.A., Kollberg, H. *et al.* (1978) Electrolytes in nails analysed by X-ray microanalysis in electron microscopy. *Acta Paediatrica Scandinavica* **67**, 89.

Seaborg, B. & Bordurtha, J. (1989) Nail size in normal infants. Establishing standards for healthy term infants. *Clinical Pediatrics* **28**, 142–145.

Serizawa, S., Nagai, T., Ito, M. & Sato, Y. (1990) Cholesterol sulphate levels in the hair and nails of patients with recessive X-linked ichthyosis. *Clinical and Experimental Dermatology* **15**, 13–15.

Silverman, R.A. (1990) Pediatric disease. In: *Nails: Therapy, Diagnosis, Surgery* (eds R.K. Scher & C.R. Daniel), pp. 82–105. W.B. Saunders, Philadelphia.

Sirota, L., Straussberg, R. & Fishman, P. (1988) X-ray microanalysis of the fingernails in term and preterm infants. *Pediatric Dermatology* 5, 184–186.

Skopp, G. & Pötsch, L. (1997) A case report on drug screening of nail clippings to detect prenatal drug exposure. *Therapeutic Drug Monitoring* 19, 386–389.

Sobolewski, S., Lawrence, A.C.K. & Bagshaw, I. (1978) Human nails and body iron. *Journal of Clinical Pathology* 31, 1068–1072.

Tarnoky, A.L., Bayliss, V.M. & Bowen, H.J.M. (1976) The use of electrolyte measurement in the detection of cystic fibrosis. *Clinica Chimica Acta* 69, 505.

## Nail plate changes

### Koilonychia

Sometimes at birth, the nail curves over the tip of the digit towards the pulp; physiological clubbing may be seen in this age group. In childhood the nail is thin, flexible and transparent. Its surface is smooth, shiny and almost flat and the lunula is seldom visible. Koilonychia is often present as a normal variant affecting the big toe (Fig. 3.1a). There is however an increased prevalence of koilonychia attributed to microtrauma associated with barefoot walking and frequent water immersion (Yinnon & Matalon 1988). Although koilonychia is common in healthy infants, it still has an association with iron deficiency and may be used as a clinical clue which may be noted before other clinical and laboratory signs of anaemia develop (Hogan & Jones 1970). Weak nails may result from selenium deficiency (Vinton *et al.* 1987).

### References

Hogan, G.R. & Jones, B. (1970) The relationship of koilonychia and iron deficiency in infants. *Journal of Pediatrics* 77, 1054–1057.

Vinton, N.E., Dahlstrom, K.A., Strobel, C.T. *et al.* (1987) Selenium deficiency. *Journal of Pediatrics* 111, 711–718.

Yinnon, A.M. & Matalon, A. (1988) Koilonychia of the toenails in children. *International Journal of Dermatology* 27, 685–687.

### Lamellar splitting

Lamellar splitting is a common finding in early infancy (Fig. 3.1b).

### Oblique markings

In early childhood, fingernails often have oblique ridges which converge towards the centre distally (Fig. 3.2). These disappear in early adult life (Pinkus 1976). The appearance has been termed 'Chevron Nail' (Shuster 1996; Zaiac *et al.* 1998) and 'Herring Bone Nail' (Parry *et al.* 1995). It is not clear whether

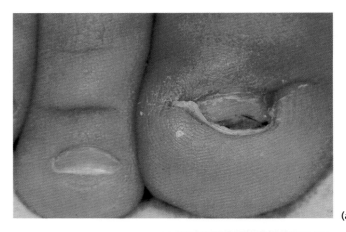

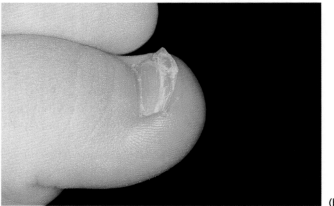

**Fig. 3.1** (a) Koilonychia of the great toenail. (b) Lamellar splitting of the nail.

the distinction is of any real significance, although Shuster proposed that chevron was a preferable term because it does not imply the central spine implicit in the term herring-bone. The semantics is debatable. Whilst of no apparent medical significance, the pattern is difficult to explain in terms of matrix behaviour and pattern formation. The author favours the possibility that there is a limited transverse component to nail plate growth in childhood, in addition to the recognized longitudinal growth. Their combination results in narrow regions of oblique patterning which are not always symmetrical around a central longitudinal axis.

### Transverse depressions

In the studies carried out by Turano (1968), 92% of normal infants between 8 and 9 weeks of age had a single transverse depression (Beau's line) of the fingernails; this first appeared at the proximal portion of the nail as early as 4 weeks of age and grew out to the distal edge by 14 weeks of age. Beau's lines of this type could be the result of malnutrition or other physiological disturbance, occurring during birth. Wolf *et al.* (1982) reported Beau's lines in all 20 nails of a female infant soon after

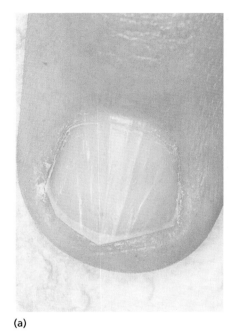

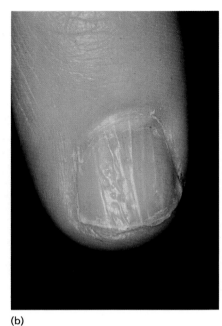

**Fig. 3.2** (a) Herring-bone nail. (b) Temporary, oblique ridges of early childhood converging towards the centre distally, here associated with pits.

(a)

(b)

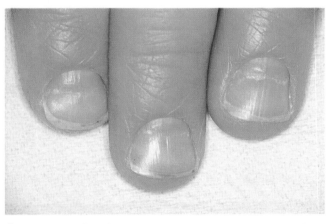

**Fig. 3.3** Transverse depressions.

birth; the transverse depressions extended through the entire thickness of the nail which separated into two and gave rise to latent onychomadesis. The condition appears to have resulted from intrauterine distress (Fig. 3.3).

In childhood, cancer chemotherapy may produce serial Beau's lines or transverse leuconychia reflecting the periodicity of treatment regimens.

Lamellar dystrophy is a common finding in children, although it has not been the subject of any reports. It is seen both at birth and later, particularly in the thumb and big toe-nail. It is unclear whether the change arises due to prolonged bathing and frequent wetting, which are considerations when the condition develops in adults. However, it may be limited to the thumb alone if it is habitually sucked. Thumb sucking can also contribute to chronic paronychia, which in turn may

result in irregular transverse ridges and depressions in the nail plate.

Malalignment can occur in the big toe, as do a range of patterns of ingrowing. All these tend to alter the contour and thickness of the nail plate and are dealt with later in the chapter.

## References

Parry, E.J., Morley, W.N. & Dawber, R.P.R. (1995) Herringbone nails: an uncommon variant of nail growth in childhood? *British Journal of Dermatology* **132**, 1021–1022.

Pinkus, H. (1976) *Cancer of the Skin* (eds R. Andrade, S.L. Gumport, G.L. Popkin & T.D. Rees). W.B. Saunders, Philadelphia.

Shuster, S. (1996) The significance of chevron nails. *British Journal of Dermatology* **135**, 144–161.

Turano, A.F. (1968) Transverse nail ridging in early infancy. *Pediatrics* **41**, 996.

Wolf, D., Wolf, R. & Golberg, M.D. (1982) Beau' lines. A case report. *Cutis* **29**, 141.

Zaiac, M.N., Glick, B.P. & Zaias, N. (1998) Chevron nail. *Journal of the American Academy of Dermatology* **38**, 773.

## Soft tissue features

### Nail fold capillaries

The adult nail fold capillary pattern matures rapidly during the first 3 months of life (Maricq 1965); the loops appear in the neonatal period and their evolution during the first 3 months depends on weight (i.e. neonatal maturity) (Syme & Riley 1970). The normal nail fold capillary network in children resembles that observed in adults with some differences, such as lower number of loops per millimetre, a higher subpapillary venous plexus visibility (PVS) score and a higher frequency of atypical loops (Terreri *et al.* 1999).

### References

Maricq, H.R. (1965) Nailfold capillaries in normal children. *Journal of Nervous and Mental Disease* **141**, 197–203.

Syme, J. & Riley, I.D. (1970) Nail fold capillary loop development in the infant of low birth weight. *British Journal of Dermatology* **83**, 591.

Terreri, M.T., Andrade, L.E., Puccinelli, M.L. *et al.* (1999) Nail fold capillaroscopy: normal findings in children and adolescents. *Seminars in Arthritis and Rheumatism* **29**, 36–42.

### Blistering diseases

Vesiculobullous lesions involving the nail apparatus are an infrequent occurrence and necessitate sterile puncture for Gram stain, Tzanck smear, bacterial and viral culture, in order to rule out staphylococcal or herpetic infections, as both of these infections carry a high mortality during the neonatal period if left untreated (Silverman 1990).

#### Self-inflicted bullous lesions

This bullous eruption in the newborn infant is always present from the time of birth, beginning *in utero* (Murphy & Langley 1963). It may appear on the dorsum of the thumb or index finger. The bullae measure from 0.5 cm to 1.5 cm in diameter. The fluid is clear, light yellow and sterile. These lesions are presumed to be self-inflicted (*in utero*) as a consequence of a vigorous sucking reflex in otherwise normal newborns.

The differential diagnosis (Murphy & Langley 1963) includes epidermolysis bullosa, incontinentia pigmenti and congenital syphilis. Staphylococcal and streptococcal bullae generally do not occur before the 5th day of life, and vesicular eruptions due to herpes simplex do not occur before the 6th day.

### References

Murphy, W.F. & Langley, A.L. (1963) Common bullous lesion—presumably self inflicted—occurring in the utero in the new infant. *Pediatrics* **32**, 1099.

Silverman, P.A. (1990) Diseases of the nails in infants and children. In: *Advances in Dermatology*, Vol. 5 (eds J.P. Callen, M.V. Dahl, L.E. Golitz, L.A. Schachner & S.J. Stegman), pp. 153–171. Year Book Medical, Chicago.

#### Epidermolysis bullosa

There are more than 20 genetic variants of epidermolysis bullosa (EB), and nail changes in any of these is determined by a combination of the underlying epidermolysis, trauma and infection. This means that there is no fixed pattern of dystrophy

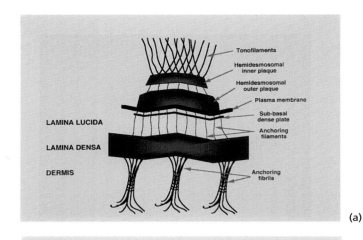

(a)

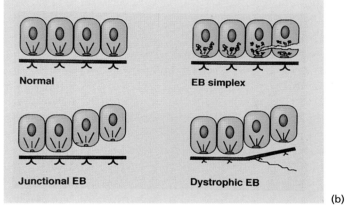

(b)

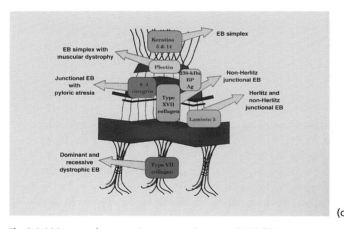

(c)

**Fig. 3.4**  (a) Structure of cutaneous basement membrane zone (BMZ). (b) Mutations in the genes encoding protein components of BMZ. (c) The ultrastrutural level of blister formation determines the broad subtype of EB. (Courtesy of J.E. Mellerio, London; from *Clinical and Experimental Dermatology* (1999) **24**, 25–32.)

according to the genotype, although some aspects are more commonly found in one variant than another (Bruckner-Tuderman *et al.* 1995). The condition is typically divided into the three main forms classified according to the level of split in the epidermis (Fig. 3.4). Epidermolysis bullosa simplex (EBS) (Fig. 3.5)

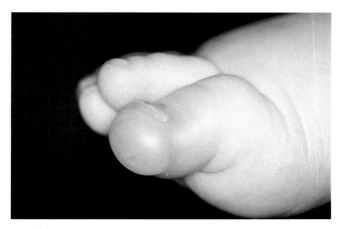

**Fig. 3.5** Epidermolysis bullosa simplex.

corresponds to a split in the basal keratinocytes and reflects a defect in keratins 5 or 14 (Corden & McLean 1996). Junctional epidermolysis bullosa (JEB) arises when there is a split in the lamina lucida which has been attributed in some instances to defects of laminin 5 (Pulkkinen *et al.* 1994). Immunohistochemical studies of the nail unit on an aborted 18-week fetus with Herlitz JEB demonstrated reduced immunostaining for the $\beta_3$ and $\alpha_3$ components of laminin 5 and absent staining for the $\gamma_2$ component (Cameli *et al.* 1996). Dystrophic epidermolysis bullosa (DEB) is due to a split beneath the basement membrane in the region of the lamina densa and defects of collagen VII appear to be responsible for the structural abnormality (Leigh *et al.* 1988). A further variant involves the presentation of epidermolysis bullosa in children with muscular dystrophy. These individuals appear to have absent plectin, which is a large cytoskeletal protein (Deng *et al.* 1998). Nail dystrophy is part of the phenotype (Patrizi *et al.* 1994; Deng *et al.* 1998).

In many forms of EBS, the nails remain normal. In some they manifest a low threshold for being shed after minor trauma and whilst they may grow back normally in early life, they may eventually become dystrophic if recurrently lost, with thickening, longitudinal ridges and onycholysis. Because trauma plays a large part in this process, it is often the big toenails that become abnormal.

JEB may present within the first weeks of life with inflammation and nail loss. Although at other sites JEB does not produce scarring, it may result in permanent anonychia, probably due to secondary bacterial infection and chronic inflammation. In one rare form of the variant, JEB progressiva, the loss of nails may be the first sign of the underlying diagnosis, presenting as late as 15 years of age (Bircher *et al.* 1993).

DEB commonly results in permanent loss of nails and this is compatible with what we understand to be the underlying defect, whereby the matrix epithelium might be lost following a split in the papillary dermis. In some localized forms of the disease, the nail changes may be the only abnormality (Fine *et al.* 1991). Fusion of fingers and toes can occur in DEB mutilans and

results in a mitten appearance associated with the loss of all nails.

Bart's syndrome has recently been characterized as a form of DEB and typically presents as areas of skin loss at birth with nails, especially toenails, absent (Zelickson *et al.* 1995). In three of 37 affected individuals from one family, nail changes were the only manifestation of the disease.

In all forms of EB affecting the nails, recurrent bullae may result in nail thinning, pterygium formation and aplasia. Sometimes the nails become thickened and onychogryphotic. Meticulous hygiene, topical antibiotics (mupirocin) and synthetic dressings may optimize nail regrowth when possible. In these patients shoes with wide-toe boxes can also be used to minimize the loss of toenails from friction (Silverman 1990).

### Epidermolysis bullosa acquisita

The immunobullous disorder, epidermolysis bullosa acquisita (EBA), may appear at any age (3 months in the case reported by McCuaig *et al.* (1989)), although no congenital cases have been reported. Distal onycholysis is a recorded feature in a 10 year old who also suffered loss of the right third fingernail. In its place was firm, vertically striated and folded skin. A few of the toenails were opaque and thickened by subungual hyperkeratosis (McCuaig *et al.* 1989).

In this autoimmune disease, the autoantibodies are directed against type VII collagen, possibly indicating common ground with the pathomechanism of DEB. The differentiation between mechanobullous and immunobullous disease in children is critical in that significant clinical benefit may be achieved in EBA with corticosteroids and/or dapsone therapy.

### References

Bircher, A.J., Lang-Muritano, M., Pfaltz, M. & Bruckner-Tuderman, L. (1993) Epidermolysis bullosa junctionalis progressiva in 3 siblings. *British Journal of Dermatology* **128**, 429–435.

Bruckner-Tuderman, L., Schnyder, U.W. & Baran, R. (1995) Nail changes in epidermolysis bullosa: clinical and pathogenetic considerations. *British Journal of Dermatology* **132**, 339–344.

Cameli, N., Picardo, M., Pisano, A. *et al.* (1996) Characterisation of the nail matrix basement membrane zone: an immunohistochemical study of normal nails and of the nails in Herlitz junctional epidermolysis bullosa. *British Journal of Dermatology* **134**, 182–184.

Corden, L.D. & McLean, W.H. (1996) Human keratin disease: hereditary fragility of specific epithelial tissues. *Experimental Dermatology* **5**, 297–307.

Deng, M., Pulkkinen, L., Smith, F.J. *et al.* (1998) Novel compound heterozygous mutations in the plectin gene in epidermolysis bullosa with muscular dystrophy and the use of protein truncation test for detection of premature termination codon mutations. *Laboratory Investigation* **78**, 195–204.

Fine, J.-D., Bauer, E.A., Briggaman, R.A. *et al.* (1991) Revised clinical and laboratory criteria for subtypes of inherited epidermolysis bullosa. *Journal of the American Academy of Dermatology* **24**, 119–135.

Leigh, I.M., Eady, R.A.J., Heagerty, A.H.M. *et al.* (1988) Type VII collagen is a normal component of epidermal basement membrane, which shows altered expression in recessive dystrophic epidermolysis bullosa. *Journal of Investigative Dermatology* **90**, 639–642.

McCuaig, C.C., Chan, L.S., Woodley, D.T. *et al.* (1989) Epidermolysis bullosa acquisita in childhood. Differentiation from hereditary epidermolysis bullosa. *Archives of Dermatology* **125**, 944–949.

Patrizi, A., Di Lernia, V., Neri, I. *et al.* (1994) Epidermolysis bullosa simplex associated with muscular dystrophy: a new case. *Pediatric Dermatology* **11**, 342–345.

Pulkkinen, L., Christiano, A.M., Airenne, T. *et al.* (1994) Mutations in the $\gamma_2$ chain gene (LAMC2) of kalinin/laminin-5 in the junctional forms of epidermolysis bullosa. *Nature Genetics* **6**, 293–298.

Silverman, P.A. (1990) Diseases of the nails in infants and children. In: *Advances in Dermatology*, Vol. 5 (eds J.P. Callen, M.V. Dahl, L.E. Golitz, L.A. Schachner & S.J. Stegman), pp. 153–171. Year Book Medical, Chicago.

Zelickson, B., Matsumara, K., Kist, D. *et al.* (1995) Bart's Syndrome: ultrastructure and genetic linkage. *Archives of Dermatology* **131**, 663–668.

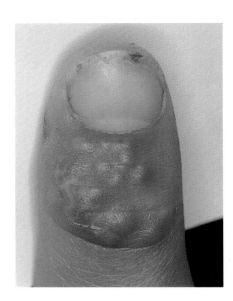

**Fig. 3.6** Herpes simplex sometimes associated with thumb or finger sucking.

## Infection

### Herpetic whitlow

Herpetic whitlow is the major diagnostic consideration when a painful blister forms around the nail in children (Feder & Long 1983). This condition presents with pain of the distal phalanx followed shortly by swelling and redness. A cluster of tapioca-like vesicles then develops and may coalesce. These lesions contain clear fluid that becomes turbid but rarely purulent over a 10-day period (in contrast to blistering distal dactylitis) (Silverman 1990). Soft tissue changes may lead to onycholysis or onychomadesis, but permanent dystrophy is exceptional.

Thumb or finger sucking is sometimes associated with localized extensions of the eruption producing a viral stomatitis combined with involvement of the digit (Fig. 3.6). Herpetic infections in patients who are less than 1 year old affect the index, the 3rd finger and the thumb, whereas in adults the most commonly infected digits are the thumb and index finger. The incidence of involvement of multiple digits is about twice the reported incidence of 10% in adults who have herpetic infection of the hand (Behr *et al.* 1987).

Tzanck smear reveals multinucleated giant cells. Unroofing of any large vesicles and subungual decompression if fluid has collected have been advocated for relieving severe pain. Topical and systemic antiviral agents are logical first-line therapy (Silverman 1990).

### References

Behr, J.T., Daluga, D.J., Light, T.R. *et al.* (1987) Herpetic infections in the fingers of infants. *Journal of Bone and Joint Surgery* **69A**, 137–139.

Feder, H.M. & Long, S.S. (1983) Herpetic whitlow: epidemiology, clinical characteristics, diagnosis and treatment. Further observation. *Clinical and Experimental Dermatology* **7**, 455–457.

Silverman, P.A. (1990) Diseases of the nails in infants and children. In: *Advances in Dermatology*, Vol. 5 (eds J.P. Callen, M.V. Dahl, L.E. Golitz, L.A. Schachner & S.J. Stegman), pp. 153–171. Year Book Medical, Chicago.

### Impetigo (Fig. 3.7)

The dorsal aspect of the distal phalanx may be involved by impetigo. It comes in two forms:
1 Vesiculopustular with its familiar honey-crusted lesions (Jacobs 1981), usually due to β-haemolytic streptococci;
2 Bullous, usually due to phage type 71 staphylococci (develops on intact skin).

The latter is characterized by the appearance of large, localized, intraepidermal bullae that persist for longer periods than the transient vesicles of streptococcal impetigo, which subsequently rupture spontaneously to form very thin crusts. The lesions of bullous impetigo may mimic the non-infectious bullous diseases such as drug-induced bullae or bullous pemphigoid.

Oral therapy of bullous impetigo with cloxacillin should be instituted and continued until the lesions resolve. Cefprozil and clarithromycin are acceptable substitutes (Darmstadt & Lane 1994). The lesions should be cleansed several times daily and topical mupirocin ointment rubbed into all the affected areas.

Poorly trimmed nails may serve as a paronychial focus for infection in children during remission induction treatment for various malignant disorders (Gutjahr & Schmitt 1984). Intense scratching of infected atopic dermatitis, coupled with minor trauma to the fingertips, have been found to create distal subungual microabscesses that spread contiguously to the underlying bone (Boiko *et al.* 1988).

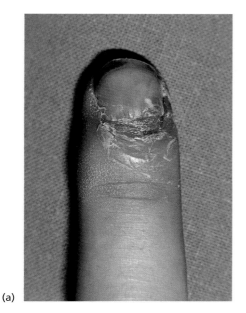

(a)

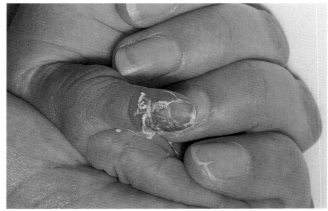

(b)

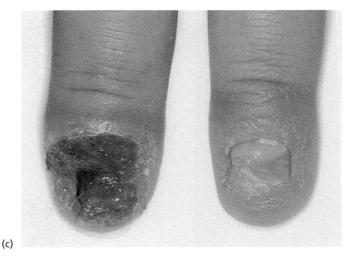

(c)

**Fig. 3.7** (a) Impetigo involving the proximal nail fold with subsequent onychomadesis. (b) Impetigo of the distal digit, surrounding the nail. (c) Honey-crusted lesion involving the nail bed, before and after 1 month of penicillinase-resistant penicillin

## References

Boiko, S., Kaufman, R.A. & Lucky, A.W. (1988) Osteomyelitis of the distal phalanges in 3 children with severe atopic dermatitis. *Archives of Dermatology* **124**, 418–423.

Darmstadt, G.L. & Lane, A.T. (1994) Impetigo: an overview. *Pediatric Dermatology* **11**, 293–303.

Gutjahr, P. & Schmitt, H.J. (1984) Caring of the nails and anticancer treatment. *European Journal of Pediatrics* **143**, 74.

Jacobs, A.H. (1981) What's new in pediatric dermatology? *Acta Dermato-Venereologica* **95** (Suppl.), 91–95.

## Blistering distal dactylitis (Fig. 3.8)

Blistering distal dactylitis (BDD) is a variant of streptococcal skin infection. This condition presents as a superficial, non-tender, blistering β-haemolytic streptococcal infection over the anterior fat pad of the distal phalanx of the finger (Hays & Mullard 1975), *Staphylococcus aureus* and *S. epidermidis* are isolated less frequently. *S. aureus* may be characterized by involvement of multiple digits (Norcross & Mitchell 1993) and is thought to be becoming more common as a cause of BDD (Woroszylski *et al.* 1996). The lesion may or may not have a paronychial extension and more than one digit is frequently involved (Schneider & Palette 1982). This blister with an erythematous base, containing thin, white pus, has a predilection for the tip of the digit. It extends to the subungual area of the free edge of the nail plate. This area may provide a nidus for bacteria and act as a focus of chronic infection (Baran 1982), similar to the rhinopharynx. Recurrent blistering dactylitis has also been reported with ingrowing toenail (Telfer *et al.* 1989). The age range of affected patients is 2–16 years. The condition is exceptionally reported in adults: a healthy fishmonger (Palomo-Arellano *et al.* 1985); an unusual case due to group B β-haemolytic streptococcus in a patient with insulin-dependent-diabetes (Benson & Solivan 1987); another case due to *S. aureus* in an immunosuppressed patient (Zemtsov

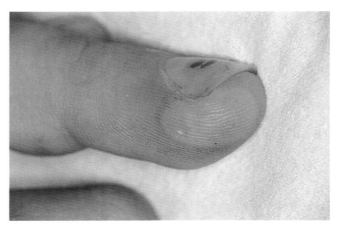

**Fig. 3.8** Blistering distal dactylitis.

& Veitschegger 1992); and a questionable publication (Parras *et al.* 1988).

Local care entails incision and drainage of thin white pus. Antiseptic soaks facilitate the response to systemic antibiotics: effective regimens include penicillin G in a single intramuscular dose, or a 10-day course of oral phenoxymethylpenicillin, erythromycin ethyl succinate or Augmentin. Antiseptic and systemic therapy combined may decrease the reservoir of streptococci by preventing spread to family contacts (McCray & Esterly 1981, 1982).

Non-blistering dactylitis may be infective or sterile. Tuberculous dactylitis has been reported in a Chinese child (Clarke 1990) and haemophilus infection superimposed on dactylitis seen in sickle cell disease is also recognized (Webb & Sergeant 1990). Sickle cell disease (Morris *et al.* 1994) and forms of juvenile or psoriatic arthritis (Petty 1994) are the main non-infective forms of dactylitis seen in childhood.

The differential diagnosis includes blisters resulting from friction, thermal and chemical burns, infectious states such as herpetic whitlow and staphylococcal bullous impetigo and Weber–Cockayne variant of epidermolysis bullosa (McCray & Esterly 1981).

## References

Baran, R. (1982) Blistering distal dactylitis. *Journal of the American Academy of Dermatology* **6**, 948.

Benson, P.M. & Solivan, G. (1987) Group B streptococcal blistering distal dactylitis in an adult diabetic. *Journal of the American Academy of Dermatology* **17**, 310–311.

Clarke, J.A. (1990) Tuberculous dactylitis in childhood. The need for continued vigilance. *Clinical Radiology* **42**, 287–288.

Hays, G.C. & Mullard, J.E. (1975) Blistering distal dactylitis: clinically recognizable streptococcal infection. *Pediatrics* **56**, 129.

McCray, M.K. & Esterly, N.B. (1981) Blistering distal dactylitis. *Journal of the American Academy of Dermatology* **5**, 592.

McCray, M.K. & Esterly, N.B. (1982) Blistering distal dactylitis. *Journal of the American Academy of Dermatology* **6**, 949.

Morris, J., Serjeant, B.E. & Serjeant, G. (1994) Sickle cell anaemia in Nigeria: a comparison between Benin and Lagos. *African Journal of Medicine and Medical Sciences* **23**, 101–107.

Norcross, M.C. Jr & Mitchell, D.F. (1993) Blistering distal dactylitis caused by *Staphylococcus aureus*. *Cutis* **51**, 353–354.

Palomo-Arellano, A., Jimenez-Reyes, J., Martin-Moreno, L. *et al.* (1985) Blistering distal dactylitis in an adult. *Archives of Dermatology* **121**, 1242.

Parras, F., Ezpelata, C., Romero, J. *et al.* (1988) Blistering distal dactylitis in an adult. *Cutis* **41**, 127–128.

Petty, R.E. (1994) Juvenile psoriatic arthritis, or juvenile arthritis with psoriasis? *Clinical and Experimental Rheumatology* **12** (Suppl. 10), S55–S58.

Schneider, J.A. & Palette, H.L. (1982) Blistering distal dactylitis: a manifestation of group A beta-hemolytic streptococcal infection. *Archives of Dermatology* **118**, 879–880.

Telfer, N.R., Barth, J.H. & Dawber, R.P.R. (1989) Recurrent blistering distal dactylitis of the great toe associated with an ingrowing toenail. *Clinical and Experimental Dermatology* **14**, 380–381.

Webb, D.K. & Sergeant, G.R. (1990) *Haemophilus influenzae* osteomyelitis complicating dactylitis in homozygous sickle cell disease. *European Journal of Pediatrics* **149**, 613–614.

Woroszylski, A., Durn, C. & Tamayo, L. (1996) Staphylococcal blistering dactylitis: report of two patients. *Pediatric Dermatology* **13**, 292–293.

Zemtsov, A. & Veitschegger, M. (1992) *Staphylococcus aureus* induced blistering distal dactylitis in adult immunosuppressed patient. *Journal of the American Academy of Dermatology* **26**, 784–785.

## Toxic shock syndrome

In this *S. aureus* infection with fever, hypotension, generalized erythema, diarrhoea, central nervous system and electrolytes abnormalities, hair and nails may shed about 2 months following the acute illness (Litt 1983).

## Reference

Litt, I.F. (1983) Toxic shock syndrome: an adolescent disease. *Journal of Adolescent Health Care* **4**, 270–274.

## *Veillonella* infection of the newborn

Forty-two epidemics of subungual infection have been described by Sinniah *et al.* (1972) among infants in postnatal wards and special care baby units (Fig. 3.9). The number of fingers affected per patient ranged from one to 10; the thumbs were less frequently involved than other digits, and the toenails were spared altogether. Three stages were found: first, a small amount of clear fluid appears under the centre of the nail, along with mild inflammation at the distal end of the finger. This initial vesicle lasts approximately 24 h; it sometimes enlarges but never to the edge of the nail. Some small lesions bypass the second, pustular stage, going directly into the third stage. As a rule

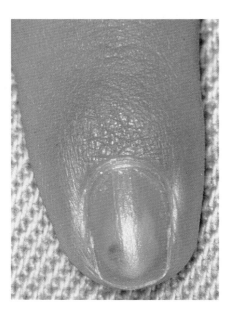

**Fig. 3.9** Subungual *Veillonella* infection.

the fluid becomes yellow after 24 h, the pus remaining for 24–48 h before gradually turning brown, and being absorbed. This colour fades progressively over a period of 2–6 weeks, leaving the nail and nail bed apparently completely normal. Subungual pus obtained by aseptic puncture of the nails showed tiny, gram-negative cocci about 0.4 μm in diameter. These organisms resembled *Veillonella*, bacteria of dubious pathogenicity and the most common anaerobes to be found in saliva of adults (Sutter 1984). In neonates, *Veillonella* is more common in the bowel of bottle-fed than breast-fed children and this is compatible with those on intensive care units (Benno *et al.* 1984). It is also found in the vagina and respiratory tract.

## Other bacterial infections

Anaerobic infections (*Bacteroides*, *Bacillus fragilis* and *Fusibacterium*) may affect many sites, including the fingers and nail beds (Hurwitz & Kahn 1983). In the newborn, nursery epidemics of staphylococcus produce cases of omphalitis, mammary abscess, dacryocystitis or paronychia. The localization is probably due to the presence of a locus minoris resistentiae, with trauma perhaps being a factor in paronychia (Koblenzer 1978).

In Leiner's disease (Fig. 3.10), recurrent paronychia infections and interdigital intertrigo (usually due to gram-negative bacteria) may be only some of the many infective episodes observed (Koblenzer 1978). Topical clindamycin is usually effective.

In childhood, local trauma, caused by onychophagia, may result in the development of opportunistic infection by the normal oropharyngeal flora resulting in acute paronychia. This may be caused by BH 1 organisms (*Eikenella corrodens*). It is uncommon in the absence of an immune deficiency (Barton & Anderson 1974).

It is important to remember that the nail matrix is very susceptible to infection in early life and may be irreversibly damaged within 48 h of the onset of acute infection. This means that rapid intervention is required and it is of value to relieve pressure developing beneath the nail if there is a collection of

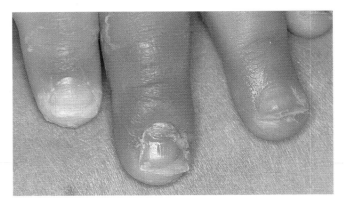

**Fig. 3.10** Leiner's disease.

pus. Not only will this reduce the chance of pressure necrosis of the matrix, but it will also give pain relief.

## References

Barton, L.L. & Anderson, L.E. (1974) Paronychia caused by HB1 organisms. *Pediatrics* **54**, 372.

Benno, Y., Sawada, K. & Mitsuoka, T. (1984) The intestinal microflora of infants: composition of fecal flora in breast-fed and bottle-fed infants. *Microbiology and Immunology* **28**, 975–986.

Hurwitz, S. & Kahn, G. (1983) IXth Postgraduate Seminar in Paediatric Dermatology. *Journal of the American Academy of Dermatology* **8**, 271.

Koblenzer, P.J. (1978) Common bacterial infections of the skin in children. *Pediactic Clinics of North America* **25**, 321.

Sinniah, D., Sandiford, B.R. & Dugdale, A.E. (1972) Subungual infection in the newborn. An institutional outbreak of unknown etiology, possibly due to Veillonella. *Clinical Pediatrics* **11**, 690.

Sutter, V.L. (1984) Anaerobes as normal oral flora. *Reviews of Infectious Diseases* **6** (Suppl. 1), S62–S66.

## Fungal infection

Candida is the most common fungus to be associated with periungual and nail changes in infancy (Chapter 4) but the nail changes may fail to fill the criteria of a true onychomycosis in terms of nail plate invasion and the reproducibility of cultures. Onychomycosis is uncommon in childhood and has been examined in a small number of studies. In a true prevalence study performed in Finland, there were no cases of onychomycosis identified in the 200 subjects under the age of 20 years of a total study size of 800 people between the age of 6 and 80 years (Heikkilä & Stubb 1995). A larger and less precise study in North America identified a prevalence of onychomycosis to be 0.16% among 2500 subjects under the age of 18 visiting a dermatologist for non-fungal disease (Gupta *et al.* 1997). Philpot and Shuttleworth (1989) identified one child out of 494 aged 5–10 years (0.2% prevalence) with onychomycosis, where the sample was taken from schools and a dermatology clinic. An average from the 11 studies of onychomycosis in children performed in the last 30 years suggests a prevalence of between 0 and 2.6% (Gupta *et al.* 1997). However, the bias towards performing the studies in dermatology clinics undermines the methodology of assessment of prevalence. Where studies have been performed in the community, prevalence has been far lower, ranging from 0 to 0.2%. When confirmed, paediatric onychomycosis tends to be associated with concomitant tinea pedis (47%) (Gupta *et al.* 1997) or tinea of the scalp. The pattern may resemble that in adults, although there is a greater incidence of superficial white infection and possibly also proximal subungual infection, which when seen in adults might suggest immune suppression (Chang & Logermann 1994).

*Trichophyton rubrum* is the most common pathogen in children (Fig. 3.11a) and adults, although superficial white infection is more commonly associated with *Trichophyton mentagrophytes* and sometimes *Candida* spp.

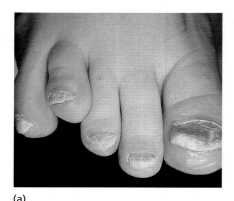

(a)

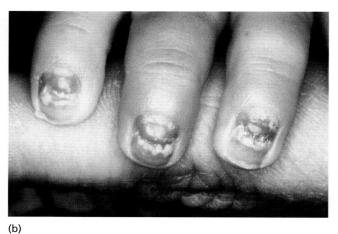

(b)

**Fig. 3.11** (a) Onychomycosis due to *Trichophyton rubrum* in a young child. (b) Congenital candidosis with onychomadesis. (Courtesy of F. Cambazard, Saint-Etienne.)

Cases of onychomycosis reported in children under 2 years of age are exceptional (Schmunes 1976; Borbujo *et al.* 1987). Both congenital (Fig. 3.11b) and neonatal candidosis have been reported (Chaland & Bouygues 1986; Perel *et al.* 1986; Kurgansky & Sweren 1990; Davis-Gibney & Siegfried 1995; Raval *et al.* 1995). In the case reported by Plantin *et al.* (1992), neonatal candidosis was limited to paronychia of all the fingers, followed by onychomadesis and distolateral subungual onychomycosis affecting some toes (Chapter 5). Generalized chronic dermatophytosis in early childhood has also been observed.

In HIV infection in childhood, candidiasis presents with nail dystrophy identical to that seen in chronic mucocutaneous candidiasis, and dermatophytosis as severe onychomycosis may appear (Silverman 1990).

Treatment of dermatophyte onychomycosis in childhood is similar to that in adults, although the experience of use of the newer systemic antifungals is limited and this is reflected in their licensed indications around the world. Consequently, there is a tendency to adopt topical therapy, such as amorolfine, cyclopiroxolamine or a topical imidazole. These may be appropriate in limited superficial white onychomycosis, but where there is cutaneous or scalp involvement, or the nail plate infection is substantial, systemic therapy may be needed. Griseofulvin is probably still the drug of choice worldwide, but it has drawbacks in terms of the prolonged treatment period and side effects (Stiller *et al.* 1993). There is increasing evidence to support the use of terbinafine, itraconazole and fluconazole where medical factors and cost allow (Chang & Logermann 1994; Goulden & Goodfield 1995; Assaf & Elewski 1996; Gupta *et al.* 1998). Given the lack of licensed indication and relatively little experience, exact dosing schedules are difficult to define. This has been attempted by Gupta *et al.* (1997) (Table 3.1). However, a two-phase treatment with bifonazole-urea, effect-

**Table 3.1** Treatment of onychomycosis in infancy. (Some agents may not be licensed for use in children.)

| Drug | Mode | Age/weight | Dose | Duration (weeks) | |
| --- | --- | --- | --- | --- | --- |
| | | | | Toes | Fingers |
| Griseofulvin | Continuous | Children <50 kg | Microsize 15–20 mg/kg/d Ultramicrosize 9.9–13.2 mg kg/d | 26–52 | 18–40 |
| Itraconazole | Pulse | <20 kg | 5 mg/kg/d: 1 week per month | 3 pulses: 3 weeks over 3 months | 2 pulses: 2 weeks over 2 months |
| | | 20–40 kg | 100 mg/d | | |
| | | 40–50 kg | 200 mg/d | | |
| | | >50 kg | 200 mg × 2 daily | | |
| Terbinafine | Continuous | <20 kg | 62.5 mg/d | 12 | 6 |
| | | 20–40 kg | 125 mg/d | | |
| | | >40 kg | 250 mg/d | | |
| Fluconazole | Pulse | Children <50 kg | 3–6 mg/kg/d once per week | 18–26 | 12–16 |

ive and safe, may represent a new therapeutic choice for onychomycosis in children (Bonifaz & Ibarra 2000), provided few nails are infected.

## References

Assaf, R.R. & Elewski, B.E. (1996) Intermittent fluconazole dosing in patients with onychomycosis: results of a pilot study. *Journal of the American Academy of Dermatology* 35, 216–219.

Bonifaz, A. & Ibarra, G. (2000) Onychomycosis in children: treatment with bifonazole-urea. *Pediatric Dermatology* 17, 310–314.

Borbujo, J.M., Fonseca, E. and Gonzalez, A. (1987) Onicomicosis por *Trichophyton rubrum* en un recién nacido. *Acta Dermato-Sifilitica* 78, 207.

Chaland, G. & Bouygues, D. (1986) Candidose cutanée congénitale. Deux observations. *Pediatrie* 41, 321–327.

Chang, P. & Logermann, H. (1994) Onychomycosis in children. *International Journal of Dermatology* 33, 550–551.

Davis-Gibney, M.D. & Siegfried, E.C. (1995) Cutaneous congenital Candidiasis: a case report. *Pediatric Dermatology* 12, 359–363.

Goulden, V. and Goodfield, M.J.D. (1995) Treatment of childhood dermatophyte infections with oral terbinafine. *Pediatric Dermatology* 12, 53–54.

Gupta, A.K., Chang, P., Del Rosso, J.Q. *et al.* (1998) Onychomycosis in children: prevalence and management. *Pediatric Dermatology* 15, 464–471.

Heikkilä, H. & Stubb, S. (1995) The prevalence of onychomycosis in Finland. *British Journal of Dermatology* 133, 699–703.

Kurgansky, D. & Sweren R. (1990) Onychomycosis in a 10-weeks-old infant [letter]. *Archives of Dermatology* 126, 1371.

Perel, Y., Taïeb, A., Fonton J. *et al.* (1986) Candidose cutanée congénitale. Une observation avec revue de la littérature. *Annales de Dermatologie et de Vénéréologie* 113, 125–130.

Philpot, C.M. & Shuttleworth, D. (1989) Dermatophyte onychomycosis in children. *Clinical and Experimental Dermatology* 14, 203–205.

Plantin, P., Jouan, N., Calligaris, C. *et al.* (1992) Onychomadèse du nourrison à *Candida albicans*. Contamination néonatale. *Annales de Dermatologie et de Vénéréologie* 119, 213–215.

Raval, D.S., Barton, L.L., Hansen, R.C. *et al.* (1995) Congenital cutaneous Candidiasis: case report and review. *Pediatric Dermatology* 12, 355–358.

Schmunes, E. (1976) Onychomycosis in a 14-month-old child. *Southern Medical Journal* 69, 1097.

Silverman, P.A. (1990) Diseases of the nails in infants and children. In: *Advances in Dermatology*, Vol. 5 (eds J.P. Callen, M.V. Dahl, L.E. Golitz, L.A. Schachner & S.J. Stegman), pp. 153–171. Year Book Medical, Chicago.

Stiller, M., Sangueza, O. & Shupack, J. (1993) Systemic drugs in the treatment of dermatophytosis. *International Journal of Dermatology* 32, 16–20.

## Miscellaneous

### Chronic paronychia (Fig. 3.12)

Candida paronychia, usually in association with oral can-

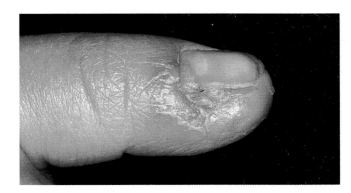

**Fig. 3.12** Chronic paronychia.

didosis, may arise as a result of chronic maceration due to thumb sucking.

Chronic paronychia is not uncommon in children. It differs from the condition seen in adults in the source of the maceration, associated diseases such as atopic dermatitis (Hanifin 1991), the clinical appearances of the lesion and the patients' responses to their symptoms (Stone & Mullins 1968). In children the lesions are generally very prominent, with total involvement of the proximal nail fold. The skin is usually erythematous and glistening due to the wet environment produced by continuous thumb sucking. This condition appears as a response to search of relief from itching. The quality of the nail substance is regularly altered, making its texture poor.

Hyperglycaemia is not an associated finding. *Candida albicans* is usually present. When the acute flare occurs, the patient with atopic dermatitis experiences pruritus and discomfort in the proximal nail fold. Children respond to this by sucking, the symptoms of chronic paronychia perpetuating the habit which initiates the maceration. The lesions tend to be more severe in children than in adults and the nail may be shed. The severity in children may reflect the irritant quality of saliva and the fact that exposure may be all night long (Stone & Mullins 1968). Also, the threshold for an irritant reaction may be less in some children than in adults; this applies particularly to atopics (Fig. 3.13). The eczematous background to many cases of paronychia emphasizes the need to treat it primarily as a localized dermatosis rather than an infection, in spite of the presence of *Candida*.

Multiple persistent and repeated paronychia in infancy can represent a more serious underlying disorder, and such infants should be investigated for endocrine disease, immune deficiency syndromes (Solomon & Esterly 1973) and systemic disease such as histiocytosis X, acrodermatitis enteropathica and Reiter's syndrome.

Therapy for childhood paronychia should first be directed at drying the affected digits. The near impossibility of preventing thumb sucking makes it difficult. Clotrimazole applied several times daily when candida is suspected and topical clindamycin solution can be helpful. The latter kills bacteria, has a bitter

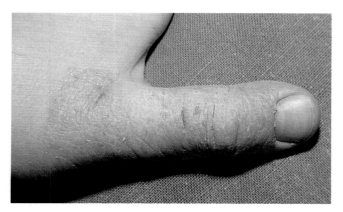

**Fig. 3.13** Atopic dermatitis involving the thumb.

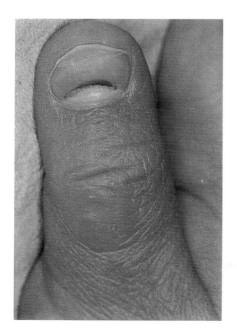

**Fig. 3.14** Thumb sucking associated with nail biting. (Subungual haemorrhage.)

taste to discourage further sucking, and has an alcohol propylene glycol vehicle that dries out residual moisture (Silverman 1990). An alternative approach employs the use of topical steroids in combination with antimicrobials; this is useful when much of the clinical complaint arises through the inflammation of the nail folds, which is slow to settle on antimicrobial therapy alone.

## References

Hanifin, J.M. (1991) Atopic dermatitis in infants and children. *Pediatric Clinics of North America* **38**, 763–790.

Silverman, P.A. (1990) Diseases of the nails in infants and children. In: *Advances in Dermatology*, Vol. 5 (eds J.P. Callen, M.V. Dahl, L.E. Golitz, L.A. Schachner & S.J. Stegman), pp. 153–171. Year Book Medical, Chicago.

Solomon, L.M. & Esterly, N.B. (1973) *Neonatal Dermatology*. W.B. Saunders, Philadelphia.

Stone, O.J. & Mullins, F.J. (1968) Chronic paronychia in children. *Clinical Pediatrics* **7**, 104.

## Finger sucking and nail biting

Finger sucking (Fig. 3.14) is usually limited to those under the age of 5 and is a normal childhood activity (Taylor & Peterson 1983). After that age opinion is not clear as to whether it represents a problem in terms of oral development, with the potential risk of altering the bite of the incisors (Josell 1995) such that they do not meet in the front. Atypical patterns of finger sucking have resulted in deformity of the digits, requiring surgical correction (Reid & Price 1984). Transfer of infection from finger to mouth and possible systemic illness are potential risks at all ages. It is seldom necessary to pursue a specific strategy to persuade a child to stop sucking his or her digit, but such strategies exist (Vogel 1998) and may be valuable when faced with intractable paronychia or relevant dental problems.

Nail biting (Fig. 3.15) is a more complicated habit with direct connotations of self-harm. In spite of this it is common. A study in primary and secondary schools in the North of England re-

vealed that 36% of children aged 5 bit their nails, rising to 57% at age 12 and falling to 31% by 16 (Birch 1955). The pattern and extent of biting rarely take the form of onychotillomania seen in adults, where the entire nail plate may be lost and psychiatric problems may be manifest (Combes & Scott 1951; Sait *et al.* 1985; Colver 1987). Simple nail biting appears unrelated to psychiatric illness (Clark 1970), although some studies have proposed that the behaviour is associated with significant stresses and anxiety (DeFrancesco *et al.* 1989). Turning the interpretation around, 31% of children with trichotillomania are also nail biters (Simeon *et al.* 1997).

In addition to disposing to periungual infection and chronic paronychia, nail biting can result in soft tissue problems in the mouth. Fragments of nail can get caught between teeth or embedded in periodontal soft tissues, provoking gingivitis. This reaction is difficult to settle unless the fragment is dislodged or there is abscess formation and liquefaction of local soft tissues (Hodges *et al.* 1994; Creath *et al.* 1995).

A study performed via orthodontic practitioners claimed that nail biters between the ages of 13 and 15 were at greater risk of tooth root resorption than non-nail biters (Odenrick & Brattström 1985). The explanation for this was that long-term repetitive biting seen in other circumstances causes root resorption and nail biting is likely to do likewise. Although this finding was determined through jaw X-rays, it is not clear to what extent it would have a clinical correlate in terms of oral health.

Other forms of nail trauma seen in adults are also occasionally seen in children. There is a single report of 'washboard nails' in an 11-year-old girl. She admitted to the habit of rubbing and picking at the thumb cuticle from the age of 5. The nail consequently developed a series of irregular transverse depres-

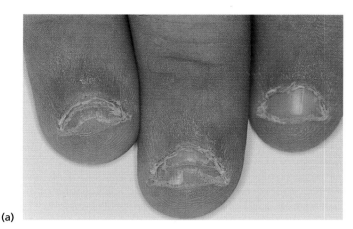

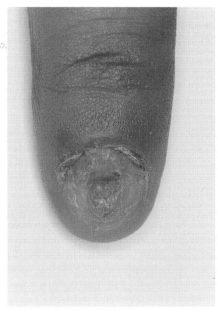

**Fig. 3.15** (a) Nail biting. (b) Nail biting and picking.

sions associated with loss of cuticle and slight bolstering of the proximal nail fold (Kinoshita *et al.* 1994).

## References

Birch, L.B. (1955) The incidence of nail biting among school children. *British Journal of Educational Psychology* **25**, 123–128

Clark, D.F. (1970) Nail biting in subnormals. *British Journal of Medical Psychology* **43**, 69–71.

Colver, G. (1987) Onychotillomania. *British Journal of Dermatology* **117**, 397–402.

Combes, F.C. & Scott, M.J. (1951) Onychotillomania. *Archives of Dermatology and Syphilology* **63**, 778–780.

Creath, C., Steinmetz, S. & Roebuck, R. (1995) A case report: gingival swelling due to fingernail biting habit. *Journal of the American Dental Association* **126**, 1019–1021.

DeFrancesco, J.J., Zahner, G.E.P. & Pawelkiewicz W. (1989) Childhood nailbiting. *Journal of Social Behaviour and Personality* **4**, 157–161.

Hodges, E.D., Allen, K.A & Durham, T. (1994) Nail-biting and foreign body embedment: a review and case report. *Pediatric Dentistry* **16**, 236–238.

Josell, S.D. (1995) Habits affecting dental and maxillofacial growth and development. *Dental Clinics of North America* **39**, 851–860.

Kinoshita, T., Johno, M., Ono, T. & Kikuchi, I. (1994) A case of nail picking. *Journal of Dermatology* **21**, 211–212.

Odenrick, L. & Brattström, V. (1985) Nail biting: frequency and association with root resorption during orthodontic treatment. *British Journal of Orthodontics* **12**, 78–81.

Reid, D.A. & Price, A.H. (1984) Digital deformities and dental malocclusion due to finger sucking. *British Journal of Dermatology* **37**, 447–452.

Sait, M.A., Reddy, B.S.N. & Garg, B.R. (1985) Onychotillomania. *Dermatologica* **171**, 200–202.

Simeon, D., Cohen, L. & Stein, D. (1997) Comorbid self-injurious behaviors in 71 female hair pullers: a survey study. *Journal of Nervous and Mental Diseases* **185**, 299–304.

Taylor, M.H. & Peterson, D.S. (1983) Effect of digit-sucking habits on root morphology in primary incisors. *Pediatric Dentistry* **5**, 61–63.

Vogel, L.D. (1998) When children put their fingers in their mouths. *New York State Dental Journal* **64**, 48–53.

## The twenty-nail dystrophy of childhood (Fig. 3.16)
(see also Chapters 2 and 5)

'Twenty-nail dystrophy' was the term coined by Hazelrigg *et al.* (1977) to describe an entity already recognized by Samman (1978) as 'excess ridging' of childhood. This is an acquired, idiopathic nail dystrophy in which all 20 nails are uniformly and simultaneously affected with excess longitudinal ridging and loss of lustre. We have designated this condition 'vertical striated sand paper twenty-nail dystrophy' (Baran & Dupré 1977). Achten and Wanet-Rouard (1974) used the term 'trachyonychia' after Alkiewicz (1950), to describe a dystrophy characterized by roughness of the nail surface and grey opacity of the nail, which becomes brittle with terminal splitting. It begins insidiously in early childhood and resolves slowly with age. The clinical presentation may fall short of all 20 nails.

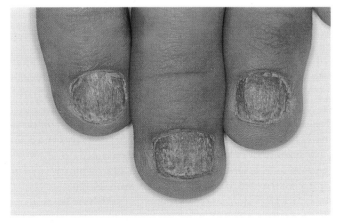

**Fig. 3.16** Twenty-nail dystrophy of childhood—sandpapered nails.

The pathogenesis is controversial (Wilkinson *et al.* 1979). Alopecia areata (Baran *et al.* 1978; Horn & Odom, 1980), less often lichen planus (Baran *et al.* 1978; Scher *et al.* 1978) or even both associated in the same patient (Fenton & Samman 1988) and rarely psoriasis (Baran *et al.* 1978) have all been associated with the twenty-nail dystrophy. Other possible causes include ichthyosis vulgaris, in association with atopic dermatitis (James *et al.* 1981), selective IgA deficiency (Leong *et al.* 1982), familial severe cases (Arias *et al.* 1982; Pavone, 1982), dark red lunulae and knuckle pads (Runne 1980) and rarely ectodermal dysplasias. This condition, reported in twins, may be a result of single localized tissue malformation (Commens 1988). An autoimmune process may be involved in some cases (Person 1984). We have presented a case of lichen planus graft-versus-host disease precipitated by an exchange transfusion in newborn (Brun *et al.* 1984).

Congenital, familial and hereditary cases have occurred in both children and adults. Morphologically there are two main types (Baran 1981). In the first type, 'vertical striated sand-papered twenty-nail dystrophy' or sand-blasted nails is most frequently associated with alopecia areata. It is difficult to demonstrate the condition adequately on photographs. In the second type, all 20 nails are shiny, opalescent and have longitudinal ridging. This fine stippled appearance reflects light and is clearly seen on photographs (Baran 1981).

Alopecia areata may occur in association with both types. In the descriptions by Hazelrigg *et al.* (1977), one case was of the second type; the majority were of the first type. Also the thumbnails and great toenails were yellow, thickened and rough; i.e. all nails were not uniformly affected despite the definition given by Hazelrigg *et al.* In a study of the clinical features of 272 children with alopecia areata, it was noted that 11.7% had trachyonychia (Tosti *et al.* 1994a). It is interesting that about 30% had pitting and this may be an indication that the disease process is in a continuum whereby increased pitting eventually roughens the entire nail surface in the form of trachyonychia.

Only some reports include histological data. We have found, in children, either vacuolated cells with intercellular and intracellular oedema in the nail bed epidermis and squamous cells of the matrix presenting with homogeneous pale staining, or changes typical of lichen planus. Scher *et al.* (1978) reported one case that showed microscopic evidence of lichen planus. Silverman and Rhodes (1984) saw a child with oral lichen planus who had twenty-nail dystrophy. Donofrio and Ayala's (1984) patient showed psoriasiform epithelial hyperplasia with hypergranulosis. Wilkinson *et al.* (1979) presented histopathological findings that were incompatible with the definition of the condition as a variant of lichen planus; there was considerable distortion of the nail matrix with a fairly dense mononuclear inflammatory infiltrate below and within the matrix epithelium, together with marked spongiosis. No basal cell liquefaction was present. These changes suggested an eczematous picture. Alkiewicz (1950) found similar histological findings in two cases in which roughness of the nails had been induced by

strong chemicals and in a third case involving all 20 nails with no obvious cause. Examination of nail biopsy specimens may therefore rule out lichen planus with its distinctive features and psoriasis restricted to the nails. Braun-Falco *et al.* (1981) reported spongiotic dermatitis of the nail matrix and the nail bed with column-like parakeratosis within the nail in trachyonychia, due to alopecia areata, atopic dermatitis and the idiopathic form. In those subjects with no obvious cause and histological evidence of eczematous changes, alopecia areata has occured in some cases. Jerasutus *et al.* (1990) studied five cases, the youngest being 15 years old. All histological sections showed distinctive changes of spongiotic inflammation of the nail matrix, suggesting they either represent a subgroup of antigenous eczema or an autoimmunological response to the matrix. Tosti *et al.* (1991) found in 11 patients that a mild to moderate lymphocytic infiltration associated with exocytosis and spongiosis is the histological hallmark of trachyonychia due to alopecia areata.

Localized nail surface changes, or splits, may be combined with lichen striatus. Whilst having trachyonychia as one of the possible features, the causal diagnosis can usually be made on clinical grounds because of the associated verrucous lichenoid rash (Samman 1968). However, this is not universally present and an isolated split or surface change on the margin of one nail or two adjacent nails in a child or adolescent should suggest the diagnosis of lichen striatus with a good prognosis for complete resolution, usually within 12 months (Tosti *et al.* 1997).

We believe that the term 'twenty-nail dystrophy' has no specific significance. It is more useful clinically to describe the morphological appearance, such as roughness and ridging, and to examine nail biopsy specimens if possible to clarify the pathogenesis. This point is underlined by the histological study carried out by Tosti, where 23 cases of idiopathic trachyonychia were biopsied yielding a cross-section of results including the histology of psoriasis, lichen planus and the spongiotic histology associated with the classic autoimmune variant of the disease (Tosti *et al.* 1994b). Since the term has come to include such a wide variety of conditions that affect all 20 nails, it has lost its diagnostic value and should therefore be discarded.

## References

Achten, G. & Wanet-Rouard, J. (1974) Atrophie unguéale et trachyonychie. *Archive Belges de Dermatologie* 30, 201–207.

Alkiewicz, J. (1950) Trachyonychie. *Annales de Dermatologie et de Syphiligraphie* 10, 136–140.

Arias, A.M., Yung, C.W., Rendler, S. *et al.* (1982) Familial severe twenty-nail dystrophy. *Journal of the American Academy of Dermatology* 7, 349–352.

Baran, R. (1981) Twenty nail dystrophy of alopecia areata. *Archives of Dermatology* 117, 1.

Baran, R. & Dupré, A. (1977) Vertical striated sand paper nails. *Archives of Dermatology* 113, 1613.

Baran, R., Dupré, A., Christol, B. *et al.* (1978) L'ongle grésé peladique. *Annales de Dermatologie et de Vénéréologie* 105, 387–392.

Braun-Falco, O., Dorn, M., Neubert, U. *et al.* (1981) Trachyonychie: 20-Nägel-Dystrophie. *Hautzart* **32**, 17–22.

Brun, P., Baran, R. & Czernielewski, Y. (1984) Dystrophie lichénienne des 20 ongles. Manifestation possible d'une maladie du greffon contre l'hôte (MGCH) chronique par exsanguino transfusion néonatale? Presented at the annual 'Journées dermatologiques de Paris', March 1984.

Commens, C.A. (1988) Twenty-nail dystrophy in identical twins. *Pediatric Dermatology* **5**, 117–119.

Donofrio, P. & Ayala, F. (1984) Twenty-nail dystrophy: report of a case and review of the literature. *Acta Dermato-Venereologica* **64**, 180–182.

Fenton, D.A. & Samman, P.D. (1988) Twenty-nail dystrophy of childhood associated with alopecia areata and lichen planus. *British Journal of Dermatology* **119** (Suppl. 33), 63.

Hazelrigg, D.E., Duncan, W.C. & Jarrett, M. (1977) Twenty nail dystrophy of childhood. *Archives of Dermatology* **113**, 73–75.

Horn, R.T. & Odom, R.B. (1980) Twenty nail dystrophy of alopecia areata. *Archives of Dermatology* **116**, 573–574.

James, W.D., Odom, R.B. & Horn, R.T. (1981) Twenty nail dystrophy and ichythyosis vulgaris. *Archives of Dermatology* **117**, 316.

Jerasutus, S., Suvanprakorn, P. & Kitchawengkul, O. (1990) Twenty nail dystrophy. *Archives of Dermatology* **126**, 1068–1070.

Leong, A.B., Gange, R.W. & O'Connor, R.D. (1982) Twenty nail dystrophy (trachyonychia) associated with selective IgA deficiency. *Journal of Pediatrics* **100**, 418–420.

Pavone, L. (1982) Hereditary twenty nail dystrophy in a Sicilian family. *Journal of Medical Genetics* **19**, 131–135.

Person, J.R. (1984) Twenty-nail dystrophy: a hypothesis. *Archives of Dermatology* **120**, 437–438.

Runne, U. (1980) Twenty-nail dystrophy mit 'Knuckle pads'. *Zeitschrift für Hautkrankheiten* **55**, 901–902.

Samman, P.D. (1978) *The Nail in Disease*, pp. 178–184. William Heinmann, London.

Samman, P.D. (1968) Nail dystrophy and lichen striatus [abstract]. *Transactions of the St John Hospital Dermatology Society* **54**, 119.

Scher, R.K., Fischbein, R. & Ackerman, A.B. (1978) Twenty-nail dystrophy. A variant of lichen planus. *Archives of Dermatology* **114**, 612–613.

Silverman, R.A. & Rhodes, A.R. (1984) Twenty-nail dystrophy of childhood: a sign of localized lichen planus. *Pediatric Dermatology* **1**, 207–210.

Tosti, A., Fanti, P.A., Morelli, R. *et al.* (1991) Trachyonychia associated with alopecia areata: a clinical and pathologic study. *Journal of the American Academy of Dermatology* **25**, 266–270.

Tosti, A., Fanti, P.A., Morelli, R. *et al.* (1994a) Prevalence of nail abnormalities in children with alopecia areata. *Pediatic Dermatology* **11**, 112–115.

Tosti, A., Bardazzi, F., Piraccini, B.M. *et al.* (1994b) Idiopathic trachyonychia (twenty nail dystrophy): a pathological study of 23 patients. *British Journal of Dermatology* **131**, 866–872.

Tosti, A., Peluso, A.M., Misciali, C. *et al.* (1997) Nail lichen striatus: clinical features and long term follow up. *Journal of the American Academy of Dermatology* **36**, 908–913.

Wilkinson, J.D., Dawber, R.P.R., Bowers, R.P. *et al.* (1979) Twenty nail dystrophy of childhood. *British Journal of Dermatology* **100**, 217–221.

## Melanonychia in children (see also Chapter 11)

Longitudinal melanonychia (LM) (Fig. 3.17) in children is less common than it is in adults. In races, such as Afro-Carribbeans, where all adults gradually acquire pigmented streaks in the nail, it is still rare to see it in children under the age of 10. In other dark-skinned races, the same pattern is seen, with an increase of prevalence of melanonychia as a benign phenomenon with age. In Caucasians and less pigmented racial groups, the concern with a pigmented streak is that it may represent an early subungual melanoma. The likelihood of this in a child is remote, but cases have been reported. One concerned a 12-month-old boy, without LM (Lyall 1967), and another a child of 3 (Kiryu 1998). The need for matrix biopsy of childhood melanonychia is controversial (Baran 1993; Tosti *et al.* 1996), but it is possible that enlarging pigmented streaks will require tissue diagnosis.

In one study of four Japanese children, pigmentation of the nail plate presented in each of them between the age of 1 month and some time in the 2nd year of life. Histology was not obtained in any case and over the follow-up period of 3–11 years the pigment changed. In all nails there was a process of evolution and subsequent regression, although it is not clear whether the pigment disappeared completely; the clinical pattern was termed 'regressing naevoid nail melanosis in childhood' (Kikuchi *et al.* 1993). In a French series of longitudinal melanonychia in children, eight children between the ages of 2 and 14 were reported, in whom melanonychia had been noted at some point from birth up to 12 years of age (Léauté-Labrèze *et al.* 1996). Five had excisional biopsy of involved matrix revealing junctional naevi. Two were left with significant postoperative nail dystrophy. Three were followed with no biopsy and there was no clinical evolution. A similar finding was made in a larger Italian study where histology was obtained from 100 patients with isolated longitudinal melanonychia (Tosti *et al.* 1996). Twenty-two of 100 lesions had histology of melanocytic naevi. Eleven of the 22 were children under the age of 14 and no alternative diagnosis was made in this age group. In two children, the pigment was noted to have faded between the initial consultation and biopsy (Tosti *et al.* 1994). In a clinical and histopathological study of 40 cases of LM in children below 16 years of age, Goettmann-Bonvallot *et al.* (1999) found a lentigo in 12 cases, a naevus in 19 cases and functional LM in nine children.

The question remains as to whether pigmented streaks with benign histology in childhood become melanomas in adulthood. None of the five melanomas identified in Tosti's series of 100 longitudinal melanonychia were congenital, but their exact history is not defined. In conclusion, pigmented nail streaks in childhood should be biopsied and excised according to the same criteria as naevi elsewhere (Léauté-Labrèze *et al.* 1996). It will remain an area in which the clinician's judgement will be important and surveillance will play a large part in management.

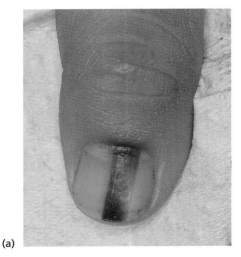

(a)

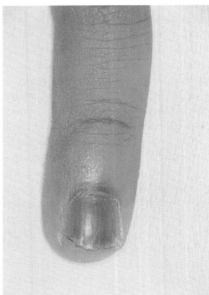

(b)

**Fig. 3.17** (a) Melanonychia in children. (b) Congenital melanonychia involving progressively the whole nail plate. (c) Congenital total melanonychia with pseudo-Hutchinson's sign.

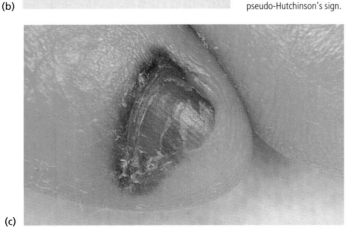

(c)

## References

Baran, R. (1993) Longitudinal melanonychia. *Dermatology* **186**, 83.

Goettmann-Bonvallot, S., André, J. & Belaich, S. (1999) Longitudinal melanonychia in children: a clinical and histopathologic study of 40 cases. *Journal of the American Academy of Dermatology* **41**, 17–22.

Kikuchi, I., Inoue, S., Sakaguchi. E. *et al.* (1993) Regressing nevoid nail melanosis in childhood. *Dermatology* **186**, 88–93.

Kiryu, H. (1998) Malignant melanoma *in situ* arising in the nail unit of a child. *Journal of Dermatology* **25**, 41–44.

Léauté-Labrèze, C., Bioulac-Sage, P. & Taïeb, A. (1996) Longitudinal melanonychia in children. A study of eight cases. *Archives of Dermatology* **132**, 167–169.

Lyall, D. (1967) Malignant melanoma in infancy. *Journal of the American Medical Association* **202**, 93.

Tosti, A., Baran, R., Morelli, R. *et al.* (1994) Progressive fading of a longitudinal melanonychia due to a nail matrix melanocytic naevus in a child. *Archives of Dermatology* **130**, 1076–1077.

Tosti A., Baran, R., Piraccini, B.M. *et al.* (1996) Nail matrix naevi: a clinical and histopathologic study of twenty two patients. *Journal of the American Academy of Dermatology* **34**, 765–771.

## Ingrowing toenail in infancy

There are five kinds of ingrowing toenail in infancy (Baran 1989a): (a) congenital hypertrophic lip of the hallux; (b) distal embedding with normally directed nail; (c) distal lateral embedding; (d) congenital malalignment of the big toenail; and (e) overcurvature of the nails.

Two peaks are observed: 0–3 years and 9–13 years. The ratio of males to females is more than 2 : 1.

Infantile ingrowing toenails may have a congenital origin or may result from acquired factors (Table 3.2).

### Congenital hypertrophic lip of the hallux (Fig. 3.18)

When they appear at birth, hypertrophic lateral nail folds are generally bilateral and symmetrical, affecting most often the medial nail fold of the hallux. They present as firm, red tender swellings (Piraccini *et al.* 2000). They enlarge progressively, sometimes covering one-third of the nail plate (Hammerton & Shrank 1988). They may be the result of asynchronism between the growth of the soft tissue and the nail, the hypertrophic lat-

**Table 3.2** Aetiology of ingrowing toenails in infancy.

Infantile ingrowing toenails may have:
 Intrauterine position
 Inherited factors
 Normal variations in the development of the great toes

Acquired factors:
 Prone position
 Constricting garments
 Unsuitable shoes
 Improper nail care

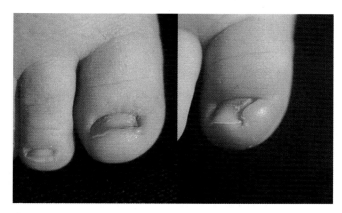

**Fig. 3.18** Congenital hypertrophic lip of the hallux.

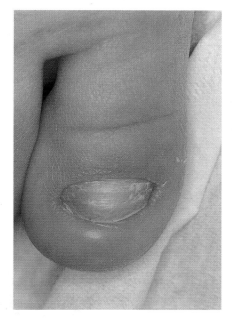

**Fig. 3.19** Distal embedding with normally directed nail.

ingrowing, and prevents the free margin of the nail from growing normally. The deformity produced by congenital hypertrophy of the distal soft tissue may sometimes be aggravated by acquired factors, such as the habit of sleeping prone in infancy (Bailie & Evans 1978). The changes in the toenail occur at the time when the child starts kicking actively and is subjected to tight-fitting clothing (jumpsuits of stretchable material) or tight shoes (Bird 1978; Walker 1979). If the big toenail is normally orientated, proper growth will be re-established by the age of 6 months in most cases, despite the previous barrier of distal tissue (Honig *et al.* 1982).

### Distal–lateral nail embedding (Fig. 3.20)

Careless cutting may leave a spicule of nail which penetrates the lateral nail fold as the nail grows forwards.

If there is excess of granulation tissue it is useful to alternate Mycolog ointment (Tri-Adcortyl) in the morning, and shaving soap in the evening, under occlusion (Blenderm tape) (Baran 1989a). In resistant cases, after paring down granulation tissue, intralesional triamcinolone (5 mg/mL) may be injected into the swollen region, in addition to systemic antibiotic therapy. A chlorhexidine-soaked cotton wool pledget introduced beneath

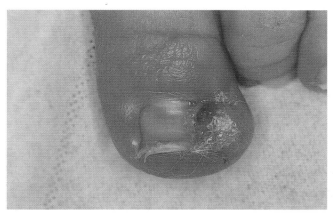

(a)

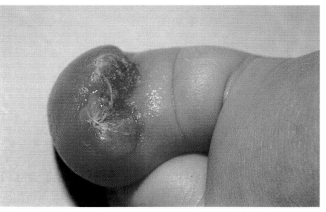

(b)

**Fig. 3.20** (a) Distal–lateral nail embedding. (b) Distal–lateral nail embedding with marked paronychia.

eral lip growing faster than the nail plate, leading to ingrowing, with pain, which increases when walking begins (Martinet *et al.* 1984). This condition, which resembles recurring digital fibrous tumour of childhood (and might be called pseudodigital fibrous tumour of the hallux), usually disappears spontaneously after several months.

### Distal embedding with normally directed nail (Fig. 3.19)

This condition should be distinguished from the ingrowing appearance of the nails of premature infants and some term infants which may be shorter than the distal digital pulp (Silverman 1990).

The infantile type of ingrowing toenail presents a rim of tissue at the distal edge of the nail and some hypertrophy of the lateral nail fold. This prominent ridge of skin at the extremity of the big toe forms an anterior nail wall, which encourages the nail plate, under general anaesthesia, has been advocated (Connolly & Fitzgerald 1988).

Paronychia must be treated conservatively. The infecting organisms should be cultured and tested for antibacterial sensitivity. Local treatment is by twice-daily application of antiseptics (Hibitane) and shaving soap covered with non-adherent gauze, such as Telfa. Systemic antibiotics appropriate to the laboratory results can be added, if necessary.

In those rare cases where permanent improvement has not been obtained by 10–12 months of age (Hendricks 1979; Bentley-Phillips & Coll 1983; Engels 1985), a circular or semicircular soft tissue resection should be performed, after X-ray has ruled out a subungual exostosis.

### Congenital malalignment of the big toenail (Fig. 3.21)

In 1978, Samman described several cases of a 'dystrophy' limited to one or both great toenails. Baran *et al.* (1979) termed this 'congenital malalignment of the big toenail'; placing the emphasis on the main characteristic of this condition the nail plate is deviated laterally with respect to the longitudinal axis of the distal phalanx. Medial deviation is rare, but possible (Baran & Bureau 1987).

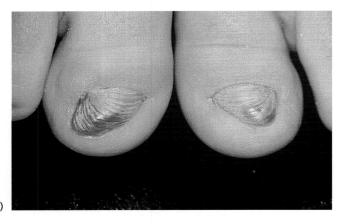

(a)

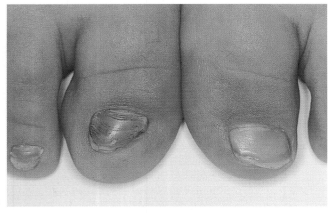

(b)

**Fig. 3.21** (a) Bilateral congenital malalignment of the big toenail. (b) Unilateral congenital malalignment.

Transverse ridging, which may be single or more often multiple, is one of the earliest signs to appear and may develop over the entire surface of the nail plate (Baran 1980). The ridges form regular waves when they are numerous. They seem to follow recurrent episodes of damage to the matrix, sometimes leading to latent onychomadesis or shedding of a large portion of the nail; the new nail is already well advanced before the old is lost.

The nail plate may be thickened with gradual tapering of the distal portion. Sometimes there is associated onycholysis, and the nail may acquire a greyish tint, a brown discoloration (due to a haemorrhage) or a greenish hue (which is due to *Pseudomonas*). This would be of minor importance if it were not for the complications that may arise both in infancy as ingrowing toenail (Baran & Bureau 1983), even congenitally (Katz 1996) as well as in the elderly (hemionychogryphosis).

The most important complication is ingrowing toenail with painful inflammation of part of the perionychial area. At this stage examination may show a nail which is short, pressing against a rim of skin at the extreme tip of the big toe and forming a lip. Primary malalignment of the nail appears then to be the main factor causing the 'nail embedding'. Because the main direction of nail growth in these patients occurs laterally, there is insufficient forward thrust to allow the nail plate to mount the heaped-up tissue in front of it, even when physiological koilonychia exists (Baran *et al.* 1979; Baran 1980; Baran & Bureau 1983). At this stage a simple surgical procedure successfully realigns the whole nail apparatus (Chapter 10) (Fig. 3.21b). The best results are obtained when the malalignment is corrected surgically before the age of 2 years (Baran 1989a,b), but we have obtained good results even in adulthood. Spontaneous improvement (Dawson 1979, 1982, 1989; Handfield-Jones & Harman 1988; Baran 1989b), or even complete resolution occurs in less than 50% of patients under 10 years of age. Careful examination of the posterolateral corner of the affected nails may reveal a bulge in some; therefore we postulate that it could result from traction upon the nail plate by the thickened dorsal expansion of the lateral ligament at the distal interphalangeal joint described by Guéro *et al.* (1994) and demonstrated on magnetic resonance imaging (MRI).

Management must depend on accurate assessment of the degree of malalignment and the associated changes (Baran 1985), since it appears impossible to foresee spontaneous realignment (Baran *et al.* 1998):

1 If the nail deviation is mild, and in the absence of complications, the nail, as it hardens, may overcome the initial slight distal embedding, and sufficient normal nail may grow to the tip of the digit to prevent further secondary traumatic changes. Treatment should be conservative.

2 If the deviation is marked and the nail is buried in the soft tissues, the patient may be disabled later on, in childhood and in adult life. Surgical rotation of the misdirected matrix (Chapter 10), usually associated with the simple section of the dorsal expansion of the lateral ligament (Baran *et al.* 1998), is then

essential in order to prevent permanent nail dystrophy, despite the possibly favourable course of some cases.

Congenital malalignment of the great toenail is an inherited condition (Barth *et al.* 1986; Harper & Beer 1986) and the 'inherited nail dystrophy principally affecting the great toenails over 3 generations' (Dawson 1979) pertains to the same dysplasia.

## Overcurvature of the nails

In this normally congenital deformity, the lateral borders of the nail plate extend down into the lateral nail grooves giving them a plicated appearance (Chapman 1973). Onset of this inherited disorder is always in the teens or early twenties.

## References

Bailie, F.B. & Evans, D.M. (1978) Ingrowing toenails in infancy. *British Medical Journal* 2, 737–738.

Baran, R. (1980) Congenital malalignment of toenail. *Archives of Dermatology* 116, 1346.

Baran, R. (1985) An inherited nail dystrophy principally affecting the great toenails [letter]. *British Journal of Dermatology* 112, 124.

Baran, R. (1989a) The treatment of ingrowing toenails in infancy. *Journal of Dermatologic Treatment* 1, 55–57.

Baran, R. (1989b) Great toenail dystrophy. *British Journal of Dermatology* 120, 139–140.

Baran, R. & Bureau, H. (1983) Congenital malalignment of the big toenail as a cause of ingrowing toenail in infancy. Pathology and treatment (a study of thirty cases). *Clinical and Experimental Dermatology* 8, 619–623.

Baran, R. & Bureau, H. (1987) Congenital malalignment of the big toenail. A new subtype [letter]. *Archives of Dermatology* 123, 437.

Baran, R., Bureau, H. & Sayag, J. (1979) Congenital malalignment of the toenail. *Clinical and Experimental Dermatology* 4, 359–360.

Baran, R., Grognard, C., Duhard, E. & Drapé, J.L. (1998) Congenital malalignment of the great toenail. An enigma resolved by a new surgical treatment. *British Journal of Dermatology* 139 (Suppl. 51), 72.

Barth, J.H., Dawber, R.P.R., Ashton, R.E. *et al.* (1986) Congenital malalignment of great toenails in two sets of monozygotic twins. *Archives of Dermatology* 122, 379–380.

Bentley-Phillips, B. & Coll, I. (1983) Ingrowing toenail in infancy. *International Journal of Dermatology* 22, 115–116.

Bird, S. (1978) Trouble with children's feet [letter]. *British Medical Journal* 4, 1297.

Chapman, R.S. (1973) Overcurvature of the nails: an inherited disorder. *British Journal of Dermatology* 89, 317–318.

Connolly, B. & Fitzgerald, R.J. (1988) Pledgets in ingrowing toenails. *Archives of Disease in Childhood* 63, 71–72.

Dawson, T.A.J. (1979) An inherited nail dystrophy principally affecting the great toenails. *Clinical and Experimental Dermatology* 4, 309–313.

Dawson, T.A.J. (1982) An inherited nail dystrophy principally affecting the great toenails; further observations. *Clinical and Experimental Dermatology* 7, 455–457.

Dawson, T.A.J. (1989) Great toenail dystrophy [letter]. *British Journal of Dermatology* 20, 139.

Engels, M. (1985) Nagelbettveänderungen im Neugeborenalter. *Pädiatrie und Pädologie* 20, 173–176.

Guéro, S., Guichard, S. & Freitag, S.R. (1994) Ligamentary structure of the base of the nail. *Surgical and Radiologic Anatomy* 16, 47–52.

Hammerton, M.D. & Shrank, A.B. (1988) Congenital hypertrophy of the lateral nail folds of the hallux. *Pediatric Dermatology* 5, 243–245.

Handfield-Jones, S.E. & Harman, R.R.M. (1988) Spontaneous improvement of the congenital malalignment of the great toenails [letter]. *British Journal of Dermatology* 118, 305–306.

Harper, K.J. & Beer, W.E. (1986) Congenital malalignment of the great toenails—an inherited condition. *Clinical and Experimental Dermatology* 11, 514–516.

Hendricks, W.M. (1979) Congenital ingrowing toenails. *Cutis* 24, 393–394.

Honig, P.J., Spitzer, A., Bernstein, R. *et al.* (1982) Congenital ingrown toenails. *Clinical Pediatrics* 21, 424–426.

Katz, A.M. (1996) Congenital ingrown toenails. *Journal of the American Academy of Dermatology* 34, 519–520.

Martinet, C., Pascal, M., Civatte, J. *et al.* (1984) Bourrelet latéro-unguéal du gros orteil du nourrisson. *Annales de Dermatologie et de Vénéréologie* 111, 731–733.

Piraccini, B.M., Parente, G.L., Varotti, E. *et al.* (2000) Congenital hypertrophy of the lateral nail folds of the hallux: clinical features and follow-up of seven cases. *Pediatric Dermatology* 17, 348–351.

Samman, P.D. (1978) Great toenail dystrophy. *Clinical and Experimental Dermatology* 3, 81–82.

Silverman, R.A. (1990) Pediatric disease. In: *Nails: Therapy, Diagnosis, Surgery* (eds R.K. Scher & C.R. Daniel), pp. 82–105. W.B. Saunders, Philadelphia.

Walker, S. (1979) Paronychia of the great toe of infants. *Clinical Pediatrics* 18, 247.

# THE NAIL IN OLD AGE

The elderly constitute a large and rapidly growing segment of the population (Beauregard & Gilchrest 1987). Some nail diseases exhibit a predilection for the aged or show a varying frequency of incidence with age (Baran & Dawber 1985). Some anomalies may persist from an earlier age but are modified by advancing years. Underlying pathology may worsen with the superimposition of degenerative changes, altered vascular supply and reduced capacity for tissue repair. The foot demonstrates the cumulative effects of trauma and mechanical distortion which usually result in thickened nails and a disposition to onychomycosis. These problems are of increasing relevance as elderly people undertake more sport in addition to the normal requirements of mobility (Gordon & Cuttic 1994). Changes in the hands are more related to diminished tissue repair and inflammatory or degenerative changes of the distal interphalangeal joint. These influences are associated with reduced rate of longitudinal nail growth, thinning of the nail plate and accentuation of longitudinal ridges, particularly noted in those with rheumatoid arthritis (Cribier *et al.* 1997).

In elderly people, distinctive changes may be noted in the nails (Baran 1982; Cohen & Scher 1992). In the foot 1st and 5th digits are involved. The nail is heaped up as a result of pressure from each side. Excessive chronic pressure may cause loss of normal lateral nail grooves and matrix distortion, subungual keratosis, onychophosis (keratotic nail grooves) and ulceration (Helfand 1989). These conditions, which can be extremely painful, may reduce stability and limit ambulation and require continuing management for relief. However, careful evaluation will often identify the cause as an anatomical or dynamic abnormality reflected in abnormal gait and resulting in repeated microtrauma (Gilchrist 1979).

Hallux valgus and overlapping toes may require moulded shoes to provide adequate shoe fit, they relieve pressure and deformed joints, distribute pressure evenly over the foot and provide comfort (Gilchrist 1979). The use of protective padding may be indicated (Baran & Dawber 1985).

Unfortunately some elderly subjects have difficulty reaching their feet, some others find their nails too thick to cut, and finally they may be deterred by poor vision (Beauregard & Gilchrest 1987). Periodic treatment should be given to relieve pain and there may be a role for specialized nursing care in the elderly with expertise in foot problems (Bryant 1995).

## Aetiology of senile changes

Senile changes may be attributed in part to arteriosclerosis even without gross evidence of obliteration of the vessel. The ability of an extremity to withstand trauma is severely limited when arterial insufficiency is present. Although a pulseless foot may have an adequate collateral circulation for ordinary metabolic demands, any break in the skin can lead to gangrene and amputation because the increased requirement for blood flow cannot be met (Bakow & Friedman 1969). All these factors, associated with the dangers to the foot that they entail, combine to make chronic infection of the foot a major problem (Tarara 1970). The histological study of Lewis and Montgomery (1955) bears out this concept, because at least minimal thickening of the

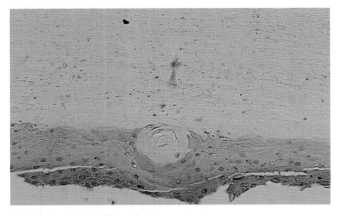

**Fig. 3.22** Pertinax body of the nail apparatus.

walls of the blood vessels was present in the nail generative areas. Alterations in elastic tissue are prominent and more diffuse in the dermis beneath the pink nail bed, and more pronounced than they are in the adjacent, glabrous perionychial skin. The change in elastic tissue, present to a lesser degree beneath the lunula, is absent from the dermis of the matrix area which is covered by the proximal nail fold. However, the whole subungual area may show thickening of the walls of blood vessels and reveal fragmentation of their elastic tissue. Parker and Diffey (1983) suggest that the nail plate acts as a very efficient sunscreen, with very low transmission in the damaging UV B range (280–315 nm). The nail plate contains an increased number of 'pertinax bodies' as compared with the normal adult nail (Fig. 3.22). They could be interpreted as remnants of nuclei of keratinocytes. Retarded nail plate growth results in larger corneocytes (Germann et al. 1980).

## Linear nail growth

Thumbnail growth measured by Orentreich and Scharp (1967) in 257 individuals decreased by an average of 38% from the 3rd to the 9th decade. The decrease was greater in females up to the 6th decade. Subsequently, no further decrease occurred until the 8th decade, by which time the rate for males decreased more rapidly. Bean (1980) observed that the average daily growth of his left thumb nail decreased from 0.123 mm a day at 32 to 0.095 mm a day at 67 years of age. Alternating 7-year cycles of constant growth rate with 7-year periods of marked decline in nail growth have been suggested (Orentreich et al. 1979). Underlying factors which may influence the rate of decline are actinic effects on the nail matrix, circulatory impairment, nutritional deficiency, hormonal changes, and local and systemic infections. Other factors may also be important (Chapter 1). According to Orentreich et al. (1979) the determination of the rate of linear nail growth may prove a useful measurement of physiological ageing.

## Variations in the contour of the nail

The normal nail plate has a double curvature, longitudinal and transverse. Modifications of the contour in old age include platonychia (flattening) and koilonychia (spooning). Most typically the convexity is increased from side to side and decreased in the longitudinal axis. 'Watch glass' nails and true clubbing are frequent in men affected by chronic pulmonary disease (Tammaro & Lampugnani 1969). The longitudinal ridges become more pronounced and numerous (Fig. 3.23). This could be due to variations in the turnover rate of the matrix cells or may be related to whorls of generative cells in the most proximal region of the nail matrix.

## Variations in the colour

Distinctive changes are noted in the nails in elderly subjects.

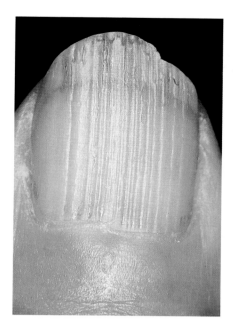

**Fig. 3.23** Longitudinal ridges—age related.

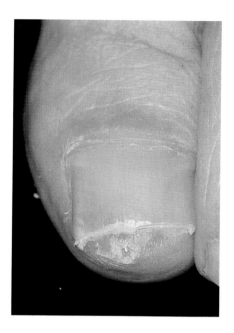

**Fig. 3.24** Distal subungual heloma.

Macroscopically, the nails appear dull and opaque. The colour varies from shades of yellow to grey. Frequently, the lunula is not visible. The white nails of old age, similar to those reported in cirrhosis, azotaemia and hypoalbuminaemia, have been termed 'neapolitan nails' because of the three bands as in neapolitan ice cream (Horan *et al.* 1982). These white changes occur without detectable protein, liver or kidney abnormalities. Nail bed capillaries show frequent distortions in normal subjects over 70 years of age, including numerous short tortuous capillary loops, and the subpapillary venous plexus is ill defined. These capillary distortions may explain the frequency in the distal one-third of splinter haemorrhages in the elderly, favoured by trauma to the nails such as the use of walking aids and intake of multiple drugs besides anticoagulants. The latter are often responsible for subungual haematomas especially in the feet, but idiopathic subungual haemorrhages are also common in patients with diabetes mellitus, chronic renal disease or recent stroke (Helfand 1989). Nevertheless, splinters appear less commonly in the elderly than in young people and represent an unhelped physical sign in the elderly (Young & Mulley 1987).

Acral arteriolar ectasia (Paslin & Heaton 1972) is a distinct vascular malformation consisting of purple serpiginous vessels on the dorsa of the digits, first arising in the 5th decade of life. The vessels are ectatic arterioles and are believed to represent a rare vascular malformation.

## Variations in thickness and consistency

The thickness of the plate may be normal, increased or decreased. The fingernail is often soft and fragile, prone to longitudinal fissuring and splitting into layers. Therefore, hands should be protected by cotton gloves during housework or

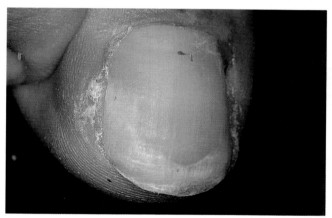

**Fig. 3.25** Onychophosis involving the lateral nail groove.

other occupations. Gloves are more comfortable worn inside out with the seams on the outside. The fingernail should never be used as a 'tool', crude traumatic tasks being done with 'finger pads' for 'finger chores'.

The toenail is usually thicker and harder with hyperkeratotic lesions in the toenail region. These are often present for several years before treatment is sought. The most common toenail deformities are hypertrophy, associated with chronic fungal infection, onychogryphosis and ingrowing toenail as residua of previous disease, trauma or deformity of adult life or childhood (Jahss 1979). Ill-fitting shoes can be the cause of onycholysis (Fig. 3.24) and the development of hyperkeratotic tissue in varying degrees on the periungual folds or in the lateral nail grooves in response to repeated minor trauma. This condition, which may be diffuse or localized as a corn, is called onychophosis (Fig. 3.25). Repeated minor trauma may produce a

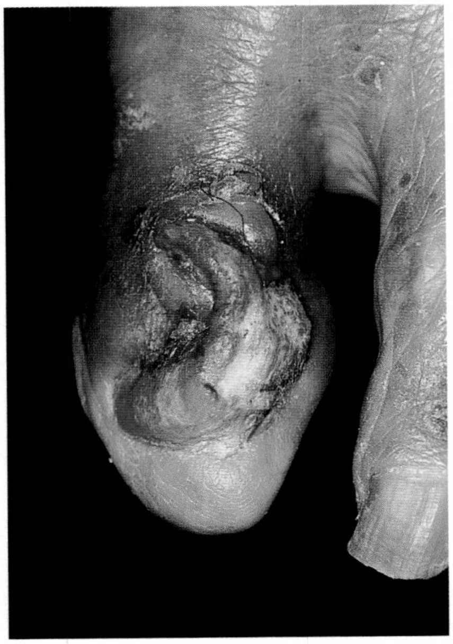

**Fig. 3.26**
Onychogryphosis
associated with ulceration
of the proximal nail fold.
(Courtesy of C. Ohata,
Japan.)

subungual corn (heloma or onychoclavus) of the distal nail bed (Fig. 3.26). Typically the corn affects the great toe and appears as a painful dark spot under the nail (Gilchrist 1979) resembling a foreign body. Treatment of subungual onychoclavus consists of removing a section of the nail and excising the hyperkeratotic tissue. In lesser toes a corn occurs under the pulp of hammertoe below the nail tip.

Onychogryphosis (Chapter 2) may interfere with shoe comfort. Hemionychogryphosis with lateral deviation of the nail plate results from congenital malalignment of the big toenail.

Although a pulseless foot may have adequate collateral circulation for ordinary metabolic needs, gangrene may supervene if minor trauma and secondary infection occurs (Bakow & Friedman 1969).

## Mechanical factors and nail changes

Hallux valgus is seen predominantly in females. It is an acquired deformity, often secondary to ill-fitting shoes, but it can also be induced by congenital, anatomical factors. It is a medial laxity of the metatarso-sesamoido-phalangeal joint with lateral dislocation or subdislocation of the sesamoid bones. The latter is maintained by a lateral retraction which is aggravated by the motor muscles of the big toe, whose action is towards valgus due to the natural angulation (Groulier 1981).

The influence of hallux valgus on the corresponding big toenail has been stressed by Fabry (1983). Progressive lateral deviation of the big toenail appears with lateral overcurvature of the nail plate.

Hammer toe is a deformity arising through increased extension at the metacarpophalangeal joint and corresponding flexion at the proximal interpahalangeal joint. In the extreme form the tip of the digit is directed downwards and develops a callous associated with thickening of the nail plate and distal nail bed. This is called a claw deformity. These abnormalities may arise due to inflammatory joint disease and are manifestations of imbalanced forces within the foot. They can be painful and may require treatment. This is available with wedges, splints, padding and modified footwear. Such conservative therapies are likely to provide relief in the majority of cases (Moraros & Hodge 1993; Gordon & Cuttic 1994). Surgical treatment may involve arthrodesis (Ohm *et al.* 1990), silicone implants (Shaw & Alvarez 1992) or phalangectomy (Newman & Fitton 1979).

## Ingrowing toenail (see also Chapter 11)

Ingrowing toenail represents an inflammation of the lateral nail folds due to the intrusion of the adjacent margin of the nail plate. Improper cutting and pressure from ill-fitting footwear are probably the major factors in the elderly. In addition, blunt or sharp protuberance of the distal tuft, mainly associated with pincer nails, results from an abnormal positional relationship between the 1st metatarsal and the hallux (Lemont & Christman 1990). Although troublesome, an ingrowing nail is usually only an inconvenience to the average sufferer. However, in an old person with impaired arterial circulation an ingrowing nail may become a serious problem, since infection and gangrene may supervene.

Three major types characterize this common problem sometimes complicated by onychomycosis:
1 Overcurvature of the nail plate (pincer nail, onychocryptosis);
2 Subcutaneous ingrowing toenail;
3 Hypertrophy of the lateral nail fold.

## Tumours in the nail area

The relative frequency of benign and malignant tumours in this area varies with age.

Myxoid pseudocysts (mucous cysts, periungual ganglion) are probably the commonest benign tumour. They occur more commonly in women. The commonest site is on the proximal nail fold of the fingers and only rarely on the toes. The lesions are usually asymptomatic, varying from soft to firm, cystic to fluctuant. Longitudinal nail grooving may result from pressure on the matrix. Clinical signs of degenerative arthritis and Heberden's nodes are associated in about 15% of cases, radiologically the majority show terminal interphalangeal joint osteoarthritis—'wear and tear' arthritis.

Carcinoma of the nail apparatus is not uncommon; about 150 cases have been reported in the literature. In a series of 58 cases of subungual epidermoid carcinoma, Attieh *et al.* (1979) reported 46 cases in the age range 50–79 years, with a peak incidence in the 7th decade. The initial manifestations of Bowen's disease and squamous cell carcinoma are difficult to differentiate in this area; there may be localized pain, swelling and inflammation. Because of the many chronic conditions which affect this region, a high index of suspicion is required for the early detection of carcinoma. A biopsy is necessary in order to confirm the diagnosis.

Patterson and Helwig (1980) reported 66 cases of subungual melanomas; 53% were found on the foot, 98% of these occurring on the big toe. Of these patients, 70% were aged between 50 and 80 years, with a peak incidence being in the 8th decade.

Although the majority of lesions in the nail area are inflammatory, infective or due to congenital or acquired deformity, neoplasia must be considered in the differential diagnosis of localized and chronic inflammatory conditions.

## Nail fungal infection

Hyperkeratosis, especially beneath the nail, may occur primarily or secondary to fungal infection of the skin. In either case, ultimately several nails become infected, particularly toenails. Chronic paronychia is related to complicating factors, such as peripheral vascular insufficiency and diabetes mellitus. The toenails often become thickened to such a degree that the wearing of shoes may trigger pain.

English and Atkinson (1974) carried out fungal examinations for onychomycosis on the thickened toenail of 168 patients attending a chiropody clinic for old age pensioners. The nails of 68 (41%) of the patients were microscopically positive. Cultures from 12% of these were negative. Of the remainder, 20 (12%) were infected by dermatophytes and 42 (25%) by non-dermatophytes. Fungi and especially non-dermatophytes (Achten et al. 1979; de Gentile et al. 1995) have a predilection for the big toenail, especially in people over the age of 60. Environmental conditions, peripheral vascular insufficiency (arterial, venous and lymphatic), orthopaedic defects (e.g. overriding of the toes) or onychogryphosis (Higashi & Matsumura 1988) may be the cause of this site preference.

The importance of onychomycosis of the toenails in the elderly is unclear and it is argued that it may contribute to reduced mobility and have a distinct morbidity in contrast with the same condition in earlier life (Scher 1996). It appears to be common in Western countries; a Finnish prevalence study revealed that 18% of people over the age of 58 examined for onychomycosis had microscopy and culture positive fungal nail infection (Heikkilä & Stubb 1995). How much this arises because of pre-existing nail dystrophy and how much the infection contributes to physical distortion is an unanswered question. There is no data on relief of symptoms in this age group brought about by treatment of onychomycosis, although all clinicians will have experience of individual patients who have found it more easy to walk once their fungal infection has been treated. Studies on the impact of onychomycosis on quality of life illustrate that most aspects of foot discomfort or nail care inconvenience are greater in those with onychomycosis when compared to disease-free controls. However, in all respects, the majority of those with onychomycosis deemed their problem to be 'insignificant' (Whittam & Hay 1997).

The management of onychomycosis in the elderly may include no therapy, palliative treatment with mechanical or chemical debridement, topical antifungal therapy (nail lacquers), new oral antifungal agents or a combination of treatment modalities (Gupta 2000). Combination therapy is our first line choice.

## References

Achten, G., Wanet-Rouard, J., Wiame, L. et al. (1979) Les onychomycoses à moisissures. Dermatologica 159 (Suppl. 1), 128.

Attieh, F.F., Shah, J., Booher, R.J. et al. (1979) Subungual squamous cell carcinoma. Journal of the American Medical Association 241, 262–263.

Bakow, R.B. & Friedman, S.A. (1969) The significance of trophic foot changes in the aged. Geriatrics 11, 135–139.

Baran, R. (1982) Nail care in the 'golden years' of life. Current Medical Research Opinion 7 (Suppl. 2), 96.

Baran, R. & Dawber, R.P.R. (1985) The ageing nail. In: Skin Problems in the Elderly (ed. L. Fry), pp. 315–330. Churchill Livingstone, Edinburgh.

Beauregard, S. & Gilchrest, B.A. (1987) A survey of skin problems and skin care regimens in the elderly. Archives of Dermatology 123, 1638–1643.

Bean, W.B. (1980) Nail growth: thirty-five years of observations. Archives of Internal Medicine 140, 73.

Bryant, J.L. (1995) Preventive foot care program: a nursing perspective. Ostomy Wound Management 41, 28–34.

Cohen, P.R. & Scher, R.K. (1992) Geriatric nail disorders: diagnosis and treatment. Journal of the American Academy of Dermatology 26, 521–531.

Cribier, B., Sibilia, J., Kuntz, J.L. et al. (1997) Nail abnormalities in rheumatoid arthritis. British Journal of Dermatology 137, 958–962.

English, M.P. & Atkinson, R. (1974) Onychomycosis in elderly chiropody patients. British Journal of Dermatology 91, 67.

Fabry, H. (1983) Haut- und Nagelveränderungen bei Hallux valgus. Aktuelle Dermatologie 9, 77–79.

de Gentile, L., Bouchara, J.P. & Le Clech, C. (1995) Prevalence of Candida ciferrii in elderly patients with trophic disorders of the legs. Mycopathologia 131, 99–102.

Germann, H., Barran, W. & Plewig, G. (1980) Morphology of corneocytes from human nail plates. Journal of Investigative Dermatology 74, 115–118.

Gilchrist, A.K. (1979) Common foot problems in the elderly. Geriatrics 34, 67–70.

Gordon, G.M. & Cuttic, M.M. (1994) Exercise and the aging foot. Southern Medical Journal 87, S36–S41.

Groulier, P. (1981) Hallux valgus—hallux rigidus. Revue Praticien 31, 1031–1032.

Gupta, A.K. (2000) Onychomycosis in the elderly. Drugs and Aging 16, 397–407.

Heikkilä, H & Stubb, S. (1995) The prevalence of onychomycosis in Finland. British Journal of Dermatology 133, 699–703.

Helfand, A.E. (1989) Nail and hyperkeratotic problems in the elderly foot. American Family Physician 39, 101–110.

Higashi, N. & Matsumura, T. (1988) The aetiology of onychogryphosis of the great toenail and of ingrowing nail. Hifu 30, 620–623.

Horan, M.A., Puxly, J.A. & Fox, R.A. (1982) The white nails of old age (Neapolitan nails). *Journal of the American Geriatric Society* **30**, 734–737.

Lemont, H. & Christman, R.A. (1990) Subungual exostosis and nail disease and radiologic aspects. In: *Nails: Therapy, Diagnosis, Surgery* (eds R.K. Scher & C.R. Daniel), pp. 250–257. W.B. Saunders, Philadelphia.

Lewis, B. & Montgomery, H. (1955) The senile nail. *Journal of Investigative Dermatology* **24**, 11.

Moraros, J. & Hodge, W. (1993) Orthotic survey. Preliminary results. *Journal of the American Podiatric Medical Association* **83**, 139–148.

Newman, R.J. & Fitton, J.M. (1979) An evaluation of operative procedures in the treatment of hammer toe. *Acta Orthopaedica Scandinavica* **50**, 709–712.

Ohm, O.W., McDonell, M. & Vetter, W.A. (1990) Digital arthrodesis: an alternate method for correction of hammer toe deformity. *Journal of Foot Surgery* **29**, 207–211.

Orentreich, N. & Scharp, N.J. (1967) Keratine replacement as an ageing parameter. *Journal of the Society of Cosmetic Chemistry* **18**, 537–547.

Orentreich, N., Markofsky, J. & Vogelman, J.H. (1979) The effect of ageing on the rate of linear nail growth. *Journal of Investigative Dermatology* **73**, 126–130.

Parker, S.G. & Diffey, B.L. (1983) The transmission of optical radiation through human nails. *British Journal of Dermatology* **108**, 11.

Paslin, D.A. & Heaton, C.L. (1972) Acral arteriolar ectasia. *Archives of Dermatology* **106**, 906–908.

Patterson, G. & Helwig, C. (1980) Subungual melanoma. *Cancer* **46**, 2074–2087.

Scher, R.K. (1996) Onychomycosis: a significant medical disorder. *Journal of the American Academy of Dermatology* **35**, S2–S5.

Shaw, A.H. & Alvarez, G. (1992) The use of digital implants for the correction of hammer toe deformity and their potential complications and management. *Journal of Foot Surgery* **31**, 63–74.

Tammaro, A.E. & Lampugnani, P. (1969) Studio del complesso ungueale nell'età senile. *Minerva Medica* **60**, 3651–3655.

Tarara, E.L. (1970) Ingrown toenail: a problem among the aged. *Postgraduate Medicine* **47**, 199–202.

Whittam, L.R. & Hay, R.J. (1997) The impact of onychomycosis on quality of life. *Clinical and Experimental Dermatology* **22**, 87–89.

Young, J. & Mulley, G. (1987) Splinter haemorrhages in the elderly. *Age and Ageing* **16**, 101–104.

# CHAPTER 4

# Fungal (onychomycosis) and other infections involving the nail apparatus

**R.J. Hay, R. Baran & E. Haneke**

In this chapter the onychomycoses are considered in detail, together with a variety of infections occasionally seen in and around the nail apparatus; some infections (see chapter contents above) are discussed, where appropriate, in other chapters.

Onychomycoses occur throughout the world but there are regional differences in incidence. Precise data as to their prevalence have only recently become available and the results again vary from country to country (Baran *et al.* 1999). The results also vary with the method of calculation of the prevalences. For instance Roberts (1992) found that by using a photographic identification method in randomly selected individuals, about 2.3% of subjects in the UK had changes in their nails compatible with onychomycosis. However, larger numbers have been found by direct examination of populations attending dermatologists in the USA and in Finland. Specific groups such as diabetics have also been found to have a higher prevalence than normal individuals (Gupta *et al.* 1998a). Sociocultural and occupational factors play an important part in the increase as well as the spread of organisms such as *Trichophyton rubrum*. In rural areas in Zaire, the incidence was found to be 0.89%, whereas in city dwellers it was 4% in men and 2.8% in women (Vanbreuseghem 1977). Fungal infections of the nails have been reported in 6.5–27% of miners (Götz & Hantschke 1965). Some 1.5% of all patients attending dermatological centres have onychomycosis (Achten & Wanet-Rouard 1981). Between 18% and 40% of all nail disorders are onychomycoses (Pardo-Castello & Pardo 1960; Achten & Wanet-Rouard 1978) and 30% of all dermatomycoses are nail infections (Langer 1957).

## Onychomycosis

Fungal infections of the nail apparatus may be classified as superficial, distal or proximal according to the site of fungal invasion (Fig. 4.1). In this chapter a new classification (Baran *et al.* 1998b) is used, which expands on previous schemes to include mycoses involving the whole nail apparatus as well as a new form, endonyx onychomycosis. The appearance of the lesion may provide clues to the likely identity of the infecting organism, although it is seldom possible to identify the species on clinical grounds alone: for instance, irrespective of right or left handedness, unilateral hand involvement is a common feature of dermatophytosis caused by *Trichophyton rubrum*; in such patients both feet are commonly infected (Vazquez *et al.* 1998) (Fig. 4.2). Similarly onychomycosis confined to the fingernails is more suggestive of a *Candida* infection, especially in paronychia and onycholysis, although infections caused by either *Scytalidium dimidiatum* (*Hendersonula toruloidea*) or *S. hyalinum* may both produce identical nail lesions. These observations contribute to the process of making the diagnosis, but this will depend ultimately on the laboratory identification of the fungus. Invasive onychomycosis can also be proved convincingly by histology. A search for infections at other sites such as the hands, feet (soles and webs) or groins, or the scalp in infants, should be instituted when there is a suspicion of onychomycosis. Discoloured dyschromic nail changes caused by fungi are considered in the section on chromonychia (page 89).

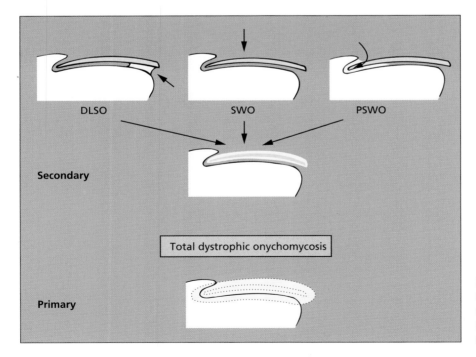

**Fig. 4.1** Diagram to show the site of invasion and types of onychomycosis. DLSO, Distal and lateral subungual onychomycosis; EO, endonyx onychomycosis; PSWO, proximal subungual white onychomycosis; SWO, superficial white onychomycosis.

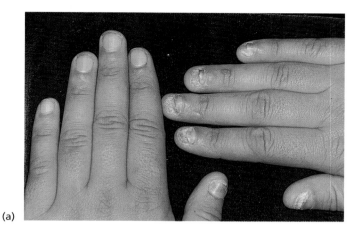

(a)

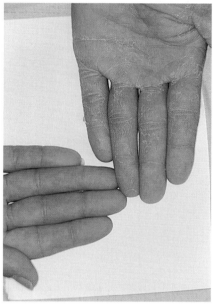

(b)

**Fig. 4.2** (a) Distal and lateral subungual onychomycosis presenting as one hand/two-foot tinea syndrome. (b) Involvement of the palm of the same hand.

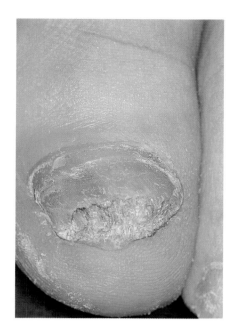

**Fig. 4.3** Distal and lateral subungual onychomycosis due to *Trichophyton rubrum*.

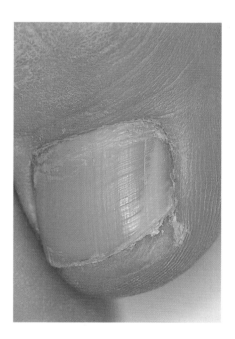

**Fig. 4.4** Distal and lateral subungual onychomycosis restricted to the medial edge due to *Trichophyton* (*mentagrophytes* var.) *interdigitale*.

## Distal and lateral subungual onychomycosis (Figs 4.3–4.10)

### Primary distal and lateral subungual onychomycosis (Table 4.1)

In this pattern of infection the onychodermal band is disrupted by infection and the fungus reaches the underside of the nail via the hyponychium, the nail bed, or the lateral nail fold where the stratum corneum is invaded. The nail bed infection in distal and lateral subungual onychomycosis (DLSO) caused by *T. rubrum* is the result of the fungus spreading from the plantar (Evans 1998) and palmar surface of the feet and hands, a pattern seen in the one-hand/two-foot tinea syndrome (Daniel *et al*. 1997). The thickened horny layer raises the free edge of the nail plate with disruption of the normal nail plate–nail bed attachment (Baran *et al*. 1998a). The disease spreads proximally and the

nail becomes opaque. Fungal invasion leads to orthokeratosis of the nail bed epithelium. In advanced nail disease a more severe inflammatory reaction affects the nail bed with penetration of mononuclear cells and polymorphonuclear leucocytes into the subungual keratin, sometimes mimicking Munro's microabscesses. Parakeratotic foci, often containing inspissated serum, may appear (Haneke 1991). In time, tunnels produced by dermatophytes and containing air, described by Alkiewicz (1948) as a transverse net, appear as opaque streaks in the nail plate. Occasionally, this may be seen more clearly

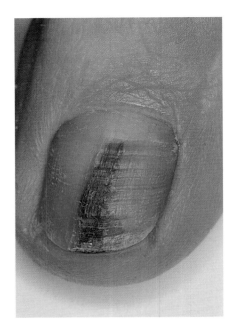

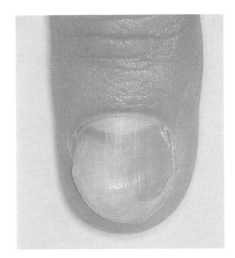

**Fig. 4.5** Distal and lateral subungual onychomycosis due to *Trichophyton rubrum nigricans* presenting with longitudinal melanonychia.

**Fig. 4.7** Onycholysis due to *Trichophyton rubrum*.

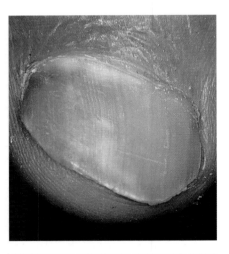

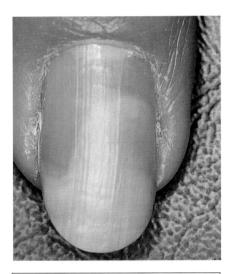

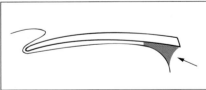

**Fig. 4.6** Onycholysis due to *Trichophyton rubrum*.

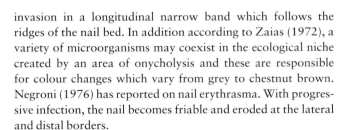

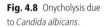

**Fig. 4.8** Onycholysis due to *Candida albicans*.

with the aid of a lens, after the nail plate has been treated with cedar oil to render it translucent. Where the network is sufficiently dense, it appears as an opaque white or yellowish zone or streak, a clinical feature often seen in dermatophyte or mould infections. Such lacunae often contain masses of fungi as well as keratin debris and their existence provides a difficult target for treatment as persistence of infection may occur at this site, possibly due to poor drug penetration. Often there is nail

invasion in a longitudinal narrow band which follows the ridges of the nail bed. In addition according to Zaias (1972), a variety of microorganisms may coexist in the ecological niche created by an area of onycholysis and these are responsible for colour changes which vary from grey to chestnut brown. Negroni (1976) has reported on nail erythrasma. With progressive infection, the nail becomes friable and eroded at the lateral and distal borders.

The clinical appearances of nail dystrophies caused by different fungi are seldom diagnostic, but there may be some useful and potentially distinctive features apart from the differences in

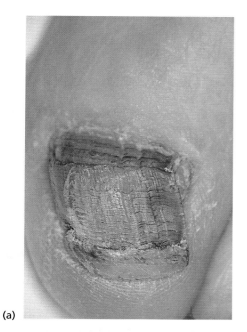

(a)

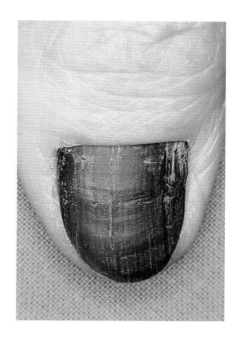

**Fig. 4.10** Black nail due to *Candida parapsilosis*. (Courtesy of O. Binet, France.)

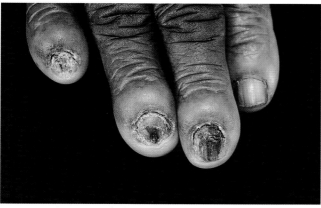

(b)

**Fig. 4.9** (a) Distal and lateral subungual onychomycosis (DLSO) due to *Scytalidium dimidiatum* in a Caucasian patient. (Courtesy of D. Jones UK.) (b) DLSO associated with paronychia due to *S. dimidiatum*.

**Table 4.1** Causes of distal and lateral subungual onychomycosis (DLSO).

| | |
|---|---|
| Dermatophytes | *Trichophyton rubrum, T. interdigitale, Epidermophyton floccosum, T. schoenleinii, T. tonsurans, T. soudanense, T. erinacei, T. verrucosum, T. concentricum, T. violaceum, M. canis* |
| Yeasts | *Candida albicans, C. parapsilosis* |
| Moulds | *Scopulariopsis brevicaulis, Scytalidium dimidiatum, S. hyalinum* |

the overall pattern of nail involvement discussed previously. For example hyperkeratosis accompanying onycholysis is a common feature of dermatophyte infections, which are the commonest causes of DLSO, whereas in *Candida* onychomycosis, gross hyperkeratosis is mainly seen in total nail plate involvement in patients with chronic mucocutaneous candidiasis; in other cases of true *Candida* onychomycosis thickening of the nail plate may be minimal. There has been some debate about the role of *Candida* as a cause of DLSO. *Candida* species are said not to produce specific keratinases and therefore they cannot invade the healthy nail plate. There does appear to be a group of patients in whom there is genuine distal and lateral invasion of the nail plate with erosion, confirmed histologic-

ally, but without significant thickening. This is mainly seen in women, patients with endogenous or exogenous Cushing's syndrome or those with Raynaud's phenomenon (Hay *et al.* 1988c). It may also occur in some tropical countries. While it is possible that some invasion is secondary to pre-existing onycholysis (see below), this is seldom possible to establish. There is often a distinctive brown- or cinnamon-coloured discoloration of nails, mainly toenails, affected by *Scopulariopsis brevicaulis*. It is caused by the presence of large numbers of pigmented conidia produced *in situ* (Belsan & Fragner 1965). Likewise brown pigmentation appearing as an irregular streak in the nail plate, often at the lateral border of the great toenail, is also a feature of infections caused by *Trichophyton interdigitale* and *T. rubrum* may sometimes present with longitudinal melanonychia (Higashi 1990; Perrin & Baran 1994). In this case the cause of the pigmentation is unknown. The nail dystrophies caused by *Scytalidium dimidiatum* (Fig. 4.9) or *Scytalidium hyalinum* are similar to dermatophyte onychomycosis (Moore 1978; Gugnani *et al.* 1986) and may be found in Caucasians (Jones *et al.* 1985). However, secondary paronychia appears to be

**Table 4.2** Organisms found in distal lateral subungual onychomycosis (DLSO) with pre-existing onycholysis.

| Dermatophytes | *Trichophyton rubrum, T. interdigitale, Epidermophyton floccosum* |
|---|---|
| Yeasts | *Candida albicans, C. parapsilosis, C. tropicalis* |
| Mould | Various species have been reported including *Aspergillus* and *Penicillium* |

commoner in fingernail infections and extensive onycholysis may also be a prominent feature of these infections. This may lead to a transverse fracture of the nail plate near the proximal nail fold and subsequent shedding of the distal plate.

### Distal and lateral subungual onychomycosis secondary to onycholysis (Table 4.2)

On occasions dermatophytes may be isolated from nails, such as the big toenail, which show idiopathic or primary onycholysis. Davies (1968) reported on 3955 samples of nails infected with *T. rubrum*. Nine per cent of the normal, healthy looking nails were positive for fungus on direct microscopy, culture or both. This was confirmed by Baran and Badillet (1982), who examined 46 samples of normal nails from patients infected in other sites with *T. rubrum* (35 cases), *T. interdigitale* (10 cases) (one patient having a mixed infection), and *Epidermophyton floccosum* (one case). *T. rubrum* was found in the nails of four of these patients, *T. interdigitale* in two and *E. floccosum* in one only. A subsequent control study was carried out on 52 outpatients seeking medical advice for reasons other than big toenail dystrophy. Dermatophytes were isolated from clinically normal big toenails in two patients, *T. rubrum* in one case and *E. floccosum* in the other. In these apparently healthy nails, the fungi were presumably acting as commensals rather than pathogens. However, they are potentially invasive, particularly in nails showing onycholysis, and may be transmitted to a different host. On the fingers, primary onycholysis is more frequently associated with secondary invasion by *Candida* and/or *Pseudomonas*. It is most common in women in whom there is repeated contact with water, soap and detergents. Contrary to the classical pattern of DLSO, which usually starts with distal hyperkeratosis, there is a reversal of the usual order of evolution of each lesion in secondary onychomycosis. For example, in the fingernails onycholysis precedes any subsequent thickening of the distal subungual area, hence the name of DLSO associated with onycholysis. Repeated episodes of friction secondary to rubbing of the nails against shoes or the repeated episodic trauma incurred during running or jogging may also create an area of traumatic onycholysis where microorganisms are also potentially but not invariably pathogenic. A variety of fungi not normally considered pathogenic may be isolated from dystrophic nails, particularly in the elderly (English & Atkinson 1974).

The usual clinical pattern of nail involvement most closely resembles DLSO. Hyperkeratosis and brown or green discoloration are common and the toenails are most commonly affected. The organisms isolated may include *Aspergillus* species such as *A. terreus* or *A. versicolor*, *Acremonium* spp., *Penicillium* spp. and *Pyrenochaeta unguium hominis* (Punithaligam & English 1975). As these organisms do not appear to be able to break down keratin, it is assumed that they are colonists of dystrophic or abnormal nails. It is however difficult to be certain that they are not contributing to the nail dystrophy. There is some evidence that some of these species (e.g. *Acremonium* spp.) produce perforating organs, specialized hyphal structures usually associated with hair invasion, analogous to those seen in dermatophytosis. Other non-dermatophyte fungi invading nails such as *S. brevicaulis* can be demonstrated by electron microscopy inside keratinized cells (Achten *et al.* 1979). *Scytalidium* species, pathogenic in humans, produce keratinases.

Other yeasts may also be isolated from the same site. These include *Candida* species such as *C. guilliermondii*. As with the moulds discussed above, it is assumed that they are secondary invaders. The distinction between nail pathogens and opportunistic organisms which inhabit nails under abnormal conditions is a tenuous one. As has been seen above, even the dermatophytes can be secondary invaders (Baran & Badillet 1983). Likewise *S. brevicaulis* is often merely a colonist.

The clinical significance of nail invasion or colonization by fungi, which are not normally pathogenic, needs to be carefully considered in the light of laboratory findings such as the results of nail biopsy. It is likely that organisms which colonize nails may play a more destructive role if the host's immune defences or the nail matrix is altered by disease or another infection. Equally their removal may simply be 'academic' if the nail dystrophy remains after antifungal therapy.

## Superficial onychomycosis

### Superficial white onychomycosis (Figs 4.11–4.13, Table 4.3)

Superficial white onychomycosis (SWO) is fairly rare and is normally confined to the toenails.

Here the surface of the nail plate is the initial site of invasion. The causative organisms produce a clinical picture of small superficial white patches with distinct edges (Zaias 1966). These later coalesce and may gradually cover the whole nail, hence the term leuconychia trichophytica (mycotica). The chalky white surface becomes roughened and the texture softer than normal. The appearance has been likened to 'paper-bark' (McAleer 1981), the affected nail plate crumbles easily and old lesions acquire a yellowish colour. The upper surface of the nail plate is the primary site of the fungal invasion. This type of nail invasion is caused by *T. interdigitale* (*mentagrophytes*) in more than 90% of the cases. Using epi-illumination microscopy the individual white flakes representing colonies of *T. interdigitale* can be observed clearly. Patches of SWO are not uncommonly

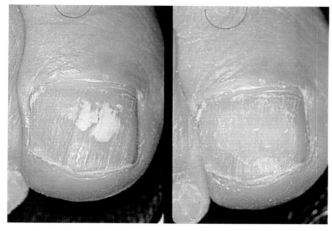

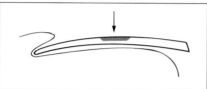

**Fig. 4.11** Superficial white onychomycosis due *to Trichophyton interdigitale.* (a) Before scraping. (b) After superficial scraping.

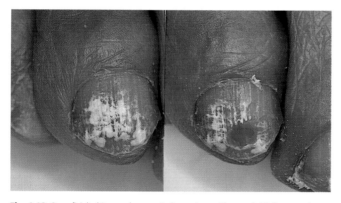

**Fig. 4.12** Superficial white onychomycosis due to *Aspergillus* spp. (a) Before scraping. (b) After scraping.

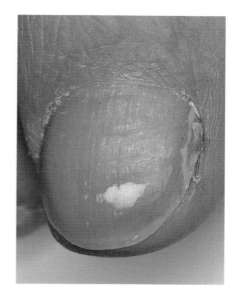

**Fig. 4.13** Superficial white onychomycosis associated with distal and lateral subungual onychomycosis due to *Trichophyton interdigitale.*

**Table 4.3** Causes of superficial white onychomycosis (SWO).

| | |
|---|---|
| Dermatophytes | *Trichophyton interdigitale* (*Microsporum persicolor, T. rubrum* * and *T. equinum*) |
| Yeasts | *Candida albicans* (only in infants, Zaias 1990a) |
| Moulds | *Acremonium* and *Fusarium* spp., *Aspergillus terreus* |

* In this case fungal elements are found deep in the nail plate.

seen in areas where the nail is occluded, for instance by an overlying adjacent toe. Infections caused by non-dermatophytes such as *Aspergillus terreus, Fusarium oxysporum* or *Acremonium* spp. are more often seen in patients in a tropical or subtropical environment. *Candida albicans* has occasionally been isolated in infants (Zaias 1990a).

### Superficial black onychomycosis (Fig. 4.14)

A similar pattern of nail plate invasion and dystrophy may be caused by dematiaceous or black fungi. These are rare but the following have been described as possible causes: *S. dimidiatum* (Badillet 1988; Meisel & Quadripur 1992); *T. rubrum* (Badillet 1988).

### Variants of superficial white onychomycosis

In HIV-infected patients SWO is not rare in finger or toenails and is due to *T. rubrum* (Chapter 6). However, here the pattern of infection is different, as there is often proximal subungual infection as well (see below).

### Endonyx onychomycosis (Fig. 4.15)

In endonyx onychomycosis (EO) infections of the fingernails due to the dermatophytes which cause endothrix scalp infections may present with less nail plate thickening, but the plate is pitted and the distal margin covered with lamellar splits (Kalter & Hay 1988). These changes have been studied in detail by Tosti *et al.* (1999) and shown to consist of areas of superficial nail plate invasion but with deep penetration, and fungal hyphae are seen within the nail plate. The nail surface has lamellar-like splits and the end of the nail plate is often friable and split. However, hyperkeratosis is minimal and dense opacification is unusual. These changes are typical of invasion caused by *Trichophyton soudanense* but similar changes have been seen with *T. violaceum.*

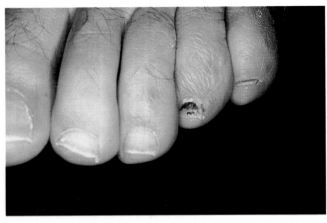

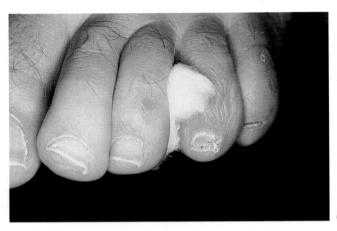

(a)                                                                                          (b)

**Fig. 4.14** Superficial black onychomycosis due to *Scytalidium dimidiatum*. (a) Before scraping. (Courtesy of G. Badillet, France.) (b) After superficial scraping.

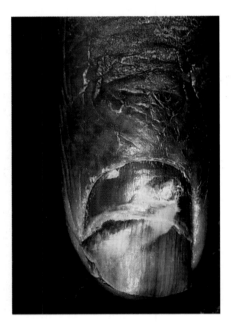

**Fig. 4.15** Endonyx onychomycosis due to *Trichophyton soudanense*.

be seen where there is a recurrence of nail infection in an incompletely treated nail.

This type of nail invasion is usually caused by *T. rubrum*; but *T. megnini*, *T. schoenleinii* or *E. floccosum* may be seen.

Recently a rapidly developing form of PWSO has been recorded in patients with AIDS. Here the infection may spread rapidly under the nail from the proximal margin of all the finger and toenails (Dompmartin *et al.* 1990). Histopathology shows that the entire nail plate is infiltrated with fungi, which are lying in a longitudinal parallel arrangement. However, the picture is complicated in that other surfaces such as the superior aspect of the plate and the distal or lateral margins may also be involved.

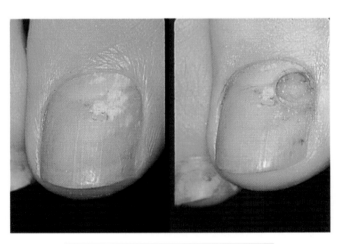

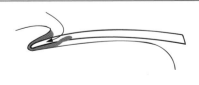

**Fig. 4.16** (a) Proximal white subungual onychomycosis. (b) Biopsy restricted to the nail plate.

## Proximal subungual onychomycosis

### Proximal white subungual onychomycosis (Figs 4.16–4.18)

Proximal white subungual onychomycosis (PWSO) is rare and affects both fingernails and toenails. This clinical pattern of nail invasion is very rare. The causative organisms penetrate via the proximal nail fold, the stratum corneum of which is the primary site of the fungal invasion. When reaching the matrix the fungus invades the undersurface of the nail plate. A white spot appears from beneath the proximal nail fold and, although it is confined initially to the lunula area, when the white spot moves distally, it still remains in the same layer of the nail plate. The fungus has to invade more distal parts of the matrix to get entrapped in the deeper layers of the nail plate. This is sometimes accompanied by slight discomfort. This pattern may also

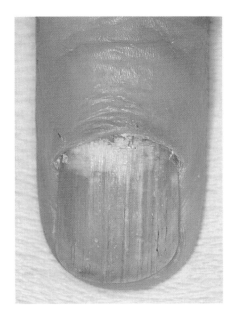

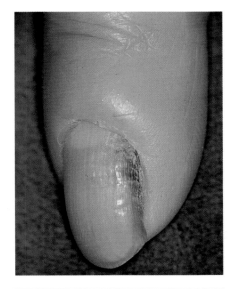

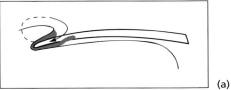

(a)

**Fig. 4.17** Proximal white subungual onychomycosis with dystrophic keratin of the superficial nail plate.

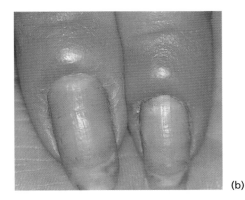

(b)

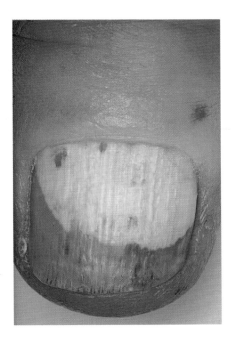

**Fig. 4.18** Proximal white subungual onychomycosis in AIDS.

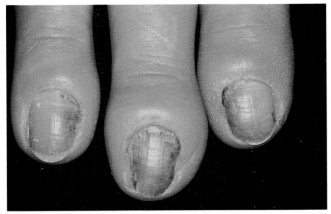

(c)

**Fig. 4.19** (a) Proximal subungual onychomycosis secondary to chronic paronychia. (b) Early stage—normal nails. (c) Gross lateral periungual inflammation and swelling with early nail plate involvement of the lateral edges. *(continued p. 138)*

Possibly because of the rapid spread these patients do not show much nail thickening (Weismann *et al.* 1988).

## Proximal subungual onychomycosis secondary to paronychia (Fig. 4.19)

Paronychia is observed mainly in adult women and affects particularly the index, middle finger and thumb of the dominant hand. Frequent manual work with carbohydrate-containing foods and moisture, maceration, occlusion, hyperhidrosis and acrocyanosis favour the disease. In children, finger sucking is a

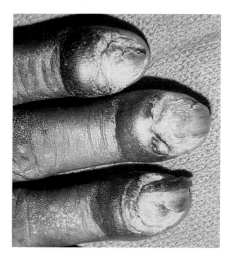

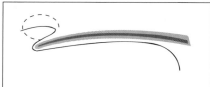

(d)

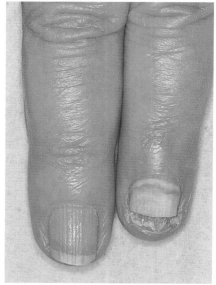

(e)

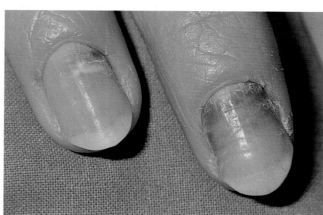

(f)

cause of paronychia (Stone & Mullins 1968). Diabetes mellitus and other hormonal disturbances and drugs such as corticosteroids, cytotoxics and antibiotics may exacerbate *Candida* paronychia. The first step in the development of chronic paronychia is mechanical infection or chemical trauma that produce cuticle damage. At that time the epidermal barrier of the ventral aspect of the proximal nail fold is destroyed and the area is suddenly exposed to a variety of environmental hazards. Irritants and allergens may then produce an inflammatory reaction of the nail fold and nail matrix, which interferes with the normal nail growth. Usually the nail fold inflammation affects the lateral portion of the matrix leading to nail plate deformity on the same side, appearing as irregular transverse ridging or a dark narrow strip down one or both lateral borders of the nail.

The thickened free end of the erythematous proximal nail fold becomes rounded, retracted and loses the ability to form a cuticle. The disease tends to run a protracted course interrupted by subacute exacerbations due to secondary *Candida* and bacterial infection with the formation of a small abscess in the space formed between the proximal nail fold and the nail plate. *Candida* spp. and bacteria are frequently isolated from beneath the proximal nail fold in patients with chronic paronychia (Daniel *et al.* 1996).

Depending on the major aetiological factors involved, chronic paronychia can be classified into the following types (Tosti & Piraccini 1997):

1 Contact allergy (topical drug ingredients, rubber, etc.) (Tosti *et al.* 1991).

2 Food hypersensitivity (a variety of immediate contact dermatitis due to foods).

3 *Candida* hypersensitivity (a similar reaction to that suggested in some patients with recurrent vaginitis).

4 Irritative reaction (irritative chronic paronychia may subsequently acquire a secondary hypersensitivity and develop chronic food hypersensitivity paronychia and/or *Candida* hypersensitivity paronychia).

5 *Candida* paronychia. True *Candida* paronychia is uncommon in temperate climates except in patients with chronic mucocutaneous candidiasis and HIV infection. In this condition proximal nail fold inflammation is usually associated with proximal onycholysis or onychomycosis due to *Candida*, which can be isolated both from the proximal nail fold and clipping of the affected nail plate. In contrast to *Candida* infection, non-dermatophyte moulds such as *Fusarium* (Fig. 4.19e) may produce subacute paronychia accompanied by proximal white onychomycosis especially in immunocompromised individuals (Baran *et al.* 1997). In *Fusarium* infection subsequent disseminated spread of the organism to affect other sites in the severely neutropenic patients may be preceded by a type of cellulitis proceeding from the nail fold (Rabodonirina *et al.* 1994).

**Fig. 4.19** (*cont'd*) (d) Chronic paronychia with total dystrophic onychomycosis. (e) Chronic leuconychia with paronychia due to *Fusarium* infection. (f) Transverse green stripe due to *Pseudomonas* infection corresponding to exacerbation of the paronychia.

*Scopulariopsis brevicaulis* may be responsible for identical features with a white or yellow discoloration of the nail plate (Tosti *et al.* 1996a). Proximal subungual onychomycosis (PSO) may also be associated with marked periungual inflammation and black discoloration of the lunula region due to *Aspergillus niger* (Tosti & Piraccini 1998).

On rare occasions other infections may involve the nail fold causing a form of paronychia. Amongst the fungi, the agents of sporotrichosis and, less commonly, chromoblastomycosis, coccidioidomycosis, paracoccidioidomycosis, blastomycosis and mycetoma may involve this area.

6 Bacterial paronychia. Bacteria may play a role in the pathogenesis of paronychia associated with *Candida* (see above). In addition, *Staphylococcus aureus* may cause an acute paronychia in an otherwise healthy patient. This generally arises as a result of an acute nail fold infection or whitlow and the nail fold may become swollen with subsequent discharge of pus via this area. Alternatively chronic paronychia caused by *S. aureus* is not infrequently seen in patients with skin disease, such as psoriasis or eczema, affecting the nail fold. Generally these are difficult to distinguish clinically from *Candida* infections. *Pseudomonas* infection of the proximal nail fold may produce transverse green stripes on the nail corresponding to exacerbations of the paronychia (Shellow & Koplon 1968) (Fig. 4.19f).

7 Paronychia caused by foreign bodies (Stone *et al.* 1964, 1975).

## Total dystrophic onychomycosis (Figs 4.20–4.26)

Total dystrophic onychomycosis (TDO) represents the most advanced form of all the four previous types described above, especially DLSO. The nail crumbles and disappears leaving a thickened and abnormal nail bed which usually retains fragments of nail plate. All 20 nails may be involved in chronic generalized dermatophytosis (Hadida *et al.* 1966; Boudghène-Stambouli & Mérad-Boudia 1998). In the new form of total nail dystrophy observed in patients with AIDS, infection appears to have spread from under the proximal nail fold (PSO) but this has not been established in all cases. The dorsum of the nail plate may also be involved. The term acute TDO might be

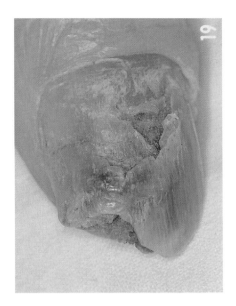

**Fig. 4.21** Total dystrophic onychomycosis due to *Trichophyton rubrum*.

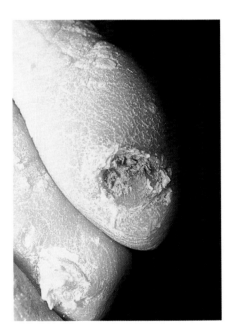

**Fig. 4.22** Total dystrophic onychomycosis due to *Trichophyton rubrum*. (Courtesy of S. Goettmann-Bonvalot, France.)

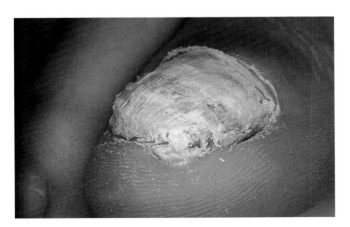

**Fig. 4.20** Total dystrophic onychomycosis due to *Scopulariopsis brevicaulis*.

appropriate for this type of infection. In contrast to secondary TDO, primary TDO is observed only in patients suffering from chronic mucocutaneous candidiasis (CMC) or in other immunodeficiency states (Table 4.4) (Coleman & Hay 1997). *Candida* invasion rapidly involves all the tissues of the nail apparatus. The thickening of the soft tissues results in a swollen distal phalanx more bulbous than clubbed. The nail plate is thickened, opaque and yellow-brown in colour. Hyperkeratotic areas secondary to *Candida* invasion may develop in skin adjacent to the nail. Oral candidiasis is generally present in these patients. This syndrome, which usually occurs in childhood or infancy, recurs despite treatment. Dual or sole infection with dermatophytes may occur in patients with CMC.

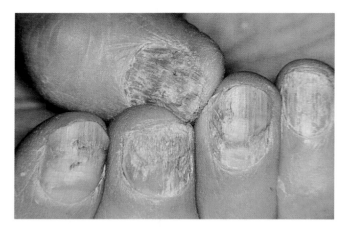

**Fig. 4.23** Isolated unilateral *Candida* total dystrophic onychomycosis.

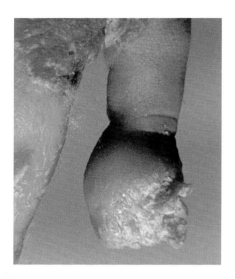

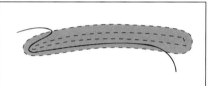

**Fig. 4.25** Chronic mucocutaneous candidiasis (primary total dystrophic onychomycosis).

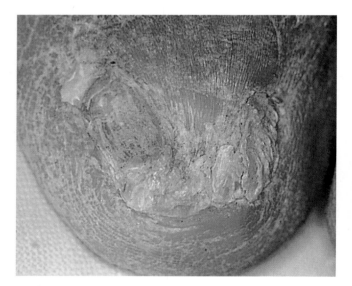

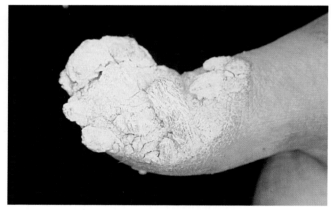

**Fig. 4.26** Chronic mucocutaneous candidiasis (primary total dystrophic onychomycosis).

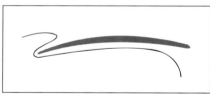

**Fig. 4.24** Total dystrophic onychomycosis secondary to *Trichophyton rubrum*.

## Laboratory investigation

### Direct microscopy

Small pieces taken from clinically infected areas of nail and particularly of subungual hyperkeratosis are treated with 10–30% potassium hydroxide. To hasten clearing of the nail the slide may be warmed over a Bunsen flame. The softened nail is flattened with gentle pressure applied to a coverslip. Zaias and Taplin (1966) recommended a formulation of potassium hydroxide and dimethylsulfoxide. Sixty millilitres of a 20% KOH solution is mixed with 40 mL of pure dimethylsulphoxide (DMSO). This technique is useful for the preservation of specimens, but globular artefacts may sometimes be seen and these must be distinguished from yeast.

There are other techniques in which stains are used to highlight the presence of fungi. These are often very useful in difficult cases. One such technique, useful in non-dermatophyte infections, is the use of an equivolume mixture of Parker Quink ink and potassium hydroxide (Milne 1989). Spores of non-dermatophyte fungi and some mycelial elements are highlighted using this technique. The stain, chlorazol black, is also useful

**Table 4.4** Subtypes of chronic mucocutaneous candidiasis (CMC)*. (From Coleman & Hay 1997 with permission.)

| Type | Pattern of inheritance | Special clinical/immunological features |
|---|---|---|
| CMC | | |
|   Without endocrinopathy (212050†) | Recessive | Childhood onset |
|   With endocrinopathy‡ (240300†) | Recessive | Childhood onset. Patients have the polyendocrinopathy syndrome |
|   Without endocrinopathy (114580†) | Dominant | Childhood onset |
|   With endocrinopathy | Dominant | Childhood onset. Associated with hypothyroidism |
| Sporadic CMC | None known | Childhood onset |
| CMC with keratitis | None known | Childhood onset. Associated with keratitis |
| Late-onset CMC§ | None known | Onset in adult life. Associated with thymoma |

* While originally severe CMC (e.g. *Candida* granuloma) was described in association with specific subtypes, it is now apparent that extensive infection, including hyperkeratotic candidiasis and dermatophytosis, is not specific to any one variety.

† McKusick numbers.

‡ The main endocrine diseases seen with this variety are hypoparathyroidism and hypoadrenalism.

§ Other late-onset types have been recorded., e.g. with systemic lupus erythematosus, but as they are usually associated with systemic corticosteroid therapy, they have been excluded as secondary candidiasis.

for highlighting hyphae in direct material taken from nails. Calcofluor white, a fluorescent whitening agent mixed with an equal volume of KOH, may also be used to highlight, non-specifically, the fungal elements in nail (Milne 1989). Fluorescent whiteners specifically bind to structural proteins of plants, for example chitin and lignin, but not to keratin and other animal proteins; the physicochemical process is called substrate binding.

The nail is examined for fungal hyphae or arthrospores. In *Candida* infections yeast forms are also present. In certain non-dermatophyte infections conidia may be formed *in situ*. This is characteristic of *Scopulariopsis* infections although it may also occur in onychomycosis caused by *Aspergillus* species. The hyphae of *S. dimidiatum* and *S. hyalinum* are very similar in appearance to those of dermatophytes although they may appear thinner, irregular and more sinuous. This is seen best with phase contrast illumination (Fig. 4.27).

At present a more specific system for immunological detection of fungi in nails, such as the use of fluorescein-conjugated antidermatophyte antibodies, has not been widely applied in medicine, although this technique (Piérard *et al.* 1994a) along with another using fluorescent lectin stains which bind differentially to different nail fungi have been assessed (see below) (Robles Martinez *et al.* 1990).

## Culture (Figs 4.28 & 4.29)

Scrapings from subungual keratosis and nails should be planted into Sabouraud's agar and incubated at 26°C. The different organisms can be recognized using morphological and or biochemical criteria. The presence of chloramphenicol or streptomycin and penicillin in the medium prevents the growth of contaminant bacteria. However, wherever possible nails should be plated on medium both with and without cycloheximide

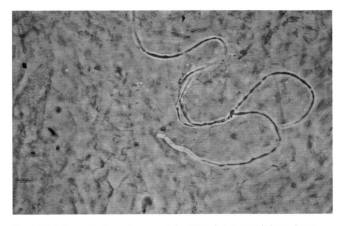

**Fig. 4.27** Subungual nail scrapings mounted in KOH solution—mycelial strands are easily visible (*Scytalium dimidiatum*).

(actidione), as it inhibits some non-dermatophytes which may cause onychomycosis.

It is sometimes difficult to isolate fungi, even from nails which are positive on direct microscopy. The problem is compounded if the patient has already received topical or systemic treatment and if the hyphae in the most accessible part of the nail plate are not viable (Gentles 1971). In order to improve the isolation rate various methods have been devised. These include the use of a grinder (Zaias *et al.* 1969; Daniel 1985) or a dental drill fitted with a suction nozzle, which collects the nail dust for microscopy and culture (English & Atkinson 1973). This latter instrument has raised the success rate of culture from microscopically positive nails from the usual rate of 50–75% to about 88%, but is not a practical procedure for the routine laboratory.

*S. brevicaulis* forms filaments as well as spores of characteristic size and morphology in nail. According to Ornsberg (1980),

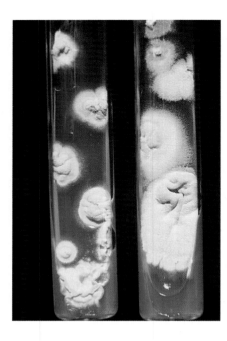

**Fig. 4.28** Fungal culture (*Scopulariopsis brevicaulis*).

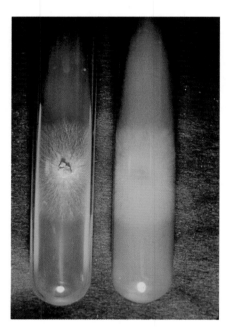

**Fig. 4.29** Fungal culture (*Epidermophyton floccosum*).

English (1976) suggested that the following criteria are helpful in determining whether a fungus is merely a commensal or whether it is truly responsible for nail dystrophy:

**1** If a dermatophyte is isolated, it is considered to be the likely pathogen.

**2** If moulds or yeast are isolated, they are thought to be significant only if mycelia, arthrospores or yeast cells are found on direct microscopic examination of the nail specimen.

**3** Final confirmation of mould infection requires isolation of the mould on at least five out of 20 inocula, in addition to the absence of dermatophytes on either actidione-containing, or actidione-free media.

Most clinicians would find these criteria too stringent although they provide a useful guideline. They are also questionable since, in onycholysis of certain nails such as the big toenail, cultured dermatophytes may be present as commensals (Baran & Badillet 1983). The clinical appearances of the nails, tortuous or 'atypical' hyphal elements in nail clippings and repeated isolations of a non-dermatophyte are all helpful clues to the possible involvement of an unusual organism. Likewise the presence of *Candida* species in material taken from under nails with onycholysis does not appear to be diagnostic of invasion of the nail plate, certainly if only yeast forms are seen on direct microscopy (Hay *et al.* 1988a); the presence of *Candida* mycelium in nail material and the growth of *C. albicans* is more likely to imply a pathogenic role for these organisms in nail dystrophy. Similarly *Malassezia* species have been described in patients with onycholysis. It has been suggested that they are pathogens in view of the treatment response of some cases to antifungal therapy (Civila *et al.* 1982). However, these observations should be interpreted with caution, as patients with idiopathic onycholysis show spontaneous remission; these lipophilic yeasts may simply be commensals of onycholytic nails. A study of the use of terbinafine showed that the clinical response of nails to treatment with terbinafine was dependent on the response of dermatophytes and that mould or yeast fungi isolated from the nails came and went but their presence had no effect on the response to treatment.

Histological examination of the nail plate, with the underlying tissue, will not only demonstrate the fungal elements but also reveal the depth of their penetration into the nail plate. This may provide further evidence of the pathogenic role of fungi isolated in culture, particularly if they can be identified *in situ* on morphological grounds, or by immunofluorescent labelling using specific antisera (see above).

## Histopathology for demonstrating fungi in the nail

(Figs 4.30–4.42) (Achten & Simonart 1963, 1965; Achten & Wanet-Rouard 1978; Achten *et al.* 1979; Scher & Ackerman 1980a; Haneke 1985, 1991; Suarez *et al.* 1991; Piérard *et al.* 1994b; Contet-Audonneau *et al.* 1995; Baral *et al.* 1996; Mehregan *et al.* 1997; Machler *et al.* 1998)

Histopathology reliably demonstrates whether a fungus is invasive or merely colonizing subungual debris.

the demonstration of *S. brevicaulis* on direct microscopy and the presence of more than 10 colonies in culture is diagnostic of infections caused by this organism. If there are less than three colonies, and *S. brevicaulis* is not seen on direct microscopy, the organism is probably present as a commensal. *S. brevicaulis* is often found in toenails infected by dermatophytes, particularly *T. rubrum* or *T. interdigitale* (Baran *et al.* 1998a). The dermatophyte responsible for the primary infection may eventually be isolated after repeated scrapings have been taken. *Aspergillus* spp. may also form conidia in nails *in vivo*.

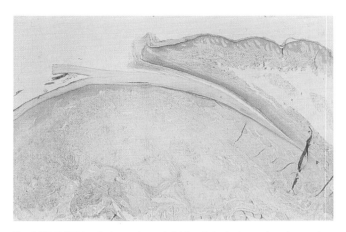

**Fig. 4.30** Nail histopathology—advanced distal and lateral subungual onychomycosis. H&E stain, × 16.

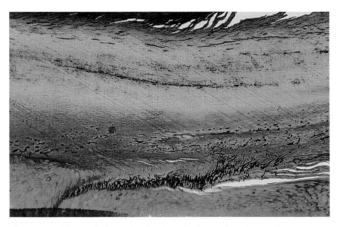

**Fig. 4.33** Nail histopathology—distal and lateral subungual onychomycosis. Grocott stain, × 100.

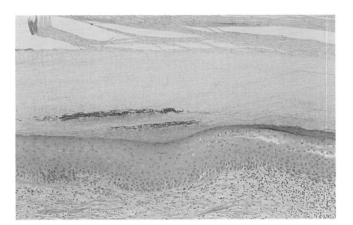

**Fig. 4.31** Nail histopathology—advanced distal and lateral subungual onychomycosis. H&E stain, × 100.

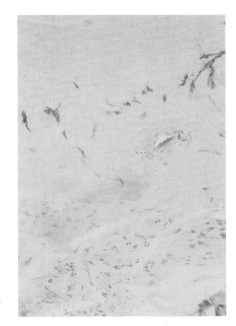

**Fig. 4.34** Nail histopathology—distal and lateral subungual onychomycosis. PAS stain, × 250.

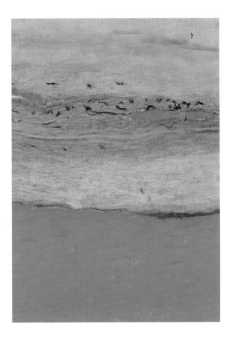

**Fig. 4.32** Nail histopathology—advanced distal and lateral subungual onychomycosis. Grocott stain, × 250.

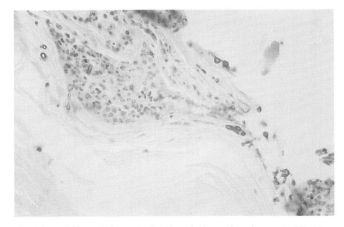

**Fig. 4.35** Nail histopathology—distal and lateral subungual onychomycosis. PAS stain, × 250.

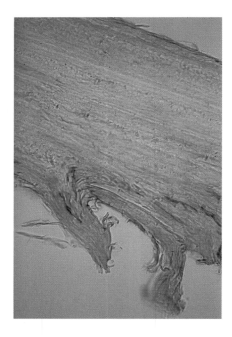

**Fig. 4.36** Nail histopathology—distal and lateral subungual onychomycosis. PAS stain, × 250.

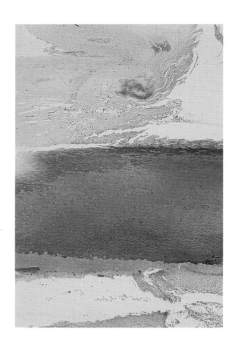

**Fig. 4.39** Nail histopathology—proximal white subungual onychomycosis showing fungal infection at the junction of the pale upper proximal nail fold and the nail plate (red).

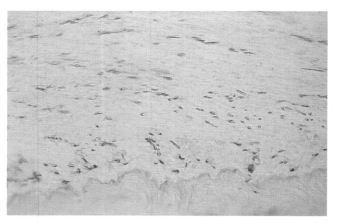

**Fig. 4.37** Nail histopathology—endonyx onychomycosis. (Courtesy of A. Tosti, Italy.)

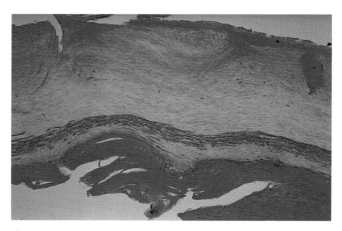

**Fig. 4.40** Nail histopathology—proximal white subungual onychomycosis.

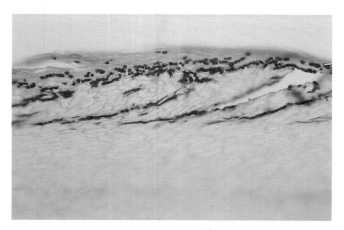

**Fig. 4.38** Nail histopathology—superficial white onychomycosis. PAS stain, × 400.

According to the site of the pathology, nail clippings should be taken from the edge, or the lateral part of the nail plate together with a shallow portion of subungual tissue (Chapter 3). They are then embedded directly into paraffin without using a fixative. The specimens are stained with haematoxylin and eosin, periodic acid–Schiff (PAS) and toluidine blue; calcofluor and Grocott's stain can also be used. The fungi can be seen in the subungual keratin and undersurface of the nail plate. Histopathological examination of nail clippings with subungual keratosis very often shows fungal elements even when cultures are repeatedly negative. Nail clippings may be embedded in paraffin without prior fixation. However, some softening techniques may be applied beforehand to facilitate sectioning. The use of a chitin-softening solution containing mercuric chloride, chromic acid, acetic acid and 95% alcohol has been

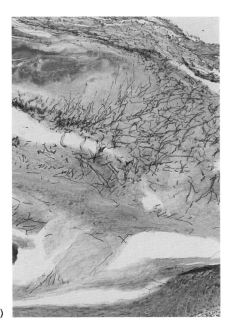

(a)

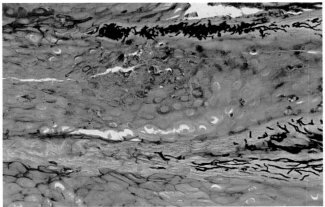

(b)

**Fig. 4.41** (a) Nail histopathology—total dystrophic onychomycosis (TDO). PAS stain, × 100. (b) Nail histopathology—TDO. Grocott stain, × 250.

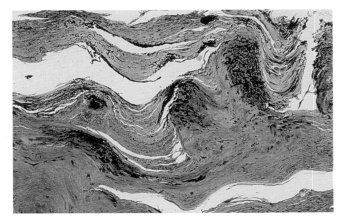

**Fig. 4.42** Nail histopathology—chronic mucocutaneous candidiasis. Grocott stain, × 100.

advocated as a means of enhancing the quality of the histological sections (Suarez *et al.* 1991). PAS stain is usually sufficient to demonstrate fungi; however, small serum inclusions may be mistaken for fungi by the inexperienced as they are also PAS positive (Haneke 1985, 1988, 1991). The methenamine silver stain (Grocott) and calcofluor are more selective (Haneke 1985, 1991). The fungi are usually located in the subungual keratosis, but may have invaded the deepest parts of the nail plate. Histopathology shows whether the fungi are invasive or only contaminants, for example spores in clefts of the subungual keratin. Fungi cannot be further identified, since both dermatophytes and moulds may produce hyphae and large, thick-walled arthrospores. However, some fungi do produce distinctive morphological features in nail which aid identification, for example yeasts plus hyphae and pseudohyphae with *Candida albicans* or rough surfaced conidiospores with *S. brevicaulis*.

Nail clippings often show abundant Munro-like abscesses in onychomycosis; since fungi may be sparse one cannot make the diagnosis of nail psoriasis from the presence of intracorneal abscesses in the absence of fungi alone. If the hyponychium is not affected, any non-dermatophyte fungi cultured from the nails should be regarded as contaminants. However, if fungi can be demonstrated histologically in the hyponychium of a nail from which fungi have not been isolated the culture result is clearly false negative. This view is supported by the therapeutic investigations reported by Gentles and Evans (1970). They have shown that treatment with griseofulvin affects the form and position of the fungus in relation to keratin in patients with microscopically visible fungi, by allowing nail growth to carry hyphal tips to the free edge of the nail. This may account for the positive results using the staining techniques described above in cases where repeated culture has been negative. For the early diagnosis of PWSO a 3-mm punch biopsy taken from the proximal white area and restricted to the nail plate is indispensable. The hyphae are located in the deeper portion of the nail plate and the keratinized cells of the adherent superficial layers of the nail plate.

The flattened filaments lie parallel to the nail surface and 'worm' their way into the intercellular spaces.

Another technique which can be used to highlight fungi in nail biopsy material is the use of a fluorescein-conjugated lectin stain (for instance concanavalin A) on nail biopsies softened with 10% KOH. Fungal elements are strongly stained with the lectin conjugate (Robles Martinez *et al.* 1990).

Histopathology of nail biopsies has given considerable information concerning the pathogenesis of onychomycoses. It also allows one to subdivide the various clinical types of onychomycoses and provides convincing evidence of the different ways of infection and ports of entry.

Distal-lateral subungual onychomycosis develops from an infection of the hyponychium and almost invariably shows fungi in the hyperkeratosis of the distal nail bed. The fungi progress towards the matrix and induce mild inflammation. This causes an 'epidermization' of the nail bed with the formation of a pronounced granular layer and a thick, mainly orthokeratotic, horny layer. The latter is protected by the overlaying nail plate, preventing its desquamation and keeping it moist and soft. This gives an ideal microenvironment for the fungi, which are often present in very large amounts. The nail plate is invaded from its undersurface with the hyphae showing a parallel, often longitudinal arrangement. High power magnification frequently shows tunnels in the nail substance, the diameter of which are considerably greater than those of the fungi; they are seen macroscopically as a transverse net (Alkiewicz 1948). The subungual keratosis may be secondarily colonized by opportunistic bacteria and fungi, which may produce discoloration, friability and loss of lustre of the nail. Longstanding fungal infections may cause severe inflammatory changes with spongiosis, exocytosis of lymphocytes and polymorphonuclear leucocytes, and papillomatosis of the nail bed. The subungual keratosis then contains globules of serum and abundant microabscesses, but the keratosis is still mainly orthokeratotic. When the nail plate is destroyed the parallel longitudinal arrangement of the fungi gets lost and the fungi criss-cross the subungual keratin and nail plate remnants in an irregular arrangement.

Bacterial colonization may be seen, mostly as a line of small basophilic coccoid organisms. In onychomycosis nigricans, the nail plate and even a portion of the subungual keratosis is diffusely yellowish-brown to dark brown, and there is no specific pigmentary change (Haneke 1986). Occasionally, a whitish-yellow longitudinal band is seen extending from the hyponychium towards the matrix; this is often left after an otherwise successful treatment of onychomycosis of the toenail and does not respond to further systemic antifungals. Histopathology reveals a PAS-positive globus consisting of a huge amount of densely packed fungal elements, mainly arthrospores but also hyphae.

Proximal subungual onychomycosis develops from infection of the proximal nail fold. Histopathology shows fungi in the cuticle, a hyperkeratotic eponychium with fungal invasion and usually a mild inflammatory infiltrate beneath the epidermis of the eponychium. The fungi may invade the nail plate surface; they are then again regularly arranged in a parallel longitudinal manner. They grow slowly towards the matrix and are then enclosed in the growing nail plate. Since the fungi are taken away from the matrix, there is only mild inflammation and progression of the pathogen from the proximal matrix to the nail bed takes a long time. Both hyphae and thick spores may be seen in different layers of the nail plate, often causing microscopic slits which may abruptly extend to a particular type of onycholysis with apparent leuconychia. In advanced PSO, there may be as severe changes as in DLSO (Haneke 1985, 1988).

In superficial white onychomycosis there are chains of round spores in the nail plate extending in between superficial splits of the nail. There is no inflammatory infiltrate in the nail bed beneath (Haneke 1985, 1991).

Primary total dystrophic onychomycosis is a characteristic feature of chronic mucocutaneous candidiasis (Haneke 1988) and both DLSO and PSO may lead to secondary total dystrophic onychomycosis (TDO).

Total dystrophic onychomycosis in chronic mucocutaneous candidiasis is characterized by a complete loss of the ordered nail structure. The proximal nail fold may have been reduced to a small rim of tissue, the cuticle is lost, matrix and nail bed are papillomatous and covered with a thick irregular keratosis and there is a heavy inflammatory infiltrate invading matrix and nail bed epithelium. Electron microscopic investigation shows composite keratohyalin granules in the matrix. Fungal elements are seen in variable amounts. When they form hyphae they are irregularly arranged, because there is no orderly nail plate growth left (Haneke 1988).

## Differential diagnosis

Subungual hyperkeratosis, onycholysis, leuconychia, splinter haemorrhages as well as dystrophy involving the whole nail plate may be seen both in dermatophytosis and in psoriasis, and it may be impossible to diagnose isolated psoriasis of the nails on clinical grounds unless there is extensive pitting and/or the oil drop sign. Nail clippings or, in total nail dystrophy, a shave biopsy from the hyperkeratotic zone of the affected nail bed, may be helpful in differentiating between psoriasis and dermatophytosis (Leyden et al. 1972; Scher & Ackerman 1980b); parakeratosis and neutrophils within this zone can be seen in both conditions (page 145). Koutselinis et al. (1982) suggested that in clinical practice, surface and subungual scrapings are satisfactory for the cytological diagnosis of psoriasis; the skin surface biopsy technique of Marks and Dawber (1971) may be used similarly (Chapter 3).

In psoriasis neither hyphae nor spores are found in the cornified cells of the nail bed nor in the lowest portion of the nail plate. However, dual pathologies do occur and psoriatic nails, particularly toenails, may be associated with commensal fungi as secondary colonization or invasion caused by *Candida* or dermatophytes. Recent studies suggest that the incidence of dermatophytosis of the nails is higher than previously thought in patients with psoriasis (Gupta et al. 1997a). Dermatophyte infections may involve the nails in Darier's disease, lichen planus and ichthyotic states such as the KID syndrome (keratosis, ichthyosis and deafness). The yellow nail syndrome may also be mistaken for a fungal infection; however, the hardness of the nail plate, its increased longitudinal curvature and the light green/yellow discoloration are all typical. The irregularly buckled nail of eczema, and the ridged or dystrophic nail of lichen planus must be distinguished from onychomycosis.

## Treatment

In the treatment of fungal nail disease the site of involvement and the identity of the organism are important factors determining the choice of therapy. The patient's choice is also important. As the rate of growth of toenails is one-third to one-half that of fingernails, therapy of the former using the classical systemic drugs, such as griseofulvin or ketoconazole, must be continued for 12–18 months, whereas fingernail infection may be cured in 6 months. This limits their value in the face of new developments. Drug effectiveness can easily be checked by Zaias' method (1983).

## Topical treatment

Historically, topical nail therapy has met with little success, due in part to the absence of effective topical products. This is regrettable since there are potential candidates for topical therapy such as for fungal infections where potent systemic therapy is undesirable because of toxic effects or drug interactions. In addition, some patients may be unable or unwilling to take oral drugs for the many months of therapy required to ensure successful therapy, especially when only a few nails are affected. Therefore effective topical therapy directly applied to the nail plate would be an attractive alternative with the additional benefit of a complete absence of systemic side effects and drug interactions. However, many of the conventional formulations of the antifungal agents (powders, solutions, creams, ointments) are not specifically adapted for use in the nails due to insufficient adhesion of the base, leading to insufficient penetration of the active ingredient through the nail into the nail bed; they are also not formulated to take account of the length of time which would be required to permit the growth of a healthy nail; they also do not remain in contact with the site of application for long enough (they are readily removed by rubbing, wiping, washing).

Improvement of the conventional formulations led to the development of an alcoholic solution containing 28% tioconazole and undecylenic acid, for instance, which has produced moderate results (Hay *et al.* 1985, 1987). Penetration of the drug tioconazole through the plate is excellent, but not matched by clinical efficacy.

## Transungual drug delivery system

A further step forward has been achieved with the development of new vehicles in the form of colourless nail lacquers known from cosmetic formulations. Two compounds, amorolfine and ciclopirox, are currently used in a lacquer base in several countries. These formulations fulfil two essential prerequisites: first, the active ingredient is in contact with the nail for long periods; second, through evaporation of the solvents, the concentration of the active ingredient in the remaining film reservoir increases, thus providing the high concentration gradient essential for maximal penetration.

The amorolfine concentration in the film-forming solution is 5%; solvent evaporation leaves a film with a final amorolfine concentration of 19.8%. The ciclopirox concentration is 8% in the nail lacquer, increasing to 34.8%.

Release can be optimized by selecting the components of the lacquer formulation (solvent, polymer, plasticizer) that help to modulate the release of the drug and maintain the antifungal at a high level in the nail plate.

Because of the additional occluding properties of these formulations, transungual water loss is reduced and thus enhances mass transport of the drug into and through the nail plate. Despite fulfilling all necessary prerequisites, diffusion may be disturbed in nails with fungal channels and splits, particularly at the border between the nail plate and the nail bed. This partially explains why cure is not always achieved.

### Amorolfine

Amorolfine belongs to a new family of antifungal drugs, the morpholines (Polak 1988; Reinel 1992). Amorolfine inhibits two steps in the pathway of ergosterol biosynthesis, namely the 14α-reductase and the 7,8Δ-isomerase, which play an important role in regulating membrane fluidity. This leads to accumulation of abnormal sterols and inhibits fungal growth. Amorolfine possesses a broad antimycotic spectrum against fungi pathogenic to plants and humans. In addition, it shows strong fungicidal activity which is dependent on both concentration and time. Amorolfine is fungicidal against yeasts, dimorphic and dematiaceous fungi, but does not appear to be active against *Aspergillus*, *Fusarium* and *Mucor*.

### Ciclopirox

Ciclopirox, a hydroxy-pyridone derivative, is incorporated in a clear nail lacquer containing poly(butyl hydrogen maleate, methoxyethylene) (1 : 1), ethylacetate and 2-propanol.

In contrast to most antifungals, it does not interfere with sterol biosynthesis. It acts as a chelating agent and primarily affects iron-dependent mitochondrial enzymes. Consequently, as ciclopirox also impairs transport mechanisms into the fungal cell and in growing cells, there is reduced synthesis of macromolecules such as proteins and nucleic acids. Ciclopirox is characterized by a comparably strong and broad fungicidal and sporicidal activity against the whole spectrum of human fungal pathogens at concentrations close to the minimum inhibitory concentration (MIC) (Ceschin-Roques *et al.* 1991).

Its spectrum includes fungi such as *Scytalidium* spp. which are resistant to many other antifungals used in the treatment of onychomycosis. At therapeutically relevant concentrations, the spectrum of activity covers, in addition, gram-positive and gram-negative bacteria.

The transungual drug delivery system (TUDDS) is a new method of delivery which leads to penetration of mycotic nail keratin more rapidly than healthy nails. However, the effectiveness of exclusively topical antimycotic treatment depends on the type of onychomycosis. PSO and TDO cannot be affected by topical treatment. This is considered to be the most appropriate therapy for subungual onychomycosis. In the case of

DLSO the cure rate depends largely upon the severity of nail infection. Where more than 60% of the nail plate is altered topical monotherapy is generally ineffective (Effendy 1995).

## Clinical studies

In the framework of three large studies 714 patients with onychomycosis without matrix involvement applied amorolfine nail lacquer once weekly for 6 months. Mycological cure including negative culture and microscopy was achieved in 52.1% of the 424 toenail, and in 64.3% of the 98 fingernail mycoses. Local adverse events, mostly skin irritation, were reported in six patients (<1%) (Zaug 1995).

In an open multicentre study in 250 practices, 5401 nails from 1239 patients were treated with the 8% ciclopirox lacquer formulation applied once daily to the affected nails over a treatment period of up to 6 months. The layer of lacquer was removed once weekly. A cure was obtained in more than 50% of cases with a 60% success rate for fingernails. Only 2% of patients complained of periungual burning and redness (Seebacher et al. 1993). In a recent study (Nolting & Ulbricht 1997) it has been shown that under normal circumstances, one or two weekly applications of ciclopirox were as efficient as the former daily treatment.

In summary, topical treatment is suitable for SWO and early DLSO. The responses of patients with non-extensive nail disease involving multiple nails are usually not as good. In addition, it is necessary to treat infected skin sites separately.

## Oral antifungal treatment

There are now a variety of drugs which can be used for the treatment of onychomycosis. Those in use in most countries are fluconazole, itraconazole and terbinafine. Griseofulvin and ketoconazole are less frequently used.

### Griseofulvin

Griseofulvin is an oral antifungal agent derived from certain *Penicillium* species such as *P. griseofulvum*. It is *only* active against dermatophytes. In nail infection it is normally given in a daily dose of 500–1000 mg for adults, although this may be increased to 2 g in recalcitrant cases. Absorption of the drug is enhanced when it is given in ultramicrosize or microsize particle form and with food. In nail infections, griseofulvin is given until there is clinical and mycological recovery. The complete replacement of infected tissue with healthy nail depends upon the rate of growth, but some patients or some nails fail to improve even after treatment of apparently adequate dose and duration.

The results of treating toenail infections are usually not satisfactory, particularly in the elderly. The overall cure rate using griseofulvin for toenail infections is generally less than 40%. Treatment is the result of the interaction of a number of factors,

including penetration of the drug into nail keratin and leakage from the nail, the rate of nail growth and the sensitivity of the organism to the drug (MIC). Resistance to griseofulvin has been correlated with treatment failure by some investigators (Artis et al. 1981), but not by others (Davies et al. 1977). It is not clear whether the higher MIC values seen in isolates from some clinically unresponsive cases are due to a permanent or reversible change in sensitivity. The latter has been demonstrated *in vitro* (Rosenthal & Wise 1960) and this may explain why previously unresponsive cases may sometimes clear after the reintroduction of griseofulvin after a drug-free interval of 6–18 months. An alternative method of enhancing the effect of griseofulvin is the use of cimetidine as an adjunct to antifungal treatment (Presser & Blank 1981). However, the true value of this combined therapy in nail infections needs more objective assessment.

Allergic reactions such as urticaria may occur during griseofulvin therapy, but the most common reasons for discontinuing treatment are headache or gastrointestinal intolerance. Griseofulvin competes with some drugs including anticoagulants and there is interference with its absorption and metabolism by phenobarbitone (Davies 1980). It may also be responsible for precipitating porphyria cutanea tarda in predisposed patients, as well as a lupus erythematosus-like eruption.

Generally griseofulvin is little used now for the management of onychomycosis.

### Ketoconazole

Ketoconazole, an imidazole drug, is an alternative to griseofulvin (Cox et al. 1982). It works by blocking the cytochrome P-450-dependent demethylation stage in the conversion of lanosterol into ergosterol in the formation of the fungal cell membrane. It is active against *Candida* as well as dermatophytes (Botter et al. 1979; Baran 1982), but has little effect on non-dermatophyte moulds such as *S. brevicaulis*. The daily adult dose is 200 mg given with food and this may be increased to 400 mg or even 600 mg in some cases. Ketoconazole is effective in *Candida* onychomycosis including chronic mucocutaneous candidiasis (Haneke 1981; Hay & Clayton 1992). It is also effective against chronic generalized dermatophyte onychomycosis. Side effects including gastrointestinal intolerance are less common than with griseofulvin. It also blocks human metabolic processes such as adrenal androgen biosynthesis dependent of cytochrome P-450, causing symptoms such as gynaecomastia in males. These effects are mainly seen at higher dose ranges (over 600 mg daily). However, a sporadic drug-induced hepatitis has been associated with the drug on rare occasions (Heiberg & Svejgaard 1981; Strauss 1982; Tkach & Rinaldi 1982); the risk of hepatitis has been assessed as 1 per 10 000 prescriptions, but appears to be slightly commoner in patients with onychomycosis (Fromtling 1988), particularly when they had been treated previously with griseofulvin. The duration of the therapy is similar to griseofulvin. Hepatic function has to be monitored regularly. Generally ketoconazole is now not much used for the management of onychomycosis in view of the risk, albeit rare, of hepatitis.

## Itraconazole

Itraconazole is a triazole antifungal drug. Although its mode of action is similar to that seen with ketoconazole (Fromtling 1988), it has not been reported to have serious side effects in man, since it binds more specifically to fungal cytochrome P-450. The main adverse reactions are nausea, gastrointestinal fullness and headache. It has been used for a variety of mycoses including onychomycosis. In onychomycosis at a dose of 100 mg daily it has been found to have activity in patients with previously treatment-unresponsive dermatophytosis as well as *Candida* nail infections (Hay *et al.* 1988c). It does not appear to be effective in *Scytalidium* infections, but it is very active against *Aspergillus* spp.

Studies of itraconazole have drawn attention to another fact, the mode of drug penetration and nail binding. Itraconazole, a lipid-soluble drug, appears to penetrate into nails and is detectable within 2 weeks of the start of the therapy. It is also detectable in this site for a considerable period thereafter; and in one study it was found in nail plate material 1 year after a 3-month period of therapy (Willemsen *et al.* 1992). Using a dose of 200 mg daily for 3 months significant recovery rates have been reported in both fingernail and toenail infection (Willemsen *et al.* 1992). However, given the long half-life of itraconazole in nail and the cost advantages of using less drug, a new regimen has been devised and assessed. The main regimen used involves giving 200 mg itraconazole twice daily for 1 week each month over 2 months for fingernails, and over 3 months for toenails. The results from published studies suggest efficacy rates of at least 70% at long-term follow up (Gupta *et al.* 1998b), although some results are less encouraging. One feature of clinical trials using pulsed itraconazole has been the range of strikingly different results produced in different clinical situations and countries. It is difficult to explain these, although variations in compliance or absorption or in the partition of itraconazole between keratinocytes in the nail plate and fungal cells may play important roles in defining the responses to treatment.

Adverse events have not been prominent. Generally the frequency of side effects with the pulsed regimen is about 5–7% and the main problems reported are nausea, vomiting, headache and dyspepsia. Hepatic reactions are very rare with itraconazole. Other rare problems recorded include thrombocytopenia, rhabdomyolysis and urticaria.

Drug interactions occur with itraconazole and these result, for instance, in the reduction of the serum levels of rifampicin. It can increase levels of digoxin, terfenadine and astemizole to toxic levels. Other interactions include cyclosporin A, tacrolimus and midazolam.

## Fluconazole

Fluconazole, another azole antifungal drug of the triazole group, is mainly used (100 mg daily) in the management of systemic disease or superficial candidiasis (Fromtling 1988), especially in patients with AIDS and in other immunosuppressed subjects. There is, however, evidence that levels detectable by bioassay are found in nails within 48 h (Hay 1988). This drug is unusual amongst the azole antifungals for its water solubility, which might account for rapid penetration into nail (Grant & Clissold 1990). It has a low frequency of mainly gastrointestinal side effects. It is considered to be less hepatotoxic than ketoconazole, but AIDS patients require careful monitoring of hepatic function because hepatotoxicity may develop (Muñoz *et al.* 1991).

In a large double-blind study of the effect of different single doses (150, 300 or 450 mg per week for 6–12 months) of fluconazole on clinical and mycological recovery rates of affected toenails or fingernails there was no difference in response rates at different doses, even though there was a trend to better recovery at higher doses and the nail plate drug levels were certainly higher at the higher doses (Ling *et al.* 1998). Penetration into nails is good and levels exceed the inhibitory concentrations (Savin *et al.* 1998). In addition, the levels persist after treatment (Faergemann & Laufen 1996). Also better results were obtained if patients receiving 150 mg per week also had a nail plate removal with 40% urea (Fräki & Heikkilä 1997). Fluconazole may provide good control of chronic mucocutaneous candidiasis, particularly in nail involvement (Rybojad *et al.* 1999).

Side effects are not common with fluconazole, occurring in 5–10% of individuals. They include nausea and headache. Gastrointestinal discomfort and diarrhoea also occur. Hepatitis is very rare. Other serious adverse events include erythroderma and toxic epidermal necrolysis, multiple birth defects and thrombocytopenia. Drug reactions are fewer than with itraconazole, although the metabolism of many of the same drugs will be affected to a lesser extent.

## Terbinafine

Terbinafine is a member of the allylamine antifungal drug group. It inhibits the epoxidation of squalene, an early step in the formation of ergosterol in the fungal cell membrane (Petranyi *et al.* 1987). This is a conversion stage which occurs earlier than that inhibited by the azoles. Terbinafine is active against a wide range of pathogenic fungi *in vitro*, but *in vivo* is only useful for dermatophytosis (250 mg daily).

One potential advantage of this drug is the fact that unlike the other oral antifungals it appears to be fungicidal *in vitro* at relatively low concentrations. In dermatophytosis of the dry type rapid responses and low relapse rates have been recorded. In onychomycosis rather similar results have been seen with mycological remission of infected fingernails occurring within

3 months of starting therapy (Goodfield *et al.* 1989). These results also suggest more rapid penetration into the nail, a fact now confirmed by studies of its distribution within nail. The possibility also exists that these responses have a lower relapse rate than with other compounds. This initial study has now been extended to a placebo-controlled trial of terbinafine 250 mg daily in dermatophyte onychomycosis (Goodfield *et al.*

1992). This has shown significant recovery rates of toenail infections at 3 months and fingernails at 6 weeks. Two studies of terbinafine have shown that the drug is better than continuous itraconazole given for 3 months at a dose of 200 mg per day (Bräutigam 1998; De Backer *et al.* 1998). In addition, a further study has found that terbinafine in doses of 250 mg daily for 12 or 16 weeks is superior for both mycological and clinical

**Table 4.5** Drug interactions with the new antifungal drugs (Brodell & Elewski 1995; Roberts 1997).

| Type of drug interacting | Itraconazole | Fluconazole | Terbinafine |
| --- | --- | --- | --- |
| Drugs increasing level of antimycotic | | Hydrochlorothiazide<br>Other thiazide diuretics? | Cimetidine |
| Drugs decreasing levels of antimycotic | Rifampicin<br>Isoniazid<br>Phenytoin<br>Phenobarbital<br>Carbamazepine<br>$H_2$ antagonist<br>Antacids<br>Didanosine (due to its high pH buffer in the tablet formulation)<br>Anticholinergic drugs | Rifampicin | Rifampicin<br>Phenobarbital |
| Drugs whose activity or levels may be increased | Phenytoin<br>Warfarin<br>$H_1$ antagonist<br>    Terfenadine<br>    Astemizole<br>Digoxin<br>Alprazolam<br>Triazolam<br>Midazolam<br>Felodipine<br>Fluoxetine<br>Nifedipine<br>Corticosteroids<br>Methylprednisolone<br>Cyclosporin A<br>Cisapride<br>Zidovudine<br>Protease inhibitors<br>Busulfan<br>Vincristine<br>Oral antidiabetic drugs (sylphonyl urea)<br>    Tolbutamide<br>    Glibenclamide<br>    Glipizide<br>Lovastatin<br>Simvastatin<br>Quinidine<br>Tacrolimus | Warfarin<br>Phenytoin<br>$H_1$ antagonist?<br>    Astemizole<br>    Terfenadine<br>Midazolam<br>Triazolam<br>Nortriptyline<br>Theophylline<br>Rifabutin<br>Zidovudine<br>Cyclosporin A | Warfarin<br>Nortriptyline<br>Nicotinamide |
| Drugs that may be decreased in activity/safety | Oral contraceptives?<br>Antipryine | Oral contraceptives? | |

*Note*: Drug interactions are usually less severe with fluconazole than with itraconazole.

recovery rates than pulsed itraconazole using either 3 or 4 pulses (200 mg bid for 1 week every month) of a similar period at long-term follow up (Evans & Sigurgeirsson 1999). A smaller study found no difference in the mycological recovery rates between the continuous dosage of terbinafine, pulsed itraconazole, in conventional doses, and a similar pulsed regimen using terbinafine at 500 mg daily for 1 week every month × 3 (Tosti *et al.* 1996b). Another feature of treatment with terbinafine is the high remission rates seen at long-term follow up, over a year post treatment (Török *et al.* 1998).

A further study has shown that the combined use of terbinafine at 250 mg daily with amorolfine nail lacquer produces better responses than terbinafine alone, although the response rates of the terbinafine arm are considerably lower than those seen in other studies (Baran *et al.* 2000).

Adverse events occur in about 5–8% and include gastrointestinal fullness and discomfort as well as nausea. Hepatitis, although reported, is very rare. Transient loss or disturbance of taste is more common and is mainly seen in the elderly and underweight individuals. Thrombocytopenia and granulocytopenia have been reported rarely, along with some skin reactions such as erythema multiforme, Stevens–Johnson syndrome and erythroderma.

Drug interations with the new antifungal drugs are shown in Table 4.5.

## Nail removal (Figs 4.43–4.46)

It may be possible to enhance results of chemotherapy by various procedures: (a) mechanical removal by cutting, filing or abrading; (b) surgical removal by total or partial nail avulsion; (c) chemical removal by keratinolysis. These techniques may shorten the duration of therapy.

Filing and trimming of the nail undertaken by the patient are seldom helpful measures for treating subungual onychomycosis. However, removal of as much diseased nail as possible by a dermatologist or podiatrist is helpful, but only as an adjunct to oral or topical antifungals (Baden 1994). It is a logical

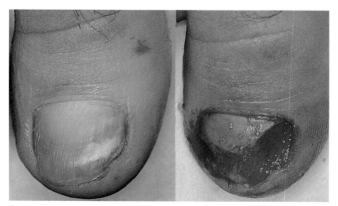

**Fig. 4.43** Partial nail removal—distal portion.

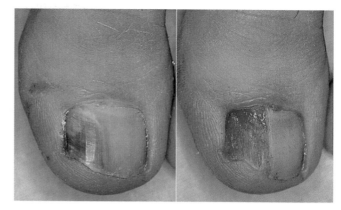

**Fig. 4.44** Partial nail removal—medial half.

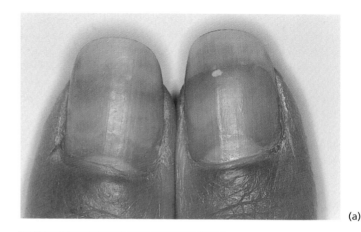

(a)

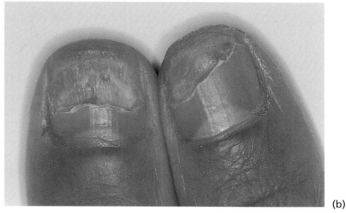

(b)

**Fig. 4.45** (a) Onycholysis due to *Candida albicans*. (b) Removal of the non-adherent nail keratin.

approach to eradication of the pathogen from lateral nail disease (Baran & De Doncker 1996) and from onycholytic pockets or canals (Hay 1986) on the undersurface of the nail, which are sometimes filled with necrotic tissue and large compact amounts of fungi (dermatophytoma) (Roberts & Evans 1998). These factors are frequently responsible for the failure of

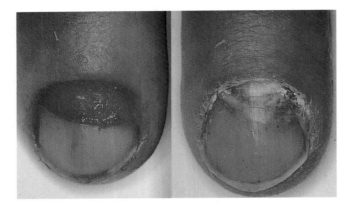

**Fig. 4.46** Partial removal of the proximal nail plate in proximal white subungual onychomycosis.

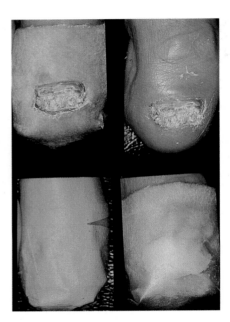

**Fig. 4.47** Urea chemical avulsion—technique.

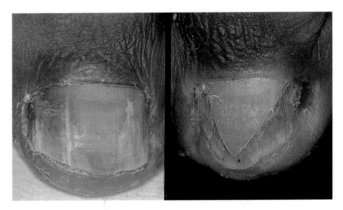

**Fig. 4.48** Urea chemical treatment—before and after removal of the affected nail keratin.

systemic antifungals. Additionally impaired host immune response, inadequate absorption or distribution of the drug and inactivation, interaction or resistance to therapy may play a part. As in the case of dermatophyte nail infections, nail plate avulsion is also helpful in treating onychomycosis caused by yeast and non-dermatophyte moulds (Rollman & Johansson 1987; Baran *et al.* 1997).

Incidental to removing the nail plate, it is imperative that the nail bed and nail grooves be debrided of subungual debris; this is best accomplished by wiping the nail bed and nail grooves with a gauze wrapped around the end of a mosquito haemostat.

Total surgical removal has to be discouraged: the distal nail bed may shrink and become dislocated dorsally. In addition, the loss of counterpressure produced by the removal of the nail plate allows expansion of the distal soft tissue and the distal edge of the regrowing nail then embeds itself. This can be largely overcome by using partial nail avulsion. However, in a small percentage of cases depending on the degree of patient discomfort, for example when total surgical removal has been decided, the patient should be instructed to use a prosthetic nail on the regrowing nail plate so that the width of the nail bed is maintained and subsequent ingrowth is avoided (Dominguez-Cherit *et al.* 1999).

Partial surgical nail avulsion for onychomycosis (Baran & Hay 1985) can be performed under local anaesthesia in a selected group of patients in whom the fungal infection is of limited extent. It permits the removal of the affected portion of the nail plate in one session, even when the disease has reached the buried region of the nail bed beneath the proximal nail fold.

The diseased nail plate including a margin of normal appearing nail is cut with an English nail splitter or a double action bone rongeur, then removed with a sturdy forceps as for total avulsion.

### Chemical avulsion (Figs 4.47 & 4.48)

Chemical avulsion is a painless method which has superseded partial surgical avulsion. It may be repeated as often as necessary. The formulation used is shown in Table 4.6 (Farber & South 1978).

Urea ointment is applied to the nail plate after protecting the surrounding skin, for example with adhesive dressing. The entire distal digit is then wrapped for a week. Urea ointment appears to focus its action on the bond between the nail keratin and the diseased nail bed; it spares only the normal nail tissue. Afterwards, blunt dissection using a nail elevator and nail clipper leaves the remaining portion of normal nail plate intact. Generally the nail is soft enough for removal after about 8 h and becomes sequentially softer with each successive application. Clinical experience has shown that this topical treatment is successful when no more than three to five nails are affected.

Following removal of the diseased part of the nail, topical antifungal agents (imidazoles, tolnaftate, haloprogin, ciclopirox) should be applied, at least, for 2 months under occlusion, especially if there is no associated systemic therapy. Combination

**Table 4.6** Urea ointment formulation.

| | |
|---|---|
| Urea | 40% |
| White beeswax (or paraffin) | 5% |
| Anhydrous lanolin | 20% |
| White petrolatum | 25% |
| Silica gel type H | 10% |

20% urea and 10% salicylic acid ointment has been suggested (Buselmeier 1980). Some authors prefer using 50% potassium iodide ointment in anhydrous lanolin plus 0.5% iodochlorhydroxyquine instead of 40% urea for keratinolysis (Dorn *et al.* 1980).

A ready-made topical preparation containing 40% urea and 1% bifonazole is available (Hay *et al.* 1988b; Bonifaz *et al.* 1995). This preparation is applied under occlusion and the patient is asked to debride the nails every day for 1–2 weeks, facilitating removal of the diseased nail keratin within 1 or 2 weeks of this daily treatment. Then 1% bifonazole cream is applied once a day for 2 months to the whole nail area and rubbed onto the nail bed. In some clinical trials, the efficacy of this ointment has been demonstrated, provided that the instructions are properly followed and that strict compliance by the patient is ensured (Bonifaz *et al.* 1995). However, such treatment is difficult to apply in the elderly, tedious when several digits are affected and/or ineffective when the proximal portion of the nail plate is invaded by fungal organisms beneath the nail fold. Once again, the treatment is more suitable for limited and early nail disease. The unpleasant odour following the use of urea ointment, especially when left for 1 week, has led to the development of a new formulation still under investigation, which may resolve most of the problems due to the chemical keratinolysis.

## Rationale for a new approach to therapy

Besides the five main considerations for choosing a drug—efficacy, safety, cost, compliance and availability (Gupta *et al.* 1997b)—choice of treatment depends on many factors, including the patient's age and preference, infecting fungus, number of nails affected, degree of nail involvement, whether toenails or fingernails are infected and when other drugs are taken (Denning *et al.* 1995). In order to improve on efficacy, some investigators still suggest that one management approach would be to check the mycological status 6 months after the start of systemic therapy and then to repeat treatment for those with positive results with the same antifungal: terbinafine (Watson *et al.* 1995; Tausch *et al.* 1997) or itraconazole (Haneke *et al.* 1997), or with fluconazole after a course of terbinafine (De Cuyper 1998).

However, by following such strategies we move away from one of the considerations of great importance nowadays, i.e. cost effectiveness.

It is important to recognize that fungal invasion of certain sites, for example the lunula, the lateral edge of the nail and the subungual area (which may lead to extensive onycholysis), may affect recovery (Table 4.7). Therefore, a rationale for a staged-therapy approach in treating onychomycosis is suggested.

Early infections with involvement of the distal two-thirds of the nail plate of up to two to four digits may be treated with topical monotherapy using the nail lacquers that act as transungual drug delivery systems. The shorter the length of nail plate invasion, the better the treatment response. Such treatment of distal subungual onychomycosis at the beginning of the fungal invasive process solves the problem of retaining the active agent in contact with the substrate for long enough to produce the desired antifungal action. Should there be no significant clinical success after a period of 6 months, a short course with systemic antifungal agents should be added.

Topical monotherapy is ineffective in more extensive infections, including those with the local factors already mentioned, i.e. where the nail plate is no longer in contact with the subungual tissue (as this interrupts the transport of the drug from the nail into the nail bed). Equally, this drawback is also encountered with the new systemic antifungal drugs which usually penetrate the nail via the nail bed, thereby interrupting the transport process of the drug from the nail bed into the ventral nail plate. Even though these drugs still enter the nail keratin through the matrix, the clinical and mycological response may be diminished. One potential solution to the management of these more extensive infections involves using antifungal nail lacquer and oral therapy with one of the newer drugs, for example terbinafine (Baran *et al.* 2000), itraconazole (Nolting & Ulbricht 1997) or fluconazole, from the start. The use of combined topical and systemic therapy may be expensive in some countries, but where this is not an issue, it is a logical clinical choice.

This combination is potentially beneficial, because topical treatment may eradicate fungal foci in the nail plate and systemic antifungals treat the nail bed and tinea pedis which usually precedes onychomycosis. Chemical or partial surgical nail avulsion may also be used to supplement the treatment to eliminate the factors encouraging chronicity, such as the development of irregularities of the nail bed. Such a combination also minimizes the risk of adverse effects from systemic drugs, which might have to be given for a long period.

Antifungal combinations may increase the magnitude and rate of microbial killing *in vivo*, shorten the total duration of therapy, prevent the emergence of drug resistance, expand the spectrum of activity, and decrease drug-related toxicity by using lower doses of antifungals (Polak-Wyss 1995; Polak 1996; Ghannoum 1997).

Biochemical studies have identified a number of potential targets for antifungal chemotherapy, including cell wall synthesis, membrane sterol biosynthesis, nucleic acid synthesis, metabolic inhibition and macromolecular biosynthesis (Polak-Wyss 1995).

The inhibition of cell wall synthesis would be, in theory, highly specific since only fungal cells build their cell wall with chitin and glucan. Because the modern systemic azoles and allylamines as well as the topical amorolfine act very specifically on the ergosterol biosynthesis in the cell membrane, as a rational partner for combination therapy one may prefer to combine the new systemic drugs with ciclopirox which acts by a completely different mechanism. As yet there is no suitable preparation of the new cell wall antagonists, such as the echinocandins, currently in development.

## Management of various subtypes

In *primary onycholysis* of the big toenails, associated with dermatophyte invasion, measures should be taken to relieve the effects of pressure and trauma, such as the provision of fitted shoes, padding or toe shields (Table 4.7). Daily topical treatment with antifungal therapy and repeated trimming of the non-adherent portion of nails should be started.

Nails affected by dermatophyte superficial white onychomycosis should be abraded after confirming the diagnosis by taking scrapings. When the culture is negative a tangential piece of the nail plate, using the shave excision technique, or a 3-mm punch biopsy of the nail plate, is taken for histopathology. This will avoid unnecessary systemic therapy since topical treatments alone are effective. Alternatively a 10% glutaraldehyde solution (Cidex), which tints the nail bronze, may be used for both dermatophytes and mould infections (Suringa 1970). Coexistence of white superficial onychomycosis and distal and lateral subungual onychomycosis is an indication for oral therapy. In the elderly or those with isolated lesser toenail involvement, treatment may be unnecessary and control of nail thickening by chiropody may be the best alternative. The 40% urea–1% bifonazole ointment may be used, combining the advantages of considerable nail softening with antimycotic action on the infectious keratotic debris from under the nail. It is wise to avoid salicylic acid in combination with urea if there is peripheral circulatory insufficiency.

### Non-dermatophyte mould onychomycosis

Assuming that the pathogenic role of mould fungi isolated from the affected nails has been confirmed using the criteria discussed previously, three patterns of infection must be considered:
1 Superficial white onychomycosis caused by *Acremonium*, *Aspergillus* or *Fusarium* spp.
2 Distal and lateral subungual onychomycosis caused by *S. brevicaulis* and certain other moulds such as *Pyrenochaeta unguium-hominis* (Punithaligam & English 1975; English 1980);
3 *S. dimidiatum* previously known as *Hendersonula toruloidea* (Gentles & Evans 1970; Campbell *et al.* 1973) (Fig. 4.9) or *Nattrassia mangiferae* (Sutton & Dyko 1989) and *S. hyalinum* (Campbell & Mulder 1977).

**Table 4.7** Causes of failure of onychomycosis treatment. (Modified after de Doncker *et al.* Poster 187 AAD 1998.)

*Poor compliance*

*Misdiagnosis*
Laboratory tests neglected
Dual pathology
Bacterial association (Elewski 1997)

*Dietary mistakes* (itraconazole and ketoconazole intake)
Lower gastric acidity/achlorhydria (e.g. in AIDS or neutropenic patients), should be compensated by intake with acidic fruit juice
Empty stomach, since absorption of these drugs (as well as griseofulvin) is influenced by presence of fat-containing meal

*Clinical variants*
Extensive onycholysis
Lateral nail fungal infection
Dermatophytoma
Paronychia

*Mycological variants*
Presence of arthroconidia with thicker cell walls
Dematiaceous fungi
*Trichophyton rubrum nigricans* (Perrin & Baran 1994)
Development of yeast resistance in immunocompromised patients as well as replacement of the most common
*Candida* spp. resistant to treatment (Roberts 1997)

*Bioavailability of drug interactions*

*Local factors*
Reduced linear nail growth
Wearing improperly fitted shoes

*Systemic factors*
Peripheral circulation impairment
Endocrine diseases (diabetes, Cushing)
Ageing with multiple-associated factors

*Host response*
Endogenous immunological factors:
  AIDS
  CMC
  Chronic dermatophytosis
Exogenous immunological factors:
  Immunosuppressive therapy (transplant patients)
  Chemotherapy

Superficial white onychomycosis caused by non-dermatophytes may respond to abrasion of the nail surface followed by topical therapy with imidazole agents, particularly those with better *in vitro* activity against mould fungi such as econazole, clotrimazole or 28% tioconazole, amorolfine, ciclopiroxolamine, 8% ciclopirox nail lacquer, and 10% glutaraldehyde may also be effective. However, topical therapy may be useful for the other categories of early or mild infection. Repeated chemical removal of the nails, followed by local applications of keratolytics and antifungal agents, may also be tried. Although there is evidence that some cases of onychomycosis due to mould fungi respond to single oral antifungal treatment such as itraconazole or terbinafine (Tosti *et al.* 1996a; Gupta *et al.* 1998b), the response is not predictable and some combination of nail removal and oral/topical therapy is usually necessary. There is also evidence that the clinical progress during the treatment of nails containing both mould fungi as well as dermatophytes is determined by the response of the dermatophytes alone (Ellis *et al.* 1997).

### *Candida* onychomycosis

Nail dystrophy caused by *Candida* can be treated with oral itraconazole, fluconazole or ketoconazole, or chemical removal followed by local antifungal treatment. If these methods are unsuccessful, combined avulsion and chemotherapy should be used. In chronic mucocutaneous candidiasis, the dose of ketoconazole may have to be increased to 400 mg or 600 mg daily. When remission is induced, treatment should be stopped. Resistance has been reported where low dose (200 mg daily) therapy is continued. Itraconazole is another effective alternative in this condition and resistance to this drug has not been recorded. Other antifungals such as low-dose amphotericin B, intravenous miconazole or oral clotrimazole have been used in the past with limited success (Hay 1981). Liposome-associated amphotericin B may be another alternative offering less toxicity.

### Onycholysis with *Candida* colonization

This variety often coexists with bacterial infection (*Pseudomonas* or *Proteus*). The patient should be advised to wear thin cotton gloves, which are regularly cleaned, under rubber gloves used for all wet work and to avoid excessive immersion in hot water, even when wearing protective gloves. After hand washing, the nail fold area must be dried carefully—in some cases the use of a hair-dryer is recommended to keep the nail plate–nail bed space as dry as possible. The nail plate has to be trimmed as far back as possible: if the patient is anxious, local anaesthesia may be required. Scissors are used to separate the nail plate proximal to the onycholytic area; then the nail bed should be debrided with a piece of gauze wrapped around a stick. Four per cent thymol in chloroform or 15% sulphacetamide in 70% ethyl alcohol may be applied twice daily to the space to suppress growth of *Candida* and *Pseudomonas*. The specific antifungals (i.e. miconazole, clotrimazole) may supplement this treatment. Thorough trimming should be repeated at intervals of 4 weeks until the nail reattaches. 'Green nails' deserve the same treatment despite good but inconstant results obtained by Zaias (1990b) with Clorox, diluted 1 in 4, a few drops being applied three times a day. Polymyxin B is no longer used for *Pseudomonas* infections; brushing the nail area with 2% acetic acid is an alternative method. The patient should be warned against cleaning with a nail file or orange wood stick under an area of onycholysis as this may increase the split. Removal of organisms in patients with onycholysis may improve the appearance of the nails but will not produce healing of the split between nail plate and nail bed.

### Chronic *Candida* paronychia

As in all varieties of paronychia, protection of the hands from water (as for onycholysis) is an indispensable part of management. Topical antifungal agents active against *Candida* must be applied to the groove between the nail plate and the proximal fold at least twice daily. Solution formulations of these drugs are much more effective than creams or ointments for paronychia. Treatment usually has to be continued for at least 3 months and until the nail fold lies flat against the nail plate. Warm compresses with Burrow's solution (1 : 40 dilution) for 10 min three times a day may also decrease the inflammatory reaction. If there are frequent acute episodes, combined treatment using intralesional or systemic steroid therapy and systemic antibiotics such as erythromycin 1 g daily, or tetracycline 1 g daily for 1 week, may be useful. Systemic therapy, such as ketoconazole, works in this condition but is no more efficacious than topical treatment. Fluconazole (50 mg/day) was, however, effective in the management of chronic *Candida* paronychia according to Amichai and Shiri (1999).

Treatment should not be considered complete until the cuticle has regrown. Reattachment of the proximal nail fold to the nail can be encouraged by dabbing the groove with a toothpick dipped into 80% phenol. All the affected areas of the nail plate should be clipped away or abraded. An alternative is the use of azole antifungal lotions applied along the nail fold and allowed to seep under this area. Chemical removal is an alternative for completely dystrophic nails. Low-voltage X-ray therapy has been suggested using 1 Gy (100 rad) given three times at weekly intervals with a 50-kV 1-mm Al filter, and may produce good results on the paronychial inflammation. Surgical therapy is seldom necessary (Chapter 10).

## Complications associated with the treatment of onychomycosis

Among 100 consecutive patients treated for onychomycosis in a private medical practice, 37 of them developed paronychia ranging from simple pain to a severe inflammatory response with redness, drainage and granuloma formation. Of these, 19 patients required surgical procedures to control onychocryptotic symptoms. Consequently, physicians should be aware that ingrowing toenails may be an adverse consequence of effective treatment for onychomycosis (Connelley *et al.* 1999; Weaver & Jespersen 2000).

## References

Achten, G. & Simonart, J. (1963) L'ongle. Etude histologique et mycologique. *Annales de Dermatologie et de Syphiligraphie* 90, 569–586.

Achten, G. & Simonart, J. (1965) Kératine unguéale et parasites fongiques: mycopathologie. *Mycologia* **27**, 193–199.

Achten, G. & Wanet-Rouard, J. (1978) Onychomycoses in the laboratory. *Mykosen* **1** (Suppl.), 125.

Achten, G. & Wanet-Rouard, J. (1981) *Onychomycosis. Mycology no. 5.* Cilag Ltd, Brussels.

Achten, G., Wanet-Rouard, J., Wiame, L. & Van Hoff, F. (1979) Les onychomycoses à moisissures: champignons 'opportunistes'. *Dermatologica* **159** (Suppl. 1), 128.

Alkiewicz, J. (1948) Transverse net in the diagnosis of onychomycosis. *Archives of Dermatology and Syphilis* **58**, 385.

Amichai, B. & Shiri, J. (1999) Fluconazole 50 mg/day therapy in the management of chronic paronychia. *Journal of Dermatological Treatment* **10**, 199–200.

Artis, W.M., Odle, B.M. & Jones, H.E. (1981) Griseofulvin-resistant dermatophytosis correlates with *in vitro* resistance. *Archives of Dermatology* **117**, 16–19.

Baden, H.P. (1994) Treatment of distal onychomycosis with avulsion and topical antifungal agents under occlusion. *Archives of Dermatology* **130**, 558–559.

Badillet, G. (1988) Mélanonychies superficielles. *Bulletin de la Société Française Mycological Medicine* **17**, 335–340.

Baral, J., Fusco, F., Kahn, H. *et al.* (1996) The use of nail clippings for detecting fungi in nail plates. *Dermatopathology Practical and Conceptual* **2**, 266–268.

Baran, R. (1982) Treatment of severe onychomycosis with ketoconazole. A new oral antifungal drug. In: *XVI Congressus Internationalis Dermatologiae, 1982, Tokyo*, p. 298.

Baran, R. & Badillet, G. (1982) Primary onycholysis of the big toenails; a review of 113 cases. *British Journal of Dermatology* **106**, 529–534.

Baran, R. & Badillet, G. (1983) Un dermatophyte unguéal est-il nécessairement pathogène? *Annales de Dermatologie et de Vénéréologie* **110**, 619–631.

Baran, R. & De Doncker, P. (1996) Lateral edge nail involvement indicates poor prognosis for treating onychomycosis with the new systemic antifungals. *Acta Dermato-Venereologica* **75**, 82–83.

Baran, R. & Hay, R. (1985) Partial surgical avulsion of the nail in onychomycosis. *Clinical and Experimental Dermatology* **10**, 413–418.

Baran, R., Tosti, A. & Piraccini, B.M. (1997) Uncommon clinical patterns of *Fusarium* nail infection: report of three cases. *British Journal of Dermatology* **136**, 424–427.

Baran, R., Haneke, E. & Tosti, A. (1998a) *Trichophyton rubrum* demonstrating three different entry sites in adolescent's toenails. *Mikologia Lekarska* **5**, 47.

Baran, R., Hay, R.J., Tosti, A. & Haneke, E. (1998b) A new classification of onychomycosis. *British Journal of Dermatology* **119**, 567–571.

Baran, R., Hay, R., Haneke, E. & Tosti, A. (1999) *Onychomycosis— The Current Approach to Diagnosis and Therapy.* Martin Dunitz, London.

Baran, R., Feuilhade, M., Datry, A. *et al.* (2000) A randomized trial of amorolfine 5% solution nail lacquer associated with oral terbinafine compared with terbinafine alone in the treatment of dermatophytic toenail onychomycoses affecting the matrix region. *British Journal of Dermatology* **142**, 1177–1183.

Belsan, I. & Fragner, P. (1965) Onychomykosen, hervorgerufen durch *Scopulariopsis brevicaulis. Hautarzt* **16**, 258.

Bonifaz, A., Guzman, A., Garcia, C. *et al.* (1995) Efficacy and safety of bifonazole urea in the two-phase treatment of onychomycosis. *International Journal of Dermatology* **34**, 500–503.

Botter, A.A., Dethier, F., Mertens, R.L.J. *et al.* (1979) Skin and nail mycoses: treatment with ketoconazole, a new oral antimycotic agent. *Mykosen* **22**, 274–278.

Boudghène-Stambouli, O. & Mérad-Boudia, A. (1998) Maladie dermatophytique: hyperkératose exubérante avec cornes cutanées. *Annales de Dermatologie et de Vénéréologie* **125**, 705–707.

Bräutigam, M. (1998) Terbinafine versus itraconazole: a controlled clinical comparison in onychomycosis of the toenails. *Journal of the American Academy of Dermatology* **38**, S53–S56.

Brodell, R.T. & Elewski, B.E. (1995) Clinical pearl: antifungal drugs and drug interactions. *Journal of the American Academy of Dermatology* **33**, 259–260.

Buselmeier, F.J. (1980) Combination urea and salicylic acid ointment nail avulsion in non dystrophic nails: follow-up observation. *Cutis* **25**, 393–405.

Campbell, C.K. & Mulder, J.L. (1977) Skin and nail infection by *Scytalidium hyalium* sp. *Sabouraudia* **15**, 161–166.

Campbell, C.K., Kurwa, H., Abdel-Aziz, A.H.M. *et al.* (1973) Fungal infections of skin and nails by *Hendersonula toruloidea. British Journal of Dermatology* **89**, 45–52.

Ceschin-Roques, C.G., Hänel, H., Pruja-Bougaret, S.M. *et al.* (1991) Ciclopirox nail lacquer 8%: *in vivo* penetration into and through nails and *in vitro* effect on pig skin. *Skin Pharmacology* **4**, 89–94.

Civila, E.S., Cont-Diaz, I.A., Vignale, R.A. *et al.* (1982) Onixis por Malassezia (*Pityrosporum ovalis*). *Medicina Cutanea Ibero-Latino-Americana* **10**, 343–346.

Coleman, R. & Hay, R.J. (1997) Chronic mucocutaneous candidosis associated with hypothyroidism: a distinct syndrome? *British Journal of Dermatology* **136**, 24–29.

Connelley, L.K., Dinehart, S.M. & McDonald, R. (1999) Onychocryptosis associated with the treatment of onychomycosis. *Journal of the American Podiatric Medical Association* **89**, 424–426.

Contet-Audonneau, N., Salvini, O., Basile, A.M. *et al.* (1995) Les onychomycoses à moisissures. Importance diagnostique de la biopsie unguéale. Fréquence des espèces pathogènes. Sensibilité aux principaux antifongiques. *Nouvelle Dermatologie* **14**, 330–340.

Cox, F.W., Stiller, R.L. & South, D.A. (1982) Oral ketoconazole for dermatophyte infections. *Journal of the American Academy of Dermatology* **6**, 455–462.

Daniel, C.R. (1985) Nail micronizer. *Cutis* **36**, 118.

Daniel, C.R., Daniel, M.P., Daniel, C.M. *et al.* (1996) Chronic paronychia and onycholysis. A thirteen-year experience. *Cutis* **58**, 397–401.

Daniel, C.R. III, Gupta, A.K., Daniel, M.P. & Daniel, C.M. (1997) Two feet–one hand syndrome: a retrospective multicenter survey. *International Journal of Dermatology* **36**, 658–660.

Davies, R.R. (1968) Mycological test and onychomycosis. *Journal of Clinical Pathology* **21**, 729–730.

Davies, R.R. (1980) Griseofulvin. In: *Antifungal Chemotherapy* (ed. D.C.E. Speller), pp. 149–182. John Wiley, Chichester, UK.

Davies, R.R., Everall, J.D. & Hamilton, E. (1977) Mycological and clinical evaluation of griseofulvin for chronic onychomycosis. *British Medical Journal* iii, 464.

De Backer, M., De Vroey, C., Lesaffre, E. *et al.* (1998) Twelve weeks of continuous oral therapy for toenail onychomycosis caused by dermatophytes: a double-blind comparative trial of terbinafine 250 mg/day versus itraconazole 200 mg/day. *Journal of the American Academy of Dermatology* **38**, S57–S63.

De Cuyper, C. (1998) Therapeutic approach of recalcitrant toenail onychomycosis. In: *Fifth International Summit on Cutaneous Antifungal Therapy. Singapore.* Abstract 26.

Denning, D.W., Evans, E.G., Klibber, C.C. *et al.* (1995) Fungal nail disease: a guide to good practice. *British Medical Journal* **311**, 1271–1281.

Dominguez-Cherit, J., Teixera, F. & Arenas, R. (1999) Combined surgical and systemic treatment of onychomycosis. *British Journal of Dermatology* **140**, 778–780.

Dompmartin, D., Dompmartin, A., Deluol, A.M. *et al.* (1990) Onychomycosis and AIDS. Clinical and laboratory findings in 62 patients. *International Journal of Dermatology* **29**, 337–339.

Dorn, M., Kienitz, T. & Ryckmanns, F. (1980) Onychomykose: Erfahrungen mit atraumatisches Nagelabsölung. *Hautarzt* **31**, 30.

Effendy, I. (1995) Therapeutic strategies in onychomycosis. *Journal of the European Academy of Dermatology and Venereology* **4** (Suppl. 1), S3–S10.

Elewski, B.E. (1997) Bacterial infection in a patient with onychomycosis. *Journal of the American Academy of Dermatology* **37**, 493–494.

Ellis, D.H., Marley, J.E., Watson, A.B. *et al.* (1997) Significance of nondermatophyte moulds and yeasts in onychomycosis. *Dermatology* **194** (Suppl. 1), 40–42.

English, M.P. (1976) Nails and fungi. *British Journal of Dermatology* **94**, 697–701.

English, M.P. (1980) Infection of the finger-nail by *Pyrenochaeta unguis-hominis*. *British Journal of Dermatology* **103**, 91–93.

English, M. & Atkinson, R. (1973) An improved method for the isolation of fungi in onychomycosis. *British Journal of Dermatology* **88**, 273.

English, M.P. & Atkinson, R. (1974) Onychomycosis in elderly chiropody patients. *British Journal of Dermatology* **91**, 67.

Evans, E.G.V. (1998) Causative pathogens in onychomycosis and the possibility of treatment resistance: a review. *Journal of the American Academy of Dermatology* **38**, S32–S36.

Evans, E.G.V. & Sigurgeirsson, B. (1999) Double blind, randomised study of continuous terbinafine compared with intermittent itraconazole in treatment of toenail onychomycosis. *British Medical Journal* **318**, 1031–1035.

Faergemann, J. & Laufen, H. (1996) Levels of fluconazole in normal and diseased nails during and after treatment of onychomycoses in toenails with fluconazole 150 mg once weekly. *Acta Dermato-Venereologica* **76**, 219–221.

Farber, E. & South, D.A. (1978) Urea ointment in the non surgical avulsion of nail dystrophies. *Cutis* **22**, 689.

Fräki, J.E., Heikkilä, H.T., Matti, O. *et al.* (1997) An open-label, noncomparative, multicenter evaluation of fluconazole with or without urea nail pedicure for treatment of onychomycosis. *Current Therapeutic Research* **58**, 481–491.

Fromtling, R.A. (1988) Overview of medically important antifungal azole derivatives. *Clinical Microbiology Reviews* **1**, 187–217.

Gentles, J.C. (1971) Laboratory investigations of dermatophyte infections of nails. *Sabouraudia: Journal of International Society of Human and Animal Mycology* **9**, 149.

Gentles, J.C. & Evans, E.G.V. (1970) Infection of the feet and nails with *Hendersonula toruloidea*. *Sabouraudia* **8**, 72–75.

Ghannoum, M.A. (1997) Future of antimycotic therapy. *Dermatological Therapy* **3**, 104–111.

Goodfield, M.J.D., Rowell, N.R., Forster, R.A. *et al.* (1989) Treatment of dermatophyte infections of the finger or toe nails with terbinafine (SFG 86–327, Lamisil) an orally active fungicidal agent. *British Journal of Dermatology* **121**, 753–757.

Goodfield, M.J.D., Andrew, L. & Evans, E.G.V. (1992) Short term treatment of dermatophyte onychomycosis with terbinafine. *British Medical Journal* **304**, 1151–1154.

Götz, H. & Hantschke, D. (1965) Einblicke in die Epidemiologie der Dermatomykosen im Kohlenbergbau. *Hautarzt* **16**, 543.

Grant, S.M. & Clissold, S.P. (1990) Fluconazole. A review of its pharmacodynamic and pharmacokinetic properties and therapeutic potential in superficial and systemic mycoses. *Drugs* **39**, 877–916.

Gugnani, H.C., Nzelibe, F.K. & Osunkwo, I.C. (1986) Onychomycosis due to *Hendersonula toruloidea* in Nigeria. *Journal of Medical and Veterinary Mycology* **24**, 239–241.

Gupta, A.K., Lynde, C.Q., Jain, H.C. *et al.* (1997a) A higher prevalence of onychomycosis in psoriatics compared with non psoriatics: a multicentre study. *British Journal of Dermatology* **136**, 786–789.

Gupta, A.K., Scher, R.K. & De Doncker, P. (1997b) Current management of onychomycosis. *Dermatologic Clinics* **15**, 121–135.

Gupta, A.K., Konnikof, N., MacDonald, P. *et al.* (1998a) Prevalence and epidemiology of toenail onychomycosis in diabetic subjects: a multicentre survey. *British Journal of Dermatology* **139**, 665–671.

Gupta, A.K., De Doncker, P., Scher, R.K. *et al.* (1998b) Itraconazole for the treatment of onychomycosis. *International Journal of Dermatology* **37**, 303–308.

Hadida, E., Schousboe, A. & Sayag, J. (1966) Dermatophyties atypiques. *Bulletin de la Société Française de Dermatologie et de Syphiligraphie* **73**, 917.

Haneke, E. (1981) Ketoconazole treatment of dermatomycoses. In: *Current Chemotherapy and Immunotheray*, Vol. II (eds P. Periti & G.G. Grass), pp. 1012–1013. American Society of Microbiology, Washington, DC.

Haneke, E. (1985) Nail biopsies in onychomycosis. *Mykosen* **28**, 473–480.

Haneke, E. (1986) Differential diagnosis of mycotic nail diseases. In: *Advances in Topical Antifungal Therapy* (ed. R.J. Hay), pp. 94–101. Springer, New York.

Haneke, E. (1988) The nails in chronic mucocutaneous candidosis. Presented at the 15th Annual Meeting, Society of Cutaneous Ultrastructure Research. Nice, France. Abstract.

Haneke, E. (1991) Fungal infections of the nail. *Seminars in Dermatology* **10**, 41–51.

Haneke, E., Ring, J. & Abeck, D. (1997) Efficacy of itraconazole pulse treatment in onychomycosis. *Zeitschrift für Hautkrankheiten* **72**, 737–740.

Hay, R.J. (1981) Management of chronic mucocutaneous conditions. *Clinical and Experimental Dermatology* **6**, 515–519.

Hay, R.J. (1986) Chronic dermatophyte infections. In: *Superficial Fungal Infections* (ed. J. Verbov), pp. 23–24. MTP Ltd, Lancaster, UK.

Hay, R.J. (1988) New oral treatments for dermatophytosis. *Annals of the New York Academy of Sciences* **544**, 580–585.

Hay, R.J. & Clayton, Y.M. (1992) The treatment of patients with chronic mucocutaneous conditions and *Candida* onychomycosis with ketoconazole. *Clinical and Experimental Dermatology* **7**, 155–162.

Hay, R.J., Mackie, R.M. & Clayton, Y.M. (1985) Tioconazole (28%) nail solution: an open study of its efficacy in onychomycosis. *Clinical and Experimental Dermatology* **10**, 152–157.

Hay, R.J., Clayton, Y.M. & Moore, M.K. (1987) A comparison of tioconazole 28% nail solution versus base as an adjunct to oral griseofulvin in patients with onychomycosis. *Clinical and Experimental Dermatology* **12**, 175–177.

Hay, R.J., Baran, R., Moore, M.K. & Wilkinson, J.D. (1988a) *Candida* onychomycosis—an evaluation of the role of *Candida* in nail disease. *British Journal of Dermatology* **118**, 47–58.

Hay, R.J., Roberts, D., Doherty, V.R. *et al.* (1988b) The topical treatment of onychomycosis using a new combined urea/imidazole preparation. *Clinical and Experimental Dermatology* **17**, 164–167.

Hay, R.J., Clayton, Y.M., Moore, M.K. *et al.* (1988c) An evaluation of itraconazole in the management of onychomycosis. *British Journal of Dermatology* **119**, 359–366.

Heiberg, J.K. & Svejgaard, E. (1981) Toxic hepatitis during ketoconazole treatment. *British Medical Journal* **283**, 825–826.

Higashi, N. (1990) Melanonychia due to tinea unguium. *Hifu* **32**, 377–380.

Jones, S.K., White, J.E., Jacobs, P.H. *et al.* (1985) *Hendersonula toruloidea* infection of the nails in Caucasians. *Clinical and Experimental Dermatology* **10**, 444–447.

Kalter, D.C. & Hay, R.J. (1988) Onychomycosis due to *Trichophyton soudanense*. *Clinical and Experimental Dermatology* **13**, 221–227.

Koutselinis, H., Aronis, K. & Stratigos, J. (1982) Cytology as an aid in the diagnosis of psoriasis of nails. *Acta Cytologica* **26**, 422–424.

Langer, H. (1957) Epidemiologische und klinische Untersuchungen bei Onychomykosen. *Archiv für Klinische und Experimentelle Dermatologie* **204**, 624.

Leyden, J.J., Decherd, J.W. & Goldschmidt, H. (1972) Exfoliative cytology in the diagnosis of psoriasis of nails. *Cutis* **10**, 701.

Ling, M.R., Swinyer, L.J., Jarratt, M.T. *et al.* (1998) Once-weekly fluconazole (450 mg) for 4, 6, or 9 months of treatment for distal subungual onychomycosis of the toenail. *Journal of the American Academy of Dermatology* **38**, S95–S102.

McAleer, R. (1981) Fungal infections of the nails in Western Australia. *Mycopathologica* **73**, 115.

Machler, B.C., Kirsner, R.S. & Elgart, G.W. (1998) Routine histologic examination for the diagnosis of onychomycosis: an evaluation of sensitivity and specificity. *Cutis* **61**, 217–219.

Marks, R. & Dawber, R.P.R. (1971) Skin surface biopsy—an improved technique for the examination of the horny layer. *British Journal of Dermatology* **84**, 117–123.

Mehregan, D.A., Mehregan, D.R. & Rincker, A. (1997) Onychomycosis. *Cutis* **59**, 247–248.

Meisel, C.E. & Quadripur, S.A. (1992) Onychomycosis due to *Hendersonula toruloidea*. *Hautnah Mykologie* **6**, 232–234.

Milne, L.J.R. (1989) Direct microscopy. In: *Medical Mycology—A Practical Approach* (eds E.G.V. Evans & M.D. Richardson), pp. 17–45. IRL Press. Oxford.

Moore, M.K. (1978) Skin and nail infections caused by non-dermatophyte filamentous fungi. *Mykosen* **1** (Suppl.), 128–132.

Muñoz, P., Moreno, S., Berengues, J. *et al.* (1991) Fluconazole-related hepatotoxicity in patients with AIDS. *Archives of Internal Medicine* **151**, 1020–1021.

Negroni, P. (1976) Erythrasma of the nails. *Medicina Cutanea Ibero-Latino-Americana* **5**, 349.

Nolting, S. & Ulbricht, H. (1997) Untersuchungen zur Applikationsfrequenz von Ciclopirox-Lack (8%) bei der Behandlung von Onychomykosen. *Jatros Dermatologie* **11**, 20–26.

Ornsberg, P. (1980) Scopulariopsis brevicaulis in nails. *Dermatologica* **161**, 259.

Pardo-Castello, V. & Pardo, O.A. (1960) *Diseases of the Nails*. CC Thomas, Springfield, IL.

Perrin, C. & Baran, R. (1994) Longitudinal melanonychia caused by *Trichophyton rubrum*. *Journal of the American Academy of Dermatology* **31**, 311–316.

Petranyi, G., Meingassner, J.G. & Mieth, H. (1987) Antifungal activity of the allylamine derivative, terbinafine, *in vitro*. *Antimicrobial Agents and Chemotherapy* **31**, 1365–1368.

Piérard, G.E., Arrèse, J.E., Pierre, S. *et al.* (1994a) Diagnostic microscopique des onychomycoses. *Annales de Dermatologie et de Vénéréologie* **121**, 25–29.

Piérard, G.E., Pierard-Franchimont, C. & Arrèse, J.E. (1994b) Onychomycosis may be caused by facultative pathogenic molds. *Dermatopathology* **4**, 131–132.

Polak, A. (1988) Mode of action of morpholine derivatives. *Annals of the New York Academy of Sciences* **544**, 221–228.

Polak, A. (1996) A combination therapy for systemic mycosis. *Infection* **17**, 203–209.

Polak-Wyss, A. (1995) Mechanism of action of antifungals and combination therapy. *Journal of the European Academy of Dermatology and Venereology* **4** (Suppl. 1), S11–S16.

Presser, S.E. & Blank, H. (1981) Cimetidine; adjunct in treatment of tinea capitis. *Lancet* **i**, 108.

Punithalingham, E. & English, M.P. (1975) *Pyrenochaeta unguishominis* sp. nov. on human toenails. *Transactions of the British Mycological Society* **64**, 539.

Rabodonirina, M., Piens, M.A., Monier, M.F. *et al.* (1994) Fusarium infections in immuno-compromised patients: case report and literature review. *European Journal of Clinical Microbiology and Infectious Diseases* **13**, 152–162.

Reinel, D. (1992) Topical treatment of onychomycosis with amorolfine 5% nail lacquer: comparative efficacy and tolerability of once and twice weekly use. *Dermatology* **184** (Suppl.), 21–24.

Roberts, D.T. (1992) Prevalence of dermatophyte onychomycosis in the United Kingdom: results of an omnibus survey. *British Journal of Dermatology* **126** (Suppl. 39), 23–27.

Roberts, D.T. (1997) The risk/benefit ratio of modern antifungal pharmacological agents. In: *Cutaneous Infection and Therapy* (eds R. Aly, K.R. Beutner & H. Maibach), pp. 183–190. Marcel Dekker, New York.

Roberts, D.T. & Evans, E.G.V. (1998) Subungual dermatophytoma complicating dermatophyte onychomycosis. *British Journal of Dermatology* **138**, 189–190.

Robles Martinez, W., Bhogal, B., Morrell, C.A. *et al.* (1990) The use of fluorescent lectine stains to identify fungi in clinical material from skin. *British Journal of Dermatology* **123** (Suppl. 37), 64.

Rollman, O. & Johansson, S. (1987) *Hendersonula toruloidea* infection: successful response of onychomycosis to nail avulsion and topical ciclopiroxolamine. *Acta Dermato-Venereologica* **67**, 506–510.

Rosenthal, S.N. & Wise, R.S. (1960) Studies concerning the development of resistance to griseofulvin by dermatophytes. *Archives of Dermatology* **81**, 684.

Rybojad, M., Abimelec, P., Feuilhade, M. *et al.* (1999) Candidose mucocutanée chronique familiale associée à une polyendocrinopathie auto-immune. *Annales de Dermatologie et de Vénéréologie* **126**, 54–56.

Savin, R.C., Drake, L., Babel, D. *et al.* (1998) Pharmacokinetics of three once-weekly dosages of fluconazole (150, 300, or 450 mg) in distal subungual onychomycosis of the fingernail. *Journal of the American Academy of Dermatology* **38**, S110–S116.

Scher, R.K. & Ackerman, B.A. (1980a) The value of nail biopsy for demonstrating fungi not demonstrated by microbiologic techniques. *American Journal of Dermatopathology* **2**, 55.

Scher, R.K. & Ackerman, B.A. (1980b) Histologic differential diagnosis of onychomycosis and psoriasis of the nail unit from cornified cells of the nail bed alone. *American Journal of Dermatopathology* **21**, 255.

Seebacher, C., Ulbricht, H. & Wörz, K. (1993) Results of a multicentre with ciclopirox nail lacquer in patients with onychomycosis. *Hautnah Mykologie* **3**, 80–84.

Shellow, W.R. & Koplon, B.S. (1968) Green striped nails: chromonychia due to *Pseudomonas aeruginosa*. *Archives of Dermatology* **97**, 149–153.

Stone, O.J. (1975) Chronic paronychia in which hair was a foreign body. *International Journal of Dermatology* **9**, 661.

Stone, O.J. & Mullins, F.J. (1968) Chronic paronychia in children. *Clinical Pediatrics* **7**, 104–107.

Stone, O.J., Mullins, J.F. & Head, E.S. (1964) Chronic paronychia. Occupational material. *Archives of Environmental Health* **9**, 585–588.

Strauss, J.S. (1982) Ketoconazole and the liver. *Journal of the American Academy of Dermatology* **6**, 546.

Suarez, S.M., Silvers, D.N., Scher, R.K. *et al.* (1991) Histologic evaluation of nail clippings for diagnosing onychomycosis. *Archives of Dermatology* **127**, 1517–1519.

Suringa, D.W.R. (1970) Treatment of superficial onychomycosis with topically applied glutaraldehyde. *Archives of Dermatology* **102**, 163–167.

Sutton, B.C. & Dyko, B.J. (1989) Revision of Hendersonula. *Mycological Research* **93**, 466–488.

Tausch, I., Bräutigam, M. & Weidinger, G. (1997) Evaluation of 6 weeks treatment of terbinafine in tinea unguium in a double-blind trial comparing 6 and 12 weeks therapy. *British Journal of Dermatology* **136**, 737–742.

Tkach, J.R. & Rinaldi, M.G. (1982) Severe hepatitis associated with ketoconazole therapy for mucocutaneous candidosis. *Cutis* **29**, 482–484.

Török, I., Simon, G., Dobozy, A. *et al.* (1998) Long-term post-treatment follow-up of onychomycosis treated with terbinafine: a multicentre trial. *Mycoses* **41**, 63–65.

Tosti, A. & Piraccini, B.M. (1997) Paronychia. In: *Contact Urticaria Syndrome* (eds S. Amin & H.I. Maibach), pp. 267–278. CRC Press, Boca Raton, FL.

Tosti, A. & Piraccini, B.M. (1998) Proximal subungual onychomycosis due to *Aspergillus niger*. Report of two cases. *British Journal of Dermatology* **139**, 152–169.

Tosti, A., Fanti, P.A., Guerra, L. *et al.* (1991) Role of foods in the pathogenesis of chronic paronychia. Poster 41. 50th American Academy of Dermatology Meetings, Dallas, TX.

Tosti, A., Piraccini, B.M., Stinchi, C. *et al.* (1996a) Onychomycosis due to *Scopulariopsis brevicaulis*: clinical features and response to systemic antifungals. *British Journal of Dermatology* **135**, 799–802.

Tosti, A., Piraccini, B.M., Stinchi, C. *et al.* (1996b) Treatment of dermatophyte nail infections: an open randomized study comparing intermittent terbinafine therapy with continuous terbinafine treatment and intermittent itraconazole therapy. *Journal of the American Academy of Dermatology* **34**, 595–600.

Tosti, A., Baran, R., Piraccini, B.M. *et al.* (1999) Endonyx onychomycosis: a new modality of nail invasion by dermatophytic fungi. *Acta Dermato-Venereologica* **79**, 52–53.

Vanbreuseghem, R. (1977) Prévalence des onychomycoses au Zaïre particulièrement chez les coupeurs de canne à sucre. *Annales de la Societé Belge de Médécine Tropicale* **57**, 7.

Vazquez, H., Leyva, J. & Arenas, R. (1998) Tinea manuum and two feet–one hand syndrome. *Dermatological Review of Mexico* **42**, 9–12.

Watson, A., Marley, J., Ellis, D. *et al.* (1995) Terbinafine in onychomycosis of the toenail: a novel treatment protocol. *Journal of the American Academy of Dermatology* **33**, 775–779.

Weaver, T.D. & Jespersen, D.L. (2000) Multiple onychocryptosis following treatment of onychomycosis with oral terbinafine. *Cutis* **66**, 211–212.

Weismann, K., Knudsen, E.A. & Pedersen, C. (1988) White nails in AIDS/ARC due to *Trichophyton rubrum* infection. *Clinical and Experimental Dermatology* **13**, 24–25.

Willemsen, M., de Doncker, P. & Willems, J. (1992) Post treatment itraconazole levels in the nail. *Journal of the American Academy of Dermatology* **26**, 731–735.

Zaias, N. (1966) Superficial white onychomycosis. *Sabouraudia* **5**, 99–103.

Zaias, N. (1972) Onychomycosis. *Archives of Dermatology* **105**, 263–274.

Zaias, N. (1990a) *The Nail in Health and Disease*, 2nd edn. Appleton & Lange, Norwalk, CT.

Zaias, N. (1990b) *The Nail in Health and Disease*, 2nd edn, p. 93. Appleton & Lange, Norwalk, CT.

Zaias, N. & Drachman, D. (1983) A method for the determination of drug effectiveness in onychomycosis. *Journal of the American Academy of Dermatology* **9**, 912.

Zaias, N. & Taplin, D. (1966) Improved preparation for the diagnosis of mycologic diseases. *Archives of Dermatology* **93**, 608.

Zaias, N., Oertel, I. & Elliot, D.F. (1969) Fungi in toe-nails. *Journal of Investigative Dermatology* **53**, 140.

Zaug, M. (1995) Amorolfine nail lacquer: clinical experience in onychomycosis. *Journal of the European Academy of Dermatology and Venereology* **4** (Suppl. 1), S23–S30.

## Other fungal infections

### Sporotrichosis (Figs 4.49 & 4.50)

Sporotrichosis is a subcutaneous fungal infection caused by the dimorphic yeast, *Sporothrix schenckii*. The infection follows implantation of the organism which is found in the environment in subtropical and tropical countries. The primary site of infection is commonly located on an exposed site and the nail fold is often involved. The area becomes oedematous and discharges pus and serous fluid. Secondary lesions along the course of draining lymphatics may develop subsequently. The best method of diagnosis is by culture, although biopsy may reveal round or oval yeast or asteroid bodies, yeast surrounded by a refractile eosinophilic halo. The usual treatment is a saturated solution of potassium iodine; oral itraconazole or terbinafine are alternatives.

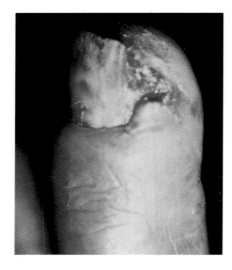

**Fig. 4.49** Sporotrichosis. (Courtesy of R. Arenas, Mexico.)

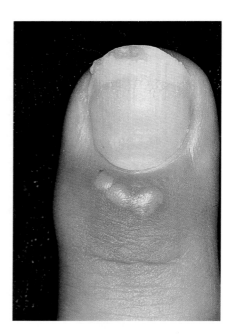

**Fig. 4.51** Herpes simplex—proximal nail fold involvement.

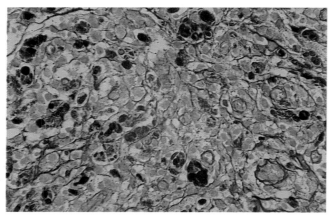

**Fig. 4.50** Sporotrichosis (*Sporothrix schenckii*). Grocott stain.

## Blastomycosis

Patients with *chromoblastomycosis* and *coccidioidomycosis* may present with a clinical picture of DLSO resulting from the invasion of the undersurface of the nail by the deep mycotic agent (Zaias 1990).

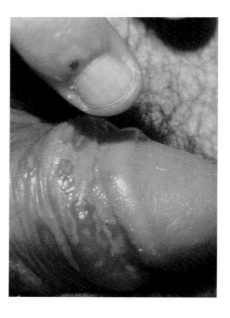

**Fig. 4.52** Herpes simplex—primary infection involving simultaneously genital mucosa and proximal nail fold of a digit.

## Other infections

### Herpes simplex (Figs 4.51–4.55)

Distal digital herpes simplex infections may affect the terminal phalanx as herpetic whitlows or start as an acute intensely painful paronychia. Recurrent forms are generally less severe and have a milder clinical course than the initial infection.

After an incubation period of 3–7 days during which local tenderness, erythema and swelling may develop, a crop of vesicles appears at the portal of entry into the skin. The vesicles typically are distributed around the paronychium and on the volar digital skin and somewhat resemble a pyogenic infection of the fingertip.

Close inspection, however, will reveal the classical pale, raised vesicles surrounded by an erythematous border. An acutely painful whitlow may develop and extend under the distal free edge of the nail and into the nail bed. A distinct predilection for the thumb and index finger was noted by La Rossa and Hamilton (1971), but any finger may be involved. Several fingers may be affected together. For 1–14 days the vesicles gradually increase in size, often coalescing into large, honey-comb-like bullae. New crops of lesions may appear during this time. Vesicular fluid is clear early in the disease but may

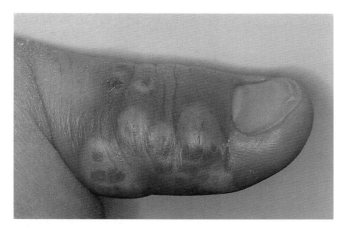

**Fig. 4.53** Herpes simplex—primary infection in a child.

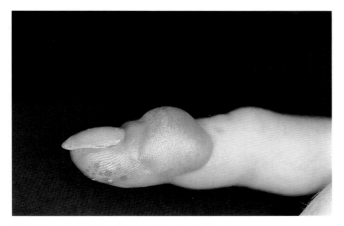

**Fig. 4.54** Herpetic whitlow. (Courtesy of S. Salasche.)

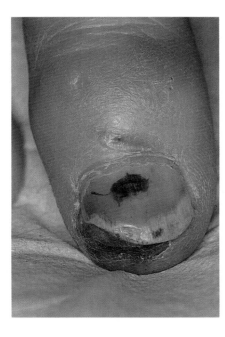

**Fig. 4.55** Subungual haemorrhage following recurrent herpes simplex.

become turbid, seropurulent or even haemorrhagic in the later stages. At times, the pale yellow colour of the vesicles will suggest pyogenic infection, yet frank pus is not usually obtained. Patients complain of tenderness and severe throbbing in the affected digit. Coexisting primary herpetic infections of the mouth and fingernails suggest autoinoculation of the virus into the nail tissues as a result of nail biting (Péchère *et al.* 1999) or finger sucking (Muller & Hermann 1970). We have seen coexisting primary herpetic infection of the penis and the index finger.

Radiating pain along the C7 distribution is sometimes noted and may predict the onset of recurrent herpetic whitlows. Lymphangitis is almost always seen in periungual herpes simplex and may even precede the vesicles by 1 or 2 days. It usually starts from the wrist and extends to the axilla with enlarged and tender lymph nodes.

Numbness and hypoaesthesia following the acute episode have been observed (Chang & Gorbach 1977). Persistent lymphoedema may also occur.

The diagnosis of herpetic infection can be made readily by examining the margin of the vesicles for the characteristic multinucleated 'balloon' giant cells, in stained smears. Characteristically, the nuclei of herpes simplex virus (HSV) infected cells appear steel-blue and homogeneous. Viral culture is confirmatory and is usually positive within 24–48 h.

Histopathology is not usually performed for periungual herpes simplex, but Tzanck smears reveal the characteristic multinucleate epidermal cells. Negative staining of blister fluid may show herpes viruses by electron microscopy. Monoclonal antibodies or polymerase chain reaction (PCR) allow confirmation of the diagnosis by immunofluorescence and also differentiation of type 1 from type 2 HSV.

In AIDS patients, recurrent herpes is severe and persistent. Herpes may be ulcerated (Garcia-Plata *et al.* 1999), destructive (Robayna *et al.* 1997) or necrotic (Gaddoni *et al.* 1994).

### Differential diagnosis

It is important to exclude primary or recurrent herpes simplex infection in the differential diagnosis of every finger infection. The typical appearance of the lesions with a disproportionate intensity of pain, the absence of pus in the confluent multiloculated vesiculopustular lesions and the lack of increased tension in the finger pulp aid in distinguishing this slow-healing infection from a bacterial infection or paronychia (La Rossa & Hamilton 1971).

Herpetic paronychia-like infection due to *Mycobacterium marinum* has been reported (Savoie 1989) (Fig. 4.56).

Herpes zoster infections, which may affect the proximal nail fold like herpes simplex, also involve the entire sensory dermatome (Fig. 4.57). The pustules of primary cutaneous *Neisseria gonorrhoeae* infection may resemble herpes simplex on the rare occasion when it occurs on the finger (Fig. 4.58). The diagnosis is established by gram stain and bacteriological culture.

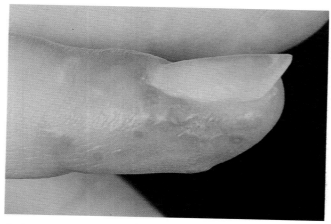

**Fig. 4.56** *Mycobacterium marinum* infection mimicking herpes paronychia. (Courtesy of J. Savoie, Canada.)

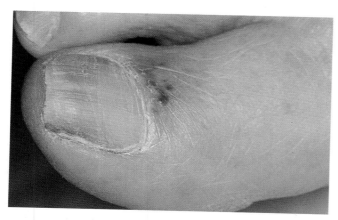

(a)

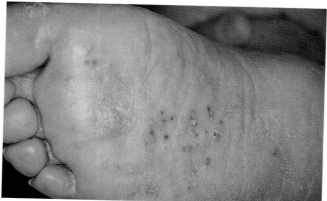

(b)

**Fig. 4.57** (a,b) Herpes zoster.

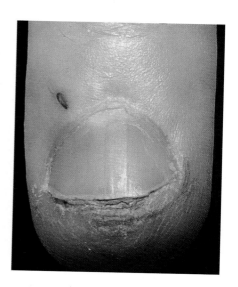

**Fig. 4.58** Primary cutaneous gonorrhoea. (Courtesy of J.E. Fitzpatrick, USA.)

## Treatment

Treatment is primarily aimed at symptomatic relief and avoidance of secondary infection. This is a preventable infection. Gloves should always be worn on both hands for procedures such as intubation, removal of dentures or providing oral care (Hamory *et al.* 1975) despite the additional costs involved

(Orkin 1975). While acyclovir may well ease the symptoms of the acute episode, a single course will not affect the chances of relapse. Continuous oral acyclovir may prevent frequent relapses in patients with recurrent herpes simplex infections, but use of this regimen may be followed by drug resistance.

## References

Chang, T. & Gorbach, S.L. (1977) Primary and recurrent herpetic whitlow. *International Journal of Dermatology* **16**, 752–754.

Gaddoni, G., Selvi, M., Resta, F. *et al.* (1994) Necrotic finger in AIDS patients. *Giornale Italiano di Dermatologia e Venereologia* **129**, 501–504.

Garcia-Plata, M.D., Moreno-Gimenez, J.C., Vexez-Garcia, A. *et al.* (1999) Herpetic whitlow in an AIDS patient. *Journal of the European Academy of Dermatology and Venereology* **12**, 241–242.

Hamory, B.H., Osterman, C.A. & Wenzel, R.P. (1975) Herpetic whitlow. *New England Journal of Medicine* **292**, 268.

La Rossa, D. & Hamilton, R. (1971) Herpes simplex infections of the digits. *Archives of Surgery* **102**, 600.

Muller, S.A. & Hermann, E.C. (1970) Association of stomatitis and paronychias due to herpes simplex. *Archives of Dermatology* **101**, 394.

Orkin, F.K. (1975) Herpetic whitlow. *New England Journal of Medicine* **292**, 648–649.

Péchère, M., Frieddi, A. & Krisher, J. (1999) Panaris multiples à herpes simplex type I. *Annales de Dermatologie et de Vénéréologie* **126**, 646.

Robayna, M.G., Herranz, P., Rubio, F.A. *et al.* (1997) Destructive herpetic whitlow in AIDS: report of 3 cases. *British Journal of Dermatology* **137**, 812–815.

Savoie, J.M. (1989) Infection à *Mycobacterium marinum* (forme sporotrichoïde). *Nouvelle Dermatologie* **8**, 524–525.

Zaias, N. (1990) *The Nail in Health and Disease*, 2nd edn. Appleton & Lange, Norwalk, CT.

## Herpes zoster (Fig. 4.57)

Herpes zoster is rarely seen around the nail. It may involve the proximal nail fold showing grouped vesicles. Nail bed involvement is particularly painful and leaves small subungual roundish haemorrhagic spots slowly growing out with the nail. Herpes zoster may produce transverse leuconychia by a uniform but temporary disturbance in the normal activity of each fingernail matrix, causing abnormal keratinization (Zigmor & Deluty 1980).

Stained Tzanck smears reveal multinucleate epidermal cells which do not allow differentiation from herpes simplex.

In AIDS, herpes zoster lesions are often verrucous.

### Reference

Zigmor, J. & Deluty, S. (1980) Acquired leukonychia striata. *International Journal of Dermatology* 19, 49–50.

### Gonorrhoea (Fig. 4.58)

The hallmark of disseminated gonococcaemia is the appearance of skin lesions (Silva & Wilson 1979). The most common is a vesicopustule which occurs juxta-articularly over the extensor surfaces of the hands, dorsal surfaces of the toes and around the nails. Haemorrhagic bullae occur in smaller numbers but in the same area. The third most common dermatological manifestation is the appearance of focal petechiae over the digits or the medial aspects of the ankles.

Primary extragenital cutaneous gonorrhoea acquired sexually is extremely rare (Fitzpatrick *et al.* 1981). It presents with a fingertip abscess extending under the nail plate with peripheral erythema from a pustular lesion. The diagnosis of gonococcal skin infection is often not entertained until the unexpected findings on the gram stain prompts further questions and culture.

Histopathology shows leucocytoclastic vasculitis with endothelial swelling, fibrinoid degeneration of vessel walls, extravasated erythrocytes and intraepidermal pustules which form from spongiform pustules.

### References

Fitzpatrick, J.E., Gramsted, N.D. & Tyler, H. (1981) Primary extragenital cutaneous gonorrhea. *Cutis* 27, 479–480.
Silva, J. & Wilson, K. (1979) Disseminated gonococcal infection. *Cutis* 24, 601–606.

### Syphilis (Figs 4.59–4.62)

Chancres of the fingers (due to occupational infection or sexual contact) may present as periungual erosion or ulceration which may sometimes involve the nail bed as in the syphilitic whitlow of Hutchinson, a paronychia, or it may resemble a pyogenic granuloma. A crusty ulceration covering the free edge of the nail in a half-moon shape or developing in one of the lateral nail folds has been reported. In this location chancres are usually painful and have a more chronic clinical course than elsewhere.

Regional lymphadenopathy accompanies the primary lesion: chancres of the fingers are associated with painless unilateral, epitrochlear and/or axillary nodes. The affected lymph nodes are discreetly enlarged, hard and non-suppurating.

Primary syphilis of the fingers accounted for 14% of extragenital chancres according to Starzycki (1983), who reported six cases. Of these, two had chancres on both their fingers and genitals resulting from sexual foreplay. Primary syphilis with exudative ulcers of the middle finger and one of the little finger of the right hand has been reported with an axillary, firm, painless lymph node (De Koning *et al.* 1977). The case of primary syphilis with multiple chancres and porphyria cutanea tarda in a HIV-infected patient is unique (Garcia-Silva *et al.* 1994).

In the secondary stage, the nail changes may be divided into two main groups; in the first group the changes due to the involvement of the matrix seem to be confined to the nails themselves; in the second group the changes are those in which the nail abnormalities are a consequence of some inflammatory condition of the peri- and subungual tissues and are without specific characteristics.

Various forms of 'dry' onychia have been described: unusual brittleness with a tendency to splitting and fissuring ('onyxis craquelé'), onycholysis, pitting with a linear arrangement of the pits from the root forwards and elkonyxis in the lunula region. Beau's lines may be seen, sometimes latent onychomadesis appears, and rarely, total nail loss. The whole nail plate may become dull, dry and thickened with a distinct line of demarcation between the affected and the distal portions which retain polish and colour, but a wedge-like thickening of the free end has been described.

Onychogryphosis may occur on the toenails. Dark or brownish pigmentation of the nail may involve the nail plate entirely

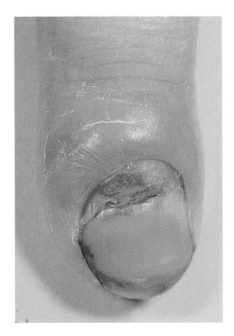

**Fig. 4.59** Primary syphilis. (Courtesy of P. de Graciansky & M. Boulle, Paris, France.)

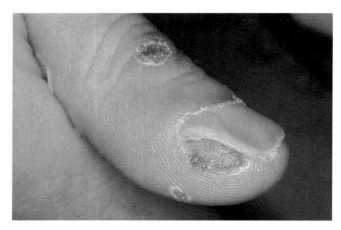

**Fig. 4.60** Secondary syphilis. (Courtesy of A. Puissant, Paris, France.)

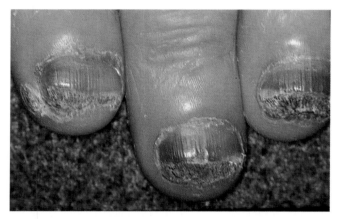

**Fig. 4.61** Secondary syphilis. (Courtesy of M. Geniaux, Bordeaux, France.)

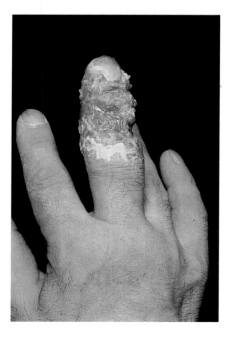

**Fig. 4.62** Tertiary syphilis. (Courtesy of G.K. Steigleider, Cologne, Germany.)

or as longitudinal pigmented streaks (Vörner 1907). The very rare amber-coloured nail plates resembling false nails were considered by Degos (1981) to be a characteristic change of late syphilis.

Pigmentation of the nail occurring over papules in the nail bed (Adamson & McDonagh 1911) is seen in the second group of syphilitic nails. The nail lesions are secondary to local inflammatory disturbances.

Milian's lilac arch (1936) located at the distal nail bed is no longer considered to be a manifestation of syphilis. It probably corresponds to a prominent onychodermal band (Baran & Gioanni 1968). The 'isolated papule of the nail bed' (Heller 1927) occurs at the time of the exanthem. A pea- to bean-sized patch appears under the normally transparent nail. At first the patch is intensely red, later yellow. The nail plate becomes thinned and fractured at this spot. This condition was said to be always limited to one finger. In fact, nearly all the fingernails may be involved (Adamson & McDonagh 1911).

In the moist forms several nails may be affected, but often only one is involved such as the thumb or the great toe. The lesion begins with erythema, swelling and pain in the proximal tissues surrounding the nail. Next the proximal and lateral nail folds separate from the nail plate, allowing discharge of the entrapped inflammatory exudate (Kingsbury *et al.* 1972). This results in a 'discharging horse-shoe-shaped ulcer'. The nail blackens and falls, exposing an unhealthy looking ulcer (Adamson & McDonagh 1911) with permanent nail deformity or anonychia. This may be the end result of untreated syphilitic paronychia. Multiple inflammatory paronychia may also occur in congenital syphilis with active manifestations (Pardo-Castello & Pardo 1960).

Danielyan and Mokrousov (1979) reported an unusual delay of 3 years before the appearance of a normal nail following adequate treatment of early secondary syphilis with penicillin. The patient was a greengrocer; there may have been minor occupational trauma which could have resulted in the Koebner phenomenon causing oxychauxis.

The differential diagnosis includes acute septic paronychia, which is generally more painful, and chronic paronychia (pages 137–139).

Tertiary syphilis very rarely affects the nail apparatus as gummata, which result in secondary necrosis with permanent nail loss when the matrix has been destroyed (Fox 1941). All individuals who have been exposed to infectious syphilis, occupationally or otherwise, within the preceding 3 months should be treated even if they show no evidence of having been infected (Felman *et al.* 1982).

## References

Adamson, H.G. & McDonagh, J.E.R. (1911) Two unusual forms of syphilitic nails: with some general remarks upon syphilis of the nails. *British Journal of Dermatology* 23, 68.

Baran, R. & Gioanni, T. (1968) Half-and-half nail. *Bulletin de la Societé Française de Dermatologie et de Syphiligraphie* **75**, 399.

Danielyan, E.E. & Mokrousov, M.S. (1979) Involvement of nail plates in a patient with secondary early syphilis. *Vestnik Dermatologii i Venerologii* **12**, 59.

Degos, R. (1981) *Précis de Dermatologie*, p. 1135. Flammarion, Paris.

De Koning, G.A.J., Blog, F.B. & Stolz, E. (1977) A patient with primary syphilis of the hand. *British Journal of Venereal Diseases* **53**, 386–388.

Felman, Y.M., Phil, M. & Nikitas, J.A. (1982) Primary syphilis. *Cutis* **29**, 122.

Fox, H. (1941) Obstinate syphilitic onychia and gumma of the nose successfully treated by fever therapy. *Archives of Dermatology* **44**, 1155.

Garcia-Silva, J., Velasco-Benito, J.A. & Peña-Penabad, C. (1994) Primary syphilis with multiple chancres and porphyria cutanea tarda in a HIV infected patient. *Dermatology* **188**, 163–165.

Heller, J. (1927) Die Krankheiten der Nägel. In: *Handbuch der Haut und Geschlechtskrankheiten*, Vol. XIII/2 (ed. J.J. Jadassohn). Springer, Berlin.

Kingsbury, D.H., Chester, E.C. & Jansen, G.T. (1972) Syphilitic paronychia, an unusual complaint. *Archives of Dermatology* **105**, 458.

Milian, G. (1936) Les maladies des ongles. In: *Nouvelle Pratique Dermatologique*, Vol. 7 (ed. J. Darier). Masson, Paris.

Pardo-Castello, V. & Pardo, O. (1960) *Diseases of Nails*, 3rd edn. C.C. Thomas, Springfield, IL.

Starzycki, Z. (1983) Primary syphilis of the fingers. *British Journal of Venereal Disease* **59**, 169–171.

Vörner, H. (1907) *Ueber Nagelpigmentation bei sekundärer Syphilis*, Muenchener Medizinische Wochenschrift, 2483.

## Pinta

See Chapter 2.

## Leprosy (Figs 4.63–4.70, Table 4.8)

Leprosy can cause many nail changes which have been observed in up to 64% of infected patients (Patki & Baran 1991).

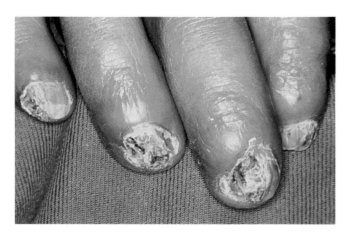

**Fig. 4.63** Lepromatous leprosy paronychia. (Courtesy of J. Delacretaz, Lausanne.)

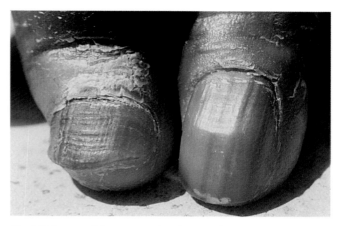

**Fig. 4.64** Racquet nail due to acroosteolysis. (Courtesy of P. Saint-André, Bamako.)

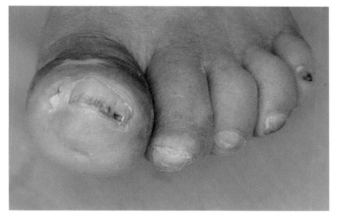

(a)

(b)

**Fig. 4.65** (a) Leprosy—shortening of the great toenail. (b) The same patient presenting with acroosteolysis.

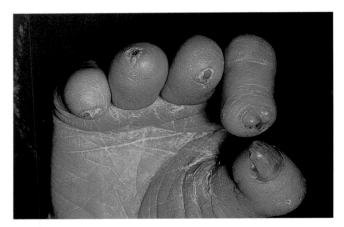

**Fig. 4.66** Leprosy—acroosteolysis involving several fingers. (Courtesy of D. Wallach, Paris.)

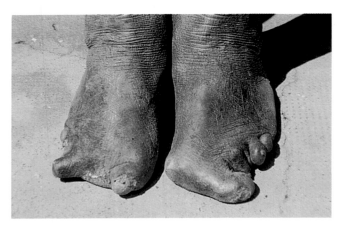

**Fig. 4.67** Leprosy—digit amputation. (Courtesy of P. Saint-André, Bamako.)

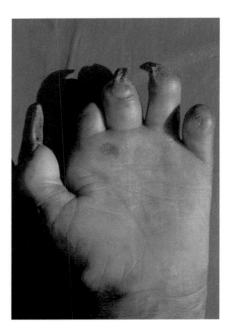

**Fig. 4.68** Leprosy—claw-like nails. (Courtesy of A.H. Patki, India.)

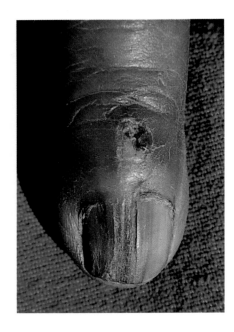

**Fig. 4.69**
Leprosy—dorsal
pterygium. (Courtesy of
A.H. Patki, India.)

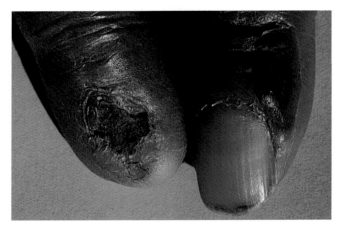

**Fig. 4.70** Leprosy—chronic ulceration of the distal dorsal soft tissues. (Courtesy of A.H. Patki, India.)

Leprosy is primarily an infection of the peripheral nervous system caused by *Mycobacterium leprae*. Clinical presentations range from a total failure of cell-mediated resistance (lepromatous) to high but incomplete resistance (tuberculoid). The skin is involved as an integral part of the expression of this disease and skin lesions are largely determined by the numbers of organisms present and the presence of effective immunological resistance. Tuberculoid or borderline tuberculoid forms where there are few organisms, and lepromatous and borderline lepromatous, the multibacillary forms, are examples of this process. The first important report on nail biopsy was written by Tachikawa (1939, 1941).

Nail changes in leprosy can be caused by neuropathy and trauma, vascular impairment and infections amongst others. Often more than one factor will be important.

**Table 4.8** Classification of nail changes in leprosy. (From Patki & Baran 1991 with permission.)

*Neuropathy and trauma*
Subungual haematoma
Onycholysis
Onychauxis
Onychogryphosis
Racquet nail
Pterygium unguis (dorsal and ventral)
Ectopic nail
Spicule nail
Complete loss—anonychia

*Vascular deficit*
Thinning
Longitudinal splits
Onychauxis
Pterygium unguis (dorsal and ventral)
Atrophy

*Infections*
Bacterial
Fungal

*Miscellaneous*
Diffusion of lunula (pseudomacrolunula)
Leuconychia
Pallor
Hapalonychia
Beau's lines

Trophic changes are responsible for modifications of the lunula in upper limbs; it becomes greyish and less sharply delineated from the rest of the subungual area, resulting in an apparent leuconychia as a pseudomacrolunula.

In tuberculoid leprosy neurological involvement is usually asymmetrical and appears early in the course of the disease, usually in areas of visible dermatological change. Nerve changes in lepromatous leprosy occur more slowly and are usually symmetrical producing a 'stocking-and-glove' anaesthesia, but paradoxically, nail changes in tuberculoid and lepromatous patients are similar, despite wide differences in pathology. Factors only associated with lepromatous disease are invasion of the bones of the terminal phalanges by lepromatous granulomas and endarteritis occurring during type 2 lepra reactions. These may result in multiple Beau's lines (Patki 1990b) and dorsal pterygium (Patki & Metha 1989).

The phalanges develop osteolysis and there is progressive telescoping of the digital bones (Queneau *et al.* 1982). When deformities such as a 'preacher's hand' occur, clawnails and other unusual appearances are produced. Dystrophic changes may occur in the nails, with progessive destruction leaving small fragments at the corner of the nail bed, or ventral pterygium (Patki 1990a).

Painless abscesses may occur periungually with destruction of the nails. This appears more often in the upper than lower limbs. Delacrétaz (1980) presented a case of lepromatous leprosy paronychia demonstrating Hansen's bacilli in a cantharidin-induced blister on the distal part of the proximal nail fold and within the proximal nail debris.

Walking barefoot, the sitting position normally assumed and the type of footwear all produce anatomical and physiological changes in the feet and legs. They may lead to pathological processes or modify those that pre- or coexist.

## References

Delacrétaz, J. (1980) Les maladies infectieuses de l'ongle. In: *Jahresversammlung der Schweizerischen Gesellschaft für Dermatologie und Venerologie*, Zürich, 3–4 October.

Patki, A.H. (1990a) Pterygium inversum in a patient with leprosy. *Archives of Dermatology* **126**, 110.

Patki, A.H. (1990b) Multiple Beau's lines due to recurrent erythema nodosum leprosum. *Archives of Dermatology* **126**, 1110–1111.

Patki, A.H. & Baran, R. (1991) Nail changes in leprosy. *Seminars in Dermatology* **10**, 77–81.

Patki, A.H. & Metha, J.M. (1989) Pterygium unguis in a patient with recurrent type 2 lepra reaction. *Cutis* **44**, 311–312.

Queneau, P., Gabbai, A., Perpoint, B. *et al.* (1982) Acro-ostéolyses au cours de la lèpre. A propos de 19 observations personnelles. *Revue de Rheumatologie* **49** (2), 111–119.

Tachikawa, N. (1939) Leprosy of the nail. Report I. *La Lepra* **10**, 183–204.

Tachikawa, N. (1941) Leprosy of the nail. Report II. *La Lepra* **12**, 111–182.

## Leishmaniasis (Fig. 4.71)

Lesions of cutaneous leishmaniasis with central granular ulceration and an elevated papular border may involve the dorsal aspect of the distal phalanx (Butler 1982). Treatment options include topical paromomycin, local, intramuscular or intravenous sodium stibogluconate, oral itraconazole or ketoconazole or intravenous amphotericin B.

In post kala-azar dermal leishmaniasis, a characteristic greyish discoloration of the skin is most noticeable on the hands, the nails and other sites, and has resulted in the condition called the 'black disease' (Moschella 1975).

## References

Butler, P.G. (1982) Levamisole and immune response phenomena in cutaneous leishmaniasis. *Journal of the American Academy of Dermatology* **6**, 1070–1077.

Moschella, S.L. (1975) Leishmaniasis. In: *Dermatology* (eds S.L. Moschella, D.M. Pillsbury & H.J. Hurley), p. 807. W.B. Saunders, Philadelphia.

## Trichinosis

Splinter haemorrhages have been known to occur in all nails simultaneously in trichinosis (Fisher 1957). Under these

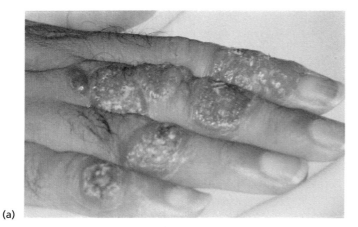

(a)

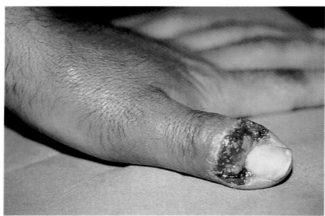

(b)

**Fig. 4.71** (a) Leishmaniasis affecting the dorsal aspect of the fingers and proximal nail fold. (Courtesy of P.G. Butler, USA.) (b) Leishmaniasis of the distal thumb. (Courtesy of C. Arroyo, Columbia.)

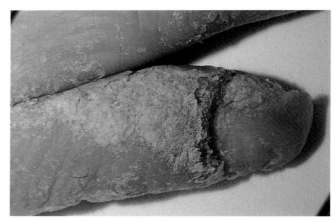

**Fig. 4.72** Norwegian scabies in Down's syndrome. (Courtesy of J. Beurey, France.)

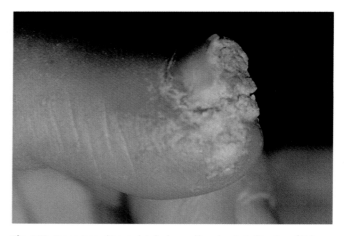

**Fig. 4.73** Norwegian scabies—isolated subungual hyperkeratosis. (Courtesy of R. De Paoli & V. Marks, USA.)

circumstances nail biopsy may be diagnostically useful (Groff 1983).

## References

Fisher, A.A. (1957) Subungual splinter haemorrhages associated with trichinosis. *Archives of Dermatology* 75, 572–573.

Groff, J.W. (1983) Organisms and associated disease. *Journal of the Association of Military Dermatology* 9, 72–75.

## Scabies (Figs 4.72 & 4.73, Table 4.9)

Norwegian scabies is a rare variety of scabies infestation of the skin in which the entire body, even the scalp, is affected by *Sarcoptes scabiei*. The lesions of Norwegian scabies have a predilection for areas of pressure and are strikingly different in clinical appearance to ordinary scabies. The hyperkeratotic lesions are accompanied by large, psoriasis-like accumulations of scales under the nails of the fingers and toes (Schiff & Ronchese 1964). This type of scabies is most often seen in the old and infirm, the mentally defective, and during therapeutic immunosuppression, as well as in AIDS.

Chronic eczematoid dermatosis, atopic eczema, lichen simplex and psoriasis may be mimicked by this condition (Haydon & Caplan 1971), and topical use of corticosteroids may alter the clinical appearance of scabies.

One of the characteristic manifestations of this condition is the existence of dystrophic nail changes. Even after seemingly successful treatment of hyperkeratotic scabies, this dystrophy persists and may be the most important marker of the persistence of this type of infestation. The mites survive in these dystrophic nails and later colonize the skin, first around the nail plates. From there they extend proximally (Kocsard 1984) and may be inoculated into all parts of the body by the scratching finger. The subungual material with abundant mites may not respond to topical therapy alone. Frequent trimming of nails and scrubbing twice daily with gamma benzene hexachloride is recommended. In resistant cases this should be supplemented

**Table 4.9** Reported associations of crusted scabies. (From De Paoli & Marks 1987 with permission.)

*Neurological or mental disorders*
Down's syndrome
Senile dementia
Syringomyelia
Tabes dorsalis
Parkinson's disease

*Nutritional disorders*
Vitamin A deficiency
Beri beri
Malnutrition

*Infectious diseases*
Leprosy
Tuberculosis
Bacillary dysentery

*Immunosuppression or impaired immunity*
Genetic:
  Bloom's syndrome
Acquired:
  Topical and systemic corticosteroids
  Immunosuppressive drugs
  Radiotherapy
  Lymphoreticular malignancies
  AIDS

*Miscellaneous*
Diabetes
Rheumatoid arthritis
Poor hygiene

by surgical scrubs using a scabicide and/or by 40% urea nail dissolution and partial nail avulsion (De Paoli & Marks 1987). Oral ivermectin has been used with great success in crusted (Norwegian) scabies, although its effects on nail involvement have not been well documented.

In the ordinary forms of scabies the clinically normal nails are not usually involved. However, the distal subungual area may provide a nidus for mites, a source for small epidemics (Scher 1983). A single case presenting with nail infestation alone has been reported in which a big toenail was raised by large accumulations of hyperkeratotic debris, containing innumerable mites and eggs (Saruta & Nakamizo 1978).

Histopathology shows that the hyponychium may be infested with *Sarcoptes hominis* (*Acarus scabiei*) in elderly people. Tangential biopsies of the hyponychial keratosis with the overlying free edge of the nail plate may show mite burrows containing mites, eggs and faeces. In Norwegian scabies, the nail may be elevated by marked subungual hyperkeratosis with alternating parakeratosis and orthokeratosis. Abundant mites are usually present. A heavy mixed infiltrate often containing many eosinophils is seen in the dermis.

## References

De Paoli, R. & Marks, V.J. (1987) Crusted (Norwegian) scabies: treatment of nail involvement. *Journal of the American Academy of Dermatology* **17**, 136–138.

Haydon, J.R. & Caplan, R.M. (1971) Epidemic scabies. *Archives of Dermatology* **103**, 168–173.

Kocsard, E. (1984) The dystrophic nail of keratotic scabies. *American Journal of Dermatopathology* **6**, 308–309.

Saruta, T. & Nakamizo, Y. (1978) Usual scabies with nail infestation. *Archives of Dermatology* **114**, 956–957.

Scher, R.K. (1983) Subungual scabies. *American Journal of Dermatopathology* **5**, 187.

Schiff, B.L. & Ronchese, F. (1964) Norwegian scabies. *Archives of Dermatology* **89**, 236.

## Pediculosis

Interestingly *pediculosis* of the foot limited to the hallux has also been reported (Diemer 1985) in a patient with onychomycosis of all toenails, which were thickened. Debridement of the right great toenail exposed multiple cavities, housing approximately 10–12 body lice. The arthropods quickly dispersed upon being disturbed, returning to the nail within minutes, disappearing into the tunnels that were present in the nail.

## Reference

Diemer, J.T. (1985) Isolated pediculosis. *Journal of the American Podiatric Medical Association* **75**, 99–101.

## Tungiasis (Figs 4.74 & 4.75)

Tungiasis is an inflammatory condition caused by the fertilized female sand flea *Tunga penetrans* and has been noted primarily in patients who have recently travelled to endemic areas.

Clinical features of tungiasis consist initially of a pruritic, tender or painful small erythematous papule with a central

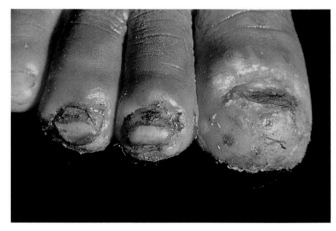

**Fig. 4.74** Tungiasis. (Courtesy of R. Pradinaud, French Guyana.)

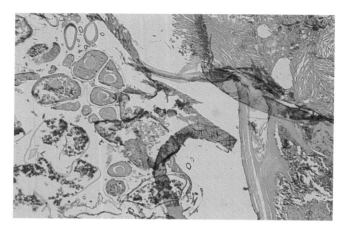

**Fig. 4.75** Tungiasis. (Courtesy of A. Carvalo, Central America.)

black dot produced by the posterior part of the flea's abdominal segments. The fully developed lesion is a white pea-sized nodule with a central black pit or plug located in the subungual and the periungual areas of the toes. Complications include cellulitis, gangrene, autoamputation of toes and tetanus (Sanusi *et al.* 1989).

Clinical differential diagnosis of tungiasis includes fire ant bite, tick sting, scabies, creeping eruption (*Ancylostoma* spp.), cercarial dermatitis and myiasis.

Definitive diagnosis rests upon demonstration of the flea using a mineral oil preparation or by examination of a biopsy specimen. This reveals an intraepidermal cystic cavity lined by an eosinophilic cuticle. The cavity contains ring-shaped portions of the organism's respiratory and digestive tracts as well as multiple round to oval eggs that may contain a pale-staining round yolk sac (Wentzell *et al.* 1986; Basler *et al.* 1988).

Treatment varies from physically removing the flea with a sterile needle to application of 4% formaldehyde solution, DDT, chloroform or turpentine. Systemic niridazole has been recommended if there are multiple sites of infection. Topical and sometimes systemic antibiotic treatment are advised in addition. Tetanus prophylaxis should be given routinely. Wearing of shoes is the primary defence against tungiasis (Basler *et al.* 1988).

## References

Basler, E.A., Stephens, J.H. & Tschen, J.A. (1988) Tunga penetrans. *Cutis* **42**, 47–48.

Sanusi, D.J., Brown, E.B., Shepard, T.G. *et al.* (1989) Tungiasis: report of one case and review of the 14 reported cases in the United States. *Journal of the American Academy of Dermatology* **20**, 941–944.

Wentzell, J.M., Schwartz, B.K. & Pesce, J.R. (1986) Tungiasis. *Journal of the American Academy of Dermatology* **15**, 117–119.

## Larva migrans (Fig. 4.76)

Intense pruritic migratory serpiginous burrows on the dorsum

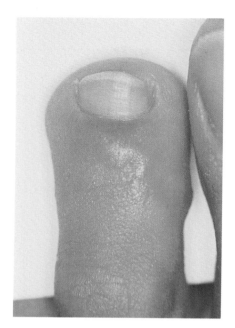

**Fig. 4.76** Larva migrans. (Courtesy of G. Cannata, Italy.)

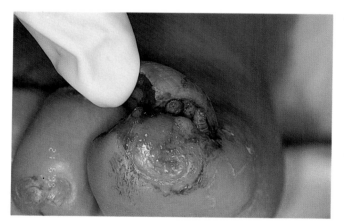

**Fig. 4.77** Subungual myiasis.

of the terminal phalanx may be observed with secondary dystrophic nail changes (Edelglass *et al.* 1982). Thiabendazole orally and topically using a 10% suspension are effective. It has been replaced recently by oral albendazole.

## Reference

Edelglass, J.W., Douglass, M.C. & Steifler, R. (1982) Cutaneous larva migrans in northern climates. *Journal of the American Academy of Dermatology* **7**, 353–358.

## Subungual myiasis (Fig. 4.77)

Infestation by larvae of *Musca domestica* is unusual in a subungual location.

Three days after a traumatic event, Muñyon and Urbanc (1978) noted a subungual haematoma of the great toenail of a Caucasian female. The portion of the haematoma underneath the proximal nail fold was found to be teeming with larval forms identified as *Musca domestica*. Another case has been reported with larvae identified as *Sarcophaga* spp. (Garcia-Doval *et al.* 2000).

## References

Garcia-Doval, I., de la Torre, C., Losada, A. *et al.* (2000) Subungual myiasis. *Acta Dermato-Venereologica* **80**, 236.

Muñyon, T.G. & Urbanc, A.N. (1978) Subungual myiasis. A case report and literature review. *Journal of the Association of Military Dermatology* **4**, 60–61.

# CHAPTER 5

# The nail in dermatological diseases

**D.A.R. de Berker, R. Baran & R.P.R. Dawber**

## Psoriasis

Psoriasis is a genetically determined hyperproliferative skin disease characterized by increased cell proliferation, glycogen accumulation and incomplete differentiation in the cells of the epidermis (Maeda *et al*. 1980). Up to 36% of psoriatic subjects have a family history of the disease; also, an association with HLA types BW17, BW16 and B13 has been established (Watson & Farber 1977). There is also a strong association with HLA-Cw6, carrying with it a 10-fold relative risk of developing psoriasis (Elder *et al*. 1994). An association with other autoimmune conditions has been suggested (Harrison *et al*. 1990).

Nail involvement in psoriasis is common and has been reported in between 50% (Zaias 1969) and 56% (Kaur *et al*. 1997) of cases. It is estimated that over a lifetime between 80% and 90% of psoriatics will suffer nail disease (Samman 1978). Over 93% of those with psoriatic nail disease consider it to be of cosmetic importance to them. However, 58% consider that it interferes with their job and 52% describe pain as a symptom (de Jong *et al*. 1996). Congenital nail psoriasis has been reported (Lerner & Lerner 1972; Farber & Jacobs 1977;

Akinduro *et al*. 1994) with nail features preceding cutaneous disease. In one case, the mother had extensive psoriasis when pregnant (Stankler 1988). Nail pits were present in 11 of 14 infants with psoriasis (Farber & Jacobs 1977). In children, nail involvement has been found to range from 7% (Puissant 1970), 13% (Asboe-Hansen 1971), 36% (Al-Fouzan & Nanda 1994) to 39% (Nanda *et al*. 1990). In a study of 50 children with juvenile psoriatic arthritis, 80% developed pitting. This was the most common clinical feature of psoriasis after the arthritis (Roberton *et al*. 1996).

Severe nail involvement may not imply severe psoriasis of the skin and the type of nail change is not associated with any particular distribution of the skin lesions (Calvert *et al*. 1963). The clinical signs of nail psoriasis can be correlated with the site of involvement of the epidermal structures of the nail. The histological changes in the nails are similar to those seen in the skin, except for the changes in the granular layer.

The main psoriatic features in the nails are, in order of frequency:
- Pitting (Fig. 5.1);
- Discoloration of the nail (Fig. 5.2);
- Onycholysis (Fig. 5.3);
- Subungual hyperkeratosis (Fig. 5.4);

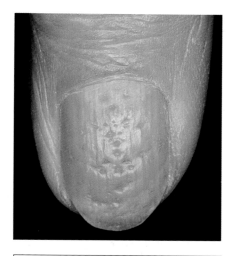

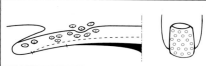

**Fig. 5.1** Psoriasis—pitting.

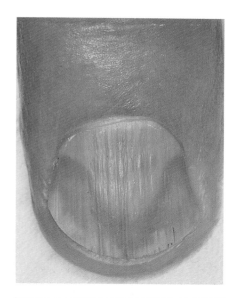

**Fig. 5.3**
Psoriasis—onycholysis with proximal brownish-red margin.

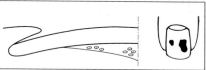

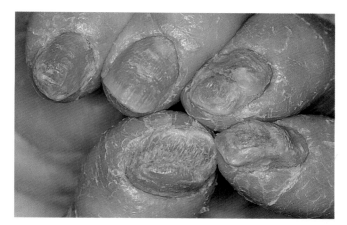

**Fig. 5.2** Psoriasis—discoloration and nail apparatus distortion.

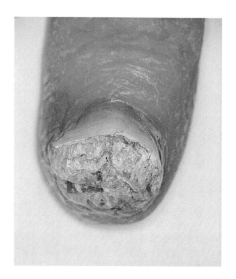

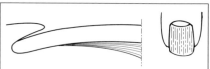

**Fig. 5.4**
Psoriasis—subungual hyperkeratosis.

- Nail plate abnormalities;
- Splinter haemorrhages (Fig. 5.5).

There may be psoriatic scaling of the proximal nail fold (Fig. 5.6) with soft tissue swelling or chronic paronychia (Ganor 1977a). The changes observed in the nail plate depend on the location and duration of the disease process. The lesions may reflect transient matrix dysfunction and be limited in extent, such as pits and transverse furrows (Fig. 5.7). Alternatively they may represent persistent disease and result in sustained nail abnormalities such as loss or thickening of the nail plate.

## Pitting and nail plate changes

Pits are punctate depressions, usually small and shallow, but they can vary in size, depth and shape (Figs 5.1 & 5.8). They

originate from focal psoriasis of the proximal matrix (Zaias 1969). Most pits are superficial, and when extensive can produce gross abnormalities in colour and texture, known as trachyonychia, where the nail is dull, rough and can be fragile (Piérard & Piérard-Franchimont 1996). Isolated deep pits are

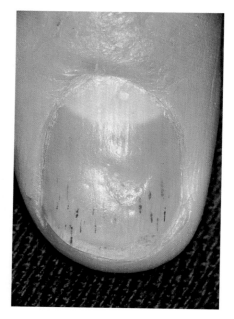

**Fig. 5.5** Psoriasis—pitting and splinter haemorrhages.

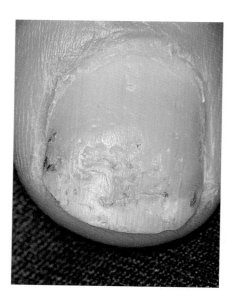

**Fig. 5.8** Psoriasis—multiple pits.

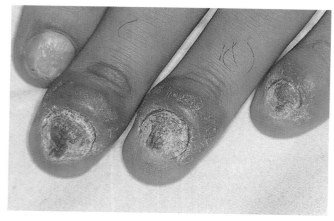

**Fig. 5.6** Psoriasis—involvement of the proximal nail fold.

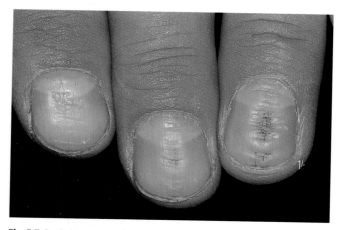

**Fig. 5.7** Psoriasis—transverse furrows.

characteristic of psoriasis (Zaias & Norton 1980). Where focal psoriasis becomes more marked, a pit may enlarge and produce a hole in the nail plate, a sign termed elkonyxis.

Pits are generally found scattered irregularly but may, as in alopecia areata (Fig. 5.7), appear as regular lines in the transverse or long axis (Samman 1978), or in a typical gridlike pattern. They grow out at the same rate as the nail. Ganor (1977b) suggested that pitting of the nails in alopecia areata might be an expression of psoriasis and less commonly of alopecia areata. Pitting is seldom observed in the toenails.

A psoriatic origin is also favoured by the presence of other multiple nail abnormalities, such as horizontal ridging and pitting. The presence of more than 20 fingernail pits suggests a psoriatic cause of the nail dystrophy. More than 60 pits per person are unlikely to be found in the absence of psoriasis.

Histologically pits represent a defect in the superficial layers of the nail plate (Fig. 5.9). They are lined by parakeratotic cells loosely adherent to one another (Alkiewicz 1948). These cells are shed with routine activity and leave a depression on the surface of the nail (Zaias 1984). This process means that pits are deeper, larger and more numerous in the distal half of the nail, although this is not proven. The persistence of parakeratotic cells may occasionally result in an opaque white scaly appearance of the pits (Tosti *et al.* 1993a), also a feature of extensive pitting disease representing trachyonychia.

Scanning electron microscopic studies of psoriatic nails (Mauro *et al.* 1975; Pfister 1981) have shown that the cells on the surface of pits are small and do not have an overlapping pattern. There are spaces between the poorly interdigitated cells. A striking feature is the presence of numerous micropits on the surface of the cells, analogous to the changes previously described in the stratum corneum (Dawber *et al.* 1972).

Serial transverse depressions are common in psoriasis, especially on the thumbs where they may mimic 'washboard' nails

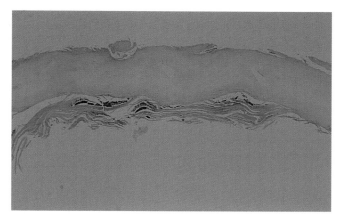

**Fig. 5.9** Psoriasis—nail plate superficial pitting. H & E stain.

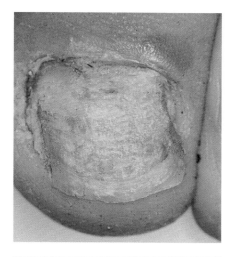

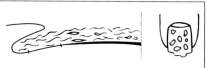

**Fig. 5.11** Psoriasis—total matrix and nail plate involvement.

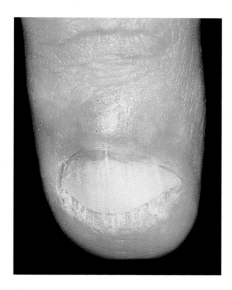

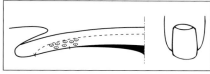

**Fig. 5.10** Psoriasis—leuconychia.

applied to nail. They differ from the subungual calcifications reported by Fischer (1982) (Chapter 11).

## Nail bed psoriasis

Nail bed and hyponychium involvement is common. Psoriasis lesions located in the nail bed produce oval, salmon-coloured, 'oily' spots of various sizes and variable duration (Fig. 5.12). These 'oily' patches less commonly occur in acropustulosis and in systemic lupus erythematosus; very large oil patches have been observed in 'lectitis purulenta et granulomatosa' (Runne & Orfanos 1981).

When oily spots affect the hyponychium medially or laterally, onycholysis occurs. The yellow colour of onycholytic nail results from a combination of an additional air : nail interface and the accumulation of squames. Onycholysis surrounded by a reddish-yellow margin visible between the normal pink nail bed and the whitish separated area, is highly suggestive of psoriasis. In all types of onycholysis, the deep surface of the nail plate retains nail bed cells (ventral matrix); Robbins *et al.* (1983) have re-emphasized this long-known fact in relation to psoriatic onycholysis in which the level of epidermal split is between the layers of neutrophil-containing parakeratotic horn of the nail bed. Onycholysis alone without previous nail injury suggests a psoriatic origin of nail dystrophy (Eastmond & Wright 1979).

The space can be colonized by microorganisms. Contaminant fungi, yeasts and *Pseudomonas* are common. In psoriatic nails the rate of dermatophyte infection is controversial. Usually dermatophytes are not found in psoriatic fingernails but they may occasionally be cultured in toenails (Zaias 1984). One study suggests that the proportion of non-dermatophyte nail

(Macaulay 1966). In the absence of psoriasis these result from the habit tic of pushing back the cuticle and represent a short-term disturbance of matrix function. Longitudinal ridges of the nail with bumps that resemble drops of melted wax are reported as common by Baden (1987). Leuconychia may be seen (Fig. 5.10) where the nail surface is normal (Alkiewicz 1948). This is sometimes seen in association with onycholysis. Concurrent proximal matrix involvement will lead to leuconychia with a rough surface (Zaias 1969), or coarse nails (Samman 1978). When the whole matrix is affected, the nail plate becomes off-white and crumbles (Zaias 1969) (Fig. 5.11).

Radio-opaque lines within the nails in psoriasis (de Graciansky *et al.* 1975) may be the result of topical substances

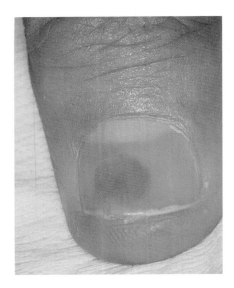

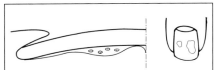

**Fig. 5.12** Psoriasis—brownish-red patch in the nail bed known as 'oil spot'.

infections is higher in psoriatic nail than in primary onychomycosis (Szepes 1986). Staberg *et al.* (1983) were not able to demonstrate any difference between the frequency of dermatophytic infections of involved psoriatic nails as compared with uninvolved psoriatic nails, or normal nails. Most recently, Gupta *et al.* (1997) reported that 27% of psoriatics with abnormal toenails had mycological evidence of onychomycosis coexistent with their psoriasis. Although it is difficult to work out what would constitute an appropriate control group for this study, the clinical implication is that onychomycosis might be the exacerbating feature of psoriasis.

Splinter haemorrhages (Fig. 5.5) are seen in the fingernails of 42% of psoriatics with nail disease and in 6% of their toenails (Calvert *et al.* 1963). The sign reflects the orientation of the capillary plexuses in the nail bed and the proliferation and fragility of these capillaries in active psoriasis.

Subungual hyperkeratosis (Fig. 5.4) is manifested as accumulated squames. The nail bed alters its keratin profile in psoriasis. Normally the keratins of terminal differentiation, k1 and k10, are absent from the healthy nail bed. However, these keratins are expressed in psoriatic nail bed combined with an increase in epidermal turnover at the same site (de Berker *et al.* 1995; de Berker & Angus 1996). These changes underlie the clinical features of subungual hyperkeratosis. When the process involves the hyponychium, the nail plate becomes raised to a variable degree and may resemble pachyonychia congenita. Sometimes a horny mass may simulate loss of the nail plate (Zaias 1969). Overcurvature of one or more nails may be seen occasionally (Samman 1978).

Special attention should be paid to chromonychia due to psoriasis of the nail. A yellow-green hue to the nail is sometimes seen in psoriasis and in *Pseudomonas* infection. The latter should be excluded (culture, Wood's lamp examination and chloroform solubility test).

The matrix is responsible for leuconychia, and subungual keratosis arising from nail bed disease causes a silvery-white colour. A yellow-green colour may be produced by the accumulation of large amounts of blood glycoprotein (Fig. 5.2), commonly seen when the hyponychium and the nail bed are involved in inflammatory processes (Zaias & Norton 1980).

### Clinical considerations in the diagnosis of nail psoriasis

#### Clinical

- Corroborating features of psoriasis at other sites
- Other causes of pitting:
    alopecia areata
    lichen planus
    eczema
    pityriasis rosea
    lichen nitidus
    pityriasis rubra pilaris.
- Other causes of onycholysis (Table 2.3)
- Other causes of nail thickening:
    trauma
    pityriasis rubra pilaris
    onychomycosis
    yellow nail syndrome
    Darier's disease
    pachyonychia congenita
    CHILD syndrome (Happle *et al.* 1980) (Fig. 5.13) or congenital homolateral epidermal hyperplasia and/or hypoplastic hemidysplasia (Laplanche *et al.* 1980)
    does nail psoriasis in a limited distribution reflect trauma or a physiological process eliciting the isomorphic reaction?, for example psoriasis in the paretic arm fingernails

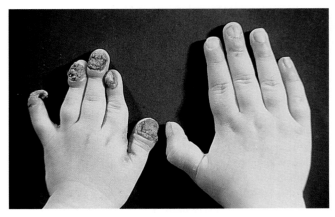

**Fig. 5.13** CHILD syndrome (courtesy of R. Happle, Germany).

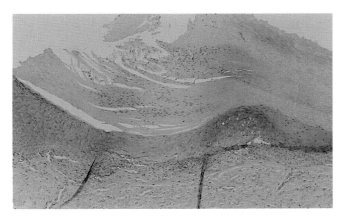

**Fig. 5.14** Psoriasis—involvement of the nail bed and nail plate. PAS stain, × 100.

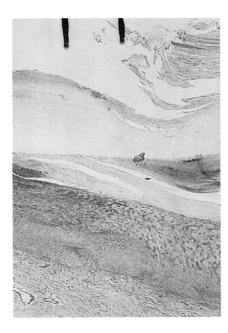

**Fig. 5.15** Psoriasis—involvement of the nail matrix and nail plate. PAS stain, × 90.

following hemiplegia (Badger *et al.* 1992) and occupational disorders leading to nail changes (Fisher & Baran 1992).

### Investigations

* Exclude fungal infection:
  clippings for microscopy and culture;
  nail plate clippings for histology;
* Formal nail biopsy for histology to exclude alternative diagnoses (Figs 5.14 & 5.15);
* X-ray to examine for psoriatic changes in the distal interphalangeal joint;
* Biopsy skin disease to confirm psoriasis at other sites.

Different forms of nail plate and nail bed biopsy have been described to help distinguish between onychomycosis and nail

psoriasis (Leyden *et al.* 1972; Scher & Ackerman 1980; Haneke 1991; Machler *et al.* 1998).

Periodic acid–Schiff (PAS) stain is helpful to rule out onychomycosis which may mimic nail psoriasis clinically and histopathologically (Haneke 1991). Both PAS and Grocott stains demonstrate fungi, neutrophils and exudate. Blancophor is a highly specific fluorochrome marker for fungi. Although psoriatic nails may be secondarily infected or colonized by dermatophytes and non-dermatophytes, parakeratosis is usually more consistent and pronounced in psoriasis than in onychomycosis.

The presence of eosinophilic masses is a common feature of exudative inflammatory nail bed disease and should not be overinterpreted.

If the diagnosis is still not clear after histological examination of a distal nail clipping, the choice then remains between a formal nail biopsy including soft tissues and a partial or complete nail avulsion, to obtain a more thorough examination of the nail plate (Grammer West *et al.* 1998). Both procedures are painful and the formal biopsy may leave scarring. However, the formal biopsy, if obtained from a site of active disease, will provide definitive information. It will help exclude other epidermal diseases such as human papilloma virus infection, squamous cell carcinoma and other infiltrative or inflammatory disorders.

### Biochemical analysis

The fingernails in psoriatic arthritis (Fig. 5.15) may be differentiated from those in rheumatoid arthritis by analysis of nail amino acids (Greaves *et al.* 1979). Clinically normal nails of patients with psoriatic and rheumatoid arthritis are significantly different with respect to threonine, proline and isoleucine content. No difference has been found between normal and dystrophic nail in psoriatic arthritis.

Three abnormal metabolites in psoriatic nails have been detected (Maeda *et al.* 1980): tetradecanoic acid octadecyl ester, hexadecanoic acid octadecyl ester and octadecanoic acid octadecyl ester. These esters could not be found in normal nails nor in ultrafiltrates of blood in cases of psoriasis. All these biochemical analyses are not routinely performed.

### Histopathology

Psoriasis may affect any or all particular parts of the nail apparatus (Lewin 1972). The proximal nail fold is virtually always affected in psoriatic arthritis of the distal interphalangeal joints, frequently also involving the eponychium and the matrix. The surface of the proximal nail fold shows typical acanthosis with drop-shaped or rectangular rete ridges, suprapapillary thinning of the epidermis, lack of granular layer and parakeratosis with pycnotic polymorphonuclear leucocytes that may be grouped to Munro's microabscesses. Neurophils also migrate through the epidermis but seldom form spongiform pustules. The capillaries of the papillary dermis are dilated and there is an inflammatory cell infiltrate around the vessels of the superficial dermis. When the proximal nail fold's distal free margin is involved, the cuticle will be lost. Involvement of the proximal nail fold's undersurface, the eponychium, induces similar changes; however, there is usually less pronounced acanthosis, but some spongiosis.

The normal nail bed and matrix have no granular layer. In psoriasis a granular layer develops, and the involved epithelium may then develop the histological features of psoriasis seen at other sites. Mounds of parakeratosis containing neutrophils are seen. The neutrophils tend to be lodged in the summits of the mounds of parakeratosis (Ackerman 1979). Foci of orthokeratotic cells are found interspersed between the mounds of parakeratotic horn which contain the neutrophils. There is usually considerable spongiosis with some exocytosis of mononuclear cells as well as—paradoxically—a focal granular layer. There may be papillomatosis of matrix and nail bed epithelium, often with spongiform pustules in the tips which then become necrotic. When this lesion involves the distal matrix and proximal nail bed, a salmon patch will be seen clinically; when it reaches the hyponychium it will lead to psoriatic onycholysis or to subungual hyperkeratosis.

Psoriasis of the most proximal portion of the matrix may cause pits. Histopathologically, a circumscribed area of matrix epithelium is affected resulting in a nidus of parakeratotic onychocytes; the width of the pit corresponds to the width of matrix involvement, its depth to the histopathological longitudinal diameter and the clinically visible length of the pit to the duration of the psoriatic lesion. In longitudinal nail biopsies one may see, under the proximal nail fold, mounds of parakeratotic cells bulging into the surface of the nail plate. When they arrive at the proximal nail fold's free margin they easily break out from the nail plate leaving the characteristic cup-shaped depression clinically known as pit.

Punctate leuconychia may arise from circumscribed psoriasis of the middle and distal matrix producing parakeratotic foci within the nail plate (Crawford 1938; White & Lapply 1952; Alkiewicz & Pfister 1976).

The use of exfoliative cytological techniques provides, according to Leyden et al. (1972), a rapid test, that can confirm an impression of psoriasis.

The severity of nail plate alteration depends on the extent of the psoriatic lesion: The more matrix is involved the more severe the alterations will be. This is easily seen in routine haematoxylin & eosin (H&E) sections, but the disorderly and irregular keratin structure is better visualized using Giemsa, Masson's trichrome stain or polarization microscopy. Small haemorrhages in the subungual keratin are demonstrated by the peroxidase reaction since they remain Prussian blue and Perl negative.

Scanning electron microscopy shows that the pits are small round depressions (Mauro et al. 1975) with their surface cells being small, separated from each other and having minute surface depressions (Dawber et al. 1972). Transmission electron microscopy of psoriatic leuconychia revealed a disorganization of keratin fibres in the onychocytes (André et al. 1988).

## Treatment

Despite recent therapeutic advances, the management of nail psoriasis remains long, tedious and sometimes unsatisfactory. Many clinicians prefer to consider it untreatable. However, a range of manoeuvres and therapies are useful (Table 5.1) and a positive and thorough approach will usually result in some improvement.

### General measures

It is important to be certain of the diagnosis to avoid pursuing a range of inappropriate measures and to ensure that an alternative diagnosis has not been missed which may have other considerations and therapies. To that end, the diagnosis should be based on clear clinical features or appropriate investigations.

### Active management

Patients and doctors need to have realistic expectations of active management and a period of patient education at the outset is important. Active management ranges from simple emollient and steroid applications to injected steroid and systemic agents. In those with minimal disease and in children it is usually best to avoid anything but the most simple therapies and to avoid the use of long-term potent topical steroid with their potential drawbacks (Deffer & Goette 1987; Requena et al. 1990; Wolf et al. 1990).

#### Topical therapies

Topical therapies are mainly for application to the base of the nail. At this site they may treat psoriasis of the nail fold and penetrate through to the underlying matrix to a limited extent. Some of the transverse ridging in psoriatic nails is associated with inflammation of the proximal nail fold. If this is reduced, the matrix function returns towards normal and nail ridging diminishes.

If onycholysis is present, the nail plate must be trimmed back to the point of separation if local medication is to be effective. Sometimes chemical avulsion may facilitate a more successful therapeutic response, particularly if the nail is very bulky. A further alternative to clipping back the nail is to use liquid scalp applications. In general this is less effective for nail bed psoriasis than direct applications of active treatment in an ointment base, although there are no published data on this topic.

#### Corticosteroid
High potency corticosteroids (i.e. flucinolone acetonide, triamcinolone acetonide, betamethasone, etc.) may be used under occlusive dressing such as non-porous tape or plastic gloves for short and repeated periods. Clobetasol proprionate (Dermovate) can be used without occlusive dressing. Side effects such as distal phalangeal atrophy have been reported (Deffer & Goette 1987; Requena et al. 1990).

**Table 5.1** Available treatments for nail psoriasis.

| Category | Therapy | References |
|---|---|---|
| Steroid | Topical | Tosti *et al.* 1998 |
| | Injected—local | Gerstein 1962; Abell & Samman 1973; Bleeker 1974, 1975; Peachey *et al.* 1976; Zaias 1990; de Berker & Lawrence 1998 |
| Calcipotriol | Injected—systemic | Arnold 1978 |
| | Topical | Kokely *et al.* 1994; Entestam & Weden 1996; Kuijpers *et al.*1996; Tosti *et al.* 1998 |
| 5-Fluorouracil | Topical | Frederiksson 1974; Fritz 1988; Tsuji & Nishumura 1991; Schissel & Elston 1998 |
| Cyclosporin | Topical | Tosti *et al.* 1990 |
| | Systemic | Arnold *et al.* 1993; Mahrle & Schulze 1995 |
| PUVA | Topical psoralen | Hofmann & Plewig 1977; Handfield-Jones *et al.* 1987 |
| | Systemic psoralen | Marks & Scher 1980 |
| Methotrexate | Systemic | Ellis & Voorhees 1987; Baran 1990; Kuijpers *et al.* 1996 |
| Radiation therapy | Grenz rays | Lindelöf 1988 |
| | Electron beam therapy | Kwang *et al.* 1994 |
| | Superficial radiotherapy | Yu & King 1992 |
| Others | Colloidal silicic acid | Lassus 1997 |
| | Nimesulide | Piraccini *et al.* 1994 |
| | Anthralin | Yamamoto *et al.* 1998 |
| | Bone marrow transplant | Yokota *et al.* 1996 |

**Table 5.2** Intralesional steroid for treating nail psoriasis. (Adapted from de Berker & Lawrence 1998.)

| | de Berker & Lawrence 1998 | Gerstein 1962 | Abell & Samman 1973 | Bleeker 1974 | Peachey *et al.* 1976 |
|---|---|---|---|---|---|
| Type of delivery | Needle | Needle | Port-o-Jet | Port-o-Jet | Port-o-Jet |
| Steroid | TA 10 mg/mL | TA 10 mg/mL | TA 5 mg/mL | TA 5 mg/mL | TA 5 mg/mL |
| Site | Matrix and nail bed | Matrix | Proximal nail fold | Proximal nail fold | Proximal nail fold |
| Regimen | 4 × 0.1 mL | 1 × 0.2 mL | 1–4 × 0.1 mL | 0.2–0.3 mL | 1 × 0.1 mL |
| | mean 1.2 doses | | weekly for 3 weeks minimum | ? No./frequency | every 4–6 weeks, 3 × |
| Follow-up (months) | 9 (3–17) | 14 | 0–24 | 5–20 | 1 |
| Patients (no.) | 19 | 4 | 58 | 400 | 28 |
| Nails (no.) | 46 | 17 | Not given | 569 | 28 |
| % digits improved at end of follow-up | | | | | |
| Onycholysis | 50% (18/36) | | 50% (17/34)* | 34% (110/322) | 19% (5/26) |
| Pits/ridges | Pits 45% (9/20) | Combined features | 91% (40/44)* | 68% (266/392) | 86 (12/14) |
| | Ridges 93% (15/16) | 35% (6/17) | | | |
| Thickening | 89% (10/12) | | No result | 11% (2/19) | No result |
| Subungual hyperkeratosis | 100% (16/16) | | No result | No result | No result |

* Patients: digits not specified.

TA, Triamcinolone acetate.

A mixture of the topical steroid combined with 5–10% benzoyl peroxide or 0.1% retinoic acid cream may give better results. Betamethasone dipropionate (64 mg/g) with salicylic acid (3%) in an ointment base is moderately effective at reducing subungual hyperkeratosis and nail plate thickening when used for 3–5 months (Tosti *et al.* 1998).

### Calcipotriol

There are several reports of nail psoriasis showing some improvement following treatment with topical calcipotriol (calcipotriene in the USA) (Kokely *et al.* 1994; Tosti *et al.* 1998). Nail plate thickness and subungual hyperkeratosis are the main features to improve (Tosti *et al.* 1998), with response more commonly seen in the fingers than the toes. Studies do not describe clinical clearance, but rather reduction of severity of psoriasis.

Calcipotriol ointment has also been used with some success in acrodermatitis continua of Hallopeau (Entestam & Wedén 1996; Kuijpers *et al.* 1996).

### 5-Fluorouracil

Frederiksson (1974) used 1% fluorouracil solution dissolved in propylene glycol applied twice daily for 6 months around the margin of the nail; it was gently massaged into the nail fold and allowed to dry. The treatment is only recommended for nails with pitting and hypertrophy as dominant symptoms and it should be used with caution when there is onycholysis, although a further single report described a good result in a patient with psoriatic trachyonychia and onycholysis (Schissel & Elston 1998); the onycholysis did not improve.

In the largest series of fluorouracil therapy, Fritz treated 59 patients in an open non-blinded study using 20% urea cream plus 1% fluorouracil (Fritz 1988). This provided an improvement of more than 50% of the clinical signs such as oil spots, subungual hyperkeratosis and combined signs. Transient rhabdomyolysis connected with topical use of 5-fluorouracil is anecdotal (Schmied & Levy 1986).

Five per cent 5-fluorouracil has been used under occlusion in acrodermatitis continua of Hallopeau to good effect (Tsuji & Nishimura 1991).

### Cyclosporin

Topical cyclosporin (Tosti *et al.* 1990) was used successfully in a single subject, applying 0.2 mL of a 10% oily preparation of cyclosporin to the nail folds over several months. However, in most settings there has been a problem with finding an effective vehicle for the delivery of cyclosporin as a topical therapy.

### Intralesional therapy

#### Corticosteroid (Table 5.2)

Intralesional injection of long-acting corticosteroids into the area of the nail matrix and/or bed is helpful, especially when these structures are affected. The injection can be delivered in several ways:
• Fine gauge needle (28) and syringe with Luer lock;
• Insulin syringe;
• Dermojet or Port-o-Jet needle-less injector.

The need for local anaesthetic will depend on the patient, the technique, the size of the needle, the volume to be injected and the tenderness of the pathology. Needle-less injectors do not require anaesthetic. When the injection needs to penetrate the matrix or go beneath the nail bed, local anaesthetic is usually required. A proximal ring block or wrist block may be used; the latter if several digits are to be treated. Distal blocks are possible, but tend to make it difficult to subsequently inject the steroid because of tissue turgor.

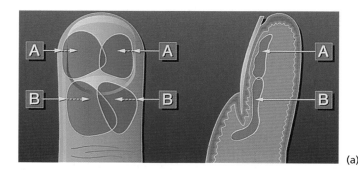

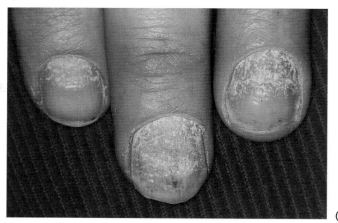

(a)

(b)

**Fig. 5.16** (a) Steroid injection technique for treating psoriatic nails. (After D.A.R. de Berker.) (b) Psoriasis—nail changes induced by lithium therapy. (Courtesy of R. Rudolph, USA.)

Many authors have abandoned jet injectors because sterilization procedures for the apparatus do not prevent contamination with hepatitis virus or retroviruses. This is because of the 'splash back' of small quantities of blood at the time of injection. Epidermoid implantation cysts, leading to amputation of a distal phalanx, were an unexpected complication in a patient of J. Mascaro (personal communication).

There are no golden rules about the strength of steroid to inject and the frequency of re-treatment. A suspension of triamcinolone acetonide is a common choice. Reports describe concentrations between 2.5 mg/mL (Norton 1982; Zaias 1990) and 10 mg/mL (de Berker & Lawrence 1998) (Fig. 5.16). In the last series, no case was treated more than three times over a mean of 9 months. No sustained tissue atrophy or other adverse side effects were noted. In the short term, subungual haemorrhage was common and two digits of 46 had short-term pain in the nail fold, possibly indicating vessel infarction by particulate steroid. Reversible atrophy at the injection sites (Peachey *et al.* 1976) was reported with use of the Port-o-Jet and periungual hypopigmentation (Bedi 1977) has also been noted.

Where response to treatment has been documented in detail, it appears that pits or ridges (Abell & Samman 1973; Bleeker 1975; Peachey *et al.* 1976) and nail thickening and subungual hyperkeratosis (de Berker & Lawrence 1998) are the features most responsive to injected steroid. Onycholysis is the most resistant. Intervals of 3–8 weeks between treatments are common, although the total number of treatments is not always defined. In the clinical setting it will typically be determined by response and a tapering regimen over a 12-month period has been described (Norton 1982). With higher doses of steroids or with frequent injections over an indefinite period, there might be concerns about atrophic side effects on local structures. However, the two cases of digital tendon rupture in the literature make this seem an unlikely complication (Gottlieb & Riskin 1989; Taras *et al.* 1995). In the first, an elderly lady received 29 steroid injections for her carpal tunnel disease (Gottlieb & Riskin 1989). In the second, a 62-year-old woman was treated 4 years before tendon rupture with two injections for a trigger thumb.

### Radiation therapies

#### Psoralen ultraviolet light A

Photochemotherapy will produce benefit in some cases within 6 months. For patients with severe nail involvement, it may be more practical, after the glabrous skin has been cleared, to continue more intensive treatment of the nail and periungual region alone (Dobson & Thiers 1981).

Hofmann and Plewig (1977) have experimented with an apparatus designed to deliver high intensity ultraviolet light A (UVA) for the treatment of psoriatic nails. The technique is time consuming and particularly valuable when only a few nails are affected, because the nails are treated one by one. However one must state that the response of psoriatic nails to photochemotherapy is not impressive. Complete clearing has been obtained (Caccialanza & Frigerio 1982) but is rare, and pitting may not respond (Marks & Scher 1980). Side effects such as subungual haemorrhage, photo-onycholysis (Mackie 1979; Baran 1990) and pigmentation of the nail plate and the nail bed may be seen and these can be avoided in the normal nails by using protective nail varnish or sunscreen preparations for non-affected nails.

Parker and Diffey (1983) suggest that the mechanisms producing resolution of psoriatic nail changes are similar to those for psoriatic plaques: approximately 2.5 times the therapeutic dose for glabrous skin would have to be delivered to the surface of the nail plate (with appropriate protection for the surrounding skin) to achieve the same effect. This factor assumes a flat action spectrum for the regression of psoriatic lesions due to psoralen photochemotherapy. If wavelengths around 330 nm prove to be effective therapeutically the factor is likely to be closer to 5 because of the differing transmission characteristics of the epidermis and the nail plate.

Müller *et al.* (1991) investigated the therapeutic effect of UV radiation with Hönle's dermalight Blue-Point on psoriasis patients with additional nail involvement. All the patients got a daily radiation of the nail matrix area for about 4 weeks except on Sunday. The range of radiation time was 5–45 s per nail. More than 60% showed improvement, with an average duration of about 10 months. Forty-two per cent of these reported a visible beginning of the restitution during their time in hospital, which generally continued after discontinuation of the therapy. Twenty-eight per cent had complete nail restitution. Handfield-Jones *et al.* (1987) advocated local psoralen ultraviolet light A (PUVA) treatment using 1% 8-methoxypsoralen (Meladin) solution applied to the proximal nail fold of affected fingers up to the terminal phalanx. The backs of the hands are exposed to a UVA source producing 3 mW/cm$^3$ at a distance of 20 cm. The initial dosage needs to be low to avoid burning, and 0.5 J increasing to a maximum of 2 J is used two to three times a week. Topical 5-MOP has been associated with photo-onycholysis (Baran & Barthelemy 1990).

#### Grenz rays

In certain rare cases, in patients over 30 years old, low-voltage X-rays may be useful. Total dose per area, per lifetime, should not exceed 10 Gy (1000 rad). Five gray of grenz rays applied on 10 occasions at intervals of 1 week (Lindelöf 1988) can be effective only when psoriatic nails are of normal thickness. This mode of treatment should not be rejected on safety grounds, since in a large-scale study of the incidence of malignant skin tumours in 14140 patients who have received Grenz ray for benign skin disorders, the risk factor was small with regards to the development of non-melanoma skin tumours (Lindelöf & Eklund 1986).

#### Superficial radiotherapy and electron beam therapy

A double-blind study of superficial radiotherapy in psoriatic nail dystrophy has demonstrated a definite, albeit temporary, benefit (Yu & King 1992). A similar temporary benefit has been demonstrated with electron beam therapy (Kwang *et al.* 1994).

### Systemic therapy

#### Retinoids

Psoriasis vulgaris has been subject to controversial reports due to its variable response. Ellis and Voorhees (1987), reporting on more than 100 patients, found the results 'very good' with a 0.2–1.2 mg/kg/day dosage range.

The authors' experience, however, suggests some caution in this evaluation. Since thinning of the nail is a common finding with etretinate, it is apparent that good results will be obtained in psoriasis patients with thick nails. By contrast, disorders such as pitting or onycholysis can become worse due to the toxic action of the drug in the nail apparatus and to the possibility of an isomorphic response. Moreover, even though thinning of thick psoriatic nails is appreciated by some patients, others complain of increased sensitivity to external pressure and an inability to use the nails in a functional way. The side effects of the retinoids on the nail (Baran 1990) are described in Chapter 7.

**Table 5.3** Exacerbating factors in nail psoriasis.

| Exacerbating factors | Mechanisms | Management |
|---|---|---|
| Long nails | The leverage upon the nail bed is increased with a long nail which exacerbates nail bed psoriasis | Keep nail short |
| Prosthetic nails | As above | If nail prostheses are kept short they can be useful in nail psoriasis. They conceal abnormalities of surface and colour |
| Trimming and manipulating the cuticle | Isomorphic reaction | Avoid manicure |
| Removing debris beneath the nail | Once the onychocorneal band has been disrupted, debris will be washed down beneath the nail into the onycholytic space. In addition squames will accumulate secondary to active psoriasis at that site. Patients will be tempted to use sharp instruments to remove this material and this will exacerbate onycholysis | Wear gloves when undertaking dirty work. Use a soft nail brush to clean the undersurface of nails |
| Irritants | Skin irritants, such as excessive washing, cleansing agent and other solvents, will exacerbate psoriasis | Avoid irritants, wear gloves when undertaking work with irritant emollient |
| Fungal infection | Co-existing pathology | Identify by mycological examination and culture followed by appropriate antifungal therapy |

### Other systemic therapies

Systemic treatment with methotrexate and cyclosporin can be expected to improve nail psoriasis, although neither are usually used for nail disease in isolation. There are no published studies examining the effect of methotrexate on nail psoriasis, but it is commonly accepted that nails may improve in tandem with the skin during methotrexate therapy (Gueissaz *et al.* 1992).

In a study of skin, nail and joint psoriasis treated with cyclosporin or acitretin for 10 weeks, both therapies produced a significant improvement in nail disease from baseline at doses of 3.0 and 0.52 mg/kg/day, respectively (Mahrle *et al.* 1995). A report of the good response of severe nail psoriasis to oral cyclosporin in a single patient required between 3 and 5 mg/kg/day (Arnold *et al.* 1993).

Cyclosporin has been reported as successful at a dose of between 2.5 and 4.4 mg/kg/day in a single case of acrodermatitis continua of Hallopeau.

Newer therapies for psoriasis may also be effective for nail manifestations, but evaluation is still at an early stage. Tacrolimus appears to work for cutaneous psoriasis when given orally, but is ineffective when used topically (Zonneweld *et al.* 1998).

### Other therapies

There are brief accounts of a range of therapies that may be worth further consideration. These include a pilot study of oral and topical colloidal silicic acid, where nail features were reported as 'cured' in half the patients after 90 days (Lassus 1997). A non-steroidal anti-inflammatory drug, nimesulide, was used orally in an uncontrolled trial of treatment in acrodermatitis continua of Hallopeau where the authors believed it was helpful (Piraccini *et al.* 1994). Although anthralin is useful elsewhere on the body, it is seldom used on the nails, partly because of the considerable staining. In one study of subjects with refractory nail psoriasis, anthralin ointment (0.4–2%) was applied as a short contact therapy to the nail bed for 30 min before washing off and the application of triethanolamine cream to help prevent staining. Moderate improvement was recorded in 60% of patients after 5 months (Yamamoto *et al.* 1998). Widespread psoriasis settled in a patient after allogenic bone marrow transplantation. The condition remained settled after the discontinuation of immunosuppressants required in the early stages of transplantation (Yokota *et al.* 1996).

Treatment of coincident fungal infection may be relevant where it is contributing to the nail disease (Gupta 1997) (Table 5.3).

## Psoriasis associated with other disorders

A number of conditions may produce clinical and/or histological nail changes similar to psoriasis or may be clinically and/or histologically related to psoriasis. Psoriasis associated with unilateral ectromelia and central nervous system anomalies has been reported by Shear *et al.* (1971), and probably belongs to the CHILD syndrome (Happle *et al.* 1980) or CHILD naevus (Happle 1987), which is a congenital homolateral epidermal hyperplasia and hypoplastic hemidysplasia (Laplanche *et al.* 1980) with ptychotropism, a pronounced affinity for the body folds (Happle 1990).

Psoriasis in AIDS tends to be much more active and resistant to most forms of therapy (Lazar & Roenigk 1988) as well as in Reiter's syndrome (Duvic *et al.* 1987). However, on an epidemiological level, psoriatic nail disease in human immunodeficiency virus (HIV) infection is not common. In one prospective study of 155 HIV-infected patients, onychomycosis was present in 30% and none were found to have features of nail psoriasis (Cribier *et al.* 1998).

**Table 5.4** Drug-induced psoriasis.

*Referenced*
Captopril (Gayrard *et al.* 1990)
Gemfibrozil (Fisher *et al.* 1988)
Lithium (Sasaki *et al.* 1989; Rudolph 1991)
Penicillins (Katz *et al.* 1987)
Terfenadine (Harrison & Stone 1988; Navaratnam & Gebauer 1990)
Timolol (ophthalmic sol. Coignet & Sayag 1990)

*Anecdotal*
Amiodarone
Antimalarials
Aspirin, salicylates
Clonidine
Corticoids
Digoxin
Indomethacin (indometacin)
Interferon alpha
Morphine
Oxyphenbutazone
Phenylbutazone
Potassium iodide
Procaine
Progesterone
Sulphonamides
Sulphapyridine trazodone

Severe exacerbation of psoriasis may be due to drugs (Abell *et al.* 1986), but in some adult patients, a significant clearing of psoriasis is associated with the initiation of zidovudine therapy (Kaplan *et al.* 1989) (Table 5.4).

The Scandinavian literature reports many cases of psoriasis aggravated β-blockers and lithium. Psoriasis-like lesions involving the nail area can appear *de novo*; they disappear after the β-blockers are discontinued (Jensen *et al.* 1976; Tegner 1976). Lithium can aggravate and/or precipitate psoriasis (Sasaki *et al.* 1989) and may even reveal isolated psoriatic nail changes (Rudolph 1991) (Fig. 5.16b). Several drugs may induce psoriasis (Nicolas *et al.* 1987).

## Psoriatic mimicry in the nail apparatus

According to Zaias (1990) psoriasiform states of the nail apparatus share: (a) a psoriasiform appearance; (b) some histopathological similarities. They differ in their clinical courses, and sometimes their involvement with other organs and sites. We have expanded this definition by adding some diseases which may present a clinical psoriasiform appearance without histological similarities. These conditions include:

1 Reiter's syndrome (page 188).
2 Pityriasis rubra pilaris (page 193).
3 Acropustulosis—acrodermatitis continua of Hallopeau.
4 Parakeratosis pustulosa (page 196).
5 Norwegian scabies (page 168).
6 Acral psoriasiform reaction to neoplasm—acrokeratosis paraneoplastica (Bolognia *et al.* 1991) (page 292).

7 Subungual hyperkeratosis when the clinical picture reminds one of psoriasis or lichen planus of the nail bed and hyponychium but with just hyperkeratosis seen histologically.
8 Keratosis cristarum (Chapter 2).
9 Hyponychial dermatitis (Fig. 5.17a–c). Contact dermatitis is suspected but all the tests are negative. Histologically a great exudation of serum-like material, also seen in other nail diseases, is the characteristic feature. PAS stain is positive.

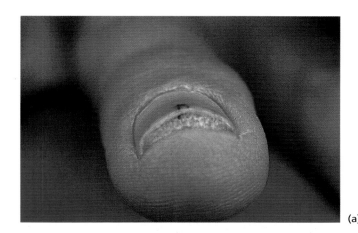

(a)

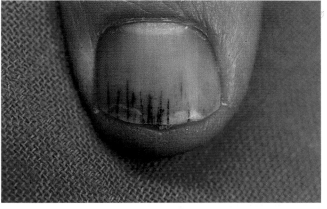

(b)

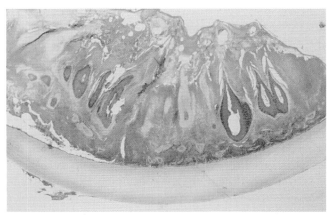

(c)

**Fig. 5.17** (a) Idiopathic distal subungual hyperkeratosis. (b) Clinical patterns—same patient. (c) Histology—same patient. (Courtesy of E. Duhard, France.)

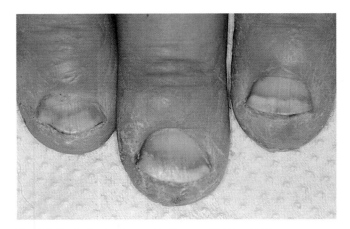

**Fig. 5.18** 'Psoriasiform' acral dermatitis. (Courtesy of B. Richert, Belgium.)

**10** Psoriasiform acral dermatitis. This term was coined by Zaias (1990). The condition looks clinically like psoriasis (Fig. 5.18), but histologically it is not.

The clinical presentation is distinctive because the patients exhibit a chronic dermatitis of the terminal phalanges and nail bed changes with onycholysis suggestive of psoriasis. There is no family history. The nail bed becomes progressively shorter and may be lost (Caputo *et al.* 1996). The fingers are described as 'sclerodermoid'. There is no Raynaud's disease and no other features of a connective tissue disorder.

Tosti *et al.* (1992) reported the pathological and immunohistochemical study of three patients. Histology shows exocytosis of lymphoid cells in the epidermis associated with marked spongiosis, parakeratosis and scale. There is an increased number of $CD1a^+CD4^+$ Langerhans cells within the epidermis and the superficial dermis. Langerhans cells are also present in the spongiotic vesicles. The monuclear infiltrate consists of mature peripheral T lymphocytes ($CD2^+CD3^+CD5^+$) with a CD4/CD8 ratio of 1/1 in the epidermis and 3/1 in the dermis. Thirty per cent of the lymphocytes expressed the interleukin 2 receptor ($CD25^+$).

There is one report of a response to the oral anti-inflammatory drug nimesulide (Caputo *et al.* 1996).

Patrizi *et al.* (1999) have observed three young patients presenting with psoriasiform acral dermatitis with concomitant presence of clinically and histologically typical skin lesions of psoriasis in other sites. They suggest that this condition is a particular variety of acral psoriasis in childhood.

**11** Punctate keratoderma with features of nail psoriasis. This description is based on two cases where onycholysis, pitting and subungual hyperkeratosis developed in tandem with palmoplantar punctate keratoderma in the absence of a personal or family history of psoriasis (Tosti *et al.* 1993b).

**12** Lichen nitidus with nail dystrophy. The main nail changes in this rare disorder are pitting and longitudinal ridging or splitting (Munro *et al.* 1993).

**13** Acral psoriasiform hemispherical papulosis (Osawa 1994) (Fig. 5.26) is probably a clinical variant of psoriasis.

## Sterile pustular conditions of the nail apparatus

There is a confusing nomenclature of sterile pustular conditions of the nail apparatus. This may reflect the unclear clinical boundaries between some of the conditions, such as acute and chronic palmoplantar pustulosis. In turn, these conditions have an unclear association with psoriasis, some manifesting in a continuum with pustular psoriasis and colleagues as a separate entity such as acrodermatitis continua of Hallopeau or subcorneal pustular dermatosis. In spite of these distinctions, chance may throw up some apparent associations; Chimenti and Ackerman (1981) describe patients with pustular lesions of subcorneal pustular dermatosis, but who had in addition stigmas suggestive of psoriasis; scaly plaques on the elbows and knees, pitted nails or arthropathy.

Moreover, some non-pustular conditions have names such as parakeratosis pustulosa where the presentation is more commonly in association with an eczematous origin and pustules are not clinically apparent.

*Localized pustular psoriasis: palmoplantar pustulosis* (Fig. 5.25a)
This chronic condition is limited to the soles and palms, with variable nail involvement. It appears genetically different from psoriasis vulgaris, lacking the association with HLA-B13 and B17 (Ward & Barnes 1978). Features of typical psoriasis elsewhere or a family history of the condition are often lacking. However, coincidence of palmoplantar pustulosis (PPP) and psoriasis vulgaris is sufficiently common to affirm that they are related (Enfors & Molin 1971). In a study of 50 patients with PPP, 30% had nail involvement. Subungual pustules was the most common feature, present in 20% of the whole group. Onycholyis, pitting and nail destruction were seen to a lesser extent (Burden & Kemmett 1996). This study examines the problem of making a clear distinction between PPP and acrodermatitis continua of Hallopeau. Previous studies have suggested that pustulation of the nail apparatus is rare in PPP and that its absence is a useful pointer to the diagnosis (Ward & Barnes 1978). Subungual pustulation seen in many of the cases reviewed by Burden and Kemmett (1996) would have been classified as acrodermatitis continua if it were not for the presence of the coincident pustules of palms and soles.

*Acrodermatitis continua of Hallopeau* (Figs 5.19 & 5.22)
The points made above illustrate how it can be difficult to distinguish acrodermatitis continua of Hallopeau (ACH) from palmoplantar pustulosis. However, typically ACH presents in a younger age group, including children, starting with a single finger or toe (Fig. 5.20). Some authorities would limit the diagnosis to a condition affecting the distal digit alone (Piraccini *et al.* 1994) and in Piraccini's study of 20 patients, 13 were women, possibly suggesting an increased incidence in females. Pustules may be studded around the nail fold and beneath the nail, where they coalesce to form lakes of pus. The nail may

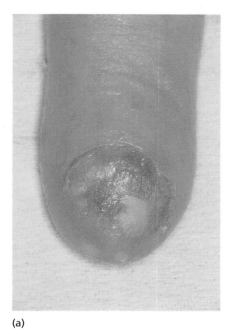

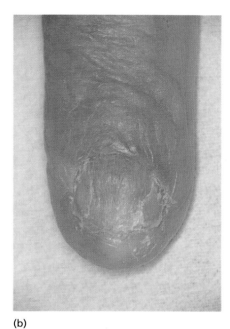

**Fig. 5.19** Psoriasis—acropustulosis, (a) before treatment and (b) after 1 month of etretinate.

(a)

(b)

gradually be lost and replaced by a mixture of scale and pustules of the nail bed.

There may be progessive loss of entire digits in the feet and loss of fingertips and fingernails (Mahowald & Parrish 1982). This illustrates a feature of severe acral inflammation associated with a spectrum of pustular disorders. Acral pustular psoriasis has been reported with resorptive osteolysis as a 'deep Koebner phenomenon' (Miller *et al.* 1971; Combemale *et al.* 1989) (Figs 5.21 & 5.22) and notable skin and subcutaneous tissue atrophy with 'tuft' osteolysis may occur, independently

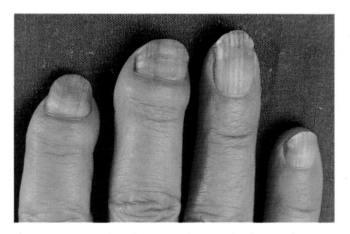

**Fig. 5.21** Psoriasis—acral pustular psoriasis with acroosteolysis. (Courtesy of P. Combemale, France.)

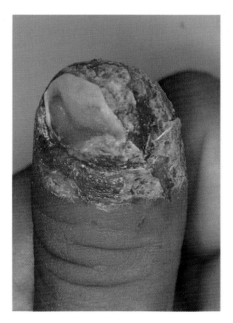

**Fig. 5.20** Psoriasis— very inflammatory acropustulosis in a 10-year-old child.

of acropustuloses and arthritis in psoriasis (Cheesbrough 1979).

Histopathology may reveal Munro–Sabouraud 'microabscesses' or the spongiform pustule of Kogoj. The pathological focus appears to be in the nail bed rather than the matrix (Piraccini *et al.* 1994) (Figs 5.23 & 5.24).

Differential diagnosis includes paronychia (Mooser *et al.* 1998) and 'acral granulomatous dermatitis' (Miyagawa *et al.* 1990), a condition which clinically resembles ACH. In contrast to the latter, however, the epidermis is histologically normal, with dermal and subcutaneous abscess formation with granulomas. The lesions respond to systemic corticosteroid therapy with residual atrophy and contractures of the fingers.

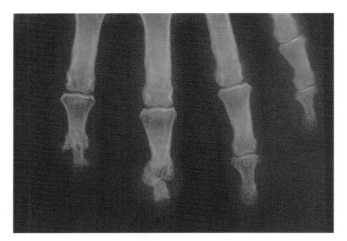

**Fig. 5.22** Psoriasis—X-ray showing 'resorptive' osteolysis (patient as in Fig. 5.21).

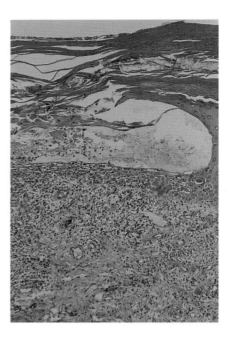

**Fig. 5.24** Psoriasis—
showing spongiform
pustule of Kogoj.

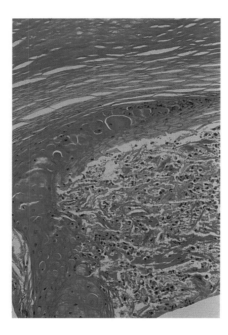

**Fig. 5.23** Psoriasis—
Munro microabscess
formation histologically.

*Acute acral pustulosis (syn. acute palmoplantar pustulosis,*
*pustular bacterid)* (Fig. 5.25b)
Acute palmoplantar pustulosis (Andrews & Machacek 1935) is
a disorder distinguished from chronic palmoplantar pustulosis
by the speed of onset and clinical signs. The large, unilocular
pustules arise on normal skin and involve the dorsa of the
hands, fingers and feet (Fig. 5.26). This condition is precipitated by infection, including systemic disease such as pneumonia or streptococcal sore throat. The pustular changes are
usually self limiting and aggressive therapy is not indicated.
There may be a background of psoriasis or chronic palmoplantar pustulosis, and a case of acute acral pustular bacterid can
evolve into the more classic chronic form (Burge & Ryan
1985). SAPHO syndrome (synovitis, acne, pustulosis, hyperostosis and osteitis), an acronym introduced by Chamot and

Kahn (1994), may be associated with subungual pustules
(Gmyrek *et al.* 1999).

*Acute generalized pustular psoriasis*
Many of the features of the nail apparatus in generalized pustular psoriasis resemble those seen in acrodermatitis continua of
Hallopeau. The setting of an acute generalized disease is the
main distinction. Lakes of subungual pus may develop and the
nails may both become thickened, yellow and be shed.

Diagnostic distinction between the different causes of sterile
pustulation of the nail apparatus relies on recognition of a
pattern of pustulation. The pathological process can be demonstrated by histology, but there is insufficient data to suggest that
this will distinguish between the disorders described above.
However, biopsy may be the only way to confirm the general
nature of a pustular and/or atrophying process of the tip of a
digit when no pustules can be seen macroscopically.

There is extensive spongiform pustule formation in the
epidermis, either with merging of the neutrophils to typical,
macroscopically visible pustules, or with necrosis of the superficial keratinocytes and thick parakeratosis stuck with Munro's
microabscesses, respectively. In the papillary dermis, there is
usually some extravasation of erythrocytes which may get into
the epidermis to eventually reach the parakeratosis; this will
add to the brownish colour of the scab.

Treatment of acute forms of acropustulosis may be directed
by the precipitating infection. In chronic forms, localized
PUVA can be of benefit. Aromatic retinoid therapy may give
good short-term results (Deichmann & Spindeldreier 1982);
but recurrences appear 1–3 months after the treatment has been
stopped (Baran 1979, 1982). Combined retinoid and PUVA

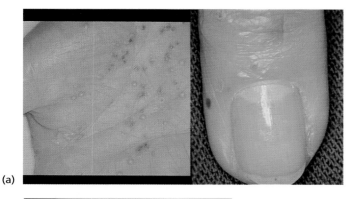

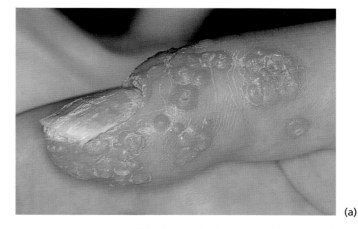

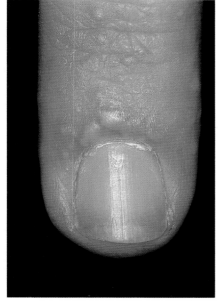

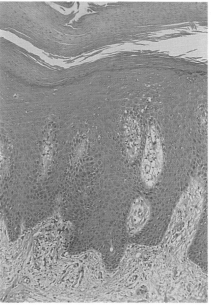

**Fig. 5.25** (a) Palmoplantar pustulosis (PPP). (b) Acute acral pustulosis (pustular bacterid).

**Fig. 5.26** (a) Acral psoriasiform hemispherical papulosis. (Courtesy of H. Osawa, Japan.) (b) Histology, same patient.

treatment delays and lowers the frequency of relapse, but recalcitrant cases may be observed (Brun *et al.* 1985). A single report of the use of calcipotriol in combination with acitretin in a right/left comparison suggests that the addition of topical calcipotriol to oral acitretin is useful (Kuijpers *et al.* 1996). Nimesulide is an oral non-steroidal anti-inflammatory drug which has been reported as useful in doses of 200 mg/day, although benefit may not be sustained when therapy is discontinued (Piraccini *et al.* 1994). It has also been used effectively in sclerodermoid psoriatic changes in a child (Caputo *et al.* 1996). Topical mechloretamine (Notowicz *et al.* 1978) and 5% fluorouracil cream (Tsuji & Nishimura 1991) have given some good results, as has intramuscular triamcinolone acetonide (Arnold 1978).

## Psoriatic arthritis

The work of Baker *et al.* (1964) showed that 83% of 53 patients with psoriatic arthritis had psoriatic involvement of fingernails or toenails at some time during the period of study. This agrees well with the finding of nail changes in 86.5% of 52 subjects with psoriatic arthritis by Lavaroni *et al.* (1994). Baker noted all types of dystrophy from mild pitting to gross distortion; these were not related to the distribution of the joint involvement. Lavaroni found subungual hyperkeratosis of the big toenail was the most common feature, followed by fingernail pitting.

Patients with the more severe types of arthritis tended to have greater nail involvement whether or not there was significant terminal interphalangeal joint disease. No topographical relationship was found between arthritis of the distal joints and psoriatic change in the nail of the same digit. These findings differ slightly from those of Jones *et al.* (1994) and Wright *et al.* (1979). Jones found nail disease in 67% of 100 subjects with psoriatic arthritis and noted a marked correlation between those with disease of the distal interphalangeal joint and disease in the adjacent nail. Wright found nail changes in all patients with distal arthritis and in 88% of patients with deforming arthritis. The concept of psoriatic 'nail matrix arthropathy' is supported by the fact that the nail matrix and the terminal interphalangeal joint share the same blood supply (Abel & Farber 1979; Farber & Nall 1992). In spite of these suggestive observations, the relationship between nail psoriasis and distal interphalangeal psoriatic joint involvement is not clear (Zaias & Norton 1980).

In childhood, Sills (1980) noted a strong correlation between nail involvement and distal arthritis. Definite juvenile psoriatic arthritis was defined by Southwood *et al.* (1989) as arthritis associated, but not necessarily coincident with, a typical psoriatic rash, or arthritis, plus at least three of four minor criteria: dactylitis, nail pitting, psoriasis-like rash or family history of psoriasis. It may, however, have more in common with juvenile rheumatoid arthritis than the seronegative spondylarthropathies with which it is traditionally associated. Where juvenile arthritis is the presenting complaint, 67% of 50 children in one study had nail pitting as the most common associated feature of psoriasis (Roberton *et al.* 1996). Only 18% went on to develop psoriatic rash within childhood.

Young females with widespread plaque-type or suberythrodermic psoriasis, with a strong family history of psoriasis, nail changes and large joint arthropathy, may form a separate subgroup of patients with a strong family history of autoimmune disease (Harrison & Stone 1988).

## Psoriatic onycho-pachydermoperiostitis (Fig. 5.27)

In this variant of psoriatic arthritis, involvement of the great toe, psoriatic nail changes and thickening of the distal soft tissues are associated with osteoperiostitis of the distal phalanx, but a normal distal interphalangeal joint. Although the condition is most commonly identified in the toes (Fournié *et al.* 1989; Boisseau-Garsaud *et al.* 1996; Schroder *et al.* 1997; Ziemer *et al.* 1998), it has also been reported in the fingers (Marghéry *et al.* 1991). Differential diagnosis includes

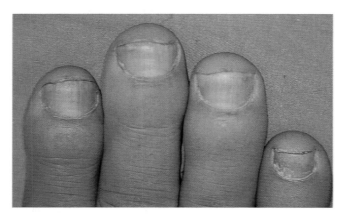

**Fig. 5.27** Psoriasis—distal interphalangeal joint arthropathy and periungual soft tissue inflammation (psoriatic acropachydermodactyly).

osteoarthritis, pachydermoperiostitis, acromegaly and hypertrophic osteoarthropathy. Clinically, diagnosis may often be delayed because there may be no overt psoriasis and pain may be a significant feature.

Prior to the definiton of psoriatic onycho-pachydermoperiostitis (POPP) as a clinical diagnosis, it was recognized that pain and swelling of the digit pulp, with nail dystrophy and osteolysis, might present in the absence of joint involvement (Buckley & Raleigh 1959; Cheesbrough 1979). In the case presented by Buckley, trauma was proposed in the context of widespread psoriasis, with bone changes representing a form of 'deep Koebner' phenomenon.

From the rheumatologist's perspective, the diagnosis of POPP may be an artificial distinction from the continuum of psoriatic arthritis. In the setting of a rheumatology clinic a radiological survey of the big toes of 202 subjects with psoriatic arthritis revealed osteoperositis in 26.2% (Goupille *et al.* 1996). In those with additional nail dystrophy, the rate of osteoperiostitis was 48.8% and severe periostitis was seen in four subjects all of whom had nail dystrophy. Destructive joint disease was also a marker for the presence of osteoperiostitis among those with psoriatic arthritis, where 54% of those with destructive joint disease were found to have osteoperiostitis in comparison to 22% of those without significant joint destruction. Osteoperiostitis was uncommon in those with psoriasis in the absence of joint disease (3/44, 6.8%), which suggests that the feature is a marker for psoriatic arthritis rather than psoriatic skin disease. Methotrexate has been recommended as the treatment of choice (Bauza *et al.* 2000).

## Reiter's syndrome

The clinical and histological features of the skin changes in patients with Reiter's syndrome may be indistinguishable from those of patients with psoriasis (Fig. 5.28a). Skin changes resembling paronychia can accompany nail involvement suggesting inflammation of the proximal nail fold. Onycholysis, ridging, splitting, greenish-yellow or sometimes brownish-red discoloration and subungual hyperkeratosis may be present. Small yellow pustules may develop and showly enlarge beneath the nail, often near the lunula. Their contents become dry and brown. The nails may be shed. Samman (1978) noted nail pitting in Reiter's syndrome, stating that deep pits and punched-out lesions can occur. According to Lovy *et al.* (1980) nail pitting may reflect a predisposition to the development of psoriasis or psoriasiform lesions dependent on the HLA-A2 and B27 antigens, as suggested by previously reported HLA typing studies. HLA-A2 and B27 were present in a 6-year-old boy who had only the nail changes which were compatible with Reiter's syndrome; HLA-A2 and B27 were also present in his father, who had uveitis, arthritis and amyloidosis (Pajarre & Kero 1977).

Antibiotics, steroids and non-steroidal anti-inflammatory drugs are without benefit. PUVA may be helpful. Aromatic retinoid therapy may clear the nails in Reiter's syndrome (Fig.

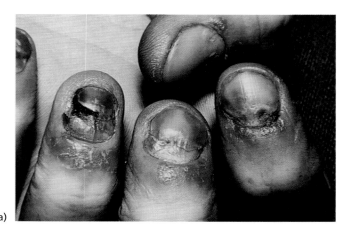

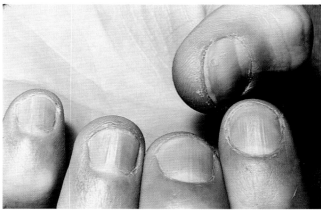

(a)

(b)

**Fig. 5.28** (a) Reiter's syndrome. (b) Reiter's syndrome—same patient, after etretinate therapy.

5.28b). Combined chemotherapy with methotrexate, aromatic retinoid and prednisolone has been suggested (Luderschmidt & Balda 1982).

Histopathology cannot definitely differentiate psoriasis from Reiter's syndrome; however, nail changes in the latter tend to be more pustular than in psoriasis vulgaris and erythrocyte extravasation is usually more pronounced.

## References

### Psoriasis

Abel, E.A., Dicicco, L.M., Ozenberg, E.K. *et al.* (1986) Drugs in exacerbation of psoriasis. *Journal of the American Academy of Dermatology* **15**, 1007–1022.

Abell, E. & Samman, P.D. (1973) Intradermal triamcinolone treatment of nail dystrophies. *British Journal of Dermatology* **89**, 191–197.

Ackerman, B. (1979) Subtle clues to diagnosis by conventional microscopy. Neutrophils within the cornified layer as clues to infection by superficial fungi. *American Journal of Dermatopathology* **1**, 69–75.

Akinduro, O.M., Venning, V.A. & Burge, S.M. (1994) Psoriatic nail pitting in infancy [letter]. *British Journal of Dermatology* **130**, 800–801.

Al-Fouzan, A.S. & Nanda, A. (1994) A survey of childhood psoriasis in Kuwait. *Pediatric Dermatology* **11**, 116–119.

Alkiewicz, J. (1948) Psoriasis of the nails. *British Journal of Dermatology* **60**, 195–200.

Alkiewicz, J. & Pfister, R. (1976) *Atlas der Nagelkrankheiten: Pathohistologie, Klinik und Differential Diagnose.* FK Schattauer, Stuttgart.

André, J., Achten, G. & Laporte, M. (1988) Normal and abnormal nails: light and electron microscopy. Dermatology in five Continents. In: *Proceedings of XVII World Congress of Dermatology*, pp. 907–908. Springer, Berlin.

Arnold, H.L. (1978) Treatment of Hallopeau's acrodermatitis with triamcinolone acetonide [letter]. *Archives of Dermatology* **114**, 963.

Arnold, W.P., Gerritsen, M.J. & van de Kerkhof, P.C. (1993) Response of nail psoriasis to cyclosporin [letter]. *British Journal of Dermatology* **129**, 750–751.

Asboe-Hansen, G. (1971) Psoriasis in childhood. In: *Psoriasis: Proceedings of the International Symposium* (eds E.M. Farber & A.J. Cox), Stanford University Press, Stanford, CA.

Baden, H. (1987) *Diseases of the Hair and Nails*, p. 48. Year Book Medical Publishers.

Badger, J., Banerjee, A.K. & McFadden, J. (1992) Unilateral subungual hyperkeratosis following a cerebrovascular incident in a patient with psoriasis. *Clinical and Experimental Dermatology* **17**, 454–455.

Baran, R. (1982) Action thérapeutique et complications du rétinoïde aromatique sur l'appareil unguéal. *Annales de Dermatologie et de Vénéréologie* **109**, 367.

Baran, R. (1990) Retinoids and the nails. *Journal of Dermatological Treatment* **1**, 151–154.

Baran, R. & Barthelemy, H. (1990) Photo-onycholyse induite par le 5-MOP (Psoraderm) et application de la méthode d'imputation des effets médicamenteux. *Annales de Dermatologie et de Vénéréologie* **117**, 367–369.

Bedi, T.R. (1977) Intradermal triamcinolone treatment of psoriatic onychodystrophy. *Dermatologica* **155**, 24–27.

de Berker, D. & Angus, B. (1996) Proliferative compartments in the normal nail unit. *British Journal of Dermatology* **135**, 555–559.

de Berker, D. & Lawrence, C.M. (1998) A simplified protocol of nail steroid injection for psoriatic nail dystrophy. *British Journal of Dermatology* **138**, 90–95.

de Berker, D., Sviland, L. & Angus, B.A. (1995) Suprabasal keratin expression in the nail bed: a marker of dystrophic nail differentiation. *British Journal of Dermatology* **133** (Suppl. 45), 16.

Bleeker, J.J. (1974) Intralesional triamcinolone acetonide using the Port-o-jet and needle injections in localised dermatoses. *British Journal of Dermatology* **91**, 479–484.

Bleeker, J.J. (1975) Intradermal triamcinolone acetonide treatment of psoriatic nail dystrophy with Port-o-jet. [letter]. *British Journal of Dermatology* **92**, 479.

Bolognia, J.L., Brewer, Y.P. & Cooper, D.L. (1991) Bazex syndrome (acrokeratosis paraneoplastica): an analytic review. *Medicine, Baltimore* **70**, 269–280.

Brun, P., Baran, R. & Juhlin, L. (1985) Acropustulose résistante à l'association Etrétinate–PUVA thérapie. *Annales de Dermatologie et de Vénéréologie* **112**, 611–612.

Burge, S.M. & Ryan, T.J. (1985) Acute palmoplantar pustulosis. *British Journal of Dermatology* **113**, 77–83.

Caccialanza, M. & Frigerio, U. (1982) Risultati della fotochemioterapia orale nel trattamento della psoriasi ungueale. *Giornale Italiano di Dermatologia e Venereologia* **117**, 251–254.

Calvert, H.T., Smith, M.A. & Wells, R.S. (1963) Psoriasis and the nails. *British Journal of Dermatology* 75, 415.

Caputo, R., Gelmetti, C., Grimault, R. & Gianotti, R. (1996) Psoriasiform and sclerodermoid dermatitis of the fingers with apparent shortening of the nail plate: a distinct entity? *British Journal of Dermatology* 134, 126–129.

Chamot, A.M. & Kahn, M.F. (1994) SAPHO syndrome. *Zeitschrift für Rheumatologie* 53, 234–242.

Coignet, M. & Sayag, J. (1990) Collyre β-bloquant et psoriasis. *Nouvelle Dermatologie* 9, 552–553.

Crawford, G.M. (1938) Psoriasis of the nails. *Archives of Dermatology and Syphilis* 38, 583–594.

Cribier, B., Mena, M.L., Partisani, M. *et al.* (1998) Nail changes in patients infected with human immunodeficiency virus. *Archives of Dermatology* 34, 1216–1220.

Dawber, R.P.R., Marks, R. & Swift, J.A. (1972) Scanning electron microscopy of the stratum corneum. *British Journal of Dermatology* 86, 272.

Deffer, T.A. & Goette, D.K. (1987) Distal phalangeal atrophy secondary to topical steroid therapy. *Archives of Dermatology* 123, 571–572.

Dobson, R. & Thiers, B.H. (1981) *Year Book of Dermatology*, p. 288. Year Book Medical Publishers, Chicago.

Duvic, M., Johnson, T., Rapini, R.P. *et al.* (1987) AIDS associated psoriasis and Reiter's syndrome. *Archives of Dermatology* 123, 1622–1632.

Elder, J.T., Henseler, T., Christophers, E. *et al.* (1994) Of genes and antigens: the inheritance of psoriasis. *Journal of Investigative Dermatology* 103, 150S–153S.

Ellis, C.N. & Voorhees, J.J. (1987) Etretinate therapy. *Journal of the American Academy of Dermatology* 16, 267–291.

Entestam, L. & Wedén, U. (1996) Successful treatment of acrodermatitis continua of Hallopeau with topical calcipotriol. *British Journal of Dermatology* 135, 644–646.

Farber, E.M. & Jacobs, A.H. (1977) Infantile psoriasis. *American Journal of Diseases of Children* 131, 1266.

Farber, E.M. & Nall, L. (1992) Nail psoriasis. *Cutis* 50, 174–178.

Fischer, E. (1982) Subunguale Verkalkungen. Frotsche. *Röntgenstr* 137, 580–584.

Fisher, A. & Baran, R. (1992) Occupational nail disorders with reference to Koebner's phenomenon. *American Journal of Contact Dermatitis* 3, 16–22.

Fisher, D., Elias, P. & Leboit, P. (1988) Exacerbation of psoriasis by the hypolipidemic agent, Germfibrozil. *Archives of Dermatology* 124, 854–855.

Frederiksson, T. (1974) Topically applied fluorouracil in the treatment of psoriatic nails. *Archives of Dermatology* 110, 735.

Fritz, K. (1988) Psoriasis of the nail. Successful topical treatment with 5-fluorouracil. *Zeitschrift für Hautkrankheiten* 64, 1083–1088.

Ganor, S. (1977a) Diseases sometimes associated with psoriasis. I, Candidosis. *Dermatologica* 154, 268.

Ganor, S. (1977b) Diseases sometimes associated with psoriasis. II, Alopecia areata. *Dermatologica* 154, 338.

Gayrard, L., Nicolas, J.F. & Thivolet, J. (1990) Erythrodermies induites par le captopril chez une patiente porteuse d'un psoriasis vulgaire. *Nouvelle Dermatologie* 9, 28.

Gmyrek, R., Grossman, M.E., Rudin, D. *et al.* (1999) Sapho syndrome: report of three cases and review of the literature. *Cutis* 64, 253–258.

Gottlieb, N.L. & Riskin, W.G. (1989) Complications of local corticosteroid injection. *Journal of the American Medical Association* 43, 1547–1548.

de Graciansky, P., Larrègue, M. & Katz, M. (1975) Opacités linéaires intra-unguéales dans le psoriasis. *Annales de Dermatologie et de Syphilis* 102, 121.

Grammer West, N.Y., Corvette, D.M., Giandoni, M.B. *et al.* (1998) Clinical pearl: nail plate biopsy for the diagnosis of psoriatic nails. *Journal of the American Academy of Dermatology* 38 (2 Part 1), 260–262.

Greaves, M.S., Fieller, N.R.J. & Moll, J.M.H. (1979) Differentiation between psoriatic arthritis and rheumatoid arthritis. A biochemical and statistical analysis of fingernails amino acids. *Scandinavian Journal of Rheumatology* 8, 33.

Gueissaz, F., Borradori, L. & Dubertret, L. (1992) Psoriasis unguéal. *Annales de Dermatologie et de Vénéréologie* 119, 57–63.

Gupta, A.K., Lynde, C.W., Jain, H.C. *et al.* (1997) A higher prevalence of onychomycosis in psoriatics compared with non-psoriatics: a multicentre study. *British Journal of Dermatology* 136, 786–789.

Handfield-Jones, S.E., Boyle, J. & Harman, R.R.M. (1987) Local PUVA treatment for nail psoriasis [letter]. *British Journal of Dermatology* 116, 280.

Haneke, E. (1991) *Onychomycosis and Psoriasis Restricted to the Nails. Distinguishable?* 50th Meeting AAD Dallas.

Happle, R. (1987) The lines of Blashko: a developmental pattern visualizing functional X-chromosome mosaicism. *Current Problems in Dermatology* 17, 5–18.

Happle, R. (1990) Ptychotropism as a cutaneous feature of the CHILD syndrome. *Journal of the American Academy of Dermatology* 23, 763–766.

Happle, R., Koch, H. & Lenz, W. (1980) CHILD syndrome: congenital hemidysplasia with erythroderma and limb defects. *European Journal of Pediatrics* 134, 27.

Harrison, P.V. & Stone, R.N. (1988) Severe exacerbation of psoriasis due to terfenadine. *Clinical and Experimental Dermatology* 13, 275.

Harrison, P.V., Khunti, K. & Morris, J.A. (1990) Psoriasis, nails, joints and autoimmunity [letter]. *British Journal of Dermatology* 122, 569.

Hofmann, C. & Plewig, G. (1977) Photochemotherapie der Nagelpsoriasis. *Hautarzt* 28, 408.

Jensen, H.A., Mikkelsen, H.I., Wadskov, V. & Sondegaard, J. (1976) Cutaneous reactions due to propanolol. *Acta Medica Scandinavica* 199, 363.

de Jong, E.M.G.J., Seegers B.A.M.P.A., Gulinck, M.K. *et al.* (1996) Psoriasis of the nails associated with disability in a large number of patients: results of a recent interview with 1728 patients. *Dermatology* 193, 300–303.

Kaplan, M., Sadick, S., Wieder, J. *et al.* (1989) Antipsoriatic effects of zidovudine in human immunodeficiency virus-associated psoriasis. *Journal of the American Academy of Dermatology* 20, 76.

Katz, M., Seidenbaum, M. & Weinrauch, L. (1987) Penicillin-induced generalized pustular psoriasis. *Journal of the American Academy of Dermatology* 17, 918–920.

Kaur, I., Handa, S. & Kumar, B. (1997) Natural history of psoriasis: a study from the Indian subcontinent. *Journal of Dermatology* 24, 230–234.

Kokely, F., Lavaroni, G., Piraccini, B.M. *et al.* (1994) Nail psoriasis treated with calcipotriol (MC903) an open study. *Journal of Dermatological Treatment* 5, 149–150.

Kuijpers, A.L.A., van Dooren-Greebe, R.J. & van der Kerkhof, P.C.M. (1996) Acrodermatitis continua of Hallopeau: response to combined treatment with acitretin and calcipotriol ointment. *Dermatology* 192, 357–359.

Kwang, T.Y., Nee, T.S. & Seng, K.T.H. (1994) A therapeutic study of nail psoriasis using electron beams. [letter]. *Acta Dermato-Venereologica* **75**, 90.

Laplanche, G., Grosshans, E. & Gebriel-Robez, O. (1980) Hyperplasie épidermique et hémidysplasie corporelle hypoplasique congénitale homolatérale. *Annales de Dermatologie et de Vénéréologie* **107**, 729.

Lassus, A. (1997) Colloidal silicic acid for the treatment of psoriatic skin lesions, arthropathy and onychopathy. A pilot study. *Journal of International Medical Research* **25**, 206–209.

Lazar, A.P. & Roenigk, H.H. (1988) AIDS can exacerbate psoriasis. *Journal of the American Academy of Dermatology* **18**, 144.

Lerner, M.R. & Lerner, A.B. (1972) Congenital psoriasis. *Archives of Dermatology* **105**, 598–601.

Lewin, K., Dewit, S. & Ferrington, R.A. (1972) Pathology of the fingernail in psoriasis. A clinicopathological study. *British Journal of Dermatology* **86**, 555.

Leyden, J.L., Decherd, J.W. & Goldschmidt, H. (1972) Exfoliative cytology in the diagnosis of psoriasis of nails. *Cutis* **10**, 701–704.

Lindelöf, B. (1988) Psoriasis of the nails treated with grenz rays: a double-blind bilateral trial. *Acta Dermato-Venereologica* **69**, 80–82.

Lindelöf, B. & Eklund, G. (1986) Incidence of malignant skin tumours in 14 140 patients after Grenz-ray treatment for benign skin disorders. *Archives of Dermatology* **122**, 1391–1395.

Macaulay, W.L. (1966) Transverse ridging of the thumbnails. *Archives of Dermatology* **93**, 421–423.

Machler, B.C., Kirsner, R.S. & Elgart, G.W. (1998) Routine histologic examination for the diagnosis of onychomycosis: an evaluation of sensitivity and specificity. *Cutis* **61**, 217–219.

Mackie, R.M. (1979) Onycholysis occurring during PUVA therapy. *Clinical and Experimental Dermatology* **4**, 111–113.

Maeda, K., Kawaguchi, S., Niwa, T., Ohki, T. & Kobayashi, K. (1980) Identification of some abnormal metabolites in psoriasis nail using gas chromatography–mass spectrometry. *Journal of Chromatography* **221**, 199.

Mahrle, G., Schulze, H.J., Farber, L. *et al.* (1995) Low-dose short-term cyclosporine versus etretinate in psoriasis: improvement of skin, nail, and joint involvement. *Journal of the American Academy of Dermatology* **32**, 78–88.

Marks, J.L. & Scher, R.K. (1980) Response of psoriatic nails to oral photochemotherapy. *Archives of Dermatology* **116**, 1023–1024.

Mauro, J., Lumpkin, L.R. & Dantzig, P.I. (1975) Scanning electron microscopy of psoriatic nail pits. *New York State Journal of Medicine* **75**, 339–342.

Mooser, G., Pillekamp, H. & Peter, R.U. (1998) Suppurative acrodermatitis continua of Hallopeau. A differential diagnosis of paronychia. *Deutsche Medizinische Wochenschrift* **123**, 386–390.

Müller, J., Kordass, D. & Boonen, H.P.T. (1991) UV-Therapie der Nagelpsoriasis. *Aktuelle Dermatologie* **17**, 166–169.

Munro, C.S., Cox, N.H., Marks, J.M. & Natarajan, S. (1993) Lichen nitidus presenting as palmoplantar hyperkeratosis and nail dystrophy. *Clinical and Experimental Dermatology* **18**, 381–383.

Nanda, A., Kaur, S., Kaur, I. *et al.* (1990) Childhood psoriasis: an epidemiologic survey of 112 patients. *Pediatric Dermatology* **7**, 19–21.

Navaratnam, A.E. & Gebauer, K.A. (1990) Terfenadine-induced exacerbation of psoriasis. *Clinical and Experimental Dermatology* **15**, 78.

Nicolas, J.F., Maudit, G., Larbre, J.P. *et al.* (1987) Psoriasis aggravés ou induits par les médicaments. *Médecine et Hygiène* **45**, 1809–1814.

Norton, L.A. (1982) Disease of the nails. In: *Current Therapy* (ed. W.B. Conn), p. 664. W.B. Saunders, Philadelphia.

Osawa, H. (1994) Acral psoriasiform hemispherical papulosis, a new entity? *Dermatology* **189**, 159–161.

Parker, S.G. & Diffey, B.L. (1983) The transmission of optical radiation through human nail. *British Journal of Dermatology* **108**, 11.

Patrizi, A., Bardazzi, F., Neri, I. *et al.* (1999) Psoriasiform acral dermatitis: a peculiar clinical presentation of psoriasis in children. *Pediatric Dermatology* **16**, 439–443.

Peachey, R.D.G., Pye, R.J. & Harman, R.R. (1976) The treatment of psoriatic nail dystrophy with intradermal steroid injections. *British Journal of Dermatology* **95**, 75–78.

Pfister, R. (1981) Die Psoriasis des Nagels. *Schweizerische Rundschau für Medizin Praxis* **70**, 1967–1173.

Piérard, G.E. & Piérard-Franchimont, C. (1996) Dynamics of psoriatic trachyonychia during low-dose cyclosporin A treatment: a pilot study on onychobiology using optical profilometry. *Dermatology* **192**, 116–119.

Piraccini, B.M., Fanti, P.A., Morelli, R. & Tosti, A. (1994) Hallopeau's acrodermatitis continua of the nail apparatus: a clinical and pathological study of 20 patients. *Acta Dermato-Venereologica* **74**, 65–67.

Puissant, A. (1970) Psoriasis in children under the age of ten: a study of 100 observations. *Gazzetta Sanita* **19**, 191.

Requena, L., Zamora, E., Martin, L. *et al.* (1990) Acroatrophy secondary to long-standing applications of topical steroids. *Archives of Dermatology* **126**, 1013–1014.

Robbins, T.D., Kouskoukis, C.E. & Ackerman, A.B. (1983) Onycholysis in psoriatic nails. *American Journal of Dermatopathology* **5**, 39–41.

Roberton, D.M., Cabral, D.A., Malleson, P.N. & Petty, R.E. (1996) Juvenile psoriatic arthritis: follow up and evaluation of diagnostic criteria. *Journal of Rheumatology* **23**, 166–170.

Rudolph, R.I. (1991) Lithium induced psoriasis of the fingernails. *Journal of the American Academy of Dermatology* **26**, 135–136.

Runne, U. & Orfanos, C.E. (1981) The human nail: structure, growth and pathological changes. *Current Problems in Dermatology* **9**, 102–149.

Samman, P. (1978) *The Nails in Disease*, 3rd edn. Heinemann, London.

Sasaki, T., Saito, S., Aihara, M. *et al.* (1989) Exacerbation of psoriasis during lithium treatment. *Journal of Dermatology* **16**, 59–63.

Scher, R.K. & Ackerman, A.B. (1980) Histologic differential diagnosis of onychomycosis and psoriasis of the nail unit from cornified cells of the nail bed alone. *American Journal of Dermatopathology* **2**, 255.

Schissel, D.J. & Elston, D.M. (1998) Topical 5-fluorouracil treatment for psoriatic trachyonychia. *Cutis* **62**, 27–28.

Schmied, E. & Levy, P.M. (1986) Transient rhabdomyolysis connected with topical use of 5-FU in a patient with psoriasis of the nails. *Dermatologica* **173**, 257–258.

Schroder, K., Goerdt, S., Siefer, J. *et al.* (1997) Psoriatic onychopachydermo-periostitis. *Hautarzt* **48**, 500–503.

Shear, C.S., Nyhan, W.L., Frost, P. & Weinstein, G.D. (1971) Psoriasis associated with unilateral ectromelia and central nervous system anomalies: skin, hair and nails. *Birth Defects Original Article Series* **8**, 197.

Staberg, B., Gammeltoft, M. & Onsberg, P. (1983) Onychomycosis in patients with psoriasis. *Acta Dermato-Venereologica* **63**, 436–438.

Stankler, L. (1988) Foetal psoriasis. *British Journal of Dermatology* **119**, 684.

Szepes, E. (1986) Mycotic infections of psoriatic nails. *Mykosen* **29**, 82–84.

Taras, J.S., Iams, G.J., Gibbons, M. & Culp, R.W. (1995) Flexor pollicis longus rupture in a thumb: a case report. *Journal of Hand Surgery* **20A**, 276–277.

Tegner, E. (1976) Reversible overcurvature of the nails after treatment with practolol. *Acta Dermato-Venereologica* **56**, 493.

Tosti, A., Guerra, L., Bardazzi, F. *et al.* (1990) Topical ciclosporin in nail psoriasis [letter]. *Dermatologica* **180**, 110.

Tosti, A., Fanti, P.A., Morelli, R. & Bardazzi, F. (1992) Psoriasiform acral dermatitis: report of three cases. *Acta Dermato-Venereologica* **72**, 206–207.

Tosti, A., Morelli, R., Bardazzi, F. *et al.* (1993a) Psoriasis of the nail. In: *Psoriasis* (ed. L. Dubertret), pp. 201–207. ISED, Brescia.

Tosti, A., Morelli, R., Fanti, P.A. & Cameli, N. (1993b) Nail changes of punctate keratoderma: a clinical and pathological study of two patients. *Acta Dermato-Venereologica* **73**, 66–68.

Tosti, A., Piraccini, B.M., Cameli, N. *et al.* (1998) Calcipotriol in nail psoriasis: a controlled double blind comparison with betamethasone dipropionate and salicylic acid. *British Journal of Dermatology* **139**, 655–659.

Tsuji, T. & Nishimura, M. (1991) Topically administered fluorouracil in acrodermatitis continua of Hallopeau. *Archives of Dermatology* **127**, 27–28.

Watson, W. & Farber, E.M. (1977) Controlling psoriasis. *Postgraduate Medicine* **61**, 103.

White, C.J. & Lapply, T. (1952) Histopathology of nail diseases. *Journal of Investigative Dermatology* **19**, 121–124.

Wolf, R., Tur, E. & Brenner, S. (1990) Coricosteroid-induced 'disappearing digit'. *Archives of Dermatology* **23**, 755–756.

Yamamoto, T., Katayama, I. & Nishioka, K. (1998) Topical anthralin therapy for refractory nail psoriasis. *Journal of Dermatology* **25**, 231–233.

Yokota, A., Hukazawa, M., Nakaseko, C. *et al.* (1996) Resolution of psoriasis vulgaris following allogenic bone marrow transplant. *Rinsho Ketsueki* **37**, 35–39.

Yu, R.C.H. & King, C.M. (1992) A double blind study of superficial radiotherapy in psoriatic nail dystrophy. *Acta Dermato-Venereologica* **72**, 134–136.

Zaias, N. (1969) Psoriasis of the nail. A clinical–pathology study. *Archives of Dermatology* **99**, 567.

Zaias, N. (1984) Psoriasis of the nail unit. *Dermatologic Clinics* **2**, 493–505.

Zaias, N. (1990) *The Nail in Health and Disease*, 2nd edn. Appleton & Lange. Norwalk, CT.

Zaias, N. & Norton, L.A. (1980) In: *Clinical Dermatology*, Vol. 1 (eds D.J. Demis, R.L. Dobson & J. McGuire), pp. 3–4.

Zonneweld, I.M., Rubins, A., Jablonska, S. *et al.* (1998) Topical tacrolimus is not effective in chronic plaque psoriasis. A pilot study. *Archives of Dermatology* **134**, 1101–1102.

## Acropustulosis

Ackerman, A.B. (1981) Is subcorneal pustular dermatosis of Sneddon and Wilkinson an entity sui generis? *American Journal of Dermatopathology* **3**, 363.

Andrews, G. & Machacek, G. (1935) Pustular bacterids of the hands and feet. *Archives of Dermatology and Syphilis* **32**, 837–835.

Baran, R. (1979) Hallopeau's acrodermatitis. *Archives of Dermatology* **115**, 815.

Baran, R. (1982) Action thérapeutique et complications du rétinoïde aromatique sur l'appareil unguéal. *Annales de Dermatologie et de Vénéréologie* **109**, 367–371.

Burden, A.D. & Kemmett, D. (1996) The spectrum of nail involvement in palmoplantar pustulosis. *British Journal of Dermatology* **134**, 1079–1082.

Cheesbrough, M.J. (1979) Osteolysis and psoriasis. *Clinical and Experimental Dermatology* **4**, 341–344.

Chimenti, S. & Ackerman, A.B. (1981) Is subcorneal pustular dermatitis of Sneddon and Wilkinson an entity sui generis? *American Journal of Dermatopathology* **3**, 363–376.

Combemale, P., Baran, R., Flechaire, A. *et al.* (1989) Acroosteolyse psoriasique. *Annales de Dermatologie et de Vénéréologie* **116**, 555–558.

Deichmann, B. & Spindeldreier, A. (1982) Aromatisches Retinoid zur Behandlung der Psoriasis pustulosa an Händen und Füssen. *Zeitschrift für Hautkrankheiten* **57**, 425.

Enfors, W. & Molin, L. (1971) Pustulosis palmaris et plantaris. A follow up study of ten year material. *Acta Dermato-Venereologica* **51**, 289–294.

Mahowald, M.L. & Parrish, R.M. (1982) Severe osteolytic arthritis mutilans pustular psoriasis. *Archives of Dermatology* **118**, 434.

Miller, J.L., Soltani, K. & Tourtellotte, C.D. (1971) Psoriatic acroosteolysis without arthritis. *Journal of Bone and Joint Surgery* **53A**, 371–374.

Miyagawa, S., Kitaoka, M., Komatsu, M. *et al.* (1990) Acral granulomatous dermatosis. *British Journal of Dermatology* **122**, 709–713.

Notowicz, A., Stolz, E. & Heuvel, N. (1978) Treatment of Hallopeau's acrodermatitis with topical mechlorethamine. *Archives of Dermatology* **114**, 129.

Tsuji, T. & Nishimura, M. (1991) Topically administrated fluorouracil in acrodermatitis continua of Hallopeau. *Archives of Dermatology* **127**, 27–28.

Ward, J.M. & Barnes, R.M.R. (1978) HLA antigens in persistent palmoplantar pustulosis and its relationship to psoriasis. *British Journal of Dermatology* **99**, 477–483.

## Psoriatic arthritis

Abel, E. & Farber, E.M. (1979) Psoriasis. In: *Clinical Dermatology*, Vol. 1 (eds D.J. Demis, R.L. Dobson & J. McGuire), pp. 1–2.

Baker, H., Golding, D.N. & Thompson, M. (1964) The nail in psoriatic arthritis. *British Journal of Dermatology* **76**, 569.

Buckley, W.R. & Raleigh, R.L. (1959) Psoriasis with acro-osteolysis. *New England Journal of Medicine* **261**, 539–541.

Cheesbrough, M.J. (1979) Osteolysis and psoriasis. *Clinical and Experimental Dermatology* **4**, 341–344.

Eastmond, C.J. & Wright, V. (1979) The nail dystrophy of psoriatic arthritis. *Annals of the Rheumatic Diseases* **38**, 226.

Goupille, P., Védère, V., Roulot, B. *et al.* (1996) Incidence of osteoperiostitis of the great toe in psoriatic arthritis. *Journal of Rheumatology* **23**, 1553–1556.

Jones, S.M., Armas, J.B., Cohen, M.G. *et al.* (1994) Psoriatic arthritis: outcome of disease subsets and the relationship of joint disease to nail and skin disease. *British Journal of Rheumatology* **33**, 834–839.

Lavaroni, G., Kokelj, F., Pauluzzi, P. & Trevisan, G. (1994) The nails in psoriatic arthritis. *Acta Dermato-Venereologica* **186** (Suppl.), 113.

Roberton, D.M., Cabral, D.A., Malleson, P.N. & Petty, R.E. (1996) Juvenile psoriatic arthritis: follow up and evaluation of diagnostic criteria. *Journal of Rheumatology* **23**, 166–170.

Sills, E.M. (1980) Psoriatic arthritis in childhood. *Johns Hopkins Medical Journal* **146**, 49–53.

Southwood, T.R., Petty, R.E., Malleson, P.N. *et al.* (1989) Psoriatic arthritis in children. *Arthritis and Rheumatism* **32**, 1007–1013.

Wright, V., Roberts, M.C. & Hill, A.G.S. (1979) Dermatological manifestations in psoriatic arthritis. A follow up study. *Acta Dermato-Venereologica* **59**, 235.

Zaias, N. & Norton, L.A. (1980) Diseases of nails. In: *Clinical Dermatology*, Vol. 1 (eds D.J. Demis, R.L. Dobson & J. McGuire), pp. 3–4.

## Psoriatic onychopachydermo-periostitis

Bauza, A., Redondo, P. & Aquerreta, D. (2000) Psoriatic onycho-pachydermo-periostitis: treatment with methotrexate. *British Journal of Dermatology* **143**, 901–902.

Boisseau-Garsaud, A.M., Beylot-Barry, M., Doutre, M.S. *et al.* (1996) Psoriatic onycho-pachydermo-periostitis. *Archives of Dermatology* **132**, 176–180.

Fournié, B., Viraben, R., Durroux, R. *et al.* (1989) L'onycho-pachydermo-périostite psoriasique du gros orteil. *Review of Rheumatism* **56**, 579–582.

Marghéry, M.C., Baran, R., Pages, M. & Bazex, J. (1991) Acropachydermie psoriasique. *Annales de Dermatologie et de Vénéréologie* **118**, 373–376.

Ziemer, A., Heider, M. & Göring, H.D. (1998) Psoriasiforme Onycho-pachydermoperiostitis der Grosszehen: Das OP3GO-Syndrom. *Hautarzt* **49**, 859–862.

## Reiter's syndrome

Lovy, M., Bluhm, G. & Morales, A. (1980) The occurrence of pitting in Reiter's syndrome. *Journal of the American Academy of Dermatology* **2**, 66.

Luderschmidt, C. & Balda, B.R. (1982) Reiter's syndrome. Case presentations. In: *XVI Congressus Internationalis Dermatologiae, Tokyo*, p. 122.

Pajarre, R. & Kero, M. (1977) Nail changes as the first manifestation of the HLA-B27 inheritance. *Dermatologica* **154**, 350.

# Pityriasis rubra pilaris

When the palms and soles are affected, as in adult acute onset type I pityriasis rubra pilaris (PRP) (Griffiths 1976), nail involvement is common (Fig. 5.29). The fingernails show well-marked changes, including terminal subungual hyperkeratosis with moderate thickening of the nail bed, splinter haemorrhages and longitudinal ridging. There is patchy parakeratosis in the nail plate suggesting a disturbance in the matrix, and the condition is sometimes attended by a distal yellow-brown discoloration in the nails. The pattern of inheritance when it does occur is usually an autosomal dominant.

Nail changes in chronic erythroderma due to Sèzary syndrome are similar to those found in patients with type I PRP,

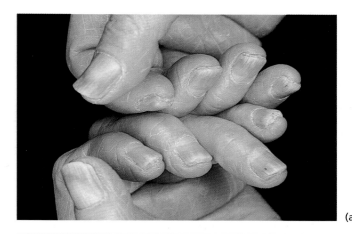

(a)

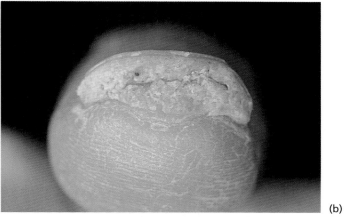

(b)

**Fig. 5.29** (a) Type I pityriasis rubra pilaris—prominent distal subungual thickening. (b) Type I pityriasis rubra pilaris—mainly distal subungual changes. (Courtesy of A. Griffiths, UK.)

suggesting a non-specific reaction to erythema (Sonnex *et al.* 1986), in addition many cases of Sézary syndrome show trachyonychia not seen in PRP. Psoriasiform pits in the nail plate are exceptionally noted, as well as onycholysis. 'Salmon patches' are not seen (Sonnex *et al.* 1986). The rate of linear nail growth is faster than normal (although not so fast as in psoriasis).

In the juvenile types of PRP, nail changes are very much less common. Lambert and Dalac (1989) have observed an unusual case with onychogryphosis of the 20 nails in a young girl afflicted by atypical juvenile type V PRP (Fig. 5.30). In localized, circumscribed juvenile type IV PRP, psoriasiform pitting may occur in the absence of any periungual abnormality (W.A.D. Griffiths, personnal communication). Parakeratotic areas are present over the nail bed epithelium, which may be thickened and show focal basal liquefaction. Keratohyalin may be seen. An inflammatory infiltrate consisting of mononuclear cells may be present in the dermis of the nail fold. The hyponychium shows both orthokeratosis and parakeratosis (Sonnex *et al.* 1986).

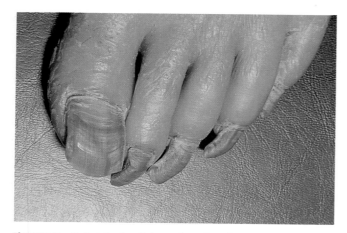

**Fig. 5.30** Type V pityriasis rubra pilaris—onychogryphotic changes. (Courtesy of D. Lambert, France.)

Nail changes have been reported in a PRP-like disease presenting in a subject with AIDS (Korman *et al.* 1997).

Good responses have been obtained with etretinate (Lauharanta & Lassus (1980) and with combined oral retinoid–PUVA therapy.

## References

Griffiths, W.A.D. (1976) Pityriasis rubra pilaris: an historical approach. 2—Clinical features. *Clinical and Experimental Dermatology* **1**, 37.

Korman, N., Nagashima Whalen, L., Briggs, J. *et al.* (1997) Pityriasis rubra pilaris: an unusual cutaneous complication of AIDS. *American Journal of Medical Science* **314**, 118–121.

Lambert, D.G. & Dalac, S. (1989) Nail changes in type V PRP. *Journal of the American Academy of Dermatology* **21**, 811–812.

Lauharanta, J. & Lassus, A. (1980) Treatment of pityriasis rubra pilaris with an oral aromatic retinoid. *Acta Dermatologica* **60**, 460–462.

Sonnex, T.S., Dawber, R.P.R., Zachary, C.B. *et al.* (1986) The nails in adult type I pityriasis rubra pilaris. A comparison with Sezary syndrome and psoriasis. *Journal of the American Academy of Dermatology* **15**, 956–960.

## Eczema

The nail apparatus is particularly vulnerable to eczematous involvement (Fig. 5.31) irrespective of the nature of the allergen or the route by which it reaches the nail apparatus. Many of the specific changes seen in non-constitutional eczema are described in Chapter 6.

The mechanism of the nail changes is obvious when the eczema is periungual. However, the cause must be sought elsewhere if, as is frequently the case, the nail disorder is unassociated with periungual eczema. General examination may reveal a specific type of eczema, for example atopic dermatitis, discoid eczema, pompholyx, etc. Modifications of the nail plate result from disturbances of the matrix. These may present as thickening with discoloration, roughness, pitting and tranverse ridging and furrowing. Nails may sometimes be shed.

Eczema of the nail bed is no longer associated with cosmetic products such as base coats, nail hardeners or hair setting lotions. False nails remain the exception (Chapter 8). The nail changes resulting from allergic contact sensitivity at this site appear hours, days or even weeks later as splinter haemorrhages, soon followed by the development of subungual hyperkeratosis; sometimes onycholysis and paronychia may also be seen, resulting from formaldehyde application. Colour changes vary from a bluish-red appearance initially, to 'rust' and finally yellow. The affected areas may be intensely painful.

Common chemical sensitizers may induce a wide range of clinical patterns in the nail area (Chapter 7). Minimal damage may simply produce onycholysis. Subungual hyperkeratosis is frequent and may be accompanied by erythema, scaling and fissuring.

It has been suggested that parakeratosis pustulosa is a variant of atopic eczema, which may also be the basis of juvenile plantar dermatitis, where the periungual tissue resembles dry eczema, but pitting is not seen, except when it is associated with atopic eczema. Allergic contact dermatitis may also be a precipitant in some instances (Tosti *et al.* 1998).

Constant rubbing and scratching of the skin, as in atopic dermatitis, causes the nails to be buffed; the surface of the nails becomes 'polished' and shiny. The subungual space is also of importance as it may harbour infection spread by scratching. The prevalence of *Staphylococcus* beneath the nails of atopics has been described as 10 times greater than that of normal controls (Nishijima *et al.* 1997). This illustrates the importance of nail care and careful cleaning when there is eczema.

When eczema involves the proximal nail fold it will often also affect the tip of the matrix. This results in surface irregularities such as ridges, furrows and pits. The nail bed, and particularly the hyponychium, may be involved with consequent subungual hyperkeratosis and loss of nail adhesion to the nail bed. Histopathology reveals spongiosis, spongiotic vesicles, variable parakeratosis and granular layer with intermittent orthokeratotic foci. The dermis shows a predominantly superficial perivascular lymphocytic infiltrate. Giemsa stain usually exhibits severe alterations in the stainability of the nail plate. The latter may become disorderly and wavy. The pits usually do not contain parakeratotic onychocytes. PAS stain may show pronounced staining of the intercellular spaces, probably due to trapping of serum glycoproteins in between the cells of the nail plate.

Treatment of the nail folds with topical corticosteroids is often helpful on top of the preventative and hand care measures that are employed in psoriatic nail disease (q.v.). An additional antimicrobial ingredient may be required. If potent steroid is used long term there may be a risk of premature closure of the underlying epiphyses in children and acroatrophy (Requena *et al.* 1990). It could be argued that steroid use would increase

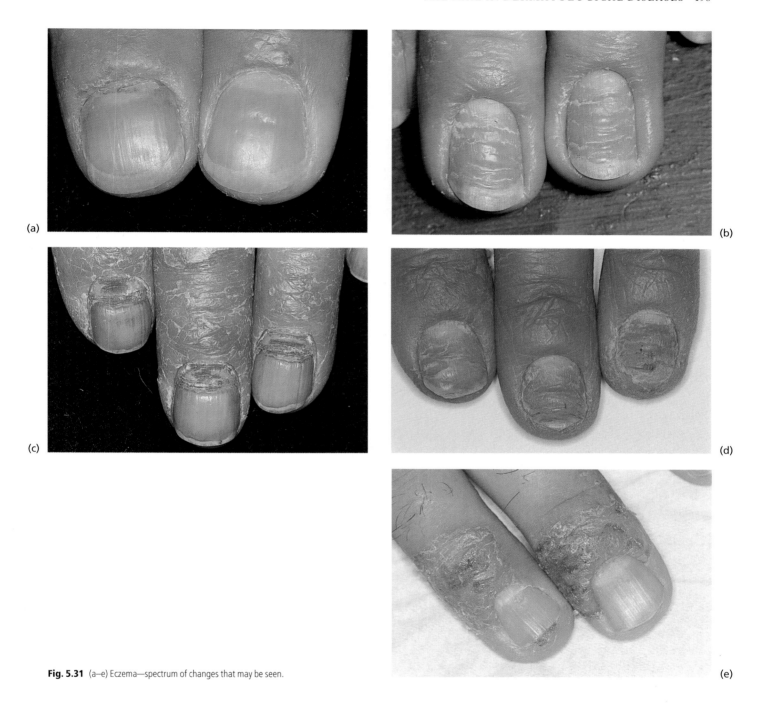

**Fig. 5.31** (a–e) Eczema—spectrum of changes that may be seen.

the risk of secondary infection such as osteomyelitis of the distal phalanges as reported in three children (Boiko *et al.* 1988); however, untreated eczema is likely to represent a risk of at least similar proportions.

## References

Boiko, S., Kaufman, R.A. & Lucky, A.W. (1988) Osteomyelitis of the distal phalanges in three children with severe atopic dermatitis. *Archives of Dermatology* **124**, 418–423.

Nishijima, S., Namura, S., Higashida, T. & Kawai, S. (1997) *Staphylococcus aureus* in the anterior nares and subungual spaces of the hands in atopic dermatitis. *Journal of International Medical Research* **25**, 155–158.

Requena, L., Zamora, E. & Martin, L. (1990) Acroatrophy secondary to long-standing applications of topical steroids. *Archives of Dermatology* **126**, 1013–1014.

Tosti, A., Peluso, A.M. & Zucchelli, V. (1998) Clinical features and long term follow up of 20 cases of parakeratosis pustulosa. *Pediatric Dermatology* **15**, 259–263.

## Pityriasis rosea

Sufficient damage may be done to the nail matrix in pityriasis rosea to produce multiple irregular indentations of the nails. These form rectangular areas of dystrophy observed in the middle third of each nail (Silver & Glickman 1964). We have seen pitting following the same condition, the pits being distributed in transverse lines.

### Reference

Silver, S.H. & Glickman, F.S. (1964) Pityriasis rosea followed by nail dystrophy. *Archives of Dermatology* 90, 31.

## Parakeratosis pustulosa (Hjorth–Sabouraud)

(Fig. 5.32)

This parakeratotic condition of the fingertips has been well described by Sabouraud (1931), and Hjorth and Thomsen (1967) who studied 91 cases, 16 of them within their own clinic. It usually occurs in girls of approximately 7 years of age. The lesions start close to the free margin of the nail. In some cases, a few isolated pustules or vesicles may be observed in the initial phase; these usually disappear before the patient presents to the doctor. Confluent eczematoid changes which cover the skin immediately adjacent to the distal edge of the nail are pink or of normal skin colour and densely studded with fine scales; there is a clear margin between the normal and affected area. The skin changes may extend to the dorsal aspect of the finger or toe, but usually only the fingertip is affected. The most striking and characteristic change is the hyperkeratosis beneath the nail tip. The nail plate, which is deformed and often thickened, is lifted up. Commonly the deformity produced is asymmetrical and limited to one corner of the distal edge, or at least more pronounced at the corners of the nail. Pitting occurs; rarely transverse ridging of the nail plate is present.

Most cases resolve within a few months but some cases persist for many years, even into adult life. Long-term follow up in a group of 20 children revealed an aetiology in 11 (55%) (Tosti *et al.* 1998). Psoriasis was implicated in 40%, atopic dermatitis in 5–10% and an allergic contact sensitivity in seven of 20 (35%), but was problably relevant in only two of 20 (10%). Recovery was seen in 12 of 20 (60%) over a period of 3 months to 3 years. The mean follow up period was 4 years.

Histological findings (de Dulanto *et al.* 1974) are of some value and include hyperkeratosis and parakeratosis, pustulation and crusts, acanthosis and mild exocytosis, papillomatosis and heavy cellular infiltrates composed mainly of lymphocytes and fibroblasts around dilated capillary loops. According to Botella *et al.* (1973), the histology presents many of the features common to psoriasis and eczema. Avci and Günes (1994) reported the presence of dyskeratotic cells in the spinous layer.

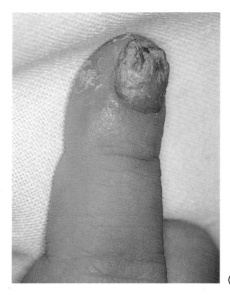

(a)

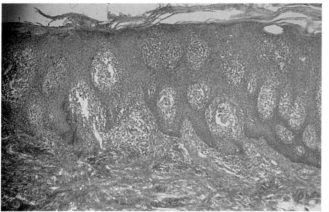

(b)

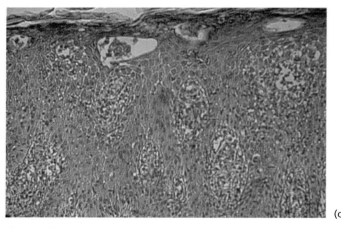

(c)

**Fig. 5.32** (a) Parakeratosis pustulosa—Hjorth–Sabouraud. (b) Parakeratosis pustulosa—histology (courtesy of J. Mascaro, Spain). (c) Parakeratosis pustulosa—histology. (Courtesy of J. Mascaro, Spain.)

In the differential diagnosis of parakeratosis pustulosa, the following points are important:

**1** Pustules are very rare and only seen in the initial stage, as distinct from pustular psoriasis or Hallopeau's disease.

**2** Patients with psoriasis develop a coarse sheet of scales and not the fine type of scaling typically seen in parakeratosis pustulosa.

**3** The age distribution differs from that found in atopic dermatitis, which may cause transverse ridging due to the involvement of the proximal nail fold.

**4** If the nail changes predominate, especially on the feet, the disorder can be mistaken for tinea. Thumb sucking, which is a predisposing factor in chronic candidal paronychia, should be ruled out when a single thumb is affected.

No single treatment makes any difference to the frequency of recurrence or the overall duration of parakeratosis pustulosa (Hjorth & Thomsen 1967). Topical steroids provide some symptomatic relief.

## References

Avci, O. & Günes, A.T. (1994) Parakeratosis pustulosa with dyskeratotic cells [letter]. *Dermatology* **189**, 413–414.

Botella, R., Martinez, C., Albero, P. & Mascaro, J.M. (1973) Parakeratosis pustulosa de Hjorth. Discussion nosologica a proposito de tres casos. *Acta Dermato-Sifilitica* **1–2**, 101.

de Dulanto, F., Armijo-Moreno, M. & Camacho-Martinez, F. (1974) Parakeratosis pustulosa: histological findings. *Acta Dermato-Venereologica* **54**, 365–367.

Hjorth, N. & Thomsen, K. (1967) Parakeratosis pustulosa. *British Journal of Dermatology* **79**, 527–532.

Sabouraud, R. (1931) Les parakeratoses microbiennes du bout des doigts. *Annales de Dermatologie et de Syphilis* **11**, 206–210.

Tosti, A., Peluso, A.M. & Zucchelli, V. (1998) Clinical features and long term follow up of 20 cases of parakeratosis pustulosa. *Pediatric Dermatology* **15**, 259–263.

## Lichen planus

The aetiology of lichen planus is unknown. There is some evidence for a genetic susceptibility with the increased frequency of HLA-A3 (Lowe *et al.* 1976) and HLA-B7 (Copeman *et al.* 1978) or HLA-A3 and HLA-A5 in familial lichen planus. Associations with HLA-DR1 (Valsecchi *et al.* 1988) and HLA-DR10 have also been demonstrated (White & Rostom 1994).

Primary immunological disturbances are another most likely hypothesis. Associations with alopecia areata and vitiligo (Aloi *et al.* 1987; Kanwar *et al.* 1993), Castleman tumour coexisting with pemphigus vulgaris (Plewig *et al.* 1990) and localized scleroderma (Brenner *et al.* 1979) or chronic liver diseases suggest that lichen planus results from an immune imbalance, often associated with systemic involvement (Cottoni *et al.* 1988).

The mechanism for the manifestation of this immune process appears to involve Langerhans' cells and T lymphocytes. It is proposed that abnormal antigen presentation by Langerhans' cells early in the disease process may result in subsequent pathological recruitment of T lymphocytes (Shiohara *et al.* 1988) and attack upon epidermal attachment (Haapalainen *et al.* 1995).

Nail involvement of one or all of the nail components occurs in 10% of patients with lichen planus (Samman 1961) and, overall, permanent nail dystrophy may be seen in one or more nails in 4% of sufferers. It is uncommon for nail involvement to be the first or single manifestation of the disease (Marks & Samman 1972; Scott & Scott 1979; Tosti *et al.* 1987). The condition is most common in the 5th or 6th decade (Tosti *et al.* 1993), although childhood onset is well recognized in isolation (Burgoon & Kostrzewa 1969; Bhargava 1975; Kanwar *et al.* 1983; Peluso *et al.* 1993), or just with scalp (de Berker & Dawber 1991) or oral mucous membrane involvement (Takeuchi *et al.* 2000). Kanwar *et al.* (1991) reported that only one child out of 17 had changes suggestive of lichen planus of the nails. Nail changes may possibly be more marked in noncaucasians (Milligan & Graham-Brown 1990; de Berker & Dawber 1991).

## Clinical features

The clinical features depend upon the site affected by the pathological process.

### Nail fold disease (Figs 5.33 & 5.34)

The dorsum of the proximal nail fold may be blue/red, with or without swelling. This indicates that the proximal nail matrix is involved and nail plate changes are likely to occur afterwards (Samman 1961).

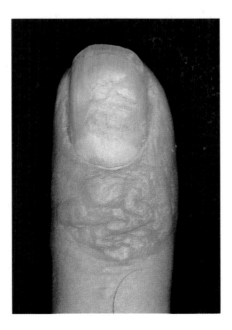

**Fig. 5.33** Lichen planus involving the dorsum of the distal phalanx and the nail plate.

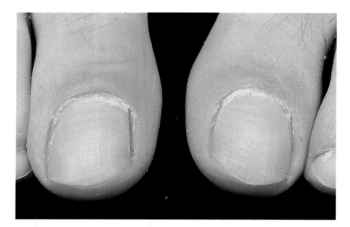

**Fig. 5.34** Lichen planus—bluish colour in the dorsal nail fold.

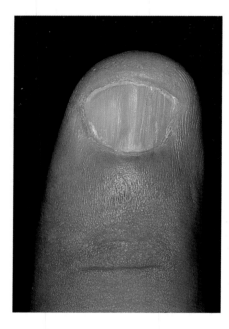

**Fig. 5.35** Lichen planus—longitudinal bulge.

## Matrix disease

A small focus of lichen planus in the matrix may present as a bulge under the proximal nail fold (Fig. 5.35). The nail gradually reflects the disease process with a longitudinal red line indicating a thinned nail plate, evolving into a distal split, where it is most fragile. The lunula may also be red, either in a focal or generalized pattern. The next stage is a complete split. At this point the matrix disease is relatively advanced and there may be pterygium formation between the underlying matrix disease and the overlying proximal nail fold. The term pterygium derives from the latin for wing and aims to evoke the clinical picture of two wings of nail divided by a spine of scar tissue. Even if the disease subsequently subsides, the scar formed during the active phase will prevent normal nail regrowth.

A broader focus of matrix involvement may result in loss of a proportionate fraction of the nail, sometimes with complete loss. The most dramatic form of matrix disease is seen in ulcerative lichen planus where complete and sometimes irreversible nail loss combines with large areas of bulla formation and erosion, usually on the soles and sometimes on the palms (Perez *et al.* 1982; Fabiero *et al.* 1989; Isogai *et al.* 1997). Lesions may be haemorrhagic and prone to residual scarring (Cram *et al.* 1966). Mucosal surfaces may be involved and there may be cicatricial alopecia. Often the eroded lesions appear on a surface that is already atrophic and the skin discoloured (Degos & Schnitzler 1967). Bullous erosive changes can occur on the feet, accompanied by more classic pterygium formation on the fingers.

Healthy skin is rarely affected. This very incapacitating condition is aggravated by the spontaneous shedding of the nail, with atrophy of the matrix, leading to permanent anonychia (Oberste-Lehn & Kühl 1954). Weidner and Ummenhofer (1979) have drawn clinical parallels between epidermolysis bullosa hereditaria dystrophica and dystrophic erosive lichen planus, stressing the different mode of blister formation.

Focal disease that does not proceed to significant scarring may leave pigmentary changes similar to lesions seen on the skin. This may appear as a longitudinal melanonychia and is transitory (Juhlin & Baran 1990). It has been reported in isolation (Fig. 5.36) (Baran *et al.* 1985, 1988) and after treatment of lichen planus by intramuscular injections of triamcinolone acetonide Kenalog (Juhlin & Baran 1989). In Afro-Carribeans, postinflammatory subungual hyperpigmentation may appear (Zaias 1970).

Longitudinal ridging (Fig. 5.37) can be a manifestation of nail lichen planus, where diffuse matrix involvement results in selective atrophy of the nail plate (Fig. 5.38). It appears that some longitudinal units of nail matrix are less susceptible to the disease. This results in a differentially thinned nail, where the most obvious feature is the resistant longitudinal ridge (Fig. 5.35) which represents less damaged nail of normal thickness. Nails thinned in this fashion are susceptible to splitting in the transverse as well as the longitudinal axis and so lamellar dystrophy and onychorrhexis may be seen (Fig. 5.36).

Pitting is a further manifestation of lichen planus of the proximal nail matrix. It may be limited in time and location and so appear as a true pit. Alternatively, the pits may be so numerous and recurrent in time that the surface of the nail takes on a more stippled appearance. This stippling is achieved through multiple small foci of matrix disturbance and abnormal nail production. Consequently, the nail may be thin and fragile. Its surface quality is changed, so that it appears dull and almost dusty (Fig. 5.39). The free edge may be ragged and split, producing onychorrhexis.

In some instances 'idiopathic atrophy of the nails' may represent the extreme form of pitting arising secondary to lichen planus (Samman 1969). The original description was at a time when nail biopsy was not performed in such cases, but histological reports in African and Asian children suggest that

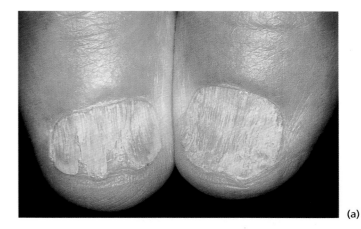

(a)

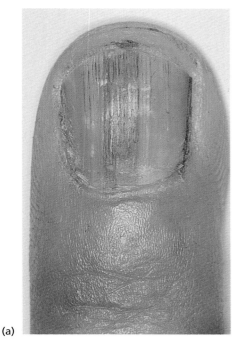

(a)

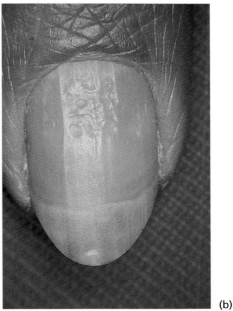

**Fig. 5.37** (a) Lichen planus—ridging, fissuring and superficial nail fragility. (b) Lichen planus—pitting.

(b)

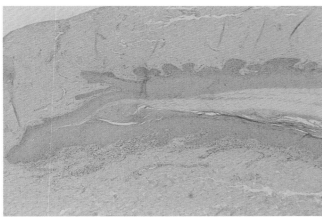

(b)

**Fig. 5.36** (a) Lichen planus—longitudinal melanonychia. (b) Histology of the matrix area in the same patient.

'idiopathic atrophy' represents a scarring atrophic variant of lichen planus of the nails (Marks & Samman 1972; Colver & Dawber 1987) in most of the cases. 'Idiopathic atrophy' with normal cuticle may represent a benign non-scarring process where lichen planus is not clearly implicated (Scher *et al.* 1978; Silverman & Rhodes 1984) and the disease may be part of a different autoimmune process (Barth *et al.* 1988). A significant proportion of those with idiopathic atrophy have a direct or indirect assocation with alopecia areata, and in that situation, the histology is usually spongiotic and non-scarring (Tosti *et al.* 1991) although scarring lichenoid features have been reported alongside alopecia areata (Kanwar *et al.* 1993). Similar congenital findings (Achten & Wanet-Rouard 1974), even in siblings, have been reported (Suarez & Scher 1990). Isolated lichen planus of the nails has been reported in association with primary biliary cirrhosis (Sowden *et al.* 1989).

### Nail bed disease

Lichen planus seldom exclusively involves the nail bed and features of nail bed disease are usually seen in combination with nail surface changes reflecting matrix pathology. Nail bed features include subungual hyperkeratosis (Fig. 5.40) and onycholysis (Fig. 5.41) (Kint & Vermander 1982), which may present alone or in combination. The 'pup tent' sign, in which the nail plate splits and elevates longitudinally and the lateral edges angle downward, is apparent when viewing the nail on end (Boyd *et al.* 1991).

### Variants of lichen planus

• Acquired leuconychia affecting all 20 nails has been found in

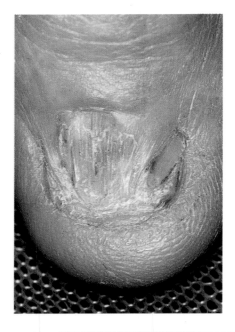

**Fig. 5.38** Lichen planus—permanent atrophy and scarring.

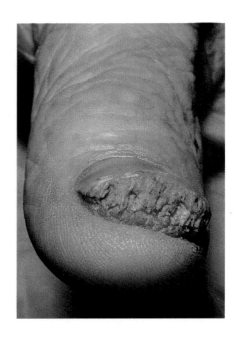

**Fig. 5.40** Lichen planus—subungual hyperkeratosis.

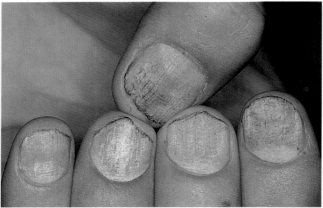

**Fig. 5.39** Lichen planus—twenty-nail dystrophy type.

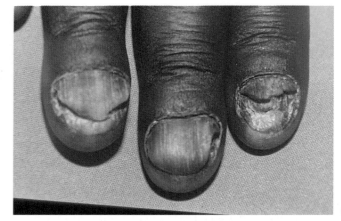

(a)

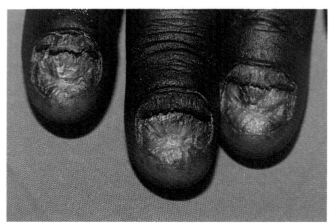

(b)

**Fig. 5.41** (a,b) Lichen planus—severe progressive form with onycholysis. (Courtesy of J.L. Bonafé, France.)

lichen planopilaris with ventral involvement of the proximal nail fold by a papule of lichen planus (Tosti *et al.* 1988).

• Lichen planus-like eruptions following bone marrow transplantation are a manifestation of graft-versus-host disease (Fig. 5.42) (Saurat & Gluckman 1977). The nail changes are identical, in some cases, to those seen in typical lichen planus with fluting and onychatrophy (Liddle & Cowan 1990), or there may be superficial ulceration in the lunula area similar to that found in ulcerative lichen planus (Fig. 5.43).

Paraneoplastic pemphigus with clinical features of erosive lichen planus may be associated with Castelman's tumour (Jansen *et al.* 1995).

• Where lichen planopilaris of the scalp is the presenting complaint, there may be associated lichenoid nail changes. In one series of 45 patients with lichen planopilaris, 25% had nail involvement at presentation and one developed nail disease subsequently (Mehregan *et al.* 1992).

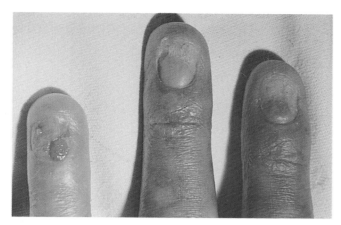

**Fig. 5.42** Lichen planus-like ulcerative changes following bone marrow transplantation (graft-versus-host disease). (Courtesy of J.H. Saurat, Switzerland.)

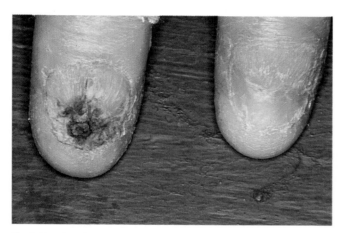

**Fig. 5.43** Lichen planus—lupus erythematosus 'overlap' syndrome.

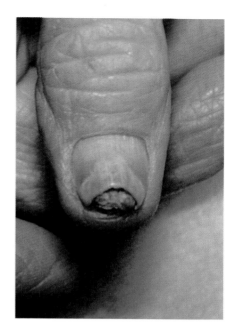

**Fig. 5.44** Lichen planus—single digit involved; subungual keratotic variety. (Courtesy of V. Lambert, USA.)

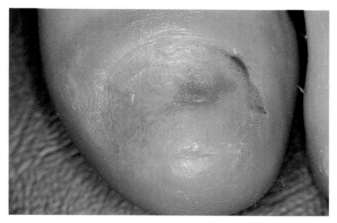

**Fig. 5.45** Lichen planus—ulcerative, scarring variety.

• Disseminated lichenoid papular dermatosis was observed in AIDS with a periungual distribution; progressively the nails become thinned with splinter haemorrhages and an irregular border of the distal margin of the lunula (Büchner *et al.* 1989).
• There are numerous drugs associated with a lichen planus-like reaction (Boyd & Nelder 1991).
• A keratotic tumour of the nail bed in a single finger is an unusual presentation (Lambert *et al.* 1988) (Fig. 5.44).
• Haneke (1983) reported a case of subungual bullous lichen planus mimicking the yellow nail syndrome of all nails.
• Permanent anonychia may be the only manifestation of ulcerative lichen planus (Cornelius & Shelley 1967) (Fig. 5.45) as well as localized lichen sclerosus (Kossard & Cornish 1998).

When lichen planus is limited to the nails, accurate clinical diagnosis may be difficult. Because of its normally destructive nature, an early nail biopsy is necessary in order to establish the diagnosis and determine whether adequate treatment is possible. The differential diagnosis of lichen planus changes in the nail include dystrophy and onychatrophy following Stevens–

Johnson syndrome, sequellae of severe bacterial infection, genetic causes, impaired peripheral circulation, radiodermatitis, mechanical trauma to the matrix area and yellow nail syndrome (Scott & Scott 1979; Norton 1982; Haneke 1983).

## Histopathology (Table 5.5)

In addition to the classical pathological features of lichen planus of the skin and mucosae such as a dense band-like lymphocytic infiltrate with epidermotropism, hydropic degeneration of basal cells, development of a stratum granulosum often consisting of several layers of cells with abundant keratohyalin granules, and a saw-tooth appearance of the epithelial rete ridges, there is often a marked spongiosis in the epithelium of the matrix and nail bed. It may be so marked as to simulate

| | Ventral aspect of the proximal nail fold | Matrix | Nail bed |
|---|---|---|---|
| Normal reference | As for normal skin | No granular layer | No granular layer |
| Granular layer | Increased | Present | Present |
| Acanthosis | Present | – | Present |
| Saw toothing | Present | Rare | Absent |
| Lichenoid infiltrate | Present | Present | Present |
| Colloid bodies | Present | Rare | Rare |
| Vacuolar degeneration | Present | Rare | Rare |

**Table 5.5** Common histological findings in nail lichen planus. (After Tosti *et al.* 1993.)

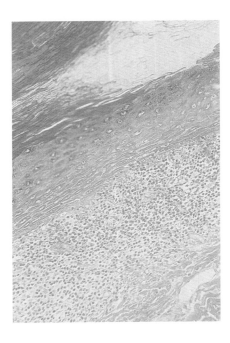

**Fig. 5.46** Lichen planus—matrix area, showing prominent, dense dermal and dermo-epidermal inflammation and epidermal (matrix) spongiosis.

allergic contact dermatitis. Due to the granular layer, normal keratin will be produced that does not adhere to the nail plate keratin, thus giving rise to subungual (hyper-) keratosis and/or onycholysis. Foci with hypergranulosis in the matrix can thus not produce nail keratin and nail plate irregularities such as ridges or even nail plate atrophy will appear. Nail biopsies have shown that in the lichen planus of the nails most commonly seen, that is with longitudinal ridges, depressions and superficial fragility (Fig. 5.46), there is usually an involvement of the eponychium, proximal tip and proximal part of the matrix—these structures are responsible for the nail plate's surface. Unusually severe liquefactive degeneration of the basal layer of the nail bed has been shown to cause isolated bullous lichen planus of the nails (Haneke 1983). Longitudinal melanonychia is a rare feature in ungual lichen planus (Baran *et al.* 1985). It is probably due to activation of melanocytes by the inflammatory process and also the melanocyte destruction in the course of lichen planus.

The observations from one series of 24 patients with nail lichen planus allows generalizations concerning histological features at the different sites in the nail unit (Tosti *et al.* 1993).

### Prognosis and treatment

The prognosis depends on the degree of matrix involvement and scarring with pterygium formation (Fig. 5.38). Complete involvement of the matrix and nail bed will produce a total loss of the nail plate and permanent atrophy with scarring if the inflammatory process is sufficiently destructive. Ulcerative lichen planus and graft-versus-host disease may result in more long-term damage than other forms of lichen planus involving the nails. Less destruction is associated with the milder clinical variants, with ridging and roughness of the nail surface. The 20-nail variant or trachyonychia seen in children can resolve spontaneously.

Even in the more aggressive forms of nail lichen planus, the treatment may play a big part in determining the long-term outcome. If the destructive process can be halted early, irreversible damage may be avoided (Tosti *et al.* 1993).

Treatment of lichen planus depends on the severity and the extension of the disease. Since there is no known specific cause, therapy is always symptomatic, for example anti-inflammatory. Since the common types of lichen planus generally resolve spontaneously within a few months of onset, very little treatment may be needed. Severe non-scarring types may be helped by potent topical treatment, with optional occlusion with plastic dressings. Intralesional triamcinolone can be used when individual digits require treatment (Norton 1982). If the condition is severe or generalized, oral steroid therapy may be needed to arrest destruction. Up to 60 mg per day may be needed and one series typically employed 0.5 mg/kg given on alternate days (Tosti *et al.* 1993). Patients with ulcerative lichen planus may benefit from grafting (Crotty *et al.* 1980). This would only be undertaken once the end stage was reached with persistent ulceration.

Oral retinoids have been reported in a single publication, with etretinate at a dose of 0.4 mg/kg in combination with 0.05% fluocinonide lotion (Kato & Ueno 1993). Oral azathioprine has been reported as successful therapy in two adults with erosive lichen planus with nail involvement (Lear & English 1996).

### References

Achten, G. & Wanet-Rouard, J. (1974) Atrophie unguéale et trachyonychie. *Archives Belges Dermatologie* **30**, 201–207.

Aloi, F.G., Colonna, S.M. & Manzoni, R. (1987) Associazone di lichen ruber planus, alopecia areata, vitiligine. *Giornale Italiano di Dermatologia e Venereologia* 122, 197–200.

Baran, R. (2000) Lichen planus of the nails mimicking the yellow nail syndrome. *British Journal of Dermatology* 143, 1117–1118.

Baran, R., Jancovici, E., Sayag, J. & Dawber, R.P.R. (1985) Longitudinal melanonychia in lichen planus. *British Journal of Dermatology* 113, 369–370.

Baran, R., Jancovici, E., Sayag, J., Dawber, R.P.R. & Pinkus, H. (1988) Lichen plan pigmentogène unguéal. *Recherche Dermatologique* 1, 36–38.

Barth, J.H., Millard, P.R. & Dawber, R.P.R. (1988) Idiopathic atrophy of the nails. A clinico-pathological study. *American Journal of Dermatopathology* 10, 514–517.

de Berker, D. & Dawber, R.P.R. (1991) Childhood lichen planus [letter]. *Clinical and Experimental Dermatology* 16, 233.

Bhargava, R.K. & Goyal, R.K. (1975) Solitary involvement of nails in lichen planus. *Indian Journal of Dermatology and Venereology* 41, 142.

Boyd, A.S. & Neldner, K.H. (1991) Lichen planus. *Journal of the American Academy of Dermatology* 25, 593–619.

Büchner, S.A., Itin, P., Ruffli, T. *et al.* (1989) Disseminated lichonoid papular dermatosis with nail changes in AIDS. *Dermatologica* 179, 99–101.

Burgoon, C.F. & Kostrzewa, R.M. (1969) Lichen planus limited to the nails. *Archives of Dermatology* 100, 371.

Colver, G.B. & Dawber, R.P.R. (1987) Is childhood idiopathic atrophy of the nails due to lichen planus? *British Journal of Dermatology* 116, 709–712.

Copeman, P.W.M., Tan, R.S.H., Timlin, D. & Samman, P.D. (1978) Familial lichen planus. Another disease or a distinct people? *British Journal of Dermatology* 98, 573.

Cornelius, C.E. & Shelley, W.B. (1967) Permanent anonychia due to lichen planus. *Archives of Dermatology* 96, 434–435.

Cottoni, F., Solinas, A., Piga, M.R. *et al.* (1988) Lichen planus, chronic liver diseases and immunologic involvement. *Archives of Dermatological Research* 280 (Suppl.), S55–S60.

Cram, D.L., Kierland, R.R. & Winkelmann, R.K. (1966) Ulcerative lichen planus of the feet. *Archives of Dermatology* 93, 692–701.

Crotty, C.P., Su, W.P.D. & Winkelmann, R.K. (1980) Ulcerative lichen planus. *Archives of Dermatology* 116, 1252.

Degos, R. & Schnitzler, L. (1967) Lichen érosif des orteils. *Annales de Dermatologie et de Syphilis* 94, 241–253.

Fabiero, J.M., Fernandez-Redondo, V., Losada, A. *et al.* (1989) Liquen ruber plano con afectacion ungueal. *Acta Dermato-Sifilitica* 80 (5), 319–321.

Haapalainen, T., Oksala, O., Kallinonen, M. *et al.* (1995) Destruction of the epithelial anchoring system in lichen planus. *Journal of Investigative Dermatology* 105, 100–103.

Haneke, E. (1983) Isolated bullous lichen planus of the nails mimicking yellow nail syndrome. *Clinical and Experimental Dermatology* 8, 425–428.

Isogai, Z., Koashi, Y., Sunohara, A. & Tsuji, T. (1997) Ulcerative lichen planus: a rare variant of lichen planus. *Journal of Dermatology* 24 (4), 270–272.

Jansen, T., Plewig, G. & Anhalt, G.J. (1995) Paraneoplastic pemphigus with clinical features of erosive lichen planus associated with Castleman's tumor. *Dermatology* 190, 245–250.

Juhlin, L. & Baran, R. (1989) Longitudinal melanonychia after healing of lichen planus. *Acta Dermato-Venereologica* 69, 338–339.

Juhlin, L. & Baran, R. (1990) On longitudinal melanonychia after healing of lichen planus. *Acta Dermato-Venereologica* 70, 183.

Kanwar, A.J., Govil, D.C. & Singh, O.P. (1983) Lichen planus limited to the nails. *Cutis* 32, 163–168.

Kanwar, A.J., Handa, S., Ghosh, S. *et al.* (1991) Lichen planus in childhood. A report of 17 patients. *Pediatric Dermatology* 8, 288–291.

Kanwar, A.J., Ghosh, S., Thami, G.P. & Kaur, S. (1993) Twenty nail dystrophy due to lichen planus in a patient with alopecia areata. *Clinical and Experimental Dermatology* 18, 293–294.

Kato, N. & Ueno, H. (1993) Isolated lichen planus of the nails treated with etretinate. *Journal of Dermatology* 20, 577–580.

Kint, A. & Vermander, F. (1982) Lichen ruber of the nails. *Dermatologica* 165, 520–521.

Kossard, S. & Cornish, N. (1998) Localized lichen sclerosus with nail loss. *Australasian Journal of Dermatology* 39, 119–120.

Lambert, D.R., Siegle, R.J. & Camisa, C. (1988) Lichen planus of the nail presenting as a tumor. Diagnosis by longitudinal nail bed biopsy. *Journal of Dermatologic Surgery and Oncology* 14, 1245–1247.

Lear, J.T. & English, J.S. (1996) Erosive and generalized lichen planus responsive to azathioprine. *Clinical and Experimental Dermatology* 21, 56–57.

Liddle, B.J. & Cowan, M.A. (1990) Lichen planus-like eruption and nail changes in a patient with graft-versus-host disease [letter]. *British Journal of Dermatology* 122, 841–843.

Lowe, N.J., Cudworth, A.G. & Woodrow, J.C. (1976) HL-A antigens in lichen planus. *British Journal of Dermatology* 95, 169–171.

Marks, R. & Samman, P.D. (1972) Isolated nail dystrophy due to lichen planus. *Transactions of the St John Hospital Dermatology Society* 58, 93–97.

Mehregan, D.A., Van Hale, H.M. & Muller, S.A. (1992) Lichen planopilaris: clinical and pathologic study of forty-five patients *Journal of the American Academy of Dermatology* 27 (6 Part 1), 935–942.

Milligan, A. & Graham-Brown, R.A.C. (1990) Lichen planus in childhood, a review of six cases. *Clinical and Experimental Dermatology* 15, 340–342.

Norton, L.A. (1982) *Diseases of the Nails: Current Therapy* (ed. H.F. Conn), p. 664. W.B. Saunders, Philadelphia.

Oberste-Lehn, H. & Kühl, M. (1954) Lichen planus pemphigoides mit Ulcerationen und Anonychie. *Zeitschrift für Haut-Geschlechtskr* 17, 195–199.

Peluso, A.M., Tosti, A., Piraccini, B.M. & Cameli, N. (1993) Lichen planus limited to the nails in childhood: case report and literature review. *Pediatric Dermatology* 10, 36–39.

Perez, A.G., Rodriguez Pichardo, A.B. & Bueno Montes, J. (1982) Liquen plano erosivo plantar con onicoatrofia. *Medicina Cutanea Ibero-Latino-Americana* 10, 89.

Plewig, G., Jansen, T., Jungblut, R.M. *et al.* (1990) Castelman-tumor, Lichen ruber und Pemphigus vulgaris: paraneoplastiche association immunologische Erkrankungen. *Hautarzt* 41, 662–670.

Samman, P.D. (1961) The nails in lichen planus. *British Journal of Dermatology* 73, 288–292.

Samman, P.D. (1969) Idiopathic atrophy of the nails. *British Journal of Dermatology* 81, 746–749.

Saurat, J.H. & Gluckman, E. (1977) Lichen planus-like eruption following bone marrow transplantation, a manifestation of the graft-versus-host disease. *Clinical and Experimental Dermatology* 2, 335–344.

Scher, R.K., Fischbein, R. & Ackerman, A.B. (1978) Twenty-nail dystrophy. A variant of lichen planus. *Archives of Dermatology* **114**, 612–613.

Scott, M.J. Jr. & Scott, M.J. Sr. (1979) Ungual lichen planus. *Archives of Dermatology* **115**, 1197–1199.

Shiohara, T., Moriya, N., Tanaka, Y. *et al.* (1988) Immunpathologic study of lichenoid skin diseases: correlation between HLA-DR positive keratinocytes or Langerhans cells and epidermotropic cells. *Journal of the American Academy of Dermatology* **18**, 67–74.

Silverman, R.A. & Rhodes, A.R. (1984) Twenty-nail dystrophy of childhood. A sign of lichen planus. *Pediatric Dermatology* **1**, 207–210.

Sowden, J.M., Cartwright, P.H., Green, J.R.B. *et al.* (1989) Isolated lichen planus of the nails associated with primary biliary cirrhosis. *British Journal of Dermatology* **121**, 659–652.

Suarez, S.M. & Scher, R.K. (1990) Idiopathic atrophy of the nails. A possible hereditary association. *Pediatric Dermatology* **7**, 39–41.

Takeuchi, Y., Iwase, N., Suzuki, M. *et al.* (2000) Lichen planus with involvement of all twenty nails and the oral mucous membrane. *Journal of Dermatology* **27**, 94–98.

Tosti, A., De Padova, M.P., Taffurelli, M. *et al.* (1987) Lichen planus limited to the nails. *Cutis* **40**, 25–26.

Tosti, A., De Padova, M.P. & Fanti, P. (1988) Nail involvement in lichen planopilaris. *Cutis* **42**, 213–214.

Tosti, A., Fanti, P.A., Morelli, R. *et al.* (1991) Trachyonychia associated with alopecia areata. A clinical and pathological study. *Journal of the American Academy of Dermatology* **25**, 266–270.

Tosti, A., Peluso, A.M., Fanti, P.A. *et al.* (1993) Nail lichen planus. Clinical and pathological study of 24 patients. *Journal of the American Academy of Dermatology* **28**, 724–730.

Tosti, A., Piraccini, B.M. & Cameli, N. (2000) Nail changes in lichen planus may resemble those of yellow nail syndrome. *British Journal of Dermatology* **142**, 848–849.

Valsecchi, R., Bontempelli, M., Rossi, A. *et al.* (1988) HLA-DR and DQ antigens in lichen planus. *Acta Dermato-Venereologica* **68**, 77–80.

Weidner, F. & Ummenhofer, B. (1979) Lichen ruber ulcerosus (dystrophicans). *Zeitschrift für Hautkrankheiten* **54**, 1088.

White, A.G. & Rostom, A.I. (1994) HLA antigens in arabs with lichen planus. *Clinical and Experimental Dermatology* **19**, 236–237.

Zaias, N. (1970) The nail in lichen planus. *Archives of Dermatology* **101**, 264–271.

## Lichen planus/lupus erythematosus/overlap syndrome

(Copeman *et al.* 1970)

Despite extensive histological and immunopathological studies (Stary *et al.* 1987), it is still not clear whether lichen planus and lupus erythematosus can coexist or whether these cases represent an unusual variant of discoid lupus erythematosus (Romero *et al.* 1977).

## References

Copeman, P.W.M., Schroeter, K.L. & Kierland, R.R. (1970) An unusual variant of lupus erythematosus or lichen planus. *British Journal of Dermatology* **83**, 269–272.

Romero, R.W., Nesbitt, L.T. & Reed, R.J. (1977) Unusual variant of lupus erythematosus or lichen planus. *Archives of Dermatology* **113**, 741–748.

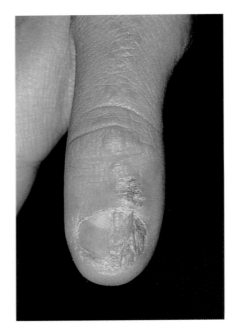

**Fig. 5.47** Lichen striatus.

Stary, A., Schwarz, T., Duschet, P. *et al.* (1987) Das lichen ruber planus—Lupus erythematodes/Overlap-Syndrom. *Zeitschrift für Hautkrankheiten* **62**, 381–394.

## Lichen striatus

This is a linear dermatosis of unknown aetiology. It is characterized by the sudden appearance of erythematous, squamous or lichenoid papules arranged in a continuous or interrupted streak involving the entire length of an extremity. It may extend along a finger or a toe as far as the proximal nail fold and affect the nail plate. The reported cases (Senear & Caro 1941, Samman 1968; Kaufman 1974; Owens 1977; Meyers *et al.* 1978; Vasili & Bhatia 1981; Yaffe 1981) illustrated several types of nail dystrophy, including fraying, longitudinal splitting (Fig. 5.47), punctate or transverse leuconychia, shredding, onycholysis and total nail loss (Baran *et al.* 1979). The nail dystrophy may precede the onset of the rash and an isolated assymetrical nail dystrophy in a young person should raise suspicion of the diagnosis (Karp & Cohen 1993). Zaias (1990) noted longitudinal dystrophy with hyperpigmentation on the lateral portion of the nail in two patients. All these lesions are transient, usually resolving in under a year (Tosti *et al.* 1997), and can probably be explained by the pathological changes observed, particularly the transitory disruption of the basal layer.

Histology obtained from five subjects with nail involvement in lichen striatus revealed a dense band-like lymphohystiocytic infiltrate involving the proximal nail fold, nail bed and nail matrix dermis. Exocytosis with slight spongiosis, focal hypergranulosis and dyskeratotic cells were detectable in the nail matrix epithelium (Tosti *et al.* 1997).

The presence of nail involvement in lichen striatus usually indicates a protracted course and the deformity of nail plate may persist for several years (Niren *et al.* 1981). In such cases, lichen striatus may appear as a variant of inflammatory linear verrucous epidermal nevus (ILVEN) (Laugier & Olmos 1976) The differential diagnosis from ILVEN may be difficult when the linear lesion involves a digit, extends to the proximal nail fold and causes dystrophic linear ridging of the nail plate (Altman & Mehregan 1971; Landwehr & Starink 1983). A periungual psoriasiform plaque, loss of cuticle and onycholysis but no pitting has also been reported in ILVEN (Cheesbrough & Kilby 1978). In linear epidermal naevus the affected nail is brown and dystrophic. Linear porokeratosis, a distinctive clinical variant of porokeratosis of Mibelli (Rahbari *et al.* 1974), should be included in the list of differential diagnosis of linear keratotic cutaneous eruption in childhood.

## References

Altman, J. & Mehregan, A.H. (1971) Inflammatory linear verrucose epidermal nevus. *Archives of Dermatology* **104**, 385–389.

Baran, R., Dupré, A., Lauret, P. & Puissant, A. (1979) Le lichen striatus onychodystrophique. A propos de 4 cas avec revue de la littérature (4 cas). *Annales de Dermatologie et de Vénéréologie* **106**, 885–891.

Cheesbrough, M.J. & Kilby, P.E. (1978) The inflammatory linear verrucous epidermal nevus. A case report. *Clinical and Experimental Dermatology* **3**, 293–298.

Hauber, K., Rose, C., Brocker, E.B. & Hamm, H. (2000) Lichen striatus: clinical features and follow-up in 12 patients. *European Journal of Dermatology* **10**, 536–539.

Karp, D.L. & Cohen, B.A. (1993) Onychodystrophy in lichen striatus [see comments]. *Pediatric Dermatology* **10**, 359–361.

Kaufman, J.P. (1974) Lichen striatus with nail dystrophy. *Cutis* **14**, 232–284.

Landwehr, A.J. & Starink, T.M. (1983) Inflammatory linear verrucous epidermal naevus, report of case with bilateral distribution and nail involvement. *Dermatologica* **166**, 107–109.

Laugier, P. & Olmos, L. (1976) Naevus linéaire inflammatoire et lichen striatus. Deux aspects d'une même affection. *Bulletin de la Société Française de Dermatologie et de Syphilis* **83**, 48–53.

Meyers, M., Storino, W. & Barsky, S. (1978) Lichen striatus with nail dystrophy. *Archives of Dermatology* **114**, 964–965.

Niren, N.M., Waldman, G.D. & Barski, S. (1981) Lichen striatus with onychodystrophy. *Cutis* **27**, 610–613.

Owens, D.W. (1977) Lichen striatus with onychodystrophy. *Archives of Dermatology* **105**, 457–458.

Rahbari, H., Cordero, A.A. & Mehregan, A.H. (1974) Linear porokeratosis. *Archives of Dermatology* **109**, 526–528.

Samman, P.D. (1968) Nail dystrophy and lichen striatus [abstract]. *Transactions of the St John Hospital Dermatology Society* **54**, 119.

Senear, F.E. & Caro, M. (1941) Lichen striatus. *Archives of Dermatology and Syphilis* **43**, 116–133.

Tosti, A., Peluso, A.M., Misciali, C. & Cameli, N. (1997) Nail lichen striatus: clinical features and long term follow up. *Journal of the American Academy of Dermatology* **36**, 908–913.

Vasili, D.B. & Bhatia, S.G. (1981) Lichen striatus. *Cutis* **28**, 442–446.

Yaffee, H.S. (1981) Letter to the editor *Cutis* **28**, 650.

Zaias, N. (1990) *The Nail in Health and Disease*, 2nd edn. Lange & Appleton. Norwalk, CT.

## Lichen nitidus

Cases have been reported demonstrating nail changes, especially as numerous pits (Fritsch 1967) or fine pitting (Munro *et al.* 1993) producing the effect of fine rippling toward the lateral border of some nails (Kellet & Beck 1983). Some nails may become brittle and ridged or have beaded surface and others may show thickening and deep ridging (Barker 1955). Rough nails with ridging and rippling were accompanied by swelling and violaceous discoloration of the posterior nail fold in a 15-year-old girl affected by lichen nitidus (Natarajan & Dick 1986). In the case of a 10-year-old boy, the presentation included marked involvement of the oral mucosa (Bettoli *et al.* 1997). Lichen planus restricted to the nails with giant cells could not be ruled out in the case reported by Fanti *et al.* (1991).

## References

Barker, L.P. (1955) Lichen nitidus, generalized, with nail changes. *Archives of Dermatology and Syphilis* **72**, 487.

Bettoli, V., De Padova, M.P., Corazza, M. & Virgili, A. (1997) Generalized lichen nitidus with oral and nail involvement in a child. *Dermatology* **194**, 367–369.

Fanti, P.A., Tosti, A., Morelli, R. *et al.* (1991) Lichen planus of the nails with giant cells, lichen nitidus? *British Journal of Dermatology* **125**, 194–195.

Fritsch, P. (1967) Der Lichen nitidus (Pinkus). *Zeitschrift für Haut-Geschlkr* **42**, 649–666.

Kellet, J.B. & Beck, M. (1983) Lichen nitidus associated with distinctive nail changes. *Clinical and Experimental Dermatology* **9**, 201–204.

Munro, C.S., Cox, N.H., Marks, J.M. & Natarajan, S. (1993) Lichen nitidus presenting as palmoplantar hyperkeratosis and nail dystrophy. *Clinical and Experimental Dermatology* **18**, 381–383.

Natarajan, S. & Dick, D. (1986) Lichen nitidus associated with nail changes. *International Journal of Dermatology* **25**, 461–462.

## Lichen aureus (Fig. 5.48)

Palleschi *et al.* (1995) reported the case of a 45-year-old man who presented with copper-coloured papules in a linear pattern affecting the proximal nail folds of the hands and feet. The lesions were symmetrical. Histology showed a lichen aureus. This entity is regarded as a variety of capillarities of unknown aetiology.

## Reference

Palleschi, G.M., Giacomelli, A. & Falcos, D. (1995) Lichen aureus acrale-bilaterale. *Giornale Italiano di Dermatologia e Venereologia* **130**, 271–274.

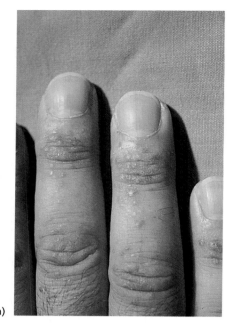

(a)

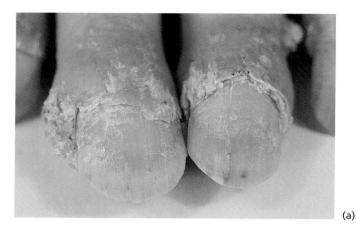

(a)

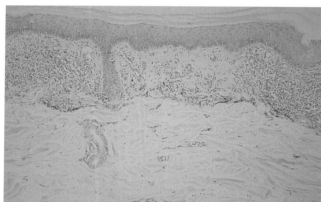

(b)

**Fig. 5.48** (a,b) Lichen aureus.

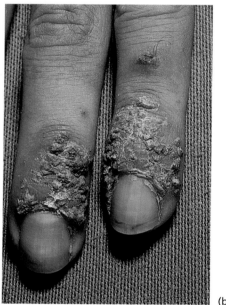

(b)

**Fig. 5.49** (a) Keratosis lichenoides chronica. Hyperkeratotic hypertrophy of the periungual tissues. (Courtesy of L. Balus, Italy.) (b) Keratosis lichenoides chronica. Hyperkeratotic hypertrophy of the periungual tissues. (Courtesy of C. Grupper, Paris, France.)

## Keratosis lichenoides chronica

The majority of patients affected by keratosis lichenoides chronica manifest three varieties of hyperkeratotic lesion:

1 Linear, lichenoid and warty;
2 Yellowish keratotic patches;
3 Raised papules with keratotic plugs.

Hence, the name lichenoid tri-keratosis proposed by Pinol-Aguade *et al.* (1974).

Keratosis lichenoides chronica may appear clinically and even histologically to be a variant of lichen planus, but is a distinct entity (Braun-Falco *et al.* 1989). About one-third of the patients have nail involvement (Panizzon & Baran 1981) with changes which may clinically resemble psoriasis, but pitting or pustulosis never occur. Hyperkeratotic hypertrophy of the periungual tissues is a distinctive sign (Fig. 5.49) (Baran 1983).

PUVA therapy and etretinate (Schnitzler *et al.* 1981; Baran *et al.* 1984) have improved some cases.

### References

Baran, R. (1983) Nail changes in keratosis lichenoides chronica are not a variant of lichen planus. *British Journal of Dermatology* **109**, 43–46.

Baran, R., Panizzon, R. & Goldberg, L.H. (1984) Nails in keratosis lichenoides chronica, characteristics and response to treatment. *Archives of Dermatology* **120**, 1471–1474.

Braun-Falco, O., Bieber, T. & Heider, L. (1989) Keratosis lichenoides chronica, Krankheitsvariante oder Krankheitsentitie. *Hautarzt* **40**, 614–622.

Panizzon, R. & Baran, R. (1981) Keratosis lichenoides chronica. *Aktuelle Dermatologie* **7**, 6–9.

Pinol-Aguade, J., De Asprer, J. & Ferrando, J. (1974) Lichenoid tri-keratosis (Kaposi–Bureau–Barrière–Grupper). *Dermatologica* **148**, 179–188.

Schnitzler, L., Bouteiller, G., Bechetoille, A. *et al.* (1981) Keratose lichénoïde chronique avec atteinte muqueuse synechiante sévère. Etude évolutive sur 18 ans. Thérapeutique par le rétinoïde aroma-tique. *Annales de Dermatologie et de Vénéréologie* **108**, 371–379.

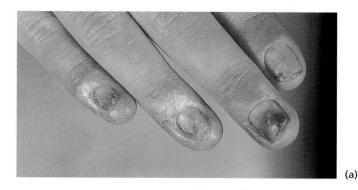

(a)

## Discoid lupus erythematosus (Fig. 5.50)

The features and histopathology of lichen planus and discoid lupus erythematosus have much in common in diseases of the appendages. In the scalp they can at times be indistinguishable, and in the digits there is considerable overlap between some of the scarring sequelae. However, nail involvement in discoid lupus is less common than in lichen planus and the focus of scarring is more on the nail fold than on the matrix. Neverthe-less, in aggressive discoid lupus of the digit, both structures may be involved and nail destruction with pterygium formation may occur as in lichen planus. Some of these more aggressive forms represent variants of systemic lupus (Hudson Peacock *et al.* 1997).

The nails present longitudinal ridging, which may be broken off in their distal part or partially split. The red-bluish colour of the nail bed may be diffuse (Kint & Van Herpe 1976) or assume the aspect of minute spots through the atrophic nail plate (Sannicandro 1960).

In 'lupus erythematosus unguium mutilans' (Heller 1906) the nail area shows a cyanotic tinge, adherent scales and only the debris of the nail plate. Subungual friable yellowish-brown material may lift up the nail plate, some nails may be entirely

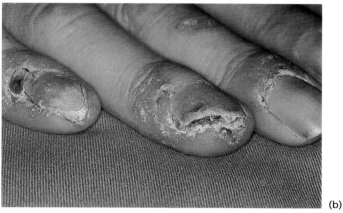

(b)

**Fig. 5.50** (a) Discoid lupus erythematosus. (Courtesy of P. Baptista, Portugal.) (b) Discoid lupus erythematosus. (Courtesy of A. Forgem.)

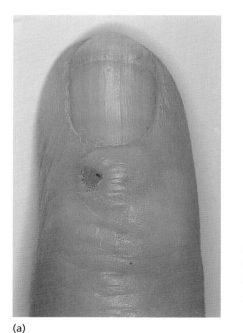

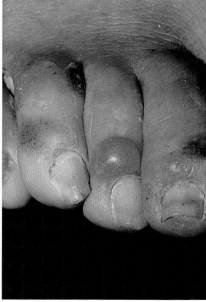

**Fig. 5.51** (a,b) Bullous pemphigoid—mainly periungual involvement.

(a)

(b)

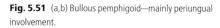

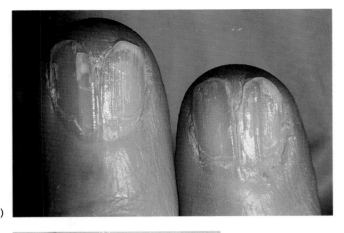

(a)

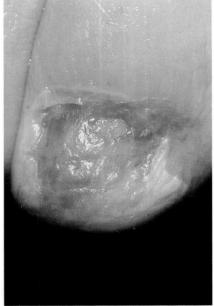

(b)

**Fig. 5.52** (a,b) Bullous pemphigoid—nail plate and nail bed changes.

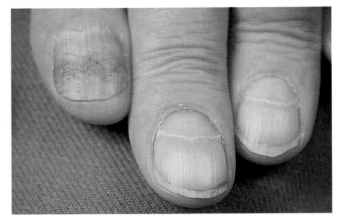

(a)

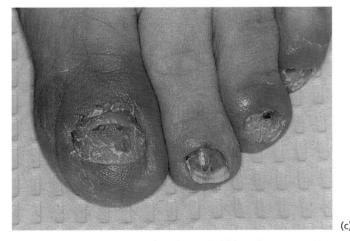

(b)

(c)

destroyed leaving the nail bed exposed as a deep red, shiny area (McCarthy 1930).

Horny growths on each finger, like a bird's claw, have been observed. They are accompanied by lack of lustre, thickening of the nails and a dirty greyish discoloration with shallow longitudinal furrows (Yang 1935).

The skin around the nails may be normal or reddish with brownish-grey adherent scales (Hekele & Mayer 1959) and sclerosis of the nail bed (Sannicandro 1960). In hypertrophic lupus erythematosus gross hyperkeratosis of the palms and soles may extend onto the dorsa of toes to surround the nails, which are longitudinally ridged with subungual hyperkeratosis (Buck *et al.* 1988).

Although the clinical signs are not pathognomonic, the diagnosis may be suspected because of the combination of typical red-blue colouring of the nail bed and alterations in the nail

**Fig. 5.53** (a) Beau's lines. (Courtesy of L. Juhlin, Sweden.) (b) Pemphigus—paronychia. (Courtesy of S. Goettmann-Bonvallot, France.) (c) Pemphigus—nail bed and periungual involvement.

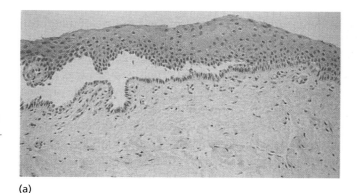

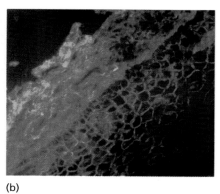

**Fig. 5.54** (a) Pemphigus vulgaris—matrix histology. (b) Pemphigus vegetans with nail dystrophy—immunofluorescence of the matrix.

(a)

(b)

plates which tend to crumble (Kint & Van Herpe 1976). In chilblain lupus erythematosus, a chronic unremitting type seen predominantly in women, there is gross distortion of the finger-tips and nail plates (Millard & Rowell 1978). Lupus erythematosus has been associated with finger clubbing (Mackie 1979).

Lupus erythematosus of the perionychium shows characteristic hyperkeratosis, liquefaction degeneration of basal cells, a predominantly lymphocytic infiltrate in the superficial dermis, and oedema with ectatic capillaries in the papillary dermis (Mackie 1973). Lupus erythematosus of the nail bed causes hyperorthokeratosis with a corresponding granular layer, thinning of the spinous layer and oedema of the basal cells, which also exhibit ill-defined borders. Hyalin bodies are observed in the superficial dermis (Kint & van Herpe 1976). These features are consistent with, but not diagnostic of, lupus erythematosus.

Potent topical steroids under occlusion may give some improvement.

## References

Buck, D.C., Dodd, H.J. & Sarkany, I. (1988) Hypertrophic lupus erythematosus. *British Journal of Dermatology* **119** (Suppl. 33), 72–74.

Hekele, K. & Mayer, A. (1959) Seltene Lokalisation des Lupus erythematodes chronicus discoides. *Dermatologische Wochenschrift* **34**, 934–940.

Heller, J. (1906) Lupus erythematosus der Nägel. *Dermatologische Zeitschrift* **13**, 613–615.

Hudson Peacock, M.J., Joseph, S.A., Cox, J. *et al.* (1997) Systemic lupus erythematosus complicating complement type 2 deficiency: successful treatment with fresh frozen plasma. *British Journal of Dermatology* **136**, 388–392.

Kint, A. & Van Herpe, L. (1976) Ungual anomalies in lupus erythematosus discoides. *Dermatologica* **153**, 298–302.

Mackie, R.M. (1973) Lupus erythematosus associated with finger clubbing. *British Journal of Dermatology* **89**, 533–535.

McCarthy, L. (1930) Lupus erythematosus unguium mutilans treated with gold and sodium thiosulphate. *Archives of Dermatology and Syphilis* **22**, 647–654.

Millard, L.G. & Rowell, N.R. (1978) Chilblain lupus erythematosus (Hutchinson). *British Journal of Dermatology* **98**, 497–506.

Sannicandro, F. (1960) Contributo alla conoscenza clinica ed istologica del lupus eritematoso cronico disseminato del complesso unguale. *Minerva Dermatologica* **35**, 32–34.

Yang, K.L. (1935) Lupus erythematosus with unusual changes in the finger tips and nails. *Acta Dermato-Venereologica* **16**, 365–369.

## Bullous pemphigoid (Figs 5.51a & 5.52b)

Nail involvement in bullous pemphigoid usually reflects blistering of an element in the nail unit which affects the nail. Typically a nail fold is involved, but blistering of the nail bed and matrix is seen. The location of the blister will determine the effect on the nail, with paronychia, onycholysis, onychomadesis or nail loss being common end points (Namba *et al.* 1999). It is difficult to judge whether the presentation of bullous pemphigoid in the nail unit is anything more than chance associated with a widespread disease. However, the subsequent evolution of Beau's lines seems to be more than chance (de Berker *et al.* 1995). Less common and unrepresentative examples of bullous pemphigoid with nail features have entered the literature because of their unusual and interesting nature. These include:
- Esterly *et al.* (1973) reported a case of dystrophic nails in a 12-year-old girl who had unequivocal bullous pemphigoid.
- Scarring nail dystrophy made up of longitudinal splits and pterygium of several fingernails, in a patient with pemphigoid, revealed in the longitudinal nail biopsy linear deposits of C3 and IgM at the basement membrane zone of the proximal nail fold and the nail bed (Barth *et al.* 1987).
- Cicatricial pemphigoid with nail dystrophy consisting of atrophia, longitudinally ridged and split nails resembling lichen planus has been reported (Burge *et al.* 1985).
- Miyagawa *et al.* (1981) reported dystrophic nails in a 59-year-old woman who had a chronic bullous disease with coexistent linear IgG and IgA at the basement membrane zone on direct immunofluorescence, and both IgG and IgA on indirect immunofluorescence. This case was thought to represent an overlap of bullous pemphigoid and dermatitis herpertiformis.
- In childhood the finding of nail dystrophy consisting of hyperkeratosis, haemorrhage and horizontal ridging (Fox *et al.* 1982) with a bullous eruption was contrary to the diagnosis of

childhood bullous pemphigoid and more in favour of epidermolysis bullosa.

## References

Barth, J.H., Wojnarowska, F., Millard, P.R. & Dawber, R.P.R. (1987) Immunofluorescence of the nail bed in pemphigoid. *American Journal of Dermatopathology* 9, 349–350.

de Berker, D., Nayar, M., Dawber, R. & Wojnarowska, F. (1995) Beau's lines in immunobullous disorders *Clinical and Experimental Dermatology* 20, 358–361.

Burge, S.M., Powell, S.M. & Ryan, T.J. (1985) Cicatricial pemphigoid with nail dystrophy. *Clinical and Experimental Dermatology* 10, 472–475.

Esterly, N.B., Gotoff, S.P., Lolekha, S. *et al.* (1973) Bullous pemphigoid and membranous glomerulonephropathy in a child. *Journal of Pediatrics* 83, 466.

Fox, B.J., Odom, R.B. & Findlay, R.F. (1982) Erythromycin therapy in bullous pemphigoid, possible anti-inflammatory effects. *Journal of the American Academy of Dermatology* 7, 504.

Miyagawa, S., Kiriyama, Y., Shirai, T. *et al.* (1981) Chronic bullous disease with coexistent circulating IgG and IgA anti-basement membrane zone antibodies. *Archives of Dermatology* 117, 349.

Namba, Y., Koizumi, H., Kumakuri, M. *et al.* (1999) Bullous pemphigoid with permanent loss of the nails. *Acta Dermato-Venereologica* 79, 480–481.

## Pemphigus (Figs 5.53a & 5.54b)

Nail involvement in pemphigus is like that in bullous pemphigoid and is usually secondary to bullae that are adjacent to the fingernails and toenails. Dystrophic changes include discoloration, subungual and splinter haemorrhages (Böckers & Bork 1987), chronic paronychia (Stone & Mullins 1966; Kim *et al.* 1996), pitting, trachyonychia (de Berker *et al.* 1993) transverse grooves and onychomadesis (Parameswara & Naik 1981). Beau's lines may appear on all 20 digits after each pemphigus flare (Lauber & Turk 1990). The lateral and proximal nail folds of all 10 fingers (Dhawan *et al.* 1990) and even 20 digits (Degos *et al.* 1955; Engineer *et al.* 2000) may present as an inflammatory painful and tender paronychia, and sero-sanguineous fluid can be expressed. This is considered by Zaias (1990) as the hallmark of this condition. The nail fold disease resembles a pyogenic granuloma.

Primary involvement of the subungual region (Baumal & Robinson 1973) is rare and results in nail shedding with a chronic, erosive process due to pemphigus. Nail bed and matrix biopsy showed suprabasilar acantholysis and intercellular deposition of immunoglobin G (IgG) and C3 in a single case (Fulton *et al.* 1983; de Berker *et al.* 1993).

In Brazilian pemphigus foliaceus, established cases initially show yellowish, or later dark discoloration of the nails (Vieira sign), onychorrhexis and onycholysis (Azulay 1982). Nail shedding is not exceptional. Pterygium and subungual hyperkeratosis and even onychogryphosis have been recorded. The nails may be rough or, in constrast, shiny due to permanent rubbing and scratching (Costa 1943).

In pemphigus vegetans of Hallopeau, the fingernails show pustules with onychatrophy. Sterile pus may be expressed from the nail folds (Leroy *et al.* 1982).

Histopathology of the involved nail shows superbasilar acantholytic clefts leading to intraepithelial blister formation in matrix (Fulton *et al.* 1983) and nail bed (Baumal & Robinson 1973). IgG and C3 (Fulton *et al.* 1983) are demonstrated in the intercellular spaces.

## References

Azulay, R.D. (1982) Brazilian pemphigus foliaceus. *International Journal of Dermatology* 21, 122–124.

Baumal, A. & Robinson, M.J. (1973) Nail bed involvement in pemphigus vulgaris. *Archives of Dermatology* 107, 751.

de Berker, D., Dalziel, K., Dawber, R. & Wojnarowska, F. (1993) Pemphigus associated with nail dystrophy. *British Journal of Dermatology* 129, 461–464.

Böckers, M. & Bork, K. (1987) Multiple gleichzeitige Hämatome der Finger—und Zehennägel mit nachfolgender Onychomadesis bei Pemphigus vulgaris. *Hautarzt* 38, 477–478.

Costa, O.G. (1943) Lesoes ungueais no penfigo foliaceo. *Anales Brasiliera de Dermatologia et Sifilitica* 18, 67–73.

Degos, R., Carteaud, A. & Delort, J. (1955) Onyxis et perionyxis du pemphigus. *Bulletin de la Société Française de Dermatologie et de Syphilis* 62, 475–476.

Dhawan, S.S., Zaias, N. & Pena, N. (1990) The nail fold in pemphigus vulgaris. *Archives of Dermatology* 126, 1374–1375.

Engineer, L., Norton, L.A. & Ahmed, R. (2000) Nail involvement in pemphigus vulgaris. *Journal of the American Academy of Dermatology* 43, 529–535.

Fulton, R.A., Campbell, L., Carlyle, D. & Simpson, N.B. (1983) Nail bed immunofluorescence in pemphigus vulgaris. *Acta Dermato-Venereologica* 63, 170–172.

Kim, B.S., Song, K.Y., Youn, J.I. & Chung, J.H. (1996) Paronychia—a manifestation of pemphigus vulgaris. *Clinical and Experimental Dermatology* 21, 315–317.

Lauber, J. & Turk, K. (1990) Beau's lines and pemphigus vulgaris. *International Journal of Dermatology* 29, 309.

Leroy, D., Lebrun, J., Maillard, V. *et al.* (1982) Pemphigus végétant à type clinique de dermatite pustuleuse chronique de Hallopeau. *Annales de Dermatologie et de Vénéréologie* 109, 549–555.

Parameswara, Y.R. & Naik, R.P.C. (1981) Onychomadesis associated with pemphigus vulgaris. *Archives of Dermatology* 117, 759.

Stone, O.J. & Mullins, J.F. (1966) Vegetative lesions in pemphigus. *Dermatologia International* 5, 137.

Zaias, N. (1990) *The Nail in Health and Disease*, 2nd edn. Lange & Appleton, Norwalk, CT.

## Alopecia areata

Nail involvement in alopecia areata is relatively common. One study in adults with alopecia areata suggests a prevalence of nail changes in those presenting with scalp disease of 20%

(Sharma *et al.* 1996a). There are two substantial prevalence studies in childhood alopecia areata. A comparison of the childhood and adult studies confirms the clinical impression that nail changes are more common in children than adults. In an Indian study, 30% of 201 cases presented with nail changes (Sharma *et al.* 1996b). The figure in an Italian study was 46% of 272 children (Tosti *et al.* 1994).

### Clinical features (Figs 5.55–5.60)

The most common feature of the nails in alopecia areata is pitting, affecting 34% in varying degrees (Tosti *et al.* 1994). Trachyonychia is the roughened stippled effect sometimes seen in alopecia areata, which is pathologically a variant of pitting. Whilst random classic pitting was the most common form, geometric patterns seldom seen in psoriasis were seen in 7%. This range of appearances accommodates the conflicts in earlier literature. According to Samman (1978), the pits are small as in psoriasis. Others described the pits as smaller and more regular than those found in psoriasis (Munro & Darley 1979). Ebling considered them larger and less deep than in psoriasis (Ebling & Rook 1979). Unlike the pits in psoriasis, they do not contain parakeratotic cells (Alkiewicz 1964).

Trachyonychia was seen in 12%. Nail loss, Beau's lines koilonychia, friable stump-like nails or onychomadesis, which can be latent before leading to shedding of the nails, are also seen. The nail plate may be thinned (commonest) or thickened.

Gross nail dystrophy is said to be proportional to the degree of hair loss (Tosti *et al.* 1994; Sharma *et al.* 1996a), especially in the early stages. The rate of onset of hair loss may also play a part. Onychodystrophy has been reported with minimal hair loss and does not necessarily imply a poor prognosis for regrowth. Sometimes nail changes may precede the involvement of the hair, but this has no bearing on the prognosis with regard to regrowth of hair. Onychodystrophy may persist or even develop subsequent to, and persist for some time after, resolution of the alopecia areata.

Leuconychia may be punctate, transverse or diffuse. Rarely, other colours may be seen—yellow, grey or brown—and the character may be opaque, and is termed asbestos nail (Van de Kerkhof 1987). Red colour changes are rare but may be seen as dusky red discoloration of the lunula or of the proximal third of all the nails (Leider 1955; Ringrose & Bahcall 1957; Misch 1981; Tosti *et al.* 1994). Bergner *et al.* (1992) reported two cases with red lunulae developed a few weeks after the acute onset of hair loss, which disappeared slowly, leaving Beau's lines. Interestingly the erythema of the fingernail lunulae of one patient migrated distally.

Mottled lunulae are frequently seen due to an irregular, spotty absence of whiteness (Shelley 1980). The spots on the lunulae appear identical in colour with the regular nail bed. These changes are reversible, coming and going for no definable reason. This phenomenon may also occur in association with psoriasis.

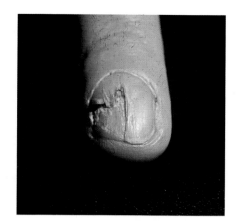

**Fig. 5.55** Alopecia areata—transverse and longitudinal fissures, with onychorrhexis. (Courtesy of Professor G. Achten, Belgium.)

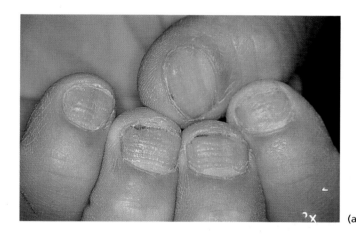

(a)

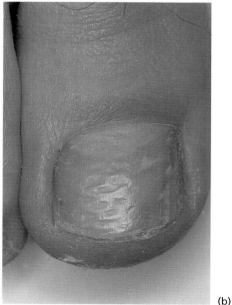

(b)

**Fig. 5.56** (a) Alopecia areata—multiple lines made of regular horizontal pits. (b) Alopecia areata—irregular pitting.

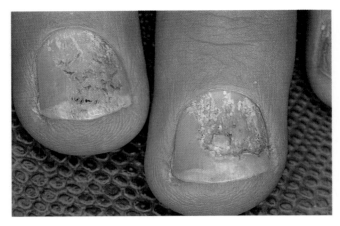

**Fig. 5.57** Alopecia areata—dull, roughened, friable nails.

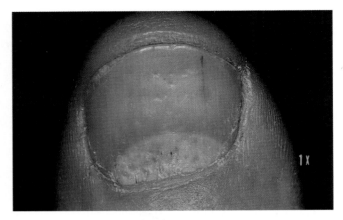

**Fig. 5.59** Alopecia areata—'spotty' lunula.

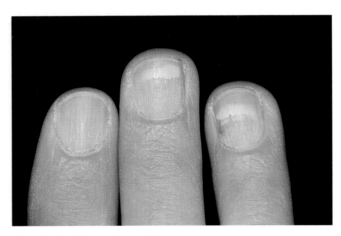

**Fig. 5.58** Alopecia areata—leuconychia.

Alopecia areata involves either some nails which may become dull, roughened, fragile and friable, or all the nails, in which case they present as a 'twenty-nail dystrophy'.

The following types can be distinguished:

1 The monomorphic twenty-nail dystrophy with thickened nails. They appear brown, irregular and masquerade as an ectodermal dysplasia or longstanding onychomycosis (Fig. 5.60a).

2 The vertical, striated, sandpaper twenty-nail dystrophy (Fig. 5.60b). This belongs to the monomorphic group—the whole nail plate gives the appearance of having been sandpapered in a longitudinal direction. Because of this 'excessive ridging', the nail lustre disappears. In sandpaper twenty-nail dystrophy an eczematous appearance of the epidermis of the nail bed with vacuolated plate-staining keratinocytes of the matrix has been reported (Baran *et al*. 1978) (page 118).

3 The monomorphic, shiny twenty-nail dystrophy (Horn & Odom 1980). In this type the opalescent nail plates present longitudinal ridging with a stippled appearance. They are thin and fragile (Fig. 5.60c).

4 The polymorphic twenty-nail dystrophy (Fig. 5.60d). Any of

the disorders mentioned above may be seen on different digits concurrently. Irrespective of the thickness of the nail plate, the nails appear fragile and friable.

### Clinical associations

Some diseases may be associated with alopecia areata. In the triad 'alopecia universalis, onychodystrophy and total vitiligo' (Demis & Weiner 1963), the nail dystrophy has the appearance of longstanding fungal infection. We believe that the pseudomycotic nail dystrophy observed in vitiligo (Milligan *et al*. 1988) may well be due to alopecia areata restricted to the nails.

The coexistence of vitiligo, alopecia areata, onychodystrophy, localized scleroderma and lichen planus has been reported (Brenner *et al*. 1979) with thickening of the nails, subungual hyperkeratoses and slight koilonychia. The coexistence of autoimmune liver disease, vitiligo, alopecia and nail dystrophy has been reported in a 7-year-old boy (Sacher *et al*. 1990), where there were autoantibodies to liver kidney microsomal antigens.

Lichen planus (Fenton & Samman 1988) or psoriasis may be associated with alopecia areata (Ehrenfeld & Silver 1966), and it has been suggested that the pitting of the nails described in alopecia areata might be an expression of psoriasis (Ganor 1977). This may explain the psoriasiform histological findings of Dotz *et al*. (1985). However in alopecia areata the rate of growth of the nail plate is reduced (cf. psoriatic nails). The differential diagnosis includes lichen planus, psoriasis and onychomycosis. Thorough clinical examination of the patient should rule out psoriasis. Involvement of the buccal and genital mucous membranes in lichen planus may be of some help in diagnosis. A nail biopsy is of great value when the disorder of the nail precedes the hair loss. When the condition is limited to the nails alone, it is impossible to determine the diagnosis with certainty. In such cases a nail biopsy affords the only chance of diagnosing conditions with a characteristic histology, such as lichen planus or psoriasis. It is interesting to note that in some

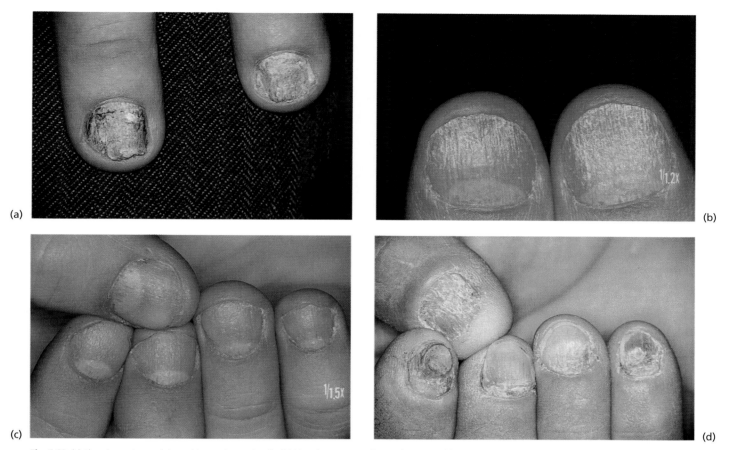

**Fig. 5.60** (a) Alopecia areata—total dystrophic pseudomycotic nails. (b) Alopecia areata—sandpapered twenty-nail dystrophy. (c) Monomorphic shiny twenty-nail dystrophy. (d) Polymorphic twenty-nail dystrophy type.

cases of 'idiopathic' twenty-nail dystrophy of childhood, the histological findings were reported as predominantly 'eczematous' (Wilkinson *et al*. 1979; Tosti *et al*. 1991).

### Histopathology

Histologically spongiotic changes appear to be a constant finding in the clinical manifestations of alopecia areata of the nails (Haneke 1984), therefore spongiotic inflammation of the nail matrix of patients with idiopathic trachyonychia suggests the possibility that it may sometimes represent a variety of alopecia areata limited to the nails (Tosti *et al*. 1991). There is a predominantly lymphocytic infiltrate with perivascular accentuation and epidermotropism. The epithelium is diffusely spongiotic and spongiotic vesicles are often seen. They extend up to the superficial epithelial layers and the proteinacous exudate may be included in the nail, it is then visible as homogeneous, eosinophilic, PAS-positive inclusions in the nail plate and subungual keratin. The nail plate keratin is wavy and irregularly arranged. Depressions are seen on the surface; however, in contrast to psoriatic pits, they do not contain parakeratotic cells (Alkiewicz 1964; Haneke 1984; Laporte *et al*. 1988; Achten *et*

*al*. 1991). It may be extremely difficult to differentiate alopecia areata of the nail when there is marked spongiosis from eczematous dermatitis. In the latter, there is usually spongiotic dermatitis of the eponychium and outer surface of the proximal nail fold. These features are not seen in alopecia areata (Haneke 1984).

Laporte *et al*. (1988) have studied light and electron microscopy of nail plate changes in alopecia areata. The upper part of the nail plate shows an architectural disorder of the corneocyte arrangement, sometimes little depressions, more often thin parallel pits giving a flaky aspect. Under electron microscopy, the cytoplasm is full of vacuoles of variable size (from 140 to 1600 nm) and electron-dense deposits of material. Keratin fibres are rarefied. The intercellular spaces become larger while the number of 'ampullar dilatations' rises. The upper portion of the nail is more affected than the lower one.

### Prognosis and treatment

Hair regrowth is generally accompanied by an improvement in the nail dystrophy, which slowly clears within a few months. Therapy with matrix injection with corticosteroids hastens resolution in some cases. Short courses of oral corticosteroids are also effective but should not be recommended for routine use. Potent topical steroids can be used to good effect over a period of a few months, but excessive use can lead to local side effects, including premature closure of the epiphyses of the distal phalanx in the young. Squaric acid dibutyl ester treatment of the scalp alone also seems to bring some improvement in the nails, but this is only temporary.

## References

Achten, G., André, J. & Laporte, M. (1991) Nails in light and electron microscopy. *Seminars in Dermatology* **10**, 54–64.

Alkiewicz, J. (1964) Pathologische Reaktionen an den epithelialen Anhangsgebilden, Nagel. In: *Handbuch der Haut- und Geschlechtskrankheiten, Ergänzungswerk*, Vol. 1/2 (ed. J.J. Jadassohn), pp. 299–343. Springer, Berlin.

Baran, R., Dupré, A., Christol, B. *et al.* (1978) L'ongle grésé peladique. *Annales de Dermatologie et de Vénéréologie* **105**, 387.

Bergner, T., Donhauser, G. & Ruzicka, T. (1992) Red lunulae in severe alopecia areata. *Acta Dermato-Venereologica* **72**, 203–205.

Brenner, W., Diem, E. & Gschnait, F. (1979) Coincidence of vitiligo, alopecia areata, onychodystrophy, localized scleroderma and lichen planus. *Dermatologica* **159**, 356.

Demis, D.J. & Weiner, M.A. (1963) Alopecia universalis, onychodystrophy, and total vitiligo. *Archives of Dermatology* **88**, 195.

Dotz, W.I., Lieber, C.D. & Vogt, P.J. (1985) Leuconychia punctata and pitted nails in alopecia areata. *Archives of Dermatology* **121**, 1452–1454.

Ebling, F.J. & Rook, A. (1979) The nails. In: *Textbook of Dermatology* (eds A. Rooks, D.S. Wilkinson & F.J. Ebling), p. 1781, 3rd edn. Blackwell Scientific Publications, Oxford.

Ehrenfeld, I.D. & Silver, H. (1966) Simultaneous occurrence of onychomycosis, psoriasis of scalp and nails, and alopecia areata. *Archives of Dermatology* **93**, 379–380.

Fenton, D.A. & Samman, P.D. (1988) Twenty-nail dystrophy of childhood associated with alopecia areata and lichen planus. *British Journal of Dermatology* **119** (Suppl. 33), 63.

Ganor, S. (1977) Diseases sometimes associated with psoriasis, II, alopecia areata. *Dermatologica* **154**, 338.

Haneke, E. (1984) Pathology of inflammatory nail diseases. In: *7th Colloquium of the International Society for Dermatopathology, Graz, Austria.*

Horn, R.T. & Odom, R.B. (1980) Twenty-nail dystrophy of alopecia areata. *Archives of Dermatology* **116**, 573.

Laporte, M., André, J., Stouffs-Vanhoof, F. & Achten, G. (1988) Nail changes in alopecia areata, light and electron microscopy. *Archives of Dermatological Research* **280** (Suppl.), 585–589.

Leider, M. (1955) Progression of alopecia areata through alopecia totalis to alopecia generalisata. Peculiar nail changes (obliteration of the lunula by erythema) while under cortisone therapy. *Archives of Dermatology* **71**, 648.

Milligan, A., Barth, J.H., Graham-Brown, R.N.C. & Dawber, R.P.R. (1988) Pseudo-mycotic nail dystrophy and vitiligo. *Clinical and Experimental Dermatology* **13**, 109–110.

Misch, K.J. (1981) Red nails associated with alopecia areata. *Clinical and Experimental Dermatology* **6**, 561.

Munro, D.D. & Darley, C.R. (1979) In: *Dermatology in General Medicine* (eds T.B. Fitzpatrick, A.Z. Eisen, K. Wolff, I.M. Freedberg & K.F. Austen), p. 403. McGraw-Hill, New York.

Ringrose, E.J. & Bahcall, C.R. (1957) Alopecia areata symptomatica with nail base changes. *Archives of Dermatology* **76**, 263.

Sacher, M., Blümel, P., Thaler, H. & Manns, M. (1990) Chronic active hepatitis associated with vitiligo, nail dystrophy, alopecia and a new variant of LKM antibodies. *Journal of Hepatology* **10**, 364–369.

Samman, P.D. (1978) *The Nails in Disease.* Heinemann, London.

Sharma, V.K., Dawn, G. & Kumar, B. (1996a) Profile of alopecia areata in Northern India. *International Journal of Dermatology* **35**, 22–27.

Sharma, V.K., Kumar, B. & Dawn, G. (1996b) A clinical study of childhood alopecia areata in Chandigarh, India. *Pediatric Dermatology* **13**, 372–377.

Shelley, W.B. (1980) The spotted lunula. *Journal of the American Academy of Dermatology* **2**, 385.

Tosti, A., Fanti, P.A., Morelli, R. *et al.* (1991) Trachyonychia associated with alopecia areata. A clinical and pathological study. *Journal of the American Academy of Dermatology* **25**, 266–270.

Tosti, A., Morelli, R., Bardazzi, F. & Peluso, A.M. (1994) Prevalence of nail abnormalities in children with alopecia areata. *Pediatric Dermatology* **11**, 112–115.

Van de Kerkhof, P.C.M. (1987) Nail changes in alopecia areata. In: *Congressus Mondialae Dermatologiae, Berlin Abstracts.* Part I, WS 33, p. 288.

Wilkinson, J.D., Dawber, R.P.R., Bowers, R.P. & Fleming, K. (1979) Twenty-nail dystrophy of childhood. *British Journal of Dermatology* **100**, 217.

## Darier's disease

Darier's disease is inherited as an autosomal dominant. Penetrance of the gene is high. The nail signs diagnostic of Darier–White disease or dyskeratosis follicularis are very common. In a study on 163 patients, they were found in 92% by Burge and Wilkinson (1992) and in 95% of a smaller number in a similar study (Munro 1992). Ronchese (1965), Bingham and Burrow (1984) and Munro and MacLeod (1991) reported the occurrence of nail changes in the absence of other evidence of disease. The number of abnormal nails ranges from two or three to all nails in a minority of patients. Toenails are involved, but less often and less severely than fingernails (Burge & Wilkinson 1992). The nails lesions (54 out of 56 patients) and palmar pitting (49 out of 56 patients) are earlier and more consistent evidence of the presence of the gene than is the characteristic rash (Munro & MacLeod 1991).

Nail features include longitudinal, subungual, red or white streaks, or both, associated with distal wedge-shaped subungual keratoses (Zaias & Ackerman 1973) (Fig. 5.61a). The single or multiple red longitudinal streaks may, with time, develop into white ones. Such changes extending through the nail and crossing the lunula are most characteristic. Where a streak meets the free edge of the nail, a V-shaped notch is usually present originating from the distal nail bed and hyponychium. The wedge-shaped subungual keratosis may massively thicken the nail plate in severe cases (Fig. 5.62) (Savin & Samman 1970). A similar clinical finding can be seen with isolated distal subungual keratoses, which are histologically multi-

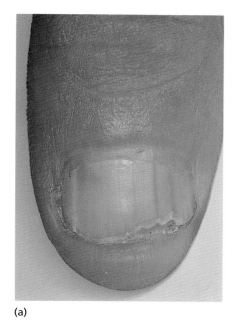

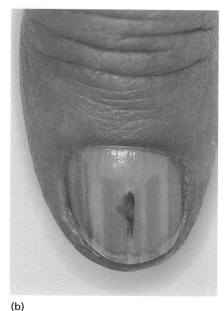

**Fig. 5.61** (a) Darier's disease—longitudinal white lines associated with two longitudinal red lines. (b) Darier's disease—longitudinal white lines associated with nail bed haemorrhage.

(a)

(b)

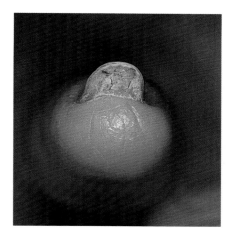

**Fig. 5.62** Darier's disease—subungual hyperkeratosis.

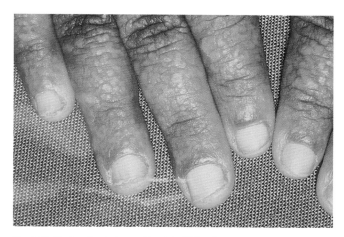

**Fig. 5.63** Hopf acrokeratosis verruciformis in childhood.

nucleate and arise in the absence of Darier's disease (Baran & Perrin 1995). Haemorrhagic Darier's disease reported in 6% of Burge and Wilkinson's patients (1992) may involve the subungual tissue (Fig. 5.61b).

The linear red abnormality represents thinned nail due to matrix disease. This is associated both directly and indirectly with fragility and ridges, which crack and develop painful splits. Splinter haemorrhages, true leuconychia resulting from epithelial hyperplasia of the matrix and keratotic papules occurring on the proximal nail fold are also seen. Secondary invasion of the nails with dermatophytes, *Candida* and *Pseudomonas* is frequent. Periungual squamous cell carcinoma has been reported (Downs *et al.* 1997). The red longitudinal streak of Darier's may also be mimicked by a warty dyskeratoma (Higashi 1990; Baran & Perrin 1997).

According to Zaias and Ackerman (1973), all constituents of the nail unit may be affected histologically in Darier's disease. The findings in the nail bed, however, differ in three respects

from those in the skin by the absence of suprabasilar clefts, the presence of multinucleated epithelial giant cells and the absence of inflammatory infiltrate. These characteristic changes lead to the diagnosis in the rare cases where Darier's disease is limited to the nails, which rarely appears before the age of 5 years (Bingham & Burrow 1984).

Differential diagnoses include occupational marks in manual labourers, lichen planus, X-ray damage, epiloia and onychomycosis (Ronchese 1965). Keratotic papules on the dorsal portion of the nail fold may resemble acrokeratosis verruciformis (Hopf) but, histologically, they demonstrate the features of Darier's disease (Zaias & Ackerman 1973). The nails in the former are pearly white in childhood (Fig. 5.63) and become horny, brown and grooved later in life (Niedelman & McKusick 1962). Red longitudinal streaks have been observed by Macfarlane *et al.* (2000) in a family presenting with

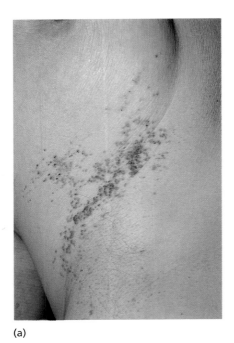

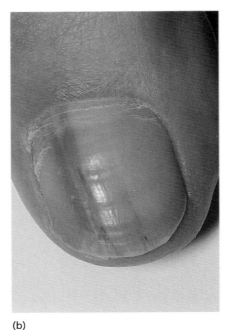

(a)                                                    (b)

**Fig. 5.64** (a) Acantholytic dyskeratotic epidermal linear naevus. (Courtesy of P.Y. Vénencie, France.) (b) Acantholytic dyskeratotic epidermal linear naevus with longitudinal reddish pigmentation of the nail. (Courtesy of N.H. Cox, UK.)

acrokeratosis verruciformis in whom they identified a mutation in the *ATP2A2* gene which is defective in Darier's disease. A solitary longitudinal white or red line may occur in persons with a tumour in the nail matrix or nail bed. More equivocal could be acantholytic epidermolysis bullosa presenting with white and red streaks mimicking bullous Darier's disease (Hoffman *et al.* 1995).

Topical breaks and distal notches of Darier's disease may be found on some fingernails or toenails in patients with unilateral keratotic papules present in streaks or in a whorled linear distribution consistent with Blaschko's lines (Munro & Cox 1992) which are thought to reflect cutaneous mosaicism. This hypothesis is supported by the report of a patient with an acantholytic dyskeratotic epidermal naevus associated with ipsilateral nail dystrophy and palmar pits, characteristic of Darier's disease (Cambiaghi *et al.* 1995). Another patient was reported, presenting unilateral keratotic papules in a distribution of Blaschko's lines associated with longitudinal white and/or red streaks and a distal notch in the three first fingernails of the same side (Vénencie & Dallot 1997) (Fig. 5.64).

Whether acantholytic dyskeratotic epidermal naevus and unilateral Darier's disease (Jorda *et al.* 1996; Tarlé *et al.* 1997) are the same condition is, however, still debatable.

In Hailey–Hailey disease, Burge (1992) observed longitudinal white bands in more than half of the 44 patients examined, but in contrast to Darier's disease, the 'sandwich' of red and white lines, pathognomonic of this condition and nail fragility, are not features and the nail changes are asymptomatic. Longitudinal leuconychia may be the first clue to the diagnosis of Hailey–Hailey disease (Kirtschig *et al.* 1992) (Fig. 5.65).

Oral aromatic retinoids are effective on the keratotic papules

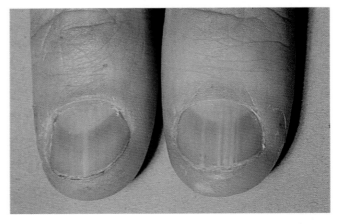

**Fig. 5.65** Hailey–Hailey disease—longitudinal white bands. (Courtesy of S. Burge, UK.)

of the proximal nail fold but the nail lesions are not improved by treatment (Burge *et al.* 1981). In some cases Darier's disease seems to be a partially immunodeficient state (Jegasothy & Humeniuk 1981), which could explain the recurrent pyoderma to which the nail area is particularly vulnerable.

The nail bed epithelium is hyperplastic, giving rise to subungual parakeratosis which may be 10–30 cells thick. The nuclei of the nail bed epithelium vary in size and shape and abundant multinucleate keratinocytes are found throughout the nail bed. In contrast to epidermal dyskeratosis follicularis lesions there are usually neither suprabasilar acantholytic clefts nor multinucleate epithelial giant cells, and the inflammatory infiltrate is nearly absent. The longitudinal red streaks are due to vasodilatation.

Matrix involvement results in parakeratotic layers in the nail plate and causes longitudinal white streaks. Multinucleate keratinocytes are included in the parakeratotic nail. The nail plate surface is altered when the most proximal part of the matrix is affected. Cleft formation may occur in the junction of the matrix and the undersurface of the proximal nail fold. Lesions on the proximal nail fold are identical to those of the epidermis.

## References

Baran, R. & Perrin, C. (1995) Localized multinucleate distal subungual keratosis. *British Journal of Dermatology* **133**, 77–82.

Baran, R. & Perrin, C. (1997) Focal subungual warty dyskeratoma. *Dermatology* **195**, 278–280.

Bingham, E.A. & Burrow, D. (1984) Darier's disease. *British Journal of Dermatology* **111** (Suppl. 26), 88–89.

Burge, S. (1992) Hailey–Hailey disease: the clinical features, response to treatment and prognosis. *British Journal of Dermatology* **126**, 275–282.

Burge, S.M. & Wilkinson, J.D. (1992) Darier–White disease: a review of the clinical features of 163 patients. *Journal of the American Academy of Dermatology* **27**, 40–50.

Burge, S.M., Wilkinson, J.D., Miller, A.J. & Ryan, T.J. (1981) The efficacy of an aromatic retinoid in the treatment of Darier's disease. *British Journal of Dermatology* **104**, 675–680.

Cambiaghi, S., Brusasco, A., Grimalt, R. *et al.* (1995) Acantholytic dyskeratotic epidermal naevus as a mosaic form of Darier's disease. *Journal of the American Academy of Dermatology* **32**, 284–286.

Downs, A.M., Ward, K.A. & Peachey, R.D. (1997) Subungual squamous cell carcinoma in Darier's disease. *Clinical and Experimental Dermatology* **22**, 277–279.

Higashi, N. (1990) Focal acantholytic dyskeratosis. *Hifu* **32**, 507–510.

Hoffman, M.D., Fleming, G. & Pearson, R.W. (1995) Acantholytic epidermolysis bullosa. *Archives of Dermatology* **131**, 586–589.

Jegasothy, B.V. & Humeniuk, J.M. (1981) Darier's disease, a partially immunodeficient state. *Journal of Investigatve Dermatology* **76**, 129–132.

Jorda, E., Revert, A., Montesinos, E. *et al.* (1996) Unilateral Darier's disease. *International Journal of Dermatology* **35**, 288–289.

Kirtschig, G., Effendy, I. & Happle, R. (1992) Leuconychia longitudinalis als ein Leitsymptom des Morbus Hailey–Hailey. *Hautarzt* **43**, 451–452.

Macfarlane, C.S., McSween, R., Sakuntabhal, A. *et al.* (2000) Acrokeratosis of Hopf is caused by mutation in *ATP2A2*, the gene which is defective in Darier's disease. *British Journal of Dermatology* **143** (Suppl. 57), 47.

Munro, C.S. (1992) The phenotype of Darier's disease: penetrance and expressivity in adults and children. *British Journal of Dermatology* **127**, 126–130.

Munro, C.S. & Cox, N.H. (1992) An acantholytic dyskeratotic epidermal naevus with other features of Darier's disease on the same site of the body. *British Journal of Dermatology* **127**, 168–171.

Munro, C.S. & MacLeod, R.I. (1991) Variable expression of the Darier's disease gene. *British Journal of Dermatology* **125** (Suppl. 38), 37.

Niedelman, M.L. & McKusick, V.A. (1962) Acrokeratosis verruciformis (Hopf), a follow-up study. *Archives of Dermatology* **86**, 779–782.

Ronchese, F. (1965) The nail in Darier's disease. *Archives of Dermatology* **91**, 617–618.

Savin, J.A. & Samman, P.D. (1970) The nail in Darier's disease. *Medical Biology Illinois* **20**, 85–88.

Tarlé, R.G., Tarlé, S.F., Neto, J.F. *et al.* (1997) Doença de Darier unilateral ou nevo epidérmico disceratosico acantolitico? *Anales Brasiliera de Dermatologia* **72**, 37–39.

Vénencie, P.Y. & Dallot, A. (1997) Acantholytic dyskeratotic epidermal nevus: a mosaic form of Darier's disease? *Annales de Dermatologie et de Vénéréologie* **126**, 829–830.

Zaias, N. & Ackerman, A.B. (1973) The nail in Darier–White disease. *Archives of Dermatology* **107**, 193–199.

## Porokeratosis of Mibelli (Fig. 5.66)

The nails, only rarely affected in this condition, may be thickened, opaque, ridged, fissured or partially destroyed. After nail loss the nail bed shows only warty debris. This appearance has been described by Respighi (1893) as 'hyperkeratosis eccentrica atrophicans'. The nail changes may also resemble those of impaired peripheral circulation (Samman & Fenton 1986). Soft atrophic nails with pigmentation of the free edges were described by Franks and Davis (1943). Involvement of a toenail resembling an onychomycosis was accompanied by lesions of buccal mucosa in a case of generalized porokeratosis of Mibelli (Kobayasi 1934).

Linear porokeratosis may involve the dorsal aspect of the digits (Rahbari *et al.* 1974).

## References

Franks, A. & Davis, J. (1943) Porokeratosis (Mibelli). *Archives of Dermatology* **48**, 50.

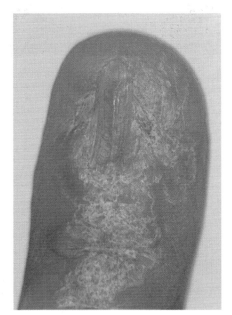

**Fig. 5.66** Porokeratosis of Mibelli. (Courtesy of J.L. Verret, France.)

Kobayasi (1934) Generalized porokeratosis of Mibelli with lesions of the buccal mucosa and of the nails. *Japanese Journal of Dermatology and Urology* **36**, 439.

Rahbari, H., Cordero, A.A. & Mehregan, A.H. (1974) Linear porokeratosis a distinctive clinical variant of porokeratosis of Mibelli. *Archives of Dermatology* **109**, 526–528.

Respighi, E. (1893) Di une ipercheratosi non ancora descritta. *Giornale Italiano di Dermatologia e Venereologia* **28**, 356.

Samman, P.D. & Fenton, D. (1986) *The Nails in Disease*, 4th edn. Heinemann, London.

## Stevens–Johnson syndrome (erythema multiforme) (Fig. 5.67)

Any drug that may induce bullae can cause nail changes or nail loss due to damage to the nail matrix. Erythema and oedema of the proximal nail often occur (Huff 1985). In some cases sloughing of the whole nail is possible with eventual regrowth (Wentz & Seiple 1947). In others, after discharge, all the nails are shed resulting in cicatricial anonychia and pterygium (Lyell 1967; Wanscher & Thomsen 1977; Hansen 1984).

In a review of 81 cases of erythema multiforme, Ashby and Lazar (1951) called attention to the fact that paronychia, as well as shedding of the nails (Fig. 5.67b), may be seen in cases of Stevens–Johnson syndrome. This was confirmed by Coursin (1966).

### References

Ashby, D.W. & Lazar, T. (1951) Erythema multiforme exsudativum major (Stevens–Johnson syndrome). *Lancet* **i**, 1091.

Coursin, D.B. (1966) Stevens–Johnson syndrome, nonspecific parasensitivity reaction. *Journal of the American Medical Association* **198**, 133.

Hansen, R.C. (1984) Blindness, anonychia and mucosal scarring as sequellae of the Stevens–Johnson syndrome. *Pediatric Dermatology* **1**, 298–300.

Huff, J.C. (1985) Erythema multiforme. *Dermatologic Clinics* **3**, 141–152.

Lyell, A. (1967) A review of toxic epidermal necrolysis in Britain. *British Journal of Dermatology* **79**, 662–671.

Wanscher, B. & Thomsen, K. (1977) Permanent anonychia after Stevens–Johnson syndrome. *Archives of Dermatology* **113**, 970.

Wentz, H.S. & Seiple, H.H. (1947) Stevens–Johnson syndrome, a variation of erythema multiforme exsudativum (Hebra). A report of two cases. *Annals of Internal Medicine* **26**, 277.

## Toxic epidermal necrolysis

In a case of junctional naevi following toxic epidermal necrolysis (Burns & Sarkany 1978), fingernails and toenails which had been shed during the acute episode failed to regrow, there was pterygium formation affecting most of the digits. Similar effects have been reported following phenylbutazone (Lyell 1967).

### References

Burns, D.A. & Sarkany, I. (1978) Junctional naevi following toxic epidermal necrolysis. *Clinical and Experimental Dermatology* **3**, 323.

Lyell, A. (1967) A review of toxic epidermal necrolysis in Britain. *British Journal of Dermatology* **79**, 662–671.

## Acroosteolysis (Fig. 5.68)

The term acroosteolysis describes the occurrence of destructive changes of the distal phalangeal bone. The cutaneous signs of acroosteolysis range from bulbous fingertips with soft tissue thickening associated with pseudoclubbing to severe destruction of the digits and metacarpal or metatarsal bones (Meyerson & Meier 1972). Shortening of the distal phalanges

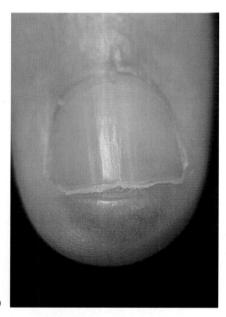

(a)

(b)

**Fig. 5.67** (a) Erythema multiforme. (b) Latent onychomadesis leading to nail shedding after Stevens–Johnson syndrome. (Courtesy of A. Krebs.)

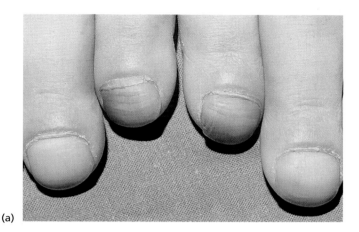

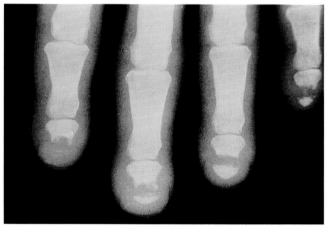

(a)

(b)

**Fig. 5.68** (a) Acroosteolysis due to vinyl chloride disease. (Courtesy of G. Moulin, France.) (b) Characteristic radiological pattern for vinyl chloride disease (same patient).

causes the nails to appear abnormally broad (acquired racquet nails). Koilonychia may be observed. Pincer nail deformity has occurred after traumatic acroosteolysis. In severe cases the nail unit can be destroyed.

Toes are frequently affected in diseases that are characterized by neurosensory loss. Deformation and destruction of the digits is commonly accompanied by trophic changes in soft tissues and ulcerations (Phelip & Pras 1975; Queneau *et al.* 1982).

Functional symptoms such as acroparaesthesia, dull pain or vasospastic changes of the digits can be early manifestations of acroosteolysis. In familial acroosteolysis, pain is a conspicuous symptom. On radiographic examination, two varieties of acroosteolysis, which may occur together or independently, may be seen—transverse acroosteolysis and longitudinal acroosteolysis (Destouet & Murphy 1983; Kemp *et al.* 1986). In transverse acroosteolysis the distal phalangeal shaft shows a transverse lytic band, while the tuft and base are preserved.

Fragmentation of the separated distal tuft can occur with near total loss of the tuft, i.e. acronecrosis. In longitudinal acroosteolysis, terminal resorption of the distal end of the

phalanx progressively results in a 'licked candystick' appearance of phalangeal, metacarpal or metatarsal bones. The transverse radiological pattern is characteristic for vinyl chloride disease, renal osteodystrophy, idopathic-non-familial acroosteolysis and familial acroosteolysis. In longitudinal acroosteolysis, which may be observed in scleroderma, hyperparathyroidism, psoriasis, neurological disorders and frostbite, cystic changes and irregularity of the distal tufts can be followed by severe bone resorption resulting in pencilling of the phalanges. Progressive destruction of the bone produces peg-shaped phalanges.

Acroosteolysis can be idiopathic (familial or non-familial) or it can occur in association with a number of metabolic, neuropathic and collagen disorders (Table 5.6). It may also be a feature of several vascular disorders including atherosclerosis, Burger's disease, ainhum and progeria.

Idiopathic acroosteolysis includes a number of different disorders which can be distinguished according to the presence or absence of genetic transmission and the association with familial renal disease, neuropathy and ulcerative skin lesion (Elias *et al.* 1978). A large number of diseases which involve neurosensory loss can result in acroosteolysis. These include lepromatous leprosy, diabetic neuropathy, tabes dorsalis, syringomyelia, familial as well as non-familial mutilant ulcerative acropathy (Thévenard's disease, Bureau–Barrière's disease) and congenital insensitivity to pain syndrome (Phelip & Pras 1975; Queneau *et al.* 1982). Acroosteolysis can also be observed in patients with infective, inflammatory, neoplastic or mechanical processes that involve the spine, Raynaud's phenomenon or scleroderma. Reversible occupational acroosteolysis that may be associated with Raynaud's phenomenon and sclerodermatous skin changes has been observed in 3–4% of the workers involved in the polymerization of vinyl chloride (Wilson *et al.* 1967). A genetic susceptibility to vinyl choride disease has been suggested by HLA studies. In addition, acrosteolysis can complicate the course of some rheumatological disorders, such as rheumatoid arthritis or psoriasic arthropathy. Acromegaly and hyperparathyroidism also cause bone resorption leading to acroosteolysis (Phelip & Pras 1975; Destouet & Murphy 1983; Kemp *et al.* 1986). The pathogenesis of acroosteolysis is still unknown. The occurrence of acroosteolysis after thermal or biomechanical injuries, as well as in association with vascular or neurological disorders, supports the view that different noxious events can induce the development of this condition. Vascular occlusion possibly plays a major role in the development of bone destruction. The hypothesis that vascular occlusion represents the common pathogenetic event for all the different varieties of acroosteolysis has been suggested (Elias *et al.* 1978; Scher 1986).

## References

Baran, R. & Tosti, A. (1993) Acroosteolysis in a guitar player. *Acta Dermato-Venereologica* 73, 64–65.

**Table 5.6** Causes of acroosteolysis. (From Baran & Tosti 1993.)

Acrodermatitis continua Hallopeau
Acromegaly
Adjuvant
Burea–Barrière's disease
Burger's disease
Carpal tunnel syndrome
Collagen disease
   Mixed connective tissue disease
   Polymyositis
   Scleroderma
   Rheumatoid arthritis
   Sjögren's syndrome
Congenital insensitivity to pain syndrome
Diabetic neuropathy
Ehlers–Danlos syndrome
Epidermolysis bullosa
Gout
Hyperparathyroidism
Ichthyosiform erythroderma
Infection
Juvenile hyalin fibromatosis
Leprosy
Metastases
Mucopolysaccharidoses
Multicentric reticulohistiocytosis
Neoplasms
Nutritional deficiencies
Pachydermoperiostosis
Physical injuries
   Burns
   Frostbite
   Fulguration
   Mechanical stress (guitar players)
Pycnodysostosis
Porphyria
Psoriatic arthritis
Progeria
Raynaud's disease
Renal osteodystrophy
Rothmund's syndrome
Sarcoidosis
Self-mutilation after spinal cord injury
Sezary's syndrome
Spine tumours
Syphilis
Syringomyelia
Tabes dorsalis
Thèvenard's disease
Vascular diseases
   Ainhum
   Atherosclerosis
   Burger's disease
Van Bogaert–Hazay syndrome
Vinyl chloride disease
Werner's syndrome

Destouet, J.M. & Murphy, W.A. (1983) Acquired acroosteolysis and acronecrosis. *Arthritis and Rheumatism* **26**, 1150–1154.

Elias, A.N., Pinals, R.S., Anderson, H.C. *et al.* (1978) Hereditary osteodysplasia with acro-osteolysis (the Hajdu–Cheney syndrome). *American Journal of Medicine* **65**, 627–636.

Kemp, S.S., Dalinka, M.K. & Schumacher, H.R. (1986) Acro-osteolysis. Etiologic and radiological considerations. *Journal of the American Medical Association* **255**, 2058–2061.

Meyerson, L.B. & Meier, G.C. (1972) Cutaneous lesions in acroosteolysis. *Archives of Dermatology* **106**, 224.

Phelip, X. & Pras, P. (1975) Les acro-ostéolyses. *Rheumatologie* **49**, 325–333.

Queneau, P., Gabbai, A., Perpoint, B. *et al.* (1982) Acro-ostéolyses au cours de la lèpre. *Revue de Rheumatisme* **49**, 111–119.

Scher, R.K. (1986) Acroosteolysis and the nail unit [letter]. *British Journal of Dermatology* **115**, 638–639.

Wilson, R.H., McCormick, W.E., Tatus, C.F. *et al.* (1967) Occupational acrosteolysis. *Journal of the American Medical Association* **201**, 577.

## Acrokeratoelastoidosis

The keratotic lesions of this rare condition may be seen over the knuckles and the nail folds (Highet *et al.* 1982).

### Reference

Highet, A.S., Rook, A. & Anderson, J.R. (1982) Acrokeratoelastoidosis. *British Journal of Dermatology* **106**, 337.

## Pityriasis lichenoides acuta (Fig. 5.69)

In a case of acute 'vasculitic' and necrotic variety of pityriasis lichenoides acuta, permanent nail dystrophy occurred.

## Punctate keratoderma

Patients with palmoplantar keratoderma may exhibit nail changes that are commonly associated with diffuse palmoplantar keratoderma. Onychogryphosis, nail thickening, subungual hyperkeratosis, longitudinal fissures and onychomadesis have all been reported (Poppa & Santini 1965; Stone & Mullins 1965; Schirren & Dinger 1966). Tosti *et al.* (1993) have observed nail abnormalities which were suggestive of psoriasis in two patients, where punctate palmoplantar keratoderma and psoriatic nail and skin changes coincided. Subungual hyperkeratosis was a prominent feature, but onycholysis, splinter haemorrhages and pitting were also present. Pathological study of the nail bed and nail matrix revealed sharply limited columns of hyperkeratosis associated with hypergranulosis and depression of the underlying nail bed epidermis.

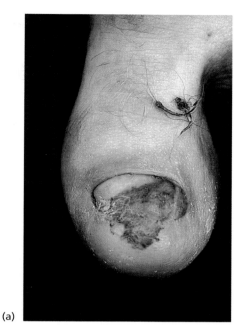

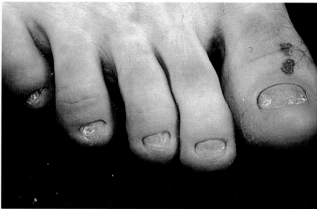

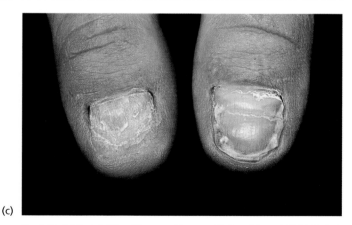

(a)

(b)

(c)

**Fig. 5.69** (a) Pityriasis lichenoides acuta. (Courtesy of R. Russell-Jones, UK.) (b) Pityriasis lichenoides acuta (same patient.) (c) Pityriasis lichenoides acuta (same patient).

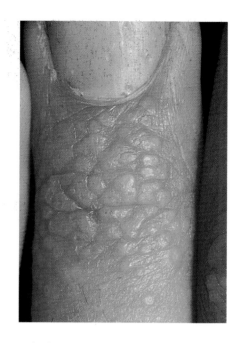

**Fig. 5.70** Granuloma annulare—perforating variety. (Courtesy of C.P. Sanlaska, USA.)

Etretinate therapy, which produced a significant improvement in the palmoplantar keratoderma, was of no apparent value in treating nail keratoderma.

### References

Poppa, A. & Santini, R. (1965) Cheratodermia plamo-plantare punctata di Brauer-Buschke-Fischer. Keratoderma dissipatum hereditarium palmo-plantare di Brauer. *Giornale Italiano di Dermatologia e Venereologia* **125**, 527–558.

Schirren, A. & Dinger, R. (1966) Untersuchunen bei Keratosis palmoplantaris papulosa. *Archives of Clinical and Experimental Dermatology* **221**, 481.

Stone, O.J. & Mullins, J.F. (1965) Nail changes in keratosis punctata. *Archives of Dermatology* **92**, 557–558.

Tosti, A., Morelli, R., Fanti, P.A. *et al.* (1993) Nail changes of punctate keratoderma, a clinical and pathological study of two patients. *Acta Dermato-Venereologica* **73**, 66–68.

### Granuloma annulare

The classical features of granuloma annulare include single or multiple flesh-coloured papules and expanding annular plaques that are composed of small papules on the extremities. Atypical changes such as pseudochromic paronychia have been observed (Fig. 5.70).

Generalized perforating granuloma annulare (Samlaska *et al.* 1992) is characterized by 1–4-mm umbilicated papules on the extremities, and is most commonly seen in children and young adults. Transepithelial elimination of mucinous, degenerating collagen fibres and surrounding palisading lymphohistiocytic granulomas are important histological features—perforating sarcoidosis may be difficult to rule out.

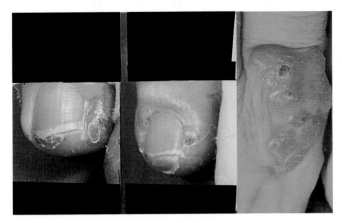

**Fig. 5.71** Erythema elevatum diutinum. (Courtesy of R. Caputo, Italy.)

## Reference

Samlaska, C.P., Sandberg, G.D., Maggio, K.L. *et al.* (1992) Generalized perforating granuloma annulare. *Journal of the American Academy of Dermatology* 27, 319–322.

## Erythema elevatum diutinum

This rare condition consists of persistent symmetrical red- or rust-coloured and purple plaques affecting the backs of the hands and other extensor surfaces overlying joints (Ryan 1992). Smaller annular lesions on the extensor aspects of the hands or lesions of the proximal nail fold have also been observed (Fig. 5.71). Subungual haemorrhage, onycholysis and paronychia have been reported in a case associated with B-cell lymphona (Futei & Konohara 2000).

## References

Futei, Y. & Konohara, I. (2000) A case of erythema elevatum diutinum associated with B-cell lymphoma: a rare distribution involving palms, soles and nails. *British Journal of Dermatology* 142, 116–119.

Ryan, T.J. (1992) Cutaneous vasculitis. In: *Rook/Wilkinson/Ebling Textbook of Dermatology* (eds R.H. Champion, J.L. Burton & F.J.G. Ebling), pp. 1893–1962, 5th edn. Blackwell Scientific Publications, Oxford.

# CHAPTER 6

# The nail in systemic diseases and drug-induced changes

## A. Tosti, R. Baran & R.P.R. Dawber

**Cardiac and circulatory disorders**

Cardiac disorders

*Clubbing (see also Chapter 2)*

*Cardiac failure*

*Bacterial endocarditis*

Circulation disorders

*Raynaud's phenomenon and Raynaud's disease*

*Acrocyanosis*

*Cutaneous reaction to cold*

*Perniosis (chilblains)*

*Erythromelalgia*

*Venous disease*

*Splinter haemorrhages*

*Gangrene*

*Ainhum and pseudoainhum*

**Connective tissue diseases**

Nail fold capillary microscopy

Systemic sclerosis

Systemic lupus erythematosus

Dermatomyositis

Rheumatoid arthritis

Antisynthetase syndrome

Wegener's granulomatosis

Periarteritis nodosa

Microscopic polyarteritis

Multicentric reticulohistiocytosis

Follicular mucinosis (alopecia mucinosa)

Fibroblastic rheumatism

Osteoarthritis

**Respiratory disorders**

Hypertrophic pulmonary osteoarthropathy

Yellow nail syndrome

Shell nail syndrome

Sarcoidosis

Bronchial carcinoma

Asthma

Smoking cessation

**Renal disorders**

Muehrcke's lines

Haemodialysis

Leuconychia and renal failure

Renal transplantation

Half-and-half nails

Henoch-Schöenlein purpura

Nail–patella syndrome

Acro-renal-ocular syndrome

Yellow nail syndrome and renal disorders

**Hepatic disorders**

Viral hepatitis

Cirrhosis

Wilson's disease

Haemochromatosis

**Gastrointestinal disorders**

Clubbing

Ulcerative colitis

Peutz–Jeghers–Touraine syndrome

Cronkhite–Canada syndrome

Plummer–Vinson (Patterson–Kelly–Brown) syndrome

Crohn's disease

Pyodermatitis-pyostomatitis vegetans

*Helicobacter pylori* infection

**Nutritional disorders and deficiencies**

Pellagra

Vitamin A deficiency

Vitamin C deficiency

Vitamin $B_{12}$ deficiency

Zinc deficiency

Selenium deficiency

Calcium deficiency

Fetal alcohol syndrome

Iron deficiency

Malnutrition

**Endocrine disorders**

Hypogonadism

Pituitary disease

Adrenal disease

Parathyroid disease

Thyroid disease

Pregnancy and menstrual factors

**Metabolic disorders**

Diabetes

Hyperoxaluria

Cystic fibrosis

Hartnup disease

Histidinaemia

Lipoid proteinosis (Urbach–Wiethe disease)

Dyslipoproteinaemias

Fabry's disease

Gout

Lesch-Nyhan syndrome

Alkaptonuria

Homocystinuria

Fucosidosis

Porphyria

Amyloidosis

**Nervous disorders**

Hereditary

Phacomatoses

Syringomyelia

Hemiplegia

Spinal cord injuries

Congenital abscence of pain

Peripheral neuropathies

Cervical rib syndrome

Carpal tunnel syndrome

Peripheral nerve injuries

Reflex sympathetic dystrophy (algodystrophy, causalgia)

Other central nervous system disorders

Migraine

Psychological and psychiatric disorders

**Immunological disorders**

Primary immunological deficiency syndromes

Therapeutic immunosuppression

Graft-versus-host disease

Behçet's disease

HIV diseases and the acquired immune deficiency syndrome

Low interleukin 2 levels

**Infectious diseases (see Chapters 4 and 7)**

Malaria

Kawasaki disease (mucocutaneous lymph node syndrome)

Hand, foot and mouth disease

Cutaneous diphtheria

**Haematological disorders**

Polycythaemia

Essential thrombocythaemia

Haemoglobinopathies

Anaemias

Hereditary haemorrhagic telangiectasia (Osler syndrome)

Leukaemias

Plasmocytoma

Lymphoma

Hodgkin's diseases

Gamma heavy chain disease

Cryoglobulinaemia

Afibrinogenaemia

Complement type 2 deficiency

Extrinsic clotting system disturbance

**Neoplastic disorders**

Langerhans' cell histiocytosis

Juvenile xanthogranuloma

Nail changes and paraneoplastic disorders

Acrokeratosis paraneoplastica of Bazex and Dupré

Glucagonoma syndrome

Lung neoplasm

Acanthosis nigricans

Digital ischaemia

Papuloerythroderma

Breast carcinoma

Leiomyosarcoma

Multicentric reticulohistiocytosis

Nasopharyngeal carcinoma

Gastrointestinal malignancy

Castleman's tumour

Cowden's disease

Metastases (see Chapter 11)

Leukaemias

Plasmocytoma

Lymphoma

HTLV-1 positive cutaneous T-cell lymphoma

Hodgkin's disease

**Systemic drugs**

Nail clipping for monitoring previous exposure to drugs or poisons

Drug-induced photoonycholysis

Nail changes associated with drug-induced erythroderma

Nail changes associated with exposure to systemic medications in early pregnancy

Drugs acting on the central nervous system

*Anticonvulsant drugs*

*Benzodiazepines*

*Tricyclic antidepressants*

*Phenothiazines*

*Lithium carbonate*

*Buspirone*

*L-Dopa*

*Clomipramine*

*Cocaine*

Retinoids

*Liarozole*

*Psoralens*

Antimicrobial agents
  *Tetracyclines*
  *Cephalosporin*
  *Chloramphenicol*
  *Clofazimine*
  *Quinolones*
  *Roxithromycin*
  *Sulphonamides*
  *Dapsone*
  *Emetine*
Antiretroviral drugs
  *Didanosine*
  *Lamivudine*
  *Azidothymidine (AZT, zidovudine)*
  *Protease inhibitors*
Antifungals
  *Itraconazole*
  *Fluconazole*
  *Ketoconazole*
  *Amorolfine*
Anti-inflammatory agents
  *Acetanilid*
  *Aspirin*
  *Benoxaprofen*
  *Ibuprofen*
  *Phenazopyridine*
Cardiovascular drugs
  *β-blockers*
  *Amiodarone*
  *Angiotensin-converting enzyme inhibitors*
  *Clonidine*
  *Calcium channel blockers*
  *Quinidine*
  *Amrinone*
  *Purgatives*
Intoxicants
  *Toxic oil syndrome*
  *Polychlorinated biphenyl intoxication*
  *Carbon monoxide*
  *Selenium*
  *Vinyl chloride*

Heavy metal intoxications
  *Arsenic*
  *Silver*
  *Mercury*
  *Gold*
  *Lead*
  *Thallium*
  *Aniline*
  *Chromium salts*
Anticoagulants
  *Warfarin*
Antimalarial agents
Hormones
  *Oral contraceptive pill*
  *Androgens*
  *Parathyroid extracts*
  *Cortisone*
  *Adrenocorticotropic hormone, melanocyte-stimulating hormone*
Cancer chemotherapeutic agents
Radiation
Pulse oximetry
Miscellaneous drugs
  *Antihistamines*
  *Carotene*
  *Cyclosporin*
  *Dimercaptosuccinic acid*
  *Diuretics*
  *Ergotamine*
  *Fluorine*
  *Gelatin, biotin, cystine, methionine*
  *Hydroquinone*
  *Iron*
  *Peloprenoic acid*
  *Penicillamine and bucillamine*
  *Phenylephrine*
  *Salbutamol*
  *L-Tryptophan*
  *Vitamin A*
  *Interferon alpha*

## Cardiac and circulatory disorders

### Cardiac disorders

**Clubbing** (see also Chapter 2)

In congenital cardiovascular diseases cyanosis and clubbing are common findings (Fig. 6.1). The regional distribution of clubbing and cyanosis (differential cyanosis) may give a clue to the identification of the specific abnormality (Chesler *et al.* 1968; Silverman & Hurst 1968) (Fig. 6.2).

Symmetrical clubbing and cyanosis of fingers and toes is diagnostic of congenital heart diseases with right to left shunt. Clubbing and cyanosis more evident on fingers than on toes

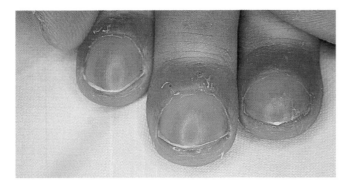

**Fig. 6.1** Congenital heart disease—clubbing with cyanosis.

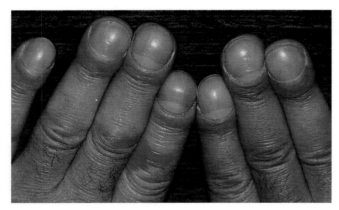

**Fig. 6.2** Clubbing of all digits with prominent Raynaud's phenomenon of the three fingers on the left. (Courtesy of L. Requena, Spain.)

suggests a complete transposition of the great vessels and a reversed shunt from the pulmonary artery into the aorta through a patent ductus arteriosus delivering oxygenated blood to the lower limbs. The anatomical proximity of the ductus to the left subclavian artery may result in differential cyanosis of the arms as well, since oxygenated blood from the pulmonary artery may enter the left subclavian artery through the ductus. The presence of coarctation or a complete interruption of the aortic arch may make the difference between upper and lower limbs more obvious. Unilateral clubbing has been reported in aneurysms of aortic arch, subclavian and innominate arteries.

Cyanosis and clubbing or hypertrophic osteoarthropathy of the lower extremities can occur secondary to a patent ductus arteriosus with reversal of blood flow. The left hand can manifest minimal cyanosis when the left subclavian artery receives unsaturated blood from the patent ductus. The right hand is normal.

Hypertrophic osteoarthropathy limited to the lower extremities can be the initial sign of an infected abdominal aortic graft associated with aortoenteric fistula (Dalinka *et al.* 1982; Sorin *et al.* 1990), but other manifestations such as Osler's nodes should be sought, because they represent another useful clue for the diagnosis of arterial graft sepsis.

In aortic regurgitation, flushing of the nail beds synchronized with the heart beat (Quincke pulsation) and the prominence of the proximal nail fold capillary loops are distinctive peripheral signs.

Red fingertips (tuft erythema) can be a sign of small or intermittent right to left shunts which cause a minimal reduction of the arterial oxygen saturation.

## References

Chesler, E., Moller, J.H. & Edwards, J.E. (1968) Anatomic basis for delivery of right ventricular blood into localised segments of the systemic arterial systemic arterial system: relation to differential cyanosis. *American Journal of Cardiology* **21**, 72–80.

Dalinka, M.K., Reginato, A.J., Berkowitz, H.D. *et al.* (1982) Hypertrophic osteoarthropathy as indication of aortic graft infection and aortoenteric fistula. *Archives of Surgery* **117**, 1355–1359.

Silverman, M.E. & Hurst, J.W. (1968) The hand and the heart. *American Journal of Cardiology* **22**, 718–728.

Sorin, S.B., Askari, A. & Rhodes, R.S. (1990) Hypertrophic osteoarthropathy of the lower extremities as a manifestation of arterial graft sepsis. *Arthritis and Rheumatism* **23**, 768–770.

## Cardiac failure

Suffusion or redness of the proximal portion of the half moons has been associated with cardiac failure (Terry 1954). Red lunulae, however, can also be observed in many other diseases, such as reumathoid arthritis, systemic lupus erythematosus, alopecia areata, hepatic cirrhosis, lymphogranuloma venereum, psoriasis, carbon monoxide poisoning, as well as reticulosarcoma and chronic obstructive pulmonary disease (Wilkerson & Wilkin 1989).

## References

Terry, R. (1954) Red half-moons in cardiac failure. *Lancet* ii, 842–844.

Wilkerson, M.G. & Wilkin, J.K. (1989) Red lunulae revisited: a clinical and histopathologic examination. *Journal of the American Academy of Dermatology* **20**, 453–457.

## Bacterial endocarditis

Petechiae are the most frequent manifestation of subacute bacterial endocarditis. Subungual splinter haemorrhages are a common sign as well, even though they are frequently observed in a wide variety of unrelated diseases (Chapter 10). Although splinter haemorrhages in subacute bacterial endocarditis have been described as painful and proximally located, sufficient data to confirm this are not available.

Osler's nodes (Fig. 6.3) can be an important clinical clue for the diagnosis of subacute bacterial endocarditis. These small red tender nodules precisely localized in the finger pulp or around the nails may develop over a period of anything from hours to days. Non-tender haemorrhagic or nodular lesions

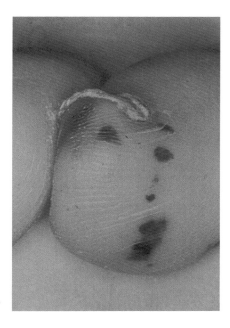

**Fig. 6.3** Bacterial endocarditis—Osler's nodes.

## References

Beylot, C., Castaing, R., Poisot, D. *et al.* (1974) 'Acral cyanosis' manifestation d'une coagulation intravasculaire disséminée au cours d'une endocardite bactérienne aigue. *Annales de Dermatologie et de Syphiligraphie* **101**, 375–382.

Cardullo, A.C., Silvers, D.N. & Grossman, M.E. (1990) Janeway lesions and Osler's nodes: a review of histopathologic findings. *Journal of the American Academy of Dermatology* **22**, 1088–1090.

Dellion, S., Cordoliani, F., Degos, C. *et al.* (1996) Cas pour diagnostic. *Annales de Dermatologie et de Vénéréologie* **123**, 125–126.

Kerr, A. & Tan, J. (1979) Biopsies of the Janeway lesion of infective endocarditis. *Journal Cutanea Pharmazeuten* **6**, 124–129.

Lerner, P.I. & Weinstein, L. (1966) Infective endocarditis in the antibiotic era. *New England Journal of Medicine* **274**, 259–266.

Parikh, S.K., Lieberman, A., Colbert, D.A. *et al.* (1996) The identification of methicillin-resistant *Staphylococcus aureus* in Osler's nodes and Janeway lesions of acute bacterial endocarditis. *Journal of the American Academy of Dermatology* **35**, 767–768.

Sahn, E.E., Bluestein, E. (1992) Purpuric palmar macule in a child with fever of unknown origin. *Archives of Dermatology* **128**, 681–686.

## Circulation disorders

In peripheral functional or organic arterial diseases the nail plates can present late dystrophic changes as a consequence of the reduced vascular supply to the fingers. Nails may become thin, brittle, longitudinally ridged and distally split. Onycholysis can be an additional feature. Platonychia or a tendency to koilonychia as well as apparent leuconychia often affect the proximal three-quarters of the nail plate. Beau's lines or even complete shedding of one or more nails (onychomadesis) can be observed. Thickening and distortion of the nail growth (onychogryphosis) may be a sign of impaired peripheral circulation in elderly persons (Samman & Strickland 1962; Sarteel *et al.* 1985).

In vasospastic conditions impaired peripheral flow may give rise to dorsal or ventral pterygium. Pterygium more frequently affects fingernails than toenails (Edwards 1948). Reduction of blood flow to less than 50% in the presence of a valid collateral supply results in irreversible damage to the microcirculation with critical ischaemia (Petruzzellis *et al.* 1997). In arterial obliteration periungual tissues are frequently involved with recurrent paronychia, fingertip ulceration or infection and pulp atrophy or gangrene. When gangrene sets in, nails usually become distorted and may finally be destroyed and replaced by scar tissue, if the digit survives.

Digital ischaemia is encountered in a large number of diseases. Many disorders give rise to digital ischaemia through vasospasm; other disorders that organically occlude the vessels often cause considerable secondary vasospasm (Edwards 1954).

In obstruction of large arteries such as in arteriosclerosis, thromboangiitis obliterans (Buerger's disease), Volkmann's contracture, neurovascular compression at the root of the upper limb (thoracic outlet or cervical rib, scalenus, costoclavicular,

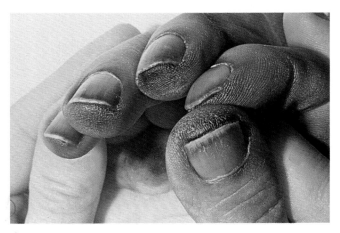

**Fig. 6.4** Acral cyanosis associated with disseminated intravascular coagulation. (Courtesy of Cl. Beylot, Bordeaux, France.)

on the palms and soles (Janeway lesions) are also suggestive of subacute bacterial endocarditis (Sahn & Bluestein 1992; Dellion *et al.* 1996). Although the pathogenesis of Osler's nodes and Janeway lesions is uncertain, septic microemboli are a possible cause. This hypothesis is supported by the pathological demonstration of neutrophilic dermal abscesses with clumps of gram-positive bacteria in the dermal vessels of typical Janeway lesions and Osler's nodes (Kerr & Tan 1979; Cardullo *et al.* 1990; Parikh *et al.* 1996). Finger clubbing may occur in 7–52% of patients. It is usually a late sign (Lerner & Weinstein 1966). Acral cyanosis (Fig. 6.4) evolving towards purpura and even necrosis has been reported during widespread intravascular coagulation complicating acute bacterial endocarditis (Beylot *et al.* 1974).

hyperabduction syndrome), neurovascular compression of the lower limb (popliteal artery entrapment syndrome), digital ischaemia and gangrene usually affect a single limb (Dorazio & Ezzet 1979; Ferrero *et al.* 1980; De Palma & Broadbent 1981; Kerdel 1984; Eagle 1996). In Buerger's disease, ulceration and gangrene can develop at the sides of the nails or the tips of the digits, especially after trauma. In early phases of the disease, painful vesicles may develop in the digit pulp with intense hyperaemia and hypersensivity of the surrounding skin (Quenneville *et al.* 1981). Pseudo-whitlow resulting from finger arteritis can occur (Thiebot *et al.* 1990). Growth abnormalities of the nails are common (Giblin *et al.* 1989). Subungual splinter haemorrhages have been reported as an early symptom of Buerger's disease (Quenneville *et al.* 1984). Intermittent blue discoloration of the left extremity was reported to be the initial symptom of thoracic outlet syndrome in a 26-year-old woman (Oriba & Lo 1990).

Ischaemia affecting a single hand, especially the left, after acute coronary ischaemia, suggests a diagnosis of shoulder–hand syndrome due to reflex vasospasm. Loss of demarcation of the margin of the lunula (pseudomacrolunulae) can be a sign of hand ischaemia. Unilateral digital ischaemia may result from repetitive use of the hypothenar eminence as a hammer, which results in damage and thrombus formation in the ulnar artery and superficial palmar arch. The hypothenar hammer syndrome most commonly affects the 2nd, 3rd, 4th and 5th digits and is usually occupational (Duncan 1996).

In chronic digital ischaemia of the lower limbs the nail plate can be distorted, thickened, rough and darkened. Nail growth is frequently reduced and onychogryphosis may occur. Periungual hyperaesthesia which can accompany severe digital ischaemia should be differentiated from an ingrown toenail. Improvement of the circulation is usually followed by nearly normal growth of the nail plate (Samman & Strickland 1962).

Microembolization to the digital arteries from aortoiliac or femoropopliteal atheromatous plaques can cause an acute digital ischaemia (blue digit syndrome) which requires immediate surgical treatment in order to prevent limb gangrene (Lee *et al.* 1984; Sperandio & McCarthy 1988). Cholesterol embolism can also produce painful ischaemia of the toes, which may eventually progress to ulceration and gangrene. The affected digit is blue-purple in colour and painful, but peripheral pulses are always preserved and the digit is not cold. Cholesterol microembolism usually results from complications of aortic surgical procedures or aortic and left heart atherosclerosis and may be associated with treatment with anticoagulants (Hyman *et al.* 1987) and fibrinolytics. Clinical manifestations of cholesterol microembolism also include livedo reticularis of the lower limbs and abdomen and renal impairment. The prognosis is poor and no treatment has been proven effective. A biopsy of the affected toe reveals cholesterol crystals in the lumen of medium calibre arterioles. The diagnosis can be confirmed by an ophthalmological examination that reveals asymptomatic microemboli of the retinal vessels. Purple toe syndrome may

**Table 6.1** Mechanism and conditions leading to symmetrical peripheral gangrene.

| | |
|---|---|
| Hypotension | Cardiac failure of different origin |
| | Treatment with β-blocking agents |
| | Shock |
| Vasoconstriction | Frosbite |
| | Secondary Raynaud's phenomenon |
| | Shock |
| | Treatment with vasoactive agents, ergotamine, vasopressin, dopamine *and* chloroquine. |
| Endothelial damage | Arterial calcification: uraemia, oxalosis |
| | Bacterial sepsis |
| | Black foot disease |
| | Carbon monoxide poisoning |
| | Kaposi's sarcoma |
| | Rickettsiosis |
| | Treatment with bleomycin |
| | Vasculitis of different origin |
| | Viral diseases: hepatitis, measles, chickenpox, AIDS |
| Obliteration | Calciphylaxis |
| | Cholesterol embolism |
| | Chronic myelogeneous leukaemia |
| | Cold haemagglutinin disease |
| | Cryoglobulinaemia |
| | Disseminated intravascular coagulation |
| | Essential thrombocythaemia |
| | Heparin-induced thrombosis |
| | Hypernatraemic dehydration |
| | Hyperviscosity states |
| | Lupus erythematosus (Yang *et al.* 1996) |
| | Malaria |
| | Paraproteinaemia |
| | Polycythaemia vera |
| | Primary hyperoxaluria |
| | Septic embolism |
| | Sickle cell anaemia |
| | Thromboembolic occlusion |
| | Venous thrombosis |

Modified from Itin *et al.* (1986).

regress spontaneously or may progress to ulceration and necrosis. Cholesterol microembolization has also been associated with punctiform subungual haemorrhages of the fingers (Calhoun 1975; Lesenne *et al.* 1996; Vanhooteghem *et al.* 1996).

Ischaemic necrosis affecting simultaneously the distal parts of two or more limbs without obstruction of the great arteries (symmetrical peripheral gangrene) can be observed in a large number of diseases (Table 6.1) (Itin *et al.* 1986). Disseminated intravascular coagulation due to bacterial septicaemia (purpura fulminans) and dehydration due to acute gastrointestinal fluid loss are the most common causes of peripheral gangrene in children (Bass & Cywes 1989). Purpura fulminans may develop during the acute or convalescent phase of several bacterial and viral infections. Ecchymoses, haemorrhagic bullae and necrosis suddenly develop on the extremities and abdomen. Peripheral gangrene commonly occurs and the disease is often fatal (Benson *et al.* 1988). Hypotension, vasoconstriction, endothelial damage and vascular obstruction are possible pathogenetic mechanisms of symmetrical peripheral gangrene. Agglutination should be suspected when distal cyanosis is difficult to relieve by elevation or stroking. Symmetrical peripheral gangrene has also been described during the blast crisis in chronic myelogenous leukaemia, small blood vessels being occluded by large non-deformable myeloblasts (Frankel *et al.* 1987). Patients with cold haemagglutinin disease develop acrocyanosis or even symmetrical peripheral gangrene on exposure to cold as a consequence of vascular occlusion due to agglutinated red cells (Shelley & Shelley 1984). Thirty-six per cent of primary hyperoxaluria patients at European dialysis centres developed distal ischaemia and gangrene (Baethge *et al.* 1988). Secondary syphilis should also be included in the differential diagnosis of blue toe syndrome (Federman *et al.* 1994).

Extensive venous thrombosis of almost the entire venous system of an extremity can cause reversible tissue ischaemia or real gangrene without arterial or capillary occlusion (Hirschmann 1987). Blood flow within the arteries is arrested as a result of the high venous and intramuscular pressure.

The association of severe pain, extensive oedema, cyanosis and prominence of the superficial veins of a single limb are diagnostic of ischaemic acute venous thrombosis. When gangrene occurs, petechiae, purpura, bullae and finally blackened skin develop (Duschet *et al.* 1993).

Persistent digital ischaemia is an uncommon paraneoplastic syndrome. Gangrene can occasionally develop (Albin *et al.* 1986).

Digital gangrene has been occasionally described after ergotamine or β-blockers, as well as after the injection of large volumes of local anaesthetic, especially when adrenaline (epinephrine) is used. Dopamine hydrochloride is also responsible for symmetrical peripheral gangrene (Park *et al.* 1997). Digital necrosis and gangrene can be a consequence of fibrinogen replacement in patients with congenital afibrinogenaemia, a rare genetic disorder characterized by the complete absence of fibrinogen in the plasma (Rupee *et al.* 1996). It can also occur as a postoperative complication of digital cyanosis secondary to poor tissue handling or bandaging technique.

In pseudoxanthoma elasticum, ischaemic symptoms as well as ischaemic resorption of the terminal phalanges (acroosteolysis) can occur (Reed & Sugarman 1974).

## References

Albin, G., Lapeyre, A.C., Click, R.L. *et al.* (1986) Paraneoplastic digital thrombosis: a case report. *Angiology* 37, 203–206.

Baethge, B.A., Sanusi, I.D., Landreneau, M.D. *et al.* (1988) Livedo reticularis and peripheral gangrene associated with primary hyperoxaluria. *Arthritis and Rheumatism* 31, 1199–1203.

Bass, D.H. & Cywes, S. (1989) Peripheral gangrene in children. *Pediatric Surgery International* 4, 408.

Benson, M.P., Lupton, G.P., James, W.D. *et al.* (1988) Purpura and gangrene in a septic patient. Purpura fulminans secondary to pneumococcal sepsis. *Archives of Dermatology* 124, 1851.

Calhoun, P. (1975) Cholesterol emboli causing gangrene of the extremities. *Archives of Dermatology* 111, 1373–1375.

De Palma, R.G. & Broadbent, R.W. (1981) Management of occlusive disease of the subclavian and innominate arteries. *American Journal of Surgery* 142, 197–202.

Dorazio, R. & Ezzet, F. (1979) Arterial complications of the thoracic outlet syndrome. *American Journal of Surgery* 38, 246–250.

Duncan, W.C. (1996) Hypothenar hammer syndrome: an uncommon cause of digital ischemia. *Journal of the American Academy of Dermatology* 34, 880–883.

Duschet, P., Seifert, W., Halbmayer, W.M. *et al.* (1993) Ischemic venous thrombosis caused by a distinct disturbance of the extrinsic clotting system. *Journal of the American Academy of Dermatology* 28, 831–835.

Eagle, K. (1996) Thromboangiitis obliterans. *Massachussetts Medical Society Tome* 334, 891.

Edwards, E.A. (1948) Nail changes in functional and organic arterial disease. *New England Journal of Medicine* 239, 362–365.

Edwards, E.A. (1954) Varieties of digital ischemia and their management. *New England Journal of Medicine* 250, 709–717.

Federman, D.G., Valdivia, M. & Kirsner, R.S. (1994) Syphilis presenting as the 'Blue toe syndrome'. *Archives of Internal Medicine* 154, 1029–1031.

Ferrero, R., Barile, C., Bretto, P. *et al.* (1980) Popliteal artery entrapment syndrome. *Journal of Cardiovascular Surgery* 21, 45–52.

Frankel, D.H., Larson, R.A. & Lorincz, A.L. (1987) Acral lividosis: a sign of myeloproliferative diseases. *Archives of Dermatology* 123, 921–924.

Giblin, W., James, W.D. & Benson, P. (1989) Buerger's disease. *International Journal of Dermatology* 28, 638–642.

Hirschmann, J.V. (1987) Ischemic forms of acute venous thrombosis. *Archives of Dermatology* 123, 933–936.

Hyman, B.T., Landas, S.K., Ashman, R.F. *et al.* (1987) Warfarin related purple toes syndrome and cholesterol microembolization. *American Journal of Medicine* 82, 1233–1237.

Itin, P., Stalder, H. & Vischer, W. (1986) Symmetrical peripheral gangrene in disseminated tuberculosis. *Dermatologica* 173, 189–195.

Kerdel, F.A. (1984) Subclavian occlusive disease presenting a painful nail. *Journal of the American Academy of Dermatology* 10, 523–525.

Lee, B.Y., Brancato, R.F., Thoden, W.R. *et al.* (1984) Blue digit syndrome: urgent indication for digital salvage. *American Journal of Surgery* 147, 418–422.

Lesenne, M., Asseman, P.H., Bauchart, J.J. *et al.* (1996) Les embolies de cholesterol: un diagnostic souvent meconnu. *Artères et Veines* 15, 167–172.

Oriba, H.A. & Lo, J.S. (1990) Blue extremity: a cutaneous manifestation of thoracic outlet syndrome. *International Journal of Dermatology* 29, 385–386.

Park, J.Y., Kanzler, M. & Swetter, S. (1997) Dopamine-associated symmetric peripheral gangrene. *Archives of Dermatology* 133, 247–248.

Petruzzellis, V., Vadalá, P. & Di Vendra, G. (1997) Acral gangrene. *European Journal of Dermatology* 7, 399–404.

Quenneville, J.G., Prat, A. & Gossard, D. (1981) Subungueal-splinter haemorrhage an early sign of thromboangiitis obliterans. *Angiology* **32**, 424–432.

Reed, W.B. & Sugarman, G.I. (1974) Thermography in the study of pseudoxanthoma elasticum. *Cutis* **13**, 423–424.

Rupee, R.A., Kind, P. & Ruzicka, T. (1996) Cutaneous manifestations of congenital afibrinogenemia. *British Journal of Dermatology* **134**, 548–550.

Samman, P.D. & Strickland, B. (1962) Abnormalities of the finger nails associated with impaired peripheral blood supply. *British Journal of Dermatology* **74**, 165–173.

Sarteel, A.M., Merlen, J.F. & Larere, J. (1985) L'ongle en pathologie vasculaire. *Journal des Maladies Vasculaires* **10**, 199–206.

Shelley, W.B. & Shelley, E.D. (1984) Acrocyanosis of cold agglutinin disease successfully treated with antibiotics. *Cutis* **33**, 556–557.

Sperandio, C.P. & McCarthy, D.J. (1988) Digital arterial embolism—true blue toe syndrome. A histopathologic analysis. *Journal of the American Podiatric Medical Association* **78**, 593–598.

Thiebot, B., Lecrocq, C., Balguerie, X. *et al.* (1990) Neuf aspects de la pathologie du doigt. *Nouvelle Dermatologie* **9**, 340–345.

Vanhooteghem, O., Papadopoulos, T., Sass, U. *et al.* (1996) Clinical manifestations of cholesterol crystal embolism with subungual haemorrhages: a possible relationship? *Dermatology* **192**, 395–397.

Yang, S.G., Kim, K.H., Park, K.C. *et al.* (1996) A case of systemic lupus erythematous showing acute gangrenous change of finger tips. *British Journal of Dermatology* **134**, 185–187.

## Raynaud's phenomenon and Raynaud's disease
(Figs 6.5–6.9)

In Raynaud's disease bilateral symmetrical involvement of multiple digits is usually observed. The classic triphasic colour changes which characterize Raynaud's phenomenon consist of pallor—'white finger syndrome' (due to acute vasoconstriction) —followed by cyanosis and finally hyperaemia. Permanent cyanosis may be present in advanced cases. The nails are frequently thin, brittle, longitudinally ridged and split at the free edge. Koilonychia can be observed. Unilateral splinter haemor-

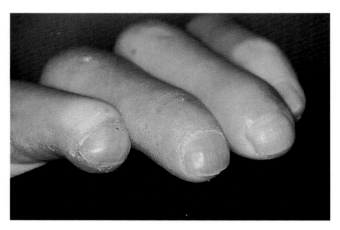

**Fig. 6.6** Raynaud's disease and acrosclerosis.

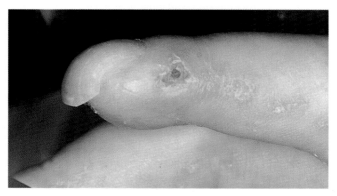

**Fig. 6.7** Raynaud's disease and acrosclerosis.

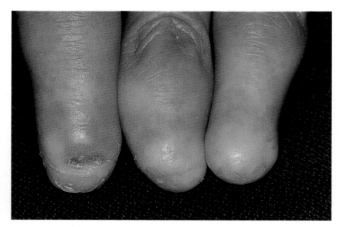

**Fig. 6.8** Severe acrosclerosis.

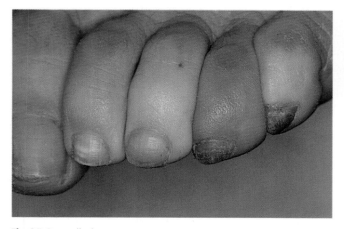

**Fig. 6.5** Raynaud's phenomenon.

rhages have been reported in two patients affected by unilateral Raynaud's phenomenon (Ramelet *et al.* 1982).

Dorsal or ventral pterygium, chronic paronychia, painful puckered ulcers of the fingertips and, rarely, gangrene are symptoms of severe Raynaud's disease. Massive digital necrosis resulting from severe Raynaud's phenomenon may be the first

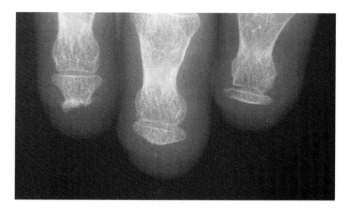

**Fig. 6.9** X-ray showing loss of terminal phalangeal bone in acrosclerosis.

manifestation of a collagen disease (Saban *et al.* 1991). The most useful signs for predicting the development of a collagen disease in patients with Raynaud's phenomenon are pitting scars of the digit pulp, puffy fingers, the presence of antinuclear antibodies and capillaroscopy changes (Mannarino *et al.* 1994). Nail fold capillaroscopy during cold exposure is able to discriminate between healthy people and patients with primary Raynaud's disease, but seems to be of minor value for follow-up evaluation of patients due to individual variations (Creutzig *et al.* 1997).

Physical examination, screening for antinuclear antibodies, capillaroscopy, and radiography of the hands and chest are useful in distinguishing Raynaud's disease from the early stage of systemic scleroderma. Asymmetrical involvement of a few digits suggests Raynaud's phenomenon secondary to arterial diseases. Other possible causes of Raynaud's phenomenon include drugs, occupation, haematological diseases, hepatitis B infection, neurovascular compression and tumours (Escudier *et al.* 1982; Kleinsmith 1985).

Management of Raynaud's disease includes avoidance of excessive exposure to cold, chemical and mechanical trauma, tobacco and consumption of some drugs such as β-blockers, ergotamine or oral contraceptives that can decrease cutaneous blood flow. So far no perfect treatment for Raynaud's disease has been developed. Biofeedback training and Pavlovian conditioning can be useful therapeutic tools (Jobe *et al.* 1985). Vasodilators such as nifedipine, prazosin, methyldopa and topical nitroglycerin can be prescribed when vasospastic phenomena are very frequent and prevent the patient from pursuing normal activities. More invasive treatments such as intra-arterial or intravenous reserpine, intravenous infusion of prostaglandin ($PGE_1$ and $PGE_2$) or low molecular weight dextran, plasmapheresis and cervicothoracic sympathectomy are still controversial. Microsurgical digital sympathectomy has been successfully utilized (Drake *et al.* 1992). Ketanserine, a selective antagonist of 5-hydroxytryptamine (5-HT, serotonin) is still experimental but might represent a hope for the future (Dowd 1986).

## References

Creutzig, A., Hiller, S., Appiah, R. *et al.* (1997) Nailfold capillaroscopy and laser Doppler fluxometry for evaluation of Raynaud's phenomenon: how valid is the local cooling test? *Vasa* **26**, 205–209.

Dowd, P.M. (1986) The treatment of Raynaud's phenomenon. *British Journal of Dermatology* **114**, 527–533.

Drake, D.B., Kesler, R.W. & Morgan, R.F. (1992) Digital sympathectomy for refractory Raynaud's phenomenon in an adolescent. *Journal of Rheumatology* **19**, 1286–1288.

Escudier, B., Barrier, J., Bletry, O. *et al.* (1982) Une cause rare d'artérite digitale avec phénomène de Raynaud et nécroses pulpaires: le virus B de l'hépatite. *Annales de Medecine Interne* **133**, 600–603.

Jobe, J.B., Beetham, W.P., Roberts, D.E. *et al.* (1985) Induced vasodilation as a home treatment for Raynaud's disease. *Journal of Rheumatology* **12**, 953–956.

Kleinsmith, D.A.M. (1985) Raynaud's syndrome: an overview. *Seminars in Dermatology* **4**, 104–113.

Mannarino, E., Pasqualini, L., Fedeli, F. *et al.* (1994) Nailfold capillaroscopy in the screening and diagnosis of Raynaud's phenomenon. *Angiology* **45**, 37–42.

Ramelet, A.A., Tscholl, R. & Monti, M. (1982) Association d'hématomes filiformes des ongles et d'un syndrome de Raynaud. *Annales de Dermatologie et de Vénéréologie* **109**, 655–659.

Saban, J., Rodriguez-Garcia, J.L., Pais, J.R. *et al.* (1991) Raynaud's phenomenon with digital necrosis as the first manifestation of undifferentiated connective tissue syndrome. *Dermatologica* **182**, 121–123.

## Acrocyanosis

In acrocyanosis persistent blue or reddish discoloration of the digits of the hands and/or feet is present. The nail bed reveals permanent cyanosis. Chronic paronychia and dystrophic changes of the nail plate can be observed. Nail fold capillary microscopy (Figs 6.10 & 6.11) shows dilated, tortuous and often thrombosed capillaries. Brittleness, roughness and transverse grooving may be present. Increased sweating favours the

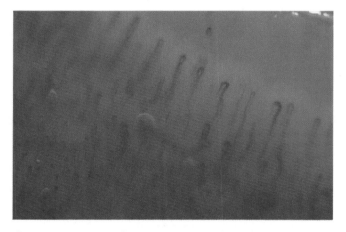

**Fig. 6.10** Acrocyanosis. Nail fold capillary microscopy—elongated, tortuous capillary loops.

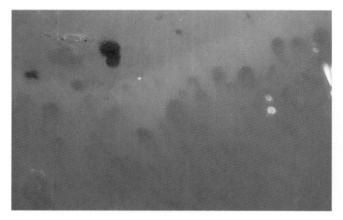

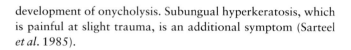

**Fig. 6.11** Acrocyanosis. Nail fold capillaries show dilatation, stasis and thrombosis of many vessels.

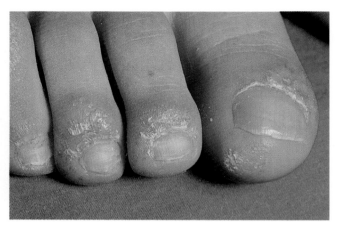

**Fig. 6.13** Chilblains (perniosis).

development of onycholysis. Subungual hyperkeratosis, which is painful at slight trauma, is an additional symptom (Sarteel *et al.* 1985).

### Reference

Sarteel, A.M., Merlen, J.F. & Larere, J. (1985) L'ongle en pathologie vasculaire. *Journal des Maladies Vasculaires* 10, 199–206.

### Cutaneous reaction to cold

Exposure to abnormal cold can damage the nail apparatus. Beau's lines and onychomadesis result from injury to the nail matrix. In severe frostbite, gangrene of the fingertips and toes may be seen (Corbett 1982) (Fig. 6.12). Epiphyseal destruction causing stunted growth and mild flexion deformity of the fingers has been described after frostbite in children (Nakazato & Ogino 1986).

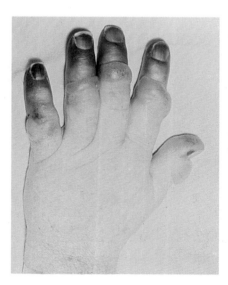

**Fig. 6.12** Gangrene due to frostbite. (Courtesy of Dr G. Webster, USA.)

### References

Corbett, D.W. (1982) Cold injuries. *Journal of the Association of Military Dermatology* 8, 34–40.
Nakazato, T. & Ogino, T. (1986) Epiphyseal destruction of children's hands after frostbite: a report of two cases. *Journal of Hand Surgery* 11A, 289–292.

### Perniosis (chilblains)

Perniosis represents an abnormal reaction to cold exposure. In acute perniosis, the lesions that are usually bilateral, symmetrical and self limiting are associated with an itching and burning sensation. Erythema, cyanosis and oedematous patches that change into tender blue nodules are seen on the extremities (Fig. 6.13). Vesicles, bullae, petechiae, haemorrhages and ulcers can occasionally occur in severe cases. In chronic perniosis the lesions begin as burning erythematous blue patches that develop into tender nodules and then into haemorrhagic bullae that rupture leaving shallow, slow-to-heal ulcers. Clinical variants of perniosis include annular, papular or pustular lesions. Herman *et al.* (1981) described painful red-purple macules, papules and plaques on the digits, predominantly on the toes, in nine women. They considered this disorder, which was histologically characterized by a lymphocytic vasculitis, to be a distinct variant of perniosis.

Elderly males presenting with perniosis should be investigated for a possible myelomonocytic leukaemia (Cliff *et al.* 1996).

### References

Cliff, S., James, S.L. & Mercieca, J.E. (1996) Perniosis—a possible association with a preleukaemic state. *British Journal of Dermatology* 135, 330–345.
Herman, E.W., Kezis, J.S. & Silvers, D.N. (1981) A distinctive variant of pernio. *Archives of Dermatology* 117, 26–28.

## Erythromelalgia

Erythromelalgia is a rate condition characterized by burning pain in the extremities associated with local erythema and warmth. Clinical symptoms are usually aggravated by exercise or warming. Acrocyanosis and gangrene of the digits can occasionally occur (Lorette & Machet 1991). Erythromelalgia may be apparently idiopathic or secondary to other conditions, most commonly myeloproliferative disorders. In secondary erythromelalgia, asymmetrical involvement of the extremities can be seen (Healsmith *et al.* 1991). Because erythromelalgia secondary to myeloproliferative disorders typically responds to a single low dose of aspirin, aspirin administration is often used for diagnostic purposes (Naldi *et al.* 1993).

## References

Healsmith, M.F., Graham-Brown, R.A.C. & Burns, D.A. (1991) Erythromelalgia. *Clinical and Experimental Dermatology* **16**, 46–48.
Lorette, G. & Machet, L. (1991) Erithromélalgie. *Annales de Dermatologie et de Vénéréologie* **118**, 739–742.
Naldi, L., Brevi, A., Cavalieri d'Oro, L. *et al.* (1993) Painful distal erythema and thrombocytosis. Erythromelalgia secondary to thrombocytosis. *Archives of Dermatology* **129**, 105–106.

## Venous disease

In chronic venous stasis and in postphlebitic venous stasis, clubbing of the toenails can be observed. Nails are thickened and darkened with a hyperplastic nail bed. Onychogryphosis frequently occurs. Nails are commonly infected by fungi, which are most often moulds (Sarteel *et al.* 1985).

## Reference

Sarteel, A.M., Merlen, J.F. & Larere, J. (1985) L'ongle en pathologie vasculaire. *Journal des Maladies Vasculaires* **10**, 199–206.

## Splinter haemorrhages

The longitudinal orientation of the capillary vessels in the nail bed explains the linear pattern of nail bed haemorrhages. The nature of Splinter haemorrhages (SH) is not clearly known (Wood 1956). They may result from emboli in the terminal vessels of the nail bed (Platts & Greaves 1958), which may be unilateral (Tobi & Kobrin 1981; Ramelet *et al.* 1982). The emboli may be septic (Fanning & Aronson 1977), or due to trauma of various types. They are more uncommon in the first three fingers of both hands.

The majority of SH originate within the distal third of the nail where the nail plate separates from the nail bed. In this region, special delicate 'spirally wound' capillaries produce the pink line normally seen through the nail, about 4 mm proximal to the tip of the finger. The rupture of these superficially located thin-walled vessels gives rise to linear haemorrhages looking

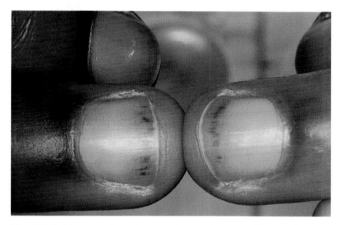

**Fig. 6.14** Splinter haemorrhages in systemic lupus erythematosus. (Courtesy of A. Pons, Paris.)

like wood splinters under the nails (Martin & Platts 1959). SH are contained in the basal layer of the nail plate and move superficially and distally with the growth of the nail; at this stage they can be scraped from the undersurface of the nail plate.

Proximal SH are rare. Although proximal splinters have been reported as a characteristic physical sign of subacute bacterial endocarditis, there are no published data to confirm this (Young *et al.* 1988).

SH involving the whole nail bed have been described in chronic mountain sickness, in cyanotic congenital heart disease, in congenital arteriovenous fistula of the lung and in a patient affected by a rectal cancer with hepatic metastasis (Alkiewicz & Paluszynski 1962; Heath *et al.* 1981). SH can be an early sign in patients with antiphospholipid syndrome (Fig. 6.14), where SH frequently develop in association with amaurosis fugax due to transient ischaemic attacks (TIA). SH are probably due to the formation of platelet thrombi within the small vessels of the nail bed (Asherson 1990; Ames *et al.* 1992; Francès *et al.* 1994a).

When first formed, SH appear as plum-coloured long thin linear structures, but darken to brown and then black in 1–2 days. SH have been observed in 26–56% of healthy subjects and trauma is the most common cause of this nail symptom. However, chronic persistence of SH independent of disease or trauma has been described (Miller & Vaziri 1979). Traumatic SH affects almost exclusively the fingernails (most commonly the right thumb) and are distally located and symptomless (Heath & Williams 1978; Monk 1980). The 'pen push' manoeuvre used in assessing pain responses is responsible for proximal nail bed haemorrhages in comatose patients (coma nails) (Pierson *et al.* 1993; Wijdicks & Schievink 1997).

There is a statistically greater incidence of SH in male patients compared with female patients, and in black people compared with white people (Kilpatrick *et al.* 1965). Although trauma is the most common cause, increased capillary fragility, microemboli and capillaritis have also been considered as possible mechanisms of SH formation (Young *et al.* 1988). The

**Table 6.2** Conditions associated with splinter haemorrhages.

Altitude (high)
Amyloidosis
Antiphospholipid syndrome
Arterial emboli
Arthritis (notably rheumatoid arthritis and rheumatic fever)
Behçet's disease
Blood dyscrasias (severe anaemia, thrombocytopenia)
Buerger's disease
Cirrhosis
Collagen diseases
Cryoglobulinaemia (with purpura)
Cystic fibrosis
Darier's disease
Diabetes mellitus
Drug reactions (especially with tetracyclines)
Eczema
Exfoliative dermatitis
Heart disease (notably uncomplicated mitral stenosis and subacute bacterial endocarditis)
Haemochromatosis
Haemodialysis and peritoneal dialysis
Hepatitis
Histiocytosis X
HIV infection
Hypertension
Hypoparathyroidism
Indwelling brachial artery cannula
Irradiation
Keratosis lichenoides chronica
Leukaemia
Malignant neoplasms
Mitral stenosis
Mycosis fungoides
Occupational hazards
Onychomycosis
Pemphigus
Peptic ulcer
Porphyria
Pityriasis rubra pilaris
Psittacosis
Psoriasis
Pterygium
Pulmonary disease
Radial artery puncture
Radiodermatitis
Raynaud's disease
Renal disease (chronic glomerulonephritis)
Osler's disease
Sarcoidosis
Scurvy
Septicaemia
Sweet's syndrome (Bochaton et al. 1997)
Thyrotoxicosis
Trauma
Trichinosis
Vasculitis

simultaneous appearance of SH in several nails, especially in females, should raise the suspicion of an underlying pathological disorder. Many conditions have been associated with the presence of SH (Table 6.2). In patients with subacute bacterial endocarditis, trichinosis or indwelling arterial catheters, SH can be associated with pain (Young *et al.* 1988). Between 10% and 30% of patients affected by trichinosis develop SH during the larval migrating phase of the infestation. Splinters, which are 2 mm wide and 4–5 mm long, appear initially red, then plum coloured and finally black (Fisher 1957). SH may result from emboli in the terminal vessels of the nail bed, for example in patients with major arterial embolus or mitral stenosis. SH associated with the hypereosinophilic syndrome may be a clinical marker of thrombosis preferentially involving the CNS (Francès *et al.* 1994b). Unilateral splinters may follow the insertion of catheters into the radial or brachial arteries even in the absence of catheter infection. SH were found to develop following radial puncture in a patient with antiphospholipid syndrome (Martens *et al.* 1996). Mountain climbers at high altitude can develop multiple SH which are probably a result of raised haemoglobin levels associated with repeated finger trauma (Heath & Williams 1978; Heath *et al.* 1981).

## References

Alkiewicz, J. & Paluszynski, J. (1962) Hématomes multiples filiformes intra-unguéaux. *Annales de Dermatologie et de Syphiligraphie* **89**, 47–51.

Ames, D.E., Asherson, R.A., Aynes, B. *et al.* (1992) Bilateral adrenal infarction, hypoadrenalism and splinter hemorrhages in the primary antiphospholipid syndrome. *British Journal of Rheumatology* **31**, 117–120.

Asherson, R.A. (1990) Subungual splinter haemorrhages: a new sign of antiphospholipid coagulopathy? *Annals of the Rheumatic Diseases* **49**, 268.

Bochaton, H., Paul, C. & Dubertret, L. (1997) Multiple subungual hemorrhages as a manifestation of Sweet's syndrome. *European Journal of Dermatology* **7**, 121–122.

Fanning, W.L. & Aronson, M. (1977) Osler node, Janeway lesions and splinter hemorrhages. *Archives of Dermatology* **113**, 648–649.

Fisher, A.A. (1957) Subungual splinter hemorrhages associated with trichinosis. *Archives of Dermatology* **75**, 752–754.

Francès, C., Piette, J.C., Saada, V. *et al.* (1994a) Multiple subungual splinter hemorrhages in the antiphospholipid syndrome. *Lupus* **3**, 123–128.

Francès, C., Aractingi, S., Bletry, O. *et al.* (1994b) Hémorragies filiformes sous-unguéales multiples sur ongles sains et hypereosinophilie: un marqueur clinique de thrombose (6 observations). *Annales de Dermatologie et de Vénéréologie* **121** (Suppl 1), S60.

Heath, D. & Williams, D.R. (1978) Nail haemorrhages. *British Heart Journal* **40**, 1300–1305.

Heath, D., Harris, P., Williams, D. *et al.* (1981) Nail haemorrhages in native highlanders of the Peruvian Andes. *Thorax* **36**, 764–766.

Kilpatrick, Z.M., Greenberg, P.A. & Sanford, J.P. (1965) Splinter haemorrhages, their clinical significance. *Archives of Internal Medicine* **115**, 730–735.

Martens, P.B., Levins, J.A. & Hunder, G.G. (1996) Splinter hemorrhages following arterial puncture. *Arthritis and Rheumatism* **39**, 169–170.

Martin, B.F. & Platts, M.M. (1959) A histological study of the nail region in normal human subjects and in those showing splinter haemorrhages of the nails. *Journal of Anatomy* **93**, 323–330.

Miller, A. & Vaziri, N.D. (1979) Recurrent atraumatic subungual splinter hemorrhages in healthy individuals. *Southern Medical Journal* **72**, 1418–1420.

Monk, B.E. (1980) The prevalence of splinter haemorrhages. *British Journal of Dermatology* **103**, 183–185.

Pierson, J.C., Lawlor, K.P. & Steck, W.D. (1993) Pen push purpura: iatrogenic nail bed hemorrhages in the extensive care unit. *Cutis* **51**, 422–423.

Platts, M.M. & Greaves, M.S. (1958) Splinter hemorrhages. *British Medical Journal* **19**, 143–144.

Ramelet, A.A., Tscholl, R. & Monti, M. (1982) Association d'hématomes filiformes des ongles et d'un Syndrome de Raynaud. *Annales de Dermatologie et de Vénéréologie* **109**, 655–659.

Tobi, M. & Kobrin, I. (1981) Splinter hemorrhages associated with an indwelling brachial artery cannula. *Chest* **80**, 767.

Wijdicks, E.F.M. & Schievink, W.I. (1997) Coma nails. *Journal of Neurology, Neurosurgery and Psychiatry* **63**, 294.

Wood, P.H. (1956) *Disease of Heart and Circulation*, 2nd edn, p. 648. Eyre and Spottiswood, London.

Young, J.B., Will, E.J. & Mulley, G.P. (1988) Splinter haemorrhages: facts and fiction. *Journal of the Royal College of Physicians, London* **22**, 240–243.

## Gangrene

Table 6.1 shows the various mechanisms and conditions associated with symmetrical peripheral gangrene.

### Ainhum and pseudoainhum (Fig. 6.15)

Ainhum affects the black population of subtropical regions of America, Africa and Asia. A painful constricting band encircles the 5th toe with eventual spontaneous amputation. It may be unilateral, but 75% of the cases are bilateral. The condition is often secondary to an abnormality in the foot vessels producing an abnormal blood supply (Dent *et al.* 1981) alone or in combination with chronic trauma, infection and hyperkeratosis. Constriction by external forces such as hair or threads is encountered in children or mentally deranged adults (and is sometimes referred to as pseudoainhum). Removal of the constricting band and performing a Z-plasty may prevent spontaneous amputation (Kamalan 1981).

### References

Dent, D.M., Fatar, S. & Rose, A.G. (1981) Ainhum and angiodysplasia. *Lancet* **ii**, 396–397.

Kamalan, A. (1981) Ainhum trichoporosis and Z-plasty. *Dermatologica* **162**, 372.

## Connective tissue diseases

In collagen diseases, the proximal nail fold is the most important site of change. Periungual ischaemic lesions resulting from small vessel necrotizing vasculitis reflect the underlying vasculopathy of collagen diseases and may be a cutaneous manifestation of several disorders, including rheumatoid arthritis, systemic lupus erythematosus, dermatomyositis, periarteritis nodosa and Wegener's granulomatosis.

Periungual erythema and telangiectasia are a common feature of patients affected by dermatomyositis, systemic lupus erythematosus or systemic sclerosis. The observation of periungual erythema is a simple and useful way to detect connective tissue diseases in clinical practice (Ohtsuka 1997). In these patients irregular capillary loops are frequently visible even without a lens. Haemorrhages of the nail fold capillaries (nail fold bleeding) can be frequently seen within the cuticle. A close relationship between these haemorrhages and nail fold capillary abnormalities has been reported (Ohtsuka 1998). Several patterns of cuticle haemorrhages have been detected in patients with collagen diseases, the band pattern being characteristic for systemic scleroderma (Maeda *et al.* 1997). Massive digital necrosis resulting from Raynaud's phenomenon can be the first manifestation of a collagen disease (Saban *et al.* 1991).

### References

Maeda, M., Kachi, H., Takagi, H. *et al.* (1997) Hemorrhagic patterns in the cuticles distal to the proximal nail folds in the fingers of patients with systemc scleroderma. *European Journal of Dermatology* **7**, 191–196.

Ohtsuka, T. (1997) The relation between periungual erythema and nailfold capillary abnormalities in patients with connective tissue diseases. *European Journal of Dermatology* **7**, 561–565.

Ohtsuka, T. (1998) The relation between nailfold bleeding and

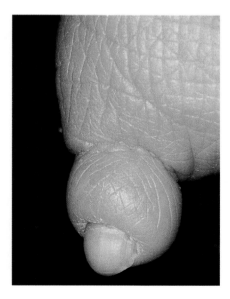

**Fig. 6.15**
Pseudoainhum.

**Table 6.3** Nail fold capillary pattern in connective tissue diseases.

| | Capillary density | Morphological changes |
|---|---|---|
| Scleroderma | Paucity of visible capillaries, avascular areas | Enlarged capillary loops |
| SLE, DLE | Normal | Tortuous capillary loops, meandering loops |
| MCTD and dermatomyositis | Paucity of visible capillaries | Enlarged capillary loops, tortuous capillary loops |
| Rheumatoid arthritis | Normal, paucity of visible capillaries | Normal, irregular capillary loops |

DLE, Discoid lupus erythematosus; MCTD, mixed connective tissue disease.

capillary microscopic abnormalities in patients with connective tissue diseases. *International Journal of Dermatology* 37, 23–26.

Saban, J., Rodriguez-Garcia, J.L., Pais, J.R. *et al.* (1991) Raynaud's phenomenon with digital necrosis as the first manifestation of undifferentiated connective tissue syndrome. *Dermatologica* **182**, 121–123.

## Nail fold capillary microscopy (Table 6.3, Figs 6.16–6.19)

Nail fold capillary microscopy is a simple, non-invasive technique which can give useful information for the early diagnosis of collagen diseases. Several instruments have been successfully used for the *in vivo* examination of the nail fold capillary bed. Portable capillaroscopes (Panasonic light scope or Micro Mike)

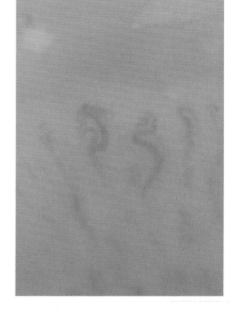

**Fig. 6.17** Dilated capillary loops in lupus erythematosus (×60).

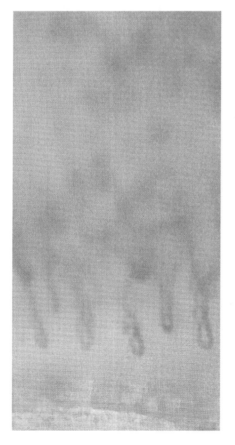

**Fig. 6.16** Capillary microscopy—normal nail fold capillary loops (×60).

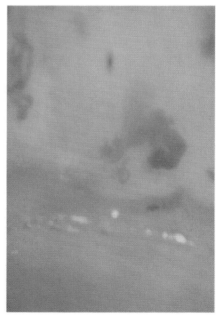

**Fig. 6.18** Dermatomyositis— obstructed and thrombosed capillaries (×60).

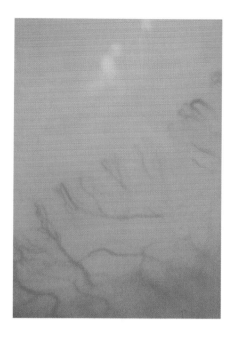

**Fig. 6.19** Rheumatoid arthritis—rather elongated capillary loops.

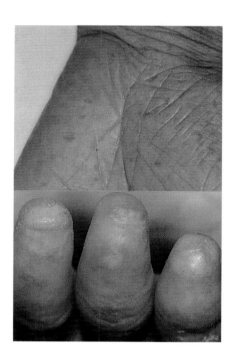

**Fig. 6.20** CREST syndrome.

and common ophthalmoscopes can be used in ordinary screening (Goldman 1981; Minkin & Rabhan 1982; Studer *et al.* 1991). A dermatoscope can also be utilized (Bauersachs & Lossner 1997). Stereomicroscopes that permit higher magnifications (×40) and photographic documentation of the nail fold capillary bed are advisable for a long-term follow-up of microangiopathic changes. Capillary videomicroscopy in connection with local cold exposure permits a more accurate assessment of the microcirculation and can be used in a large number of vasospastic conditions (Gasser & Dubler 1996). Capillary microscopy of the proximal nail fold requires the application of a thin layer of oil to the skin in order to increase its transparency. The orientation of proximal nail fold capillaries parallel to the surface of the skin permits the observation of both the arterial and the venous limbs of the capillary.

In normal subjects, nail fold capillaries are arranged in parallel rows and appear as fine regular loops with a small space between the afferent and efferent limbs. In collagen disorders, the morphology of the vascular nail bed loops may be grossly altered (Table 6.3).

An examination of the proximal nail fold in patients with scleroderma characteristically reveals capillary enlargement and loss. These capillary changes, consisting of enlarged loops and avascular areas, are present in most of the patients affected by systemic sclerosis and by its CREST variant, but not in morphoea (Minkin & Rabhan 1982; Studer *et al.* 1991) or in eosinophilic fasciitis (Herson *et al.* 1989). When patients with localized scleroderma show typical nail fold capillary abnormalities, a possible association with systemic sclerosis should be ruled out (Maricq 1992). The severity of the proximal nail fold changes has been proposed as an index of the degree of systemic involvement and it has been suggested that it reflects

the state of the total vascular system (Maricq *et al.* 1976; Schmidt & Mensing 1988). The prognostic value of capillary changes in scleroderma is, however, still being discussed (Lovy *et al.* 1985) and quantitative morphological studies have failed to confirm this evidence (Lefford & Edwards 1986; Statham & Rowell 1986). A correlation between nail fold capillary abnormalities and pulmonary arterial hypertension has recently been reported (Ohtsuka *et al.* 1997). Nail bed capillary microscopy may permit the differentiation of early scleroderma from idiopathic Raynaud's phenomenon (Carpentier *et al.* 1983), which is not generally associated with microvascular changes in the nail fold. Capillaroscopy may also be useful in distinguishing the CREST variant of systemic sclerosis (Fig. 6.20) from hereditary haemorrhagic telangiectasia, which is characterized by the presence of giant capillaries (Maire *et al.* 1986). The aetiology of reduced capillary numbers in scleroderma is unknown, but may be related to the frequent capillary thromboses observed in the nail fold in this condition. Such thromboses lead to microinfarcts that heal by scarring.

In systemic lupus erythematosus, the nail fold examination shows a normal density of capillary loops but a marked deformation of the individual capillaries. The vessel dilatation is minimal although the arrangement of the capillary loops is tortuous and can be corkscrew shaped (Redisch *et al.* 1970; Minkin & Rabhan 1982; Granier *et al.* 1986). Meandering loops that may resemble glomerular tufts can occasionally be observed. Patients with anticardiolipin antibodies (ACA) also present with capillary abnormalities similar to those observed in patients without ACA (Vayssairat *et al.* 1997). Similar proximal nail fold abnormalities have been described in discoid lupus erythematosus (Rowell 1986). In systemic lupus erythe-

**Table 6.4** Nail alterations in connective tissue diseases.

| | Periungual tissues | Nail unit |
|---|---|---|
| Scleroderma | Ischaemic lesions, ulcers, gangrene, dissolution of the terminal phalanges | Chronic paronychia, onycholysis, onychogryphosis, pterygium inversum unguis*, parrot's beak nail* |
| SLE | Digital ulcers, gangrene | Nail fold telangiectasia, cuticular haemorrhages, leuconychia, pitting, ridging, onycholysis, onychomadesis, nail bed hyperkeratosis |
| DLE | | Nail bed hyperkeratosis |
| Dermatomyositis | | Nail fold telangiectasia, cuticular haemorrhages, cuticular hyperkeratosis |
| Rheumatoid arthritis | Ischaemic lesions | Nail fold infarcts*, beading, ridging, yellow nail syndrome, red lunulae* |
| Wegener's granulomatosis | Necrotic lesions | Linear infarcts of the proximal nail fold |
| Periarteritis nodosa | Necrotic lesions | Nail fold infarcts |

* Distinctive changes.

matosus direct immunofluorescence of the proximal nail fold shows the typical lupus band test (Schnitzler *et al.* 1980).

In patients with polymyositis, dermatomyositis and mixed connective tissue disease, the capillaroscopy changes resemble those described in patients with scleroderma. Capillary dilatation and drop out are the most common findings. Tortuosity, deformation and a bushy appearance of the individual capillaries are frequently associated features (Granier *et al.* 1986; Wong *et al.* 1988). The severity of the microvascular abnormalities has been observed to decrease with prolonged disease remission (Ganczarczyk *et al.* 1988). A study of 85 cases of dermatomyositis showed severe disturbances of microcirculation including vasodilatation with megacapillaries, irregular and tortuous capillary loops, a decrease in the number of loops, an aggregation of erythrocytes, a granular and slow blood stream, a stasis in the transitional portion of the loops, a cloudy microscopic field as well as marked exudation, haemorrhages and invisibility of subpapillary blood plexus (Liu *et al.* 1991). These changes were more marked in patients with visceral disorders and when the disease was in an active stage. In childhood dermatomyositis, the presence of enlarged capillaries and avascularity correlated with more severe and persistent forms of the disease (Spencer-Green *et al.* 1983; Silver & Maricq 1989). Patients with Sjögren's syndrome may show nail fold capillary abnormalities indistinguishable from those of systemic lupus erythematosus (Ohtsuka 1997). Patients affected by rheumatoid arthritis generally do not present any alterations in the nail fold capillaries (Lefford & Edwards 1986). Tortuosity, elongation of loops, paucity of visible capillaries and increased plasma skimming have been occasionally described, however (Redisch *et al.* 1970). Although capillary microscopy is a useful complementary investigation for the evaluation of patients with collagen disorders, it should not be used as a diagnostic criterion in individual patients. In fact, some of the capillary microscopy abnormalities, which are observed in patients with collagen diseases, may occur also in normal controls.

The clinical signs in the nail apparatus associated with connective tissue diseases are outlined in Table 6.4.

## References

Bauersachs, R.M. & Lossner, F. (1997) The poor man's capillary microscope. A novel technique for the assessment of capillary morphology. *Annals of the Rheumatic Diseases* **56**, 435–437.

Carpentier, P., Franco, A., Beani, J.C. *et al.* (1983) Intéret de la capillaroscopie périunguéale dans le diagnostic précoce de la sclérodermie systemique. *Annales de Dermatologie et de Vénéréologie* **110**, 11–20.

Ganczarczyk, M.L., Lee, P. & Armstrong, S.K. (1988) Nailfold capillary microscopy in polymyositis and dermatomyositis. *Arthritis and Rheumatism* **31**, 116–119.

Gasser, P. & Dubler, B. (1996) Die Entwicklung der apparativen un mebtechnischen Aspekte für die klinische Kapillaromikroskopie. *Zeitschrift für Rheumatologie* **55**, 260–266.

Goldman, L. (1981) A simple portable capillaroscope. *Archives of Dermatology* **117**, 605–606.

Granier, F., Vayssairat, M., Priollet, P. *et al.* (1986) Nailfold capillary microscopy in mixed connective tissue disease. *Arthritis and Rheumatism* **29**, 189–195.

Herson, S., Brechignac, S., Piette, J.P. *et al.* (1989) Capillaroscopie unguéale au cours de la fasciite avec éosinophilie: un élément disinctif d'avec la sclérodermie systémique. *Annales de Medecine Interne* **140**, 440–443.

Lefford, F. & Edwards, J.C.W. (1986) Nail fold capillary microscopy in connective tissue disease: a quantitative morphological analysis. *Annals of the Rheumatic Diseases* **45**, 741–749.

Liu, C., Su, W. & Luo, Y. (1991) Changes in cutaneous microcirculation, hemorrheology and platelet aggregation function in dermatomyositis. *Journal of Dermatological Science* **2**, 346–352.

Lovy, M., MacCarter, D. & Steigerwald, J.C. (1985) Relationship between nailfold capillary abnormalities and organ involvement in systemic sclerosis. *Arthritis and Rheumatism* **28**, 496–501.

Maire, R., Schnewlin, G. & Bollinger, A. (1986) Videomikroskopische Untersuchungen von Teleangiektasien bei Morbus Osler und

Sklerodermie. *Schweizersiche Medizinische Wochenschrift* **116**, 335–338.

Maricq, H.R. (1992) Capillary abnormalities, Raynaud's phenomenon, and systemic sclerosis in patients with localized scleroderma. *Archives of Dermatology* **128**, 630–632.

Maricq, H.R., Spencer Green, G. & Le Roy, E.C. (1976) Skin capillary abnormalities as indicators of organ involvement in scleroderma (systemic sclerosis), Raynaud's syndrome and dermatomyositis. *American Journal of Medicine* **61**, 862–870.

Minkin, W. & Rabhan, N.B. (1982) Office nail fold capillary microscopy using ophthalmoscope. *Journal of the American Academy of Dermatology* **7**, 190–193.

Ohtsuka, T. (1997) Nailfold capillary abnormalities in patients with Sjögren syndrome and systemic lupus erythematosus. *British Journal of Dermatology* **136**, 94–96.

Ohtsuka, T., Hasegawa, A., Nakamo, A. *et al.* (1997) Nailfold capillary abnormality and pulmonary hypertension in systemic sclerosis. *International Journal of Dermatology* **36**, 116–122.

Redisch, W., Messina, E.J., Hughes, G. *et al.* (1970) Capillaroscopic observations in rheumatic diseases. *Annals of the Rheumatic Diseases* **29**, 244–253.

Rowell, N.R. (1986) Lupus erythematosus, scleroderma and dermatomyositis. The 'collagen' or 'connective-tissue' diseases. In: *Textbook of Dermatology* (eds A. Rook, D.S. Wilkinson, F.J.G. Ebling *et al.*), pp. 1281–1392. Blackwell Scientific Publications, Oxford.

Schmidt, K.U. & Mensing, H. (1988) Are nailfold capillary changes indicators of organ involvement in progressive systemic sclerosis? *Dermatologica* **176**, 18–21.

Schnitzler, L., Baran, R. & Verret, J.L. (1980) La biopsie du repli sus-unguéal dans les maladies dites du collagène. Etude histologique, ultrastructurale et en immunofluorescence de 26 cas. *Annales de Dermatologie et de Vénéréologie* **107**, 777–785.

Silver, R.M. & Maricq, H.R. (1989) Childhood dermatomyositis: serial microvascular studies. *Pediatrics* **83**, 278–283.

Spencer-Green, G., Schlesinger, M., Bove, K.E. *et al.* (1983) Nailfold capillary abnormalities in childhood rheumatic diseases. *Journal of Pediatrics* **102**, 341–346.

Statham, B.N. & Rowell, N.R. (1986) Quantification of the nail fold capillary abnormalities in systemic sclerosis and Raynaud's syndrome. *Acta Dermato-Venereologica* **66**, 139–143.

Studer, A., Hunziker, T., Lutolf, O. *et al.* (1991) Quantitative nailfold capillary microscopy in cutaneous and systemic lupus erythematosus and localized and systemic scleroderma. *Journal of the American Academy of Dermatology* **24**, 941–945.

Vayssairat, M., Abuaf, N., Deschamps, A. *et al.* (1997) Nailfold capillary microscopy in patients with anticardiolipin antibodies: a case-control study. *Dermatology* **194**, 36–40.

Wong, M.L., Highton, J., Palmer, D.G. (1988) Sequential nail fold capillary microscopy in scleroderma and related disorders. *Annals of the Rheumatic Diseases* **47**, 53–61.

## Systemic sclerosis (Figs 6.6–6.9 and 6.20–6.22)

A functional increase in precapillary resistance is probably responsible for the abnormal microvascular function in systemic scleroderma. Capillary blood pressure and red blood cell velocity in nail fold capillaries of patients with systemic sclerosis are significantly lower than those recorded in healthy controls.

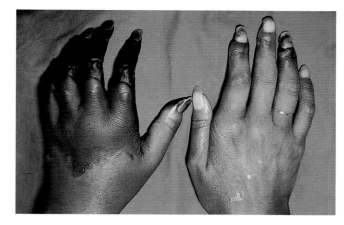

**Fig. 6.21** Systemic sclerosis—gangrenous appearance of the left hand. (Courtesy of N.R. Rowel, UK.)

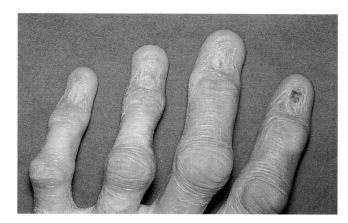

**Fig. 6.22** Acral pansclerotic morphoea. (Courtesy of N.R. Rowel, UK.)

These abnormalities are not restricted to enlarged capillaries, but are also detected in normally shaped capillaries of scleroderma patients (Hahn *et al.* 1998). Raynaud's phenomenon usually precedes the development of the other cutaneous signs of scleroderma. Swelling of the fingers can be an early symptom of systemic scleroderma. The round fingerpad sign has been recently described as a useful clinical diagnostic sign of scleroderma. This sign describes the disappearence of the peaked contour on the fingerpads and its replacement by a hemisphere-like fingerpad contour. The round fingerpad sign is most commonly found on the ring fingers. A positive sign has been observed not only in patients with scleroderma but also in patients with Raynaud's phenomenon or mixed connective tissue disease (Mizutami *et al.* 1991).

In well-developed cases of scleroderma, the fingers have a tapered appearance due to sclerosis of the overlying skin and frequently exhibit flexion contractures. Patients with hereditary sclerodactyly may resemble systemic sclerosis but there is no Raynaud's phenomenon (Eubel *et al.* 1985).

Periungual ischaemic lesions and ulcers are frequent in systemic scleroderma. Digital gangrene is occasionally seen even in the absence of severe systemic involvement (Fig. 6.21). A patient has been reported in which digital gangrene was the sole cutaneous evidence of systemic sclerosis (Barr & Robinson 1988). Unique digital skin lesions presenting as multiple, soft dome-shaped tumours along the lateral aspect of the terminal phalanges of the thumb and index finger were associated with systemic sclerosis (Marzano *et al.* 1997).

Chronic paronychia and onycholysis are common complaints and discoloration of the nail plate may be indicative of a secondary mycotic or bacterial infection. The nail folds can present ragged cuticles (Rowell 1986). Impaired peripheral circulation can lead to nail thinning and ridging. When atrophy of the terminal phalanges occurs, the nails become small and brittle. Onychogryphosis can also be observed.

Pterygium inversum unguis and Parrot's beak nail are the only distinctive nail changes of systemic scleroderma (Chapter 2). Pterygium inversum unguis was first linked to scleroderma by Patterson (1977). Although it is more frequently observed in patients with acrosclerosis and fingertip ulcerations, it aids in the diagnosis of the disease (Zaias 1990; Caputo *et al.* 1993). Pterygium inversum unguis consists of the obliteration of the normal distal separation between the ventral surface of the nail plate and the skin of the hyponychium. The resulting adhesion between the nail plate and the fingertip skin leads to pain when the nails are clipped. Pterygium inversum associated with scleroderma is probably a consequence of the fingertip ulcerations and scarring. No form of treatment for this condition has been effective.

Parrot's beak nail, otherwise known as nail beaking (Chapter 2), is a nail change that develops as a consequence of the atrophy of the fingertip soft tissues which characterizes severe acrosclerosis. The nail plate bends around the shortened fingertip. Complete destruction of the nail apparatus is the final consequence of the dissolution of the terminal phalanges which occurs in the most severely affected patients.

Systemic sclerosis-like disorders have been reported to develop following exposure to vinyl chloride, aliphatic and aromatic hydrocarbons, epoxy resins, silicon, bleomycin, L-tryptophan and toxic oil, as well as after silicone 'breast implant' (Bélangé *et al.* 1989; Connolly *et al.* 1990; Rustin *et al.* 1990). A syndrome resembling systemic sclerosis characterizes the chronic phase of graft-versus-host disease.

Although localized scleroderma is not usually associated with nail changes, complete loss of both fingernails and toenails has been reported in a patient affected by acral pansclerotic morphoea (Rowell 1987) (Fig. 6.22).

Iloprost appears useful as a treatment of imminent gangrene and ischaemic ulcers in systemic sclerosis (Zachariae *et al.* 1996). Digital calcification in systemic sclerosis may be treated effectively with good tissue preservation using the carbon dioxide laser (Bottomley *et al.* 1996).

## References

Barr, W.G. & Robinson, J.A. (1988) Systemic sclerosis and digital gangrene without scleroderma. *Journal of Rheumatology* 15, 875–877.

Bélangé, G., Chaouat, D. & Chauoat, Y. (1989) Les connectivites induites non médicamenteuses. *Revue de Medecine Interne* 10, 135–141.

Bottomley, W.W., Goodfield, M.J.D. & Sheehan-Dare, R.A. (1996) Digital calcification in systemic sclerosis, effective treatment with good tissue preservation using the carbon dioxide laser. *British Journal of Dermatology* 135, 302–304.

Caputo, R., Cappio, F., Rigoni, C. et al. (1993) Pterygium inversum unguis. Report of 19 cases and review of the literature. *Archives of Dermatology* 129, 1307–1309.

Connolly, S.M., Quimby, S.R., Griffing, W.L. et al. (1990) Scleroderma and L-tryptophan: a possible explanation of the eosinophilia myalgia syndrome. *Journal of the American Academy of Dermatology* 23, 451–457.

Eubel, R., Klose, L. & Mahrle, G. (1985) Hereditare sklerodaktylie und syndactylie. *Hautarzt* 36, 302–304.

Hahn, M., Heubach, T., Steins, A. et al. (1998) Hemodynamics in nailfold capillaries of patients with systemic scleroderma: synchronous measurements of capillary blood pressure and red blood cell velocity. *Journal of Investigative Dermatology* 110, 982–985.

Marzano, A.V., Berti, E., Gasparini, G. et al. (1997) Unique digital lesions associated with systemic sclerosis. *British Journal of Dermatology* 136, 598–600.

Mizutami, H., Mizutami, T., Okada, H. et al. (1991) Round fingerpad sign: an early sign of scleroderma. *Journal of the American Academy of Dermatology* 24, 67–69.

Patterson, J.W. (1977) Pterygium inversum unguis-like changes in scleroderma. *Archives of Dermatology* 113, 1429–1430.

Rowell, N.R. (1986) Lupus erythematosus, scleroderma and dermatomyositis. The 'collagen' or 'connective-tissue' diseases. In: *Textbook of Dermatology* (eds A. Rook, D.S. Wilkinson, F.J.G. Ebling et al.), pp. 1281–1392. Blackwell Scientific Publications, Oxford.

Rowell, N.R. (1987) Acral pansclerotic morphea with intractable pain. CVII Congressus Mundi Dermatologiae. The CMD Case Collection. In: *Berlin Clinical Dermatology* (eds D.S. Wilkinson, S.M. Masearó & C.E. Orfanos), pp. 178–180. Schattauer, Stuttgart.

Rustin, M.H.A., Bull, H.A., Ziegler, V. et al. (1990) Silica-associated systemic sclerosis is clinically, serologically and immunologically indistinguishable from idiopathic systemic sclerosis. *British Journal of Dermatology* 123, 725–734.

Zachariae H., Halkier-Sprensen L., Bjerring P. et al. (1996) Treatment of ischemic digital ulcers and prevention of gangrene with IV Iloprost in systemic sclerosis. *Acta Dermato-Venereologica* 76: 236–238.

Zaias, N. (1990) *The Nail in Health and Disease*, pp. 189–199. Appleton & Lange, Norwalk, CN.

## Systemic lupus erythematosus (Figs 6.23–6.25)

Blood vessel infarction leading to focal necrosis of the nail fold and cuticular haemorrhages are common features of systemic lupus erythematosus (SLE). Digital ulcers and/or gangrene may represent a clinical manifestation of cutaneous vasculitis but are not necessarily related to systemic involvement (Hashimoto

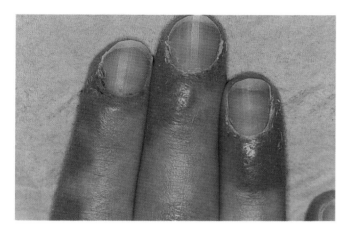

**Fig. 6.23** Systemic lupus erythematosus.

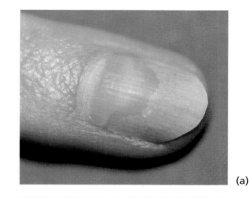

(a)

**Fig. 6.25** (a) Systemic lupus erythematosus—onycholysis due to vasculitic lesion. (Courtesy of S. Goettmann-Bonvallot, Paris.) (b) Systemic lupus erythematosus—periungual vasculitic lesion. (Courtesy of S. Goettmann-Bonvallot, Paris.)

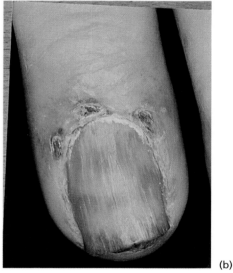

(b)

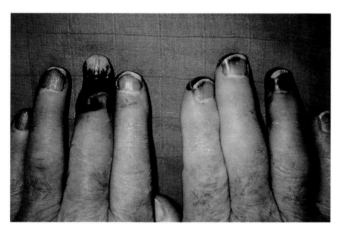

**Fig. 6.24** Systemic lupus erythematosus with gangrenous digits.

*et al.* 1983). Limb gangrene due to large or medium size arterial occlusion can occur (Yang *et al.* 1996), as well as ischaemic venous thrombosis (Duschet *et al.* 1993). Although a wide spectrum of nail abnormalities has been described in SLE, none is sufficiently distinctive to be useful in the diagnosis of the disease. Patients may, in fact, present with altered keratinization of the nail matrix leading to punctate or striate leuconychia as well as nail pitting or ridging. Onycholysis, Beau's lines or onychomadesis can occur. Onycholysis has been reported as the most frequent nail abnormality in SLE (Urowitz *et al.* 1978). Red lunulae (Jorizzo *et al.* 1983; Wilkerson & Wilkin 1989; Garcia-Patos *et al.* 1997; Wollina *et al.* 1999) as well as oil patches of the nail bed (Runne & Orfanos 1981) have been described. Nail fold hyperkeratosis, ragged cuticles and splinter haemorrhages can also be observed (Rowell 1986). In addition, splinter haemorrhages and digital infarcts have been reported in a patient with microscopic polyangiitis, a less severe variant of antineutrophil cytoplasmic antibody-associated disease (Irvine *et al.* 1996). Finger clubbing has been occasionally

reported (Mackie 1973; Menkes *et al.* 1980). Pterygium inversum unguis has been reported in seven patients affected by SLE (Caputo *et al.* 1993). A diffuse, dark blue-black pattern of hyperpigmentation intermixed with longitudinal pigmented bands was present in 52% of 33 black patients with SLE (Vaughn *et al.* 1990). In a 34-year-old Arab patient presenting with SLE and all fingernails affected by longitudinal melanonychia, transverse biopsy of the nail matrix showed a vasculitis (Skowron *et al.* 2001). A 9-year-old hispanic girl with SLE developed 'darker' nail beds and periungual areas. Longitudinal banding and diffuse blue-black nail dyschromia were evident (Baird 1994). Chronic paronychia of 10 years' duration, without any discharge of pus, was observed in a 39-year-old woman (Bories 1998).

Nail bed hyperkeratosis may be seen both in discoid lupus and in SLE. In the latter, it has been described in association with periungual and palmoplantar hyperkeratosis (Buck *et al.* 1988).

The term lupus erythematosus ungium mutilans describes a rare destructive involvement of the nails associated with decalcification and atrophy of the distal phalanges (McCarthy 1931).

In patients with antiphospholipid antibodies the formation of platelet thrombi in the smaller vessels may result in splinter haemorrhages (Asherson 1990; Ames *et al.* 1992; Wolf *et al.* 1992; Francès *et al.* 1994; Mujic *et al.* 1995). Digital ischaemia and digital gangrene are not uncommon (Asherson *et al.* 1986; Grob & Bonegrandi 1989) (Fig. 6.24). Acral erythematous, purpuric or cyanotic macules, painful nodules resembling vasculitis, haemorrhages, capillaritis, blue toe syndrome, purpura fulminans and porcelain-white scars or atrophie blanche are additional cutaneous signs observed in the antiphospholipid syndrome (Nahass 1997).

## References

Ames, D.E., Asherson, R.A., Ayres D. *et al.* (1992) Bilateral adrenal infarction, hypoadrenalism, and splinter haemorrhages in the 'primary' antiphospholipid syndrome. *British Journal of Rheumatology* **31**, 117–120.

Asherson, R.A. (1990) Subungual splinter haemorrhages: a new sign of the antiphospholipid coagulopathy? *Annals of the Rheumatic Diseases* **49**, 268–271.

Asherson, R.A., Derksen, R.H.W.M., Harris, E.N. *et al.* (1986) Large vessel occlusion and gangrene in systemic lupus erythematosus and 'lupus-like' disease: a report of six cases. *Journal of Rheumatology* **13**, 740–747.

Baird, J.S. (1994) Chromonychia with SLE. *Journal of Rheumatology* **21**, 176–177.

Bories, A. (1998) Perionyxis revélateur d'un lupus érythémateux systémique. *Nouvelle Dermatologie* **17**, 185.

Buck, D.C., Dodd, H.J. & Sarkany, I. (1988) Hypertrophic lupus erythematosus. *British Journal of Dermatology* **33** (Suppl.), 72–74.

Caputo, R., Cappio, F., Rigoni, C. *et al.* (1993) Pterygium inversum unguis. Report of 19 cases and review of the literature. *Archives of Dermatology* **129**, 1307–1309.

Duschet, P., Seifert, W., Halbmeyer, W.M. *et al.* (1993) Ischemic venous thrombosis caused by a distinct disturbance of the extrinsic clotting system. *Journal of the American Academy of Dermatology* **28**, 831–835.

Francès, C., Piette, J.C., Saada, V. *et al.* (1994) Multiple subungual splinter hemorrhages in the antiphospholipid syndrome: a report of 5 cases and review of the literature. *Lupus* **3**, 123–128.

Garcia-Patos, V., Bartralot, R., Ordi, J. *et al.* (1997) Systemic lupus erythematosus presenting with red lunulae. *Journal of the American Academy of Dermatology* **3**, 834–836.

Grob, J.J. & Bonerandi, J.J. (1989) Thrombotic skin disease as a marker of the anticardiolipin syndrome: livero vasculitis and distal gangrene associated with abnomal serum antiphospholipid activity. *Journal of the American Academy of Dermatology* **20**, 1063–1069.

Hashimoto, H., Tsuda, H., Takasaki, Y. *et al.* (1983) Digital ulcers/ gangrene and immunoglobulin classes complement fixation of Anti-dsDNA in systemic lupus erythematosus patients. *Journal of Rheumatology* **10**, 727–732.

Irvine, A.D., Bruce, I.N., Walsh, M. *et al.* (1996) Dermatological presentation of disease associated with antineutrophil cytoplasmic antibodies: a report of two contrasting cases and a review of the literature. *Journal of the American Academy of Dermatology* **134**, 924–928.

Jorizzo, J.L., Gonzalez, E.B. & Daniels, J.C. (1983) Red lunulae in a patient with rheumatoid arthritis. *Journal of the American Academy of Dermatology* **8**, 711–714.

Mackie, R.M. (1973) Lupus erythematosus in association with finger-clubbing. *British Journal of Dermatology* **89**, 533–535.

McCarthy, L. (1931) Lupus erythematosus ungium mutilans treated with gold and sodium thiosulphate. *Archives of Dermatology and Syphiligraphy* **24**, 647–654.

Menkes, C.S., Marin, A. & Delbarre, F. (1980) Rupture de tendons et hippocratisme digital au cours du lupus érythémateux disséminé. *Rheumathisme* **50**, 333–335.

Mujic, F., Lloyd, M., Cuadrado, M.J. *et al.* (1995) Prevalence and clinical significance of subungual splinter hemorrhages in patients with antiphospholipid syndrome. *Clinical and Experimental Rheumatology* **13**, 327–331.

Nahass, G.T. (1997) Antiphospholipid antibodies and the antiphospholipid antibody syndrome. *Journal of the American Academy of Dermatology* **36**, 149–168.

Rowell, N.R. (1986) Lupus erythematosus, scleroderma and dermatomyositis. The 'collagen' or 'connective-tissue' diseases. In: *Textbook of Dermatology* (eds A. Rook, D.S. Wilkinson, F.J.G. Ebling, *et al.*), pp. 1281–1392. Blackwell Scientific Publications, Oxford.

Runne, U. & Orfanos, C.E. (1981) The human nail. *Current Problems in Dermatology* **9**, 102–149.

Skowron, E., Combenale, P., Faisant, M. *et al.* (2001). Longitudinal melanonychia and systemic lupus erythematosus. *Journal of the American Academy of Dermatology* (in press).

Urowitz, M.B., Gladman, D.D., Chalmers, A. *et al.* (1978) Nail lesions in systemic lupus erythematosus. *Journal of Rheumatology* **5**, 441–447.

Vaughn, R.Y., Bailey, J.P., Field, R.S. *et al.* (1990) Diffuse nail dyschromia in black patients with systemic lupus erythematosus. *Journal of Rheumatology* **17**, 640–643.

Wilkerson, M.G. & Wilkin, J.K. (1989) Red lunulae revisited: a clinical and histopathologic examination. *Journal of the American Academy of Dermatology* **20**, 453–457.

Wolf, P., Soyer, H.P., Aver-Greumbach, P. & Kerl, H. (1992) Acral microlivedo—a clinical manifestation of the antiphospholipid syndrome. *Zeitschrift für Hautkrankheiten* **67**, 714–717.

Wollina, U., Barta, U., Unlemann, C. & Oelzner, P. (1999) Lupus erythematosus-associated red lunula. *Journal of the American Academy of Dermatology* **41**, 419–421.

Yang, S.G., Kim, K.H. Park, K.C. *et al.* (1996) A case of systemic lupus erythematosus showing acute gangrenous change of fingertips. *British Journal of Dermatology* **134**, 178–192.

## Dermatomyositis

Erythema and telangiectasia of the proximal nail fold are typical features of dermatomyositis (Fig. 6.26a). Thickness, hardness, roughness and hyperkeratosis of the cuticles are common in patients with dermatomyositis, even in the absence of nail fold abnormalities (Samitz 1974) (Fig. 6.26b). Cuticular haemorrhages are frequent. Pitting of the fingernails may be seen occasionally (Dupré *et al.* 1981; Rowell 1986). The presence of periungual ischaemic lesions might be a predictive sign of malignancy in adult dermatomyositis (Basset-Seguin *et al.* 1990) (Fig. 6.27).

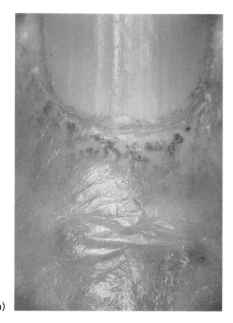

(a)

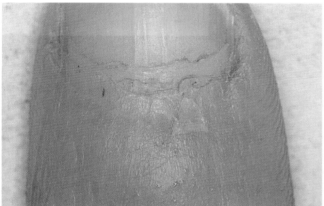

(b)

**Fig. 6.26** (a) Dermatomyositis—dilated nail fold capillaries. (b) Dermatomyositis—ragged cuticles.

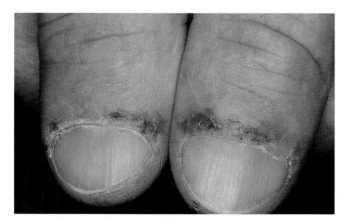

**Fig. 6.27** Periungual ischaemic lesions—predictive sign of malignancy in dermatomyositis.

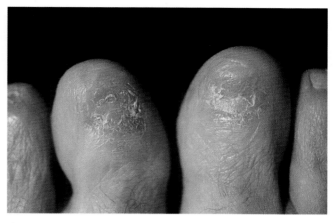

**Fig. 6.28** Dermatomyositis—complete loss of several toenails.

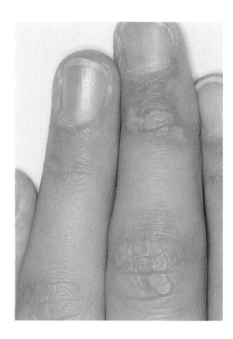

**Fig. 6.29**
Dermatomyositis—
Gottron's papules in a
child.

The complete loss of several toenails has been described in a patient with dermatomyositis (Tosti *et al.* 1987) (Fig. 6.28). Erythema and scaling of the nail bed along with nail fold erythema and telangiectasia were prominent features. Thickening of the nail cuticles was also evident. Red lunulae have been reported in a patient with dermatomyositis (Jorizzo *et al.* 1983). Two patients with pterygium inversum unguis have been reported (Caputo *et al.* 1993). Gottron's papules may be seen at the proximal area of the dorsal aspect of the terminal phalanges (Fig. 6.29).

### References

Basset-Seguin, N., Roujeau, J.C., Gheradi, R. *et al.* (1990) Prognostic factors and predictive signs of malignancy in adult dermatomyositis. A study of 132 cases. *Archives of Dermatology* **126**, 633–637.

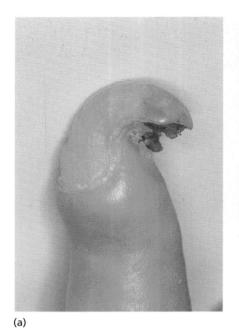

(a)

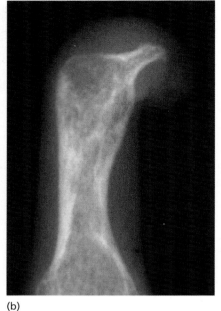

(b)

Caputo, R., Cappio, F., Rigoni, C. *et al.* (1993) Pterygium inversum unguis. Report of 19 cases and review of the literature. *Archives of Dermatology* **129**, 1307–1309.

Dupré, A., Viraben, R., Bonafe, J.L. *et al.* (1981) Zebra-like dermatomyositis. *Archives of Dermatology* **117**, 63–64.

Jorizzo, J.L., Gonzalez, E.B. & Daniels, J.C. (1983) Red lunulae in a patient with rheumatoid arthritis. *Journal of the American Academy of Dermatology* **8**, 711–714.

Rowell, N.R. (1986) Lupus erythematosus, scleroderma and dermatomyositis. The 'collagen' or 'connective-tissue' diseases. In: *Textbook of Dermatology* (eds A. Rook, D.S. Wilkinson, F.J.G. Ebling *et al.*), pp. 1281–1392. Blackwell Scientific Publications, Oxford.

Samitz, M.H. (1974) Cuticular changes in dermatomyositis. *Archives of Dermatology* **110**, 866–867.

Tosti, A., De Padova, M.P., Fanti, P. *et al.* (1987) Unusual severe nail involvement in dermatomyositis. *Cutis* **40**, 261–262.

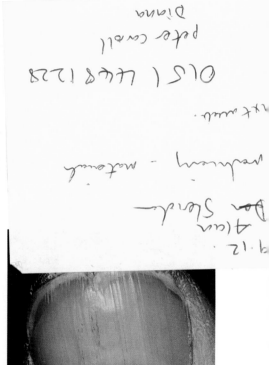

**Fig. 6.31** Rheumatoid arthritis, red lunula.

## Rheumatoid arthritis (Figs 6.30–6.34)

Palmar erythema and nail fold telangiectasia are well-known features of rheumatoid arthritis. The nail growth rate may be reduced in severe generalized rheumatoid disease (De Nicola *et al.* 1974). Longitudinal ridging with beading of the nails is commonly observed (Hamilton 1960; Michel *et al.* 1997) and does not seems to be related to the duration of the disease (Cimmino *et al.* 1994) Thumbnails and great toenails are more frequently affected. A global pattern of beading on the surface of at least six fingernails or four toenails has been reported to be highly specific for rheumatoid arthritis (predictive value of about 95%). Because nail beading is infrequent in the early phase of the disease, the diagnostic value of this nail abnormality is limited. It has been suggested that nail beading results from microvascular changes in the nail bed (Grant *et al.* 1985). Other nail abnormalities reported in rheumatoid arthritis include: hapalonychia, subungual hyperkeratosis, onychorrhexis, onychogryphosis (Fig. 6.30), clubbing, increased transverse curvature, pitting, nail thickening and discoloration as well as splinter haemorrhages (De Nicola *et al.* 1974; Daniel *et al.* 1985; Michel *et al.* 1997). Melanonychia was observed by Cimmino *et al.* (1994).

Yellow nail syndrome has been occasionally associated with rheumatoid arthritis or with penicillamine therapy in the latter condition. A pink or dusky red homogeneous discoloration of the proximal part of the lunula is characteristic of rheumatoid arthritis (Fig. 6.31). The prevalence of this alteration in rheumatoid arthritis has never been studied but red lunulae, which are more commonly observed in thumbnails and big toenails, are possibly more frequent than the literature suggests (Jorizzo *et al.* 1983). Red lunulae have also occasionally been described

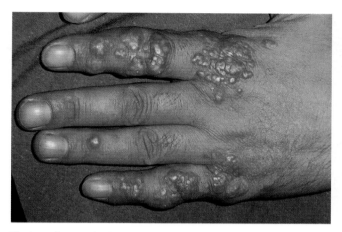

**Fig. 6.32** Rheumatoid nodules. (Courtesy of A. Rebora, Italy.)

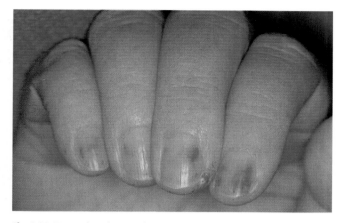

**Fig. 6.34** Wegener's syndrome—subungual purpuric lesions. (Courtesy of M.S. Daoud, USA.)

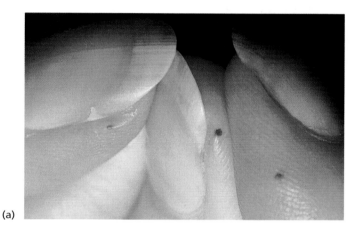

(a)

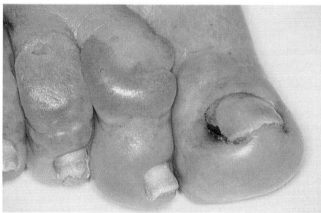

(b)

**Fig. 6.33** (a) Rheumatoid arthritis—Bywater's syndrome. (Courtesy of P.H. Normand, France.) (b) Rheumatoid arthritis—peripheral blisters and lateral periungual infarction.

in systemic lupus erythematosus, dermatomyositis, obstructive pulmonary disease and congestive heart failure (Wilkerson & Wilkin 1989).

Occasionally a 0.5–1-mm sharply demarcated deep violet area that runs parallel to the lunula at 4–5 mm from the free edge of the nails can be seen. This can also occur in some infectious diseases such as syphilis and leprosy (De Nicola *et al.* 1974).

Rheumatoid nodules (Fig. 6.32) can be localized to the terminal pads of the fingers and at the free edge of the nails. The histopathology of rheumatoid nodules shows fibrinoid necrosis surrounded by a palisade of lymphohistiocytic cells. These nodules can also occur in the absence of signs or symptoms of rheumatic disease (Rongioletti *et al.* 1990).

Nodules are reported in about 20% of patients with rheumatoid arthritis. A sudden increase in the number, size and distribution of the rheumatoid nodules after methotrexate treatment and many vasculitis lesions appearing on the nail folds was noted by Segal *et al.* (1988). Accelarated nodulosis was also reported by Abu-Shakra *et al.* (1994). Some of the patients studied by Kersten *et al.* (1992) presented with nail fold lesions and cutaneous vasculitic ulcers as well.

Nail fold and pulp lesions due to necrotizing vasculitis are not uncommon in patients with rheumatoid arthritis. Small painless infarcts of the nail fold are a characteristic feature of rheumatoid patients. The chronological evolution of these lesions has been clearly described by Bywaters and Scott (1963). Periungual swelling precedes the appearance of skin infarcts and necrosis; eschars usually disappear within a few days without scarring and this eventually results in grooving of the nail. Trauma may favour the occurrence of small ischaemic periungual lesions (Koebner phenomenon). Ischaemic areas on the nail fold can resemble an area of superficial paronychia (Fig. 6.33a) (Bywaters 1957; O'Quinn *et al.* 1965). These lesions may heal with scarring and the appearance of scars over the joints, in the nail fold and on the ends of the digits is frequent. Isolated nail fold vasculitis has a favourable prognosis compared with systemic vaculitis (Watts *et al.* 1995).

Large haemorrhages and bullae of digital pulps, as well as digital gangrene, are clinical signs of the most severe form of rheumatoid vasculitis (Fig. 6.33b).

## References

Abu-Shakra, M., Nicol, P. & Urowitz, M. (1994) Accelarated nodulois, pleural effusion and pericardial tamponade during methotrexate therapy. *Journal of Rheumatology* **21**, 934–937.

Bywaters, E.G.L. (1957) Peripheral vascular obstruction in rheumatoid arthritis and its relationship to other vascular lesions. *Annals of the Rheumatic Diseases* **16**, 84–103.

Bywaters, E.G.L. & Scott, J.T. (1963) The natural history of vascular lesions in rheumatoid arthritis. *Journal of Chronic Disease* **16**, 905–914.

Cimmino, M.A., Seriolo, B. & Accardo, S. (1994) Prevalence of nail involvement in nodal osteoarthritis. *Clinical Rheumatology* **13**, 203–206.

Daniel, R.C., Sams, W.M. & Scher, R.K. (1985) Nails in systemic disease. *Dermatologic Clinics* **3**, 465–483.

De Nicola, P.D., Morsiani, M. & Zavagli, G. (1974) *Nail Diseases in Internal Medicine.* Charles C. Thomas, Springfield, IL.

Grant, E.N., Bellamy, N., Buchanan, W.W. *et al.* (1985) Statistical reappraisal of the clinical significance of nail beading in rheumatoid arthritis. *Annals of the Rheumatic Diseases* **44**, 671–675.

Hamilton, E.B.D. (1960) Nail studies in rheumatoid arthritis. *Annals of the Rheumatic Diseases* **19**, 167–173.

Jorizzo, J.L., Gonzalez, E.B. & Daniels, J.C. (1983) Red lunulae in a patient with rheumatoid arthritis. *Journal of the American Academy of Dermatology* **8**, 711–714.

Kerstens, P.J., Boerbooms, A.M., Jeurissen, M.E. *et al.* (1992) Accelerated nodulosis during low dose methotrexate therapy for rheumatoid arthritis. An analysis of ten cases. *Journal of Rheumatology* **19**, 867–871.

Michel, C., Cribier, B., Sibilia, J. *et al.* (1997) Nail abnormalities in rheumathoid arthritis. *British Journal of Dermatology* **137**, 958–962.

O'Quinn, S.E., Kennedy, B.C. & Baker, D.T. (1965) Peripheral vascular lesions in rheumatoid arthritis. *Archives of Dermatology* **92**, 489–494.

Rongioletti, F., Cestari, R., Cozzani, E. *et al.* (1990) Nodules rhumatoides bénins chez un adulte (evaluant depuis 16 années). *Nouvelle Dermatologie* **9**, 655–656.

Segal, R., Caspi, D., Tishler, M. *et al.* (1988) Accelerated nodulosis and vasculitis during methotrexate therapy for rheumatoid arthritis. *Arthritis Rheumatism* **31**, 1182–1185.

Watts, R.A., Carruthers, D.M. & Scott, D.G. (1995) Isolated nail fold vasculitis in rheumatoid arthritis. *Annals of the Rheumatic Diseases* **54**, 927–929.

Wilkerson, M.G. & Wilkin, J.K. (1989) Red lunulae revisited: a clinical and histopathologic examination. *Journal of the American Academy of Dermatology* **20**, 453–457.

## Antisynthetase syndrome

This syndrome is characterized by lung disease, polymyositis, Raynaud's phenomenon and polyarthritis. Antiaminoacyl-transferRNAsynthetase antibodies are characteristic, the most common being anti-Jo1. Peringual ischaemic lesions and finger necrosis due to severe arteritis have been reported (Disdier *et al.* 1994).

## Reference

Disdier, P., Bolla, G., Harle, J.R. *et al.* (1994) Nécroses digitale révélatrices d'un syndrome des antisynthétase. *Annales de Dermatologie et de Vénéréologie* **121**, 493–495.

## Wegener's granulomatosis

Papular, pustular and necrotic lesions of the periungual tissues may be observed in Wegener's granulomatosis. Small linear infarcts of the nail fold have been reported in a patient affected by limited Wegener's granulomatosis (Spigel *et al.* 1983). Subungual purpuric lesions may be seen (Daoud *et al.* 1994) (Fig. 6.34). Avascular areas on nail fold capillary microscopy have been reported (Anders *et al.* 2000).

## References

Anders, H.J., Haedecke, C., Sigl, T. *et al.* (2000) Avascular areas on nail fold capillary microscopy of patients with Wegener's granulomatosis. *Clinical Rheumatology* **19**, 86–88.

Daoud, M.S., Gibson, L.E., De Remee, R.A. *et al.* (1994) Cutaneous Wegener's granulomatosis: clinical, histologic and immunopathologic features of thirty patients. *Journal of the American Academy of Dermatology* **31**, 605–612.

Spigel, G.T., Krall, R.A. & Hilal, A. (1983) Limited Wegener's granulomatosis: unusual cutaneous, radiographic and pathologic manifestations. *Cutis* **32**, 41–51.

## Periarteritis nodosa

Small infarcts of the nail fold and of the distal aspects of fingers and toes may be a feature of periarteritis nodosa. Digital gangrene can rarely occur (Broussard & Baethge 1990; Trüeb *et al.* 1999). Thinning, splitting and ridging of the fingernails and toenails associated with a blue-red rash on finger and toe tips have been reported in a patient affected by benign cutaneous periarteritis nodosa (Kassis *et al.* 1985) (Fig. 6.35). Raynaud's

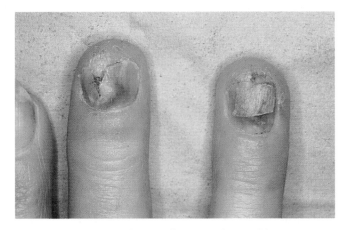

**Fig. 6.35** Periarteritis nodosa. (Courtesy of V. Kassis *et al.*, Denmark.)

phenomenon and nail dystrophy such as onychoschizia have been reported (Trüeb *et al.* 1995).

## References

Broussard, R.K. & Baethge, B.A. (1990) Peripheral gangrene in polyarteritis nodosa. *Cutis* **46**, 53–55.

Kassis, V., Kassis, E. & Thomsen, H.K. (1985) Benign cutaneous periarteritis nodosa with nail defects. *Journal of the American Academy of Dermatology* **13**, 661–663.

Trüeb, R.M., Hürlimann, A.F. & Burg, G. (1995) Periarteritis nodosa cutanea. *Hautarzt* **46**, 568–572.

Trüeb, R.M., Scheideger, E.P., Pericin, M. *et al.* (1999) Periarteritis nodosa presenting as a breast lesion: report of a case and review of the literature. *British Journal of Dermatology* **141**, 1117–1121.

## Microscopic polyarteritis

Microscopic polyarteritis is a systemic small-vessels vasculitis that primarly involves kidneys. The lung, nervous system and skin can also be affected. Ecchymotic lesions and haemorrhagic crusted macules and papules may affect periungual tissues (Homas *et al.* 1992).

## Reference

Homas, P.B., David Bajar, K.M., Fitzpatrick, J.E. *et al.* (1992) Microscopic polyarteritis. *Archives of Dermatology* **128**, 1223–1228.

## Multicentric reticulohistiocytosis (Fig. 6.36)

Multicentric reticulohistiocytosis is a rare disorder characterized by papulonodular skin lesions, a disabling polyarthritis and a typical dermal infiltration of histiocytes and multinucleated giant cells. Wart-like dark-red to flesh-coloured nodules arranged around the nail folds of fingers in a 'coral bead' configuration occur in about half of the patients (Lesher & Allen 1984). Hard and painful nodules on the fingertips have been reported. Joint destruction leads to shortening of the distal phalanges, and racket nails are characteristic (Barrow 1967). Nail brittleness, longitudinal ridging, hyperpigmentation and atrophy have also been described. Although approximately a quarter of the patients have associated malignancies, the possibility that multicentric reticulohistiocytosis is a paraneoplastic syndrome is still under discussion (Aldridge *et al.* 1984; Lesher & Allen 1984; Nunnink *et al.* 1985; Oliver *et al.* 1990). Therapy with azathioprine and prednisolone may be effective (Fedler *et al.* 1995).

## References

Aldridge, R.D., Main, R.A. & Daly, B.M. (1984) Multicentric reticulohistiocytosis and cancer. *Journal of the American Academy of Dermatology* **10**, 296–297.

Barrow, M.V. (1967) The nails in multicentric reticulohistiocytosis. *Archives of Dermatology* **95**, 200–201.

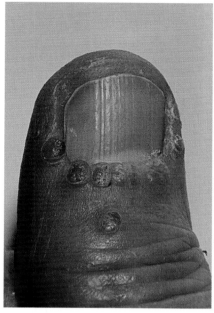

(a)

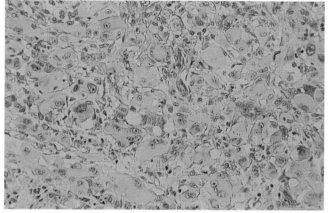

(b)

**Fig. 6.36** (a) Multicentric reticulohistiocytosis. (b) Multicentric reticulohistiocytosis—cellular infiltrate from affected area.

Fedler, R., Frantzmann, Y., Schwarze, E.W. *et al.* (1995) Die multizentrische Retikulohistiozytose. Therapie mit Azathioprin und Prednisolone. *Hautarzt* **46**, 118–120.

Lesher, J.L. & Allen, B.S. (1984) Multicentric reticulohistiocytosis. *Journal of the American Academy of Dermatology* **11**, 713–723.

Nunnink, J.C., Krusinski, P.A. & Yates, J.W. (1985) Multicentric reticulohistiocytosis and cancer: a case report and review of the literature. *Medical and Pediatric Oncology* **13**, 273–279.

Oliver, G.F., Umbert, I., Winkelmann, R.K. & Muller, S.A. (1990) Reticulohistiocytoma cutis—review of 15 cases and an association with Systemic Vasculitis in two cases. *Clinical and Experimental Dermatology* **15**, 1–6.

## Follicular mucinosis (alopecia mucinosa)

Lapiere *et al.* (1972) reported a case of follicular mucinosis with

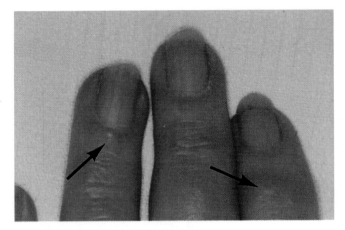

**Fig. 6.37** Fibroblastic rheumatism. (Courtesy of A. Claudy, France.)

nail involvement. All fingernails and toenails were thickened, brittle and ridged. Periungual tissues were normal. At biopsy, the nail was hollowed out by cavities running parallel to the surface and filled with amorphous material stained by mucicarmin and periodic acid–Schiff (PAS). In the nail bed a dense histiolymphocytic cell infiltrate that resembled the perifollicular infiltration separated the basal layer from the overlying keratinocytes.

### Reference

Lapiere, S., Castermans-Elias, S. & Pierard, G. (1972) Mucinose folliculaire et unguéale généralisée. *Bulletin de la Societé Française de Dermatologie et de Syphiligraphie* 79, 235–238.

### Fibroblastic rheumatism

This entity, first reported in 1980 by Chaouat *et al.*, is characterized by the association of symmetrical polyarthritis and skin nodules. The histological picture of the skin nodules is specific, revealing fibroblastic proliferation and fibrosis with thickened collagen bundles that are arranged in a 'whorl-like pattern' (Vignon-Pennamen *et al.* 1986). Cutaneous nodules are located mostly over the extensor aspect of the fingers (Fig. 6.37). The nodules are firm, flesh-coloured or yellowish, measuring from 0.5 to 1 cm in diameter. Sclerodactyly and Raynaud's phenomenon can also occur (Lévigne *et al.* 1990).

### References

Chaouat, Y., Aron-Brunietiere, R., Faures, B. *et al.* (1980) Une nouvelle entité: le rheumatisme fibroblastique. A propos d'une observation. *Reviews of Rheumatology* 47, 345–35.

Lévigne, V., Perrot, J.L., Faisant, M. *et al.* (1990) Rheumatisme fibroblastique. *Annales de Dermatologie et de Vénéréologie* 117, 199–202.

Vignon-Pennamen, M.D., Navran, B., Foldes, C. *et al.* (1986) Fibroblastic rheumatism. *Journal of the American Academy of Dermatology* 14, 1086–1088.

### Osteoarthritis

Leuconychia, longitudinal grooves and nail ridging have been reported in patients with primary interphalangeal osteoarthritis of the hand.

Osteoarthritic changes of the distal interphalangeal joints may cause nail lesions by exerting direct pressure on the nail matrix or by interfering with local blood flow. Inflammation of Heberden's nodes seems to participate in the development of the nail alterations. Mucinous (myxoid) cysts are frequently observed (Cutolo *et al.* 1990).

### Reference

Cutolo, M., Cimmino, M.A. & Accardo, S. (1990) Nail involvement in osteoarthritis. *Clinical Rheumatology* 9, 242–245.

## Respiratory disorders

Exposure to extremely high altitudes for several weeks may be followed by the development of splinter haemorrhages (page 234) and true transverse leukonychia (Hutchinson & Amin 1997). The latter may possibly result from altitude-related hypoxia and catabolic stress.

### Reference

Hutchinson, S.J. & Amin, S. (1997) Everest nails. *New England Journal of Medicine* 336, 229.

### Hypertrophic pulmonary osteoarthropathy

Hypertrophic osteoarthropathy (HO) is a syndrome consisting of digital clubbing, joint effusion and periosteal new bone formation. HO is frequently associated with intrathoracic neoplasms, either primary or metastatic, and occurs in 0.7–12% of patients with bronchogenic carcinoma (Firooznia *et al.* 1975). Lung cancer (primary or metastatic) accounts for 80% of the cases, pleural tumours for 10% and other intrathoracic tumours for 5% (Coury 1960). It can also be observed in patients with chronic intrathoracic suppurative diseases, such as bronchiectasis empyema, lung abscesses, pulmonary blastomycosis, pulmonary aspergillosis and rarely pulmonary tuberculosis.

HO can also occur in association with a variety of extrapulmonary abnormalities including inflammatory bowel disease, chronic methaemoglobinaemia, liver disorders, gastrointestinal neoplasms and cyanotic congenital heart diseases. Occasionally it is idiopathic or hereditary. HO limited to the lower limbs can be the initial symptom of an infected abdominal graft associated with aortoenteric fistula.

The complete clinical manifestations of HO include:
1 Digital clubbing accompanied by acromegalic features of the upper and lower extremities.

2 Painful swelling and tenderness of the distal third of the arms and legs and adjacent joints.

3 Joint effusions.

4 Bilateral proliferative periostitis of the long bones of the extremities at X-ray and scintigraphic examinations.

Mechanisms involved in the pathogenesis of HO are still unknown. A neural reflex initiated by the lung and mediated by the vagus nerve has been suggested by the fact that the symptoms are dramatically relieved by intrathoracic or cervical vagotomy (Holling 1967).

HO can be either an early or a late symptom of pulmonary tumours and removal of the malignant neoplasm usually results in the resolution of clinical manifestations (Stenseth *et al.* 1967; Krischer & Donath 1994).

Clubbing of the fingers is discussed more fully in the chapter on modifications of the normal nail form (Chapter 2).

## References

Coury, C. (1960) Hippocratic fingers and hypertrophic osteoarthropathy: Study of 350 cases. *British Journal of Diseases of the Chest* **54**, 202–209.

Firooznia, H., Seliger, G., Genieser, N.B. *et al.* (1975) Hypertrophic pulmonary osteoarthropathy in pulmonary metastases. *Radiology* **115**, 269–274.

Holling, H.E. (1967) Pulmonary hypertrophic osteoarthropathy. *Annals of Internal Medicine* **66**, 232–234.

Krischer, U. & Donath, G. (1994) Hypertrophic pulmonal osteoarthropathy: rare different diagnosis of unclear polyarthritis. *Aktuelle-Rheumatologie* **19**, 99–102.

Stenseth, J.H., Clagett, O.T. & Woolner, L.B. (1967) Hypertrophic pulmonary osteoarthropathy. *Diseases of the Chest* **52**: 62–68.

## Yellow nail syndrome (Fig. 6.38)

The yellow nail syndrome (YNS) is an uncommon disorder of unknown aetiology characterized by the triad of yellow nails, lymphoedema and respiratory tract involvement. This term (Samman & White 1964) was originally used to describe the association of slow-growing yellow nails with primary lymphoedema. Pleural effusion (Emerson 1966) was later recognized as an additional sign of the syndrome. Since then other respiratory conditions such as bronchiectasis, sinusitis, bronchitis and chronic respiratory infections have been associated with the disorder. Although all the three signs which classically characterize the triad of YNS do not occur in every patient, the presence of typical nail alterations should be considered an absolute requirement for the diagnosis.

The time between the development of the various manifestations may range from months to years.

YNS is more common in adults but it can also occur in children (Paradisis & Van Asperen 1977; Magid *et al.* 1987), males and females being equally affected.

Nail changes are characteristic, usually affecting both fingernails and toenails, and are associated with a very slow growth

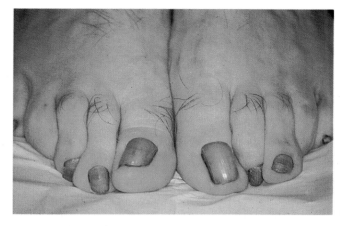

(a)

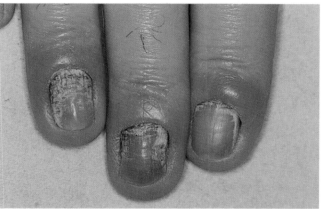

(b)

**Fig. 6.38** (a) Yellow nail syndrome. (b) Yellow nail syndrome—periungual swelling.

rate (less than 0.2 mm week) (Samman & White 1964). Nails are thickened with increased transverse curvature, so that coverage of the lateral ridges by the surrounding soft tissues is less than normal and the cuticles are deficient. Hardness of the nails (scleronychia) makes it difficult to take a biopsy through the nail plate. Erythema and oedema of the proximal nail fold can be present. Chronic paronychia can occasionally be observed. The entire nail plate shows a diffuse pale yellow to dark yellow-green discoloration. The edges of the nails are occasionally darker than the remainder and the proximal part of the nail plate can sometimes maintain a normal colour. Nails are frequently opaque so that the lunulae are no longer visible. The nail surface is usually smooth but transverse ridging due to periodic variations in the growth rate can be present. Onycholysis may occur and extend far enough toward the matrix to cause complete shedding, the nails are replaced extremely slowly. Partially separated nails sometimes show a distinctive hump.

The pathogenesis of nail and systemic manifestations of YNS is unresolved. Impaired lymphatic drainage is thought to be the underlying defect responsible for the various clinical findings in patients with YNS. While lymphoangiograms have shown abnormal findings such as atresia, hypoplasia and varicose abnormalities of peripheral lymphatics in some patients, this has not been a consistent finding. It has been suggested that a widespread lymphatic abnormality that is adequate early in life becomes deficient following inflammation or stress. Results of quantitative lymphoscintigraphy of 17 subjects with YNS suggest that the lymphatic impairment is not due to anatomical abnormalities, but rather to a functional disorder. This hypothesis is confirmed by reversibility of lymphoedema in this condition (Bull *et al.* 1996).

Defective lymph drainage in the nail regions can be responsible for the slow nail growth and for the thickened yellow nails that characterize the syndrome. Lymphatic obstruction resulting from sclerosis in the subungual stroma has been recently postulated (De Coste *et al.* 1990). The appearance of the nails probably depends on the slow growth rate. The resolution of the nail changes is, in fact, always associated with resumption of normal nail growth. Abnormal nail keratinization has been suggested by the presence of keratohyalin granules in the nail plate (Pavlidakey *et al.* 1984). The deposition of an acetone soluble yellow substance (Ohkuma 1982) has not been confirmed (Reynes *et al.* 1984). Accumulation of lipofuscin pigments may be the source of the nail colour (Norton 1985).

Evidence of lymphoedema or respiratory manifestations may not become evident for years after the nails have become involved. Lymphoedema is usually more obvious in the ankles and the legs, but the hands or even the face can be affected. It can rarely be generalized. Malek *et al.* (1996) reported a young patient with YNS associated with diffuse lymphangiectasia involving the whole small bowel. Congenital lymphoedema has also been reported in association with YNS.

Respiratory manifestations of YNS include pleural effusion or other signs of upper and lower respiratory disease such as sinusitis, bronchitis and bronchiectasis (Hiller *et al.* 1972). YNS has been reported to occur on several occasions in patients with thyroiditis, rheumatoid arthritis, nephrotic syndrome, underlying malignancies and immune deficiencies (Malliet *et al.* 1985; Nordkild *et al.* 1986). Occasional reports indicate that YNS has occurred along with a large variety of disorders, including mental retardation, sleep apnoea, connective tissue diseases, breasts of unequal size, hypoplastic kidney, myocardial infarction, increased susceptibility to skin and soft tissue infections, chronic pulmonary and hepatic tuberculosis, chylothorax, D-penicillamine therapy and even extremely hard ear wax. A case of reversible YNS in association with chronic graft versus host reaction has been reported (Mascaro & Martin-Ortega 1993).

The term YNS has been improperly used to describe yellow discoloration of the nails in patients with human immunodeficiency virus (HIV) infection (Chernosky & Finley 1985). These patients did not present the characteristic nail changes of YNS (Daniel 1986; Haas & Dover 1986; Scher 1988).

Improvement, or clearing, of nail changes concomitant with the resolution of systemic manifestations has been reported in a number of cases of YNS. In a patient with YNS associated with rheumatoid arthritis, the nail abnormalities completely regressed after gold therapy for arthritis (Launay *et al.* 1997). Spontaneous improvement of the nails can also occur (Samman 1973; Venencie & Dicken 1984). Intradermal triamcinolone injections in the proximal nail matrix have been reported to be useful. The topical use of vitamin E solution in dimethyl sulfoxide (DMSO) has been shown successful in the treatment of nail changes in YNS (Williams *et al.* 1991). Vitamin E at dosages ranging from 600 to 1200 international units daily can induce a complete clearing of the nail changes (Ayres & Mihau 1973; Norton 1985; Rommel *et al.* 1985; Tosti *et al.* 1997). Although the mechanism of action of vitamin E in YNS is still unknown, antioxidant properties of α-tocoferol may account for its efficacy. Pulse therapy with itraconazole (400 mg/daily for 1 week a month for 4–6 months) improves the YNS by stimulating nail growth (Luyten *et al.* 1996; A. Tosti, unpublished data).

In the patient reported by Arroyo and Cohen (1992), total resolution of yellow nails and lymphoedema was observed following oral zinc supplementation for 2 years. A 'Brownish black nail syndrome' in a Nigerian patient has been described as the equivalent of YNS in Caucasians (Somorin & Adesugba 1978).

## References

Arroyo, J.F. & Cohen, M.L. (1992) YNS cured by zinc supplementation. *Clinical and Experimental Dermatology* **18**, 62–64.

Ayres, S. & Mihan, R. (1973) Yellow nail syndrome. Response to vitamin E. *Archives of Dermatology* **108**, 267–268.

Bull, R.H., Fenton, D.A. & Mortimer, P.S. (1996) Lymphatic function in the yellow nail syndrome. *British Journal of Dermatology* **134**, 307–312.

Chernosky, M.E. & Finley, V.K. (1985) Yellow nail syndrome in patients with acquired immunodeficiency disease. *Journal of the American Academy of Dermatology* **13**, 731–736.

Daniel, C.R. (1986) Yellow nail syndrome and acquired immunodeficiency disease. *Journal of the American Academy of Dermatology* **14**, 844–845.

De Coste, S., Imber, M.J. & Baden, H.P. (1990) Yellow nail syndrome. *Journal of the American Academy of Dermatology* **22**, 608–611.

Emerson, P.A. (1966) Yellow nails, lymphoedema and pleural effusions. *Thorax* **21**, 247–253.

Haas, A. & Dover, J.S. (1986) Yellow nail syndrome and acquired immunodeficiency disease. *Journal of the American Academy of Dermatology* **14**, 845.

Hiller, E., Rosenow, E.C. & Olsen, A.M. (1972) Pulmonary manifestations of the yellow nail syndrome. *Chest* **61**, 452–458.

Launay, D., Hebbar, M., Louyot, J. *et al.* (1997) Syndrome des ongles jaunes associé à une polyarthrite rhumatoïde. Régression sous chrysothérapie. *Revue de Medecine Interne* **18**, 494–496.

Luyten, C., André, J., Walraevens, C. *et al.* (1996) Yellow nails syndrome and onychomycosis. *Dermatology* **192**, 406–408.

Magid, M., Esterly, N.B., Prendiville, J. *et al.* (1987) The yellow nail syndrome in an 8-year-old girl. *Pediatric Dermatology* **4**, 90–93.

Malek, N.P., Ocran, K., Tietge, U.J. *et al.* (1996) A case of the yellow nail syndrome associated with massive chylous ascites, pleural and pericardial effusions. *Zeitschrift für Gastroenterologie* **34**, 763–766.

Malliet, C., Marcucilli, A., Aubin, B. *et al.* (1985) Syndrome des ongles jaunes. *Semaine des hopitaux de Paris* **61**, 2871–2876.

Mascaro, J.M. & Martin-Ortega, E. (1993) Nail alterations in graft-versus-host disease and other immunological disorders. In: *Dermatology Progress and Perspectives*, pp. 393–394. The Parthenon Publishing Group, New York.

Nordkild, P., Kromann-Andersen, H. & Struve-Christensen, E. (1986) Yellow nail syndrome—the triad of yellow nails, lymphedema and pleural effusions. *Acta Medica Scandinavica* **219**, 221–227.

Norton, L. (1985) Further observations on the yellow nail syndrome with therapeutic effects of oral alpha-tocopherol. *Cutis* **6**, 457–462.

Ohkuma, M. (1982) Studies on yellow nails. In: *Proceedings of the XVIth International Congress on Dermatology* (eds A. Kukita & M. Seiji) Tokyo Univ Press, Tokyo.

Paradisis, M. & Van Asperen, P. (1997) Yellow nail syndrome in infancy. *Journal of Pediatrics and Child Health* **33**, 454–457.

Pavlidakey, G.P., Hashimoto, K. & Blum, D. (1984) Yellow nail syndrome. *Journal of the American Academy of Dermatology* **11**, 509–512.

Reynes, J., Bernard, E., Dellamonica, P. *et al.* (1984) Un cas de syndrome des ongles jaunes. *Annales de Dermatologie et de Vénéréologie* **111**, 273–275.

Rommel, A., Havet, M., Ball, M. *et al.* (1985) Syndrome des ongles jaunes: réponse a la vitamine E. *Annales de Dermatologie et de Vénéréologie* **12**, 625–627.

Samman, P.D. (1973) The yellow nail syndrome (report on 55 cases). *Transactions of the St Johns Hospital Dermatology Society* **59**, 37–38.

Samman, P.D. & White, W.F. (1964) The yellow nail syndrome. *British Journal of Dermatology* **16**, 153–157.

Scher, R.K. (1988) Acquired immunodeficiency syndrome and yellow nails. *Journal of the American Academy of Dermatology* **18**, 758–759.

Somorin, A.O. & Adesugba, A.J. (1978) The yellow nail syndrome associated with sinusitis, bronchiectasis and transitory lymphoedema in a Nigerian patient. *Clinical and Experimental Dermatology* **3**, 31–33.

Tosti, A., Guidetti, M.S., Lorenzi, S. *et al.* (1997) La sindrome delle unghie gialle. Esperienza di nove casi. *Giornale Italiano di Dermatologia e Venereologia* **132**, 255–258.

Venencie, P.Y. & Dicken, C.H. (1984) Yellow nail syndrome: report of five cases. *Journal of the American Academy of Dermatology* **10**, 187–192.

Williams, B.C., Buffham, R. & du Vivier, A. (1991) Successful use of topical vit E solution in the treatment of nail changes in yellow nail syndrome. *Archives of Dermatology* **127**, 1023–1028.

## Shell nail syndrome

This term was coined to describe a peculiar nail deformity which occurred in a 37-year-old woman affected by bronchiectasis (Cornelius & Shelley 1967). All fingernails and big toenails showed a similar dystrophy characterized by excessive longitudinal curvature of the nail plate associated with atrophy of the distal nail bed. A small shell-like space was present between the curved thickened nail plate and the atrophic nail bed. X-rays of fingers showed thinning of the distal phalanges with complete loss of tufting. These changes seem to be the reverse of clubbing. There is atrophy of the nail bed instead of bulbous soft tissue proliferation and bony atrophy instead of new bone formation and chronic periostitis as found in clubbing.

## Reference

Cornelius, C.E. & Shelley, W.B. (1967) Shell nail syndrome associated with bronchiectasis. *Archives of Dermatology* **96**, 694–695.

## Sarcoidosis (Fig. 6.39, Table 6.5)

Nail involvement in sarcoidosis is rare and almost always associated with evidence of bone changes in the underlying phalanges (Leibowitz *et al.* 1985). It is more commonly observed in patients with chronic and multisystem disease. Although nail involvement is commonly associated with lupus pernio of the digits or with sarcoidal dactylitis, it can also occur without apparent involvement of the adjacent soft tissue. Sarcoid dactylitis occurs in 0.2% of patients with sarcoidosis. Fusiform swelling can involve single or numerous digits (Micalizzi *et al.* 1997). It is usually painful. Digital swelling and pain can precede changes in routine radiographs (Lovy 1981; Pitt *et al.* 1983). A necrotizing variety of sarcoid dactylitis characterized by finger ulcerations and dystrophic nails has been reported in black South Africans (Leibowitz *et al.* 1985).

Nail plate alterations include thickening, onychogryphosis (Cohen & Lester 1999), brittleness, fragility, longitudinal ridging, cracking, layering and pitting (Cox & Gawkrodger 1988; Saada & Elbez 1990). Onycholysis of fingernails and toenails has also been reported (Davies & McGavin 1996), as well as splinter haemorrhages and red or brown discoloration of the nail bed. Pterygium or even partial or complete atrophy of the nails can also occur (Kalb & Grossman 1985). Nail abnormalities result from impairment of the nail matrix keratinization as a consequence of compression of the nail matrix from granulomas localized in the dermis of the proximal nail fold (Wakelin & James 1995; Tosti *et al.* 1997). These may occasionally produce destruction of the nail matrix. Granulomatous involvement of the nail bed and the hyponychium can also occur (Losada-Campa *et al.* 1995). The nail changes may clear after treatment with oral prednisone and chloroquine phosphate (Patel & Sharma 1983). Finger clubbing is very rarely associated with pulmonary sarcoidosis (Yancey 1972). It may be unidigital or asymmetrical (Hashmi & Kaplan 1992). Acquired painful clubbing of all fingers and toes without evidence of cyanosis has been reported in a patient with diffuse chronic sarcoidosis (West *et al.* 1981). A normal radiography was associated with subungual hyperkeratosis of the toenails (Fujji *et al.* 1997) with discrete epithelioid granulomas in the superficial dermis. Subungual and periungual plaques and nodules of big toenails due to sarcoid granuloma have been observed in a 46-year-old patient (Guillet *et al.* 1984).

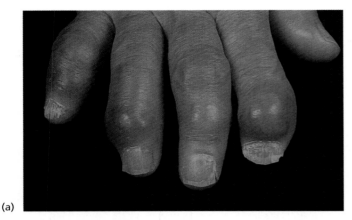

(a)

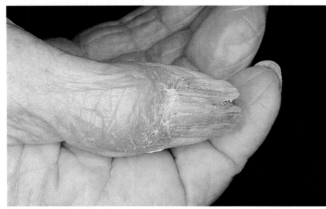

(b)

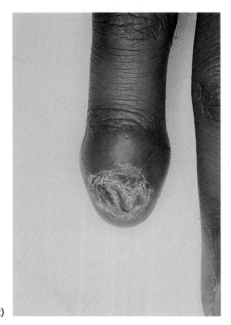

(c)

**Fig. 6.39** (a) Sarcoidosis. (b) Sarcoidosis with nail dystrophy. (c) Sarcoidosis with painful clubbing.

**Table 6.5** Nail changes reported in sarcoidosis. (After Cohen & Lester 1999.)

Atrophy

Clubbing

Dystrophy

Fragility, cracking

Irregular pink and brown macular discoloration

Lamellar splitting

Longitudinal ridging

Onycholysis

Opacity

Pitting and brittleness

Pterygium formation

Splinter haemorrhages

Subungual hyperkeratosis and hyperkeratotic verrucous lesions of the hyponychium

Thickening

## References

Cohen, P.D. & Lester, R.S. (1999) Sacoidosis presenting as nail dystrophy. *Journal of Cutaneous Medicine and Surgery* 6, 302–305.

Cox, H.N. & Gawkrodger, D.J. (1988) Nail dystrophy in chronic sarcoidosis. *British Journal of Dermatology* 118, 697–701.

Davies, M.G. & McGavin, C.R. (1996) Onycholysis in sarcoidosis—a previously undescribed association. *British Journal of Dermatology* 135, 330–345.

Fujii, K., Kanno, Y. & Ohgon, N. (1997) Subungual hyperkeratosis due to sarcoidosis. *International Journal of Dermatology* 36, 125–127.

Guillet, G., Labouche, F., Guillet, J. *et al.* (1984) La scintigraphie au citrate de Gallium (67 Ga) dans la Sarcoidose. *Annales de Dermatologie et de Vénéréologie* 111, 1023–1027.

Hashmi, S. & Kaplan, D. (1992) Asymmetric clubbing as a manifestation of sarcoid bone disease. *American Journal of Medicine* 93, 471.

Kalb, R.E. & Grossman, M.E. (1985) Pterygium formation due to sarcoidosis. *Archives of Dermatology* 121, 276–277.

Leibowitz, M.R., Essop, A.R., Schamroth, C.L. *et al.* (1985) Sarcoid dactilitis in Black South African patients. *Seminars in Arthritis and Rheumatism* 14, 232–237.

Losada-Campa, A., De la Torre-Fraga, C., Gomez de Liaño, A. *et al.* (1995) Histopathology of nail sarcoidosis. *Acta Dermato-Venereologica* 75, 404–413.

Lovy, M.R. (1981) Sarcoidosis presenting as subacute polydactilitis. *Journal of Rheumatology* 8, 350–352.

Micalizzi, C., Parodi, A. & Rebora, A. (1997) Nail dystrophy in sarcoidosis. *European Journal of Dermatology* 7, 509–510.

Patel, K.B. & Sharma, O.P. (1983) Nails in sarcoidosis: response to treatment. *Archives of Dermatology* 119, 277–278.

Pitt, P., Hamilton, E.B.D., Innes, E.H. *et al.* (1983) Sarcoid dactilitis. *Annals of the Rheumatic Diseases* 42, 634–639.

Saada, V. & Elbez, P. (1990) Sarcoidose unguéale. A propos d'un cas. *Review of European Dermatology. MST* 2, 157–160.

Tosti, A., Peluso, A.M., Misciali, C. *et al.* (1997) Systemic sarcoidosis presenting with nail dystrophy. *European Journal of Dermatology* 7, 69–70.

Yancey, J. (1972) Clubbing of the fingers in Sarcoidosis. *Journal of the American Medical Association* 222, 582.

Wakelin, S.H. & James, M.P. (1995) Sarcoidosis: nail dystrophy without underlying bone changes. *Cutis* 55, 344–346.

West, S.G., Gilbreath, R.E. & Lawless, O.J. (1981) Painful clubbing and sarcoidosis. *Journal of the American Medical Association* 246, 1338–1339.

## Bronchial carcinoma (see also 'Clubbing' above)

Onycholysis involving all the fingernails has been described in a patient affected by squamous cell carcinoma of the lung (Hickmann 1977). Another case has been reported by Cliff and Mortimer (1996).

### References

Cliff, S. & Mortimer, D.S. (1996) Onycholysis associated with cancer of the lung. *Clinical and Experimental Dermatology* 21, 244.

Hickmann, J.W. (1977) Onycholysis associated with carcinoma of the lung. *Journal of the American Medical Association* 238, 1246–1247.

## Asthma

Minimal digital clubbing may rarely occur in children with uncomplicated asthma (Sly *et al.* 1972). Significant clubbing has also been seen in children with severe asthma requiring long-term corticosteroids. In addition, all cases had atopic eczema. Complete disappearance of the clubbing followed improvement of the asthma (Rao *et al.* 1981).

### References

Rao, M., Victoria, M.S., Maraya, R. *et al.* (1981) Digital clubbing in children with chronic asthma—a clinical experience at Kings County Hospital. *Asthma* 18, 49–56.

Sly, R.M., Fuqua, G., Matta, E.G. *et al.* (1972) Objective assessment of minimal digital clubbing in asthmatic children. *Annals of Allergy* 30, 575–578.

## Smoking cessation

Yellow pigmentation of the nail plate—referred to as the 'nicotine nail'—is common. The sudden cessation of smoking due to an intercurrent disease leads to the development of a distinct line of demarcation between the distal pigmented nail and the newly emerging proximal non-pigmented nail. The term 'harlequin nail' (Verghese *et al.* 1990) or 'quitter's nail' (Verghese *et al.* 1994) have been proposed for this curious physical sign.

### References

Verghese, A., Krish, G., Howe, D. *et al.* (1990) The Harlequin nail. A marker for smoking cessation. *Chest* 97, 236–237.

Verghese, A. (1994) Quitter's nail. *New England Journal of Medicine* 330, 974.

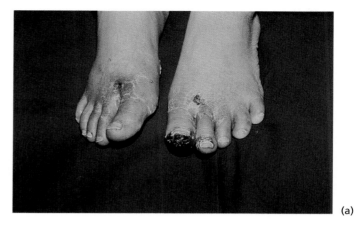

(a)

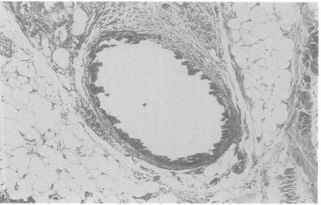

(b)

**Fig. 6.40** (a) Calciphylaxis—gangrene. (Courtesy of P. Chang, Guatemala.) (b) Calciphylaxis—histology. (Courtesy of L. Requena, Spain.)

## Renal disorders

Nail clippings from patients with chronic renal failure reveal elevated levels of creatinine. Measurement of creatinine from the nails can therefore be utilized for differentiating acute from chronic renal failure (Levitt 1966; Li *et al.* 1995; Shand *et al.* 1977). Uraemic patients can present with thickening and yellow or grey discoloration of fingernails and toenails. Onycholysis has also been reported (Bencini *et al.* 1987).

Acral necrosis due to calciphylaxis may involve several digits (Fig. 6.40) (Scheinman *et al.* 1991; Farina *et al.* 1997). Calciphylaxis has also occurred in patients undergoing renal transplantation (Fox *et al.* 1983) and in patients undergoing long-term peritoneal dialysis and haemodialysis (Gibstein *et al.* 1976).

### References

Bencini, P.L., Valeriani, D.E., Bianchini, F.E. *et al.* (1987) Alterazioni cutanee nell'uremia. *Giornale Italiano di Dermatologia e Venereologia* 122, 407–412.

Farina, M.C., Desequera, P., Soriano, M.L. *et al.* (1997) Calcifilaxis. *Acta-Dermosifilitica* 88, 333–336.

Fox, R., Banowsky, L.H. & Cruz, K.B. (1983) Post-renal transplant calciphylaxis. *Journal of Urology* **129**, 362–363.

Gibstein, R.M., Cobrun, J.W. & Adams, D.A. (1976) Calciphylaxis in man: a syndrome of tissue necrosis and vascular calcification in 11 patients with chronic renal failure. *Archives of Internal Medicine* **136**, 1273–1280.

Levitt, J.I. (1966) Creatine concentration of human fingernails and toenail clippings. *Annals of Internal Medicine* **64**, 312–327.

Li, J., Yu, H., Han, J. *et al.* (1995) The measurement of fingernail creatinine in the differentiation of acute from chronic renal failure. *Clinical Nephrology* **45**, 241–243.

Scheinman, I.L., Helm, K.F. & Fairley, J.A. (1991) Acral necrosis in a patient with chronic renal failure. *Archives of Dermatology* **127**, 247–252.

Shand, B.I., Bailey, M.A. & Bailey, R.R. (1997) Fingernail creatinine as a determinant of the duration of renal failure. *Clinical Nephrology* **47**, 135–136.

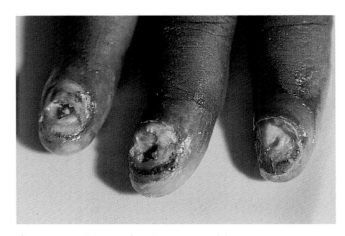

**Fig. 6.41** Haemodialysis pseudoporphyria—erosive nail changes.

## Muehrcke's lines (see Chapter 2)

Muehrcke's lines of the fingernails represent an important cutaneous sign of chronic severe hypoalbuminaemia (Muehrcke 1956). Muehrcke's lines that belong to the group of apparent leuconychia appear as paired narrow white transverse bands in the nail bed. The two bands that run parallel to the lunula are non-palpable and separated from the lunula and from each other by normal pink nail. Bands do not move distally with the growth of the nails and compression of the fingertips will cause the lines to disappear temporarily.

Muehrcke's lines are more commonly observed on the 2nd, 3rd and 4th fingers. They are rarely seen on the thumbs. The distal white band may be slightly wider than the proximal band.

Muehrcke reported these lines in the nail beds of patients with persistent severe hypoalbuminemia (below 2.2 g/100 mL). Muehrcke's lines appear to be more pronounced in patients who have had serum albumin levels of under 1.8 g/100 mL for at least 4 months. Muehrcke's lines usually disappear when albumin level returns to normal limits (above 2.2 g/100 mL) (Nabai 1998). Although Muehrcke's lines are most frequently observed in patients with nephrotic syndrome, they can also occur in association with other diseases causing hypoalbuminaemia. Conn and Smith (1965) found myoedema and Muehrcke's line useful 'bedside' indicators of the serum albumin level. The pathogenesis of Muehrcke's lines is still uncertain. Oedematous changes in the nail bed connective tissue (Lewin 1965) or alteration of the nail plate to nail bed attachment have been offered as possible explanations for the nail discoloration. Muehrcke's lines have also been described in patients submitted to combination chemotherapy for malignant neoplasms in the absence of decreased albumin levels (Schwartz & Vickerman 1979).

## References

Conn, R.D. & Smith, R.H. (1965) Malnutrition, myoedema and Muehrcke's lines. *Archives of Internal Medicine* **116**, 875–878.

Lewin, K. (1965) The finger nail in general disease. *British Journal of Dermatology* **77**, 431–438.

Muehrcke, R.C. (1956) The finger-nails in chronic hypoalbuminemia. *British Medical Journal* **1**, 1327–1328.

Nabai, H. (1998) Nail changes before and after transplantation: personal observation by a physician. *Cutis* **61**, 31–32.

Schwartz, R.A. & Vickerman, C.E. (1979) Muehrcke's lines of the fingernails. *Archives of Internal Medicine* **139**, 242.

## Haemodialysis

Splinter haemorrhages can be observed in patients receiving regular haemodialysis (Blum & Aviram 1978) or peritoneal dialysis (Kilpatrick *et al.* 1965). Brittle nails, platonychia and koilonychia have also been reported. Absence of lunula is commonly observed (Tercedor *et al.* 2001). Half-and-half nails frequently occur in chronic haemodialysis patients (Lubach *et al.* 1982). Onycholysis and pachyonychia with severe psoriasiform lesions have been reported in continuous ambulatory peritoneal dialysis and automated peritoneal dialysis patients (Lebrun-Vignes *et al.* 1999).

Sixteen per cent of patients undergoing chronic dialysis develop self-limited bullous lesions that resemble porphyria cutanea tarda (pseudoporphyria) on the dorsal side of the hands and other sun-exposed areas. Foot involvement can rarely occur (Black & Frenske 1982; Reguera *et al.* 1999). A black patient who developed severe photo-onycholysis followed by loss of the nail plates and ulceration of the nail beds has been described (Guillaud *et al.* 1990) (Fig. 6.41). Deep-seated, thick-walled, burn-like blisters of the volar fingertips have been described in a patient after haemodialysis. The condition has been referred to as a variant of bullous dermatosis of haemodialysis (Shelley & Shelley 1989). Reversible nail abnormalities consisting of acute pseudoclubbing of all fingernails followed by onychomadesis have been reported in a patient on peritoneal dialysis 2 months after *Acinetobacter* peritonitis (Caputo *et al.* 1997).

## References

Black, J.R. & Frenske, N.A. (1982) Bullous dermatosis of haemodialysis in the foot and hand. *Journal of the American Pediatrics Association* **72**, 399–401.

Blum, M. & Aviram, A. (1978) Splinter haemorrhages in patients receiving regular haemodialysis. *Journal of the American Medical Association* **239**, 47.

Caputo, R., Gelmetti, C. & Cambiaghi, S. (1997) Severe self-healing dystrophy in a patient on peritoneal dialysis. *Dermatology* **195**, 274–275.

Guillaud, V., Moulin, G., Bonnefoy, M. *et al.* (1990) Photo-oncholyse bulleuse au course d'une pseudoporphyrie des hémodialysés. *Annales de Dermatologie et de Vénéréologie* **117**, 723–725.

Kilpatrick, Z.M., Greenberg, P.A. & Sanford, J.P. (1965) Splinter haemorrhages: their clinical significance. *Archives of Internal Medicine* **115**, 730–735.

Lebrun-Vignes, B., Queffeulou, G., Marck, Y. *et al.* (1999) Toxidermies psoriasiformes à l'icodextrine. *Annales de Dermatologie et de Vénéréologie* **126**, 2S1-77.

Lubach, D., Strubbe, J. & Schmdt, J. (1982) The half and half nail phenomeneon in chronic haemodialysis. *Dermatologica* **164**, 350–353.

Reguera, M.M., Matiauda, G., Romiti, R. *et al.* (1999) Fotoonicolise bolhosa em paciente hemodialisado. *Anales Brasiliera de Dermatologia* **74**, 383–386.

Shelley, W.B. & Shelley, D. (1989) Blisters of the fingertips: a variant of bullous dermatosis of haemodialysis. *Journal of the American Academy of Dermatology* **21**, 1049–1051.

Tercedor, J., Lopez-Hernandez, B. & Rodenas, J.M. (2001) Nail diseases in haemodialysis patients: case–control study. *British Journal of Dermatology* **144**, 445–446.

## Leuconychia and renal failure

After the treatment of acute or chronic renal failure, six patients developed a single 1–2-mm-wide transverse white band affecting all fingernails. The white bands which presented regular borders and a colour similar to the lunula completely crossed the nail. White lines were more prominent in the patients who had been most ill and their distance from the proximal nail fold reflected the approximate time of renal failure. The transverse true leuconychia disappeared with outward growth of the nails (Hudson & Dennis 1966).

## Reference

Hudson, J.B. & Dennis, A.J. (1966) Transverse white lines in the fingernails after acute and chronic renal failure. *Archives of Internal Medicine* **117**, 276–279.

## Renal transplantation

Onychoschizia lamellina was observed in 11 of 32 children who had a kidney transplant. Onychoschizia involved the toenails (from two to 10 nails) in all patients. The fingernails were affected in only one case. No apparent relationship was present between onychoschizia and immunosuppressive treatment.

Two of the 32 children presented pigmented transverse striae of the toenails. These were probably related to uraemia (Menni *et al.* 1991).

Transverse true leuconychia has been associated with acute rejection of renal transplants (Linder 1978; Held *et al.* 1989). Leuconychia was observed in one of 67 kidney transplant recipients treated with cyclosporin and methylprednisolone (Bencini *et al.* 1986). Lugo-Janer *et al.* (1991) found a high prevalence of onychomycosis, including *Candida* onychomycosis and chronic or subacute paronychia in a group of 82 kidney transplant recipients. A case of subcutaneous phaeohyphomycosis caused by *Exophiala jeanselmei* with periungual involvement has been reported in a kidney transplant patient (McCown & Sahn 1997). Skin cancers have been reported as the predominant malignant neoplasm in immunosuppressed patients after kidney transplantation. A patient developed a verrucous nonpigmented malignant melanoma of the nail bed 7 years after kidney transplantation (Merkle *et al.* 1991).

## References

Bencini, P.L., Montagnino, G., Sala, F. *et al.* (1986) Cutaneous lesions in 67 cyclosporin-treated renal transplant recipients. *Dermatologica* **172**, 24–30.

Held, J.L., Chew, S., Grossman, M.E. *et al.* (1989) Transverse striate leukonychia associated with acute rejection of renal allograft. *Journal of the American Academy of Dermatology* **20**, 513–514.

Linder, M. (1978) Striped nails after kidney transplant. *Annals of Internal Medicine* **88**, 809.

Lugo-Janer, G., Sanchez, J.L. & Santiago-Delpin, E. (1991) Prevalence and clinical spectrum of skin diseases in kidney transplant recipients. *Journal of the American Academy of Dermatology* **24**, 410–414.

McCown, H.F. & Sahn, E.E. (1997) Subcutaneous phaeohyphomycosis and nocardiosis in a kidney transplant patient. *Journal of the American Academy of Dermatology* **36**, 863–866.

Menni, S., Beretta, D., Piccinno, R. *et al.* (1991) Cutaneous and oral lesions in 32 children after renal transplantation. *Pediatric Dermatology* **8**, 194–198.

Merkle, T., Landthaler, M., Eckert, F. *et al.* (1991) Acral verrucous melanoma in an immunosuppressed patient after kidney transplantation. *Journal of the American Academy of Dermatology* **24**, 505–506.

## Half-and-half nails (see Chapter 2)

A reddish discoloration of the distal nail was first reported by Bean (1963) in two patients with azotaemia. Lindsay (1967) introduced the term 'half-and-half nails' to describe the same condition that he believed to be a distinctive uraemic onychopathy.

Half-and-half nails are characterized by a red, pink or brown discoloration of the distal nail bed occupying 20–60% of the nail length. Half-and-half nails can be observed both in fingernails and toenails (Stewart & Raffle 1972; Lubach *et al.* 1982).

The proximal portion of the nails can either have a dull whitish ground glass appearance or a normal colour. Distal and proximal portions of each nail are always sharply demarcated. The longitudinal length of the distal band is not correlated with the severity of azotaemia (Lindsay 1967; Lubach *et al.* 1982). Although the distal arc does not disappear with nail growth, when pressure is applied the discoloration does not fade completely. A slow rate of nail growth has been recorded (Leyden & Wood 1972). The reported occurrence of half-and-half nails in patients with established chronic renal diseases is 9–50% (Stewart & Raffle 1972; Daniel *et al.* 1985). They were not seen in patients with acute renal failure and are very rarely detected in other disease states. A precise clinical differentiation between half-and-half nails and Terry's nails (in cirrhosis) can at times be difficult. Occasional overlap of the width of the distal discoloured zone in half-and-half nails and Terry's nails is unquestioned. The term erythematous crescent has been coined to describe a reddish discoloration of the distal nail involving less than 40% of the nail bed (Daniel *et al.* 1985).

Erythematous crescents have been reported in healthy subjects and occur frequently in patients with chronic medical illnesses including renal failure. There is no correlation between the presence or absence of pigmented nail arcs and the degree of renal function impairment or serum creatinine levels. Once present, half-and-half nails usually persist unchanged and are not influenced by haemodialysis (Lubach *et al.* 1982).

The complete disappearance of nail discoloration has been observed after successful kidney transplantation (Lubach *et al.* 1982; Daniel *et al.* 1985; Bencini *et al.* 1986).

The pathogenesis of half-and-half nails is still unknown. Stimulation of nail melanocytes by increased levels of plasma melanotrophic hormone has been suggested. Substantially higher levels of circulating melanotrophic hormone have been found in patients treated by maintenance dialysis for chronic renal failure (Gilkes *et al.* 1975). Melanin granules in the basal layer of the nail bed epidermis (Stewart & Raffle 1972) or in the distal portion of the nail plate (Leyden & Wood 1972) have been detected on the nail biopsies of three patients. Kint *et al.*, who found an increase in the number of capillaries and a distinct thickening of their walls in the nail bed of two deceased patients, did not confirm the presence of pigment (Kint *et al.* 1974). The deposition of lipochrome in the nail plate has also been suggested (Stewart & Raffle 1972).

## References

Bean, W.B. (1963) A discourse on nail growth and unusual fingernails. *Transactions of the American Clinical and Climatological Association* 74, 132–167.

Bencini, P.L., Montagnino, G., Sala, F. *et al.* (1986) Cutaneous lesions in 67 cyclosporin-treated renal transplant recipients. *Dermatologica* 172, 24–30.

Daniel, C.R., Sams, W.M. & Scher, R.K. (1985) Nails in systemic disease. *Dermatologic Clinics* 3, 465–483.

Gilkes, J.J.H., Eady, R.A.J., Rees, L.H. *et al.* (1975) Plasma immunoreactive melanotrophic hormones in patients on maintenance haemodialysis. *British Medical Journal* 1, 656–658.

Kint, A., Bussels, L., Fernandes, M. *et al.* (1974) Skin and nail disorders

in relation to chronic renal failure. *Acta Dermato-Venereologica* 54, 137–140.

Leyden, J.J. & Wood, M.G. (1972) The half-and-half nail. *Archives of Dermatology* 105, 591–592.

Lindsay, P.G. (1967) The half-and-half nail. *Archives of Internal Medicine* 119, 583–587.

Lubach, D., Strubbe, J. & Schmdt, J. (1982) The half and half nail phenomenon in chronic haemodialysis. *Dermatologica* 164, 350–353.

Stewart, W.K. & Raffle, E.J. (1972) Brown nail-bed arcs and chronic renal disease. *British Medical Journal* 1, 784–786.

## Henoch–Schöenlein purpura

Dilated nail fold capillary loops have been reported in Henoch–Schöenlein purpura (Greenberg 1983).

## Reference

Greenberg, L.W. (1983) Nailfold capillary abnormalities in Henoch–Schoenlein purpura. *Journal of Pediatrics* 103, 665–666.

## Nail–patella syndrome (see Chapter 9)

Asymptomatic proteinuria is found in about 60% of patients with nail–patella syndrome. Forty per cent of all cases of nail–patella syndrome develop nephropathy. In 5.5–8% of the cases the disease leads to the necessity of haemodialysis because of renal insufficiency.

Electron microscopy studies have revealed characteristic electronlucent areas and collagen fibril-like deposits in the glomerular basement membrane (Browning *et al.* 1988). Similar changes have been found in the nail matrix vessels (Bonner & Keeling 1991).

The nails show a variable degree of hypoplasia ranging from nail plate thinning to anonychia. The thumbs are usually more severely affected, and when several fingernails are involved the severity of the nail lesions progressively decreases from the 1st to the 5th digit. Nail atrophy is always more marked on the ulnar side of the nail. Another characteristic abnormality is the presence of triangular lunulae (Daniel *et al.* 1980). Less specific nail changes include koilonychia, onychorrhexis, nail brittleness and nail ridging (Lucas & Opitz 1966).

The presence of limb and kidney defects in *LmX1b* mutant mice suggests that the nail–patella syndrome might result from mutations in the human *LMX1B* gene (Chen *et al.* 1998).

## References

Bonner, M.V. & Keeling, J.H. (1991) Nail Patella Syndrome. Presented at the 50th Annual Meeting of the American Academy of Dermatology, Dallas, 1991.

Browning, M.C., Weidner, N. & Lorentz, W.B. (1988) Renal histopathology of the nail patella syndrome in a two-year-old-boy. *Clinical Nephrology* 29, 210–213.

Chen, H., Lun, X., Ovchinnikov, D. *et al.* (1998) Limb and kidney defects in LmX1b mutant mice suggest an involvement of LMX1B in human nail patella syndrome. *Nature Genet* 19, 51–55.

Daniel, C.R., Osment, L.S. & Noojin, R.O. (1980) Triangular lunulae. *Archives of Dermatology* **116**, 448–449.

Lucas, G.L. & Opitz, J.M. (1966) The nail–patella syndrome. *Journal of Pediatrics* **68**, 273–288.

## Acro-renal-ocular syndrome

Seven individuals from three generations of a French–Canadian family presented mild to severe thumb hypoplasia in association with renal and ocular defects (Halal *et al.* 1984).

### Reference

Halal, F., Homsy, M. & Perreault, G. (1984) Acro-renal-ocular syndrome. Autosomal dominant thumb hypoplasia, renal ectopia and eye defect. *American Journal of Medical Genetics* **17**, 753–762.

## Yellow nail syndrome and renal disorders

YNS has been reported in association with nephrotic syndrome and xanthogranulomatous pyelonephritis. The nail abnormalities improved with treatment of the underlying renal disorder (Cockram & Richards 1979; Danenberg *et al.* 1995).

### References

Cockram, C.S. & Richards, P. (1979) Yellow nails and nephrotic syndrome. *British Journal of Dermatology* **101**, 707–709.

Danenberg, H.D., Eliashar, R., Flusser, G. *et al.* (1995) Yellow nail syndrome and xanthogranulomatous pyelonephritis. *Postgraduate Medical Journal* **71**, 110–111.

# Hepatic disorders

Erythema at the base of the nails can be observed in hepatic diseases (Sarkany 1987). Multiple pigmented bands of the nail plate have been reported in patients with hyperbilirubinaemia (Aplas 1957). A yellow colour of the nail bed is a clinical sign of jaundice.

## Viral hepatitis

Periungual erythema and teleangiectasia have recently been associated with hepatitis C virus (HCV) infection, both in HIV-positive and HIV-negative patients (page 282) (Osaer *et al.* 1966). Clubbing as well as white nails and splinter haemorrhages can occur in patients with chronic active hepatitis (Sarkany 1987).

## Cirrhosis (see Chapter 2)

Nail clippings from patients with liver cirrhosis contain an increased Na, Mg and P content and a decreased S and Cl content (Djaldetti *et al.* 1987).

Curved nails with or without clubbing and cyanosis of the fingers have been reported in cirrhotics (Ratnoff & Patek 1942; Djaldetti *et al.* 1987; Berman & Lamkin 1989). Hypertrophic osteoarthropathy has been described in biliary as well as portal cirrhosis (Buchan & Mitchell 1967; Han & Collins 1968). Improvement in hypertrophic hepatic osteoarthropathy after liver transplantation is unique (Vickers *et al.* 1988). Flattening of the fingernails can also be observed. In the hepatopulmonary syndrome, associated with liver cirrhosis, clubbing is typically associated with cyanosis (Folwaczny *et al.* 1994). Nails lose their curvature and become flat; the nail beds are usually whitish or light pink, possibly due to anaemia (Kleeberg 1951). Longitudinal ridging and nail thickening have been reported as well (Terry 1954). Splinter haemorrhages can occur.

Terry's nails have been described as a common sign of liver cirrhosis which has been found in 82% of the patients (Terry 1954). Terry's nails were originally reported as white fingernails exhibiting a ground-glass-like opacity of almost the entire nail bed except for a 1–2-mm distal band of normal pink colour. The distal pink band that corresponds to the onychodermal band (Terry 1955) can occasionally be wider (Holzeberg & Walker 1984). The distal margin of the white nail bed can present a central or lateral peaking (Morey & Burke 1955). The lunula may or may not be distinguishable.

Symmetrical distribution of nail bed whiteness is characteristic and thumbs and forefingers frequently present more marked changes. Nail discoloration does not vary with nail growth. Compression of the middle phalanx accentuates the contrast between the white nail bed and the distal pink zone that becomes congested. The presence or absence of Terry's nails does not correlate with severity of cirrhosis. Terry's nails are not specific to hepatic cirrhosis and they have been observed in a variety of other diseases that include chronic congestive heart failure, adult-onset diabetes mellitus, thyrotoxicosis, rheumatoid arthritis, malignancies, disseminated sclerosis, pulmonary tuberculosis, pulmonary eosinophilia, malnutrition and actinic keratosis. They have also been frequently detected in young children and adolescent females.

In normal adults the frequency of Terry's nails has been reported to increase with ageing. The possibility of an increased risk of systemic diseases in young patients with Terry's nails has been suggested (Holzeberg & Walker 1984).

Multiple transverse white bands preceded the development of white nails in one patient (Jensen 1981).

The following have been forwarded as explanations for clinical changes observed in Terry's nails: abnormal steroid metabolism, abnormal ratio of oestrogens to androgens, increased digital blood flow (Holzeberg & Walker 1984), alteration of the nail bed to nail plate attachment (Terry 1954) and overgrowth of the connective tissue between the nail and bone (Sarkany 1987). The pathological findings of three patients showed the presence of telangiectases in the upper dermis of the distal band (Holzeberg & Walker 1984). The association between primary biliary cirrhosis and the CREST variant of systemic sclerosis was first described by Reynolds *et al.* (1971). A 20% prevalence of biliary cirrhosis among patients with CREST syndrome has been reported (Dubois *et al.* 1978). Primary biliary cirrhosis may be associated with nail lichen planus (Sowden *et al.* 1989; Gant & Camisa 1994).

## Wilson's disease

The nails of patients with hepatolenticular degeneration can present an increased copper content (Djaldetti *et al.* 1987). Bluish discoloration of the lunulae has been reported in the fingernails of patients with Wilson's disease. The azure-blue discoloration can fade proximally and be more intense at the distal margins of the lunulae (Bearn & McKusik 1958). The differential diagnosis includes blue discoloration of the lunulae due to argyria, phenolphthalein, busulphan (busulfan) and antimalarial drugs (Koplan 1966).

## Haemochromatosis

Diffuse grey or brown nail plate pigmentation can be observed in haemochromatosis (Daniel 1985). Abnormal greyish or bronze-brown hyperpigmentation of the periungual area is very frequent. Black-coal pigmentation of the lower extremities has been reported in an alcoholic patient with haemochromatosis (Pierard & Reginster 1986).

Koilonychia has been observed in 49% of patients, mainly involving the thumb, index and middle fingers. Longitudinal striations, brittleness and true or apparent leuconychia have also been described (Chevrant-Breton *et al.* 1977). Similar physical signs may be evident in Kashin–Beck disease, a poorly understood disorder seen in Asia that has been attributed to excessive amounts of iron in the water supply (Fairbanks & Fairbanks 1971).

## References

Aplas, V. (1957) Hyperbilirubinamische melanonychia. *Zeitschrift für Hautkrankheiten* **22**, 303.

Bearn, A.G. & McKusick, V.A. (1958) An unusual change in the finger-nails in two patients with hepatolenticular degeneration (Wilson's disease) 'Azure lunulae'. *Journal of the American Medical Association* **166**, 904–906.

Berman, J.E. & Lamkin, B.C. (1989) Hepatic disease and the skin. *Dermatologic Clinics* **7**, 435–447.

Buchan, D.J. & Mitchell, D.M. (1967) Hypertrophic osteoarthropathy in portal cirrhosis. *Annals of Internal Medicine* **66**, 130–135.

Chevrant-Breton, J., Simon, M., Bourel, M. *et al.* (1977) Cutaneous manifestations of idiopathic haemochromatosis. *Archives of Dermatology* **113**, 161–165.

Daniel, C.R. (1985) Nail pigmentation abnormalities. *Dermatologic Clinics* **3**, 431–443.

Djaldetti, M., Fishman, P., Harpaz, D. *et al.* (1987) X-ray microanalysis of the fingernails in cirrhotic patients. *Dermatologica* **174**, 114–116.

Dubois, A., Jourdan, J., Blotman, F. *et al.* (1978) L'association calcinose sous-cutanée, syndrome de Raynaud, sclérodactylie et télangiectasies (CREST syndrome): intérêt en hépatologie. *Gastroenterologie Clinique et Biologique* **2**, 805–809.

Fairbanks, V.F. & Fairbanks, G.E. (1971) Haemosiderosis and haemochromatosis. In: *Clinical Disorders of Iron Metabolism* (ed. E. Beutter, p. 399. Grune & Stratton, New York.

Folwaczny, C., Weber, M., Screiner, J. *et al.* (1994) Zyanose und Uhrglasnägel bei chronischer *Leberkrankheiten Internis* **35**, 1066–1068.

Gant, G.S. & Camisa, C. (1994) Ulcerative and oral lichen planus associated with sicca syndrome and primary biliary cirrhosis. *Cutis* **53**, 249–250.

Han, S.Y. & Collins, L.C. (1968) Hypertrophic osteoarthropathy in cirrhosis of the liver: Report of two cases. *Radiology* **91**, 795–796.

Holzeberg, M. & Walker, H.K. (1984) Terry's nails: revised definition and new correlations. *Lancet* **i**, 896–899.

Jensen, O. (1981) White fingernails preceded by multiple transverse white bands. *Acta Dermato-Venereologica* **61**, 261–262.

Kleeberg, J. (1951) Flat finger-nails in cirrhosis of the liver. *Lancet* **ii**, 248–249.

Koplan, B.S. (1966) Azure lunulae due to argyria. *Archives of Dermatology*, **94**, 333–334.

Morey, D.A.J. & Burke, J.O. (1955) Distinctive nail changes in advanced hepatic cirrhosis. *Gastroenterology* **29**, 258–261.

Osaer, F., Aubin, F., Bresson-Hadni, S. *et al.* (1996) Red fingers syndrome in a HIV-negative woman with hepatitis C cirrhosis. *British Journal of Dermatology* **138**, 188–203.

Pierard, G.E. & Reginster, M. (1986) Hémochromatose et mélanose mouchetée noire. *Nouvelle Dermatologie* **5**, 423.

Ratnoff, O.D. & Patek, A.J. (1942) The natural history of Laennec's cirrhosis of the liver: Analysis of 387 cases. *Medicine* **21**, 207.

Reynolds, T.B., Denison, E.K., Frankl, M.D. *et al.* (1971) Primary biliary cirrhosis with scleroderma, Raynaud's phenomenon and telangiectasia. *American Journal of Medicine* **50**, 301–312.

Sarkany, I. (1987) Cutaneous manifestations of hepatobiliary disease. In: *Dermatology in General Medicine* (eds T.B. Fitzpatrick, A.Z. Eisen, K. Wolff *et al.*), pp. 1947–1964. McGraw Hill, New York.

Sowden, J.M., Cartwright, P.H., Green, J.R.B. *et al.* (1989) Isolated lichen planus of the nails associated with primary biliary cirrhosis. *British Journal of Dermatology* **121**, 659–662.

Terry, R.B. (1954) White nails in hepatic cirrhosis. *Lancet* **i**, 757–759.

Terry, R.B. (1955) The onychodermal band in health and disease. *Lancet* **i**, 179–181.

Vickers, C., Herbert, A., Neuberger, J. *et al.* (1988) Improvement in hypertrophic hepatic osteoarthropathy after liver transplantation. *Lancet* **2**, 968.

## Gastrointestinal disorders

Splinter haemorrhages have occurred in peptic ulcer. They can be painful in trichinosis (De Nicola *et al.* 1974). Nail brittleness has been described in coeliac disease. Patients with steatorrhoea commonly exhibit thin, brittle and deformed nails. Beau's lines have been reported (Simpson 1954). Transverse leuconychia involving the 20 digits appeared in a patient with multiple intestinal parasitic infections (Hepburn *et al.* 1997). Hereditary leuconychia can be associated with duodenal ulcer and gallstones (Ingegno & Yatto 1982). A possible correlation between pincer nails and gastrointestinal diseases has been reported by Jemec *et al.* (Jemec *et al.* 1995; Jemec & Thomsen 1997).

## References

De Nicola, P., Morsiani, M. & Zavagli, G. (1974) *Nail Diseases in Internal Medicine*, p. 54. Charles C. Thomas, Springfield, IL.

Hepburn, M.J., English, J.C., Meffert, J.J. (1997) Mees' lines in a patient with multiple parasitic infections. *Cutis* 59, 321–323.

Ingegno, A.D. & Yatto, R.P. (1982) Hereditary white nails (leukonychia totalis), duodenal ulcer and gallstones: genetic implications. *New York State Journal of Medicine* 82, 1797–1800.

Jemec, G.B.E., Kollerup, G., Jensen, L.B. *et al.* (1995) Nail abnormalities in nondermatologic patients: prevalence and possible role as diagnostic aids. *Journal of the American Academy of Dermatology* 32, 977–981.

Jemec, G.B. & Thomsen, K. (1997) Pincer nails and alopecia as markers of gastrointestinal malignancy. *Journal of Dermatology* 24, 479–481.

Simpson, J.A. (1954) Dermatological changes in hypocalcemia. *British Journal of Dermatology* 66, 1–15.

## Clubbing

Finger clubbing or hypertrophic osteoarthropathy have been observed in association with a large number of diseases that involve tissues with a vagus nerve supply. Finger clubbing has been described in ulcerative colitis (**14%** of the cases), multiple polyposis, chronic bacillary dysentery, amoebic dysentery, Crohn's disease (**30%** of the cases), tuberculosis, Hodgkin's disease, intestinal lymphoma, carcinoma, coeliac disease, ascariasis, whipworm infestation, duodenal ulcer with pyloric stenosis, gastro-oesophageal reflux with protein-losing enteropathy and idiopathic steatorrhoea (Young 1966; Bowie *et al.* 1978; Kitis *et al.* 1979). Clubbing of the fingers and toes has been reported in children affected by Crohn's disease of the jejunum (Chrispin & Tempany 1967). Hypertrophic osteoarthropathy has occurred in association with chronic ulcerative colitis, Crohn's disease, multiple polyposis and upper gastrointestinal neoplasms (Singh *et al.* 1960; Hollis 1967; Farman *et al.* 1971; Ullal 1972). Regression of clubbing has been reported after the eradication of ascariasis or whipworm infestation (Bowie *et al.* 1978). Reversible clubbing of the fingers and toes has been described in association with purgative abuse (Silk *et al.* 1975; Levine *et al.* 1981). Finger clubbing was present in 77% of patients with kwashiorkor and may have been related to diarrhoea (Amla & Marayan 1968). Diffuse thickening of the gastric mucosal folds has been reported in patients with pachydermoperiostosis (Venencie *et al.* 1988).

## References

Amla, I. & Marayan, J.V. (1968) Finger nail clubbing in Kwashiorkor. *Indian Journal of Pediatrics* 35(240), 19–22.

Bowie, M.D., Morrison, A., Ireland, J.D. *et al.* (1978) Clubbing and whipworm infestation. *Archives of Disease in Childhood* 53, 411–413.

Chrispin, A.R. & Tempany, E. (1967) Crohn's disease of the Jejunum in children. *Archives of Disease in Childhood* 42, 631–635.

Farman, J., Effman, E.L. & Grnja, V. (1971) Crohn's disease and periostal new bone formation. *Gastroenterology* 61, 513–522.

Hollis, W.C. (1967) Hypertrophic osteoarthropathy secondary to upper-gastrointestinal-tract neoplasm. *Annals of Internal Medicine* 66, 125–130.

Kitis, G., Thompson, H. & Allan, R.N. (1979) Finger clubbing in inflammatory bowel disease its prevalence and pathogenesis. *British Medical Journal* 2, 825–828.

Levine, D., Goode, A.W. & Wingate, D.L. (1981) Purgative abuse associated with reversible cachexia, hypogammaglobulinaemia, and finger clubbing. *Lancet* i, 919–920.

Silk, D.B.A., Gibson, J.A. & Murray, C.R.H. (1975) Reversible finger clubbing in a case of purgative abuse. *Gastroenterology* 68, 790–794.

Singh, A., Jolly, S.S. & Bansal, B.B. (1960) Hypertrophic osteoarthropathy associated with carcinoma of the stomach. *British Medical Journal* 2, 581–582.

Ullal, S.R. (1972) Hypertrophic osteoarthropathy and leiomyoma of the esophagus. *American Journal of Surgery* 123, 356–358.

Venencie, P.Y., Boffa, G.A., Delmas, P.D. *et al.* (1988) Pachydermoperiostosis with gastric hypertrophy, anemia and increased serum bone Gla-protein levels. *Archives of Dermatology* 124, 1831–1834.

Young, J.R. (1966) Ulcerative colitis and finger-clubbing. *British Medical Journal* 1, 278–279.

## Ulcerative colitis

Patients with ulcerative colitis occasionally experience painful haemorrhages in the nail bed. Rarely, this is followed by a liquefaction and necrosis at the site. Vesicular, tender erythematous areas developing at the base of the volar surface of the digits have also been reported (Kelly 1968; Daniel 1985).

Finger clubbing has been detected in seven of 77 patients affected by ulcerative colitis with involvement of that part of the colon innervated by the vagus nerve (the proximal two-thirds of the transverse colon). Clubbing did not occur in patients with the disease limited to the distal colon (Young 1966).

Hypertrophic osteoarthropathy has also been associated with ulcerative colitis. Zaun (1980) described Terry's nails in a young man with ulcerative colitis. A patient with ulcerative colitis, sclerosing cholangitis and pyoderma gangrenosum involving the tip of the great toe has been reported (Shelley & Shelley 1988).

Pyogenic granulomas of the nail beds in a 17-year-old female with a history of ulcerative colitis has been reported 2 months prior to presenting—she developed clubbing of the nails due to growths of her nail beds. This affected all nails bilaterally, especially those of the thumb and great toes. Biopsy demonstrated a pyogenic granuloma-like lesion. This responded to the flashlamp pulsed dye laser (wavelength 585 nm), although improvement may have been due to the natural course of the disease (Max & Shwayder 1999).

## References

Daniel, C.R. (1985) Nail pigmentation abnormalities. *Dermatologic Clinics* 3, 431–443.

Kelly, M.L. (1968) Purulent mucocutaneous lesions associated with ulcerative colitis. *Medical Radiography and Photography* 44(2), 39–41.

Max, J.E. & Shwayder, T.A. (1999) Pyogenic granulomas of the nail beds in a patient with ulcerative colitis. In: 57th Annual Meeting AAD Poster Abstract Book, Poster 255. 19–24 March, 1999.

Shelley, E.D. & Shelley, W.B. (1988) Cyclosporine therapy for pyoderma gangrenosum associated with sclerosing cholangitis and ulcerative colitis. *Journal of the American Academy of Dermatology* 18, 1084–1088.

Young, J.R. (1966) Ulcerative colitis and finger-clubbing. *British Medical Journal* 1, 278–279.

Zaun, H. (1980) Milchglasnagel: hinweis auf intestinale erkrankungen. *Aktuelle Dermatologie* 6, 107–108.

## Peutz–Jeghers–Touraine syndrome

Pigmented macules on the fingers and toes are a distinctive sign of Peutz–Jeghers–Touraine syndrome. Longitudinal pigmented bands of fingernails and toenails due to melanin deposits in the nail plate have been reported (Valero & Sherf 1965). Punctate brown pigmentation of the nail has also been described (Daniel 1985). Differential diagnosis should rule out Laugier–Hunziker syndrome (Baran & Barriere 1986).

## References

Baran, R. & Barriere, H. (1986) Longitudinal melanonychia with spreading pigmentation in Laugier–Hunziker syndrome: a report of two cases. *British Journal of Dermatology* 115, 707–710.

Daniel, C.R. (1985) Nail pigmentation abnormalities. *Dermatologic Clinics* 3, 431–443.

Valero, A. & Sherf, K. (1965) Pigmented nails in Peutz–Jeghers Syndrome. *American Journal of Gastroenterology* 43, 56–58.

## Cronkhite–Canada syndrome

This rare syndrome is characterized by non-familial gastrointestinal polyposis associated with macular hyperpigmentation, patchy or diffuse hair loss and nail dystrophy (Cronkhite & Canada 1955). The syndrome usually affects middle-aged to elderly adults who develop fatigue, diarrhoea and weight loss. Nail changes occur in about 98% of patients (Herzberg & Kaplan 1990). In typical cases the proximal half of the nails shows a thin and soft triangular area, bordered by a thick, hard and ridged nail plate (Fig. 6.42) (Cunliffe & Anderson 1967; Daniel *et al.* 1982; Peart *et al.* 1984). However the proximal part may be soft and spongy with distal fingernails ragged and nearly absent (Bruce *et al.* 1999). Nail colour may vary from white to yellow to brown-black. Onycholysis and onychomadesis are frequently reported and complete loss of all

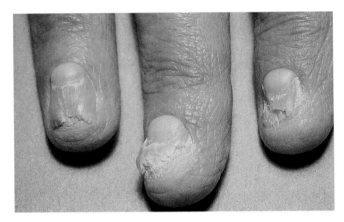

**Fig. 6.42** Cronkhite–Canada syndrome.

fingernails and toenails is not rare (Cunliffe & Anderson 1967; Daniel *et al.* 1982; Peart *et al.* 1984; Freeman *et al.* 1985; Aanestad *et al.* 1987; Bächer *et al.* 1997; Allbritton *et al.* 1998). Partial or total regeneration of nails can occur spontaneously or during remission (Daniel *et al.* 1982; Peart *et al.* 1984). Koilonychia has also been reported (Orimo *et al.* 1969).

Nail regeneration may occur in spite of acute disease. In some patients, the biochemical deficiencies have been corrected and yet the nail changes persisted.

## References

Aanestad, O., Raknerud, N., Aase, S.T. *et al.* (1987) The Cronkhite–Canada Syndrome. Case report. *Acta Chirurgica Scandinavica* 153, 143–145.

Allbritton, J., Simmons-O'Brien, E., Hutchens, D. *et al.* (1998) Cronkhite–Canada syndrome: report of two cases, biopsy findings in the associated alopecia, and a new treatment. *Cutis* 61, 229–232.

Bruce, A., Ng, C.S., Wolfsen, H.C. *et al.* (1999) Cutaneous clues to Cronkhite–Canada syndrome: a case report. *Archives of Dermatology* 135, 212.

Bächer, T.H., Schönekäs, H., Steuer, K.T. *et al.* (1997) Das Cronkhite–Canada-Syndrom. *Deutsche Medizinische Wochenschrift* 122, 676–681.

Cronkhite, L.W. & Canada, W.J. (1955) Generalized gastrointestinal polyposis: an unusual syndrome of polyposis, pigmentation, alopecia and onychoatrophia. *New England Journal of Medicine* 252, 1011–1015.

Cunliffe, W.J. & Anderson, J. (1967) Case of Cronkhite–Canada syndrome with associated jejunal diverticulosis. *British Medical Journal* 4, 601–602.

Daniel, E.S., Ludwig, S.L., Lewin, K.J. *et al.* (1982) The Cronkhite–Canada syndrome. An analysis of clinical and pathological features and therapy in 55 patients. *Medicine* 61, 293–309.

Freeman, K., Anthony, P.P., Miller, D.S. *et al.* (1985) Cronkhite–Canada syndrome: a new hypothesis. *Gut* 26, 531–536.

Herzberg, A.J. & Kaplan, D.L. (1990) Cronkhite–Canada syndrome: light and electron microscopy of the cutaneous pigmentary abnormalities. *International Journal of Dermatology* 29, 121–125.

Orimo, H., Fujita, T., Yoshikawa, M. *et al.* (1969) Gastrointestinal polyposis with protein-losing enteropathy, abnormal skin pigmentation and loss of hair and nail. *American Journal of Medicine* **47**, 445–449.

Peart, A.G., Sivak, M.V., Rankin, G.B. *et al.* (1984) Spontaneous improvement of Cronkhite–Canada syndrome in a postpartum female. *Digestive Diseases and Sciences* **29**, 470.

## Plummer–Vinson (Patterson–Kelly–Brown) syndrome

This syndrome describes the association of chronic dysphagia with atrophic changes in the oral mucosa and hypochromic anaemia. Koilonychia occurs in 40–50% of patients and usually involves the first three digits of the hands but spares the toenails. Nail brittleness is also frequent. Nail changes as well as the other clinical manifestations of Plummer–Vinson syndrome are reversible with iron therapy (Archard 1987).

### Reference

Archard, H.O. (1987) Disorders of mucocutaneous integument. In: *Dermatology in General Medicine* (eds T.B. Fitzpatrick, A.Z. Eisen, K. Wolff *et al.*), pp. 1152–1239. McGraw Hill, New York.

## Crohn's disease

Nail fold capillary microscopy of patients with Crohn's disease may reveal microcirculatory abnormalities (Gasser & Affolter 1990). An increased occurrence of psoriasis in patients with Crohn's disease has been reported (Lee *et al.* 1990).

### References

Gasser, P. & Affolter, H. (1990) Pathogenesis of Crohn's disease. *Lancet* **335**, 551.

Lee, F.I., Bellary, S.V. & Francis, C. (1990) Increased occurrence of psoriasis in patients with Crohn's disease and their relatives. *American Journal of Gastroenterology* **85**, 962–963.

## Pyodermatitis-pyostomatitis vegetans

Pyodermatitis-pyostomatitis vegetans is a rare, benign, eosinophilic pustular and vegetating mucocutaneous disease which should be differentiated from pemphigus vegetans. This condition should be considered as a marker for inflammatory chronic bowel disease (Storwick *et al.* 1994), usually ulcerative colitis. Crohn's disease has been reported with periungual pustules of the finger, leading to nail loss (Fig. 6.43) (Delaporte *et al.* 1998).

Histology shows epithelial hyperplasia, intra- and subepithelial granulocytes, microabcesses and polymorphous infiltration of the superficial dermis with numerous neutrophils and eosinophils. Pyodermatitis-pyostomatitis vegetans may belong to a spectrum of neutrophilic dermatoses (Delaporte *et al.* 1998) or be considered as a form of pyoderma gangrenosum (Powell *et al.* 1996).

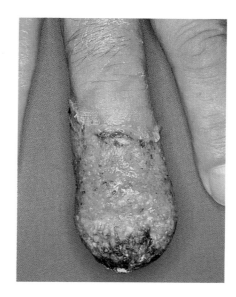

**Fig. 6.43**
Pyodermatitis—pyostomatitis vegetans. (Courtesy of E. Delaporte, France.)

### References

Delaporte, E., Viget, N., Pasturel-Michon, U. *et al.* (1998) Pyostomatite-Pyodermite végétante révélatrice d'une maladie de Crohn. *Annales de Dermatologie et de Vénéréologie* **125**, 331–334.

Powell, F.C., Su, W.P.D. & Perry, H.O. (1996) Pyoderma gangrenosum: classification and management. *Journal of the American Academy of Dermatology* **34**, 395–409.

Storwick, G.S., Prihoda, M.B., Fulton, R.J. *et al.* (1994) Pyodermatitis-pyostomatitis vegetans. A specific marker for inflammatory bowel disease. *Journal of the American Academy of Dermatology* **31**, 336–341.

## *Helicobacter pylori* infection

Oral carriage of *Helicobacter pylori* may play a role in the transmission of infection and the hand may be instrumental in this transmission (Dowsett *et al.* 1999).

### Reference

Dowsett, S.A., Archila, L., Segreto, V.A. *et al.* (1999) *Helicobacter pylori* infection in indigenous families of Central America: serostatus and oral and fingernail carriage. *Journal of Clinical Microbiology* **37**, 2456–2460.

# Nutritional disorders and deficiencies

## Pellagra

Transverse leukonychia is described in pellagra and may be associated with a general loss of nail translucency (Brownson 1915). Poikilodermatous skin and onycholysis can also be observed (Zaias 1990).

## References

Brownson, W.C. (1915) An unusual condition of the nails in pellagra. *Southern Medical Journal* 8, 672–675.

Zaias, N. (1990) *The Nail in Health and Disease*, 2nd edn, pp. 189–199. Appleton & Lange, Norwalk, CT.

## Vitamin A deficiency

The presence of 'eggshell' nail changes in vitamin A deficiency has been observed (Bereston 1950).

## References

Bereston, E.S. (1950) Diseases of the nails. *Clinical Medicine* 238–240.

## Vitamin C deficiency

Subungual haemorrhages can occur in scurvy (Miller 1989).

## Reference

Miller, S.J. (1989) Nutritional deficiency and the skin. *Journal of the American Academy of Dermatology* 21, 1–30.

## Vitamin B$_{12}$ deficiency

Reversible hyperpigmentation of the skin can be observed in patients with megaloblastic anaemia due to vitamin B$_{12}$ or folate deficiency. Skin hyperpigmentation is particularly pronounced over the knuckles and terminal phalanges. Bluish-black discoloration of fingernails and toenails can rarely occur. Uniform nail hyperpigmentation as well as longitudinal or transverse pigmented bands have been reported. Pigment changes are reversible with vitamin B$_{12}$ administration (Baker *et al.* 1963; Ridley 1977; Carmel 1985; Marks *et al.* 1985). It has been suggested that vitamin B$_{12}$ deficiency results in a decreased amount of intracellular-reduced glutathione, which normally inhibits tyrosinase activity in melanogenesis (Marks *et al.* 1985; Noppakun & Swasdikul 1986).

## References

Baker, S.S., Ignatius, M., Johnson, S. *et al.* (1963) Hyperpigmentation of skin. A sign of vitamin B$_{12}$ deficiency. *British Medical Journal* 1, 1713–1715.

Carmel, R. (1985) Hair and fingernail changes in acquired congenital pernicious anaemia. *Archives of Internal Medicine* 145, 484–485.

Marks, V.J., Briggaman, R.A. & Wheeler, C.E. (1985) Hyperpigmentation in megaloblastic anaemia. *Journal of the American Academy of Dermatology* 12, 914–917.

Noppakun, N. & Swasdikul, D. (1986) Reversible hyperpigmentation of skin and nails with white hair due to vitamin B$_{12}$ deficiency. *Archives of Dermatology* 122, 896–899.

Ridley, C.M. (1977) Pigmentation of fingertips and nails in vitamin B$_{12}$ deficiency. *British Journal of Dermatology* 97, 105–107.

## Zinc deficiency

Acrodermatitis enteropathica is a rare and inherited disease due to a specific deficit of zinc absorption. Diarrhoea, alopecia and acral dermatitis are the characteristic manifestations of the disorder. Nail involvement such as longitudinal ridging, striations, brittleness and grey discoloration of the nails has been reported in 96% of the patients. Chronic paronychia as well as vesicobullous and erosive or psoriasiform lesions on the dorsal aspect of the terminal phalanges are distinctive symptoms of the disease. The lesions have an increased occurrence around the nails and between the fingers and toes. Beau's lines can occasionally be observed after recurrences (Wells & Winkelmann 1961; Weismann 1977; Miranda *et al.* 1986). A transient symptomatic zinc deficiency may occasionally occur in breast-fed premature infants. Clinical symptoms closely resemble acrodermatitis enteropathica and include chronic paronychia. A low breast-milk zinc content has been detected in some cases (Munro *et al.* 1989).

An acute zinc deficiency associated with an acrodermatitis enteropathica-like syndrome can occur in patients submitted to total parenteral nutrition for inflammatory or neoplastic gastrointestinal disorders. Paronychia (Nurnberger 1987) and purpuric blisters of the proximal nail fold have been described (Zaias 1990). Histologically the bullous lesions were characterized by intraepidermal vacuolar changes with massive ballooning, leading to intraepidermal vesiculation and blistering, with prominent epidermal necrosis and without acantholysis (Borroni *et al.* 1992). Transverse paired white bands, which resemble the Muerhrcke's lines of chronic hypoalbuminaemia or Beau's lines, can be observed after recovery from acute zinc deficiency (Weismann 1977; Brazin *et al.* 1979; Ferràndez *et al.* 1981; Nurnberger 1987). Because 85% of serum zinc is bound to albumin, the hypothesis that Muerhrcke's lines may actually represent a marker for zinc deficiency has been put forward (Pfeiffer & Jeuney 1974; Ferràndez *et al.* 1981). Periungual brown discoloration and thickened irregular cuticles have been observed in a patient with acute zinc deficiency due to total parenteral nutrition (Brazin *et al.* 1979). A necrolytic migratory erythema-like rash has also been described in patients with zinc deficiency (Sinclair & Reynolds 1997).

Isoleucine deficiency may be the cause of an acrodermatitis enteropathica-like syndrome (Bosch *et al.* 1998).

## References

Brazin, S.A., Johnson, W.T. & Abramson, L.J. (1979) The acrodermatitis enteropathica-like syndrome. *Archives of Dermatology* 115, 597–599.

Borroni, G., Brazzelli, V., Vignati, G. *et al.* (1992) Bullous lesions in acrodermatitis enteropatica. Histopathologic findings regarding two patients. *American Journal of Dermatopathology* 14, 304–309.

Bosch, A.M., Sillevis Smitt, J.H., Van Gennip, A.H. *et al.* (1998) Iatrogenic isolated isoleucine deficiency as the cause of an acrodermatitis enteropathica-like syndrome. *British Journal of Dermatology* **139**, 488–491.

Ferràndez, C., Henkes, J., Peyri, J. *et al.* (1981) Acquired zinc deficiency syndrome during total parenteral alimentation. *Dermatologica* **163**, 255–266.

Miranda, M., Polanco, I., Fonseca, E. *et al.* (1986) Acrodermatitis enteropatica y dermatitis hipozinquémica en la infancia. *Acta Dermato-Sifilitica* **77**, 655–668.

Munro, C.S., Lazaro, C. & Lawrence, C.M. (1989) Symptomatic zinc deficiency in breast-fed premature infants. *British Journal of Dermatology* **121**, 773–778.

Nurnberger, F. (1987) Zinkmangel bei Kunstlicher ernahrung. *Zeitschrift für Hautkrankheiten* **62** (Suppl. 1), 104–110.

Pfeiffer, C.C. & Jenney, E.H. (1974) Fingernail white spots: possible zinc deficiency. *Journal of the American Medical Association* **228**, 157.

Sinclair, S.A. & Reynolds, N.J. (1997) Necrolytic migratory erythema and zinc deficiency. *British Journal of Dermatology* **136**, 783–785.

Weismann, K. (1977) Lines of Beau: possible markers of zinc deficiency. *Acta Dermato-Venereologica* **57**, 88–90.

Wells, B.T. & Winkelmann, R.K. (1961) Acrodermatitis enteropathica. *Archives of Dermatology* **84**, 90–102.

Zaias, N. (1990) *The Nail in Health and Disease*, 2nd edn., pp. 189–199. Appleton & Lange, Norwalk, CT.

## Selenium deficiency

Four children receiving long-term total parenteral nutrition developed macrocytosis, loss of hair and skin pigmentation, elevated transaminase and creatine kinase activities as well as profound muscle weakness. Selenium levels were low. Nail strengthening was observed after selenium supplementation (Vinton *et al.* 1987).

### Reference

Vinton, N.E., Dahlstrom, K.A., Strobel, C.T. *et al.* (1987) Macrocytosis and pseudoalbinism: manifestations of selenium deficiency. *Journal of Pediatrics* **111**, 711–717.

## Calcium deficiency

Simpson (1954) has observed a calcium level below normal in several cases of leuconychia.

### Reference

Simpson, J.A. (1954) Dermatological changes in hypocalcemia. *British Journal of Dermatology* **66**, 1–15.

## Fetal alcohol syndrome

Absence or dysplasia of the fingernails and toenails was found in more than 20% of patients (Crain *et al.* 1983).

### Reference

Crain, L.S., Fitzmaurice, N.E. & Mondry, C. (1983) Nail dysplasia and fetal alcohol syndrome. Case report of a heteropaternal sibship. *American Journal of Diseases of Children* **137**, 1069–1072.

## Iron deficiency

Brittle nails, koilonychia and longitudinal ridging can be observed in iron deficiency anaemia. The iron content of the fingernails is not an indication of the iron levels in iron-deficient patients (Djaldetti *et al.* 1987).

### Reference

Djaldetti, M., Fishman, P. & Hart, J. (1987) The iron content of fingernails in iron deficient patients. *Clinical Science* **72**, 669–672.

## Malnutrition

Abnormal nail growth (Daniel *et al.* 1985) and multiple pigmented bands (Bisht & Singh 1962) have been described in malnutrition. Soft and brittle nails are frequently observed in cachexia (Runne & Orfanos 1981). Persons with marasmus can often exhibit fissured nails (Miller 1989). Fingernails and toenails are severely dystrophic in kwashiorkor (Albers *et al.* 1993).

### References

Albers, S.E., Brozena, S.J. & Fenske, N.E. (1993) A case of kwashiorkor. *Cutis* **51**, 445–446.

Bisht, D.B. & Singh, S.S. (1962) Pigmented bands on nails: a new sign in malnutrition. *Lancet* **i**, 507–508.

Daniel, C.R., Sams, W.M. & Scher, R.K. (1985) Nails in systemic disease. *Dermatologic Clinics* **3**, 465–483.

Miller, S.J. (1989) Nutritional deficiency and the skin. *Journal of the American Academy of Dermatology* **21**, 1–30.

Runne, U. & Orfanos, C.E. (1981) The human nail. *Current Problems in Dermatology* **9**, 102–149.

# Endocrine disorders

## Hypogonadism

Reversible onychauxis of the fingernails has been reported in a eunuchoid (Lisser 1924). Infantile, longitudinally striated, small nails have been described in adipose genital syndrome (De Nicola *et al.* 1974).

### References

De Nicola, P., Morsiani, M. & Zavagli, G. (1974) *Nail Diseases in Internal Medicine*, pp. 67–70. Charles, C. Thomas, Springfield, IL.

Lisser, H. (1924) Onychauxis in a eunuchoid. *Archives of Dermatology and Syphiligraphy* **10**, 180–182.

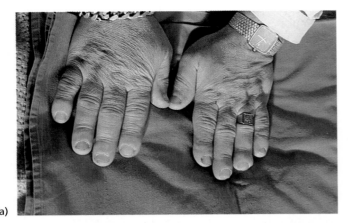

(a)

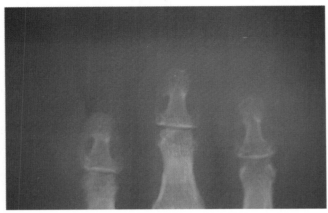

(b)

**Fig. 6.44** (a) Acromegaly. (Courtesy of D. Wendling, France.) (b) Acromegaly—Patient shown in (a), showing anchor-like shape of the lateral aspect of the distal phalanges.

## Pituitary disease

The hypertrophy of the soft tissues of the fingers that characterizes acromegaly causes the nails to appear short and broad (Haneke 1989); fingers assume a blunted shape (Fig. 6.44a). Lunulae can be absent. Nail brittleness, koilonychia and macronychia have been described, but nail thickening and hardening can also occur (Freinkel & Freinkel 1987). Chronic paronychia and ingrowing fingernails have been described in a patient affected by acromegaly (Keefe *et al.* 1987). Generalized hyperpigmentation of nails and digits is occasionally seen. Investigation by X-ray may show an anchor-like shape of the lateral aspect of the distal phalanges (Fig. 6.44b) (Wendling & Guidet 1993).

Thin and brittle nails have been noted in three adolescent patients affected by cerebral gigantism (Sotos Syndrome) (Wit *et al.* 1985). Disappearance of the lunulae, brown spots, as well as long and thin nails have been described in hypopituitarism (De Nicola *et al.* 1974). Nail thickening, fragility and striation, along with Beau's lines of the thumbnails occurred in a patient with Sheehan's syndrome (Biava 1974). Thickening of the nail plates was reported in a female pati-

ent with hypopituitarism and a feminine genotype (Hollander 1920).

## References

Biava, L. (1974) Le alterazioni ungueali nel morbo di Sheehan. *Chronice Dermatologice* **3–4**, 814–818.

De Nicola, P., Morsiani, M. & Zavagli, G. (1974) *Nail Diseases in Internal Medicine*. Charles C. Thomas, Springfield, IL.

Freinkel, R.K. & Freinkel, N. (1987) In: *Dermatology in General Medicine* (eds T.B. Fitzpatrick, A.Z. Eisen, K. Wolff *et al.*), pp. 2063–2081. McGraw Hill, New York.

Haneke, E. (1989) Nagelveranderungen bei hormonellen Storungen. *Medizinische Monatsschrift für Pharmazeuten* **12**(6), 173–178.

Hollander, L. (1920) Onychauxis due to hypopituitarism. *Archives of Dermatology Syphiligraphie* **2**, 35–43.

Keefe, M., Chapman, R.S. & Peden, N.R. (1987) Ingrowing fingernails: an unusual complication of acromegaly successfully treated by conservative means. *Clinical and Experimental Dermatology* **12**, 343–344.

Wendling, D. & Guidet, M. (1993) Les dysacromélies. *Est Medecine* **7–9**, 23–25.

Wit, J.M., Beemer, F.A., Barth, P.G. *et al.* (1985) Cerebral gigantism (Sotos syndrome). Complied data of 22 cases. Analysis of clinical features, growth and plasma somatomedin. *European Journal of Pediatrics* **144**, 131–140.

## Adrenal disease

Cutaneous and mucosal hyperpigmentation is one of the most characteristic signs of chronic adrenal insufficiency. Longitudinal pigmented bands in fingernails and toenails are occasionally observed. Nail hyperpigmentation progressively disappears after replacement therapy (Allenby & Snell 1996; Bissel *et al.* 1971). Cutaneous hyperpigmentation due to a pituitary tumour (Nelson's syndrome) occurs in about 10% of patients treated by bilateral adrenalectomy for Cushing's syndrome. Longitudinal pigmented bands in fingernails and toenails have been described (Bondy & Harwick 1969). Primary distal and lateral onycholysis as well as chronic paronychia due to *Candida* have been described in association with Cushing's syndrome (Hay *et al.* 1988; Haneke 1989).

## References

Allenby, C.F. & Snell, P.H. (1966) Longitudinal pigmentation of the nails in Addison's disease. *British Medical Journal* **1**, 1582–1583.

Bissel, G.W., Surakomol, K. & Greenslet, F. (1971) Longitudinal banded pigmentation of nails in primary adrenal insufficiency. *Journal of the American Medical Association* **215**, 1666–1667.

Bondy, P.K. & Harwick, H.J. (1969) Longitudinal banded pigmentation of nails following adrenalectomy for Cushing's syndrome. *New England Journal of Medicine* **281**, 1056–1057.

Haneke, E. (1989) Nagelveranderungen bei hormonellen Storungen. *Medizinische Monatsschrift für Pharmazeuten* **12**(6), 173–178.

Hay, R.S., Baran, R., Moore, M.K. *et al.* (1988) Candida onychomycosis—an evaluation of the role of Candida species in nail diseases. *British Journal of Dermatology* **118**, 45–58.

## Parathyroid disease

Nail and hair changes can precede other clinical manifestations of hypocalcaemia. Characteristic nail changes have been described in hypoparathyroidism. The distal half of the nail plate becomes brittle and then crumbles. The proximal nail plate is covered with irregular longitudinal grooves. Thinning, fragility and splitting at the distal free edge of the nails is commonly observed. Nail changes usually disappear when serum calcium is restored to normal levels (Simpson 1954). All 20 nails can occasionally appear opalescent, thin and brittle with fine longitudinal ridges (Yuzuk *et al.* 1986). Splinter haemorrhages have also been reported.

Secondary *Candida* infection of the nails is frequently observed. A defect in cell-mediated immunity, combined with the nail changes that favour yeast invasion, is a possible explanation for the increased susceptibility to *Candida* infection.

Shortening and thickening of the fingernails and toenails along with overgrowth of the periungual tissues have been reported in a patient suffering from idiopathic hypoparathyroidism (Emerson *et al.* 1941). Nail brittleness and Beau's lines can occur 4–6 weeks after a severe attack of acute hypocalcaemia. Shedding of the nails and necrosis of the nail beds have also been described (Simpson 1954). Impaired circulation caused by spasm in the nail bed capillary loops has been detected in latent tetany. Calcium administration can prevent angiospasm (Simpson 1954).

In polyglandular type I autoimmunity syndrome, chronic mucocutaneous candidiasis is associated with hypoparathyroidism and adrenal insufficiency (Ahonen *et al.* 1990). An inherited defect in cell-mediated immunity has been recognized.

Brachydactyly is a common feature of pseudohypoparathyroidism. Pseudo-pseudohypoparathyroidism, which appears as a variant of pseudohypoparathyroidism without hormonal resistance phenomenon, may be associated with ingrowing toenails secondary to the soft tissue and skeletal abnormalities (D. de Berker, personal communication). In hyperparathyroidism, acroosteolysis due to calcium mobilization can occur. Shortening of the distal phalanges causes the nails to appear abnormally broad (acquired racquet nails) (Fig. 6.45) (Fairris & Rowell 1984). Nail shedding has been reported after treatment with parathyroid extracts (Perrot *et al.* 1973).

## References

Ahonen, P., Myllarniemi, S., Sipila, I. *et al.* (1990) Clinical variation of autoimmune polyendocrinopathy-candidiasis-ectodermal dystrophy (APECED) in a series of 68 patients. *New England Journal of Medicine* **322**, 1829–1836.

Emerson, K., Walsh, F.B. & Howard, J.F. (1941) Idiopathic hypoparathyroidism; a report of two cases. *Annals of Internal Medicine* **14**, 1256–1270.

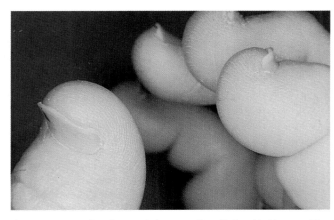

**Fig. 6.45** Hyperparathyroidism acquired racquet nails and koilonychia. (Courtesy of B. Schubert, France.)

Fairris, G.M. & Rowell, N.R. (1984) Acquired racket nails. *Clinical and Experimental Dermatology* **9**, 267.

Perrot, H., Tourniere, J. & Fournier, M. (1973) Onychopathie induite par la parathormone. *Bulletin de la Societé Française de Dermatologie et de Syphiligraphie* **80**, 313.

Simpson, J.A. (1954) Dermatological changes in hypocalcemia. *British Journal of Dermatology* **66**, 1–15.

Yuzuk, S., Keren, G., Lobel, D. *et al.* (1986) Primary cutaneous manifestation in a child with idiopathic hypoparathyroidism. *International Journal of Dermatology* **25**, 531–532.

## Thyroid disease

Nail changes are seen in approximately 5% of hyperthyroid patients. Brittle nails and onycholysis are common signs of hyperthyroidism. Koilonychia is occasionally observed (Mullin & Elastern 1986). A variable brown colour can be present in the nail plate (Daniel 1985).

In thyrotoxicosis, a characteristic onycholysis occurs in which the free edge of the nail is undulated and curved upward (Plummer's nails). The 4th digits of the hands are initially involved but the alteration may affect any and all of the fingernails and toenails. Plummer's nails are reversible with treatment of the hyperthyroidism (Luria & Asper 1958).

Diamond syndrome, which is a rare manifestation of Graves' disease, describes the association of finger clubbing (thyroid acropachy) with ophthalmopathy and pretibial myxoedema.

In hypothyroidism, the nails can appear dry, flat, brittle and longitudinally ridged. Onycholysis is occasionally observed (Keipert & Kelly 1978; Baran 1986; Orteu & Rustin 1996). Thick, hard and lusterless nails have also been described (Haneke 1989; Zaias 1990; O'Donovan 1996; Nakatsui & Lin 1998) and may develop while undergoing therapy for hypothyroidism. The nail growth rate is decreased.

In patients with hyperthyroidism only minor changes in capillary blood flow velocity could be detected, which is in contrast to patients with hypothyroidism. In the latter, the skin microvascular autoregulatory mechanisms are disturbed (Pazos-Moura *et al.* 1998).

## References

Baran, R. (1986) Les onycholyses. *Annales de Dermatologie et de Vénéréologie* **113**, 159–170.

Daniel, C.R. (1985) Nail pigmentation abnormalities. *Dermatologic Clinics* **3**, 431–443.

Haneke, E. (1989) Nagelveranderungen bei hormonellen Storungen. *Medizinische Monatsschrift für Pharmazeuten* **12**(6), 173–178.

Keipert, J.A. & Kelly, R. (1978) Acquired juvenile hypothyroidism presenting with nail changes. *Australian Journal of Dermatology* **19**, 89–90.

Luria, M. & Asper, S. (1958) Onycholysis in hyperthyroidism. *Annals of Internal Medicine* **49**, 102–108.

Mullin, G.E. & Eastern, J.S. (1986) Cutaneous consequences of accelerated thyroid function. *Cutis* **37/2**, 109–114.

Nakatsui, T. & Lin, A.N. (1998) Onycholysis and thyroid disease; report of three cases. *Journal of Cutaneous Medical Surgery* **3**, 40–42.

O'Donovan, D.K. (1996) Hypothyroid nails and evolution. *Lancet* **347**, 1262–1263.

Orteu, C.H. & Rustin, M.H.A. (1996) 20 thickened, fragile nails. *Lancet* **347**, 662.

Pazos-Moura, C.C., Moura, E.G., Breitenbach, M.M. *et al.* (1998) Nail fold capillaroscopy in hypothyroidism and hyperthyroidism: blood flow velocity during rest and post occlusive reactive hyperemia. *Angiology* **49**, 471–476.

Zaias, N. (1990) *The Nail in Health and Disease*, 2nd edn, pp. 189–199. Appleton & Lange, Norwalk, CN.

## Pregnancy and menstrual factors

Nail growth is accelerated in pregnancy and slowed during lactation (Runne & Orfanos 1981). Although Beau's lines, increased brittleness and softening as well as subungual keratosis and onycholysis can occur in pregnancy, they are probably not related to hormonal factors (Wong & Ellis 1984). Hyperpigmentation is very common in pregnancy and can be associated with longitudinal melanonychia (Texier 1980; Fryer & Werth 1992). Beau's lines have been associated with dysmenorrhoea but they can also occur physiologically with each menstrual cycle (Colver & Dawber 1984). Transverse leuconychia has also been associated with menstruation (Baran 1981).

## References

Baran, R. (1981) Modifications of colour. In: *The Nail* (ed. M. Pierre), pp. 30–39. Edinburgh. Churchill Livingston.

Colver, G.B. & Dawber, R.P.R. (1984) Multiple Beau's lines due to dysmenorrhoea? *British Journal of Dermatology*, **111**, 111–113.

Fryer, J.M. & Werth, V.P. (1992) Pregnancy-associated hyperpigmentation: longitudinal melanonychia. *Journal of the American Academy of Dermatology* **26**, 493–494.

Runne, U. & Orfanos, C.E. (1981) The human nail. *Current Problems in Dermatology* **9**, 102–149.

Texier, L. (1980) Chromonychie en bandes longitudinales de la grossesse. Presented at the Meeting of the Société Française de Dermatologie. Filiale du sud-ouest, Bordeaux, France, 21 June.

Wong, R.C. & Ellis, C.N. (1984) Physiologic skin changes in pregnancy. *Journal of the American Academy of Dermatology* **10**, 929–940.

## Metabolic disorders

### Diabetes

Furosine and fructose-lysine values in the nails are indicators of non-enzymatic glycosylation associated with diabetic hyperglycaemia. A significant correlation exists between nail glycosylation and glycosylated haemoglobin as well as fasting blood glucose levels in diabetics (Bakan & Bakan 1985). Furosine and fructose-lysine levels in the nails reflect the blood glucose levels within 3–5 months before nail clipping and can therefore be utilized for assessing diabetic control in the previous months (Oimomi *et al.* 1986). No correlations have been detected between furosine values of stratum corneum, nails and the prevalence of cutaneous manifestations in diabetics (Nozaki *et al.* 1988).

Periungual erythema and telangiectasia can be a very early manifestation of diabetes mellitus. Proximal nail fold capillaroscopy can show venous dilatation and tortuosity. The former has been suggested to be an indicator of functional microangiopathy and of long-term blood glucose control. Tortuosity, by contrast, has been related to long-term microangiopathy (Huntley 1989). Skin capillary aneurysms, detected by indocyanine green in type I diabetes, are an important morphological feature of diabetic microangiopathy (Zaugg-Vesti *et al.* 1995). Haemorrhages and ischaemic areas can also be present.

Scleroderma-like skin changes (diabetic cheiroarthropathy) involving the fingers and dorsum of the hands occur in 20–30% of diabetic patients. Thickening of the skin on the dorsum of the fingers causes the skin on the periungual regions and knuckles to have a pebbled or rough appearance (Huntley 1989). Diabetic cheiroarthropathy is more common in patients with insulin-dependent diabetes and has been linked with a high risk of microvascular complications (Cropley 1993). Chronic paronychia and onycholysis due to *Candida* are frequently observed in diabetics. Onychomycosis is also common. A recent study shows that the risk odds ratio for diabetic subjects to have toenail onychomycosis was 2.7 times greater compared with normal individuals. Toenail onychomycosis was present in 26.2% of the diabetics (Gupta *et al.* 1997). A positive correlation has been detected between blood glucose levels and the percentage of positive fungal cultures in toenails (Greene & Scher 1987).

The toenails of diabetic patients may show mild surface abnormalities. An optical profilometric study of the microrelief of toenail surface revealed that toenails of diabetics are signi-

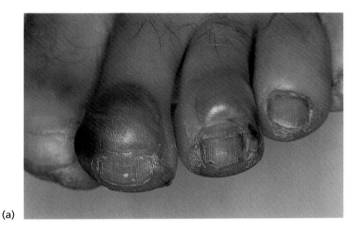

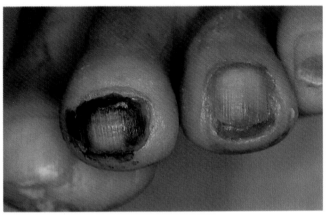

**Fig. 6.46** (a) Diabetic foot—periungual blisters. (b) Same patient—nail thickening, periungual haemorrhage and ulceration.

ficantly more rough than toenails of non-diabetics. A seasonal variation in the nail surface of diabetics was also observed, with more prominent roughness during the winter time. This suggests that environmental conditions together with diabetic microangiopathy and vasomotor dysregulation are involved (Piérard-Franchimont *et al.* 1996). Smooth thickened toenails of yellow or yellowish-green colour have been described in diabetics. The great toes usually manifest prominent changes and the yellow discoloration is most often evident on the distal aspect of the nails (Lithner 1976). Multiple Beau's lines have also been reported (Sweren & Burnett 1992). Clear, non-scarring spontaneous blisters on the tips of the toes or involving finger proximal nail folds, can occasionally be observed. They are often symmetrical (Jelinek 1994). Toenail thickening or onychogryphosis can result from diabetic angiopathy and neuropathy. Neuropathic ulcers, ischaemic ulceration of the nail bed and gangrene are major complications of diabetic feet (Fig. 6.46) (Gfesser *et al.* 1994). Mononeuritis multiplex involving both ulnar nerves produced short, fragile and discoloured nails in both hands with motor changes (Mann & Burton 1982). Infections are frequent, and are also the most likely cause of foot amputation (Brodsky & Schneidler 1991).

Large hands and feet and clubbing have been described in congenital lipodystrophic diabetes with acanthosis nigricans (Seip–Lawrence syndrome) (Reed *et al.* 1965).

## References

Bakan, E. & Bakan, N. (1985) Glycosylation of nail in diabetics: possible marker of long-term hyperglycemia. *Clinica et Chimica Acta* **147**, 1–5.

Brodsky, J.W. & Schneideler, C. (1991) Diabetic foot infection. *Orthopedic Clinics of North America* **22**, 473–489.

Cropley, T.G. (1993) The diagnostic challenge of diabetic hands. *Archives of Dermatology* **129**, 40–41.

Gfesser, M., Worret, W.I., Schneider, J. *et al.* (1994) Das diabetische Fuss syndrom. *Zeitschrift für Hautkrankheiten* **69**, 581–584.

Greene, R.A. & Scher, R.K. (1987) Nail changes associated with diabetes mellitus. *Journal of the American Academy of Dermatology* **16**, 1015–1021.

Gupta, A.K., Konnikow, N., MacDonald, P. *et al.* (1997) Prevalence of onychomycosis in diabetics: a North American Survey. *Journal of the European Academy of Dermatology and Venereology* **9** (Suppl. 2) (abstract).

Huntley, A.C. (1989) Cutaneous manifestations of diabetes mellitus. *Dermatologic Clinics* **7**, 531–546.

Jelinek, J.E. (1994) Cutaneous manifestations of diabetes mellitus. *Journal of Dermatology* **33**, 605–617.

Lithner, F. (1976) Purpura, pigmentation and yellow nails of the lower extremities in diabetics. *Acta Medica Scandinavica* **199**, 203–208.

Mann, R.J. & Burton, J.L. (1982) Nail dystrophy due to diabetes neuropathy. *British Medical Journal* **284**, 1445.

Nozaki, S., Sueki, H., Fujisawa, R. *et al.* (1988) Glycosylated proteins of stratum corneum, nail and hair in diabetes mellitus: correlation with cutaneous manifestations. *Journal of Dermatology* **15**, 320–324.

Oimomi, M., Nishimoto, S., Kitamura, Y. *et al.* (1986) Increased fructose-lysine of nail protein and blood glucose control in diabetic patients. *Hormone Metabolism Research* **18**, 827–829.

Piérard-Franchimont, C., Jebali, A., Ezzine, N. *et al.* (1996) Seasonal variations in polymorphic nail surface changes associated with diabetes mellitus. *Journal of the European Academy of Dermatology and Venereology* **7**, 182–183.

Reed, W.B., Dexter, R., Corley, C. *et al.* (1965) Congenital lipodystrophic diabetes with acanthosis nigricans. *Archives of Dermatology* **91**, 326–334.

Sweren, R.J. & Burnett, J.W. (1992) Multiple Beau's lines. *Cutis* **29**, 41–42.

Zaugg-Vesti, B.R., Franzeck, U.K., Von Ziegler, C. *et al.* (1995) Skin capillary aneurysms detected by indocyanine green in type I diabetes with and without retinal microaneurysms. *International Journal of Microcirculation: Clinical and Experimental* **15**, 193–198.

## Hyperoxaluria

Primary hyperoxaluria is a rare genetic disorder of glyoxalate metabolism characterized by hyperoxaluria, recurrent calcium oxalate nephrolithiasis, chronic renal failure and early death from uraemia. Subungual oxalate granuloma has been reported (Sina & Lutz 1990).

Acrocyanosis and Raynaud's phenomenon, livido reticularis, loss of distal pulses, peripheral gangrene and cutaneous calcifications of the digits have also been reported (Baethge *et al.* 1988; Villada *et al.* 1990).

## References

Baethge, B.A., Sanusi, I.D., Landreneau, M.D. *et al.* (1988) Livedo reticularis and peripheral gangrene associated with primary hyperoxaluria. *Arthritis and Rheumatism* **31**, 1199–1202.

Sina, B. & Lutz, L.L. (1990) Cutaneous oxalate granuloma. *Journal of the American Academy of Dermatology* **22**, 316–317.

Villada, G., Bressieux, J.M., Schillinger, F. *et al.* (1990) Manifestations cutanées d'une oxalose par hyperoxalurie primitive. *Annales de Dermatologie et de Vénéréologie* **117**, 844–846.

## Cystic fibrosis

Nail clippings from patients with cystic fibrosis show an elevated sodium and chloride content (Runne & Orfanos 1981; Chapman *et al.* 1985). Periungual telangiectasia and splinter haemorrhages can occur (Zaias 1990).

## References

Chapman, A.L., Fegeley, B. & Cho, C.T. (1985) X-ray microanalysis of chloride in nails from cystic fibrosis and control patients. *European Journal of Respiratory Diseases* **66**: 218–223.

Runne, U. & Orfanos, C.E. (1981) The human nail. *Current Problems in Dermatology* **9**, 102–149.

Zaias, N. (1990) *The Nail in Health and Disease*, 2nd edn. Appleton & Lange, Norwalk, CN.

## Hartnup disease

Nail 'streaks' have been described in Hartnup disease (Daniel *et al.* 1985).

## Reference

Daniel, C.R., Sams, W.M. & Scher, R.K. (1985) Nails in systemic disease. *Dermatologic Clinics* **3**, 465–483.

## Histidinaemia

Pachyonychia, indistinct lunulae, onychoschizia and Beau's lines have been reported in a patient affected by histidinaemia (Pravatà *et al.* 1987).

## Reference

Pravatà, G., Amato, S. & Corrao, A. (1987) Ipotricosi, onicopatia distrofica, anomalie dentarie in un caso di istidinemia. *Giornale Italiano di Dermatologia e Venereologia* **122**, 361–336.

## Lipoid proteinosis (Urbach–Wiethe disease)

In patients with lipoid proteinoisis nail growth can be arrested (Konstantinov *et al.* 1992).

## Reference

Konstantinov, K., Kabakchiev, P., Karchev, T. *et al.* (1992) Lipoid proteinosis. *Journal of the American Academy of Dermatology* **27**, 293–297.

## Dyslipoproteinaemias

Nail clippings from patients with type IV and V hyperlipoproteinaemia contain significant amounts of Sudan IV positive substances. A relationship between lipids found in the nail plate and the status of circulating triglycerides has been suggested (Salamon *et al.* 1988).

Plane xanthomas on the tips of the fingers can occur in patients with types III and IV hyperlipoproteinaemia (Fine & Moschella 1985). Extensive tuberous xanthomas on the fingers have been described in a patient with type III hyperlipoproteinaemia (Brewer & Fredrickson 1987). Tendon xanthomas of extensor tendons of the fingers occur in cerebrotendinous xanthomatosis (Rodman 1981), in sitosterolaemia and familial hypercholesterolaemia. Periungual pseudo-Koenen's tumours of the 2nd and the 3rd toes have been reported in a patient affected by familial hypercholesterolaemia (Keller 1960).

## References

Brewer, H.B. & Fredrickson, D.S. (1987) Dyslipoproteinemias and xantomatoses. In: *Dermatology in General Medicine* (eds B. Fitzpatrick, A.Z. Eisen, K. Wolff *et al.*), pp. 1722–1738. McGraw Hill, New York.

Fine, J.D. & Moschella, S.L. (1985) Diseases of nutrition and metabolism. In: *Dermatology* (eds S.L. Moschella & H.J. Hurley), pp. 1422–1532. W.B. Saunders, Philadelphia.

Keller, P.H. (1960) Hypercholesterinamische Xanthomatose. *Dermatologische Wochenschrift* **141**, 336.

Rodman, O. (1981) The spectrum of cerebrotendinous xanthomatosis. *Journal of the Association of Military Dermatology* **7**, 8–11.

Salamon, T., Nikuln, A., Grujic, M. *et al.* (1988) Sudan IV-positive material of the nail plate related to plasma triglycerides. *Dermatologica* **176**, 52–54.

## Fabry's disease

'Bushy' nail fold capillaries abnormalities have been described in one patient with Fabry's disease (Frank *et al.* 1996). Telangiectatic hyperkeratotic papules can be localized on the distal finger (Shelley *et al.* 1995), the pulp of the fingernails and toenails. A 'turtle-back' configuration of the fingernails has been reported (Fine & Moschella 1985), and a distal purpuric-like border has been observed in the fingernails of a patient with Fabry's disease (Carsuzaa *et al.* 1985).

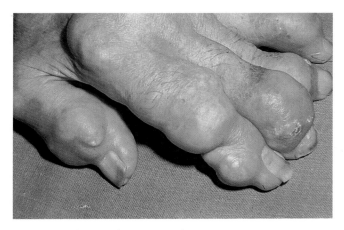

**Fig. 6.47** Gout. (Courtesy of L. Simon, France.)

## References

Carsuzaa, F., Rommel, A., Geniaux, M. *et al.* (1985) Maladie de Fabry. *Annales de Dermatologie et de Vénéréologie* **112**, 635–638.

Fine, J.D. & Moschella, S.L. (1985) Diseases of nutrition and metabolism. In: *Dermatology* (eds S.L. Moschella & H.J. Hurley), pp. 1422–1532. W.B. Saunders, Philadelphia.

Frank, J., Jansen-Genzel, W., Lentner, A. *et al.* (1996) Angiokeratoma corporis diffusum universale (Fabry disease). *Hautarzt* **47**, 776–779.

Shelley, E.D., Shelley, W.B. & Kurezynski, T.W. (1995) Painful fingers, heat intolerance and telangiectases of the ear: easily ignored childhood signs of Fabry's disease. *Pediatric Dermatology* **12**, 215–219.

## Gout

Tophi can occasionally have a periungual location and cause distortion of the nail apparatus (Fig. 6.47). Longitudinal striations, brittleness and crumbling of the nails have been described (Rail 1969). These nail changes, which closely resemble nail psoriasis, can be of diagnostic importance in atypical joint diseases (Runne & Orfanos 1981). Onychogryphosis has been reported as a common manifestation of hyperuricaemia, occurring in 45–73% of hyperuricaemic patients (Harvàth & Vecék 1986). In hereditary hyperuricaemia, the nails can show thickening, splitting and dystrophic changes (Gospos 1976).

## References

Gospos, C. (1976) Gicht subacute periarticulare knotige hautgicht der endphalangen mit nageldystrophie. *Zeitschrift für Hautkrankheiten* **51**, 29.

Harvàth, G. & Vecék, F. (1986) Uricaemia and onychogryphosis. *Ceskoslovenska Dermatologie* **61**, 338–390.

Rail, G.A. (1969) Nail changes in gout. *British Medical Journal* **2**, 782–783.

Runne, U. & Orfanos, C.E. (1981) The human nail. *Current Problems in Dermatology* **9**, 102–149.

## Lesch–Nyhan syndrome

Lesch–Nyhan syndrome, an X-linked inborn error of metabolism, is characterized by hyperuricaemia, mental retardation, spastic cerebral palsy, choreoathetosis and compulsive self biting of the lips, fingers and hands. The enzyme defect has been identified as a deficiency in hypoxanthine-guanine phosphoribosyltransferase. The neuropsychiatric manifestations of the disease have recently been related to a deficit in the dopaminergic nerve terminals and cell bodies (Ernst *et al.* 1996).

## Reference

Ernst, M., Zametkin, A.J., Matochik, J.A. *et al.* (1996) Presynaptic dopaminergic deficits in Lesch–Nyhan disease. *New England Journal of Medicine* **334**, 1568–1572.

## Alkaptonuria

Alkaptonuria is a rare autosomal recessive metabolic disorder caused by the deficiency of homogentisic acid oxidase. This leads to deposition of oxidized homogentisic acid pigment in connective tissues. The clinical manifestations of alkaptonuria include distinctive skin pigmentation (ochronosis) (Fig. 6.48), arthritis and dark urine. Extensor tendons of the hands and finger nail beds can appear as bluish-grey, bluish-black or brown (Goldsmith 1987).

## Reference

Goldsmith, L.A. (1987) Cutaneous changes in errors of aminoacid metabolism: alkaptonuria. In: *Dermatology in General Medicine* (eds T. Fitzpatrick, A.Z. Eisen, I.M. Freedberg *et al.*), pp. 1642–1646. McGraw Hill, New York.

## Homocystinuria

Periungual telangiectasia can be observed in homocystinuria.

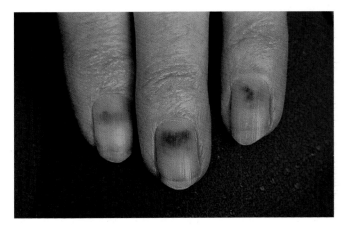

**Fig. 6.48** Ochronosis. (Courtesy of E.J. ter Bors, The Netherlands.)

Longitudinal ridging in the absence of nail fragility has also been reported (Baden & Zaias 1987).

## Reference

Baden, H.P. & Zaias, N. (1987) Nails. In: *Dermatology in General Medicine* (eds T. Fitzpatrick, A.Z. Eisen, I.M. Freedberg *et al.*), pp. 651–666. McGraw Hill, New York.

## Fucosidosis

Purple nail bands can be a feature of type III fucosidosis, an autosomal recessive metabolic disorder, which mimics Fabry's disease (Epinette *et al.* 1973). The disease is caused by deficiency of the lysosomial enzyme α-L-fucosidase.

## Reference

Epinette, W.W., Norins, A.L. & Drew, A.L. (1973) Angiokeratoma corporis diffusum with alpha-L-fucosidase deficiency. *Archives of Dermatology* **107**, 754–757.

## Porphyria (Fig. 6.49)

Increased levels of porphyrins in hair and fingernails have been detected in patients with porphyria cutanea tarda (Alberdi *et al.* 1991). In congenital erythropoietic porphyria (Gunther's disease), severe mutilating deformities of the fingers result from repeated episodes of blistering. In two patients with late-onset congenital erythropoietic porphyria, koilonychia preceded the onset of the skin manifestation (Deybach *et al.* 1981). Red fluorescence of the nail plate with Wood's light has been described in erythropoietic porphyria (Daniel 1985). Total leukonychia and opaque blue-grey or brownish fingernails with absent lunulae have also been reported (Redeker & Bronow 1964; Thivolet *et al.* 1968).

Photoonycholysis is a possible manifestation of erythropoietic porphyria, porphyria cutanea tarda, variegate porphyria and Bantu porphyria (Duterque *et al.* 1983). Local pain, tenderness and sensation of fluid accumulation beneath the nail plate is followed by onycholysis that can result in loss of the fingernail (Schmitd *et al.* 1974; Marsden & Dawber 1977). Nail involvement can be a prominent symptom of the disease in black people (Bovenmyer 1976). Photoonycholysis associated with digital and subungual bullae has also been reported in porphyria cutanea tarda-like syndrome of haemodialysis (Guillaud *et al.* 1990). Onycholysis was the presenting sign of contraceptive pill-induced porphyria cutanea tarda in a patient (Byrne *et al.* 1976).

Yellow, black or brown discoloration of the nail, finger clubbing and loss of the lunula have been reported in porphyria cutanea tarda. Splinter haemorrhages, koilonychia and longitudinal pigmented bands or distal hemitorsion of the nail plate can also occur (Puissant *et al.* 1971; Baran 1981; Pizzino *et al.* 1988). Mutilating scarring deformities of fingers are seen in hepatoerythropoietic porphyria.

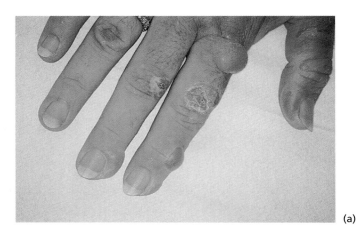

(a)

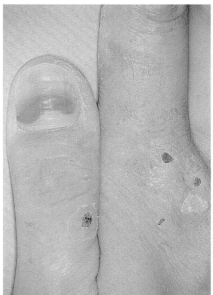

(b)

**Fig. 6.49** (a) Porphyria cutanea tarda, digital blistering. (b) Porphyria cutanea tarda, onycholysis and blistering.

## References

Alberdi, Y., Jeronimo, E., Stella, A.M. *et al.* (1991) Pofirinas en pelos y unas de pacientes con porfiria cutanea tardia en tratamiento con cloroquina y de ratas intoxicadas con hexaclorobenceno. *Revista Argentina Dermatologia* **72**, 70–79.

Baran, R. (1981) The nail in dermatological disease. In: *The Nail* (ed. M. Pierre), pp. 46–53. Churchill Livingstone, Edinburgh.

Bovenmyer, D.A. (1976) Erythropoietic protoporphyria: first report of cases in the American Negro. *Cutis* **18**, 277–280.

Byrne, J.P.H., Boss, J.M. & Dawber, R.P.R. (1976) Contraceptive pill-induced porphyria cutanea tarda presenting with onycholysis of the fingernails. *Postgraduate Medical Journal* **52**, 535–538.

Daniel, C.R. (1985) Nail pigmentation abnormalities. *Dermatologic Clinics* **3**, 431–443.

Deybach, J.C., De Verneuil, H., Phung, N. *et al.* (1981) Congenital erythropoietic porphyria (Gunther's disease): enzymatic studies on two cases of late onset. *Journal of Laboratory and Clinical Medicine* **97**, 551–558.

Duterque, M., Civatte, J., Jeaumougin, M. *et al.* (1983) Porphyrie érythropoiétique de Gunther de revelation tardive. *Annales de Dermatologie et de Vénéréologie* **110**, 709–710.

Guillaud, V., Moulin, G., Bonnefoy, M. *et al.* (1990) Photo-onycholyse bulleuse au cours d'une pseudoporphyrie des hémodialysés. *Annales de Dermatologie et de Vénéréologie* **117**, 723–725.

Marsden, R.A. & Dawber, R.P.R. (1977) Erythropoietic protoporphyria with onycholysis. *Proceedings of the Royal Society of Medicine* **70**, 572–574.

Pizzino, D., De Padova, M., Labanca, M. *et al.* (1988) Patologia degli annessi cutanei nella porfiria cutanea tarda. *Giornale Italiano di Dermatologia e Venereologia* **123**, 607–608.

Puissant, A., David, V., Lachiver, D., *et al.* (1971) Formes clinique atypiques de la porphyrie cutanée tardive. *Bollettino dell Istituto Dermatologico San Gallicano* **7**, 19.

Redeker, A.G. & Bronow, R.S. (1964) Erythropoietic protoporphyria presenting as hydroa aestivale. *Archives of Dermatology* **89**, 104–109.

Schmitd, H., Snitker, G., Thomsen, K. *et al.* (1974) Erythropoietic protoporphyria. *Archives of Dermatology* **110**, 58–64.

Thivolet, J., Freycon, J., Perrot, H. *et al.* (1968) Protoporphyrie érythropoiétique. *Bulletin de la Societé Française de Dermatologie et de Syphiligraphie* **75**, 829–841.

## Amyloidosis (Fig. 6.50)

Dystrophic nail changes are a possible early manifestation both of primary and myeloma-associated systemic amyloidosis (Breathnach & Black 1979; Breathnach *et al.* 1979; Wheeler & Barrows 1981; Blanc *et al.* 1982; Ostlere *et al.* 1995; Bedlow *et al.* 1999). Nail abnormalities can closely mimic nail lichen planus. The nails appear uniformly thinned, brittle, longitudinally ridged and distally split (Fanti *et al.* 1991; Derrick & Price 1995). Nail flattening, cracking, crumbling and even partial or complete anonychia can occur (Jones *et al.* 1972; Breathnach 1988). Narrow pink longitudinal subungual striations as well as splinter haemorrhages (Desirello *et al.* 1988) and subungual haematomas (Bluhm *et al.* 1980) have occasionally been reported. Yellow discoloration of the nail plate, subungual papillomatosis and onycholysis have also been described. Scleroderma-like diffuse infiltration of the hands and fingertip ulcerations can occur (Brownstein & Helwig 1970). At nail biopsy typical amyloid deposits are detectable in the superficial dermis and around blood vessels (Pineda *et al.* 1988; Fanti *et al.* 1991). Chronic ulceration of distal extremities due to neuropathic changes can be observed in heredofamilial amyloid polyneuropathy (Brownstein & Helwig 1970). Smooth, thickened yellow toenails and black nail beds have also been described (Lithner 1976). Chronic paronychia is unusual (Ahmed *et al.* 2000).

Shaw *et al.* (1983) described a case of macular cutaneous amyloidosis with autosomal dominant nail changes consisting of marked thickening and yellow discoloration. These nail changes resolved during the 3rd and 4th decades of life.

## References

Ahmed, I., Cronk, J.S., Crutchfield, C.E. *et al.* (2000) Myeloma-associated systemic amyloidosis presenting as chronic paronychia and palmodigital erythematous swelling and induration of the hands. *Journal of the American Academy of Dermatology* **42**, 339–342.

Bedlow, A.J., Sampson, S.A. & Holden, C.A. (1999) Primary systemic amyloidosis of the hair and nails. *Clinical and Experimental Dermatology* **23**, 298–299.

Blanc, D., Kienzler, J.L., Faivre, R. *et al.* (1982) Amylose systématisée primitive avec alopécie et onychodystrophie généralisées. *Annales de Dermatologie et de Vénéréologie* **109**, 877–880.

Bluhm, J.F., Johnson, S.C. & Norbach, D.H. (1980) Bullous amyloidosis. *Archives of Dermatology* **116**, 1164.

Breathnach, S.M. (1988) Amyloid and amyloidosis. *Journal of the American Academy of Dermatology* **18**, 1–16.

Breathnach, S.M. & Black, M.M. (1979) Systemic amyloidosis and the skin: a review with special emphasis on clinical features and therapy. *Clinical and Experimental Dermatology* **4**, 517–536.

Breathnach, S.M., Wilkinson, J.D. & Black, M.M. (1979) Systemic amyloidosis with underlying lymphoproliferative disorder. Report of a case in which nail involvement was a presenting feature. *Clinical and Experimental Dermatology* **4**, 495–499.

Brownstein M.H. & Helwig, E.B. (1970) The cutaneous amyloidosis. *Archives of Dermatology* **102**, 20–28.

Derrick, E.K. & Price, M.L. (1995) Primary systemic amyloid with nail dystrophy. *Journal of the Royal Society of Medicine* **88**, 290–291.

Desirello, G., Nazzari, G., Stradini, D. *et al.* (1988) Amiloidosi primaria. *Giornale Italiano di Dermatologia e Venereologia* **123**, 99–101.

Fanti, P.A., Tosti, A., Morelli, R. *et al.* (1991) Nail changes as the first sign of systemic amyloidosis. *Dermatologica* **183**, 44–46.

Jones, N.F., Hilton, P.J., Tighe, J.R. *et al.* (1972) Treatment of 'primary' renal amyloidosis with melphalan. *Lancet* **ii**, 616–619.

Lithner, L. (1976) Skin lesions of the legs and feet and skeletal lesions of the feet in familial amyloidosis with polyneuropathy. *Acta Medica Scandinavica* **199**, 197–202.

Ostlere, L.S., Stevens, H., Metha, A. *et al.* (1995) Nail dystrophy. *Archives of Dermatology* **131**, 951–956.

Pineda, M.S., Herrero, C., Palou, J. *et al.* (1988) Nail alterations in systemic amyloidosis: report of one case, with histologic study. *Journal of the American Academy of Dermatology* **18**, 1357–1359.

Shaw, M., Jurecka, W., Beack, M.M. *et al.* (1985) Macular amyloidosis associated with familial nail dystrophy. *Clinical and Experimental Dermatology* **2**, 363–368.

Wheeler, G.E. & Barrows, G.H. (1981) Alopecia universalis. A manifestation of occult amyloidosis and multiple myeloma. *Archives of Dermatology* **117**, 815–816.

## Nervous disorders

Hauser (1983) believes that localization of nail diseases only to certain nails may be caused by visceral-cutaneous reflexes that produce alterations in the terminal vascular system.

## Reference

Hauser, W. (1983) Zur Lokalization und Pathogenese von Nagelkrankungen. *Aktuelle Dermatologie* **9**, 70–74.

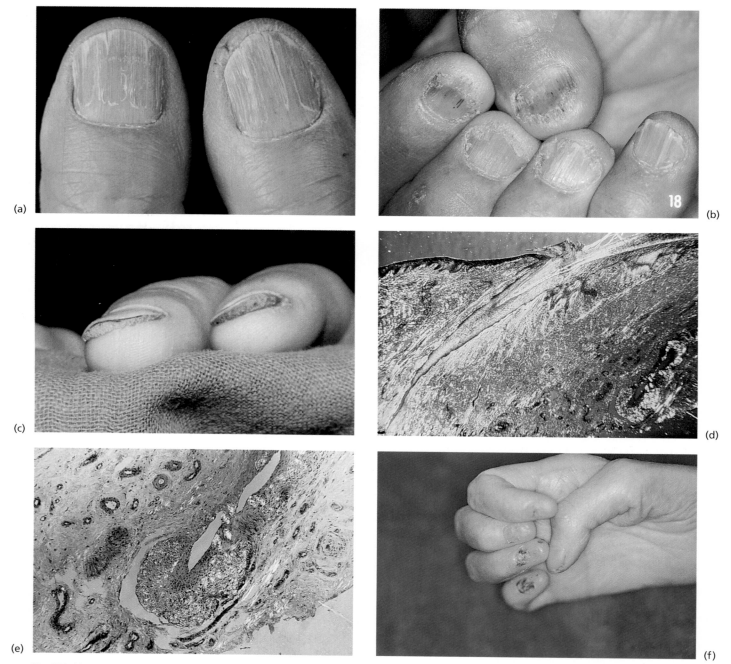

**Fig. 6.50** (a) Systemic amyloidosis—onychoschizia and distal splitting. (b) Systemic amyloidosis—koilonychia and splinter haemorrhages. (c) Systemic amyloidosis—subungual papillomatosis. (d) Typical amyloid deposit. (Courtesy of J.M. Mascaro, Spain.) (e) Typical amyloid deposit. (Courtesy of J.M. Mascaro, Spain.) (f) Heredofamilial amyloid polyneuropathy. (Courtesy of B. Fouilloux, France.)

## Hereditary

Thick, hard nails with onychogryphosis occur in Morgagni–Stewart–Morel syndrome (Kupp 1958). Onychomadesis is seen in Bogaert–Scherer–Epstein syndrome (cerebrotendinous xanthomatosis) and nail plate disorders are a feature of Divry–Van Bogaert syndrome (meningeal angiomatosis). Polydactyly and polyonychia occur as part of the Lawrence–Moon–Biedl syndrome. Self-mutilation occurs in the Lesch–Nyhan syndrome.

## Reference

Kupp, J. (1958) Beiträge zu dem hypothalamischen zentralregulie rund sorgan des Nagelsystem. *Zentralblatt für Allgemeine Pathologie und Pathologische Anatomie* **98**, 290–293.

## Phacomatoses

Supernumerary digits and congenital enlargement of limbs or digits can occur in neurofibromatosis (Chao 1961). Plexiform neurofibroma can produce hypertrophic fingers or toes with dislocation of the nails. Macrodactyly of the foot associated with plexiform neurofibroma of the digital branches of the medial plantar nerve was the sole manifestation of von Recklinghausen's neurofibromatosis in one patient (Turra *et al.* 1986). A patient with pterygium inversum unguius-like changes has also been reported (Patterson 1977).

Periungual fibromas (Koenen's tumours) are a pathognomonic sign of tuberous sclerosis (Chapter 11). They occur in approximately 50% of patients and are usually noticed after puberty but continue to develop with age. They appear as pedunculated, smooth, firm, flesh-coloured, pointed, grain-shaped growths that originate in the periungual groove and usually extend outward over the nail plate. The nail plate frequently shows longitudinal ridging and grooving resulting from pressure on the matrix. Partial or complete atrophy of the nail plate can also occur. Pachyonychia may be observed in toenails. Cuticular hyperkeratosis, which may indicate a subclinical Koenen tumour, has been observed in some cases (Colomb *et al.* 1976). Nail plate abnormalities can also occasionally be seen in digits without a Koenen's tumour. Histologically, Koenen's tumours can be considered fibrokeratomas that originate from the proximal nail fold or the surrounding connective tissue (Kint & Baran 1988). Extensive subungual fibromas that disrupt the entire nail bed have been reported (Nickel & Reed 1962). Cyst-like lesions and periosteal thickening of the phalanges are frequently observed. Macrodactyly can also occur.

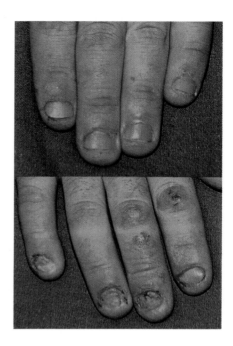

**Fig. 6.51** Syringomyelia. (Courtesy of Cl. Beylot, France.)

## References

Chao, D.H.C. (1961) Congenital neurocutaneous syndromes in childhood. *Journal of Pediatrics* **59**, 189–199.

Colomb, D., Racouchot, J. & Jeunne, R. (1976) Les lésions des ongles dans la sclérose tubéreuse de Bourneville isolées on associées aux tumeurs de Koenen. *Annales de Dermatologie et de Vénéréologie* **103**, 431–437.

Kint, A. & Baran, R. (1988) Histopathologic study of Koenen tumours. *Journal of the American Academy of Dermatology* **18**, 369–372.

Nickel, W.R. & Reed, W.B. (1962) Tuberous sclerosis. *Archives of Dermatology* **85**, 209–226.

Patterson, J.W. (1977) Pterygium inversum unguius-like changes in scleroderma. *Archives of Dermatology* **113**, 1429–1430.

Turra, S., Frizziero, P., Cagnoni, G. *et al.* (1986) Macrodactyly of the foot associated with plexiform neurofibroma of the medial plantar nerve. *Journal of Pediatric Orthopedics* **6**, 489–492.

## Syringomyelia (Fig. 6.51)

Segmental loss of pain and temperature sensation in the hands and arms is the principal clinical feature of syringomyelia. Thickening and callosities of the skin on the fingers and knuckles result from repeated minor trauma. Swelling and oedema of the hands are frequent. Macrodactyly of either or both the index and medial fingers can be present (Ambrosetto 1965). Nails can be deformed and slow growing. Longitudinal striations can occur. Painless ulceration of the fingers, painless ulceration and crusting of periungual tissue resembling chronic paronychia as well as painless whitlows are commonly observed (Adams 1987). Resorption or spontaneous amputation of the terminal phalanges can also occur (Tosti *et al.* 1994). Asymmetric anonychia has been reported in one patient (Leopold & Wassilew 1988). Many of these changes correspond to the syndrome of Morvan, in which analgesic whitlows with dermal changes of these types affect the upper extremities.

Differential diagnosis includes leprosy and hereditary sensory neuropathy.

## References

Adams, R.D. (1987) Neurocutaneous diseases. In: *Dermatology in General Medicine* (eds T.B. Fitzpatrick, A.Z. Eisen, K. Wolff *et al.*), p. 2053. McGraw Hill, New York.

Ambrosetto, C. (1965) La patologia della mano in neurologia, II parte. *Relazioni Clinico Scientifiche* **90** (XVII), 10–17.

Leopold, A. & Wassilew, S.W. (1988) Cutaneous changes in syringomyelie. *Zeitschrift für Hautkrankheiten* **6**, 494–496.

Tosti, A., Peluso, A.M., Morelli, R. *et al.* (1994) Cutanous amputation of the terminal phalanges in syringomyelia. *Dermatology* **189**, 185–187.

## Hemiplegia

The nail growth rate is retarded on the affected side in hemiplegia. Overcurvature and narrowing of the nails have been reported (Lewis & Pickering 1935). Longitudinal and transverse striations or onychomadesis can occur. Unilateral pterygium inversum unguis involving the right fingers and toes has been described in a patient affected by a paresis of the entire right side after a cerebrovascular accident. Mild subungual hyperkeratosis was also present (Morimoto & Gurevitch 1988). Neapolitan's nails only occurred unilaterally on the hemiparetic side in some patients who previously had had strokes (Horan *et al.* 1982). A patient with a longstanding history of psoriasis developed progressive nail changes consisting of subungual hyperkeratosis and accelerated nail growth confined to his left hand 2 years after a mild left side hemiparesis due to a cerebrovascular event (Badger *et al.* 1992).

## References

Badger, J., Banerjee, A.K. & McFadden, J. (1992) Unilateral sub-ungual hyperkeratosis following a cerebrovascular incident in a patient with psoriasis. *Clinical and Experimental Dermatology* 17, 454–455.

Horan, M.A., Puxty, J.A. & Fox, R.A. (1982) The white nails of old age (neapolitans nails). *Journal of the American Geriatric Society* 30, 734–737.

Lewis, T. & Pickering, G.W. (1935) Circulatory changes in the fingers in some diseases of the nervous system, with special reference to the digital atrophy of peripheral nerve lesions. *Clinical Science* 2, 149–183.

Morimoto, S.S. & Gurevitch, A.W. (1988) Unilateral pterygium inversum unguis. *International Journal of Dermatology* 27, 491–494.

## Spinal cord injuries (Fig. 6.52)

Thickening of the toenails and onychogryphosis are very common in patients with spinal cord injuries. The occurrence of nail hypertrophy is not related to the neurological level of injury (Stover *et al.* 1994). Ingrowing toenails, which usually occur after the initial period of bed rest, are also very common in patients with a spinal cord injury. Tetraplegics appear to be more frequently affected than paraplegics. Nail brittleness, atrophic skin changes and toe flexor spasms have been considered the main predisposing factors in the development of ingrowing toenails in patients with spinal injuries (Jaffray & El Masri 1985). Marked periungual and palmar erythema has also been associated to tetraplegia (Stover *et al.* 1994). Progressive self-biting of the fingers and hands resulting in multiple finger amputations has been described in two patients following C4 complete spinal cord injury. Stress, isolation and loss of sensation were responsible for this self-abusive behaviour (Dahlin *et al.* 1985). Acroosteolysis of the fingers as the result of self-mutilation has been observed in a quadriplegic patient after a spinal cord injury at the C5–C6 level (Marmolya *et al.* 1989).

Unilateral nail dystrophy after C4 complete spinal cord injury presented as transverse white bands on the right ring and little fingernails. They moved distally as the nails grew and the proximal newly formed nail in the affected fingers became

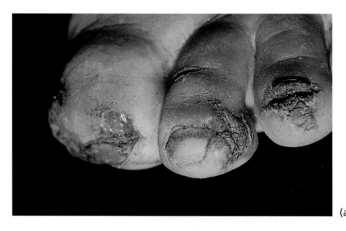

(a)

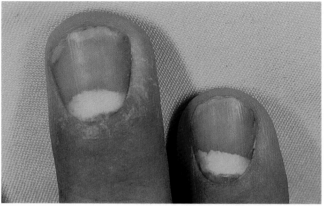

(b)

**Fig. 6.52** (a) Spinal cord injury. (b) Unilateral nail dystrophy 1 month after C4 spinal cord injury. (Courtesy of S. Burge, UK.)

brittle and dystrophic over a 5-month period (Harris *et al.* 1996). Unilateral hyperhidrosis, callosities and nail dystrophy appeared in a boy with tethered spinal cord syndrome (Wollina *et al.* 1998).

## References

Dahlin, P.A., Van Buskirk, N.E., Novotny, R.W. *et al.* (1985) Self-biting with multiple finger amputations following spinal cord injury. *Paraplegia* 23, 306–318.

Harris, A.J., Burge, S.M. & Gardener, B.P. (1996) Unilateral nail dystrophy after C4 complete spinal cord injury. *British Journal of Dermatology* 135, 855–856.

Jaffray, D. & El Masri, W. (1985) Ingrowing toenails and tetraplegia. *Paraplegia* 23, 176–181.

Marmolya, G., Yagan, R. & Freehafer, A. (1989) Acro-osteolysis of the fingers in a spinal cord injury patient. *Spine* 14, 137–139.

Stover, S.L., Hale, A.M. & Buell, A.B. (1994) Skin complications other than pressure ulcers following spinal cord injury. *Archives of Physical Medicine and Rehabilitation* 75, 987–993.

Wollina, U., Mohr, F. & Schier, F. (1998) Unilateral hyperhidrosis, callosities and nail dystrophy in a boy with tethered spinal cord syndrome. *Pediatric Dermatology* 15, 486–487.

## Congenital absence of pain

There are two varieties of congenital absence of pain: congenital indifference to pain and congenital insensitivity to pain (Winkelmann et al. 1962). In congenital indifference to pain children discriminate painful stimulations, but are not able to integrate pain sensation into conscious experience. This is possibly due to a dysfunction in the central structures where pain is integrated. Patients with congenital insensitivity to pain, on the other hand, have abnormalities of the peripheral nerves of central sensory pathways leading to an inability to recognize and avoid noxious stimuli (Serratrice 1992). In congenital insensitivity to pain syndrome with anhidrosis, congenital analgesia is associated with inability to sweat, which leads to defective thermoregulation with recurrent episodes of hyperthermia (Okuno et al. 1990; Guidetti et al. 1996).

Patients with congenital absence of pain usually present early mucocutaneous signs that first appear at the time of tooth eruption (Piñol Aguadé et al. 1973; Thompson et al. 1980; Hatzis et al. 1992; Ozbarlas et al. 1993). Autoextraction of teeth is also common in these children. Hand lesions, due to chewing of the fingers, include periungual ulcerations, nail deformities and even severe finger mutilations (Person et al. 1977; Hatzis et al. 1992; Ozbarlas et al. 1993; Domingues et al. 1994). Trauma may lead to gangrene and toes may have to be amputated (Rosenberg et al. 1994). Scarring is a common sequela of tongue and finger chewing. X-ray studies of the fingers may show partial resorption of the terminal phalanges (Ozbarlas et al. 1993).

Compulsive self-biting of the lips, fingers and hands in the absence of sensory deficits is a typical symptom of Lesch–Nyhan syndrome (see page 269).

## References

Domingues, J.C., Moreno, A., Mariano, A. et al. (1994) Congenital sensory neuropathy with anhidrosis. Pediatric Dermatology 11, 231–236.

Hatzis, J., Gourgiotou, K., Koumelas, D. et al. (1992) Congenital sensory neuropathy with anhidrosis (hereditary sensory neuropathy type IV). Australian Journal of Dermatology 33, 103–107.

Guidetti, M.S., Piraccini, B.M., Misciali, C. et al. (1996) Congenital insensitivity to pain with anhidrosis. European Journal of Dermatology 6, 278–279.

Okuno, T., Inoue, A., & Izumo, S. (1990) Congenital insensitivity to pain with anhidrosis. Journal of Bone and Joint Surgery 72A, 279–282.

Ozbarlas, N., Sarikayalar, F. & Kale, G. (1993) Congenital insensitivity to pain with anhidrosis. Cutis 51, 373–374.

Person, J.R., Rogers III, R.S. & Rhodes, K.H. (1977) Congenital sensory neuropathy: report of an atypical case. Archives of Dermatology 113, 954–957.

Piñol Aguadé, J., Ferrando, J., Estrach, T. et al. (1973) Indiferencia congénita al dolor con anhidrosis eliperlaxitud articular. Medicina Cutanea Ibero-Latino-Americana 3, 185–203.

Rosenberg, S., Wagahashi Marie, S.K. & Kliemann, S. (1994) Congenital insensitivity to pain with anhidrosis. Pediatric Neurology 11, 50–56.

Serratrice, G. (1992) Indifférence et insensibilité congénitales à la douleur. Bulletin de l'Academie Nationale de Medicine 176, 609–618.

Thompson, C.C., Park, R.I. & Prescott, G.H. (1980) Oral manifestations of the congenital insensivity-to-pain syndrome. Oral Surgery Oral Medicine Oral Pathology 50, 220–225.

Winkelmann, R.K., Lambert, E.H. & Hayles, A.B. (1962) Congenital absence of pain. Archives of Dermatology 85, 325–339.

## Peripheral neuropathies (Fig. 6.53)

Congenital and acquired sensory neuropathies that produce analgesia are frequently associated with recurrent painless acral skin ulcers. Spontaneous amputation of the digits can occasionally occur. Acropathia ulcero-mutilans acquisita (Bureau–Barrière's syndrome) is an acquired unilateral or bilateral polyneuropathy which starts in middle age and mainly affects the lower limbs in man. The onset and development can be precipitated by chronic trauma, alcohol intake and diabetes. It is very rarely accompanied by lesions on the upper limbs (Vanhooteghem et al. 1999). In non-familial Bureau–Barrière's syndrome, mutilant ulcer acropathy, annular constriction (pseudo-ainhum) leading to spontaneous loss of the digits, are

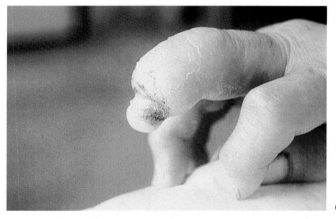

(a)

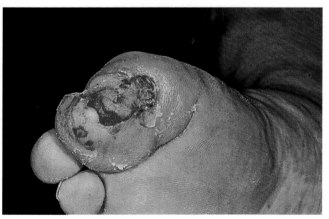

(b)

**Fig. 6.53** (a) Acropathia ulceromutilans. (Courtesy of O. Vanhooteghen, Belgium.) (b) Acropathia ulceromutilans. (Courtesy of H. Barrère, France.)

one of the most frequent symptoms (Torres Cortijo 1973, 1982; Eichorn & Schauder 1989). In leprosy neurological involvement can produce severe dystrophic changes and acroosteolysis of the fingers (De Las Agnas 1973).

## Cervical rib syndrome

In cervical rib syndrome, compression of subclavian vessels and the brachial plexus can produce cutaneous changes of the affected limb. Deficient vascular supply can cause fingertip ulceration, cyanosis and gangrene. Nail grooving, pachyonychia and onycholysis can also be present. Thinning, discoloration, ridging and shortening of the nails have been reported in the absence of symptoms of peripheral ischaemia (Rubin & Cipollaro 1939). In Volkmann syndrome, thinning and tapering of the fingers as well as overcurvature of the nails can occur (Ambrosetto 1965).

## Carpal tunnel syndrome (Fig. 6.54)

In carpal tunnel syndrome, blistering (Cox *et al.* 1995), and ulceration of the fingertip and subungual regions combined with dystrophic nail changes may be seen in either or both index and medial fingers. Nail abnormalities include onychomadesis, Beau's lines, striate leuconychia and severe dystrophy. Gangrene, spontaneous amputation and acroosteolysis of the terminal phalanges have been described (Bouvier *et al.* 1979; Treves *et al.* 1980; Adoue *et al.* 1984; Geffray *et al.* 1984; Tosti *et al.* 1993). The condition can be bilateral (Romani *et al.* 1996). In a case of carpal tunnel syndrome, the skin changes included anhidrosis, alopecia, nail dystrophy and episodes of acute necrosis. The nail changes involved the left 3rd finger, with a longitudinal black streak in the nail plate along with a hyperkeratotic cuticle and transverse grooving. Moreover, the

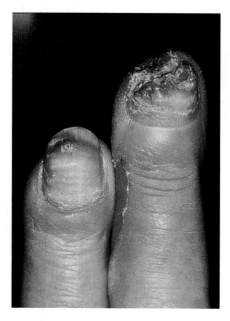

**Fig. 6.54** Carpal tunnel syndrome.

same finger had a necrotic bulla on the dorsal aspect of the distal phalanx (Aratari *et al.* 1984). A 70-year-old man affected by squamous cell carcinoma developed carpal tunnel syndrome and acrokeratosis paraneoplastica of Bazex. Both conditions improved after treatment of the tumour. This suggests that carpal tunnel syndrome was a paraneoplastic phenomenon (Poskitt & Duffil 1992).

Koilonychia limited to the 2nd and 3rd fingernails of both hands has also been reported; nail changes completely regressed after surgical treatment (Beurey *et al.* 1984).

## Peripheral nerve injuries

Retarded growth of the fingernails usually follows damage to the median or ulnar nerves. However, increased nail growth has also been reported after median nerve injuries (Ambrosetto 1965). Fingerpads become atrophic and nails can appear narrowed and clawlike. The bones of the affected fingers become less dense and in longstanding cases can decrease in size (Lewis & Pickering 1935). Unidigital clubbing has been described with trauma to the digit or median nerve (Stoll & Beetham 1954). Unilateral Beau's lines following hand injury were first reported by Ward *et al.* in 1988 and related to damage to flexor tendons and digital nerves of the affected fingers (Ward *et al.* 1988). However, in some patients unilateral Beau's lines and onychomadesis occur after hand trauma in the absence of signs of nerve injury. Unilateral Beau's lines may be associated with pyogenic granuloma of the same fingers (Price *et al.* 1994). Cast immobilization of the wrist and hand may contribute to the development of Beau's lines and pyogenic granuloma of the proximal nail fold (Harford *et al.* 1995; Tosti *et al.* 2001).

Marked nail changes following median nerve injury have been reported (Ross & Ward 1987). A bilateral ulnar neuropathy produced shortening, fragility and yellow discoloration of the nails on the ring and little finger of both hands in a diabetic patient affected by mononeuritis multiplex (Mann & Burton 1982). Onycholysis occurred after collateral palmar nerve injury (Waintraub *et al.* 1937). Symptomatic pterygium inversum unguis has been associated with lesions of the peripheral nerves in the fingers and toes (Runne & Orfanos 1981).

Three patients developed onychomadesis and focal haemorrhage of multiple proximal nail folds after major peripheral or major peripheral and central neurological deficit (Baran & Goettmann 1993).

In POEMS syndrome (Crow–Fukase syndrome) the acronym indicates the association of polyneuropathy with organomegaly, endocrinopathy, M proteins and skin changes. The skin changes of POEMS syndrome include hyperpigmentation, hypertrichosis, haemangioma and skin thickening that resembles scleroderma. Clubbing of the fingers occurs in 44% of cases. Apparent leuconychia (Terry's nails) (Fig. 6.55), acrocyanosis and Raynaud's phenomenon have also been reported (Tang *et al.* 1983; Shelley & Shelley 1987; Dereure *et al.* 1990). This multisystem disease is generally associated with a plasmocytoma or with an osteosclerotic myeloma.

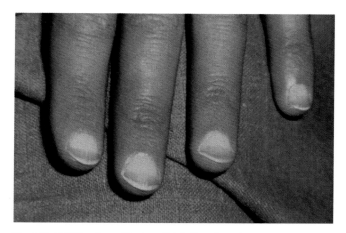

**Fig. 6.55** POEMS syndrome. (Courtesy of J.J. Guilhou, France.)

Arnold (1979) described sympathetic leuconychia in nails adjacent and controlateral to an injured nail.

## References

Adoue, D., Arlet, P., Giraud, P. *et al.* (1984) Syndrome du canal carpien avec ulcérations digitales chez un insuffisant rénal en hémodialyse périodique. *Annales de Dermatologie et de Vénéréologie* **111**, 1019–1021.

Ambrosetto, C. (1965) La patologia della mano in neurologia, II parte. *Relazioni Clinico Scientifiche* **90** (XVII), 10–17.

Aratari, E., Regesta, G. & Rebora, A. (1984) Carpal tunnel syndrome appearing with prominent skin symptoms. *Archives of Dermatology* **120**, 517–519.

Arnold H.L. (1979) Sympathetic symmetric punctate leukonychia. *Archives of Dermatology* **115**, 495–496.

Baran, R. & Goettmann, S. (1993) Nail bleeding associated with neurological deficits. *Dermatology* **187**, 197–199.

Beurey, J., Weber, M., Barthelme, D. *et al.* (1984) Koilonychie et syndrome du canal carpien. *Annales de Dermatologie et de Vénéréologie* **111**, 49–52.

Bouvier, M., Lejeune, E., Rouillat, M. *et al.* (1979) Les formes ulcéro-mutilantes du syndrome du canal carpien. *Revue du Rhumatisme* **46**, 169–176.

Cox, N.H., Large, D.M. & Ive, F.A. (1995) Cutaneous manifestations of carpal tunnel syndrome. *Journal of the American Academy of Dermatology* **32**, 682.

De Las Agnas, J.T. (1973) *Lecciones de Leprologia*, p. 251. Fontille, Spain.

Dereure, O., Guillot, B., Dandurand, M. *et al.* (1990) Les signes cutanés du syndrome POEMS. A propos de 3 observations et revue de la littérature. *Annales de Dermatologie et de Vénéréologie* **117**, 283–290.

Eichhorn, K. & Schauder, S. (1989) Nicht familiare Akroosteopathia ulcero-mutilans der Fube. *Hautarzt* **40**, 316–318.

Geffray, L., Leman, C., Dehais, J. *et al.* (1984) Deux cas de syndrome du canal carpien avec ulcérations digitales et acro-ostéolyse. *Revue du Rhumatisme* **51**, 45–47.

Harford, R.R., Cobb, M.W. & Banner, N.T. (1995) Unilateral Beau's lines associated with a fractured and immobilized wrist. *Cutis* **56**, 263–264.

Lewis, T. & Pickering, G.W. (1935) Circulatory changes in the fingers in some diseases of the nervous system, with special reference to the digital atrophy of peripheral nerve lesions. *Clinical Science* **2**, 149–183.

Mann, R.J. & Burton, J.L. (1982) Nail dystrophy due to diabetic neuropathy. *British Medical Journal* **284**, 1445.

Poskitt, B.L. & Duffil, M.B. (1992) Acrokeratosis paraneoplastica of Bazex presenting with carpal tunnel syndrome. *British Journal of Dermatology* **127**, 544–545.

Price, M.A., Bruce, S., Waidhofer, W. *et al.* (1994) Beau's lines and pyogenic granulomas following hand trauma. *Cutis* **54**, 248–249.

Romani, J., Puig, L., de Miguel, G. *et al.* (1996) Carpal tunnel syndrome presenting as sclerodactyly, nail dystrophy and acro-osteolysis in a 60-year-old woman. *Dermatology* **195**, 159–161.

Rubin, L.C. & Cipollaro, A.C. (1939) Onychodystrophy caused by cervical rib. *Archives of Dermatology* **39**, 430–433.

Ross, J.K. & Ward, C.M. (1987) An abnormality of nail growth associated with median nerve damage. *Journal of Hand Surgery* **12B**, 11–13.

Runne, U. & Orfanos, C.E. (1981) The human nail. *Current Problems in Dermatology* **9**, 102–149.

Shelley, W.B. & Shelley, E.D. (1987) The skin changes in the Crow–Fukase (POEMS) Syndrome. *Archives of Dermatology* **123**, 85–87.

Stoll, B.A. & Beetham, W.R. (1954) Unidigital clubbing with report of a case. *Medical Journal of Australia* **825**, 5.

Tang, L.M., Hsi, M.S., Ryu, S.J. *et al.* (1983) Syndrome of polyneuropathy, skin hyperpigmentation, oedema and hepatosplenomegaly. *Journal of Neurology, Neurosurgery and Psychiatry* **46**, 1108–1114.

Torres Cortijo, A. (1973) Constricturas anulares ainhum y pseudoainhum. *Medicina Cutanea Ibero-Latino-Americana* **2**, 95–102.

Torres Cortijo, A.V. (1982) Annular constriction (pseudo-ainhum) as first symptom of Bureau-Barriere's mutilant ulcer acropathy. Case presentation. In: *XVI Congressus Mundi Dermatologiae, Tokyo*, pp. 58–59.

Tosti, A., Morelli, R., D'Alessandro, R. *et al.* (1993) Carpal tunnel syndrome presenting with ischemic skin lesions, acroosteolysis and nail changes. *Journal of the American Academy of Dermatology* **29**, 287–290.

Tosti, A., Piraccini, B.M. & Camacho, F. (2001) Onychomadesis and pyogenic granuloma following cast immobilization. *Archives of Dermatology* **137**, 231–232.

Treves, R., Arnaud, J.P., Benabbou, M. *et al.* (1980) Ulcerations digitales an cours d'un syndrome du canal carpien avec Syndrome de Reynaud. *Revue du Rhumatisme* **47**, 578–579.

Vanhooteghem, O., Lateur, N., Hautecoeur, P. *et al.* (1999) Acropathia ulcero-mutilans acquisita of the upper limbs. *British Journal of Dermatology* **140**, 334–337.

Waintraub, L.C., Charaf, E. & Laudan, M. (1937) Un cas de troubles trophique unguéal d'origine traumatique. *Revue Française de Dermatologie et de Vénéréologie* **13**, 14–16.

Ward, D.J., Hudson, I. & Jeffs, J.V. (1988) Beau's lines following hand trauma. *Journal of Hand Surgery* **13B**, 411–414.

## Reflex sympathetic dystrophy (algodystrophy, causalgia) (Fig. 6.56)

Reflex sympathetic dystrophy (RSD) is a neurovascular disorder that results from minor nerve injuries producing a paradoxical sympathetic activity. Most commonly RSD is precipitated by

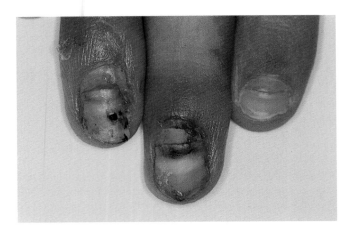

**Fig. 6.56** Reflex sympathetic dystrophy.

myocardial infarction or traumatic events, but other factors such as frostbite, phlebitis, tumours and infections have occasionally been responsible. Two cases of RSD after a fingernail biopsy have also been reported (Ingram *et al.* 1987; Haneke 1992). Wrist fractures are the most frequent causes of sympathetic dystrophy of the hand (Subbarao & Stillwell 1981). The clinical course of RSD is typically characterized by three stages. The cutaneous signs of the inflammatory stage, which is associated with intense and persistent pain, usually consist of erythema and swelling. The 2nd stage, which is often evident by the 3rd month after injury, is characterized by dystrophic skin changes associated with cyanosis and hyperhidrosis. Pain may or may not still be present. The 3rd stage is characterized by sclerotic and atrophic skin changes and tendon contractures.

Changes in the nail growth rate occurs in 66% of patients (Veldman *et al.* 1993). Increased nail growth and excessive transverse curvature of the nail plate have been reported during the 1st stage of RSD; nail brittleness can be observed in the 2nd and 3rd stages (Cony & Geniaux 1990; Shelton & Lewis 1990). Unilateral clubbing, acute periungual inflammatory changes, leuconychia and Beau's lines have also been described (Saunders & Hanna 1988; Tosti *et al.* 1993; O'Toole *et al.* 1995; Studer *et al.* 1996; Vanhooteghem *et al.* 1998). Acute whitlow-like inflammatory nail changes may result from recurrent atopic dermatitis of the hands (Camacho & Ordonez 1996). In a patient on peritoneal dialysis a severe nail dystrophy developed consisting of acute pseudoclubbing, elkonyxis, Beau's lines and onychomadesis. Spontaneous recovery occurred within 4 months (Caputo *et al.* 1997).

## References

Camacho, F. & Ordonez, E. (1996) Reflex sympathetic dystrophy with nail involvement. Its role in atopic dermatitis. *European Journal of Dermatology* 6, 172–174.

Caputo, R., Gelmetti, C. & Cambiaghi, S. (1997) Severe self-healing nail dystrophy in a patient on peritoneal dialysis. *Dermatology* 195, 274–275.

Cony, M. & Geniaux, M. (1990) Signes cutanés de l'algodystrophie. *Review of European Dermatology MST* 2, 281–88.

Haneke, E. (1992) Sympathische Reflexdystrophie, (Sudeck-dystrophie) nach nagelbiopsie. *Zentralblatt für Haut und Geschlechtskrankheiten* 160, 263.

Ingram, G.J., Scher, R.K. & Lally, E.V. (1987) Reflex sympathetic dystrophy following nail biopsy. *Journal of the American Academy of Dermatology* 16, 253–256.

O'Toole, E.A., Gormally, S., Drumms, B. *et al.* (1995) Unilateral Beau's lines in childhood reflex sympathetic dystrophy. *Pediatric Dermatology* 12, 245–247.

Saunders, P.R. & Hanna, M. (1988) Unilateral clubbing of fingers associated with causalgia. *Medical Journal* 297, 1635.

Shelton, R.M. & Lewis, C.W. (1990) Reflex sympathetic dystrophy: a review. *Journal of the American Academy of Dermatology* 22, 513–520.

Studer, E.M., Harms, M., Masouyé, I. *et al.* (1996). Nagelveränderungen in Rahmen einer Reflexdystrophie. *Hautartz* 47, 206–208.

Subbarao, S. & Stillwell, G.K. (1981) Reflex sympathetic dystrophy of the upper extremity: analysis of total outcome of management of 125 cases. *Archives of Physical and Medical Rehabilitation* 62, 549–554.

Tosti, A., Baran, R., Peluso, A.M. *et al.* (1993) Reflex sympathetic dystrophy with prominent involvement of the nail apparatus. *Journal of the American Academy of Dermatology* 29, 865–868.

Vanhooteghem, O., André, J., Halkin, V. *et al.* (1998) Leuconychia in reflex sympathetic dystrophy: a chance association? *British Journal of Dermatology* 139, 355–356.

Veldman, P.H.J., Reynen, H.M. & Arntz, I.E. (1993) Signs and symptoms of reflex sympathetic dystrophy: prospective study of 829 patients. *Lancet* 342, 1012–1016.

## Other central nervous system disorders

The paralysed limbs of patients with anterior poliomyelitis can exhibit toes or fingers that are considerably diminished in size and have retarded nail growth (Lewis & Pickering 1935). Hyponychial haemorrhages, horizontal ridging, onycholysis and onychomadesis have also been described.

Multiple sclerosis can produce longitudinal striations.

In multiple system atrophy, Siragusa *et al.* (1998) observed fingernails with a single, well-defined, transverse, reddish band occupying the central area of all of them.

'Coma nails' refer to bilateral subungual haematoma from nail bed compression with a pencil to monitor the response to pain (Wijdicks & Schievink 1997).

Increased nail growth rate as well as hyponychial haemorrages have been reported in Parkinson's disease. Onycholysis and onychomadesis have been described in tabes dorsalis; the latter also occurs in patients with rabies encephalomyelitis and epilepsy. Beau's lines may follow a severe epileptic convulsion.

Multiple paronychia has been recorded in epidemic encephalitis (Schirmer 1924).

## References

Lewis, T. & Pickering, G.W. (1935) Circulatory changes in the fingers in some diseases of the nervous system, with special reference to the digital atrophy of peripheral nerve lesions. *Clinical Science* 2, 149–183.

Schirmer, O. (1924) Ueber trophische Nagelveranderungen (multiple Panaritien) bei einem Fall von encephalitis epidemica. *Schweizersiche Medizinische Wochenschrift* 54, 984–985.

Siragusa, M., Del Gracco, S., Elia, M. *et al.* (1998) Peculiar dyschromic changes of finger nails in a patient with multiple system atrophy. *International Journal of Dermatology* 37, 156–160.

Wijdicks, E. & Schievink, W.I. (1997) Coma nails. *Journal of Neurology, Neurosurgery and Psychiatry* 63, 294.

## Migraine

Nail fold video-microscopy can be useful for monitoring the response to prophylactic treatment in migraine patients and testing new antimigraine drugs (Hegyalijai *et al.* 1997).

## Reference

Hegyalijai, T., Meienberg, O., Dubler, B. *et al.* (1997) Cold-induced acral vasospasm in migraine as assessed by nailfold video-microscopy: prevalence and response to migraine prophylaxis. *Angiology* 48, 345–349.

## Psychological and psychiatric disorders

Nail biting affects up to 60% of children and 45% of teenagers (Odenrick & Brattstrom 1985). The prevalence in adults is much less.

Whether nail biting in adults should be categorized as a psychological or psychiatric disease-associated sign is controversial. Although nail biting has been associated with sociopathy, anxious and obsessional symptoms, as well as aggressive needs, no evidence indicates a direct relationship between this habit and an underlying mental disorder. Patterns of nail biting vary among patients and may involve one, many or all nails (Singer & Gibson 1988; Guillet & Sassolas 1998).

Nail biting, which makes nails short and irregular, frequently induces secondary bacterial infections of periungual tissues. Longitudinal melanonychia due to matrix melanocyte stimulation can be a further consequence (Baran 1990; Salmon-Ehr *et al.* 1999). Picking, breaking or chewing of the skin over the posterior nail fold is frequently associated with nail biting. The terms perionychophagia and perionychomania have been coined for describing this autodestructive habit. According to Hirsch (1991) the symptom is not only regarded as a tension-reducing measure but also as a protosymbolically created surrogate of the early mother–child unit in which skin, hand and mouth play a dominant role.

Periungual warts commonly afflict nail biters. Apical root resorption (Oderick & Brattstrom 1985) or nail pterygium are uncommon complications of this habit. Osteomyelitis has also been reported as a complication of nail biting (Waldman & Frieden 1990; Tosti *et al.* 1993; Sagerman *et al.* 1995).

When nail biting persists in adult life it is usually severe and associated with a poor prognosis.

Self-induced trauma to the nails commonly causes nail deformities (Chapter 10).

The tick habit of grinding or horizontally stroking the edge of the second or third nail plate across both or either the proximal thumb nail plate and nail fold produces the characteristic deformity of multiple transverse lines associated with central nail depression on the thumbnails (Samman 1963). Although onychotillomania is usually a sign of an underlying psychological or psychiatric illness, self-induced nail changes are occasionally claimed to be due to occupational exposure (Norton 1987). Compulsive rubbing, picking or tearing of the nails can result in their gradual destruction (Sait & Garg 1985). Instruments such as scissors, knives, pliers and razor blades have been used by patients for causing self-inflicted damage (Colver 1987).

The clinical presentation of onychotillomania can mimic other nail disorders or have bizarre features. Preservation of the nail folds is usual. Self-inflicted onycholysis, splinter haemorrhages and subungual haematoma can be confused with other more common nail diseases. Traumatic picking or cutting of the corners of the nail plate can lead to ingrown toenails or fingernails. Nail plate depressions, scratches and even hollows may result from gouging nails with an instrument. Nail pterygium is the result of severe destruction and scarring. Picking and tearing of the exposed nail bed can follow nail plate destruction with pustular infection of the nail bed and proximal nail fold and produce nail bed destruction (Corraze 1965).

Although most patients deny manipulating their nails, some patients do admit their habit but give an unreliable explanation for it. Parasitophobia has been reported in some patients (Sait & Garg 1985; Colver 1987). Treatment of the underlying psychological disorders and occlusive dressings should be carried out in order to prevent irreversible changes. Behavioural therapy can be helpful (Peterson *et al.* 1994). Fluoxetine and its derivatives may be effective in the treatment of onychotillomania as well as of other obsessive-compulsive disorders (Vittorio & Phillips 1997).

A double-edged nail can be observed in patients with psychoses (Daniel *et al.* 1985). An acute psychotic episode may be accompanied by broad white banding in the nails (Pfeiffer & Jenney 1974).

The subpapillary plexus of the proximal nail fold is clearly visible and extensive in many schizophrenic patients. A significant correlation has been reported between the visibility of the subpapillary plexus and the family history, duration and severity of schizophrenia. Patients with nail fold changes frequently present glossy, smooth, thin-looking skin on the terminal phalanges. Capillary haemorrhages as well as long and straight sweat ducts in the nail fold area have also been commonly detected (Maricq 1969).

Transverse leuconychia has been described in patients with manic-depressive illness. Brittle hair and nails are frequently observed in anorexia nervosa. They may be due to the hypothyroid state that results from starvation. Finger clubbing associated with laxative abuse has also been reported (Gupta *et al.* 1987).

## References

Baran, R. (1990) Nail biting and picking as a possible cause of longitudinal melanonychia. *Dermatologica* **181**, 126–128.

Colver, G.B. (1987) Onychotillomania. *British Journal of Dermatology* **117**, 397–402.

Corraze, M.J. (1965) Un cas de pathomimie inhabituel: périonyxis pustuleux. *Bulletin de la Société Française de Dermatologie* **72**, 191–192.

Daniel, R.C., Sams, W.M. & Scher, R.K. (1985) Nails in systemic disease. *Dermatologic Clinics* **3**, 465–483.

Guillet, G. & Sassolas, B. (1998) Une onychopathie compulsive peu banale: l'onychophagie des vingt ongles. *Cutis & Psyché* **6**, 14–15.

Gupta, M.A., Gupta, A.K. & Haberman, H.F. (1987) Dermatologic signs in anorexia nervosa and bulimia nervosa. *Archives of Dermatology* **123**, 1386–1390.

Hirsch, M. (1991) Perionychomanie und perionychophagie oder habituelles nagelbettreiben. *Forum of Psychoanalysis* **7**, 127–135.

Maricq, H.R. (1969) Association of a clearly visible subpapillary plexus with other peculiarities of the nailfold skin in some schizophrenic patients. *Dermatologica* **138**, 148–154.

Norton, L.A. (1987) Self induced trauma to the nails. *Cutis* **40**, 223–227.

Odenrick, L. & Brattstrom, V. (1985) Nailbiting: frequency and association with root resorption during orthodontic treatment. *British Journal of Orthodontics* **12**, 78–81.

Pfeiffer, C.C. & Jenney, E.H. (1974) Fingernail white spots: possible zinc deficiency. *Journal of the American Medical Association* **228**, 157.

Peterson, A.L., Campise, R.L. & Azrin, N.H. (1994) Behavioral and pharmacological treatments for tic and habit disorders: a review. *Journal of Developmental and Behavioral Pediatrics* **15**, 430–441.

Sait, M.A. & Garg, R.B.R. (1985) Onychotillomania. *Dermatologica* **171**, 200–202.

Sagerman, S.D. & Lourie, G.M. (1995) Eikenella osteomyelitis in a chronic nail biter: a case report. *Journal of Hand Surgery* **20A**, 71–72.

Salmon-Ehr, V., Mohn, C. & Bernard, P. (1999) Melanonychies longitudinales secondaires à une onychophagie. *Annales de Dermatologie et de Vénéréologie* **126**, 44–45.

Samman, P.D. (1963) A traumatic nail dystrophy produced by habit tick. *Archives of Dermatology* **88**, 895–899.

Singer, P. & Gibson, G.H. (1988) Unilateral onychodystrophy secondary to nail biting. *Cutis* **42**, 191–192.

Tosti, A., Peluso, A.M., Bardazzi, F. *et al.* (1993) Phalangeal osteomyelitis due to nail biting. *Acta Dermato-Venereologica* **74**, 206–207.

Vittorio, C.C. & Phillips, K.A. (1997) Treatment of habit tic deformity with fluoxetine. *Archives of Dermatology* **133**, 1203–1204.

Waldman, B.A. & Frieden, I.J. (1990) Osteomyelitis caused by nail biting. *Pediatric Dermatology* **7**, 189–190.

# Immunological disorders

## Primary immunological deficiency syndromes

Susceptibility to infections is a typical feature of congenital hypogammaglobulinaemias. Pyoderma can affect periungual tissues causing acute paronychia. A 10-month-old boy affected by trachyonychia involving all fingernails and toenails (twenty-nail dystrophy) and selective IgA deficiency has been reported (Leong *et al.* 1982). Chronic mucocutaneous candidiasis and pyoderma are frequently found in severe combined immunodeficiency (Roberts & Weismann 1986). Diffuse and severe chronic warts unresponsive to therapy have also been reported in a patient with combined immunodeficiency (Asadullah *et al.* 1997). Dystrophic nails are a feature of Zinsser–Engman–Cole syndrome and koilonychia has been described in the Nezelof syndrome (Roberts & Weismann 1986). In biotin-responsive multiple carboxylase deficiencies *Candida* paronychia and onychodystrophy may occur. Patients with immunodeficiency and short-limbed dwarfism exhibit short, stubby hands and extremities (Ammann 1987). In Wiskott–Aldrich syndrome, characterized by the triad of thrombocytopenia, atopic eczema and recurrent infections, acute paronychia as well as nail pitting and transverse ridging due to atopic eczema can occur. Intense scratching results in a polished shiny surface of the nails.

Persistent *Candida* infections of the skin, nails and mucous membranes occur in chronic mucocutaneous candidiasis. Nail involvement can occasionally be the sole manifestation of the condition (Ammann 1987). Chronic paronychia is commonly observed. *Candida* invasion of the nail plate produces thickening, distortion and fragmentation of the nail plate (Palestine *et al.* 1983). A combination of dermatophyte and *Candida* infection can be seen. Fingertips can show a bulbous appearance (Goslen & Kobayashi 1987).

Elevated levels of IgE, eczematous skin lesions and recurrent cold staphylococcal abscesses are the characteristic features of Job's syndrome (Hyper-IgE syndrome) where acute paronychia, atrophic changes, mild clubbing and chronic candidal infection of the fingernails can occur (Davis *et al.* 1966; Zachary 1986).

Osteomyelitis of the distal phalanges has been reported in three children with severe atopic dermatitis. The insidious onset of distal wedge-shaped subungual black macules was followed by oedema, erythema and pain in the involved fingers (Boiko *et al.* 1988). The occurrence of osteomyelitis can be a consequence of the decreased cutaneous resistance to bacteria in atopic dermatitis coupled with repetitive scratching of infected skin with accumulation of necrotic keratin and bacteria beneath the distal nail plate.

## References

Ammann, A.J. (1987) Cutaneous manifestations of immunodeficiency disorders. In: *Dermatology in General Medicine* (eds T.B.

Fitzpatrick, A.Z. Eisen, K. Wolff *et al.*), pp. 2507–2522. McGraw-Hill, New York.

Asadullah, K., Renz, H., Wolf-Dietrich, D. *et al.* (1997) Verrucosis of hands and feet in a patient with combined immune deficiency. *Journal of the American Academy of Dermatology* 36, 850–852.

Boiko, S., Kaufman, R.A. & Lucky, A.W. (1988) Osteomyelitis of the distal phalanges in three children with severe atopic dermatitis. *Archives of Dermatology* 124, 418–423.

Davis, S.D., Schaller, J. & Wedgwood, R.J. (1966) Job's syndrome. *Lancet* i, 1013–1015.

Goslen, J.B. & Kobayashi, G.S. (1987) Fungal diseases with cutaneous involvement. In: *Dermatology in General Medicine* (eds T.B. Fitzpatrick, A.Z. Eisen, K. Wolff *et al.*), pp. 2193–2248. McGraw-Hill, New York.

Leong, A.B., Gange, R.W. & O'Connor, R.D. (1982) Twenty-nail dystrophy (trachyonychia) associated with selective Ig-A deficiency. *Journal of Pediatrics* 100, 418–419.

Palestine, R.F., Su, W.P.D. & Liesegang, T.J. (1983) Late-onset chronic mucocutaneous and ocular candidiasis and malignant thymoma. *Archives of Dermatology* 119, 580–586.

Roberts, S.O.B. & Weismann, K. (1986) The skin in systemic disease. In: *Textbook of Dermatology* (eds A. Rook, D.S. Wilkinson, F.J.G. Ebling *et al.*), pp. 2343–2347. Blackwell Scientific Publications, Oxford.

Zachary, C.B. (1986) Hyper IgE syndrome case history. *Clinical and Experimental Dermatology* 11, 403–408.

## Therapeutic immunosuppression

Paronychia, onychomycosis and Norwegian scabies can be seen in patients undergoing therapeutic immunosuppression. Blistering distal dactylitis due to haemolytic *Staphylococcus aureus* has been described in an adult patient taking high doses of systemic steroids for the treatment of Crohn's disease (Zemtsov & Veitschegger 1992).

## Reference

Zemtsov, A. & Veitschegger, M. (1992) *Staphylococcus aureus* induced blistering distal dactylitis in adult immunosuppressed patient. *Journal of the American Academy of Dermatology* 26, 784–785.

## Graft-versus-host disease (Table 6.6)

Acral erythema is a frequent manifestation of acute cutaneous graft-versus-host disease (GVHD) and may first appear as reddening of the tips of the fingers and periungual skin (Horwitz & Dreizen 1990; Farmer & Hood 1987). Onychomadesis is possible.

In chronic GVHD nail changes can closely resemble nail lichen planus. Longitudinal ridging, brittleness splitting, roughness and even partial or complete atrophy of the nails may be observed as well as pterygium formation (Liddle & Cowan 1990; Müller-Serten & Vakilzadeh 1994). Superficial ulcerations of the lunula (elkonyxis) have been described. Nail plate

**Table 6.6** Nail alterations in graft-versus-host disease. (Courtesy of J. Mascaro, Barcelona.)

| Nail alteration | Acute GVHD N/N (total 12) | Chronic GVHD N/N (total 28) |
|---|---|---|
| Leuconychia | 3/12 | 3/28 |
| Melanonychia | 2/12 | 2/28 |
| Yellow nail syndrome | 0/12 | 1/28 |
| Loss of brightness | 0/12 | 13/28 |
| Bed haemorrhages | 1/12 | 3/28 |
| Cuticular haemorrhages | 0/12 | 2/28 |
| Bed erythema | 6/12 | 6/28 |
| Periungual erythema | 11/12 | 22/28 |
| Fingertip erythema | 7/12 | 8/28 |
| Dorsal pterygium | 0/12 | 4/28 |
| Subungual hyperkeratosis | 0/12 | 6/28 |
| Cuticular hyperkeratosis | 6/12 | 3/28 |
| Onychomadesis | 2/12 | 5/28 |
| Onycholysis | 5/12 | 13/28 |
| Nail atrophy | 0/12 | 4/28 |
| Pachyonychia | 0/12 | 3/28 |
| Trachyonychia | 2/12 | 19/28 |
| Onychorrhexis | 3/12 | 15/28 |
| Onychoschizia | 0/12 | 5/28 |
| V-shaped onychoschizia | 0/12 | 1/28 |
| Longitudinal ridges | 7/12 | 28/28 |
| Transversal ridges | 2/12 | 6/28 |
| Beau's lines | 0/12 | 4/28 |
| Pitting | 0/12 | 1/28 |
| Bed erosions | 0/12 | 3/28 |
| Onychomycosis (*C. albicans*) | 0/12 | 1/28 |

opacification, thickening and onycholysis can also occur (James & Odom 1983), as well as koilonychia (Chosidow *et al.* 1992). Cuticular telangiectasia may be seen in the scleroderma-like changes resulting from GVHD. Mascaro and Martin-Ortega (1993) reported a series of 40 patients with nail disease of GVHD (Table 6.6) Nail changes were more frequent in the chronic lichenoid phase and were associated with cutaneous or oral lesions of GVHD. Secondary fungal infections are not uncommon. Immunophenotyping of inflammatory cells performed on the nail biopsy of a child who developed a severe lichen planus-like onychodystrophy after transfusion of non-irradiated blood, showed a prevalence of T-suppressor lymphocytes and epidermal expression of HLA-Dr (Ia) antigens (Brun *et al.* 1985).

White superficial onychomycosis due to *Trichophyton rubrum* was the initial cutaneous presentation of chronic GVHD in Basuk and Scher's patient (1987). Differential diagnosis of cutaneous and nail manifestations of chronic GVHD includes dyskeratosis congenita, a rare genodermatosis that frequently requires bone marrow transplantation because of pancytopenia (Ling *et al.* 1985; Esterly 1986).

## References

Basuk, P.J. & Scher, R.K. (1987) Onychomycosis in graft versus host disease. *Cutis* **40**, 237–241.

Brun, P., Baran, R., Desbas, C. *et al.* (1985) Dystrophie lichénienne isolée des 20 ongles. Etude en immunofluorescence par les anticorps monoclonaux. Conséquences pathologiques. *Annales de Dermatologie et de Vénéréologie* **112**, 215.

Chosidow, O., Bagot, M., Vernant, J.P. *et al.* (1992). Sclerodermatous chronic graft-versus host-disease. *Journal of the American Academy of Dermatology* **26**, 49–55.

Esterly, N.B. (1986) Nail dystrophy in dyskeratosis congenita and chronic graft-versus-host disease. *Archives of Dermatology* **22**, 506–507.

Farmer, E.R. & Hood, A.F. (1987) Graft-versus-host disease. In: *Dermatology in General Medicine* (eds T.B. Fitzpatrick, A.Z. Eisen, K. Wolff *et al.*), pp. 1344–1352. McGraw-Hill, New York.

Horwitz, L.J. & Dreizen, J. (1990) Acral erythema induced by chemotherapy and graft-versus-host disease in adults with hematogenous malignancies. *Cutis* **46**, 397–404.

James, W.D. & Odom, R.B. (1983) Graft-versus-host disease. *Archives of Dermatology* **119**, 683–689.

Liddle, B.J. & Cowan, M.A. (1990) Lichen planus-like eruption and nail changes in a patient with graft-versus-host disease. *British Journal of Dermatology* **122**, 841–843.

Ling, N.S., Fenske, N.A., Julius, R.L. *et al.* (1985) Dyskeratosis congenita in a girl simulating chronic graft-versus-host disease. *Archives of Dermatology* **121**, 1424–1428.

Mascaro, J.M. & Martin-Ortega, E. (1993) Nail alterations in graft versus host disease and other immunological disorders. In: *Dermatology Progress and Perspectives*. The Parthenon Publishing Group, New York.

Müller-Serten, B. & Vakilzadeh, F. (1994) Chronische sklerodermiforme Graft-versus-Host Disease. *Hautarzt* **45**, 772–775.

## Behçet's disease

Proximal nail fold capillaroscopy of patients with Behçet's disease frequently reveals non-specific abnormalities (Wechsler *et al.* 1984; Vaiopoulos *et al.* 1995). Subungual flame-shaped haemorrhagic lesions that are probably due to nail bed vasculitis have also been described (O'Duffy *et al.* 1971; Casanova *et al.* 1986; Cornelis *et al.* 1989). Sabin *et al.* (1990) reported a patient who had Behçet's disease and half-and-half nails.

## References

Casanova, J.M., Delgado, S., Menendez, F. *et al.* (1986) Hemorragias subungueales en el curso de la enfermedad de Behcet. *Acta Dermato-Sifilitica* **77**, 137–141.

Cornelis, F., Sigal-Nahum, M., Gaulier, A. *et al.* (1989) Behçet's disease with severe cutaneous necrotizing vasculitis: response to plasma exchange. Report of a case. *Journal of the American Academy of Dermatology* **21**, 576–579.

O'Duffy, J.D., Carney, J.A. & Deodhar, S. (1971) Behçet's disease. Report of 10 cases, 3 with new manifestations. *Annals of Internal Medicine* **75**, 561–570.

Sabin, A.A., Kalyoncu, A.F., Toros, Z. *et al.* (1990) Beçhet's disease with half-and-half nail and pulmonary artery aneurysm. *Chest* **97**, 1277.

Vaiopoulos, G., Pangratis, N., Samarkos, M. *et al.* (1995) Nail fold capillary abnormalities in Behçet's disease. *Journal of Rheumatology* **22**, 1108–1111.

Wechsler, B., Huong Du, L.T., Mouthon, J.M. *et al.* (1984) Aspects capillaroscopiques péri-unguéaux au cours de la maladie de Behçet. *Annales de Dermatologie et de Vénéréologie* **111**, 543–550.

## HIV diseases and the acquired immune deficiency syndrome

Increased nail and hair growth have been found by Harindra *et al.* (1993) in patients with AIDS.

Periungual erythema has been described in HIV patients (Péchere *et al.* 1996). The erythema, which can involve the fingers and the toes, may be painful (Battegay & Itin 1996). Capillary microscopy of these lesions only shows dilated capillaries. The pathology reveals an increased number of dilated blood vessels in the superficial dermis (Ruiz-Avila *et al.* 1995). The pathogenesis of periungual erythema in AIDS is still discussed. Angiogenic factors produced by HIV have been implicated (Ruiz-Avila *et al.* 1995). Liver impairment induced by hepatitis viruses has been suggested by the presence of viral hepatitis in most of the affected patients. Red finger syndrome associated with necrotizing vasculitis in an HIV-infected patient with hepatitis B is an example (Abajo *et al.* 1998).

Onychophagia and onychotillomania are probably not uncommon in patients with AIDS (Valenzano *et al.* 1988).

Fungal, viral and bacterial infections may affect the nails either primarily or secondarily in patients with AIDS (Daniel *et al.* 1992). Mucocutaneous candidiasis is a common manifestation of HIV infection.

Acute and chronic paronychia as well as total dystrophic onychomycosis due to *Candida albicans* are frequently observed in AIDS patients (Kaplan *et al.* 1987; Tosti *et al.* 1998).

A case of cryptococcal whitlow (Fig. 6.57a,b), in an unusual clinical presentation of an HIV-positive patient, has been reported by Verneuil *et al.* (1995). The mycological culture was positive for *Cryptococcus neoformans* serotype D. The lesion resolved with fluconazole (400 mg/day, during 2 months).

Gaddoni *et al.* (1994) reported two cases of finger necrosis in AIDS. In the first patient, ulcerative, necrotic lesions due to *C. albicans* were localized to terminal phalanges of both thumbs. The second patient was characterized by relapsing infections involving some fingers of both hands, with ulceration, necrosis and destruction of subcutaneous tissue in the terminal phalanges that presumably were caused by herpes simplex virus type I. Herpes simplex infections of the digits frequently produce atypical cutaneous manifestations in patients with AIDS. These include chronic ulcerative lesions, sometimes hyperkeratotic, crusted or necrotic, leading to finger gangrene (Belinchon & Ramos 1994) and even amputation of the distal phalanx. These are often complicated by bacterial superinfections (Fig. 6.57c). Recurrence is frequent if acyclovir treatment is not prolonged (Baden *et al.* 1991; Robayna *et al.* 1997). Atypical herpes zoster has also been reported with hyperkeratotic lesions (Fig. 6.57d) responding only with intravenous foscarnet

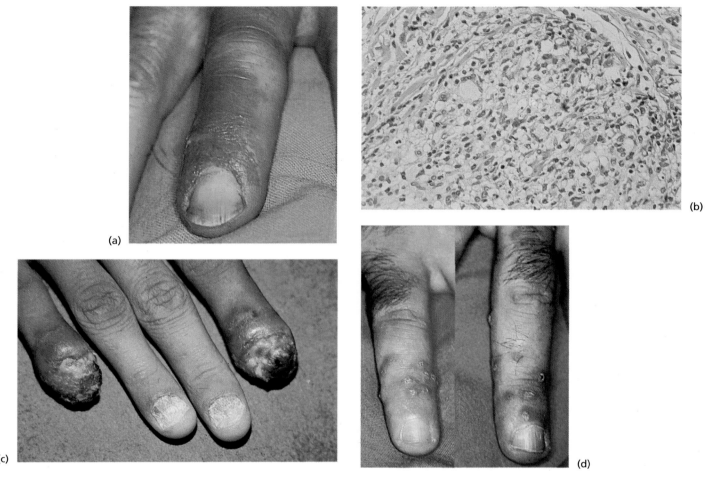

**Fig. 6.57** (a,b) Cryptoccocal whitlow. (Courtesy of D. Leroy, France.) (b) Same patient. (c) Herpetic whitlow in AIDS patient. (Courtesy of M.M.S. Nico & E.A. Rivitti, Brazil.) (d) Herpes zoster in AIDS. (Courtesy of M. Casado, Spain.)

(Fernandez-Diaz *et al*. 1995). Onychomycosis due to dermatophytes is also frequent and *Trichophyton rubrum* is the most common isolated organism; fungal invasion may even involve periungual tissues (Fischer & Warner 1987; Kaplan *et al*. 1987; Torssander *et al*. 1988; Prose 1990). Proximal white subungual onychomycosis due to *Trichophyton rubrum* is common in AIDS (Dompmartin *et al*. 1990). This clinical form of onychomycosis, which is rarely encountered in HIV-negative patients, starts as an irregular white patch that appears from beneath the proximal nail fold and progressively extends distally to involve the whole nail plate (Noppakun & Head 1986; Weismann *et al*. 1988). The infection, more frequent when the CD4+ cell count is less than 450 cells/mm³, may spread to all the fingers (even over the paronychium) (Kaplan *et al*. 1987) and toenails and is caused by prexisting *Trichophyton rubrum* tinea pedis that predates immunosuppression. This mycotic leuconychia should be differentiated from apparent leuconychia present in more than 10% of HIV-infected patients (Cribier *et al*. 1998).

Onychomycosis due to non-dermatophytic moulds is also common in AIDS. *Scopulariopsis brevicaulis* infection leading to destruction of the fingernails and toenails has been reported. Proximal subungual onychomycosis due to *Fusarium* sp. may be the source of disseminated fusariosis (Baran *et al*. 1997). *Pityrosporum ovale* was the only microorganism isolated in two patients with AIDS who presented a total dystrophic onychomycosis of all fingernails (Dompmartin *et al*. 1990).

Fingernail lesions due to recurrent infection by *Staphylococcus aureus* have been reported in association with hyper IgE (Raiteri *et al*. 1993). Periungual warts are common and frequently recur after removal. A severe herpetic whitlow may also be the first sign of the disease (Cockerell 1990), and it has also been described in children with AIDS (Prose 1990).

Norwegian scabies can occur in patients with HIV infection and causes dystrophic nails with subungual crusting (Jucowics *et al*. 1989; Inserra & Bickley 1990; Aricó *et al*. 1992). In HIV patients, psoriasis is about twice as common as in the general population. Nail abnormalities may be associated with widespread skin psoriasis or be the sole manifestation of the disease (Weitzul & Duvic 1997). Typical nail changes of Reiter's syndrome and psoriasis are therefore frequently observed in patients with HIV infection (Fischer & Warner 1987; Cockerell 1990). Splinter haemorrhages have also been seen (Kaplan *et al.* 1987). Digital clubbing has been reported in infants with AIDS (Scott *et al.* 1984; Graham *et al.* 1997; Katz 1997; Smyth *et al.* 1997). It can also occur in adults (Boonen *et al.* 1996; Belzunegui *et al.* 1997). Pityriasis rubra pilaris (PRP) is an unusual cutaneous complication of AIDS (Bonomo *et al.* 1997). It presents with different clinical features (development of nodulocystic and lichen spinulosis lesions) and has a poorer prognosis than the classical adult type. Miralles *et al.* (1995) propose the designation of a new category of PRP (type 6). In their patients, all the nails showed paronychia, subungual hyperkeratosis and hyperplastic cuticles.

Yellow discoloration of the distal portion of some nails is a frequent finding in HIV-infected patients. Although originally described under the diagnosis of yellow nail syndrome (Chernosky & Finley 1985), the yellow discoloration of the nails observed in patients with HIV infection is a different condition. Typical nail changes of YNS such as reduced nail growth, nail plate overcurvature, scleronychia and loss of cuticles are not observed. Colour changes can be preceded by opacification and decreased size or loss of the lunulae. Onycholysis at the distal part of the lateral nail folds as well as transverse and/or longitudinal ridging can be present. Great toenails are most commonly involved whereas fingernails are only rarely affected. Asymmetrical involvement of several nails is usual. Yellow toenail changes have been considered together with seborrhoeic dermatitis, hairy leukoplakia and oral candidiasis as possible indicators of progression to established AIDS in HIV-positive patients (Morfeld-Manson *et al.* 1989). Although dermatophytes have been suggested as a contributing factor in the development of yellow nails, bacterial and mycological cultures usually fail to reveal any infectious microorganisms.

A lichenoid dermatitis associated with nail changes has been described in a 39-year-old man with AIDS. The nail plates were thinned and the distal margin of the lunula presented an irregular border associated with longitudinal bands. Splinter haemorrhages and periungual lichenoid papules were also present (Buchner *et al.* 1989).

Generalized lichen spinulosus was accompanied by extensive onychodystrophy in an HIV-positive male (Cohen & Dicken 1991).

Patients with AIDS or an AIDS-related complex may develop Beau's lines following episodes of severe illness (Prose *et al.* 1992).

Non-vasculitic neutrophilic dermatosis is a rare complication of HIV infection. In one case violaceous annular and arcuate bullous lesions with crusting involved the distal thumb (Berger *et al.* 1994). Few cases of vasculitis have been described in cases of HIV infection. Enelow *et al.* (1992) reported a patient with vasculitis associated with eosinophilia and digital gangrene.

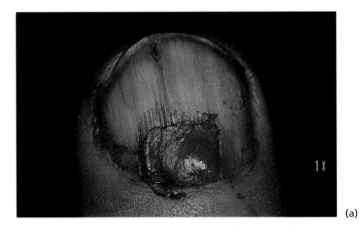

(a)

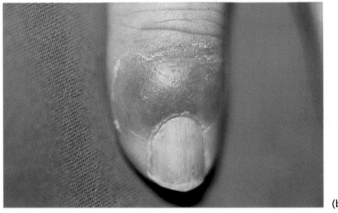

(b)

**Fig. 6.58** (a) (AIDS—Kaposi sarcoma, subungual location. (b) AIDS—Kaposi's sarcoma in periungual location. (Courtesy of S. Goettmann-Bonvalot, France.)

Diffuse nail pigmentation as well as longitudinal or transverse hyperpigmented bands are frequently seen in HIV-positive patients receiving AZT (zidovudine). Multiple longitudinal melanonychia as well as hyperpigmented macules on the palms, soles and mucous membranes unrelated to AZT treatment have also been described in AIDS (Granel *et al.* 1997). The serum levels of $\alpha$-MSH were significantly increased in one patient (Fisher & Warner 1987; Gallais *et al.* 1992). Mild bluish pigmentation of fingernails and toenails has also been described in two black patients with HIV infection (Panwalker 1987; Chandrasekar 1989; Glaser & Remlinger 1996).

Kaposi's sarcoma can involve the nail area (Friedman-Kien & Saltzam 1989; Dompmartin *et al.* 1990) (Fig. 6.58a). A periungual Kaposi's sarcoma resembling a chronic paronychia has been reported in a patient with AIDS (Fig. 6.58b) (Fischer & Warner 1987). Subungual squamous cell carcinoma has been frequently reported in AIDS, often in association with HPV 16 infection (Daniel 1993; Tosti *et al.* 1994).

## References

Abajo, P., Porras-Luque, J.L., Buezo, G.F. *et al.* (1998) Red finger syndrome associated with necrotizing vasculitis in an HIV infected patient with hepatitis B. *British Journal of Dermatology* **139**, 154–155.

Aricõ, M., Nato, G., La Rocca, E. *et al.* (1992) Localised Crusted Scabies in the acquired immunodeficiency syndrome. *Clinical and Experimental Dermatology* **17**, 339–341.

Baden, L.A., Bigby, M. & Kwan, T. (1991) Persistent necrotic digits in a patient with the acquired immunodeficiency syndrome. *Archives of Dermatology* **127**, 113–114.

Baran, R., Tosti, A. & Piraccini, B.M. (1997) Uncommun clinical patterns of *Fusarium* nail infection: report of three cases. *British Journal of Dermatology* **136**, 424–427.

Battegay, M. & Itin, P.H. (1996) Red fingers syndrome in HIV patients. *Lancet* **348**, 763.

Belinchon, I. & Ramos, J.M. (1994) Lesion en la uña del dedo pulgar de un paciente con sida. *Enf Inf Microbiol Clin* **12**, 167–168.

Belzunegui, J., Gonzales, C. & Figueroa, M. (1997) Clubbing in patients with human immunodeficiency virus infections. *British Journal of Rheumatology* **36**, 142–143.

Berger, T.G., Dhar, A. & McCalmont, T.H. (1994) Neutrophilic dermatoses in HIV infection. *Journal of the American Academy of Dermatology* **31**, 1045–1047.

Boonen, A., Schrey, G. & Van der Linden, S. (1996) Clubbing in human immunodeficiency virus infection. *British Journal of Rheumatology* **35**, 292–294.

Bonomo, R.A., Korman, N., Nagashima-Whalen, L. *et al.* (1997) Pityriasis rubra pilaris: an unusual cutaneous complication of AIDS. *American Journal of Medical Science* **314**, 118–121.

Buchner, S.A., Itin, P., Rufli, T. *et al.* (1989) Disseminated lichenoid papular dermatosis with nail changes in acquired immunodeficiency syndrome: clinical, histological and immunohistochemical considerations. *Dermatologica* **179**, 99–101.

Chandrasekar, P.H. (1989) Nail discoloration and human immunodeficiency virus infection. *American Journal of Medicine* **86**, 506–507.

Chernosky, M.E. & Finley, V.K. (1985) Yellow nail syndrome in patients with acquired immunodeficiency disease. *Journal of the American Academy of Dermatology* **13**, 731–736.

Cockerell, C.J. (1990) Cutaneous manifestations of HIV infection other than Kaposi's sarcoma: clinical and histologic aspects. *Journal of the American Academy of Dermatology* **22**, 1260–1269.

Cohen, S.J. & Dicken, C.H. (1991) Generalized lichen spinulosus in a HIV-positive man. *Journal of the American Academy of Dermatology* **25**, 116–118.

Cribier, B., Leiva Mena, M., Rey, D. *et al.* (1998) Nail changes in patients infected with HIV. *Archives of Dermatology* **134**, 1216–1220.

Daniel, C.R. (1992) Nail disease in patients with HIV infection. In: *Dermatology Progress and Perspectives, 1809 World Congress* (eds W.H.C. Burgdary & S.I. Katz), pp. 382–385. Parthenon Publishing Group, New York.

Daniel, C.R., Norton, L.A. & Scher, R.K. (1992) The spectrum of nail diseases in patients with HIV infection. *Journal of the American Academy of Dermatology* **27**, 93–97.

Dompmartin, D., Dompmartin, A., Deluol, A.M. *et al.* (1990) Onychomycosis and AIDS. Clinical and laboratory findings in 62 patients. *International Journal of Dermatology* **29**, 337–339.

Enelow, R.S., Hussein, M., Grant, K. *et al.* (1992) Vasculitis with eosinophilia and digital gangrene in a patient with acquired immunodeficiency syndrome. *Journal of Rheumatology* **19**, 1813–1816.

Fernandez-Diaz, M.L., Herranz, P., de Lucas, R. *et al.* (1995) Atypical herpes zoster in a patient with AIDS. *Journal of the European Academy of Dermatology and Venereology* **5**, 62–66.

Fisher, B.K. & Warner, L.C. (1987) Cutaneous manifestations of the acquired immunodeficiency syndrome. *International Journal of Dermatology* **276**, 615–630.

Friedman-Kien, A.E. & Saltzman, B.R. (1990) Clinical manifestations of classical, endemic African and epidemic AIDS-associated Kaposi's sarcoma. *Journal of the American Academy of Dermatology* **22**, 1237–1250.

Gaddoni, G., Selvi, M., Resta, F. *et al.* (1994) Necrotic finger in AIDS patients. *Giornale Italiano di Dermatologia e Venereologia* **129**, 501–504.

Gallais, V., Lacour, J.P., Perrin, C. *et al.* (1992) Acral hyperpigmented macules and longitudinal melanonychia in AIDS. *British Journal of Dermatology* **126**, 387–391.

Glaser, D.A. & Remlinger, K. (1996) Blue nails and acquired immunodeficiency syndrome: not always associated with azidothymidine use. *Cutis* **57**, 243–244.

Graham, S.M., Dley, H.M. & Ngwira, B. (1997) Finger clubbing and HIV in Malawian children. *Lancet* **349**, 31.

Granel, F., Truchetet, F. & Grandidier, M. (1997) Pigmentation diffuse (unguéale, buccale, cutanée) associée à une infection par le virus de l'immunodéficience humaine (VIH). *Annales de Dermatologie et de Vénéréologie* **124**, 460–462.

Harindra, V., Sivapalan, S. & Basu Roy, R. (1993) Increased hair and nail growth in patients with AIDS. *British Journal of Clinical Practice* **4**, 215–216.

Inserra, D.V. & Bickley, L.K. (1990) Crusted scabies in acquired immunodeficiency syndrome. *International Journal of Dermatology* **29**, 287–289.

Jucowics, P., Ramon, M.E., Don, P.C. *et al.* (1989) Norwegian scabies in an infant with acquired immunodeficiency syndrome. *Archives of Dermatology* **125**, 1670–1671.

Kaplan, M.H., Sadick, N., McNutt, S. *et al.* (1987) Dermatologic findings and manifestations of acquired immunodeficiency syndrome. *Journal of the American Academy of Dermatology* **16**, 485–506.

Katz, B.Z. (1997) Finger clubbing as a sign of HIV infection in children. *Lancet* **349**, 575.

Miralles, E.S., Nuñez, M., De Las Heras, M.E. *et al.* (1995) Pityriasis rubra pilaris and human immunodeficiency virus infection. *British Journal of Dermatology* **133**, 990–993.

Morfeld-Manson, L., Julander, I. & Nillson, B. (1989) Dermatitis of the face, yellow toe nail changes, hairy leukoplakia and oral candidiasis are clinical indicators of progression to AIDS opportunistic infection in patients with HIV infection. *Scandinavian Journal of Infectious Diseases* **21**, 497–505.

Noppakun, N. & Head, E. (1986) Proximal white subungual onychomycosis in a patient with acquired immune deficiency syndrome. *International Journal of Dermatology* **25**, 586–587.

Panwalker, A. (1987) Nail pigmentation in the acquired immunodeficiency syndrome (AIDS). *Annals of Internal Medicine* **107**, 943–944.

Pechère, M., Krischer, J., Rosay, A. *et al.* (1996) Red fingers in patients with HIV and hepatitis C infection. *Lancet* **348**, 196–197.

Prose, N.S. (1990) HIV infection in children *Journal of the American Academy of Dermatology* **22**, 1223–1231.

Prose, N.S., Abson, K.G. & Scher, R.K. (1992) Disorders of the nails and hair associated with human immunodeficiency virus infection. *International Journal of Dermatology* **31**, 453–457.

Raiteri, R., Sinico, A., Gioanirini, P. *et al.* (1993) Job's-like-syndrome in HIV-1 infection. *European Journal of Dermatology* **3**, 355–363.

Robayna, M.G., Herranz, P. & Rubio, F.A. (1997) Destructive herpetic whitlow in AIDS: report of cases. *British Journal of Dermatology* **137**, 812–815.

Ruiz-Avila, P., Tercedor, J., Fuentes, E. *et al.* (1995) Painful periungual teleangiectasias in a patient with acquired immunodeficiency syndrome. *International Journal of Dermatology* **34**, 199–200.

Scott, G.B., Buck, B.E., Laterman, J.G. *et al.* (1984) Acquired immunodeficiency syndrome in infants. *New England Journal of Medicine* **310**, 76–81.

Smyth, A., Roberts, N., Parker, S. *et al.* (1997) Finger clubbing as a sign of HIV infection in children. *Lancet* **249**, 575.

Torssander, J., Karlsson, A., Morfeld-Manson, L. *et al.* (1988) Dermatophytosis and HIV infection. *Acta Dermato-Venereologica* **68**, 53–56.

Tosti, A., La Placa, M., Fanti, P.A. *et al.* (1994) Human papillomavirus type 16-associated periungual squamous cell carcinoma in a patient with acquired immunodeficiency syndrome. *Acta Dermato-Venereologica* **74**, 478–479.

Tosti, A., Piraccini, B.M., Lorenzi, S. *et al.* (1998) Candida onychomycosis in HIV infection. *European Journal of Dermatology* **8**, 173–174.

Valenzano, L., Giacalone, B., Grillo, L.R. *et al.* (1988) Compromissione ungueale in corso di AIDS. *Giornale Italiano di Dermatologia e Venereologia* **123**, 527–528.

Verneuil, L., Dompmartin, A., Duhamel, C. *et al.* (1995) Panaris cryptococcique chez un malade VIH positif. *Annales de Dermatologie et de Vénéréologie* **122**, 688–691.

Weismann, K., Knudsen, E.A. & Pedersen, C. (1988) White nails in AIDS/ARC due to *Trichophyton rubrum* infection. *Clinical and Experimental Dermatology* **13**, 24–25.

Weitzul, S. & Duvic, M. (1997) HIV-related psoriasis and Reiter's syndrome. *Seminars in Cutaneous Surgery* **16**, 213–218.

## Low interleukin 2 level

Interleukin 2 secretion by phytohaemagglutinin-stimulated mononuclear leucocytes was deficient in a 21-year-old woman with a lifelong history of widespread friable vascular nodules and plaques resembling chronic mucocutaneous candidiasis (Helm *et al.* 1993). Thickening and induration of the proximal and lateral nail folds suggested chronic paronychia and cultures revealed *Candida*.

## Reference

Helm, T.N., Calabrese, L.H., Longworth, D.L. *et al.* (1993) Vascular nodules and plaques resembling chronic mucocutaneous candidiasis in a patient with a low interlukin 2 level. *Journal of the American Academy of Dermatology* **29**, 473–477.

## Infectious diseases (see also Chapters 4 & 7)

Acute febrile illness and some systemic diseases may produce transverse linear grooves (Beau's lines) with slightly elevated proximal ridging resulting from matrix damage. All nails of the fingers and toes are usually involved but this change may occasionally be restricted to the thumbs and great toes. In severe cases the nail becomes detached but usually the grooves are superficial. The lines appear from under the cuticle at about 1 month after the acute illness and grow forward as the nail grows, thereby giving a way of assessing the date of the illness. Transverse leuconychia may have the same significance as Beau's lines.

## Malaria

Changes in nail colour occur during acute episodes. Immediately prior to the fever, the nails become pale grey and this is maintained throughout the pyrexia, nail bed pallor was 85% sensitive in identifying parasitaemic children and 41% specific (Redd *et al.* 1996). Subungual haemorrhages, striate leuconychia and koilonychia are described in quartan malaria, as are multiple transverse, dark brown lines and furrows. Beau's lines may occur following infection with *Plasmodium vivax* malaria (Glew & Howard 1973).

## References

Glew, R.H. & Howard, W.A. (1973) Transverse furrows of the nails associated with *Plasmodium vivax* malaria. *Johns Hopkins Medical Journal* **132**, 61–64.

Redd, S.C., Kazembe, P.N., Luby, S.P. *et al.* (1996) Clinical algorithm for treatment of *Plasmodium falciparum* malaria in children. *Lancet* **347**, 223–227.

## Kawasaki disease (mucocutaneous lymph node syndrome) (Fig. 6.59)

Kawasaki disease mainly affects children from 6 months to 10 years of age and rarely adults (Butler *et al.* 1987; Porneuf *et al.* 1996). Beau's lines develop in the nail plate 1 or 2 months after onset of the illness in 94% of patients (Bures 1984; Porneuf *et al.* 1996), and complete shedding of the nails and telogen effluvium can be seen (Traedwell 1987). Transient apparent leuconychia has been reported by Iosub and Gromish (1984) in three patients with desquamation of the skin of most fingernails and toenails. It characteristically appeared 14 days after the onset of symptoms at the skin–nail junctions. This sign is the major feature used to distinguish mucocutaneous lymph node Syndrome (MCLS) from other similar entities (Kawasaki *et al.* 1974). Late changes include fissuring of the nail beds and peeling of fingernails (Levin & Dillon 1992). Ischaemic necrosis of the extremities is a rare complication (Ames *et al.* 1985). Acquired pincer nail deformity in an infant with Kawasaki's disease affected all the digits of her hand and to a milder extent her toes. The deformities slowly resolved over the ensuing 2 months (Vanderhooft & Vanderhooft 1999).

## References

Ames, E.L., Jones, J.S., Van Dommelen, B. *et al.* (1985) Bilateral hand necrosis in Kawasaki syndrome. *Journal of Hand Surgery* **10A**, 391–395.

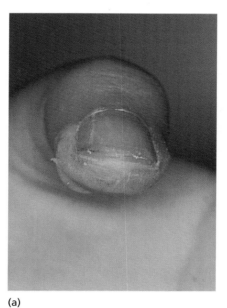

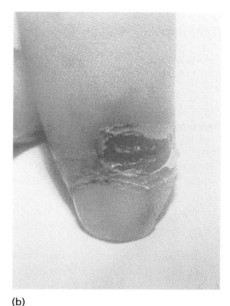

**Fig. 6.59** (a) Kawasaki syndrome, 14 days.
(b) Cutaneous diphtheria.

(a)

(b)

Bures, F.A. (1981) Beau's lines in mucocutaneous lymph node syndrome. *American Journal of Disease in Childhood* **135**, 383.

Butler, D.F., Hough, D.R., Friedman, S.J. *et al.* (1987) Adult Kawasaki syndrome. *Archives of Dermatology* **123**, 1356–1361.

Iosub, S. & Gromish, D.S. (1984) Leukonychia partialis in Kawasaki disease. *Journal of Infectious Diseases* **150**, 617–618.

Kawasaki, T., Kosaki, F. & Okawa, S. (1974) A new infantile acute febrile mucocutaneous lymph node syndrome prevailing in Japan. *Paediatrics* **54**, 271–276.

Levin, M. & Dillon, M.J. (1992) Kawasaki disease. In: *Recent Advances in Dermatology* (eds R. Champion & R.J. Pye). Churchill Livingstone, Edinburgh.

Porneuf, M.D., Sotto, A., Barbuat, C. *et al.* (1996) Kawasaki syndrome in an adult AIDS patient. *International Journal of Dermatology* **35**, 292–294.

Treadwell, P.A. (1987) Kawasaki disease. In: *Advances in Dermatology*, Vol. 2 (eds S.P. Callen, H.V. Dahl, L.E. Golitz *et al.*), pp. 112–116. Year Book Medical Publisher, Chicago.

Vanderhooft, S.L. & Vanderhooft, J.E. (1999) Pincer nail deformity after Kawasaki's disease. *Journal of the American Academy of Dermatology* **41**, 341–342.

## Hand, foot and mouth disease

Onychomadesis involving several or all the nails may follow hand, foot and mouth disease. Nail shedding, which may be associated with palmoplantar desquamation, is due to nail matrix injury during the viral eruption (Bernier *et al.* 1998).

## Reference

Bernier, V., Labrèze, C. & Taïeb, A. (1998) Onychomadesis and 'Hand, foot and mouth' disease. *Annales de Dermatologie et de Vénéréologie* **125** (Suppl. 1), 178.

## Cutaneous diphtheria

Cutaneous diphtheria has become a rare disease following widespread immunization, however cases of cutaneous diphtheria have recently been reported in travellers to endemic areas (Antos *et al.* 1992) and in a patient with AIDS (Halioua *et al.* 1992).

The disease typically begins as a pustule, and then becomes a slightly depressed round-shaped ulceration varying in size from 0.5 cm to a few centimetres in diameter, with inflammatory edges covered with a false membrane which bleeds after being scraped off. The natural anaesthetic nature of the lesion is emphasized by most of authors. Within 1–3 weeks, the false membrane becomes a blackish scab, which rapidly falls off giving way to an atrophic scar. Cutaneous diphtheria is usually found on the lower and upper limbs. Differential diagnosis includes impetigo, echthyma and eczema (Livingood *et al.* 1946; Bixby 1948).

Thus, cutaneous diphtheria most often appears on preexisting dermatological lesions, such as traumatic wounds, burns, insect bites and infection.

## References

Antos, H., Mollison, L.C., Richards, M.J. *et al.* (1992) Diphtheria: another risk of travel. *Journal of Infection* **25**, 307–310.

Bixby, E.W. (1948) Cutaneous diphtheria, *Archives de Dermatology et de Syphiligraphie* **58**, 381–384.

Halioua, B., Patey, O., Casciani, D. *et al.* (1992) Diphtérie cutanée chez un patient infecté par le virus de l'immunodeficience humaine (VIH). *Annales de Dermatologie et de Vénéréologie* **119**, 874–877.

Livingood, C.S., Perry, D.J. & Forrester, J.S. (1946) Cutaneous diphtheria: a report of 140 cases. *Journal of Investigative Dermatology* **7**, 341–364.

## Haematological disorders

Brittle nails and Terry's nails are the most common nail abnormalities in patients with blood disorders (Jemec *et al.* 1995).

### Reference

Jemec, G.B.E., Kollerup, G., Jensen, L.B. *et al.* (1995) Nail abnormalities in nondermatologic patients: prevalence and possible role as diagnostic aids. *Journal of the American Academy of Dermatology* **32**, 977–981.

### Polycythaemia

Red nail beds are seen in polycythaemia. Ischaemic acral necrosis and/or ulcers can be caused by peripheral arterial occlusions (Fagrell & Mellstedt 1978). A lamellar dystrophy of the nails has been reported in two patients affected by polycythaemia rubra vera. In one of them, improvement of the dystrophy was noticed after treatment of polycythaemia (Graham-Brown & Holmes 1980). Erythromelalgia can occur in association with polycythaemia. Koilonychia has been reported by De Nicola *et al.* (1974).

### References

De Nicola, P., Morsinai, M. & Zavagli, G. (1974) *Nail Diseases in Internal Medicine*, p. 79. Charles C. Thomas, Springfield, IL.

Fagrell, B. & Mellstedt, H. (1978) Polcythaemia vera as a cause of ischemic digital necrosis. *Acta Chir Scandinavica* **144**, 129–132.

Graham-Brown, R.A.C. & Holmes, R. (1980) Polycythaemia rubra vera with lamellar dystrophy of the nails: a report of two cases. *Clinical and Experimental Dermatology* **5**, 209–212.

### Essential thrombocythaemia

Cutaneous manifestations of essential thrombocythaemia include erythromelalgia, livedo reticularis and microvascular occlusive events that may lead to gangrene of toes and fingers (Itin & Winkelmann 1991).

Painful ulceronecrotic lesions are especially observed on the distal parts of limbs, in particular the toes (Velasco *et al.* 1991). Acrocyanosis and Raynaud's phenomenon have also been reported (Itin & Winkelmann 1991).

### References

Itin, P.H. & Winkelmann, R.K. (1991) Cutaneous manifestations in patients with essential thrombocythaemia, *Journal of the American Academy of Dermatology* **24**, 59–63.

Velasco, J.A., Santos, J.C., Bravo, J. *et al.* (1991) Ulceronecrotic lesions in a patient with essential thrombocythaemia. *Clinical and Experimental Dermatology* **16**; 53–54.

## Haemoglobinopathies

Symmetrical peripheral gangrene can be observed in patients with sickle cell anaemia. Phalangeal osteomyelitis has been also described (Haltalin & Nelson 1965). Mee's lines have been reported by Hudson and Dennis (1966). Cyanosis of the lunulae is a typical sign of nigraemia, a rare hereditary disease that is associated with the presence of an abnormal haemoglobin (haemoglobin M) (Tamura 1964).

### References

Haltalin, K.C. & Nelson, J.D. (1965) Hand-foot syndrome due to streptococcal infections. *American Journal of Diseases of Children* **109**, 156–159.

Hudson, J.B. & Dennis, A.J. (1966) Transverse white lines in the fingernails after acute and chronic renal failure. *Archives of Internal Medicine* **117**, 276–279.

Tamura, A. (1964) Nigremia. *Japanese Journal of Human Genetics* **9**, 183–192.

### Anaemias

Pallor of the nail bed and reduction or absence of the lunula are frequently observed in anaemias with decrease of the linear nail growth rate (De Nicola *et al.* 1974). Splinter haemorrhages can occur. Nail brittleness, ridging and koilonychia are commonly reported in hypochromic anaemia (see also page 263). Reversible shedding of fingernails and toenails has been described in one patient (Handfield-Jones & Kennedy 1988). Bluish-black discoloration of fingernails and toenails rarely appears in patients with megaloblastic anaemia (Carmel 1985) (page 262). Transverse leuconychia of fingernails and toenails has been reported in a patient with immunohaemolytic anaemia associated with warm-reacting antibodies (Marino 1990). Nail fold capillary abnormalities with enlarged and ramified capillaries with a 'bushy' aspect have been described in patients with sickle cell anaemia (Bachir *et al.* 1993).

### References

Bachir, D., Maurel, A., Portos, J.L. *et al.* (1993) Comparative evaluation of laser Doppler flux metering, bulbar conjunctival angioscopy, and nail fold capillaroscopy in sickle cell disease. *Microvessels Research* **45**, 20–32.

Carmel, R. (1985) Hair and fingernail changes in acquired and congenital pernicious anaemia. *Archives of Internal Medicine* **145**, 484–485.

De Nicola, P., Morsiani, M. & Zavagli, G. (1974) *Nail Diseases in Internal medicine*, pp. 79–80. Charles C. Thomas, Springfield, IL.

Handfield-Jones, S.E. & Kennedy, C.T.C. (1988) Nail dystrophy associated with iron deficiency anaemia. *Clinical and Experimental Dermatology* **13**, 54.

Marino, M.T. (1990) Mees' lines. *Archives of Dermatology* **126**, 827–828.

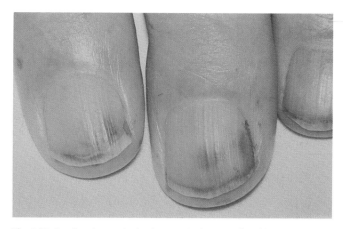

**Fig. 6.60** Hereditary haemorrhagic telangiectasia. (Courtesy of L. Juhlin, Uppsala, Sweden.)

## Hereditary haemorrhagic telangiectasia (Osler syndrome) (Fig. 6.60)

Subungual telangiectasia and haemorrhages occur in patients with Osler syndrome (De Nicola 1974). Capillaroscopy of the proximal nail fold can reveal the presence of giant capillaries (Maire *et al*. 1986).

### References

De Nicola, P., Morsiani, M. & Zavagli, G. (1974) *Nail Diseases in Internal Medicine*, pp. 79–80. Charles C. Thomas, Springfield IL.

Maire, R., Schnewlin, G. & Bollinger, A. (1986) Videomikroskopische Untersuchungen von Teleangiektasien bei Morbus Osler und Sklerodermie. *Schweiz Med Wochenschr* **116**, 335–338.

## Leukaemias

See page 298.

## Plasmocytoma

See page 299.

## Lymphoma

See page 300.

## Hodgkin's disease

See page 302.

## Gamma heavy chain disease

This condition, which mainly occurs in association with lymphoproliferative and autoimmune disorders, is characterized by the presence in serum and urine of a structurally abnormal heavy chain devoid of light chains. Cutaneous lesions are the most frequent extrahaematopoietic manifestations of the disease. A patient with gamma heavy chain disease developed cutaneous nodules, livedo reticularis and digital necrosis caused by necrotizing vasculitis (Lassoned *et al*. 1990).

### Reference

Lassoned, K., Picard, C., Danon, F. *et al*. (1990) Cutaneous manifestations associated with gamma heavy chain disease. *Journal of the American Academy of Dermatology* **23**, 988–991.

## Cryoglobulinaemia (Fig. 6.61)

Subungual haemorrhage of all the digits with decrease of linear nail growth was seen in a patient with purpura (Leyh 1967).

Livedo reticularis, Raynaud's phenomenon and painful digital necrosis can be observed in cryoglobulinaemia, particu-

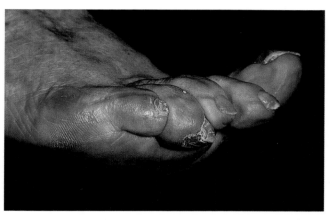

(a)

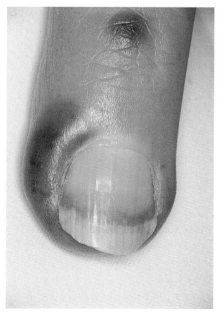

(b)

**Fig. 6.61** (a) Cryoglobulinaemia. (b) Cryoglobulinaemia—bullous purpura.

larly in patients with type 1 or type 2 cryoglobulinaemia (Garceau *et al.* 1990).

Rallis *et al.* (1995) reported a patient whose fingers and toes were cold to the touch and demonstrated decreased capillary refill. This was associated with purplish discoloration of the distal third of all fingertips, becoming more intense in the proximal nail beds. Essential mixed cryoglobulinaemia was found.

### References

Garceau, S., Gilbert, M., Marceau, D. *et al.* (1990) A propos d'un cas de nécrose d'un doigt. *Review of European Dermatology MTS* 2, 590–593.

Leyh, F. (1967) Purpura cryoglobunaemia. In: *XIII Congressus Internationalis Dermatologiae, Münich*, pp. 90–94.

Rallis, T.M., Kadunce, D.P., Gerwels, J.W. *et al.* (1995) Cryoglobulineamia. *Archives of Dermatology* 131, 341.

### Afibrinogenaemia

Complete congenital absence of fibrinogen led to dark blue discoloration of the toes followed by ischaemic necrosis with ulceration and life-threatening haemorrhage after skin biopsy (Rupec *et al.* 1996).

### Reference

Rupec, R.A., Kind, P. & Ruzicka, T. (1996) Cutaneous manifestations of congenital afibrinogenaemia. *British Journal of Dermatology* 134, 548–550.

### Complement type 2 deficiency

Systemic lupus erythematosus may complicate complement type 2 deficiency with destructive nail dystrophy affecting all digits; fresh frozen plasma produced a successful treatment (Hudson-Peacock *et al.* 1997).

### Reference

Hudson-Peacock, M.J., Joseph, S.A., Cox, J. *et al.* (1997). Complement type 2 deficiency. *British Journal of Dermatology* 136, 388–392.

### Extrinsic clotting system disturbance

Ischaemic venous thrombosis (previously described as phlegmasia coerulea dolens) leading to necrosis of four toes was due to a serum protein with inhibitory properties in the extrinsic coagulation system *in vitro*. Systemic steroids led to rapid clinical resolution paralleled by normalization of the prothrombin time and disappearance of the inhibitor (Duschet *et al.* 1993).

### Reference

Duschet, P., Seifert, W., Halb-Meyer, W.M. *et al.* (1993) Ischemic venous thrombosis caused by a distinct disturbance of the extrinsic clotting system. *Journal of the American Academy of Dermatology* 28, 831–835.

## Neoplastic disorders

### Langerhans' cell histiocytosis (Fig. 6.62)

Nail involvement in histiocytosis X (Langerhans' cell histiocytosis) is rare (Esterly *et al.* 1985) and it has been considered to represent an unfavourable prognostic sign (Timpatanapong *et al.* 1984; Holzberg *et al.* 1985). However, other reported cases have remitted spontaneously (Ellis 1985) or responded to treatment with vinblastine and steroids or etoposide (de Berker *et al.* 1994) or cotrimazole every 12 h (Jain *et al.* 2000).

Nail involvement has been reported both in patients with Letterer–Siwe disease and in those with Hand–Schueller–Christian disease, but not in patients with eosinophilic granuloma of bone. Nail changes can be observed in fingernails and toenails.

Erythema and swelling of periungual tissues resembling chronic paronychia along with subungual hyperkeratosis and onycholysis are the most common findings. Small pustules of the nail bed and subungual haemorrhages or purpuric macules can occur (Harper & Staughton 1983). Paronychia with subungual purpura is quite specific for histiocytosis X. Nail pitting, longitudinal grooving, distal splitting as well as nail plate thickening, elkonyxis and onychomadesis have also been reported (de Berker *et al.* 1994). Specific infiltration by CD1+ histiocyte-like cells produced persistent and progressive destruction of the thumbnail plates in a patient with Hand–Schuller–Christian disease (Alsina *et al.* 1991). The fact that nail involvement by Langerhans' cells is usually multiple suggests that the abnormal cells 'home' to these tissues (Munro & Morton 1998).

Involvement of the nails is histologically characterized by a dermal infiltrate of atypical histiocytes with reniform nuclei and usually abundant cytoplasm. These cells migrate into the epidermis causing slight spongiosis and intraepithelial cell accumulations. There is usually dermal oedema and admixture of lymphocytes and a variable number of eosinophils. The atypical histiocytes express the CD1– antigen (OKT6), protein S-100 and are stained with peanut agglutinin. Electron microscopy usually reveals abundant Langerhans' cells (Birbeck) granules which sometimes are in continuity with the cell membrane.

Focal collections of atypical histiocytes with large hyperchromatic and pleomorphic nuclei were detected in the proximal nail fold, matrix and nail bed of a 21-month-old child affected by Letterer–Siwe disease. Electron microscopy and S-100 protein staining confirmed that the infiltration was formed by Langerhans' cells (Holzberg *et al.* 1985).

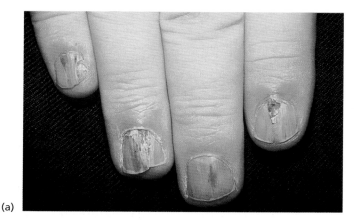

(a)

(b)

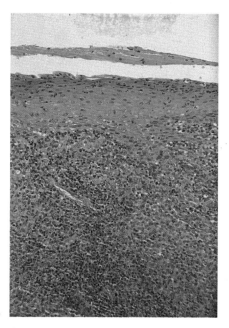

(c)

**Fig. 6.62** Langerhans' cells histiocytosis. (a) Childhood. (b) Adult. (c) Histology. (Courtesy of J.M. Mascaro.)

Nail changes occasionally respond to antineoplastic therapy but usually recur when the disease progresses (Timpatanapong *et al.* 1984). A child is reported who, despite severe nail involvement, showed spontaneous remission of her disease (Ellis 1985).

### References

Alsina, M.M., Zamora, E., Ferrando, J. *et al.* (1991) Nail changes in histiocytosis-X. *Archives of Dermatology* **127**, 1741.

de Berker, D., Lever, L.R. & Windebank, K. (1994) Nail features in Langerhans' cell Histiocytosis. *British Journal of Dermatology* **130**, 523–527.

Ellis, J.P. (1985) Histiocytosis-X—unusual presentation with nail involvement. *Journal of the Royal Society of Medicine* **78** (Suppl. 11), 3–5.

Esterly, N.B., Maurer, H.S. & Gonzalez-Crussi, F. (1985) Histiocytosis-X: a seven-year experience at a children's hospital. *Journal of the American Academy of Dermatology* **13**, 481–496.

Harper, J.I. & Staughton, R. (1983) Letter to the editor. *Cutis* **31**, 493–494.

Holzberg, M., Wade, T.R., Buchanan, I.D. *et al.* (1985) Nail pathology in histiocytosis-X. *Journal of the American Academy of Dermatology* **13**, 522–523.

Jain, S., Seghal, V.N. & Bajaj, P. (2000) Nail changes in Langerhans' cell histiocytosis. *Journal of the European Academy of Dermatology and Venereology* **14**, 212–215.

Munro, C.S. & Morton, R. (1998) Nail and scalp lesions in a man with diabetes insipidus Langerhans' cell histiocytosis. *Archives of Dermatology* **134**, 1477–1478, 1480–1481.

Timpatanapong, P., Hathirat, P. & Isarangkura, P. (1984) Nail involvement in histiocytosis-X. A 12-year retrospective study. *Archives of Dermatology* **120**, 1052–1056.

## Juvenile xanthogranuloma

Juvenile xanthogranuloma can rarely affect the fingers (Sonoda *et al.* 1985; Yamashita *et al.* 1990). A solitary xanthogranuloma of the 2nd left toenail has been reported in an 18-month-old boy. The nail appearance resembled onychogryphosis (Frumkin *et al.* 1987). We have observed a case in a 30-month-old white boy, presenting in the distal region of his right index finger a 0.5-cm nodule with an ill-defined border lifting up the nail plate, partially destroyed by the tumour. This was skin coloured and not tender under pressure (Chang *et al.* 1996) (Fig. 6.63).

### References

Chang, P., Baran, R., Villanueva, C. *et al.* (1996) Juvenile xanthogranuloma beneath a fingernail. *Cutis* **58**, 173–174.

Frumkin, A., Roytman, M. & Johnson, S.F. (1987) Juvenile xanthogranuloma underneath a toenail. *Cutis* **40**, 244–245.

Sonoda, T., Hashimoto, H. & Enjoji, M. (1985) Juvenile xanthogranuloma. Clinico-pathologic analysis and immunohistochemical study of 57 patients. *Cancer* **56**, 2280–2286.

Yamashita, J.T., Rotta, O., Michalany, N.S. *et al.* (1990) Xanthogranulome juvénile du majeur chez un nourrisson. *Annales de Dermatologie et de Vénéréologie* **117**, 295–296.

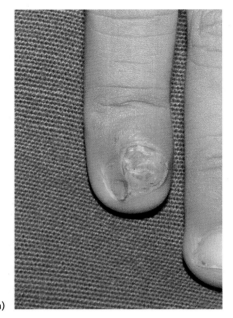

(a)

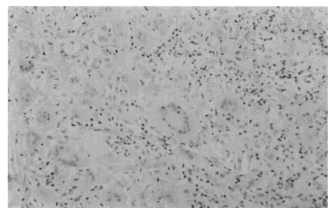

(b)

**Fig. 6.63** (a) Juvenile xanthogranuloma. (b) Histology. (Courtesy of P. Chang de Chang, Guatemala.)

## Nail changes and paraneoplastic disorders

Nail abnormalities can occur in association with numerous paraneoplastic syndromes such as glucagonoma syndrome, malignant acanthosis nigricans, Bazex syndrome, pachydermoperiostosis, palmoplantar keratoderma and dermatomyositis. Finger clubbing and pachydermoperiostosis are well-known signs of primary or metastatic intrathoracic neoplasms.

Yellow nail syndrome and shell nail syndrome have been described in patients with bronchial tumours. Koilonychia due to hypochromic anaemia can be a sign of haemorrhagic gastrointestinal neoplasms. Terry's nails have been described in pancreatic carcinoma with hepatic metastases. White banding of the nails has been observed in patients with carcinoid tumours.

In paraneoplastic pemphigus (Izaki *et al.* 1996), paronychia and onychomadesis due to proximal nail fold involvement

have been reported. In childhood paraneoplastic pemphigus associated with Castleman's tumour (Lemon *et al.* 1997), the nail folds were swollen and violaceous and the nails had been shed. The spectrum of paraneoplastic pemphigus includes cases that may present clinically and histologically as a lichen-plano-pemphigoides-like eruption (Jansen *et al.* 1995).

## References

Izaki, S., Yoshizava, Y., Hashimoto, T. *et al.* (1996) Paraneoplastic pemphigus: report of a case. *Journal of Dermatology* **23**, 397–404.

Jansen, T., Plewig, G. & Anhalt, G.J. (1995) Paraneoplastic pemphigus with clinical features of erosive lichen planus associated with Castleman's tumor. *Dermatology* **190**, 245–250.

Lemon, M.A., Weston, W.L. & Huff, J.C. (1997) Childhood paraneoplastic pemphigus associated with Castleman's tumour. *British Journal of Dermatology* **136**, 115–117.

## Acrokeratosis paraneoplastica of Bazex and Dupré
(Fig. 6.64)

Acrokeratosis paraneoplastica has now been observed in numerous countries: USA (Witkowski & Parish 1982; Pecora *et al.* 1983); Canada (Richard & Giroux 1987; Mounsey & Brown 1992); Germany (Van Hintzenstern *et al.* 1990); UK (Wishart 1986; Douglas *et al.* 1991); Italy (Scarpa *et al.* 1971); and Denmark (Jacobsen *et al.* 1984). Curiously, most of the patients are French. About 65 cases, mostly in white men over 40, two cases in Afrocaribbeans (Boudoulas & Camisa 1986) and only four cases in women (Scarpa *et al.* 1971; Grimwood & Le Ran 1987; Martin 1989 *et al.* Scarpa 1971; O'Brien 1995) have been reported.

Acrokeratosis paraneoplastica (Bazex *et al.* 1965, 1973) occurs in association with malignant epitheliomas of the upper respiratory or digestive tracts. It has been reported in malignancy of the pharyngolaryngeal area-pyriform fossa, tonsillar area, epiglottis, hard and soft palate, vocal cords, tongue, lower lip, oesophagus and the upper third of the lungs and pancreas (Martin *et al.* 1995); exceptionally in liver, prostate, stomach, thymus, uterus and vulva (Bolognia *et al.* 1991). It also occurs with metastases to the cervical and upper mediastinal lymph nodes. This 'paraneoplasia' may precede the signs of the associated malignancy (several months), disappear when the tumour is removed or reappear with its recurrence. However, the nail involvement does not always benefit from total recovery, in contrast to the other lesions (Cahuzac *et al.* 1981). The lesions are erythematous, violaceous, keratotic and have ill-defined borders. They are symmetrically distributed, affecting hands, feet, ears and occasionally the nose. The toenails suffer more severely than the fingernails. Roughened, irregular, keratotic, fissured and warty excrescences are found equally on the terminal phalanges of both fingers and toes. An association with lichen planus pigmentosus has been reported (Sassolas *et al.* 1994).

The nails are invariably involved and are typically the earliest manifestation of the disease (Baran 1977). In mild forms, the

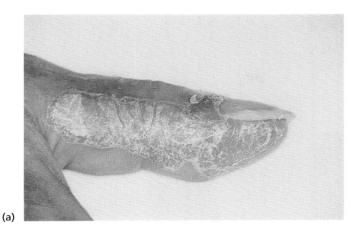

(a)

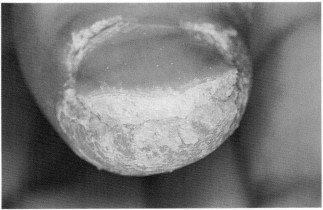

(b)

**Fig. 6.64** (a,b) Acrokeratosis paraneoplastica.

nail involvement is discrete; the affected nails are thin, soft and may become fragile and crumble. In more established disease, the nails are flaky, irregular, whitened and the free edge is raised by subungual hyperkeratosis. In severe forms, the lesions resemble advanced psoriatic nail dystrophy and may progress to complete loss of the diseased nails. The nail bed is eventually replaced by a smooth epidermis to which the irregular horny vestiges of the nail adhere. The periungual skin shows an erythemato-squamous eruption, predominantly on the dorsum of the terminal phalanges, and there may be associated chronic paronychia with occasional, acute suppurative exacerbations (Bureau *et al.* 1971). Skin and nail hyperpigmentation preceded the onset of typical skin lesions in the patient reported by Espasandin and Vignale (1990). Hyperkeratosis or warty thickening of the nail folds with ridging of the nails were observed in the cases reported by Handfield-Jones *et al.* (1992).

The two extremes of the disease may co-exist. In these cases, the proximal third of the nail is atrophic and the distal two-thirds exhibits hypertrophic changes (Thiers *et al.* 1973). The histopathological changes are non-specific. They show an ill-defined lymphocytic infiltrate around the upper dermal vessels which does not reach the dermo-epidermal junction. There is mild acanthosis and hyperkeratosis with scattered parakera-

totic foci. In some cases fibrinoid degeneration in the superficial capillaries is seen. The infiltrate usually contains a few pycnotic neutrophils resembling allergic vasculitis. Other changes reported include eosinophilic hyalinization of individual prickle cells and scattered vacuolar degeneration (Bazex & Griffiths 1980). Amino acid analysis of the hyperkeratotic and friable nails has shown that they differed from normal and other investigated diseased nails—an increase in the percentage residues of lysine, methionine and glycine, accompanied by a decrease of arginine, threonine, proline and cysteine (Juhlin & Baran 1984). Differential diagnosis includes psoriasis, Reiter's disease, onychomycosis, acrodermatitis continua, secondary syphilis, keratoderma palmaris and plantaris. Whether the paraneoplastic syndrome of Nazzaro *et al.* (1974) is a different entity from Bazex's is debatable. It resembles pityriasis rubra, keratosis pilaris, Kyrle's disease and acrokeratosis paraneoplastica. All the nails are thickened and show multiple Beau's lines.

Topical steroids (Bazex & Griffiths 1980), systemic steroids (Martin *et al.* 1989) and etretinate (Wishart 1986) have been reported to improve the eruption.

## References

Baran, R. (1977) Paraneoplastic acrokeratosis of Bazex. *Archives of Dermatology* **113**, 2613.

Bazex, A. & Griffiths, A. (1980) Acrokeratosis paraneoplastica. A new cutaneous marker of malignancy. *British Journal of Dermatology* **102**, 304.

Bazex, A., Salvator, R., Dupré, A. *et al.* (1965) Syndrome paranéoplasique à type d'hyperkératose des extrémités. Guérison après traitement de l'épithélioma laryngé. *Bulletin de la Societé Française de Dermatologie et de Syphiligraphie* **72**, 182.

Bazex, A., Dupré, A., Christol, B. *et al.* (1973) Onychose paranéoplasique, forme localisée d'acrokératose paranéoplasique. *Bulletin de la Societé Française de Dermatologie et de Syphiligraphie* **80**, 117.

Bolognia, J.L., Brewer, Y. & Cooper, D.L. (1991) Bazex's syndrome. Analytic review. *Medicine* **70**, 269–280.

Boudoulas, O. & Camisa, C. (1986) Paraneoplastic acrokeratosis. Bazex syndrome. *Cutis* **37**, 49–453.

Bureau, Y., Barrière, H., Litoux, P. *et al.* (1971) Acrokeratose paranéoplasique de Bazex. Importance des lésions unguéales. A propos de 2 observations. *Bulletin de la Societé Française de Dermatologie et de Syphiligraphie* **78**, 79.

Cahuzac, P., Faure, M. & Thivolet, J. (1981) Onychoatrophie résiduelle au cours d'une acrokératose paranéoplasique de Bazex. *Annales de Dermatologie et de Vénéréologie* **108**, 773.

Douglas, W.S., Bisland, D.J. & Howatson, R. (1991) Acrokeratosis paraneoplastica of Bazex. A case in the UK. *Clinical and Experimental Dermatology* **165**, 297–299.

Espasandin, J. & Vignale, R.A. (1990) Acroqueratosis paraneoplasica de Bazex. Un caso clinico con hyperpigmentacion. *Medicina Cutanea Ibero-Latino-Americana* **18**, 257–262.

Grimwood, R.E. & Lekan, C. (1987) Acrokeratosis paraneoplastica with esophageal squamous cell carcinoma. *Journal of the American Academy of Dermatology* **17**, 685–686.

Handfield-Jones, S.E., Matthes, C.N.A., Ellis, J.P. *et al.* (1992) Acrokeratosis paraneoplastica of Bazex. *Journal of the Royal Society of Medicine* **85**, 548–550.

Jacobsen, F.K., Abildtrup, N. & Laursen, S.O. (1984) Acrokeratosis neoplastica (Bazex syndrome). *Archives of Dermatology* **120**, 502–504.

Juhlin, L. & Baran, R. (1984) Abnormal aminoacid composition of nails in Bazex' paraneoplastic acrokeratosis. *Acta Dermato-Venereologica* **64**, 31–34.

Martin, R.W., Cornitiu, T.G., Naylor, M.F. *et al.* (1989) Bazex' syndrome in a woman with pulmonary adenocarcinoma. *Archives of Dermatology* **125**, 847–848.

Martin, S., Modiano, P., Barbaud, A. *et al.* (1995) Forme bulleuse d'acrokératose de Bazex révélatrice d'un adénocarcinome pancréatique. *Annales de Dermatologie et de Vénéréologic* **122** (Suppl. 1), 118.

Mounsey, R. & Brown, D.H. (1992) Bazex syndrome. *Otolaryngology—Head and Neck Surgery* **107**, 475–477.

Nazzaro, P., Argentieri, R., Balus, L. *et al.* (1974) Syndrome paranéoplasique avec lésions papulokératosiques des extremités et kératose pilaire spinulosique diffuse. *Annales de Dermatologie et de Vénéréologie* **101**, 411–413.

O'Brien, T. (1995) Bazex syndrome (acrokeratosis paraneoplastica). *Australian Journal of Dermatology* **36**, 91–93.

Pecora, A.L., Landsman, L., Imgrund, S.P. & Lambert, W.C. (1983) Acrokeratosis paraneoplastica (Bazex syndrome). *Archives of Dermatology* **119**, 820–826.

Richard, M. & Giroux, J.M. (1987) Acrokeratosis paraneoplastica (Bazex syndrome). *Journal of the American Academy of Dermatology* **16**, 178–183.

Sassolas, B., Zagnoli, A., Leroy, J.P. *et al.* (1994) Lichen planus pigmentosus associated with acrokeratosis of Bazex. *Clinical and Experimental Dermatology* **19**, 70–73.

Scarpa, C., Nini, G., Pasqua, M.C. *et al.* (1971) Singolare osservazione di eritro-acrocheratosi paraneoplastica. *Giornale Italiano di Dermatologia e Venereologia* **46**, 17–25.

Thiers, H., Moulin, G., Haguenauer, J.P. *et al.* (1973) Acrokeratose paraneoplastique. *Bulletin de la Societé Française de Dermatologie et de Syphiligraphie* **80**, 129.

Von Hintzenstern, J., Kiesewetter, F., Simon, M. *et al.* (1990) Paraneoplastische Akrokeratose Bazex-verlang under palliativer therapie eines Zungengrund Karzinoms. *Hautarzt* **41**, 490–493.

Wishart, J.M. (1986) Bazex paraneoplastic acrokeratosis, a case report and response to Tigason. *British Journal of Dermatology* **115**, 595–596.

Witkowski, J.A. & Parish, L.C. (1982) Bazex syndrome. *Journal of the American Medical Association* **248**, 2883–2884.

## Glucagonoma syndrome (Fig. 6.65)

Necrolytic migratory erythema, stomatitis, weight loss and diabetes are the characteristic signs of this syndrome. Erythema, fissuring and swelling of periungual tissues resembling chronic paronychia are frequently observed (Guillausseau *et al.* 1982; Rappersberger *et al.* 1987). Fingertips can also be affected with distal onycholysis. Paronychia and pyogenic granulomas of the 1st and 3rd left toes have been reported by Picard *et al.* (1988). The nail may show fragility, crumbling, longitudinal striations or pitting (Becker *et al.* 1942; Mallinson *et al.* 1974). A skin eruption similar to necrolytic migratory erythema has been

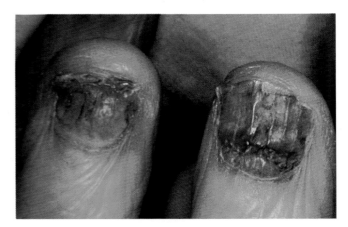

**Fig. 6.65** Glucagonoma syndrome. (Courtesy of J. Hewitt, France.)

described in zinc deficiency (Haneke 1983; Maillard *et al.* 1994; Sinclair & Reynolds 1997).

## References

Becker, S.W., Kabn, D. & Rothman, S. (1942) Cutaneous manifestations of internal malignant tumors. *Archives of Dermatology Syph* **45**, 1069–1080.

Guillausseau, P.J., Guillausseau, C., Villet, R. *et al.* (1982) Les glucagonomes. *Gastroenterologie Clinique et Biologique* **6**, 1029–1041.

Haneke, E. (1983) Imitation einer Glocagonom-Dermatitis durch erworbenen Zinkmangel. *Zeitschrift für Hautkrankheiten* **59**, 902–908.

Maillard, H., Celerier, P., Maisoneuve, C. *et al.* (1994) Erythème nécrolytique migrateur sans glucagonome. *Annales de Dermatologie et de Vénéréologie* **121** (Suppl. 1), S 123.

Mallinson, C.N., Bloom, S.R., Warin, A.P. *et al.* (1974) A glucagonoma syndrome. *Lancet* **ii**, 1–5.

Picard, C., Mazer, J.M., Bilet, S. *et al.* (1988) Syndrome du glucagonome. *Annales de Dermatologie et de Vénéréologie* **115**, 1142–1145.

Rappersberger, K., Wolff-Schreiner, E., Konrad, K. *et al.* (1987) Das glukagonom-syndrom. *Hautarzt* **38**, 589–598.

Sinclair, S.A. & Reynolds, N.J. (1997) Necrolytic migratory erythema and zinc deficiency. *British Journal of Dermatology* **136**, 783–785.

## Lung neoplasm

Hypertrophic pulmonary osteoarthropathy and finger clubbing are commonly seen in patients with primitive or secondary pulmonary neoplasms. Onycholysis of the fingernails has been observed in a 45-year-old man affected by a poorly differentiated squamous cell carcinoma of the lung who had received radiotherapy (Hickman 1977); this is probably not coincidental as another case has been reported (Cliff & Mortimer 1996).

## References

Cliff, S. & Mortimer, P.S. (1996) Onycholysis associated with carcinoma of the lung. *Clinical and Experimental Dermatology* **21**, 244.

Hickman, J.W. (1977) Onycholysis associated with carcinoma of the lung. *Journal of the American Medical Association* **238**, 1246.

## Acanthosis nigricans (Figs 6.66 & 6.67)

Nail ridging and brittleness can be associated with palmar hyperkeratosis in some patients with malignant acanthosis nigricans (Von Fischer 1949; Ebling *et al.* 1979); patchy (Ive 1963) or complete leuconychia and nail thickening have also been reported (Azizi *et al.* 1980). Hypertrophic pulmonary osteoarthropathy and bullous pemphigoid can occasionally be associated with acanthosis nigricans (Ive 1963). Warty excrescences present around the free margin of a thumbnail have been reported (Baker & Barth 1983).

## References

Azizi, E., Trau, H., Schewach-Millet, M. *et al.* (1980) Generalized malignant acanthosis nigricans. *Archives of Dermatology* **116**, 381.

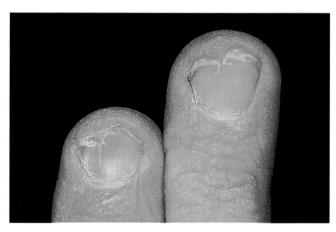

**Fig. 6.66** Malignant acanthosis nigricans. (Courtesy of H. Baker, UK.)

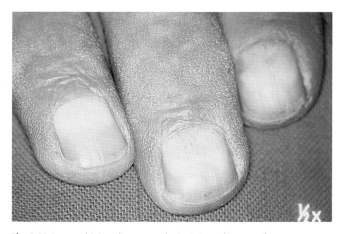

**Fig. 6.67** Leuconychia in malignant acanthosis nigricans. (Courtesy of A. Puissant, France.)

Baker, H. & Barth, J.H. (1983) Acanthosis nigricans. *British Journal of Dermatology* **109** (Suppl.), 101–103.

Ebling, F.J.G., Marks, R. & Rook, A. (1979) Disorders of keratinization. In: *Textbook of Dermatology* (eds A. Rook, D.S. Wilkinson, F.J.G. Ebling *et al.*), pp. 1393–1468. Blackwell Scientific Publications, Oxford.

Ive, F.A. (1963) Metastatic carcinoma of cervix with acanthosis nigricans, bullous pemphigoid and hypertrophic pulmonary osteoarthropathy. *Proceedings of the Royal Society of Medicine* **56**, 910.

Von Fischer, F. (1949) Acanthosis nigricans. *Dermatologica* **98**, 319–320.

## Digital ischaemia

Raynaud's phenomenon and digital necrosis can be early signs of an occult neoplasm (Hawley *et al.* 1967; Van der Meulen *et al.* 1978; Vayssairat *et al.* 1978). The onset of symptoms is not related to cold exposure. Pain and paraesthesia of fingers may precede the development of digital ischaemia. Splinter haemorrhages were also observed in three patients (Palmer 1974). Digital necrosis associated with a lupus syndrome may reveal a breast cancer relapse (Noyon *et al.* 1996). Digital ischaemia was also found to be the presenting sign in Hodgkin's disease (Halpern *et al.* 1994).

Gastrointestinal, genital (Mahler *et al.* 1999), ovarian (Maurice 1996; Legrain *et al.* 1999) and blood malignancies have been associated with digital ischaemia which may progress to gangrene. The removal of neoplasms is usually followed by an improvement of ischaemic signs (Barriere 1984; Garioch *et al.* 1991). The mechanism of digital ischaemia associated with malignancy is probably multifactorial. Metastatic involvement of the sympathetic ganglia, hypergammaglobulinaemia, production of cryoglobulins, hypercoagulable states, production of catecholamine or other neurohumoral factors have been implicated (Albin *et al.* 1986).

Fingertip necrosis appeared during chemotherapy with bleomycin, vincristine and methotrexate for HIV-related Kaposi's sarcoma (Pechère *et al.* 1996).

## References

Albin, G., Lapeyre, A.C., Click, R.L. *et al.* (1986) Paraneoplastic digital thrombosis: a case report. *Angiology* **37**, 203–206.

Barriere, H. (1984) Syndromes cutanés para-néoplasiques. *Annales de Medecine Interne* **135**, 662–668.

Garioch, J.J., Todd, P., Soukop, M. *et al.* (1991) T-cell lymphoma presenting with severe digital ischaemia *Clinical and Experimental Dermatology* **16**, 202–203.

Halpern, S.M., Todd, P. & Kirby, J.D. (1994) Hodgkin's disease presenting with digital ischaemia. *Clinical and Experimental Dermatology* **19**, 330–331.

Hawley, P.R., Johnston, A.W. & Rankin, J.T. (1967) Association between digital ischemia and malignant disease. *British Medical Journal* **2**, 208.

Legrain, S., Raguin, G. & Piette, J.C. (1999) Digital necrosis revealing ovarian carcinoma. *Dermatology* **199**, 183–184.

Mahler, V., Neureiter, D., Kirchner, T. *et al.* (1999) Digitale ischämie als Paraneoplasie bie metastarierenden Adenokarzinom des Endometrium uteri. *Hautarzt* 50, 748–752.

Maurice, P.D.L. (1996) Ovarian carcinoma and digital ischaemia. *Clinical and Experimental Dermatology* 21, 381–382.

Noyon, V., Le Hir-Garreau, I., Adamski, H. *et al.* (1996) Nécroses digitiales et syndrome lupique révélant la récidive d'un adénocarcinome mammaire. *Nouvelle Dermatologie* 15, 148.

Palmer, H.M. (1974) Digital vascular disease and malignant disease. *British Journal of Dermatology* 91, 476.

Pechère, M., Zulian, G.B., Vogel, J.J. *et al.* (1996) Fingertip necrosis during chemotherapy with bleomycin, vincristine and methotrexate for HIV-related Kaposi sarcoma. *British Journal of Dermatology* 134, 378–379.

Van der Meulen, J., The, T.H. & Wouda, A.A. (1978) Le phénomène de Raynaud: un syndrome paranéoplasique? *Nouvelle Presse Médicale* 7, 3935.

Vayssairat, M., Fiessinger, J.N., Bordet, F. *et al.* (1978) Rapports entre nécroses digitales du membres supérieur et affections malignes. *Nouvelle Presse Médicine* 7, 1279–1282.

## Papuloerythroderma (Fig. 6.68)

Papuloerythroderma is a clinically distinctive entity associated with blood eosinophilia characterized by a pruritic eruption that quickly develops into a papular erythroderma with notable sparing of compressed abdominal folds (deck chair sign) (Ofuji *et al.* 1984). Splinter haemorrhages in the nails were noted by Grob *et al.* (1989). Thrombosed capillaries in the nail folds were a striking feature in the case of Staughton *et al.* (1987). Multiple causative factors (lymphoma, gastric and lung cancer, etc.) underlie the pathogenesis of papuloerythroderma (Ofuji 1990). Langerhan's cells may possibly have a central role in the pathogenesis of this condition (Wakeel *et al.* 1991).

### References

Grob, J.J., Collet-Villette, A.M., Herchowski, N. *et al.* (1989) Papuloerythroderma. Report of a case with T-cell skin lymphoma and discussion of the nature of the disease. *Journal of the American Academy of Dermatology* 20, 927–931.

Ofuji, S. (1990) Papuloerythroderma. *Journal of the American Academy of Dermatology* 22, 697.

Ofuji, S., Furukawa, F., Miyachi, Y. *et al.* (1984) Papuloerythroderma. *Dermatologica* 169, 125–130.

Staughton, R., Laugry, J., Rowland-Payne, C. *et al.* (1987) Papuloerythroderma: the first European case In: *Clinical Dermatology* (eds D.S. Wilkinson, J.M. Mascaro & C.E. Orfanos, pp. 181–182. The CDM Case Collection, Berlin. Stuttgard, Schattawer.

Wakeel, R.A., Keefe, M. & Chapman, R.S. (1991) Papuloerythroderma. *Archives of Dermatology* 127, 96–98.

## Breast carcinoma

Longitudinal hyperpigmented nail banding unrelated to chemotherapy occurred in a 49-year-old woman with breast carcinoma (Krutchik *et al.* 1978). Leukonychia striata of all

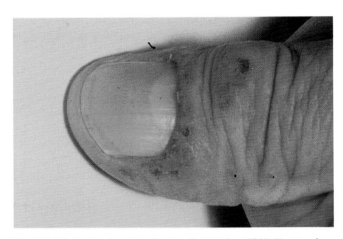

**Fig. 6.68** Papuloerythroderma-thrombosed capillaries in the nail folds. (Courtesy of R. Staughton, UK.)

fingernails has been reported in a 67-year-old woman with breast cancer (Hortobagyi 1983).

### References

Hortobagyi, G.N. (1983) Leukonychia striata associated with breast carcinoma. *Journal of Surgical Oncology* 23, 60–61.

Krutchik, A.N., Tashima, C.K., Buzdar, A.U. *et al.* (1978) Longitudinal nail banding associated with breast carcinoma unrelated to chemotherapy. *Archives of Internal Medicine* 138, 1302–1303.

## Leiomyosarcoma

Facial and nail hyperpigmentation occurred in a 47-year-old man affected by intestinal leiomyosarcoma. Skin and nail pigmentation faded dramatically 3 months after surgery (Suda *et al.* 1985). Finger clubbing was the presenting symptom of a gastric leiomyosarcoma in a 33-year-old woman. Clubbing regressed after tumour excision (Rabast 1997).

### References

Rabast, U. (1997) Trommelschlegelfinger bei einem niedrig malignen Leiomyosarkom mit gemischtet Hiatuschernie. *Deutsche Medizinische Wochenschrift* 122, 1207–1212.

Suda, M., Ishii, H., Kashiwazaki, K. *et al.* (1985) Hyperpigmentation of skin and nails in a patient with intestinal leiomyosarcoma. *Digestive Diseases and Sciences* 30, 1108–1111.

## Multicentric reticulohistiocytosis (see page 247)

A large number of malignancies have been reported in association with multicentric reticulohistiocytosis.

## Nasopharyngeal carcinoma

Thirty-two of 1300 patients affected by nasopharyngeal carcinoma developed a paraneoplastic syndrome. Hypertrophic osteo-arthropathy was observed in 17 patients whereas 13 patients exhibited finger clubbing. One patient had dermatomyositis and one patient had myeloma. Pulmonary metastases were present in 15 of the 17 patients with hypertrophic osteoarthropathy and in all of the 13 patients with finger clubbing. Most of the patients with a paraneoplastic syndrome were young and had undifferentiated nasopharyngeal carcinoma with lung meta-stases (Maalej *et al.* 1985).

## Reference

Maalej, M., Ladgham, A., Ennouri, A. *et al.* (1985) Le syndrome paranéoplasique du cancer du nasopharynx. *Presse Medicale* **14**, 471–474.

## Gastrointestinal malignancy (Fig. 6.69)

Pronounced pincer nails and universal alopecia developed in asso-ciation with a metastasizing adenocarcinoma of the sigmoid colon (Jemec & Thomson 1997).

## Reference

Jemec, G.B.E. & Thomsen, K. (1997) Pincer nails and alopecia as markers of gastrointestinal malignancy. *Journal of Dermatology* **24**, 479–481.

## Castleman's tumour (Figs 6.70 & 6.71)

There is a remarkable association between Castleman's tumours and skin diseases. A 45-year-old patient with a retro-peritoneal Castleman's tumour developed severe lichen planus involving the skin and mouth, with erosive nail bed changes and secondary loss of many fingernails and toenails. In addi-tion, pemphigus vulgaris affected the oral cavity. Both derma-

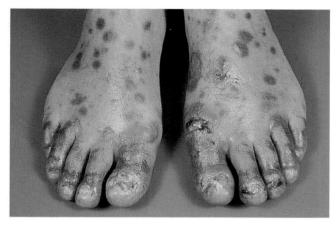

**Fig. 6.70** Castleman's tumour. (Courtesy of G. Plewig, Germany.)

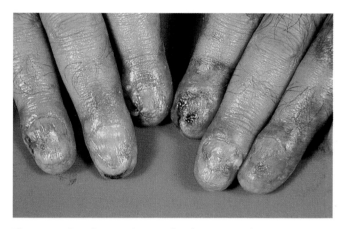

**Fig. 6.71** Castleman's tumour. (Courtesy of G. Plewig, Germany.)

toses regressed after surgical removal of the tumour (Plewig *et al.* 1990; Jansen *et al.* 1995). In a 13-year-old boy paraneo-plastic pemphigus was associated with Castleman's tumour. His nail folds were swollen and violaceous, the nails had been shed (Lemon *et al.* 1997). POEMS syndrome has also been also associated with Castleman's disease (Thajeb *et al.* 1989).

## References

Jansen, T., Plewig, G. & Anhalt, G.J. (1995) Paraneoplastic pemphigus with clinical features of erosive lichen planus associated with Castleman's tumour. *Dermatology* **190**, 245–250.

Lemon, M.A., Weston, W.L. & Huff, J.C. (1997) Childhood paraneo-plastic pemphigus associated with Castleman's tumour. *British Journal of Dermatology* **136**, 115–117.

Plewig, G., Jansen, T., Jungblut, R.M. *et al.* (1990) Castleman-Tumour, lichen ruber und pemphigus vulgaris: paraneoplastische association immunologischer erkrankungen? *Hautarzt* **41**, 662–670.

Thajeb, P., Chee, C.Y., Lo, S.F. *et al.* (1989) The POEMS syndrome among Chinese: association with Castleman's disease and some immunological abnormalities. *Acta Neurology Scandinavica* **80**, 492–500.

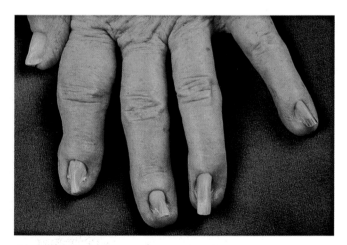

**Fig. 6.69** Pincer nails induced by gastrointestinal malignancy. (Courtesy of G.B.E. Jemec & K. Thomsen, Denmark.)

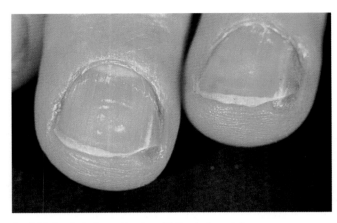

**Fig. 6.72** Cowden's disease. (Courtesy of R. Happle, Germany.)

## Cowden's disease (Fig. 6.72)

A linear nail dystrophy with changes resembling median canaliform dystrophy of Heller that extends distally from the cuticle to the edge of the nail plate has been described in a patient with Cowden's disease, an autosomal dominant genodermatosis (Lazar 1986). Siegel (1974) reported a patient with Cowden's disease who presented a solitary subungual fibrotic nodule on the great toe of the right foot and a similar lesion starting under a fingernail. Linear subungual hyperkeratosis resembling longitudinal leukonykia may involve several fingers (Happle 1989).

### References

Happle, R. (1989) Genodermatosen an Handen und Fusser. In: *Handsymposium Dermatologische Erkrankungen der Hande und Fusse* (eds P. Altmeyer, U. Schultz-Ehrenburg & H. Luther), pp. 109–111. Springer-Verlag, Berlin.

Lazar, A.P. (1986) Cowden's disease (multiple hamartoma and neoplasia syndrome) treated with isotretinoin. *Journal of the American Academy of Dermatology* **14**, 142–143.

Siegel, J. (1974) Tuberous sclerosis (form fruste) vs. Cowden syndrome. *Archives of Dermatology* **110**, 476–477.

## Metastases (see Chapter 11)

Metastases to the terminal phalanx are said to be rare. However, in 1994 we reported 118 published cases (Baran & Tosti 1994) and since then several more have been found. The lung is the most frequent primary site for metastases to the fingers, whereas the genitourinary tract is the most frequent primary site for metastases to the toes (Baran *et al.* 1998). Clinically, the affected digit shows marked swelling with diffuse inflammation of periungual tissues resembling acute paronychia.

### References

Baran, R. & Tosti, A. (1994) Metastatic bronchogenic carcinoma to the terminal phalanx with review of 116 non-melanoma metastatic tumors to the distal digit. *Journal of the American Academy of Dermatology* **31**, 251–263.

Baran, R., Guillot, P. & Tosti, A. (1998) Metastasis from carcinoma of the bronchus to the distal aspect of two digits. *British Joural of Dermatology* **138**, 708.

## Leukaemias

Splinter haemorrhages as well as subungual and periungual haematomas can occur in patients with leukaemia. Pallor of the nail bed due to anaemia can also be observed. A nail dystrophy is a common symptom in longstanding erythroderma independent of its aetiology and may therefore be observed as a non-specific lesion in about 25% of patients with chronic lymphocytic leukaemia (Beek 1948). Non-tender swelling of the proximal nail fold mimicking chronic paronychia has been reported in a patient affected by chronic lymphocytic leukaemia. All fingers except the thumbs were affected. Fingernails were mildly dystrophic with brownish discoloration. Histopathological findings of leukaemia cutis were present in the skin biopsy. Lesions dramatically resolved after irradiation (High *et al.* 1985).

Clubbing and distal digital periosteal bone destruction due to leukaemic infiltration of the distal phalanges have also been reported (Hirschfeld 1925). A patient presented spatulate fingers due to marginal and dorsal leukaemic infiltration and subungual deposits that caused bulbous tips and splintered nails. Onychogryphosis of the toenails was also present (Calvert & Smith 1955). A patient developed subungual tumours involving several fingers and the left toenail early in the course of chronic lymphocytic leukaemia. The affected nails showed an increased curvature as well as an elevation of the nail plates (Simon *et al.* 1990) (Fig. 6.73). Histopathology showed a

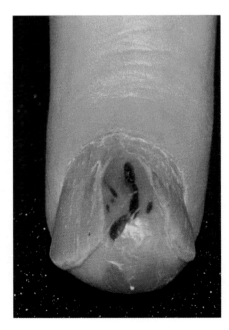

**Fig. 6.73** Leukaemic infiltrate in the nail apparatus. (Courtesy of W.P.D. Su, USA.)

massive leukaemic infiltrate in the reticular dermis and sub-cutaneous tissue sparing a grenz zone in the papillary dermis of the nail bed. The epidermis was normal.

Leukaemic infiltration in the distal phalanx of the thumb resulting in a chronic whitlow with bone involvement has been reported in a patient affected by acute monomyelocytic leukaemia (Chang *et al.* 1975). A syndrome resembling pachy-dermoperiostosis has also been described in this condition (Mackenzie 1986).

Perniotic lesions on fingers, toes, nose and ears have been reported during the preleukaemic phase of myelomonocytic leukaemia (Marks *et al.* 1969; Kelly & Dowling 1985; Cliff *et al.* 1996). Norwegian scabies was the presenting symptom of adult-T-cell leukaemia in two members of a Japanese family (Egawa *et al.* 1992).

Acute undifferentiated myeloblastic leukaemia was revealed by haemorrhagic bullous lesions with red margins noted on the dorsal aspect of hand and fingers of patients (Ochonisky *et al.* 1993).

## References

Beck, C.H. (1948) Skin manifestations associated with lymphatic leukaemia. *Dermatologica* **96**, 350–356.

Calvert, R.J. & Smith, E. (1955) Metastatic acropachy in lymphatic leukemia. *Blood* **10**, 545–549.

Chang, Y.D., Whitaker, L.A. & La Rossa, D. (1975) Acute monomyelocytic leukemia presenting as a felon. *Plastic and Reconstructive Surgery* **56**, 623–624.

Cliff, S., James, S.L., Mercieca, J.E. *et al.* (1996) Perniosis—a possible association with a preleukemic state. *British Journal of Dermatology* **135**, 330–345.

Egawa, K., Johno, M., Hayashibara, T. *et al.* (1992) Familial occurrence of crusted (Norwegian) scabies with adult T-cell leukaemia. *British Journal of Dermatology* **127**, 57–59.

High, D.A., Luscombe, H.A. & Kauh, Y.C. (1985) Leukemia cutis masquerading as chronic paronychia. *International Journal of Dermatology* **24**, 595–597.

Hirschfeld, H. (1925) Leukamic und verewandte zustande. In: *Handbook der Krankheiten der Blutbildenen Organe*, Vol. 1 (ed. A. Schittenhelm), p. 258. Springer, Berlin.

Kelly, J.W. & Dowling, J.P. (1985) Pernio: a possible association with chronic myelomonocytic leukaemia. *Archives of Dermatology* **121**, 1048–1052.

Mackenzie, C.R. (1986) Pachydermoperiostosis: a paraneoplastic syndrome. *New York State Journal of Medicine* 153–154.

Marks, R., Lim, C.C. & Borrie, P.F. (1969) A perniotic syndrome with monocytosis and neutropenia: a possible association with a preleukaemic state. *British Journal of Dermatology* **81**, 327–332.

Ochonisky, S., Aractingi, S., Dombret, H. *et al.* (1993) Acute undifferentiated myeloblastic leukemia revealed by specific hemorrhagic bullous lesions. *Archives of Dermatology* **129**, 512–513.

Simon, C.A., Su, W.P.D. & Li, C.Y. (1990) Subungual leukemia cutis. *International Journal of Dermatology* **29**, 636–639.

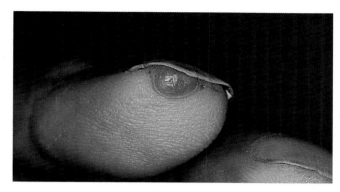

**Fig. 6.74** Plasma cell dyscrasia with polyneuropathy and endocrine disorder. (Courtesy of Y. Shindo, Japan.)

## Plasmocytoma (Fig. 6.74)

A painless subungual nodule of 2 month's duration was present on the right thumb in a 48-year-old man. Osteolytic areas in the distal phalanx were associated with osteolytic lesions in the skull and vertebrae. Histological examination of the nodule showed a dense infiltrate of immature plasma cells in the lower part of the dermis and in subcutaneous tissue (Rodriguez *et al.* 1996).

Multiple large tumours involving the digits of the hands may represent the initial symptom of multiple myeloma in a patient (Pobanz *et al.* 1955). Nail changes can be observed in patients with systemic amyloidosis secondary to plasmocytoma (page 271).

Clinical symptoms of hyalinosis cutis et mucosae occurred in a 66-year-old patient affected by plasmocytoma with monoclonal IgG light chain gammopathy. A severe onychodys-trophy characterized by onychoschisis and onycholysis was also present (Von der Helm *et al.* 1989). Digital ischaemia due to cryoglobulins can occur in patients with Waldenström's macroglobulinaemia or multiple myeloma. Finger clubbing and Terry's nails have been described in patients with POEMS syndrome associated with plasmocytoma (page 276).

## References

Pobanz, D.M., Condon, J.V. & Baker, L.A. (1955) Plasma-cell myelomatosis. *Archives of Internal Medicine* **96**, 828–832.

Rodriguez, J., Bosch, M., Castro, V. *et al.* (1996) Subungual nodule as manifestation of multiple myeloma. *International Journal of Dermatology* **35**, 661–662.

Von der Helm, D., Ring, J., Schmoeckel, C. *et al.* (1989) Erworbene hyalinosis cutis et mucosae bei Plasmozytom mit monoklonaler IgG-lambda-Gammopathie. *Hautarzt* **40**, 153–157.

## Lymphoma (Figs 6.75–6.77)

Cutaneous B-cell lymphomas rarely affect the nails. A 70-year-old patient affected by chronic lymphocytic leukaemia developed nail lesions that clinically resembled onychomycosis

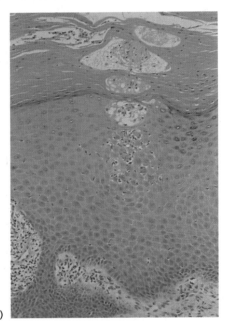

(a)

(b)

**Fig. 6.75** (a) T-cell lymphoma of nail apparatus. (b) Same case as (a) showing nail dermal infiltrate and epidermotropism.

associated with slowly growing pink tumours in the toenails. A nail biopsy established the diagnosis of non Hodgkin's, B-cell type centrocytic/centroblastic malignant lymphoma. Treatment with chlorambucil and prednisolone produced striking effects (Moller & Pedersen 1992).

The nail abnormalities observed in patients with cutaneous T-cell lymphoma may be non-specific or may be a direct consequence of the localization of the neoplastic cells in the nail constituents.

Onychodystrophy has been reported to occur in 32% of patients affected by Sézary syndrome (Wieselthier & Koh 1990). The nail changes may be indistinguishable from the onychodystrophy of other erythrodermic conditions such as pityriasis rubra pilaris, psoriasis or actinic reticuloid (Toonstra et al. 1985; Sonnex et al. 1986). Nail abnormalities reported

in association with mycosis fungoides including onycholysis, nail bed hyperkeratosis (Tomsick 1982) along with nail plate, thickening and discoloration (Trathner et al. 1990) are the most common clinical features. Ridging, roughness, Beau's lines (Singh & Kaur 1986) and onychomadesis with subsequent shedding can also occur (Fleming et al. 1996). Nail biopsy can reveal a lymphomatous infiltration of the nail apparatus (Dalziel et al. 1989; Tosti et al. 1990; Zaias 1990).

In mycosis fungoides of the digits, nail changes are not uncommon and have been reported even in childhood (Wilson et al. 1991). The nail changes occasionally improve during chemotherapy. Gangrene of the right finger due to cutaneous T-cell lymphoma has been described by Lund et al. (1990). A T-cell lymphoma which presented with sudden severe digital ischaemia has been reported. Combination chemotherapy produced complete remission of digital ischaemia (Garioch et al. 1991).

An elephantiasis-like tumescence of the 3rd left finger associated with multiple nodular lesions on several other fingers and dystrophic nail changes were the unusual manifestations of mycosis fungoides in a 56-year-old patient (Voigtlander et al. 1988). Yellow nail syndrome has been reported in a 72-year-old patient suffering from mycosis fungoides (Stosiek et al. 1993).

## References

Dalziel, K.L., Telfer, N.R. & Dawber, R.P.R. (1989) Nail dystrophy in cutaneous T-cell lymphoma. *British Journal of Dermatology* 120, 571–574.

Fleming, C.J., Hunt, M.J., Barnetson, R. St C. (1996) Mycosis fungoides with onychomadesis. *British Journal of Dermatology* 135, 1012.

Garioch, J.J., Todd, P., Soukop, M. et al. (1991) T-cell lymphoma presenting with severe digital ischaemia. *Clinical and Experimental Dermatology* 16, 202–203.

Lund, K.A., Parker, C.M., Norins, A.L. et al. (1990) Vesicular cutaneous T cell lymphoma presenting with gangrene. *Journal of the American Academy of Dermatology* 23, 1169–1170.

Moller Pedersen, L., Nordin, H., Nielsen, H. et al. (1992) Non Hodgkin malignant lymphoma in the nails in the course of a chronic lymphocytic leukemia. *Acta Dermato-Venereologica* 72, 277–278.

Singh, M. & Kaur, S. (1986) Chemotherapy induced multiple Beau's lines. *International Journal of Dermatology* 25, 590–591.

Sonnex, T.S., Dawber, R.P.R., Zachary, C.B. et al. (1986) The nails in adult type 1 pityriasis rubra pilaris. *Journal of the American Academy of Dermatology* 15, 956–960.

Stosiek, N., Peters, K.P., Hiller, D. et al. (1993) Yellow nail syndrome in a patient with mycosis fungoides. *Journal of the American Academy of Dermatology* 28, 792–794.

Tomsick, R.S. (1982) Hyperkeratosis in mycosis fungoides. *Cutis* 29, 621–623.

Toonstra, J., Van Weelden, H., Gmelin Meyling, F.H.J. et al. (1985) Actinic reticuloid simulating Sézary syndrome. Report of two cases. *Archives of Dermatological Research* 277, 159–166.

Tosti, A., Fanti, P.A. & Varotti, C. (1990) Massive lymphomatous nail involvement in Sézary syndrome. *Dermatologica* 181, 162–164.

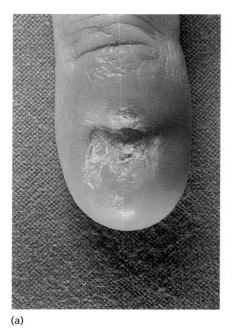

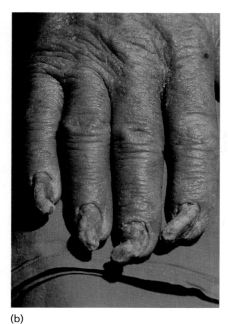

**Fig. 6.76** (a) Mycosis fungoides—tumour of the nail apparatus. (b) Sezary syndrome. (Courtesy of O. Binet, France.)

(a)

(b)

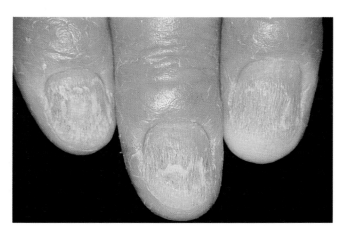

**Fig. 6.77** Mycosis fungoides after electron beam therapy.

Trathner, A., Ingber, A. & Sandbank, M. (1990) Nail pigmentation resulting from PUVA treatment. *International Journal of Dermatology* **29**, 310.

Voigtlander, V., Hartmann, A.A., Adam, W. *et al.* (1988) Mycosis fongoïde. Etiologie inattendue d'un eczéma chronique des mains avec gigantisme digital. *Annales de Dermatologie et de Vénéréologie* **115**, 1212–1214.

Wieselthier, J.S. & Koh, H.K. (1990) Sézary syndrome: diagnosis, prognosis, and critical review of treatment options. *Journal of the American Academy of Dermatology* **22**, 381–401.

Wilson, K.G., Cotter, F.E., Lowe, D.G. *et al.* (1991) Mycosis fungoides in childhood: an unusual presentation. *Journal of the American Academy of Dermatology* **25**, 370–372.

Zaias, N. (1990) *The Nail in Health and Disease*, 2nd edn, p. 227. Appleton & Lange, Norwalk, CN.

## HTLV-1 positive cutaneous T-cell lymphoma

A 34-year-old German woman noticed painless swelling and blackish discoloration which had developed within 2 weeks on several fingernails and toenails. The nails were blackish-red, thickened and leathery. An unusual haemorrhagic, epidermotropic lymphocytic infiltrate with T-cell pattern and numerous large Pautrier's abscesses, transepithelial elimination and infiltration of the subungual keratin and nail plate was seen histologically. The nail changes resolved completely within 4 months and did not recur although she later developed opportunistic infections and eventually died. HTLV-1 was confirmed serologically whereas HIV-1 and HIV-2 were negative (Wolter *et al.* 1991).

## Reference

Wolter, M., Schleussner-Samuel, P. & Marsh, W. (1991) HTLV-1-Infektion: unguales T-Zell-Lymphom als Primarmanifestation. *Hautarzt* **42**, 50–52.

## Hodgkin's disease

In a review of 50 patients with Hodgkin's disease, four patients (three males and one female) showed transverse leuconychia. All four patients had from one to three transverse white lines; one patient had dark brown discoloration of the distal part of the affected nail. All changes were more marked in the finger rather than in the toenails. In these patients the nail changes reflected a poor diagnosis, death occurring within 4 months of the development of leuconychia. No relationship between nail anomalies and chemotherapy or radiotherapy was evident (Shahani & Blackburn 1973).

A 52-year-old man with primary Raynaud's disease developed increasingly severe vasospasm with digital ischaemia in all limbs, and gangrene in two digits of the left hand. He was subsequently found to have Hodgkin's disease (Halpern *et al.* 1994).

## References

Halpern, S.M., Todd, P. & Kirby, J.D. (1994) Hodgkin's disease presenting with digital ischaemia. *Clinical and Experimental Dermatology* **19**, 330–331.

Shahani, R.T. & Blackburn, E.K. (1973) Nail anomalies in Hodgkin's disease. *British Journal of Dermatology* **89**, 457–458.

## Systemic drugs

### Nail clipping for monitoring previous exposure to drugs or poisons

Like scalp and body hair, nails are biological matrices in which drugs tend to accumulate. Although nails are exposed to external contamination, they are an interesting substrate for the investigation of drug use and for forensic studies (Pichini *et al.* 1996). Nail clippings can therefore be utilized to confirm previous intake of drugs and trace elements or exposure to poisons in the months before the examination. The great toenail is usually utilized for this purpose.

Drugs that can be measured in the nail include: amphetamines and their metabolite metamphetamine (Cirimele *et al.* 1995), chloroquine (Ofori-Adjei & Ericsson 1985), cocaine and its metabolite benzoylecigonine (Skopp & Potsch 1997) and other drugs of abuse (Engelhart *et al.* 1998; Lemos *et al.* 1999). The antifungals fluconazole, itraconazole and terbinafine can also be detected. Nail clippings can be used for monitoring levels of numerous trace elements, including iron, zinc and selenium (Garland *et al.* 1996). Arsenic, lead, copper, chromium and thallium poisoning may be confirmed by detecting the metal in nail clippings (Massey *et al.* 1984; Bu-Olayan *et al.* 1996; Kubis *et al.* 1997).

## References

Bu-Olayan, A.H., Al-Jakoob, S.N. & Alhazeem, S. (1996) Lead in drinking water from water coolers and in fingernails from subjects in Kuwait City, Kuwait. *Science of the Total Environment* **181**, 209–214.

Cirimele, V., Kintz, P. & Mangin, P. (1995) Detection of amphetamines in fingernails: an alternative to hair analysis. *Archives of Toxicology* **70**, 68–69.

Engelhart, D.A., Lavins, E.S. & Sutheiner, C.A. (1998) Detection of drugs of abuse in nails. *Journal of Analytical Toxicology* **22**, 314–318.

Garland, M., Morris, J.S., Colditz, G.A. *et al.* (1996) Toenail trace elements levels and breast cancer: a prospective study. *American Journal of Epidemiology* **144**, 653–660.

Kubis, N., Talamon, C., Smadja, D. *et al.* (1997) Neuropathie périphérique par intoxication au thallium. *Revue Neurologique (Paris)* **153**, 599–601.

Lemos, N.P., Anderson, R.A., Robertson, J.R. (1999) Nail analysis for drugs of abuse: extraction and determination of cannabis in fingernails by RIA and GC-MS. *Journal of Analytical Toxicology* **23**, 147–152.

Massey, W., Wold, D. & Heyman, A. (1984) Arsenic: homicidal intoxication. *Southern Medical Journal* **77**, 848–851.

Ofori-Adjei, D. & Ericsson, O. (1985) Chloroquine in nail clippings. *Lancet* **ii**, 331.

Pichini, S., Altieri, I., Zuccaro, P. *et al.* (1996) Drug monitoring in nonconventional biological fluids and matrices. *Clinical Pharmacokinetics* **30**, 211–228.

Skopp, G. & Potsch, L. (1997) A case report of screening of nail clippings to detect prenatal drug exposure. *Therapeutic Drug Monitoring* **19**, 386–389.

### Drug-induced photoonycholysis (Fig. 6.78)

Numerous drugs have occasionally been incriminated to cause photoonycholysis. These include trypaflavine, acriflavine hydrochloride, chloramphenicol, chlorpromazine, thiazides, clorazepate dipotassium, systemically administered 5-fluorouracil, oral contraceptives, benoxaprofen, thorazine, practolol, captopril, quinine sulphate and quinolones (flumequine, nalidixic acid, pefloxacine, ofloxacine) (Baran 1986; Baran & Brun 1986).

Drug-induced photoonycholysis, however, most commonly occurs with the use of tetracycline or psoralens, both with natural sunlight (Zala *et al.* 1977) and with artificial light sources in psoralen and ultraviolet A (PUVA) treatment (Ortonne & Baran 1978; Mackie 1979; Morgan *et al.* 1992). The development of photoonycholysis is not related to the cumulative UV dose (Segal 1963; Baran & Barthélémy 1990).

Three different clinical varieties of drug-induced photoonycholysis have been described. In all three varieties the lateral margins of the nails are never involved by the process and thumbs are only rarely affected (Baran 1986; Baran & Juhlin 1987). In the first variety, the detachment is half-moon shaped, variably pigmented and presents a well-demarcated proximal convex border. This is the most frequent clinical variety of drug-induced photoonycholysis and usually involves several digits. In the second variety, which usually involves only one nail, the proximal border of the detachment presents a well-defined, distally opened circular notch that is surrounded by a proximal brownish margin. In the third variety, which usually affects several digits, the detachment is localized in the central part of the pink nail bed showing initially a round yellow stain which turns in to a reddish colour after several days (photohaemorrhage). It may be seen initially as part of Segal's triad: photosensitivity followed by discoloration of the nails and onycholysis (Segal 1963). Photoonycholysis due to tetracycline derivatives or psoralens can be painful (Mackie 1979), and pain may occasionally precede onycholysis (Zala *et al.* 1977). The development of photoonycholysis can be preceded or followed

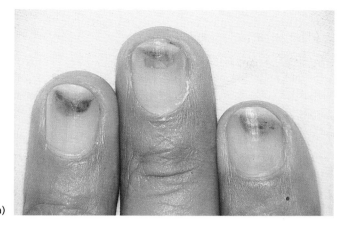

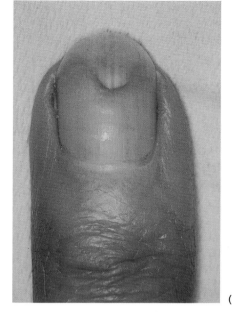

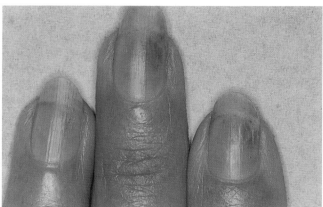

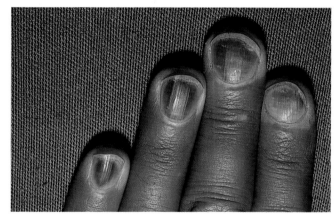

**Fig. 6.78** (a) Photoonycholysis, type I. (b) Photoonycholysis, type II. (c) Photoonycholysis, type III. (d) Photoonycholysis, type III—late stage.

by a sunburn reaction on sun-exposed areas (Segal 1963). Painful bullae under the nails have been reported with tetracycline-hydrochloride after 1 month of intensive sun bathing (Ibsen & Andersen 1983).

Photoonycholysis can occur early in treatment as well as after prolonged therapy. Interruption of the drug does not prevent the onset of onycholysis, which may be delayed even by 1 month. Long-term persistence of the drug in the skin has been suggested to explain such delayed onset of photoonycholysis in some patients (Baran & Barthélémy 1990).

Attempts to experimentally induce photoonycholysis have been unsuccessful and onycholysis does not necessarily recur with readministration of the drug. Psoralen-induced photoonycholysis is not an indication for discontinuing treatment, because the nail changes spontaneously resolve even if the therapy is not stopped (Mackie 1979). A single layer of opaque

adhesive strapping or the liberal application of coloured nail varnish has been shown to prevent the development of nail changes. The mechanism of drug-induced photoonycholysis remains undetermined (Baran & Juhlin 1987). Concentration of UV irradiation by the nail plate has been proposed. The possible role of melanin in the prevention of photoonycholysis is suggested by the observation that Afro-Caribbean or Mongoloid individuals are not apparently affected.

Because skin lipids can reduce UV transmission, the absence of sebaceous glands in the subungual area may also be important. UV irradiation between 310 and 313 nm has been suggested to have a major role in inducing the reaction. The observation that 3–20% of irradiation with wavelengths 313–500 nm can penetrate normal nails but not psoriatic nails possibly explains the poor effect of psoralens with UVA in nail psoriasis.

The origin of pigmentation observed in most cases of photo-onycholysis is poorly understood. Haemosiderin deposits due to blood extravasation and keratin dust have been implicated.

## References

Baran, R. (1986) Les onycholyses. *Annales de Dermatologie et de Vénéréologie* 113, 159–170.

Baran, R. & Barthélémy, H. (1990) Photo-onycholyse induite par le 5-MOP (Psoraderm) et application de la méthode d'imputation des effets medicamenteux. *Annales de Dermatologie et de Vénéréologie* 117, 367–369.

Baran, R. & Brun, P. (1986) Photo-onycholysis induced by the fluoro-quinolones pe-floxacine and ofloxacine. *Dermatologica* 176, 185–188.

Baran, R. & Juhlin, L. (1987) Drug induced photo-onycholysis. Three subtypes identified in a study of 15 cases. *Journal of the American Academy of Dermatology* 17, 1012–1016.

Ibsen, H.H. & Andersen, B.L. (1983) Photo-onycholysis due to tetracycline-hydrochloride. *Acta Dermato-Venereologica* 63, 555–557.

Mackie, R.M. (1979) Onycholysis occurring during PUVA therapy. *Clinical and Experimental Dermatology* 4, 111–113.

Morgan, J.M., Weller, R. & Adams, S.J. (1992) Onycholysis in a case of atopic eczema treated with PUVA photochemotherapy. *Clinical and Experimental Dermatology* 17, 65–66.

Ortonne, J.P. & Baran, R. (1978) Photo-onycholyse induite par la photochimiothérapie orale. *Annales de Dermatologie et de Vénéréologie* 105, 887–888.

Segal, B.M. (1963) Photosensivity, nail discoloration, and photo-onycholysis: side effects of tetracycline therapy. *Archives of Internal Medicine* 112, 165–167.

Zala, L., Omar, A. & Krebs, A. (1977) Photo-onycholysis induced by 8-methoxypsoralen. *Dermatologica* 154, 203–215.

## Nail changes associated with drug-induced erythroderma

Beau's lines and onychomadesis are commonly observed in drug-induced erythroderma. A distinctive nail abnormality, which has been referred to as 'shoreline nails', has been described in three patients. All fingernails and toenails presented a transverse line of discontinuity in the nail plate that was preceded by a transverse band of leukonychia. This indicates that the drug reaction initially caused a defective keratinization of the nail matrix which was followed by a total matrix arrest. Thickened toenails showed less dramatic changes. Readministration of the drug caused the appearance of multiple bands in one patient (Shelley & Shelley 1985).

## Reference

Shelley, W.B. & Shelley, E.D. (1985) Shoreline nails: sign of drug-induced erythroderma. *Cutis* 35, 220–224.

## Nail changes associated with exposure to systemic medications in early pregnancy

The occurrence of malformations depends on the time of fetal exposure and the dose of teratogen. Nails are infrequently affected except in complete expression of each syndrome. Hydantoin, trimethadione, carbamazepine (page 305), alcohol and warfarin (page 319) are all reported to cause hypoplastic nails. Valproic acid has been associated with hyperconvex nails (page 305).

## Drugs acting on the central nervous system

### Anticonvulsant drugs

Newborn infants who have been exposed to anticonvulsant drugs during gestation have a significant increase in major malformations, including fingernail hypoplasia (Holmes *et al.* 1994). Hypoplasia of the fingernails and terminal phalanges of the fingers and sometimes the toes can occur in children whose mothers have been treated with trimethadione (Kosem & Lightner 1978) or diphenylhydantoin during the first months of pregnancy (Hanson & Smith 1975; Runne & Orfanos 1981; Oskinay *et al.* 1998). Nail hyperpigmentation may also be seen (Johnson & Goldsmith 1981). Phenytoin may cause an acute lichen planus-like eruption with nail involvement (Haneke, unpublished). A unique case of acquired acromelanosis showed diffuse pigmentation sparing the nail (Kanwar *et al.* 1997). A case of serum sickness-like disease and onychodystrophy was associated with lamotrigine (Gücüyener *et al.* 1999).

Fingernail and toenail hypoplasia has been described in the newborn of a 29-year-old epileptic woman who had been treated with carbamazepine during gestation. Regression of nail hypoplasia was observed during the first months of life (Niesen & Froscher 1985). Reversible onychomadesis is a possible side effect of carbamazepine (Prabhakara & Krupa-Shankar 1996).

Reversible onychomadesis with subsequent development of bluish-black discoloration of the nails has been reported in a 31-year-old Indian man treated with carbamazepine for a generalized partial seizure disorder. A band of longitudinal melanonychia was also present in three fingernails (Mishra *et al.* 1989).

Digital abnormalities with long, thin, partly overlapping fingers and toes, and hyperconvex nails have been reported in infants of women with epilepsy who were receiving valproic acid monotherapy (Jager-Roman *et al.* 1986). Generalized onycholysis has appeared in a 2-year-old male on sodium valproate therapy (Grech & Vella 1999).

## References

Grech, V. & Vella, C. (1999) Generalized onycholysis associated with sodium valproate therapy. *European Neurology* 42, 64–65.

Gücüyener, K., Türkas, I., Serdaroglu, A. *et al.* (1999) Suspected allergy to lamotrigine. *Allergy* **54**, 767–768.

Hanson, J.W. & Smith, D.W. (1975) The fetal hydantoin syndrome. *Journal of Pediatrics* **87**, 285–290.

Holmes, L.B., Harvey, E.A., Brown, K.S. *et al.* (1994) Anti-convulsant teratogenesis: I. A study design for newborn infants. *Teratology* **49**, 202–207.

Jager-Roman, E., Deichl, A., Jakob, S. *et al.* (1986) Fetal growth, major malformations, and minor anomalies in infants born to women receiving valproic acid. *Journal of Pediatrics* **108**, 997–1004.

Johnson, R.B. & Goldsmith, L.A. (1981) Dilantin digital defects. *Journal of the American Academy of Dermatology* **5**, 191.

Kanwar, A.J., Jaswal, R., Thami, G.P. *et al.* (1997) Acquired acro-melanosis to phenytoin. *Dermatology* **194**, 373–374.

Kosem, R.C. & Lightner, E.S. (1978) Phenotypic malformations in association with maternal trimethadione therapy. *Journal of Pediatrics* **92**, 240.

Mishra, D., Singh, G. & Pandey, S.S. (1989) Possible carbamazepine-induced reversible onychomadesis. *International Journal of Dermatology* **28**, 460–461.

Niesen, M. & Froscher, W. (1985) Finger and toenail hypoplasia after carbamazepine monotherapy in late pregnancy. *Neuropediatrics* **16**, 167–168.

Oskinay, F., Yenigün, A., Kantar, M. *et al.* (1998) Two siblings with fetal hydantoin syndrome. *Turkish Journal of Pediatrics* **40**, 273–278.

Prabhakara, V.G. & Krupa-Shankar, D.S. (1996) Reversible ony-chomadesis induced by carbamazepine. *International Journal of Dermatology, Venereology and Leprosy* **62**, 256–257.

Runne, U. & Orfanos, C.E. (1981) The human nail. *Current Problems in Dermatology* **9**, 102–149.

## Benzodiazepines

Photoonycholysis and subungual haemorrhages occurred in a 36-year-old woman treated with clorazepate dipotassium 10 mg/day for several weeks (Torras & Mascaro 1989).

## Reference

Torras, H. & Mascaro, J.M. (1989) Photo-onycholysis caused by clorazepate dipotassium. *Journal of the American Academy of Dermatology* **21**, 1304–1305.

## Tricyclic antidepressant

Leukonychia has been reported in patients treated with trazo-done hydrochloride (Longstreth & Hershman 1985; Gupta *et al.* 1987).

## References

Gupta, M.A., Gupta, A.K. & Ellis, C.N. (1987) Antidepressant drugs in dermatology. *Archives of Dermatology* **123**, 647–652.

Longstreth, G.F. & Hershman, J. (1985) Trazodone-induced hepato-toxicity and leukonychia. *Journal of the American Academy of Dermatology* **13**, 149–150.

## Phenothiazines

High doses of chlorpromazine and related substituted pheno-thiazines taken for prolonged periods produce pigmentation on exposed areas of skin, ranging from tan or slate blue to a deep blue-black or purple colour. In severe cases the nail beds are also involved (Satanove 1965). The pigmentation is cumulative and increases in intensity in the summer months, fading only slightly in the winter. The mechanism is thought to be due to increased melanin deposition. Rarely, photoonycholysis may be caused by phenothiazines.

## Reference

Satanove, A. (1965) Pigmentation due to phenothiazines in high and prolonged dosage. *Journal of the American Medical Association* **191**, 263–268.

## Lithium carbonate

Lithium therapy may induce a rich golden colour in the nail plate distally, the proximal part remaining pink (Hooper 1971). Nail growth alteration occurs on reducing the dose of lithium. Transverse brown-black pigmented bands of the fingernails fol-lowed by latent onychomadesis have also been reported (Don & Silverman 1988). Psoriasis is often aggravated or precipitated by lithium treatment. Rudolph (1991) has observed a case of psoriatic trachyonychia of the fingernails as the sole manifesta-tion of lithium ingestion (Fig. 6.79). Lithium-induced Darier's disease is so far unique (Rubin 1995).

## References

Don, P.C. & Silverman, R.A. (1988) Nail dystrophy induced by lithium carbonate. *Cutis* **84**, 19–21.

Hooper, J.F. (1971) Lithium carbonate and toenails. *American Journal of Psychiatry* **138**, 1519.

Rubin, M.R. (1995) Lithium induced-Darier's disease. *Journal of the American Academy of Dermatology* **32**, 674–675.

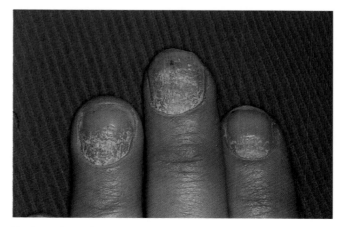

**Fig. 6.79** Lithium-induced nail dystrophy. (Courtesy of R.I. Rudolph, USA.)

Rudolph, R.I. (1991) Lithium induced psoriasis of the fingernails. *Journal of the American Academy of Dermatology* **26**, 135–136.

## Buspirone

Nail thinning can be a consequence of buspirone treatment (Daniel & Scher 1990).

### Reference

Daniel, C.R. & Scher, R.K. (eds) (1990) Nail changes secondary to systemic drugs or ingestants. In: *Nails: Therapy, Diagnosis, Surgery*, pp. 192–201. W.B. Saunders, Philadelphia.

## L-Dopa

Accelerated nail growth and hardness of the nail has been described in patients treated with L-dopa for Parkinson's disease (Miller 1973).

### Reference

Miller, E. (1973) Levodopa and nail growth. *New England Journal of Medicine* **208**, 916.

## Clomipramine

A band-like brownish discoloration developed in nails (Serdaroglu *et al.* 1995).

### Reference

Serdaroglu, S., Kosen, V. & Ozboya, T. (1995) Band-like discoloration in nail. *Deri-Hast-Frengi-Ars* **29**, 153–154.

## Cocaine

A patient developed livedo reticularis, acrocyanosis, generalized myalgias and proximal muscle weakness after the inhalation of cocaine in a base pipe. Periungual erythema, microinfarctions and diffuse swelling of the fingers were the prominent features (Zamora-Quezada *et al.* 1988).

Nasal inhalation of cocaine hydrochloride is facilitated by many devices used to transfer the cocaine to the nose. These devices include coke straw rolled paper bills and coke spoons. Some individuals grow long finger nails (typically the 5th) to use as personal coke spoons (Nolte 1995).

### References

Nolte, K.B. (1995) *Demis*, Vol. 4, unit 29–10, pp. 1–12.

Zamora-Quezada, J.C., Dineman, H., Stadecker, M.J. *et al.* (1988) Muscle and skin infarction after free-basing cocaine (crack). *Annals of Internal Medicine* **108**, 564–566.

## Retinoids (Fig. 6.80)

Synthetic retinoids have evident effects on nail keratinization. Most of the side-effects induced by retinoids on the nail apparatus can be explained as a part of the general desquamative process. The delay in the appearance of nail complications ranges from 2 weeks to 18 months after the commencement of therapy. Their occurrence is unpredictable, but the changes are far more frequent in psoriatic patients than in other subjects. Sometimes the nail changes are transient even when medication is continued (Baran 1982, 1986, 1990). Linear nail growth may be normal or more frequently decreased (Baran 1982). Accelerated fingernail growth has however been documented in patients with psoriasis (Galosi *et al.* 1985).

Nail thinning, splitting, softening and fragility are commonly seen during etretinate treatment (Ellis & Voorhees 1987). A nail biopsy obtained from a patient who developed softening, thinning and depression of the proximal nail plate showed inadequate keratinization of the nail plate in the absence of inflammatory changes (Lindskov 1982).

Although thinning of the nails can be regarded as a positive result in patients with thick psoriatic nails, some patients complain of increased sensitivity to external pressure and inability to use the nails in a functional way (Ellis & Voorhees 1987). Beau's lines, latent or complete onychomadesis, proximal onychoschizia and transverse leukonychia are possible consequences of nail matrix damage (Baran *et al.* 1983; Ferguson *et al.* 1983; Garioch & Simpson 1989).

Progressive onychoatrophy may lead to nail loss (Baran 1986). Onycholysis is an uncommon complication of etretinate therapy and even rarer with isotretinoin (Orfanos *et al.* 1978; Baran 1982; Bigby & Stern 1988). Elkonyxis has also been reported (Cannata & Gambetti 1990). A 35-year-old female treated with etretinate 0.25 mg/kg/day developed distal hemitorsion of the nail plates of several fingernails. This unusual side effect of etretinate has been referred to as 'curly nails' (Griffiths 1990). Median nail dystrophy associated with isotretinoin therapy is unusual (Bottomley & Cunliffe 1992; Dharmagunawardena & Charles-Holmes 1997).

Chronic paronychia originating from periungual psoriatic foci frequently occurs in patients with psoriasis treated with etretinate related to retention of scales on the undersurface of the proximal nail fold (Baran 1986). Pyogenic granuloma-like lesions of the nail folds may be associated with chronic paronychia or may occur separately (Hodak *et al.* 1984). Increased skin fragility along with nail plate brittleness resulting in fine spicules that break through the lateral nail grooves are possibly responsible for this peculiar side effect (Baran 1990). Pyogenic granuloma-like lesions can also occur during isotretinoin treatment (Blumental 1984; De Raeve *et al.* 1986). Ingrowing nails can occasionally be observed.

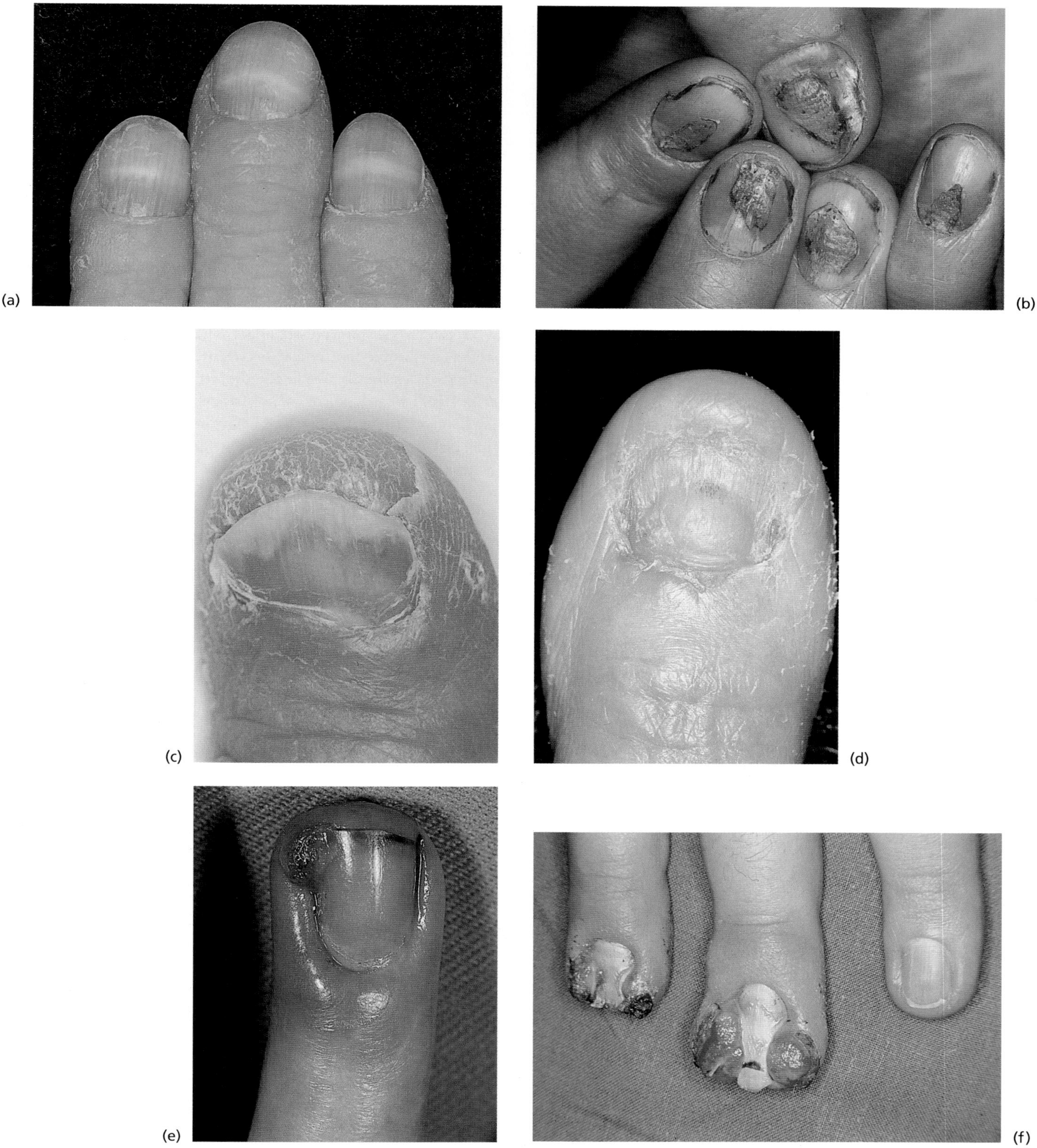

**Fig. 6.80** Nail changes due to etretinate. (a) Transverse leuconychia. (b) Proximal onychoschizia. (c) Fingertip peeling and onycholysis. (d) Nail shedding. (e) Paronychia associated with pyogenic granuloma. (Courtesy of H. Zaun, Hamburg, Germany). (f) Pyogenic granuloma. (Courtesy of J. Delescluses, Brussels.)

## References

Baran, R. (1982) Action thérapeutique et complications du rétinoide aromatique sur l'appareil unguéal. *Annales de Dermatologie et de Vénéréologie* **109**, 367–371.

Baran, R. (1986) Etretinate and the nails (study of 130 cases): possible mechanisms of some side-effects. *Clinical and Experimental Dermatology* **11**, 148–152.

Baran, R. (1990) Retinoids and the nails. *Journal of Dermatologic Treatment* **1**, 151–154.

Baran, R., Brun, P. & Juhlin, L. (1983) Leuconychie transversale induite par étrétinate. *Annales de Dermatologie et de Vénéréologie* **110**, 657.

Bigby, M. & Stern, R.S. (1988) Adverse reactions to isotretinoin. *Journal of the American Academy of Dermatology* **18**, 543–552.

Blumental, G. (1984) Paronychia and pyogenic granuloma-like lesions with isotretinoin. *Journal of the American Academy of Dermatology* **4**, 677–678.

Bottomley, W.W. & Cunliffe, W.J. (1992) Median nail dystrophy associated with isotretinoin therapy. *British Journal of Dermatology* **127**, 447–448.

Cannata, G. & Gambetti, M. (1990) Elkonyxis: une complication méconnue de l'étrétinate. *Nouvelle Dermatologie* **9**, 251.

Dharmagunawardena, B., Charles-Holmes, R. (1997) Median canaliform dystrophy following isotretinoin therapy. *British Journal of Dermatology* **137**, 646–647.

De Raeve, L., Willemsen, M., De Coninck, A. *et al.* (1986) Paronychie et formation de tissu granuleux au cours d'un traitement par isotrétinoine. *Dermatologica* **172**, 278–280.

Ellis, C.N. & Voorhees, J.J. (1987) Etretinate therapy. *Journal of the American Academy of Dermatology* **16**, 267–291.

Ferguson, M.M., Simpson, N.B. & Hammersley, N. (1983) Severe nail dystrophy associated with retinoid therapy. *Lancet* **ii**, 974.

Galosi, A., Plewig, G. & Braun-Falco, O. (1985) The effect of aromatic retinoid RO 10-9359 (Etretinate) on fingernail growth. *Archives of Dermatological Research* **277**, 138–140.

Garioch, J. & Simpson, N.B. (1989) Etretinate and severe nail plate dystrophies. *Clinical and Experimental Dermatology* **14**, 261–262.

Griffiths, W.A.D. (1990) 'Curly nails'—an unusual side-effect of etretinate. *Journal of Dermatologic Treatment* **1**, 265–266.

Hodak, E., David, M. & Feuerman, E.J. (1984) Excess granulation tissue during etretinate therapy. *Journal of the American Academy of Dermatology* **11**, 1166–1167.

Lindskov, R. (1982) Soft nails after treatment with aromatic retinoids. *Archives of Dermatology* **118**, 535–536.

Orfanos, C.E., Landes, E. & Bloch, P.H. (1978) Traitement du psoriasis pustuleux par un nouveau rétinoide aromatique (RO 10-9359). *Annales de Dermatologie et de Vénéréologie* **105**, 807–811.

## Liarozole

Liarozole, the first retinoic acid metabolism-blocking agent used for advanced prostate cancer, is responsible for nail disorders (16% of patients reported by Debruyne *et al.* 1998).

## Reference

Debruyne, F.J.M., Murray, R., Fradet, Y. *et al.* (1998). Liarozole—a novel treatment approach for advanced prostate cancer. Results of a large randonized trial versus cyproteron-acetate. *Urology* **52**, 72–81.

## Psoralens

Photoonycholysis can develop in patients undergoing PUVA therapy or treated with sunlight and orally administered psoralens (Briffa & Warin 1977). It is often painful and has been reported after the administration of both 8-methoxypsoralen (Zala *et al.* 1977; Mackie 1979; Balato *et al.* 1984) and 5-methoxypsoralen (Baran & Barthélémy 1990). Fingernails are more commonly affected than toenails. Splinter haemorrhages and subungual haematoma may be seen with onycholysis (Zala *et al.* 1977; Balato *et al.* 1984). The nail biopsy of a patient who developed photoonycholysis after 8-methoxypsoralen treatment showed multinucleate cells in the nail epithelium and multinucleate fibroblasts in the dermis of the nail bed (Zala *et al.* 1977). Beau's lines have been occasionally associated with photoonycholysis (Rau *et al.* 1978; Mackie 1979). Longitudinal melanonychia can also be seen in the fingernails of patients treated with 8-methoxypsoralen or 5-methoxypsoralen and ultraviolet irradiation (Naik & Singh 1979; Weiss & Sayegh-Carreno 1989). Pigmentation of the proximal portion of fingernail plates has been reported by Hann *et al.* (1989).

## References

Balato, N., Giordano, C., Montesano, M. *et al.* (1984) 8-methoxypsoralen-induced photo-onycholysis. *Photodermatology* **1**, 202–203.

Baran, R. & Barthélémy, H. (1990) Photo-onycholyse induite par le 5-MOP (Psoraderm) et application de la méthode d'imputation des effets medicamenteux. *Annales de Dermatologie et de Vénéréologie* **117**, 367–369.

Briffa, D.V. & Warin, A.P. (1977) Photo-onycholysis caused by photochemotherapy. *British Medical Journal* **2**, 1150.

Hann, S.K., Hwang, S.Y. & Park, Y.K. (1989) Melanonychia induced by systemic photochemotherapy. *Photodermatology* **6**, 98–99.

Mackie, R.M. (1979) Onycholysis occurring during PUVA therapy. *Clinical and Experimental Dermatology* **4**, 111–113.

Naik, R.P.C. & Singh, G. (1979) Nail pigmentation due to oral 8-methoxypsoralen. *British Journal of Dermatology* **100**, 229–230.

Rau, R.C., Flowers, F.P. & Barrett, J.L. (1978) Photo-onycholysis secondary to psoralen use. *Archives of Dermatology* **114**, 448.

Weiss, E. & Sayegh-Carreno, R. (1989) PUVA-induced pigmented nails. *International Journal of Dermatology* **28**, 188–189.

Zala, L., Omar, A. & Krebs, A. (1977) Photo-onycholysis induced by 8-methoxypsoralen. *Dermatologica* **154**, 203–215.

## Antimicrobial agents

### Tetracyclines

Yellow fluorescence of the lunulae under Wood's lamp examination can be seen in patients taking tetracyclines hydrochloride in dosages of 1 g or more daily. It can be useful for monitoring patient compliance. A reversible yellow pigmentation of the lunulae occurred in a 26-year-old man treated with tetracycline hydrochloride for acne. The yellow lunulae fluoresced on Wood's lamp examination (Hendricks 1980). Yellow discoloration of the entire nail plate has also been reported during tetracycline treatment. Reddish nail fluorescence may follow demethylchlortetracycline therapy (Zaun & Dill-Müller 1999).

Photoonycholysis is a possible side effect of treatment with tetracyclines (page 302). Among the tetracycline group, demethylchlortetracycline is the most common cause followed by doxycycline (Orentreich *et al.* 1961; Cavens 1981; Jeanmougin *et al.* 1982). Minocycline has been occasionally incriminated whereas oxytetracycline and tetracycline hydrochloride rarely induce this side effect. Beau's lines and subungual haemorrhages can occur in association with photoonycholysis (Harris 1950; Domonkos 1973). A patient who developed Raynaud's phenomenon of the left middle finger and photoonycholysis of the left hand after treatment with demethylchlortetracycline has been reported (Carter 1966). Onycholysis that is not sun related can also occur in patients on tetracycline (Daniel & Scher 1984).

Minocycline can occasionally cause abnormal pigmentation of the skin, thyroid, nails, bone, sclera, conjunctiva as well as permanent discoloration of the teeth (Poliak *et al.* 1985; Pepine *et al.* 1993). Nail pigmentation during minocycline treatment is rare and is seen accompained by cutaneous pigmentation. A blue-grey or slate-grey discoloration of the proximal portion of the nail bed (Fig. 6.81) as well as longitudinal brown pigmented bands or diffuse darkening and hyperpigmentation of the nail plate have been reported (Angeloni *et al.* 1987). Pigmentation of the proximal nail folds can also occur (Mooney & Bennet 1988). An iron chelate of minocycline has been suggested as the cause of the nail pigmentation. Elemental analysis of nail clippings from a minocycline-treated patient showed the presence of a large amount of iron in pigmented areas of the nail but not in the adjacent normal nail. The possibility that nail polish is the source of iron in the pigmented nails is supported by the observation that minocycline-induced nail pigmentation occurs almost exclusively in women (Gordon *et al.* 1985).

Pigment deposits in eyes and light-exposed skin may appear during long-term methacycline therapy (Dyster-Aas *et al.* 1974). Under Wood's light, within the first proximal millimetres there is a yellow-green fluorescence. The nail plate distal to the lunula may develop a spontaneous cyanotic appearance.

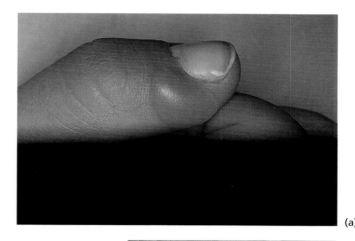

(a)

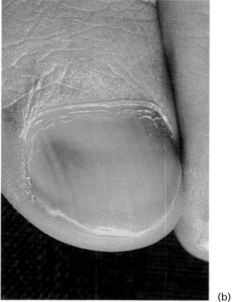

**Fig. 6.81** (a) Tetracycline—fixed bullous eruption. (b) Minocycline-induced nail pigmentation.

(b)

## References

Angeloni, V.L., Salasche, S.J. & Ortiz, R. (1987) Nail, skin and scleral pigmentation induced by minocycline. *Cutis* **40**, 229–233.

Carter, W.I. (1966) Disorders of the nails. *British Medical Journal* **2**, 1198–1199.

Cavens, T.R. (1981) Onycholysis of the thumbs probably due to a phototoxic reaction from doxycycline. *Cutis* **27**, 53–54.

Daniel, C.R. & Scher, R.K. (1984) Nail changes secondary to systemic drugs or ingestants. *Journal of the American Academy of Dermatology* **10**, 250–258.

Domonkos, A.N. (1973) Phototoxic onycholysis. *Archives of Dermatology* **108**, 733.

Dyster-Aas, K., Hanson, H., Miörner, G. *et al.* (1974) Pigment deposits in eyes and light exposed skin during longterm methacycline therapy. *Acta Dermato-Venereologica* **54**, 209–222.

Gordon, G., Sparano, B.M. & Iatropoulos, M.J. (1985) Hyperpigmentation of the skin associated with minocycline therapy. *Archives of Dermatology* **121**, 618–623.

Harris, H.J. (1950) Aureomycin and chloramphenicol in brucellosis. *Journal of the American Medical Association* **142**, 161–165.

Hendricks, A.A. (1980) Yellow lunulae with fluorescence after tetracycline therapy. *Archives of Dermatology* **116**, 438–440.

Jeanmougin, M., Morel, P. & Civatte, J. (1982) Photoonycholyse induite par la doxycycline. *Annales de Dermatologie et de Vénéréologie* **109**, 165–166.

Mooney, E. & Bennett, R.G. (1988) Periungual hyperpigmentation mimicking Hutchinson's sign associated with minocycline administration. *Journal of Dermatologic Surgery and Oncology* **14**, 1011–1013.

Orentreich, N., Harber, L.C. & Tromovitch, T.A. (1961) Photosensitivity and photo-onycholysis due to demethylchlortetracycline. *Archives of Dermatology* **83**, 730–737.

Pepine, M., Flowers, F.P. & Ramos-Caro, F. (1993) Extensive cutaneous hyperpigmentation caused by minocycline. *Journal of the American Academy of Dermatology* **28**, 292–295.

Poliak, S.C., Di Giovanna, J.J., Gross, E.G. *et al.* (1985) Minocycline-associated tooth discoloration in young adults. *Journal of the American Medical Association* **254**, 2930–2932.

Zaun, H. & Dill-Müller, D. (1999) *Krankhafte Veränderungen des Nagels*, p. 60, 7th edn. SpittaVerlag, Balingen.

## Cephalosporin

A periungual inflammatory reaction resembling acute paronychia has been described in two fingers of a patient taking cephalexine (Fig. 6.82). The reaction resolved without residual pigmentation but recurred after readministration of the drug (Baran & Perrin 1991). Shedding of the nails resulted from the administration of large doses of cephaloridine and cloxacillin in patients on maintenance haemodialysis (Eastwood *et al.* 1969).

### References

Baran, R. & Perrin, C. (1991) Fixed drug eruption presenting as an acute paronychia. *British Journal of Dermatology* **125**, 592–595.

Eastwood, J.B., Curtis, J.R., Smith, E.K.M. *et al.* (1969) Shedding of nails apparently induced by the administration of large amounts of cephaloridine and cloxacillin in two anephric patients. *British Journal of Dermatology* **81**, 750–752.

## Chloramphenicol

Onycholysis and photoonycholysis are rare complications of chloramphenicol treatment (Runne & Orfanos 1981).

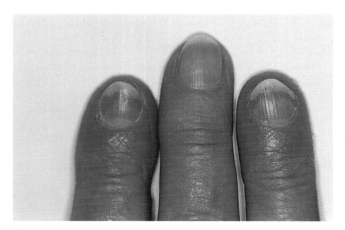

**Fig. 6.82** Acute paronychia due to cephalexine involving the 2nd and 4th fingers.

### Reference

Runne, U. & Orfanos, C.E. (1981) The human nail. *Current Problems in Dermatology* **9**, 102–149.

## Clofazimine

Two patients developed brown discoloration of the nail plate, subungual hyperkeratosis and onycholysis during treatment with clofazimine at high doses for lepromatous leprosy (Dixit *et al.* 1989). Clofazimine crystals were demonstrated in the nail plate and in the nail bed. The nail changes regressed when the dose of drug was reduced. Reversible melanonychia has also been reported in a 55-year-old man treated with 300 mg/day of clofazimine for 6 months because of granuloma faciale (Tosti *et al.* 1992).

### References

Dixit, V.B., Chaudhary, S.D. & Jain, V.K. (1989) Clofazimine induced nail changes. *International Journal of Leprosy* **61**, 476–478.

Tosti, A., Piraccini, B.M., Guerra, L. *et al.* (1992) Reversible melanonychia due to clofazimine. In: *18th World Congress of Dermatology, Book of Abstracts*, 183A. Springer Verlag. Berlin.

## Quinolones

Photoonycholysis has been reported after treatment with flumequine, pefloxacine and ofloxacine (Revuz & Pouget 1983; Baran & Brun 1986). Subungual haemorrhage was associated with photoonycholysis in one patient (Baran & Brun 1986).

### References

Baran, R. & Brun, P. (1986) Photoonycholysis induced by the fluoroquinolones pefloxacine and ofloxacine. *Dermatologica* **176**, 185–188.

Revuz, J. & Pouget, F. (1983) Photo-onycholyse à l'apurone. *Annales de Dermatologie et de Vénéréologie* **110**, 765.

## Roxithromycin

A brownish discoloration of both thumbs followed after a second course of roxithromycin by fresh pigmentation over other fingernails (Dawn *et al.* 1995).

### Reference

Dawn, G., Kanvar, A.J. & Dhar, S. (1995) Nail pigmentation due to roxithromycin. *Dermatology* **191**, 342–343.

## Sulphonamides

Onychomadesis, Beau's lines, paronychia, partial leuconychia and reduction of the nail growth may occur in patients who develop a photosensitivity reaction during sulphonamide treatment (Baran & Témime 1973). Trimethoprim–sulphamethoxazole (sulfamethoxazole) was suspected for loss of all nails in a case reported by Slaughenhoupt *et al.* (1999).

## References

Baran, R. & Témime, P. (1973) Les onychodystrophies toxi-medicamenteuses et les oncholyses. *Concours Medical* 95, 1007–1023.

Slaughenhoupt, B.L., Adeagbo, S. & Van Savage, J.G. (1999) A suspected case of trimethoprim-sulfamethoxazole-induced loss of finger and toenails. *Pediatric Infectious Disease Journal* 18, 76–77.

## Dapsone

Beau's lines occurred in a 35-year-old female with borderline lepromatous leprosy who developed dapsone hypersensitivity with erythroderma (Patki & Mehta 1989). A severe but temporary hair loss and the appearance of transverse grooves followed the dapsone syndrome (high temperature, morbilliform rash, lymphadenopathy and hepatitis) (Kromann *et al.* 1982).

## References

Kromann, N.P., Vilhelmsen, R. & Stahl, D. (1982) The dapsone syndrome. *Archives of Dermatology* 118, 531–532.

Patki, A.K. & Mehta, J.M. (1989) Dapsone-induced erythroderma with Beau's lines. *Leprosy Review* 60, 274–277.

## Emetine

White nails have been described in patients treated with emetine (de Nicola *et al.* 1974). They may become atrophic and brittle (Manson-Bahr 1945).

## References

Manson-Bahr, P. (1945) *Manson's Tropical Diseases*. Williams & Wilkins Baltimore.

De Nicola, P., Morsiani, M. & Zavagli, G. (1974) *Nail Diseases in Internal Medicine*, p. 54. Charles Thomas, Springfield, IL.

## Antiretroviral drugs

Nucleotide analogue reverse transcriptase inhibitors

## Didanosine

A painful acral erythema resembling the painful desquamating erythema of the palms and soles has been reported in HIV patients taking didanosine. The eruption cleared spontaneously without discontinuation of treatment (Pedailles *et al.* 1993).

## Lamivudine

Paronychia and pseudopyogenic granulomas affecting the toenails and the fingernails have been reported during lamivudine treatment (Zerboni *et al.* 1998; Tosti *et al.* 1999). Longitudinal melanonychia of the fingernails appeared 4 weeks after treatment with 300 mg daily. The streaks disappeared after the drug was stopped and reappeared on rechallenge (Schattenkirchner *et al.* 1995).

## Azidothymidine (AZT, zidovudine)

Various patterns of nail pigmentation have been described in patients receiving azidothymidine (Fig. 6.83). Black or heavily pigmented patients more commonly develop nail hyperpigmentation, which has been estimated to occur in about 12–67% of the patients using the drug (Groark *et al.* 1989; Don *et al.* 1990; Tosti *et al.* 1990). Bluish to brown diffuse nail discoloration as well as transverse or longitudinal banding have been described (Furth & Kazakis 1987; Panwalker 1987; Azon-Masoliver *et al.* 1988). A faint blue pigmentation of the lunulae was found by Greenberg and Berger (1990). Fingernails seem to be more commonly affected than toenails. Nail pigmentation usually occurs within 8 weeks but could occur after 1 year of therapy. It appears to be reversible when the use of AZT is discontinued or the dosage is reduced significantly. Histological studies have shown that AZT-induced nail pigmentation is due to melanin deposition (Grau-Massanes *et al.* 1990; Tosti *et al.* 1990). Nail matrix toxicity induced by the drug may result in matrix melanocyte stimulation (Fisher & McPoland 1989; Groark *et al.* 1990).

Slow nail growth has also been reported (Fischer & McPoland 1989).

Severe paronychia of the great toes developed in a 4-week-old baby treated with AZT following perinatal HIV exposure. Microbiology revealed *Candida albicans* and *Escherichia coli*, while laboratory tests showed anaemia and neutropenia. Paronychia resolved after treatment with oral fluconazole and topical antiseptics (Russo *et al.* 1999).

## References

Azon-Masoliver, A., Mallolas, J., Gatell, J. *et al.* (1988) Zidovudine-induced nail pigmentation. *Archives of Dermatology* 124, 1570–1571.

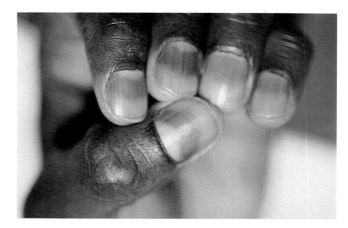

**Fig. 6.83** AZT (azidothymidine, zidovudine)-induced nail pigmentation.

Don, P.C., Fusco, F., Fried, P. *et al.* (1990) Nail dyschromia associated with zidovudine. *Annals of Internal Medicine* 112, 145–146.

Fisher, C.A. & McPoland, P.R. (1989) Azidothymidine-induced nail pigmentation. *Cutis* 43, 552–554.

Furth, P.A. & Kazakis, A.M. (1987) Nail pigmentation changes associated with azidothymidine (zidovudine). *Annals of Internal Medicine* 107, 350–351.

Grau-Massanes, M., Millan, F., Febrer, M.I. *et al.* (1990) Pigmented nail bands and mucocutaneous pigmentation in HIV-positive patients treated with zidovudine. *Journal of the American Academy of Dermatology* 22, 687–688.

Greenberg, R.G. & Berger, T.G. (1990) Nail and mucocutaneous hyperpigmentation with azidothymidine therapy. *Journal of the American Academy of Dermatology* 22, 327–330.

Groark, S.P., Hood, A.F. & Nelson, K. (1990) Nail pigmentation associated with zidovudine. *Journal of the American Academy of Dermatology* 21, 1032–1033.

Panwalker, A.P. (1987) Nail pigmentation in the acquired immunodeficiency syndrome (AIDS). *Annals of Internal Medicine* 107, 943–944.

Pedailles, S., Launay, V., Surbled, M. *et al.* (1993) Erythème acral survenant après prise de didanosine (Videx). *Annales de Dermatologie et de Vénéréologie* 120, 837–840.

Russo, F., Collantes, C. & Guerrero, J. (1999) Severe paronychia due to zidovudine-induced neutropenia in a neonate. *Journal of the American Academy of Dermatology* 40, 322–324.

Schattenkircher, S., Koschitzki, C. & Rasokat, H. (1995) Streifenförmige Nagelverfärbung unter Lamiduvine. *Zeitschrift für Hautkrankheiten* 70, 915–916.

Tosti, A., Gaddoni, G., Fanti, P.A. *et al.* (1990) Longitudinal melanonychia induced by 3′-azidodeoxythymidine. *Dermatologica* 180, 217–220.

Tosti, A., Piraccini, B.M., D'Antuono, A. *et al.* (1999) Periungual inflammation and pyogenic granulomas during treatment with the antiretroviral drugs Lamivudine and Indinavir. *British Journal of Dermatology* 140, 1165–1168.

Zerboni, R., Angius, A.G., Cusini, M. *et al.* (1998) Lamivudine-induced paronychia. *Lancet* 351, 1256.

## Protease inhibitors

Paronychia, ingrowing nails, onycholysis and pseudopyogenic granulomas of the great toes have been reported in 42 AIDS patients receiving multiple antiretroviral therapy. In all patients the nail lesions developed after the introduction of the protease inhibitor indinavir (Bouscarat *et al.* 1998).

## Reference

Bouscarat, F., Bouchard, C. & Bouhour, D. (1998) Paronychia and pyogenic granuloma of the great toes in patients treated with indinavir. *New England Journal of Medicine* 338, 1776–1777.

## Antifungals

### Itraconazole

Itraconazole treatment may produce an increase in the nail growth rate. This may be due to the antioxidant effects of itraconazole and its metabolite hydroxy-itraconazole (Guerra *et al.* 1997). Accelerated nail growth has been associated with the development of longitudinal beading of the nail plate (de Doncker & Pierard 1994). This property of itraconazole has been successfully utilized for treating patients with the yellow nail syndrome (Luyten *et al.* 1996; A. Tosti *et al.* unpublished data).

## References

de Doncker, P. & Pierard, G.E. (1994) Acquired nail beading in patients receiving itraconazole—an indicator of faster nail growth? A study using optical profilometry. *Clinical and Experimental Dermatology* 19, 404–406.

Guerra, L., Tosti, A., Ver Donck, K. *et al.* (1997) Effects of itraconazole on *in vitro* cultured nail matrix keratinocytes. *Australasian Journal of Dermatology* 36 (Suppl. 2), 283.

Luyten, C., André, J., Walraevens, C. *et al.* (1996) Yellow nail syndrome. Experience with itraconazole pulse therapy combined with vitamin E. *Dermatology* 192, 406–408.

### Fluconazole

Accelerated nail growth has been reported after treatment with fluconazole (Shelley & Shelley 1992). Longitudinal melanonychia appeared after 1 month's treatment. The band remained for 3 months after cessation of fluconazole (Kar 1998).

## References

Kar, H.K. (1998) Longitudinal melanonychia with fluconazole therapy. *International Journal of Dermatology* 37, 719–720.

Shelley, W.B. & Shelley, E.D. (1992) Portrait of a practice. *Cutis* 49, 386.

### Ketoconazole

Splinter haemorrhages and longitudinal pigmented bands have been described in patients taking ketoconazole (Positano *et al.* 1989).

## Reference

Positano, R.G., DeLauro, T.M. & Berkowitz, B.J. (1989) Nail changes secondary to environmental influences. *Clinics in Podiatric Medicine and Surgery* 6, 417–429.

### Amorolfine

Bluish or yellow-brown discoloration of the nail plate has been reported in patients who erroneously applied amorolfine 5% nail lacquer on a daily, rather than weekly, basis. The pigmentation does not occur in all patients and is possibly due to oxidation of one of the constituents of the formulation (Rigopoulos *et al.* 1996).

## Reference

Rigopoulos, D., Katsambas, A., Antoniou, C. et al. (1996) Discoloration of the nail plate due to the misuse of amorolfine 5% nail lacquer. *Acta Dermato-Venereologica* 76, 83–84.

## Anti-inflammatory agents

### Acetanilid

Acetanilid can produce purple discoloration of the nails (Positano et al. 1989).

## Reference

Positano, R.G., DeLauro, T.M. & Berkowitz, B.J. (1989) Nail changes secondary to environmental influences. *Clinics in Podiatric Medicine and Surgery* 6, 417–429.

### Aspirin

Purpura of the nail bed can be seen in patients taking aspirin.

### Benoxaprofen

Benoxaprofen is a non-steroidal anti-inflammatory agent that has been withdrawn from the market because of its serious side effects. Photoonycholysis was a common side effect of benoxaprofen treatment (McCormack et al. 1982). Benoxaprofen-induced photosensitivity and onycholysis are possibly related to the ability of the drug to stimulate spontaneous oxidative metabolism and degranulation of human leucocytes (Anderson & Anderson 1982). Onycholysis was seen in toes, without photoonycholysis (Fenton 1982). Accelerated nail growth has been reported in patients treated with benoxaprofen (Fenton et al. 1982; Fenton & Wilkinson 1983). Koilonychia has also been described.

## References

Anderson, R. & Anderson, I.F. (1982) The possible value of retinoic acid in the treatment of benoxaprofen-induced photosensitivity and onycholysis. *African Medical Journal* 26, 985.

Fenton, D.A. (1982) Side effects of benoxaprofen. *British Medical Journal* 284, 1631.

Fenton, D.A. & Wilkinson, J.D. (1983) Milia, increased nail growth and hypertrichosis following treatment with benoxaprofen. *Journal of the Royal Society of Medicine* 76, 525–527.

Fenton, D.A., English, J.S. & Wilkinson, J.D. (1982) Reversal of male-pattern baldness, hypertrichosis, and accelerated hair and nail growth in patients receiving benoxaprofen. *British Medical Journal* 284, 1228–1229.

McCormack, L.S., Elgart, M.L. & Turner, M.L. (1982) Benoxaprofen-induced photo-onycholysis. *Journal of the American Academy of Dermatology* 7, 678–680.

### Ibuprofen

Longitudinal melanonychia has been reported by Daniel and Scher (1990).

## Reference

Daniel, C.R. & Scher, R.K. (1990) Nail changes secondary to systemic drugs or ingestant. In: *Nails: Therapy, Diagnosis, Surgery* (eds R.K. Scher & C.R. Daniel), pp. 192–201. W.B. Saunders, Philadelphia.

### Phenazopyridine

Deep lemon-yellow discoloration of the nails has been reported in a patient taking phenazopyridine 300 mg/day for more than 3 years. Although the patient was also mildly icteric, nail discoloration was not related to hyperbilirubinaemia, but was possibly due to drug toxicity (Amit & Halkin 1997).

## Reference

Amit, G. & Halkin, A. (1997) Lemon-yellow nails and long-term phenazopyridine use. *Annals of Internal Medicine* 127, 1137.

## Cardiovascular drugs

### β-Blockers

β-Blockers have been implicated in the cause of psoriasiform skin eruptions and the exacerbation of pre-existing psoriasis (Gold et al. 1988). Histopathology in a case with mucous membrane, scrotal and nail involvement showed a mixed psoriasiform and lichenoid reaction. There was a mild acanthosis of matrix and nail bed epithelium, a spongiosis with mononuclear exocytosis, hypergranulosis and hyperorthokeratosis. Some polymorphonuclear leucocytes were found just beneath the hyperkeratosis. A band-like, mainly lymphocytic, infiltrate was found in the papillary dermis. Although some basal cells were swollen, hydropic degeneration of the basal layer was not a pronounced feature (E. Haneke, unpublished data). Psoriasis-like nail changes have been reported during treatment with the β-blocker agent practolol. Reversible pincer nails occurred in a 48-year-old woman treated with practolol. Painful narrowing of the nail bed and excessive transverse overcurvature were associated with subungual hyperkeratosis, onycholysis and brownish discoloration of the nail plate (Tegner 1976).

Pitting, thickening and discoloration of the nail plate (Fig. 6.84) have been described during propanolol treatment. Tiny periungual pustules can also occur (Jensen et al. 1976). Beau's lines and alopecia have been reported during metoprolol treatment (Graeber & Lapkin 1981).

Cold extremities and Raynaud's phenomenon are possible side effects of β-blocker treatment of hypertension. Pterygium inversum unguis can also occur. Peripheral ischaemia leading to digital gangrene is a rare complication of β-blocker treat-

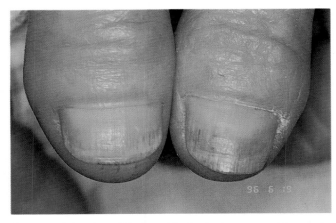

**Fig. 6.84** Nail plate pitting, thickening and discoloration due to propranolol treatment.

ment, which almost exclusively occurs in patients with hypertension. Although both cardioselective (atenolol, metoprolol, acebutolol) and non-selective (propanolol, timolol, oxyprenol) β-blockers can cause digital necrosis, propanolol is more commonly responsible (Stringer & Bentley 1980; Dompmartin *et al.* 1988). Reversion of symptoms do not always follow withdrawal of the drug and digital or limb amputation has been the final outcome in several patients.

The occurrence of acral skin necrosis is related to the twofold effect of β-blockers on the peripheral circulation. In fact, the reflex vasoconstriction (mediated by β-adrenoreceptors), which occurs in response to the reduction in cardiac output, can not be compensated by vasodilatation because of the β-receptors blockage. Elderly and hypertensive patients who have an acquired deficiency of β-receptors are more sensitive to the ischaemic effects of β-blockers.

A patient with phaeochromocytoma developed acral skin necrosis along with splinter haemorrhages and periungual telangiectases after taking atenolol. Her skin biopsy showed epidermal and sweat-gland necrosis (Naeyaert *et al.* 1987). Reversible symmetrical brown discoloration of the fingernails and toenails has been reported in a 56-year-old woman affected by glaucoma who was treated with timolol maleate 0.5% eyedrops (Feiler-Ofry *et al.* 1981).

## References

Dompmartin, A., Le Maitre, M., Letessier, D. *et al.* (1988) Nécroses digitales sous beta-bloquants. *Annales de Dermatologie et de Vénéréologie* **115**, 593–596.

Feiler-Ofry, V., Godel, V. & Lazar, M. (1981) Nail pigmentation following timolol maleate therapy. *Ophthalmologica* **182**, 153–156.

Graeber, C.W. & Lapkin, R.A. (1981) Metoprolol and alopecia. *Cutis* **28**, 633–634.

Gold, M.H., Holy, A.K. & Roenigk, H.H. Jr (1988) Beta-blocking drugs and psoriasis: a review of cutaneous side-effects and retrospective analysis of their effects on psoriasis. *Journal of the American Academy of Dermatology* **19**, 837–841.

Jensen, H.A.E., Mikkelson, H.I., Wadskov, S. *et al.* (1976) Cutaneous reactions to propanolol (Inderal). *Acta Medica Scandinavica* **199**, 363–367.

Naeyaert, J.M., Deram, E., Santosa, S. *et al.* (1987) Sweat-gland necrosis after beta-adrenergic antagonist treatment in a patient with pheochromocytoma. *British Journal of Dermatology* **117**, 371–376.

Stringer, M.D. & Bentley, P.G. (1986) Peripheral gangrene associated with β-blockade. *British Journal of Surgery* **73**, 1008.

Tegner, E. (1976) Reversible overcurvature of the nails after treatment with practolol. *Acta Dermato-Venereologica* **56**, 493–495.

## Amiodarone

Cases of hypothyroidism and hyperhyroidism have been associated with amiodarone therapy. Nail abnormalities have been reported in patients with clinical hypothyroidism secondary to amiodarone treatment (Khanderia *et al.* 1993).

## Reference

Khanderia, U., Jaffe, C.A. & Theisen, V. (1993) Amiodarone-induced thyroid dysfunction. *Clinical Pharmacology* **12**, 774–779.

## Angiotensin-converting enzyme inhibitors

Nail abnormalities have been associated with treatment with the antihypertensive drugs captopril and enalapril (Jacobs *et al.* 1992). Reversible onycholysis has been reported in patients treated with captopril (Brueggemeyer & Ramirez 1984). A lichenoid skin eruption associated with hair loss, ageusia and nail dystrophy occurred in a patient with renal insufficiency treated with captopril (Smit *et al.* 1983) (Fig. 6.85).

## References

Brueggemeyer, C. & Ramirez, G. (1984) Onycholysis associated with captopril. *Lancet* i, 1352–1353.

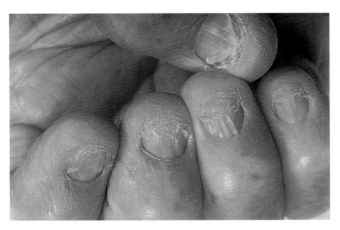

**Fig. 6.85** Captopril nail atrophy (lichen planus-like).

Jacobs, M.C., Tennstedt, D., Gengoux, P. *et al.* (1992) Eruption psori-asiforme atypique induite par le lisinopril. *Nouvelles Dermatolog-iques* **11**, 763–766.

Smit, A.J., Hoorntje, S.J. & Donker, A.J.M. (1983) Zinc deficiency dur-ing captopril treatment. *Nephron* **34**, 196–197.

## Clonidine

Raynaud's syndrome is a possible side effect of clonidine treat-ment (Delanoe & Puissant 1974).

### Reference

Delanoe, J. & Puissant, A. (1974) Les principaux medicaments respons-able des toxidermies. *La Revue de Medicine* **19**, 1199–1212.

## Calcium channel blockers

A 'nail dystrophy' has been reported in association with nifedipine, verapamil or diltiazem treatment (Stern & Khalsa 1989). A high frequency of psoriasiform eruptions is stressed by Kitamura *et al.* (1993). Pemphigoid nodularis resulted from nifedipine administration and produced pterygium unguis of the fingers and toes (Ameen *et al.* 2000).

### References

Ameen, M., Harman, K.E. & Black, M.M. (2000) Pemphigoid nodu-laris associated with nifedipine. *British Journal of Dermatology* **142**, 575–576.

Kitamura, K., Kanasashi, M., Suga, C. *et al.* (1993) Cutaneous reactions induced by calcium channel blocker. High frequency of psoriasiform eruptions. *Journal of Dermatology* **20**, 279–286.

Stern, R. & Khalsa, J.H. (1989) Cutaneous adverse reactions asso-ciated with calcium channel blockers. *Archives of Internal Medicine* **149**, 829–832.

## Quinidine

Horizontal blue-grey discoloration of the nail bed has been described in the fingernails and toenails of an 83-year-old man receiving quinidine (Mahler *et al.* 1986). This antiarrhythmic agent is the D isomer of quinine and has structural similarities with synthetic antimalarials (page 319).

### Reference

Mahler, R., Sissons, W. & Watters, K. (1986) Pigmentation induced by quinidine therapy. *Archives of Dermatology* **122**, 1062–1064.

## Amrinone

Nail discoloration has been observed during amrinone therapy (Wilsmhurst & Webb-Peploe 1983).

### Reference

Wilsmhurst, P.T. & Webb-Peploe, M.M. (1983) Side effects of amrin-one therapy. *British Heart Journal* **49**, 447–451.

## Purgatives

A bluish discoloration of the lunulae can be observed in patients treated with phenolphthalein (Campbell 1931). Paronychia-like changes and nail plate ridging have also been described (Wise & Sulzberger 1933). The differential diagnosis includes azure lunulae due to argyria or to Wilson's disease. Reversible finger clubbing has been reported in purgative abuse (page 259).

### References

Campbell, G.G. (1931) Peculiar pigmentation following the use of a purgative containing phenolphthalein. *British Journal of Dermato-logy* **43**, 186–187.

Wise, F. & Sulzberger, M.B. (1933) Drug eruptions. *Archives of Dermatology Syphiligraphie* **27**, 549–567.

## Intoxicants

### Toxic oil syndrome

In 1981 a multisystem disease occurred in Spain, after inges-tion of denatured rapeseed oil. Raynaud's phenomenon and scleroderma-like changes were commonly observed during the chronic phase of the disease (Noriega *et al.* 1982; Alonso-Ruiz *et al.* 1984).

### References

Alonso-Ruiz, A., Zea-Mendoza, A.C., Gonzales-Lanza, M. *et al.* (1984) Digital tuft alterations in toxic oil syndrome. *Lancet* **ii**, 520–521.

Noriega, A.R., Gomez-Reino, J., Lopez-Encuentra, A. *et al.* (1982) Toxic epidemic syndrome, Spain, 1981. *Lancet* **ii**, 697–702.

### Polychlorinated biphenyl intoxication

Nail pigmentation has been reported in polychlorinated biphenyl- (PCB)-exposed workers. Nail deformities occurred in 68% of patients with PCB poisoning due to the consumption of rice-bran cooking oil contaminated by large amounts of polychlorinated biphenyls and congeners. Flattened nails were noted in a quarter of Urabe and Asahi's patients (1984), ingrowing nails and lamellar dystrophy were also common.

Dark brown pigmentation was frequently seen on the finger-nails and toenails (Wong *et al.* 1982). Nail deformities were also frequently observed in children born from a few months to several years after maternal PCB poisoning. Nail deformities included koilonychia, transverse grooves, ridging, thinning, longitudinal splitting, onychauxis and transverse overcurva-ture. Hyperpigmentation of the nail plate and bed was also observed. Toenails were affected more than fingernails (Gladen *et al.* 1990).

Eighty-eight children born to mothers living in Yu-Cheng who were poisoned by PCB-contaminated cooking oil were examined by Hsu *et al.* (1995). Among the dermatological manifestations were nail abnormalities in about one-third of the exposed patients. Transverse grooves, irregular depressions, koilonychia and nail flattening were significantly more frequent than in the control group. This study indicates that the nail changes are the most persistent abnormality and their occurrence may indicate developmental retardation of the fetal nail matrix. Such a finding might suggest that PCB remaining in the mother could exert an effect on nail growth in children born several years after the intoxication event.

## References

Gladen, B.C., Taylor, J.S., Wu, Y.C. *et al.* (1990) Dermatological findings in children exposed transplacentally to heat-degraded polychlorinated biphenyls in Taiwan. *British Journal of Dermatology* **122**, 799–808.

Hsu, M.M., Mak, C.P. & Hsu, C.C. (1995) Follow-up of skin manifestations in Yu-Cheng children. *British Journal of Dermatology* **132**, 427–432.

Urabe, H. & Asahi, M. (1984) Past and current dermatological status of Yusho patients. *American Journal of Industrial Medicine* **5**, 5–12.

Wong, C.K., Chen, C.J., Cheng, P.C. *et al.* (1982) Mucocutaneous manifestations of polychlorinated biphenyls (PCB) poisoning: a study of 122 cases in Taiwan. *British Journal of Dermatology* **107**, 317–323.

## Carbon monoxide

A cherry red discoloration of the nail bed is a symptom of carbon monoxide intoxication (Baran 1981). Superficial cutaneous necrosis of the distal phalanges involving pulps and periungual region, ears and nose followed carbon monoxide poisoning (Del Guidice *et al.* 1995).

## References

Baran, R. (1981) Modifications of colour: chromonychias or dyschromias. In: *The Nail* (ed. M. Pierre), pp. 30–38. Churchill Livingstone, Edinburgh.

Del Guidice, P., Lacour, J.P., Bahadoran, P. *et al.* (1995) Nécrose cutanée des extrémités au cours d'une intoxication par le monoxyde de carbone. *Annales de Dermatologie et de Vénéréologie* **122**, 780–782.

## Selenium

Following white transverse streaking of the fingernails, tenderness and swelling of the fingertip and purulent discharge, nail loss has been described in selenium intoxication (Jenssen & Closson 1984).

## Reference

Jenssen, R. & Closson, W. (1984) Selenium intoxication. *Journal of the American Medical Association* **251**, 1938.

## Vinyl chloride

Clubbing-like nail changes in the fingers have been observed in vinyl chloride disease (Runne & Orfanos 1981). Scleroderma-like changes and acroosteolysis can also occur.

## Reference

Runne, U. & Orfanos, C.E. (1981) the human nail. *Current Problems in Dermatology* **9**, 102–149.

## Heavy metal intoxications

### Arsenic (Fig. 6.86)

Colorimetry polarography, atomic absorption and neutron activation analysis can be used to detect arsenic in body tissues, hairs and nails. Nail samples containing more than $3 \, \mu g/g$ arsenic are diagnostic for arsenic intoxication (Massey *et al.* 1984).

Mees' lines are a typical sign of arsenic poisoning. They appear as transverse white bands (Thomas 1964) that move distally with nail growth (true leuconychia). A single broad band is usually seen (Welter *et al.* 1982), but multiple lines are occasionally observed (Aldrich 1904). These bands typically appear 4–6 weeks following an acute episode of arsenic poisoning. While multiple lines may be due to multiple episodes of arsenic ingestion, an alternative theory suggests that they may be band-like precipitations of arsenic within the nail matrices (Liesegang's phenomenon) (Conomy 1972). However, any number of cases of accidental rat poisoning did not show with transverse grooves, and transverse white lines were never seen on the nails during the intense arsenical antiluetic therapy.

Beau's lines, onychomadesis, longitudinal brown hyperpigmented bands as well as diffuse blackish-brown discoloration of the nail plate have also been described in arsenic intoxication with keratoses (De Nicola *et al.* 1974).

An endemic peripheral vascular disorder resembling Buerger's disease has been described in a limited area of southern Taiwan. The disorder, which has been referred to as 'black foot disease', results in gangrene of the extremities. It has been associated with drinking artesian well water containing both arsenic and chemically unknown fluorescent substances. A similarity between fluorescent substances and ergot alkaloids has been suggested (Yu *et al.* 1984).

## References

Aldrich, C.J. (1904) Leuconychia striata arsenicalis transversus with report of 3 cases. *American Journal of Medical Sciences* **127**, 702–709.

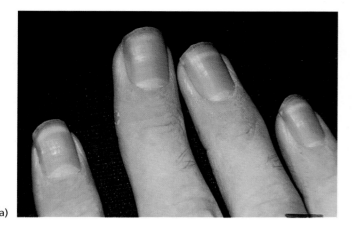

(a)

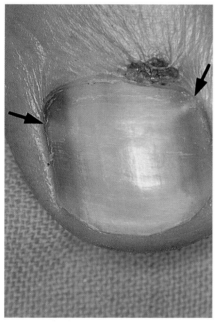

(b)

**Fig. 6.86** (a) Arsenic poisoning—transverse white band (Mees' lines). (Courtesy of J.M. Mascaro, Barcelona.) (b) Arsenic poisoning—periungual and subungual keratoses. (Courtesy of D. Leroy, France.)

Conomy, J.P. (1972) A succession of Mees' lines in arsenical neuropathy. *Postgraduate Medicine* **52**, 97–99.

De Nicola, P., Morsiani, M. & Zavagli, G. (1974) *Nail Diseases in Internal Medicine*. Charles C. Thomas, Springfield, IL.

Massey, W., Wold, D. & Heyman, A. (1984) Arsenic: homicidal intoxication. *Southern Medical Journal* **77**, 848–851.

Thomas H.M. (1964) Transverse bands in fingernails. *Bulletin of the Johns Hopkins Hospital* **115**, 238–244.

Welter, A., Michaux, M. & Blondel, A. (1982) Lignes de Mees dans un cas d'intoxication aigue à l'arsenic. *Dermatologica* **165**, 482–483.

Yu, H.S., Sheu, H.M., Ko, S.S. *et al.* (1984) Studies on blackfoot disease and chronic arsenism in Southern Taiwan. *Journal of Dermatology* **11**, 361–370.

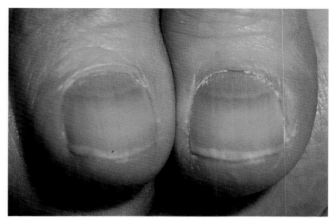

**Fig. 6.87** Argyria (silver), showing slate blue, mainly lunular, pigmentation.

## Silver

A bluish-black pigmentation of the skin of sun-exposed areas including the periungual regions is a cardinal feature of argyria. A slate-blue discoloration of the proximal nail beds is typical, the pigmentation being more evident in the lunulae (Fig. 6.87). The toes are not usually involved. The pigmentation is permanent (Plewig *et al.* 1977; Tanner & Gross 1990).

Differential diagnosis includes azure lunulae observed in patients with Wilson's disease and bluish discoloration occurring after the systemic administration of phenophthalein. Deposition of silver granules in the dermal tissue can be detected both in light-exposed and non-exposed areas of patients with argyria. The reduction of colourless silver salts to black metallic silver under the influence of light has been suggested to explain the pathogenesis of skin and nail pigmentation in argyria (Shelley *et al.* 1987).

## References

Plewig, G., Lincke, H. & Wolff, H.H. (1977) Silver-blue nails. *Acta Dermato-Venereologica* **57**, 413–419.

Shelley, W.B., Shelley, E.D. & Burmeister, V. (1987) Argyria: the intradermal 'photograph', a manifestation of passive photosensitivity. *Journal of the American Academy of Dermatology* **16**, 211–217.

Tanner, L.S. & Gross, D.J. (1990) Generalized argyria. *Cutis* **45**, 237–239.

## Mercury

Acrodynia is a rare disorder that principally occurs in infancy and is due to chronic exposure to mercury. Excruciating pain in the hands and feet together with intermittent pink discoloration of the tips of the fingers, toes and nose is an early manifestation of the disease (Dinehart *et al.* 1988). Ridging, fragility and dark discoloration of the nail plates is frequently observed. Alopecia and nail loss have been reported in severe cases. Gangrene of the extremities may develop (Boissière 1971).

Oral treatment with DMPS (sodium-dimercapto-propane-sulfphonate) has been successfully used in a child with acrodynia (Bockers *et al.* 1984).

A greysh-brown discoloration of the nails can occur after chronic exposure to topical preparations containing mercury (Butterworth & Stream 1963). Hair loss and brown pigmentation of the distal portion of the fingernails occurred in a patient with chronic mercury poisoning caused by the use of mercury-containing cosmetic bleaches. The mercury content of the patient's nails was extremely high (Wustner & Orfanos 1975). A similar case has been also reported by Bockers *et al.* (1985).

A case of systemic lichen planus due to mercury in dental amalgam was observed by Higashi *et al.* (1995). It showed pitting and scaling of the proximal portion of the toenails.

## References

Bockers, M., Schonberger, W. & Neumann, P. (1984) Klinik und Therapie der Akrodynie infolge inhalative Quecksilberintoxikation. In: *International Congress of the European Society of Pediatric Dermatology, Munster Dia-Klinik*, pp. 24–25.

Bockers, M., Wagner, R. & Oster, O. (1985) Nageldyscromie als leitsymptom einer chronischen Quecksilberintoxication Durch ein Kosmetisches Bleichmittel. *Zeitschrift für Autkz* 60, 821–829.

Boissière, H. (1971) Les gangrènes cutanèes du nourrisson. *Le Concours Medical* 24, 3138–3154.

Butterworth, T. & Strean, L.P. (1963) Mercurial pigmentation of nails. *Archives of Dermatology* 88, 55–57.

Dinehart, S.M., Dillard, R., Raimer, S.S. *et al.* (1988) Cutaneous manifestations of acrodynia (Pink disease). *Archives of Dermatology* 124, 107–109.

Higashi, N., Sano, S., Kume, A. (1995) A case of systemic lichen planus with nail deformity due to mercury in dental amalgam. *Skin Research* 37, 252–256.

Wustner, H. & Orfanos, C.E. (1975) Nagelverfarbung und haaranusfall. *Deutsche Medizinische Wochenschrift* 100, 1694–1697.

## Gold

Gold levels in skin, hair and nails do not appear to correlate with gold toxicity (Gottlieb *et al.* 1974). Yellow to dark brown nail plate pigmentation can occur after parenteral gold therapy (Fam & Paton 1984; Aste *et al.* 1994). Nail thinning, softening, fragility, onycholysis and onychomadesis can also be seen (Voigt & Holzegel 1977). Slow nail growth has been reported by Sertoli (1956).

## References

Aste, N., Pau, M., Carcassi, M. *et al.* (1994). Nail pigmentation during chrysotherapy: 'Gold nails'. *Chronica Dermatologica* 4, 647–651.

Fam, A.G. & Paton, T.W. (1984) Nail pigmentation after parenteral gold therapy for rheumatoid arthritis: 'gold nails'. *Arthritis and Rheumatism* 27, 119–120.

Gottlieb, N.L., Smith, P.M., Penneys, N.S. *et al.* (1974) Gold concentrations in hair, nail and skin during chrysotherapy. *Arthritis and Rheumatism* 17, 56–62.

Sertoli, P. (1956) Fisiopatologia del complesso ungueale. *Edizioni Minerva Medica* 250.

Voigt, K. & Holzegel, K. (1977) Bleibende Nagelveranderungen nach goldtherapie. *Hautarzt* 28, 121–123.

## Lead

Leuconychia, onychomadesis and onychalgia have been reported in lead poisoning (Pardo Castello & Pardo 1960). Diffuse hyperpigmentation of the fingernails and toenails occurred in a 55-day-old boy after the use of an astringent powder with a high lead content (Wenyuan & Mingyu 1989). Partial leuconychia and nail bed hyperkeratosis have also been described (Sertoli 1956; Baran 1981).

## References

Baran, R. (1981) Modifications of colour: chromonychias or dyschromias. In: *The Nail* (ed. M. Pierre), pp. 30–38. Churchill Livingstone, Edinburgh.

Pardo Castello, V. & Pardo, O. (1960) *Diseases of the Nails*, 3rd edn, p. 244. Charles C. Thomas, Springfield, IL.

Sertoli, P. (1956) Fisiopatologia del complesso ungueale. *Edizioni Minerva Medica* 250.

Wenyuan, Z. & Mingyu, X. (1989) Hyperpigmentation of the nail from lead deposition. *International Journal of Dermatology* 28, 273–275.

## Thallium

Diffuse or partial brownish discoloration of the nails has been described in thallium poisoning. Onychorrhexis and transverse leuconychia can be observed in acute intoxication (Herrero *et al.* 1995). Dry scaling of the distal parts of the extremities can also occur (Heyl & Barlow 1989).

Thallium intoxication may mimic systemic lupus erythematosus. The nails may occasionally show a diffuse or banded brown or yellow discoloration; universal alopecia and striated yellowish nails developed in one of five patients with connective tissue disease after thallium poisoning (Alarcon-Segovia *et al.* 1989).

## References

Alarcon-Segovia, D., Del Carmen Amigo, M. & Reyes, P.A. (1989) Connective tissue disease features after thallium poisoning. *Journal of Rheumatology* 16, 171–174.

Herrero, F., Fernandez, E., Gomez, J. *et al.* (1995) Thallium poisoning presenting with abdominal colic, paresthesia and irritability. *Journal of Toxicology. Clinical Toxicology* 33, 261–264.

Heyl, T. & Barlow, R.J. (1989) Thallium poisoning: a dermatological perspective. *British Journal of Dermatology* 121, 787–792.

## Aniline

A purplish-blue discoloration of the nail bed due to cyanosis has been reported in aniline poisoning (Baran 1981). Softening of the nail plate can also occur (Sertoli 1956).

## References

Baran, R. (1981) Modifications of colour: chromonychias or dyschromias. In: *The Nail* (ed. M. Pierre), pp. 30–38. Churchill Livingstone, Edinburgh.

Sertoli, P. (1956) Fisiopatologia del complesso ungueale. *Edizioni Minerva Medica* 250.

## Chromium salts

Dichromates produce a yellow ochre colour of the nails (Baran 1981) (see Chapter 7).

## Reference

Baran, R. (1981) Modifications of colour: chromonychias or dyschromias. In: *The Nail* (ed. M. Pierre), pp. 30–38. Churchill Livingstone, Edinburgh.

## Anticoagulants

Nail growth can be reduced during heparin treatment (Ludwig 1965). Transverse red banding, separated from the lunula by a pink area, and subungual haematoma are also recognized signs of anticoagulation (Varotti *et al.* 1997). Ross (1963) noted intermittent diffuse, orange-coloured staining of the fingernails in patients submitted to long-term treatment with phenindione.

### Warfarin

The purple toes syndrome is a rare complication of treatment with warfarin or related compounds. Patients develop a painful purple discoloration of the toenails and plantar surface and sides of the toes. The discoloration, which typically fades on moderate pressure or with leg elevation, usually develops 3–8 weeks after the initiation of therapy (Feder & Auerbach 1961; Lebsack & Weilbert 1982). The pathogenesis of the purple toes syndrome is still discussed. Pathological evidence, however, suggests that the purple toes are a consequence of cholesterol microembolization and may herald diffuse arterial obstruction by microembolic disease. Warfarin may induce cholesterol emboli by interfering with the healing of ulcerated atherosclerotic plaques and should be immediately discontinued to avoid risk of fatal outcome (Hyman *et al.* 1987).

Hypoplasia of the fingernails and terminal phalanges, associated with stippled epiphyses, can occur in children whose mothers have been treated with warfarin during the first trimester of pregnancy (Pettifor & Benson 1975).

## References

Feder, W. & Auerbach, R. (1961) 'Purple toes'; an uncommon sequela of oral coumarin drug therapy. *Annals of Internal Medicine* 55, 911–917.

Hyman, B.T., Landas, S.K., Ashman, R.F. *et al.* (1987) Warfarin-related purple toes syndrome and cholesterol microembolization. *American Journal of Medicine* 82, 1233–1237.

Lebsack, C.S. & Weilbert, R.T. (1982) Purple toes syndrome. *Postgraduate Medicine* 71, 81.

Ludwig, E. (1965) Nebenwirkungen der heparinoide auf haare und nagel. In: *Webenwirkungen und Bluntingen bei Antikoagulation und Fibrinolytika* (eds L. Zukschwerd & H.A. Thies). Schattauer-Verlag, Stuttgart.

Pettifor, J.M. & Benson, R. (1975) Congenital malformation with the administration of oral anticoagulants during pregnancy. *Journal of Pediatrics* 86, 459–462.

Ross, J.B. (1963) Side effects of phenindione. *British Medical Journal* 1, 866.

Varotti, C., Ghetti, E., Piraccini, B.M. *et al.* (1997) Subungual hematomas in a patient treated with an oral anticoagulant (warfarin sodium). *European Journal of Dermatology* 7, 395–396.

## Antimalarial agents

Because chloroquine is stored in the fingernails over a long period, determination of chloroquine in toenail clippings can be useful in assessing drug intake dating back at least 1 year (Ofori-Adjei & Ericsson 1985).

Chloroquine and hydroxychloroquine may induce or exacerbate psoriasis. A case of psoriatic onychoperiostitis precipitated by hydroxychloroquine has been reported (Sibilia *et al.* 1995). The development of pigmentary changes, which is most commonly observed in Caucasians, is a characteristic side effect of antimalarials usage (Tuffanelli *et al.* 1963). A bluish-black or bluish-brown pigmentation of the nail beds (Fig. 6.88) can be seen following prolonged treatment with amodiaquine, mepacrine (quinacrine) and chloroquine (Baden & Zaias 1987; Dodd & Sarkany 1988). Diffuse nail bed pigmentation as well as transverse hyperpigmented bands can occur. The nature of the pigment is still undetermined but both melanin and haemosiderin deposits appear to be present (Tuffanelli *et al.* 1963). The presence of a complex containing the antimalarial has also been suggested.

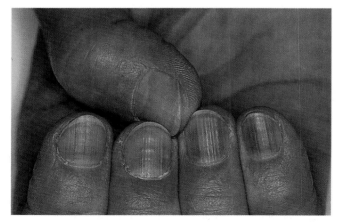

**Fig. 6.88** Antimalarial diffuse nail pigmentation. (Courtesy of J.L. Verret, Angers, France.)

Nail pigmentation usually takes several months to decrease in intensity after the cessation of therapy and it may not disappear completely. An increased incidence of retinopathy has been noted in patients with cutaneous hyperpigmentation (Tuffanelli *et al*. 1963).

Nail discoloration varying from white, diffuse yellow or lemon-green to blue-green or grey has been described in patients taking mepacrine. Blue and yellow discoloration of the nail bed may be seen together (Baran & Temine 1973). A characteristic green-yellow or whitish fluorescence of the nails under the Wood's light is also commonly observed during mepacrine treatment (Kierland *et al*. 1946). Nail pitting, ridging and shedding can occur in association with mepacrine treatment (Baran & Témime 1973).

Photoonycholysis associated with a lichenoid eruption has been described in a 66-year-old man receiving quinine sulphate (Tan *et al*. 1989).

## References

Baran, R. & Témime, P. (1973) Les onychodystrophies toxi-médicamenteuses et les onycholyses. *Le Concours Medical* **95**, 1007–1023.

Baden, H. & Zaias, N. (1987) Nails. In: *Dermatology in General Medicine* (eds T.B. Fitzpatrick, A.Z. Eisen, K. Wolff *et al*.), pp. 651–666. McGraw Hill, New York.

Dodd, H.J. & Sarkany, I. (1988) Chronic discoid lupus erythematosus with mepacrine pigmentation bands in the nails. *British Journal of Dermatology* **119** (Suppl. 33), 74–75.

Kierland, R.R., Sheard, C., Mason, H.L. *et al*. (1946) Fluorescence of nails from quinacrine hydrochloride. *Journal of the American Medical Association* **131**, 809–810.

Ofori-Adjei, D. & Ericsson, O. (1985) Chloroquine in nail clippings. *Lancet* **ii**, 331.

Sibilia, J., Cribier, B., Javier, R.M. *et al*. (1995) Recurrent psoiatic onychoperiostitis induced by hydroxychloroquine. *Reviews in Rheumatology English Edition* **62**, 795–797.

Tan, S.V., Berth-Jones, J. & Burns, D.A. (1989) Lichen planus and photo-onycholysis induced by quinine. *Clinical and Experimental Dermatology* **14**, 335.

Tuffanelli, D., Abraham, R.K. & Dubois, E.I. (1963) Pigmentation from antimalarial therapy. *Archives of Dermatology* **88**, 113–120.

## Hormones

### Oral contraceptive pill

Some postmenopausal women on the oral contraceptive pill report an increased growth rate of nails and reduced splitting and 'chipping' (Knight 1974). Photoonycholysis may occur in patients with porphyria who take the oral contraceptive pill, thus revealing an underlying occult porphyria cutanea tarda or variegata (Byrne *et al*. 1976). Nail shedding has also been reported following oral contraceptive treatment.

## References

Byrne, J.P.H., Boss, J.M. & Dawber, R.P.R. (1976) Contraceptive-pill-induced porphyria cutanea tarda presenting with onycholysis of the fingernails. *Postgraduate Medical Journal* **52**, 535–538.

Knight, J.F. (1974) Side benefits of the pill. *Medical Journal of Australia* November, 680.

### Androgens

Features resembling half-and-half nails have been described in a breast cancer patient after androgen therapy (Nixon *et al*. 1981).

## Reference

Nixon, D.W., Pirrozi, D., York, R.M. *et al*. (1981) Dermatologic changes after systemic cancer therapy. *Cutis* **27**, 181.

### Parathyroid extracts

Onychomadesis has been reported with parathyroid extract medication (Perrot *et al*. 1973).

## Reference

Perrot, H., Tourniaire, J. & Fournier, M. (1973) Onychopathie induite par la parathormone. *Bulletin de la Societé Française de Dermatologie et de Syphiligraphie* **80**, 313.

### Cortisone

Topical steroids can produce distal phalangeal atrophy. The so-called 'disappearing digit' may result from the frequent application of potent local steroids even without occlusion (Wolf *et al*. 1990). There may be atrophic tapering of the fingertip after only 1 month of treatment (Deffer & Goette 1987). This gives the finger a sharpened pencil appearence. Striking atrophy of the terminal phalanges of the fingers was noted in both hands in a case reported by Requena *et al*. (1990), showing a sharp limitation at the level of the proximal interphalangeal joints. The affected areas were characterized by severe thinning, erythema and scaling. The nails exhibited diffuse yellow discoloration and subungual hyperkeratosis whereas the nails of both thumbs were lost. After discontinuing fluorinated corticosteroids with occlusion, it took 2 years to recover a relatively normal appearance of the hands with slight persistence of some degree of acroatrophy.

Intralesional steroids might be used in the treatment of psoriasis and lichen planus. Side effects include hypopigmentation (Bedi 1977) and intramatricial haemorrhages, which may be unsightly when they appear on the nail plate. Permanent damage to the matrix may result from injections given either too frequently or in a dosage too concentrated.

### Dermojet steroids injection

Mascaro (personal communication) observed a psoriatic patient who was treated with steroids by dermojet; this produced multiple implantation epidermoid cysts which necessitated the amputation of some of the distal phalanges.

### Systemic steroids

A white woman developed a single band of transverse leuconychia in all fingernails and toenails after cortisone administration (Thomas 1964). Transverse melanonychia due to prednisone has been described by Thomsen (personal communication).

## References

Bedi, T.R. (1977) Intradermal triamcinolone treatment of psoriatic onychodystrophy. *Dermatologica* 155, 24–27.

Deffer, T.A. & Goette, K. (1987) Distal phalangeal atrophy secondary to topical steroid therapy. *Archives of Dermatology* 123, 571–572.

Requena, L., Zamora, E. & Martin, L. (1990) Acroatrophy secondary to long-standing applications of topical steroids. *Archives of Dermatology* 126, 1013–1014.

Thomas, H.M. (1964) Transverse bands in fingernails. *Bulletin of the Johns Hopkins Hospital* 115, 238–244.

Wolf, R., Tur, E. & Brenner, S. (1990) Corticosteroid induced 'disappearing digit'. *Journal of the American Academy of Dermatology* 23, 755–756.

## Adrenocorticotropic hormone, melanocyte-stimulating hormone

Transverse hyperpigmented bands have been described in patients taking adrenocorticotropic hormone (ACTH) or melanocyte-stimulating hormone (MSH) (Thomas 1964).

## Reference

Thomas, H.M. (1964) Transverse bands in fingernails. *Bulletin Johns Hopkins Hospital* 115, 238–244.

## Cancer chemotherapeutic agents (Fig. 6.89, Table 6.7)

Patients receiving cancer chemotherapeutic agents frequently exhibit nail abnormalities (Malacarne & Zavagli 1977; Dunagin 1982; Delaunay 1989). Nail pigmentation is the most frequent change. This has been reported following treatment with numerous antineoplastic agents including cyclophosphamide, doxorubicin, bleomycin sulphate, methotrexate, nitrogen mustard, nitrosurea, dacarbazine, 5-fluorouracil, daunorubicin hydrochloride, melphalan hydrochloride, etoposide, tegafur and hydroxyurea. The pigmentation, which is more common and intense in heavily pigmented than in fair-skinned individuals, usually appears 3–8 weeks after the initiation of chemotherapy. It is more commonly observed with combination chemotherapy than with the use of a single drug (Nixon 1976). The pigmentation of either the nail plate or the nail bed may occur as horizontal or longitudinal bands or as diffuse darkening, even in the same patient (Hernández-Martin *et al.* 1999).

The same chemotherapeutic agent can cause different patterns of nail pigmentation and the simultaneous presence of any type on the same nails is possible. Pigmentation may affect hands or feet or both and may involve one or more digits. Hyperpigmentation of the skin, especially over the finger joints, is commonly associated with nail pigmentation. Patients submitted to intermittent therapy can develop transverse pigmented bands that correspond to the time of drug administration and are separated by bands of normal colour (Jeanmougin *et al.* 1982). The pigmentation disappears 6–8 weeks after the discontinuation of treatment.

The mechanism of hyperpigmentation produced by chemotherapeutic agents remains obscure. Stimulation of melanocyte activity in the nail matrix and epidermis probably accounts for most of the pigmentary changes. It seems independent of both MSH and ACTH activity (Arakawa *et al.* 1978) as well as ultraviolet light. A possible genetic predisposition has been suggested by the occurrence of the pigmentation in some consanguineous patients and by the high incidence seen in patients from Sardinia (Sulis & Floris 1980) leading to nail shedding (Cetin *et al.* 1998).

Beau's lines, and onychomadesis reflect transitory inhibition of the nail matrix. They occur most frequently after short and intensive chemotherapy, especially combined chemotherapy. Damage to the nail matrix by chemotherapy can also produce true transverse leuconychia. There is no specific cancer chemotherapeutic drug, combination of drugs or drug class that causes transverse leuconychia, however cyclophosphamide, adriamycin and vincristine are the therapeutic agents most frequently involved (Jeanmougin *et al.* 1982; Kochupillai *et al.* 1983; Tucker & Church 1984; Singh & Kaur 1986; Shetty 1988; Bader-Meunier *et al.* 1990; Hogan *et al.* 1991; Requena 1991; Miles & Rubens 1995, Chapman & Cohen 1997; Lombart-Cussac *et al.* 1997; Shelley & Humprey 1997). Transverse white bands limited to ipsilateral fingernails have been reported after isolated cytostatic perfusion of the affected arm (Zaun & Omlor 1992). Apparent leuconychia is another side effect of cancer chemotherapy. Both transverse white bands of the nail bed, resembling Muehrcke's lines and half-and-half nails, have been occasionally reported (Schwartz & Vickerman 1979; Nixon *et al.* 1981; James & Odom 1983; Bianchi *et al.* 1992; Unamino *et al.* 1992). However, apparent leuconychia may be explained by haematological involvement. Toxicity to the nail bed may produce onycholysis associated with nail bed haemorrhage (Vanhooteghem *et al.* 1997; Roussou *et al.* 1998; Flory *et al.* 1999). The cytotoxic agent docetaxel produces onycholysis in 19% of patients. This drug has been reported to produce nail abnormalities in up to 41% of patients (Huinink *et al.* 1994; Jacob & Frunza-Patten 1998). Onycholysis

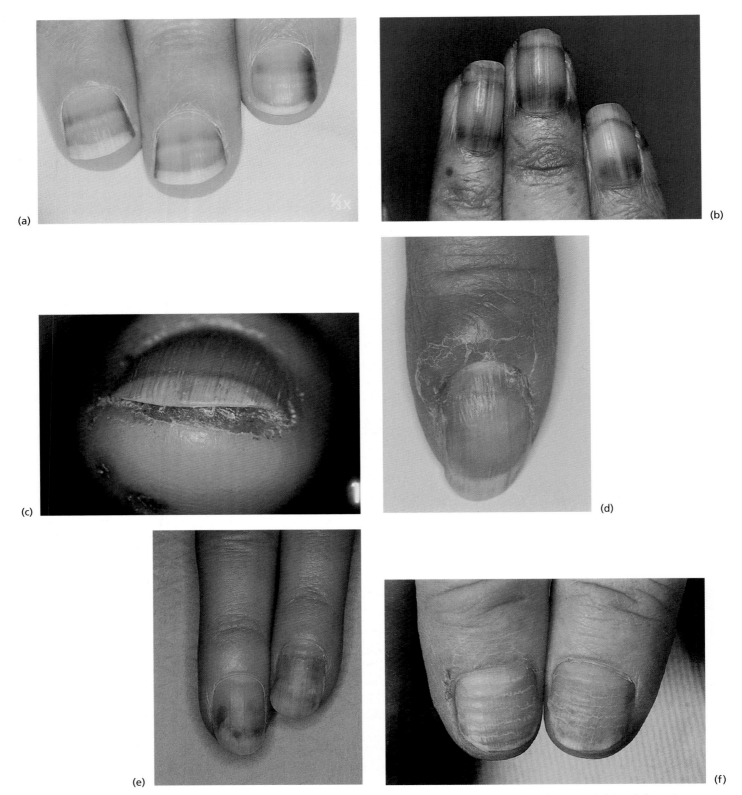

**Fig. 6.89** (a) Cancer chemotherapy—pigmentation and transverse leuconychia. (b) Cancer chemotherapy—pigmentation. (c) Cancer chemotherapy—onycholysis and inflammation. (Courtesy of E. Grosshans, France.) (d) Cancer chemotherapy—paronychial inflammation. (e) Cancer chemotherapy (taxol)—subungual haemorrhage. (Courtesy of L. Laroche, France.) (f) Beau's line after chemotherapy. (Courtesy of P. Slee, The Netherlands.)

**Table 6.7** Cancer chemotherapeutic agents—nail changes.

| Drug | Colour change | Pattern* | Site* | Remarks |
|---|---|---|---|---|
| Adriamycin (doxorubicin) | Bluish grey brown, black | D, L, H | NP, NB | Hyperpigmentation of mouth, palms, soles and dorsum of the hands, painful desquamating erythema of palms and soles, onycholysis (Pratt & Shanks 1974; Priestman & James 1975; Morris *et al.* 1977; Levine & Greenwald 1978; Runne *et al.* 1980; Sulis & Floris 1980; Daniel & Scher 1984; Lokich & Moore 1984; Curran 1990) |
| Azathioprine | Pink | D | Lu | Reduced nail growth (Dawber 1970; Koranda *et al.* 1974) |
| Bleomycin (systemic or Intralesional) | Brown | L, H | NP, NB | Brittleness, Beau's lines, onycholysis, onychomadesis, thickening of the nail bed, dark cuticles, Raynaud's phenomenon, acropachy, gangrene, sclerodermatous changes (Halnan *et al.* 1972; Ohnuma *et al.* 1972; Shetty 1977; Norton 1980; Nixon *et al.* 1981; Snauwaert & Degreff 1984; Baran 1985; Gonzales *et al.* 1986; Veraldi *et al.* 1987; Epstein 1991). Fingertip necrosis (Pechère *et al.* 1996); progressive systemic-like scleroderma (Behrens *et al.* 1998) |
| 5-Bromodeoxyuridine and radiation | Yellow, brown, white | H | | Beau's lines, onychomadesis (McCuaig *et al.* 1989) |
| Busulphan (busulfan) | Brown | L | NB | Skin pigmentation in 5–10% of the patients (Levantine & Almeyda 1974; Malacarne 1978; Baran 1981) |
| Cisplatin | Black | | | Digital necrosis (Marie *et al.* 2000) |
| Cyclophosphamide | Brown, black | D, L, H | NP, NB | Reduced nail growth, pigmentation of palms, soles, dorsum of hands and teeth (Harrison & Wood 1972; Markenson *et al.* 1975; Shah *et al.* 1978; Sulis & Floris 1980). Erythema of the onychodermal band and proximal nail folds due to cyclophosphamide and/or vincristine (Kowal-Vern & Eng 1993) |
| Cytosine arabinoside | | | | Painful desquamating erythema of palms and soles (Horwitz & Dreizen 1990) |
| Daunorubicine | Brown, black | H | NP | Reduced nail growth (De Marinis *et al.* 1978) |
| Dacarbazine (DTIC) | Brown | H | NB | (Nixon *et al.* 1981) |
| Docetaxel | | | | Scleroderma-like changes of lower extremities (Battafarrano *et al.* 1994). Active drug for squamous cell carcinoma (Dreyfuss *et al.* 1996). Active for refractory solid tumours (Blaney *et al.* 1997). Painful haemorrhagic onycholysis (Vanhooteghem *et al.* 1997; Jacob & Frunza-Patten 1998) |
| Etoposide | Brown | | NB | (Wong *et al.* 1984) |
| 5-Fluorouracil (systemic or topical) | Blue, brown, half and half nails | D, L, H | NP, NB | Nail brittleness and cracking, pigmentation of dorsum of the hands and skin overlying the veins used for infusion, Beau's lines, paronychia, onycholysis, half-and-half nail-like changes, onychomadesis, painful desquamating eyrthema of palms and soles; superficial blue hue can be scraped off (Falkson & Schulz 1962; Goldman *et al.* 1963; Hrushesky 1976; Levine & Greenwald 1978; Katz & Hansen 1979; Nixon *et al.* 1981; Baran & Laugier 1985, Guillaume *et al.* 1988) |
| Hydroxyurea | Melanic, slate, brown | L, H | NP, NB, Lu | Brittle atrophic nails, onychoschizia, pigmentation of flexural pressure areas, onycholysis, acral erythema, dermatomyositis-like eruption (Barety *et al.* 1975; Kennedy *et al.* 1975; Richard *et al.* 1989; Vomvouras *et al.* 1991; Kelsey 1992; Kwong 1996; Hernández-Martin *et al.* 1999) |
| Ifosfamide | Brown | D | NP | (Teresi *et al.* 1993) |
| Melphalan | Brown | L | NP | Beau's lines (Malacarne & Zavagli 1977; Malarcarne 1978) |
| Methotrexate | Brown | H | NB | Horizontal hyperpigmented bands of the hair, acute paronychia, onychomadesis, reduced nail growth (Dawber 1970; Wantzin & Thomsen 1983; Wheeland *et al.* 1983) |
| Mercaptopurine | | | | Onychomadesis, periungual erythema, painful desquamating erythema of palms and soles (Daniel & Scher 1984; Cox & Robertson 1986) |
| Mitotane (O, *p*-DDD) | | | | Painful desquamating eythema of palms and soles, onychomadesis (Levine & Greenwald 1978) |
| Mitoxantrone | Blue | D | | Nail softening and splitting, painful onycholysis (Creamer *et al.* 1995; Roussou *et al.* 1998), nail bed haemorrhages (Speechly-Dick & Owen 1988; Scheithauer *et al.* 1989) |
| Nitrogen mustard | Brown | H | | (Nixon *et al.* 1981) |
| Nitrosurea | Brown | H | | (Nixon *et al.* 1981) |
| Paclitaxel | | | NP | Nail bed purpura, pus formation, onycholysis (Flory *et al.* 1999) |
| Razoxane | | | | Beau's lines (Tucker & Church 1984) |
| Tegafur | Brown, black | D | NP | Spotted hyperpigmentation of lips, palms, soles and glans penis (Llistosella *et al.* 1991) |

* Pattern: D, Diffuse; L, Longitudinal; H, Horizontal. Site: NP, Nail plate; NB, Nail bed; Lu, Lunulae.

and paronychia due to cytotoxic drugs may sometimes be painful (Katz & Hansen 1979; Cunningham *et al.* 1985; Van Belle *et al.* 1989). Mitozantrone-induced onycholysis has a predilection for the large toenail (Creamer *et al.* 1995). A high-dose methotrexate and leucovorin calcium regimen can cause an acute severe bullous dermatitis associated with onycholysis, which can be serious enough to require a modification in the treatment programme (Chang 1987). Acute paronychia in toenails has also been reported with high-dose methotrexate and leucovorin calcium therapy (Wantzin & Thomsen 1983).

Onycholysis can occur following the topical use of 5-fluorouracil with occlusive dressing for warts located around the nails. It may be associated with tenderness, swelling, maceration and oozing of the proximal nail fold (Goldman *et al.* 1963; Goettmann & Belaich 1995).

Raynaud's phenomenon and sclerodermatous changes are possible consequences of systemic bleomycin therapy (Snauwaert & Degreef 1984; Behrens *et al.* 1998). They can also occur after intralesional bleomycin for periungual warts (Bovenmyer 1985; Epstein 1985, 1991; Smith *et al.* 1985). In a retrospective study of 60 patients, Vogelzang *et al.* (1981) found an incidence of 37%. Fingertip gangrene can occur in severe cases. These side effects usually occur from 3 months to 2 years after bleomycin injections and are irreversible. Bleomycin damages the matrix dermis which can result in scarring nail dystrophy. The drug is capable of stimulating the synthesis of collagen and glucosaminoglycans both *in vivo* and *in vitro* which may play a part in this process (Snauwaert & Degreef 1984). Intralesional bleomycin treatment of periungual warts can result in onychomadesis and permanent onychodystrophy (Baran 1985; Gonzales *et al.* 1986).

Painful desquamating erythema of the palms, soles and periungual regions of the hands is a common complication of continuous infusion of cytosine arabinoside, adriamicin or 5-fluorouracil (Lokich & Moore 1984; Guillaume *et al.* 1988; Horwitz & Dreizen 1990). It has also been occasionally reported with other cytotoxic agents (Cox & Robertson 1986). In chemotherapy-induced acral erythema, tingling on the palms and soles usually precedes the development of painful, symmetrical, well-defined swelling and erythema, often more pronounced over the pads of the distal phalanges. After several days the indurated erythematous plaques become dusky and develop areas of pallor that subsequently blister and desquamate. The desquamation is frequently more obvious than the original erythema. Periungual areas and nails can also be affected (Baack & Burgdorf 1991).

Beside nail pigmentation (Barety *et al.* 1975; Pirard *et al.* 1994; Michel *et al.* 1996), hydroxyurea may produce a dermatomyositis-like eruption (Senet *et al.* 1995; Suehiro *et al.* 1998) or lichenoid eruption (Daoud *et al.* 1999).

Splinter haemorrhages and subungual haematoma can occur as a consequence of thrombocytopenia. Shortening or complete disappearance of the lunulae have also been described. Delayed onychomadesis of all the fingernails and some toenails occurred in a series of 25 patients affected by malignant astrocytomas treated with continuous intracarotid 5-bromodeoxyuridine radiosensitization and radiotherapy for $8^{1}/2$ weeks. Nail shedding was preceded by the formation of a depressed transverse white band with slight discoloration superimposed. Completely normal nail regrowth occurred within 6 months. All patients also experienced ipsilateral facial dermatitis, epilation of eyebrows and eyelashes, ocular irritation and scalp alopecia (McCuaig *et al.* 1989).

## References

Arakawa, S., Takamatsu, T., Imashuku, S. *et al.* (1978) Plasma ACTH and melanocyte-stimulating hormone in nail pigmentation. *Archives of Disease in Childhood* 53, 249–258.

Baack, B.R. & Burgdorf, W.H.C. (1991) Chemotherapy-induced acral erythema. *Journal of the American Academy of Dermatology* 24, 457–461.

Bader-Meunier, B., Garel, D., Dommergues, J.P. *et al.* (1990) Leuconychies transversales et chimiothérapie antileucémique. *Annales de Pediatric (Paris)* 37, 337–338.

Baran, R. (1981) Modifications of colour: chromonychias or dyschromias. In: *The Nail* (ed. M. Pierre), pp 30–38. Churchill Livingstone, Edinburgh.

Baran, R. (1985) Onychodystrophie induite par injection intralésionnelle de bléomycine pour verrue périunguéale. *Annales de Dermatologie et de Vénéréologie* 112, 463–464.

Baran, R. & Laugier, P. (1985) Melanonychia induced by topical 5-fluorouracil. *British Journal of Dermatology* 112, 621–625.

Barety, M., Audoly, P. & Migozzi, B. (1975) Pigmentation unguéale et cutanée au cours d'un traitment par hydroxyurée. *Bulletin de la Societé Française de Dermatologie et de Syphiligraphie* 82, 208.

Battafarrano, D.F., Zimmerman, G.C., Older, S.A. *et al.* (1994) Docetaxel (taxotere) associated scleroderma-like changes of the lower extremities. *Cancer* 76, 110–115.

Behrens, S., Reuther, T., von Kobyletzki, G. *et al.* (1998) Bleomycin-induzierte PSS-artige Pseudosklerodermie. *Hautarzt* 49, 725–729.

Bianchi, L., Iraci, S., Tomassoli, M. *et al.* (1992) Coexistence of apparent transverse leukonychia (Muehrcke's lines-type) and longitudinal melanonychia after 5-fluorouracil/adriamycin/cyclophosphamide chemotherapy. *Dermatologica* 185, 216–217.

Blaney, S.M., Seibel, N.M., O'Brien, M. *et al.* (1997) Phase I trial of docetaxel administered as a 1-hour infusion in children with refractory solid tumors: a collaborative pediatric branch, national cancer institute and children's cancer group trial. *Journal of Clinical Oncology* 15, 1538–1543.

Bovenmyer, D.A. (1985) Persistent Raynaud's phenomenon following intralesional bleomycin treatment of finger warts. *Journal of the American Academy of Dermatology* 13, 470–471.

Cetin, M., Utas, S., Unal, A. *et al.* (1998) Shedding of the nails due to chemotherapy (onychomadesis). *Journal of the European Academy of Dermatology and Venereology* 11, 193–194.

Chang, J.C. (1987) Acute bullous dermatosis and onycholysis due to high-dose methotrexate and leucovorin calcium. *Archives of Dermatology* 123, 990–992.

Chapman, S. & Cohen, P.R. (1997) Transverse leukonychia in patients receiving cancer chemotherapy. *Southern Medical Journal* 90, 395–398.

Cox, G.J. & Robertson, D.B. (1986) Toxic erythema of palms and soles associated with high-dose mercaptopurine chemotherapy. *Archives of Dermatology* 122, 1413–1414.

Creamer, J.D., Mortimer, P.S. & Powles, T.J. (1995) Mitozantrone-induced onycholysis. A series of five cases. *Clinical and Experimental Dermatology* 20, 459–461.

Cunningham, D., Gilchrist, N.L., Forrest, G.J. et al. (1985) Onycholysis associated with cytotoxic drugs. *British Medical Journal* 290, 675–676.

Curran, C.F. (1990) Onycholysis in doxorubicin-treated patients. *Archives of Dermatology* 126, 1244.s

Daoud, M.S., Gibson, L.E. & Pittelkow, M.R. (1997) Hydroxyurea dermopathy: a unique lichenoid eruption complicating long-term therapy with hydroxyurea. *Journal of the American Academy of Dermatology* 36, 178–182.

Daniel, C.R. & Scher, R.K. (1984) Nail changes secondary to systemic drugs or ingestants. *Journal of the American Academy of Dermatology* 10, 250–258.

Dawber, R.P.R. (1970) The effect of methotrexate, corticosteroids and azathioprine on fingernail growth in psoriasis. *British Journal of Dermatology* 83, 680–683.

Delaunay, M. (1989) Effects cutanés indésirables de la chimiothérapie antitumorale. *Annales de Dermatologie et de Vénéréologie* 116, 347–361.

De Marinis, M., Hendricks, A. & Stoltzner, G. (1978) Nail pigmentation with daunorubicin therapy. *Annals of Internal Medicine* 89, 516–517.

Dreyfuss, A.I., Clark, J.R., Norris, C.M. et al. (1996) Docetaxel: an active drug for squamous cell carcinoma of the head and neck. *Journal of Clinical Oncology* 14, 1672–1678.

Dunagin, W.G. (1982) Clinical toxicity of chemotherapeutic agents dermatologic toxicity. *Seminars in Oncology* 9, 14–22.

Epstein, E. (1985) Persisting Raynaud's phenomenon following intralesional bleomycin treatment of finger warts. *Journal of the American Academy of Dermatology* 13, 468–469.

Epstein, E. (1991) Intralesional bleomycin and Raynaud's phenomenon. *Journal of the American Academy of Dermatology* 24, 785–786.

Falkson, G. & Schulz, E.J. (1962) Skin changes in patients treated with 5 fluorouracil. *British Journal of Dermatology* 74, 229–236.

Flory, S., Solimando, D.A., Webster, G. et al. (1999) Onycholysis associated with weekly administration of paclitaxel. *Annals of Pharmacotherapy* 33, 584–586.

Goettmann, S. & Belaich, S. (1995) Onycholyse polydactylique sévère au cours d'un traitement par 5 FU topique pour des verrues périunguéale. *Annales de Dermatologie et de Vénéréologie* 122 (Suppl. 1), S111–S112.

Goldman, L., Blaney, D.J. & Cohen, W. (1963) Onychodystrophy after topical 5 fluorouracil. *Archives of Dermatology* 88, 529–530.

Gonzales, F.U., Del Carmen Cristobal Gil, M., Martinez, A.A. et al. (1986) Cutaneous toxicity of intralesional bleomycin administration in the treatment of periungual warts. *Archives of Dermatology* 122, 974–975.

Guillaume, J.C., Carp, E., Rougier, P. et al. (1988) Effets secondaires cutanéo-muqueux des perfusions continues de 5 fluorouracile: 12 observations. *Annales de Dermatologie et de Vénéréologie* 115, 1167–1169.

Halnan, K.E., Bleehen, N.M., Brewin, T.B. et al. (1972) Early clinical experience with bleomycin in the United Kingdom in series of 105 patients. *British Medical Journal* 2, 635–638.

Harrison, B.N. & Wood, C.B.S. (1972) Cyclophosphamide and pigmentation. *British Medical Journal* 1, 352.

Hernández-Martin, A., Ros-Forteza, S. & de Unamuno, P. (1999) Longitudinal, transverse and diffuse nail hyperpigmentation induced by hydroxyurea. *Journal of the American Academy of Dermatology* 40, 333–334.

Hogan, P.A., Krafchik, B.R. & Boxall, L. (1991) Transverse striate leukonychia associated with cancer chemotherapy. *Pediatric Dermatology* 8, 67–68.

Horwitz, L.J. & Dreizen, S. (1990) Acral erythemas induced by chemotherapy and graft-versus-host diseases in adults with hematogenous malignancies. *Cutis* 46, 397–404.

Hrushesky, W.J. (1976) Serpentine supravenous 5-fluorouracil hyperpigmentation. *Cancer Treatment Reports* 60, 639.

Huinink, W.W.B., Prove, A.M., Piccart, M. et al. (1994) A phase II trial with docetaxel (taxotere) in second line treatment with chemotherapy for advanced breast cancer. *Annals of Oncology* 5, 527–532.

Jacob, C.I. & Frunza-Patten, S. (1998) Nail bed dyschromia secondary to docetaxel therapy. *Archives of Dermatology* 134, 1167–1168.

James, W.D. & Odom, R.B. (1983) Chemotherapy-induced transverse white lines in the fingernails. *Archives of Dermatology* 119, 334–335.

Jeanmougin, M., Civatte, J., Bonvalet, D. et al. (1982) Chromonychies et chimiothérapie anti-cancéreuse. *Annales de Dermatologie et de Vénéréologie* 109, 169–172.

Katz, M.E. & Hansen, T.W. (1979) Nail plate–nail bed separation. *Archives of Dermatology* 115, 860–861.

Kelsey, P.R. (1992) Multiple longitudinal pigmented bands during hydroxyurea therapy. *Clinical and Laboratory Haematology* 14, 337–338.

Kennedy, B.J., Smith, L.R. & Goltz, R.W. (1975) Skin changes secondary to hydroxyurea therapy. *Archives of Dermatology* 111, 183–187.

Kochupillai, V., Prabhu, M. & Bhide, N.K. (1983) Cancer chemotherapy and nail loss (onychomadesis). *Acta Haematologica* 70, 137.

Koranda, F.C., Dehemel, E.M., Kahn, G. et al. (1974) Cutaneous complications in immunosuppressed renal homograft recipients. *Journal of the American Medical Association* 229, 419.

Kowal-Vern, A. & Eng, A. (1993) Unusual erythema of the proximal nail fold and onychodermal band. *Cutis* 52, 43–49.

Kwong, Y.L. (1996) Hydroxyurea-induced nail pigmentation. *Journal of the American Academy of Dermatology* 35, 275–276.

Levantine, A. & Almeyda, J. (1974) Cutaneous reactions to cytostatic agents. *British Journal of Dermatology* 90, 239–242.

Levine, N. & Greenwald, E.S. (1978) Mucocutaneous side effects of cancer chemotherapy. *Cancer Treatment Reviews* 5, 67–84.

Llistosella, E., Codina, A., Alvarez, R. et al. (1991) Tegafur-induced acral hyperpigmentation. *Cutis* 48, 205–207.

Lokich, J.J. & Moore, C. (1984) Chemotherapy-associated palmar-plantar erythrodysesthesia syndrome. *Annals of Internal Medicine* 101, 798–800.

Lombart-Cussac, A., Pivot, X. & Spielman, M. (1997) Docetaxel chemotherapy induces transverse superficial loss of the nail plate. *Archives of Dermatology* 133, 1466–1467.

Malacarne, P. (1978) Chemioterapia antineoplastica e melanonichia striata. *Giornale Italiano di Dermatologia e Venereologia* 113, 223–226.

Malacarne, P. & Zavagli, G. (1977) Melphalan-induced melanonychia striata. *Archives of Dermatological Research* **258**, 81–83.

Marie, I., Levesque, H., Plissonnier, D. *et al.* (2000) Digital necrosis related to cisplatin in systemic sclerosis. *British Journal of Dermatology* **142**, 833–834.

Markenson, A.L., Chandra, M. & Miller, D.R. (1975) Hyperpigmentation after cancer chemotherapy. *Lancet* **ii**, 1128.

McCuaig, C.C., Ellis, C.N., Greenberg, H.S. *et al.* (1989) Mucocutaneous complications of intraarterial 5-bromodeoxyuridine and radiation. *Journal of the American Academy of Dermatology* **21**, 1235–1240.

Michel, J.L., Perrot, J.L., Thomas, L. *et al.* (1996) Complications cutanées de l'hydroxyuree: 17 cas. *Annales de Dermatologie et de Vénéréologie* **123** (Suppl. 1), S127–S128.

Miles, D.W. & Rubens, R.D. (1995) Transverse leukonychia. *New England Journal of Medicine* **33**, 100.

Morris, D., Aisner, J. & Wiernik, P.H. (1977) Horizontal pigmented banding of the nails in association with adriamycin chemotherapy. *Cancer Treatment Reports* **61**, 499–501.

Nixon, D.W. (1976) Alterations in nail pigment with cancer chemotherapy. *Archives of Internal Medicine* **136**, 1117–1118.

Nixon, D.W., Pirrozi, D., York, R.M. *et al.* (1981) Dermatologic changes after systemic cancer therapy. *Cutis* **27**, 181.

Norton, L.A. (1980) Nail disorders. *Journal of the American Academy of Dermatology* **22**, 451–467.

Ohnuma, T., Selawry, O.S., Holland, J.F. *et al.* (1972) Clinical study with bleomycin: tolerance to twice weekly dosage. *Cancer* **30**, 914–922.

Pechère, M., Zulian, G.B., Vogel, J.J. *et al.* (1996) Fingertips necrosis during chemotherapy with bleomycin, vincristine and methotrexate for HIV-related Kaposi's sarcoma. *British Journal of Dermatology* **134**, 372–382.

Pirard, C., Michaux, J.L. & Bourlond, A. (1994) Mélanonychie en bandes longitudinales et hydroxyurée. *Annales de Dermatologie et de Vénéréologie* **121**, 106–109.

Pratt, C.B. & Shanks, E.C. (1974) Hyperpigmentation of nails from doxorubicin. *Journal of the American Medical Association* **228**, 460.

Priestman, T.J. & James, K.W. (1975) Adriamycin and longitudinal pigmented banding of fingernails. *Lancet* **i**, 1337–1338.

Requena, L. (1991) Chemotherapy-induced transverse ridging of the nails. *Cutis* **48**, 129–130.

Richard, M., Truchetet, F., Friedel, J. *et al.* (1989) Skin lesions simulating chronic dermatomyositis during long-term hydroxyurea therapy. *Journal of the American Academy of Dermatology* **21**, 797–799.

Roussou, P., Ilias, I. & Foufopoulou, E. (1998) Onycholysis after chemotherapy in a patient with lymphoma. *Acta Dermato-Venereologica* **78**, 303.

Runne, U., Pleiff, B. & Mitrenga, D. (1980) Braunes nagelbett und onycholyse durch adriamycin; schwellung, pigmentierung und hyperkeratosen durch bleomycin. *Zeitschrift für Hautkrankheiten* **55**, 1590–1593.

Scheithauer, W., Ludwig, H., Kotz, R. *et al.* (1989) Mitoxantrone-induced discoloration of the nails. *Experimental Journal of Cancer and Clinical Oncology* **25**, 763–765.

Schwartz, R.A. & Vickerman, C.E. (1979) Muehrcke's lines of the fingernails. *Archives of Internal Medicine* **139**, 242.

Senet, P., Aractingi, S., Porneuf, M. *et al.* (1995) Hydroxyurea-induced dermatomyositis-like eruption. *British Journal of Dermatology* **133**, 455–459.

Shah, P.C., Rao, K.R.P. & Patel, A.S. (1978) Cyclophosphamide induced nail pigmentation. *British Journal of Dermatology* **98**, 675–680.

Shelley, W.B. & Humprey, G.B. (1997) Transverse leukonychia (Mees' lines) due to daunorubicin chemotherapy. *Pediatric Dermatology* **14**, 144–145.

Shetty, M.R. (1977) Case of pigmented banding of the nail caused by bleomycin. *Cancer Treatment Reports* **61**, 501.

Shetty, M.R. (1988) White lines in the fingernails induced by combination chemotherapy. *British Medical Journal* **297**, 1635.

Singh, M. & Kaur, S. (1986) Chemotherapy-induced multiple Beau's lines. *International Journal of Dermatology* **25**, 590–591.

Smith, E.A., Harper, F.E. & LeRoy, E.C. (1985) Raynaud's phenomenon of a single digit following local intradermal bleomycin sulphate injection. *Arthritis and Rheumatism* **28**, 459–461.

Snauwaert, J. & Degreef, H. (1984) Bleomycin-induced Raynaud's phenomenon and acral sclerosis. *Dermatologica* **169**, 172–174.

Speechly-Dick, M.E. & Owen, E.R.T.C. (1988) Mitozantrone-induced onycholysis. *Lancet* **i**, 113.

Suehiro, M., Kishimoto, S., Wakabayashi, T. *et al.* (1998) Hydroxyurea dermopathy with a dermatomyositis-like eruption and a large leg ulcer. *British Journal of Dermatology* **139**, 738–759.

Sulis, E. & Floris, C. (1980) Nail pigmentation following cancer chemotherapy. A new genetic entity? *European Journal of Cancer* **16**, 1317–1319.

Teresi, M.E., Murri, D.J. & Coznelius, A.S. (1993) Ifosamide-induced hyperpigmentation. *Cancer* **71**, 2873–2875.

Tucker, W.F.G. & Church, R.E. (1984) Beau's lines after razoxane therapy for psoriasis. *Archives of Dermatology* **120**, 1140.

Unamino, P., Fernandez-Lopez, E. & Santos, C. (1992) Leukonychia due to cytostatic agents. *Clinical and Experimental Dermatology* **17**, 273–274.

Van Belle, S.J.P., Dehou, M.F., De Bock, V. *et al.* (1989) Nail toxicity due to the combination adriamicyn-mitoxantrone. *Cancer Chemotherapy and Pharmacology* **24**, 69–70.

Vanhooteghem, O., André, J., Vindevoghel, A. *et al.* (1997) Docetaxel-induced subungual hemorrhage. *Dermatology* **194**, 419–420.

Veraldi, S., Renzi, D., Schianchi, R. *et al.* (1987) Ungual hyperpigmentation as the only sign of bleomycin poisoning. *Giornale Italiano di Dermatologia e Venereologia* **122**, 443–445.

Vogelzang, J.N., Bosl, G.J., Johnson, K. *et al.* (1981) Raynaud's phenomenon: a common toxicity after combination chemotherapy for testicular cancer. *Annals of Internal Medicine* **95**, 288–292.

Vomvouras, S., Pakula, A.S. & Shaw, J.M. (1991) Multiple pigmented nail bands during hydroxyurea therapy: an uncommon finding. *Journal of the American Academy of Dermatology* **24**, 1016–1017.

Wantzin, G.L. & Thomsen, K. (1983) Acute paronychia after high-dose methotrexate therapy. *Archives of Dermatology* **119**, 623–624.

Wheeland, R.G., Burgdorf, W.H.C. & Humphrey, G.B. (1983) The flag sign of chemotherapy. *Cancer* **51**, 1356–1358.

Wong, L.C., Choo, Y.C. & Ma, H.K. (1984) Oral etoposide in gesttional trophoblastic disease. *Cancer Treatment Reports* **68**, 775–777.

Zaun, H. & Omlor, G. (1992) Einseitige leukopathia unguis toxica und diffuser haarasfall nach zytostatischer extremitatenperfusion. *Hautarzt* **43**, 215–216.

## Radiation

Melanonychia striata has been reported after UVB and UVA phototherapy (Beltrani & Scher 1991). In this case one finger developed a subungual melanoma and a second finger was affected by benign melanocytic hyperplasia.

Onychomadesis, Beau's lines and nail hyperpigmentation can be consequences of X-ray therapy (Shelley *et al.* 1964; Runne & Orfanos 1981). Nail ridging has been reported in six patients who developed late chronic radiation changes after electron beam therapy (Price 1978).

### References

Beltrani, V.P. & Scher, R.K. (1991) Evaluation and management of melanonychia striata in a patient receiving phototherapy. *Archives of Dermatology* **127**, 319–320.

Price, N.M. (1978) Radiation dermatitis following electron beam therapy. *Archives of Dermatology* **114**, 63–66.

Runne, U. & Orfanos, C.E. (1981) The human nail. *Current Problems in Dermatology* **9**, 102–149.

Shelley, W.B., Rawnsley, H.M. & Pillsbury, D.M. (1964) Postirradiation melanonychia. *Archives of Dermatology* **90**, 174–176.

## Pulse oximetry

Digital skin necrosis can be a complication of pulse oximetry monitoring of critically ill or anaesthetized patients. Lesions are caused by pressure necrosis and occur at the site of application of the probe sensor (Stogner *et al.* 1991; Pettersen *et al.* 1992). On the one hand inaccuracy of the oxygen saturation determinations can be due to excessively long nails (Tweedie 1989), on the other hand unpolished acrylic nails, do not interfere with pulse oximetry (Peters 1997).

### References

Pettersen, B., Konsgaard, V. & Aune, H. (1992) Skin injury in an infant with pulse oxymetry. *British Journal of Anaesthesia* **69**, 204–205.

Peters, S.M. (1997) The effect of acrylic nails on the measurement of oxygen saturation as determined by pulse oxymetry. *American Anesthetic Journal* **65**, 361–363.

Stogner, S.W., Owens, M.J. & Baethge, B.A. (1991) Cutaneous necrosis and pulse oximetry. *Cutis* **48**, 235–237.

Tweedie, I.E. (1989) Pulse oximeters and long fingernails. *Anesthesia* **44**, 268.

## Miscellaneous drugs

### Antihistamines

Exacerbation of psoriasis, liver dysfunction and thrombocytopenia have been associated with mebhydrolin treatment (McKenna & McMillan 1993).

### Reference

McKenna, K.E. & McMillan, J.C. (1993) Exacerbation of psoriasis, liver dysfunction and thrombocytopenia associated with mebhidrolin. *Clinical and Experimental Dermatology* **18**, 131–132.

### Carotene

Long-term treatment with carotene can produce yellow discoloration of the nails.

### Cyclosporin

Two patients experienced Raynaud's phenomenon 2 days after treatment with cyclosporin 10 mg/kg/day was started. The therapy was interrupted in one patient who developed Raynaud's phenomenon again after reintroduction of the drug at a dose of 5 mg/kg/day (Deray *et al.* 1986). An increase of linear nail growth has been noticed by Baran (personal observation) and excess granulation tissue by Wakelin and Emmerson (1994) and Higgins *et al.* (1995). Repeated ingrowing toenails were noted in a 14-year-old boy. They did not recur when cyclosporin was stopped (Olujohungbe *et al.* 1993). Transverse leuconychia with marked nail pitting was observed in a psoriatic patient on cyclosporin (Siragusa & Alberti 1999).

### References

Deray, G., Lehoang, P., Achour, L. *et al.* (1986) Cyclosporine and Raynaud's phenomenon. *Lancet* **ii**, 1092–1093.

Higgins, E.M., Hughes, J.R., Snowden, S. *et al.* (1995) Cyclosporin-induced periungual granulation tissue. *British Journal of Dermatology* **132**, 829–830.

Olujohungbe, A., Cox, J., Hammon, M.D. *et al.* (1993) Ingrowing toenails and cyclosporin. *Lancet* **342**, 1111.

Siragusa, M. & Alberti, A. (1999) Mees' lines due to cyclosporin. *British Journal of Dermatology* **140**, 1198–1199.

Wakelin, S.H. & Emmerson, R.W. (1994) Excess granulation tissue development during treatment with cyclosporin. *British Journal of Dermatology* **131**, 147–148.

### Dimercaptosuccinic acid

A 16-year-old boy developed longitudinal nail striations after dimercaptosuccinic acid (DMSA) administration for mercury poisoning therapy (Thomas *et al.* 1987).

## Reference

Thomas, G., Fournier, L., Garnier, R. *et al.* (1987) Nail dystrophy and dimercaptosuccinic acid. *Journal de Toxicologie Clinique et Experimentable (Paris)* **7**, 285–287.

## Diuretics

Thiazide diuretics have been reported to produce onycholysis (Krull 1981).

## Reference

Krull, E. (1981) Fingernail abnormalities as indicators of systemic disease. *Topics in Dermatology* March.

## Ergotamine

Peripheral gangrene leading to limb amputation is a well-known complication of ergotamine overdosage (Cranley *et al.* 1963). It can also occur after the administration of standard dosages of the drug to patients presenting contraindications to its use. These include peripheral vascular disease, hypertension, coronary disease, pregnancy, thyrotoxicosis, sepsis, hepatic and renal disease, as well as anaemia and treatment with macrolides (Cameron & French 1960). Fingertip necrosis was due to sclerosis (Hahne & Balda 1998).

## References

Cameron, E.A. & French, E.B. (1960) St Anthony's fire rekindled: gangrene due to therapeutic dose of ergotamine. *British Medical Journal* **2**, 28–30.

Cranley, J.J., Krause, R.J., Strasser, E.S. *et al.* (1963) Impending gangrene of four extremities secondary to ergotism. *New England Journal of Medicine* **269**, 727–729.

Hahne, T. & Balda, B.R. (1998) Fingerkuppennekrosen nach dihydroergotaminmedikation bei limitierter systemischer sklerodermie. *Hautartz* **49**, 722–724.

## Fluorine

Prolonged fluorine ingestion produces changes in the skin and its appendages including teeth, nails and hair. Various nail dystrophies occur including brittleness, longitudinal striations (onychorrhexis), Beau's lines, as well as pitting, punctate and transverse leuconychia producing 'mottled' nails of both fingers and toes (Spira 1943, 1946).

## References

Spira, L. (1943) Mottled nails as an early sign of fluorosis. *Journal of Hygiene (Cambridge)* **43**, 69–71.

Spira, L. (1946) Disturbance of pigmentation in fluorosis. *Acta Medica Scandinavica* **126**, 65–84.

## Gelatin, biotin, cystine and methionine

These drugs have been claimed to accelerate nail growth (Runne & Orfanos 1981).

## Reference

Runne, U. & Orfanos, C.E. (1981) The human nail. *Current Problems in Dermatology* **9**, 102–149.

## Hydroquinone

A reversible brown or orange-brown pigmentation of the nails can be a consequence of topical hydroquinone treatment for melasma or actinic lentigines of the hands with a relationship to light exposure (Mann & Harman 1983).

## Reference

Mann, R.J. & Harman, R.R.R. (1983) Nail staining due to hydroquinone skin-lightening creams. *British Journal of Dermatology* **108**, 363–365.

## Iron

A patient experienced an exogenous brown discoloration of all nails and hair consequent to the use of water with a high iron content (Platschek & Lubach 1989).

## Reference

Platschek, H. & Lubach, D. (1989) Braune Haar- und Nagelverfärbungen durch eisenhaltiges Wasser. *Hautarzt* **40**, 441–442.

## Peloprenoic acid

Nail fragility was observed in psoriatics treated with peloprenoic acid derivatives (Ohkido, personal communication).

## Penicillamine and bucillamine

Longitudinal ridging, onychoschizia, elkonyxis and Beau's lines have been reported during penicillamine treatment. Absence of the lunulae and leukonychia can also be seen (Thivolet *et al.* 1968; Levy *et al.* 1983; Bjellerup 1989). Nail changes are reversible with cessation of treatment. Yellow nail syndrome has been described in patients taking penicillamine (Lubach & Marghescu 1979; Ilchyshyn & Vickers 1983). Isolated yellow nails were induced by bucillamine whose structure and chemical action are similar to those of D-penicillamine (Ishizaki *et al.* 1995).

## References

Bjellerup, M. (1989) Nail-changes induced by penicillamine. *Acta Dermato-Venereologica* **69**, 339–341.

Ilchyshyn, A. & Vickers, C.F.H. (1983) Yellow nail syndrome associated with penicillamine therapy. *Acta Dermato-Venereologica* **63**, 554–555.

Ishizaki, C., Sucki, H., Kohsokabe, S. *et al.* (1995) Yellow nail induced by bucillamine. *International Journal of Dermatology* **34**, 493–494.

Levy, R.S., Fisher, M. & Alter, J.N. (1983) Penicillamine: review and cutaneous manifestations. *Journal of the American Academy of Dermatology* **8**, 548.

Lubach, D. & Marghescu, S. (1979) Yellow-nail-syndrome durch d-Penizillamin. *Hautarzt* **30**, 547–549.

Thivolet, J., Perrot, H. & François, R. (1968) Glossite, stomatite et onychopathie provoquées par la pénicillamine. *Bulletin de la œdilla Societé Française de Dermatologie et de Syphiligraphie* **75**, 61–63.

## Phenylephrine

Purpura of the nail bed has been reported (Baran & Temime 1973).

## Reference

Baran, R. & Témime, P. (1973) Les onychodystrophies toxi-medicamenteuses et les onycholyses. *Concours Medical* **95**, 1007–1023.

## Salbutamol

Periungual and palmoplantar erythema has been described in pregnant women treated with salbutamol (Lacour *et al.* 1987).

## Reference

Lacour, J.P., Reygagne, P., Grimaldi, M. *et al.* (1987) Erythème pseudo-lupique des extrémités au cours de grossesses pathologiques traitées par salbutamol. *Presse Médicale* **32**, 1599.

## L-Tryptophan

Eosinophilic myalgia syndrome has been linked to L-tryptophan ingestion. Eosinophilic fasciitis (Gordon *et al.* 1991) as well as a reversible scleroderma-like illness (Connolly *et al.* 1990) has been reported after the ingestion of L-tryptophan for the treatment of insomnia (Connolly *et al.* 1990).

## References

Connolly, S.M., Quimby, S.R., Griffing, W.L. *et al.* (1990) L-Tryptophan: a possible explanation of the eosinophilia-myalgia-syndrome. *Journal of the American Academy of Dermatology* **23**, 451–457.

Gordon, M.L., Lebwohl, M.G., Phelps, R.G. *et al.* (1991) Eosinophilic fasciitis associated with tryptophan ingestion. *Archives of Dermatology* **127**, 217–220.

## Vitamin A

Nail dystrophy and brittle nails have been described with vitamin A treatment (Positano *et al.* 1989).

## Reference

Positano, R.G., DeLauro, T.M. & Berkowitz, B.J. (1989) Nail changes secondary to environmental influences. *Clin Pod Med Surg* **6**, 417–429.

## Interferon α

Necrosis of finger and toenails during treatment with interferon α has led to amputation of the digits (Backmeyer *et al.* 1996).

## Reference

Backmeyer, C., Farge, D., Miclea, J.M. *et al.* (1996). Nécroses digitales au cours de traitment par interferon alpha. *Annales de Dermatologie et de Vénéréologie* **123** (Suppl. 1), S124.

CHAPTER 7

# Occupational abnormalities and contact dermatitis

**R.J.G. Rycroft & R. Baran**

Cosmetic chemical sensitizers or irritants (see Chapter 8)
Discoloration of the nail plate (see Chapters 2 and 8)

**Nail protection at work**
**Nail cosmetic hazards at work**

## Definition

Occupational nail disorders represent those abnormalities of the nail apparatus produced or aggravated by the working environment.

The predisposing factors are those for occupational disorders elsewhere, that is:
• inexperienced workers;
• inadequate personal hygiene;
• excess use of irritants;
• temperature and humidity;
• inadequate protection.
  Accurate diagnosis depends on:
• appearance;
• disappearance and relapse of the nail condition;
• location of the lesion;
• patient's history.

## Diagnosis of occupational nail disorders

The fingernails are used as 'tools' in many occupations (Ronchese 1953, 1955, 1969) and the way they look is of importance in all occupations where personal contact occurs. Nail disorders can therefore be more disabling at work than might at first appear. Most nail disorders are confined to the hands.

The subject of the first part of this chapter is the wide range of nail disorders that are primarily caused by the working environment. Some of these look very like certain endogenous (constitutional) nail disorders. This makes their diagnosis more difficult. Nail changes in dermatoses such as psoriasis, tinea and lichen planus may be misinterpreted as being caused by work. Conditions such as psoriasis of the nails may, however, be exacerbated by occupational trauma or this may even precipitate an underlying tendency to the disease (isomorphic phenomenon); in patients with rheumatoid arthritis, lichen planus and secondary syphilis an identical phenomenon may occur (Fisher & Baran 1992). Atopic dermatitis should always be looked for and the most important aspect in a history for pre-employment screening is that of severe childhood eczema (English 1998).

## Aetiology

Frequently the causes of occupational nail disorders are multi-factorial. They can occur at any age, but there is widely thought to be a bimodal distribution of peaks in incidence of dermatitis, the first occurring in the early years of the job and the second in middle age. In women their frequency is twice as high as in men (English 1998).

In assessing a nail condition suspected of being occupational:
1 Visualize what the hands do at work.
2 Look for functional distribution (commonly, the first three fingers of the dominant hand).
3 Check for occupational stigmas of the nails.
4 Examine the whole of the skin surface. This should never be omitted. The correct diagnosis may be evident at a site very distant from the nails.
5 Ask about the presence of similar nail conditions in co-workers and about hobbies with potential chemical or metal exposure (Kern 1990).

Thorough investigations are necessary to identify the allergens and/or irritants that may be causing the nail disorders. Although still a research tool, estimation of the levels of metals such as arsenic and nickel in the fingernails may be a useful indicator of occupational exposure (Agahian *et al.* 1990; Peters *et al.* 1991).

There are also some laboratory tests, such as mycological and bacteriological examinations, which are essential diagnostic aids. A punch biopsy of the nail can sometimes additionally assist. An X-ray of the terminal phalanx is occasionally relevant, for example exostosis of occupational origin.

The final diagnosis may require a workplace visit.

## Handicap, impairment and disability

Handicap describes the effect on the patient's normal functioning in society as a result of the disability, while impairment is the effect of the disease process on the diseased organ (e.g. persisting fissures on the fingertips). Disability describes the functional effect of this impairment and so, in the above example, the disability might be that the patient could not use a keyboard because of the pain and disordered sensation of the fingers resulting from the disease (Finlay & Ryan 1996).

## Clinical reaction patterns

Reaction patterns that can be seen clinically include:
• changes in the texture and contour of the nail plate, ony-chauxis, worn-down nail plate (*usure des ongles*), brittle nails, koilonychia, clubbing and pseudo-clubbing;

- changes in the surface of the nail plate and its attachments, resulting from direct trauma, matrix involvement or paronychia with sometimes onychomadesis leading to nail shedding;
- changes in the surrounding tissue (pulpitis);
- changes in colour with nail plate staining or subungual alteration;
- distal bony phalanx anomalies.

## Occupational nail hazards

### Traumatic abnormalities

One of the most important groups of occupational disorders, which includes major trauma, repeated microtrauma and foreign body injury.

#### Acute major trauma

The level of the nail bed injury is the critical factor in deciding the requirement for nail bed management. Nail stability requires at least 5 mm of healthy nail bed, distal to the lunula, for nail adherence (Rosenthal 1983). Acute injury may be associated with partial or total haematoma (25% of the surface of the visible nail plate), lacerating wounds, fractures of the terminal phalanx, denudation of the distal phalanx and foreign bodies.

#### Delayed postacute traumatic deformities

These may be associated with onycholysis, dorsal pterygium, split nail deformity, various nail dystrophies and hooked nail.

#### Repeated microtrauma

This may be associated with koilonychia, finger nail fragility, toenail dystrophy and onycholysis of mechanical origin, and may be caused by foreign bodies.

*Friction and pressure* gradually wear down the nail and are characteristic of particular occupations such as guitar players (Fig. 7.1a,b) (occupational stigmas). Pottery workers (Fig. 7.1c) and workers who repeatedly lift heavy bags (Schubert *et al.* 1977) (Fig. 7.2) are other examples. Onycholysis, koilonychia, longitudinal splitting and occasional splinter haemorrhages may also be seen. Subungual haemorrhages have been reported from the USA in three inexperienced male dishwashers using heavy rubber gloves while working (Long 1958), and are frequent in sportsmen's toes (Gibbs 1973; Baran 1978) and in the toes of dancers, where there may be associated subungual exostosis (Sebastian 1977). Slaughterhouse workers, manually skinning cattle, develop a rectangular onycholysis of the central

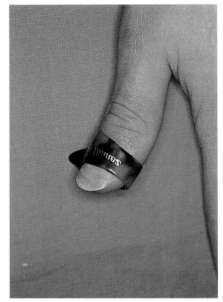

(a)

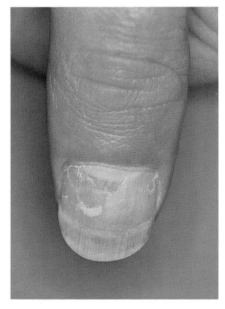

(b)

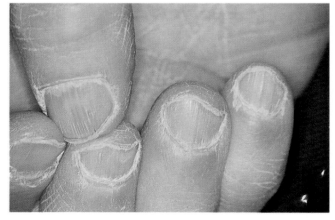

(c)

**Fig. 7.1**  (right) (a,b) Occupational stigmas in a guitar player. (Courtesy of C. Romaguera, Spain). (c) Worn-down nails due to occupational friction and pressure (pottery worker).

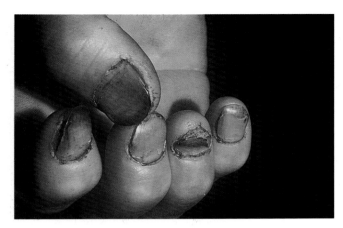

**Fig. 7.2** Nail dystrophy due to lifting heavy plastic bags.

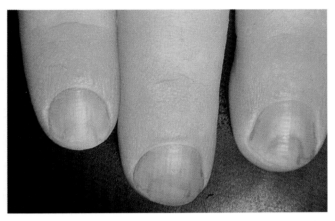

**Fig. 7.3** 'Rectangular' onycholysis—slaughterhouse workers' dystrophy. (Courtesy of T. Menne, Denmark.)

nail plate and, in one case, necrosis of the nail bed was reported (Menné *et al.* 1985) (Fig. 7.3).

Transverse leuconychia has been described in Japan from the mechanical pressure of keypunching (Honda *et al.* 1976).

*Repeated low-grade frictional trauma* occurs in a multitude of occupations (Freeman & Rosen 1990). In a carpenter, for example, scaling, erythema and fissuring involved the left thumb and both index fingers on areas corresponding to those used to grip the nails and screws.

Mechanical trauma associated with thermal injury has produced fissured, scaly patches on the pulps of toast-makers' fingers (Brooke & Coulson 1998).

*Vibrating power tools*, such as pneumatic drills and chainsaws, cause nail thickening, brittleness and splitting of the free edges. Yellow-white longitudinal bands may extend distally from the lunula, sometimes becoming confluent. Distally the nails become darkly tinged and may turn black. The nail plate may develop ridging and eventually be shed entirely (Kulcsár 1966). The same stimulus causes Raynaud's phenomenon in the skin (vibration white finger), especially when vibrating power tools are operated in cold climates (Taylor 1982; Yu *et al.* 1988), or in carpal tunnel syndrome (Boyle *et al.* 1988; Veccherini-Blineau & Guiheneuc 1988). The hand that holds and guides the tool is often more severely affected. Raynaud's phenomenon has also been seen in typists, violinists and pianists. Ekenvall (1987) has usefully reviewed the clinical assessment of patients between attacks.

Sports-related traumas are frequent. In *golfer's nails*, distal splinter haemorrhages are seen, especially in the fingers used most strongly in the golf grip hand (Ryan & Goldsmith 1995).

Catching a frisbee may produce repeated minor damage to the nail plate—*frisbee nail* (Jillson 1979).

*Judo* can be responsible for trachyonychia. The frequent grabbing of the opponent's jacket accounts for the rough 'judo' nails (Shelley & Shelley 1995).

*Karate* may produce clubbing; in addition professional and recreational karate enthusiasts are likely to injure the nail matrix as a consequence of the sharp, strong blows to which their fingernails and toenails are prone. Clinically, this presents as leuconychia, usually in transverse bands (Scher 1988).

*Tennis* and *squash* players, where sudden, abrupt changes in foot direction occur, develop tennis toe and may exhibit subungual haemorrhages.

*Soccer* players and joggers can suffer the same complications.

### Musician-related trauma

The piano can produce a vasospastic white finger disease as well as paronychia. The harp can also be responsible for paronychia associated with onycholysis and subungual haemorrhages (Harvell & Maibach 1992). The violin may induce paronychia.

Friction as a cause of irritant contact dermatitis may be observed in guitar players whose fingers are used to pluck the strings. (Freeman & Rosen 1990). Acroosteolysis associated with pain in the distal fingers has been reported (Baran & Tosti 1993).

### Foreign body injury

Exposure to certain *plants and woods* may cause foreign body injury. Thorns, thistles and sharp-edged leaves may injure the nails, especially cactus thorns in desert areas. Secondary infection is a likely complication.

*Hyacinth and narcissus bulbs* possess raphide cells containing bundles of needle-shaped crystals of calcium oxalate. These crystals readily penetrate the periungual skin causing erythema and oedema with pain and itching (Hjorth & Wilkinson 1968). Recently, paronychia associated with daffodil pickers' rash has been reported (Julian & Bowers 1997).

*Glass fibre*, above approximately 5 μm in diameter, mechanically irritates the periungual tissue. Paronychia may result from the penetration of glass spicules beneath the proximal nail fold. It may also cause onycholysis with darkening of the nail plate (Rogaïlin *et al.* 1975). Implantation of *hair* beneath the nail may produce onycholysis (de Berker *et al.* 1994; Buendia-Eisman *et al.* 1997), and even subungual trichogranuloma (Hogan 1988). Chronic paronychia which sometimes appears in hairdressers (Stone 1975) may deserve surgical management in recalcitrant cases (Baran & Bureau 1981).

*Victualler's thumbnail*, a condition of subungual osmotrauma, is the consequence of small foreign bodies of dehydrated food becoming embedded below the nails (Head 1984).

## Physical hazards

*Burns*, when mild, cause onycholysis. When severe, disfiguring scars, pterygium and fissured nails may result.

Prolonged exposure to *cold* may result in injury to the nail matrix, leading to derangement of the nail plate ranging from Beau's lines to complete shedding. Cold injury, particularly to peripheral parts, is common among such groups as soldiers on active service—adequate protective measures now make this rarer than in the past; conditions such as trench foot (Fairbairn *et al.* 1972), acute pernio (chilblains) and frostbite (Washburn 1962) may damage the nail apparatus. Seasonal koilonychia in Ladakh, in North-west India, is due to exposure to cold water while hand washing clothes (Murdoch 1993) and to wet mud while repairing walls and irrigation canals (Dolma *et al.* 1990). Frostbite, the freezing of tissues in response to cold air, metals or liquids, may cause tissue loss due to vasospasm with thrombus formation and extracellular ice crystal formation. Venous pressure increases, capillary perfusion decreases and intravascular 'sludging' is evident. Depending on the acuteness of the cold injury to the nail apparatus, changes akin to chilblains, Raynaud's phenomenon or disease and early acrosclerosis may be seen, including necrosis or gangrene of skin or deeper tissues. Numbness of the tip of the right index finger and thumb has been noted as a side-effect of cryotherapy in the treating physician. It would seem that even brief contact with the nitrogen-cooled nozzle of a cryosurgical unit is sufficient to induce superficial neural damage in the fingertips, provided that exposure occurs repeatedly (Heidenheim & Jemec 1991). It should be noted that the nail apparatus possesses a good anastomotic blood supply and large numbers of glomus bodies, which help to protect against all but the worst of cold injuries.

*Ionizing radiation* may cause the loss of nails (Gallaghar *et al.* 1955), and the late changes of chronic radiodermatitis (Messite *et al.* 1957) may give rise to Bowen's disease or skin cancer (De Dulanto & Camacho 1979) up to 30 years after exposure. The earliest signs are brittleness and longitudinal ridging (Figs 7.4 & 7.5). Later the nail plates become dull and slightly opaque with a brownish hue. The skin at a corresponding stage shows atrophy, telangiectasia and keratoses. The thumb is never involved in X-ray dermatitis. A verrucous lesion appearing on the hyponychium or adjacent nail bed may herald the development of malignant change (Fig. 7.6). Minute black

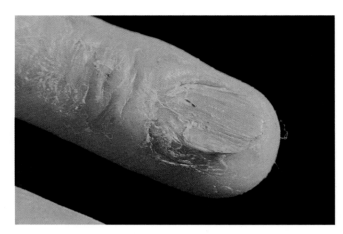

**Fig. 7.4** X-irradiation nail changes—brittleness and longitudinal ridging.

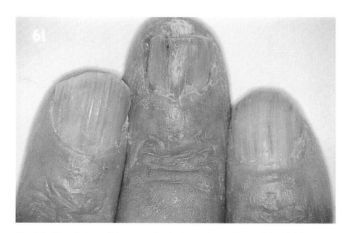

**Fig. 7.5** X-irradiation nail damage—distal subungual warty lesion of the third finger.

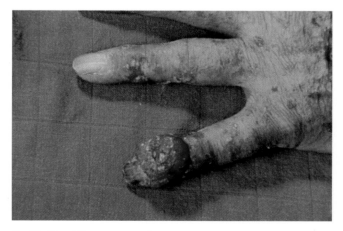

**Fig. 7.6** X-irradiation squamous carcinoma.

spots, known as 'coal spots', appear beneath the nail plate and slowly spread over large areas of nail, often in longitudinal bands. A chronic relapsing paronychia commonly occurs. Occupational radiodermatitis from Ir192 exposure was reported in three Spanish industrial radiologists (Condé-Salazar *et al.* 1986). After a brief episode of acute radiodermatitis, which may elude diagnosis, an asymptomatic period of many months may precede the typical picture of chronic radiodermatitis.

*Microwave radiation* can cause transverse ridging, onycholysis and other plate dystrophies. Brodkin and Bleiberg (1973) reported nail damage in restaurant workers exposed to a faulty microwave oven. They emphasized that the nail matrix may be damaged by microwave-induced thermal injury without the sensation of heat being felt by the oven user.

## Sensitizers

While it is debatable whether contact sensitization ever occurs through the nail plate, rather than via periungual skin, the nail plate can certainly be altered by subsequent allergic contact dermatitis. A true, positive patch test typically shows that erythema, papules or vesicles may spread beyond the test site (English 1998). Sensitizers causing occupational allergic contact dermatitis in the nail area are discussed next.

### Plants and flowers

*Alstroemeria* dermatitis can result in onycholysis, in addition to dermatitis of the thumbs and index fingers (Rycroft & Calnan 1981).

*Hydrangea* dermatitis may present with a clinical picture which includes chronic paronychia and associated nail dystrophy (Bruynzeel 1986).

*Nasturtium*, a common plant used in salads, may produce fingertip dermatitis (Derrick & Darley 1997).

The wooden *orange stick* traditionally used for applying cuticle remover has been responsible for a persistent eczema of the right hand in a manicurist (Brun 1978).

*Rhus dermatitis* (from poison ivy, oak and sumac) may result in onycholysis and a yellowish discoloration of the nail plate (Fulghum 1972).

*Tabernaemontana coronaria* has produced a unique fingertip dermatitis of the thumb, index and middle finger of both hands with itching, erythema, scaling, severe fissuring and exudation (Bajaj *et al.* 1996).

'Tulip fingers' (Fig. 7.7) is a painful, dry, fissured, hyperkeratotic eczema caused by contact with tulip bulbs. It starts beneath the free margin of the nails and extends to the fingertips and periungual regions. Suppurative granulating erosions may be seen on the fingertips in longstanding cases. At times the face, hands, forearms and genitals may also become involved. The highest concentration of the allergen, α-methylene-γ-butyrolactone, is to be found in the outermost cell layers of the inner bulb scales (Hausen 1982; Gette & Marks 1990; Bruynzeel 1997).

*Turpentine*, the oleoresin from pine trees, is now a much less common sensitizer than it used to be, owing to its gradual replacement as a solvent by less expensive substitutes. In craft

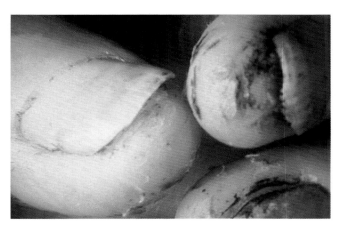

**Fig. 7.7** 'Tulip fingers' dystrophy. (Courtesy of the late N. Hjorth, Denmark.)

workers, it can still occasionally cause an eczema of the periungual tissues and fingers with subungual hyperkeratosis.

### Chemicals

*Acrylics*, the methacrylate and acrylate compounds developed during the 1930s, found extensive application in plastic glass for aircraft, paints, coatings and printing inks, as well as in dentistry. Today, acrylates have a broad area of application in various products, such as: the manufacture of dental prostheses and tooth fillings; printing colours; lacquers; paints; orthopaedic prostheses and splints; soft contact lenses; histological preparations; floor waxes; floor coatings; surface treatments of leather, textiles and paper products; nail cosmetics; and as glues, sealants and adhesives (Kanerva *et al.* 1997b). Repeated contact with acrylic materials, especially the sensitizing liquid monomers, has long been known to be responsible for contact dermatitis in dental staff (Rustemeyer & Frosch 1996) and orthopaedic surgeons (Rycroft 1977).

More recently a wider public has been affected by the practice of wearing sculptured artificial nails (Freeman *et al.* 1995). Sculptured nails are marketed as a kit containing an artificial nail called the template, a liquid monomer and a powdered polymer (Chapter 9). By mixing the monomer and polymer together polymerization is effected because of the presence of an organic peroxide catalyst and an accelerator. The material can be moulded onto the client's natural nail and hardening occurs at room temperature or in a photobonding box (Kanerva *et al.* 1996). First the natural nail is roughened with a burr. Then it is painted with the acrylic compound to produce, on hardening, an artificial nail. This is gradually enlarged and elongated by repeated applications. The prosthesis can be filed and manicured to the desired shape, and as the nail plate grows out further infillings of acrylic can be made to maintain the natural contour.

After a few months of application, patients may begin to show an allergic contact dermatitis, usually of the dorsal aspects

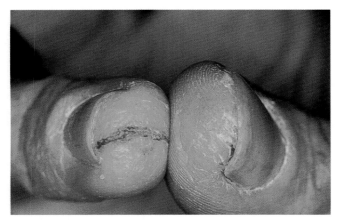

**Fig. 7.8** Fingertip dermatitis with chronic paronychia in a dentist. (Courtesy of L. Kanerva, Finland.)

of some of the fingers and paronychial tissue, the face and the eyelids, but sometimes more extensively (Fitzgerald & English 1994). Pain and persistent paraesthesia has been reported in a dental nurse (Kanerva *et al.* 1998), but permanent paraesthesia may occur without an allergic reaction (Baran & Schibli 1990). Paronychial inflammation may be quite severe: dentist's occupational allergic paronychia associated with severe fingertip dermatitis can be caused by acrylics (Fig. 7.8). In some cases, sensitization may produce significant economic and mental stress in affected patients (Kanerva *et al.* 1997d). Interestingly, no difference in the occurrence of skin problems was observed between individuals using gloves and individuals who did not use gloves while handling acrylates (Mürer *et al.* 1995). Nail discoloration may occur and the nail bed itself usually becomes dry and thickened. Onycholysis of the natural nail occurs with thinning and splitting (Goodwin 1976). This disfiguration of the nail plate can last for many months.

On patch testing the patients react strongly to the liquid acrylic monomer but not to the polymer. However (meth)-acrylate-containing products regularly contain undeclared (meth)acrylate compounds (Kanerva *et al.* 1997a). Until recently methyl methacrylate was used, but in 1976 the Food and Drug Administration in the USA banned its use. Since then, other methacrylates as well as acrylates, dimethacrylates and trimethacrylates have been used instead (Rosenzweig & Scher 1993), which also sensitize (Marks *et al.* 1979; Freeman *et al.* 1995; Kanerva *et al.* 1996).

Manicurists, who apply these artificial nails to clients, may become sensitized. The thumb and index (Condé-Salazar *et al.* 1986) or middle fingers of the left hand are constantly exposed as the manicurist holds the client's finger during the building-up process of the sculptured nails. Even exposure to the vapour from open bottles may subsequently elicit dermatitis in highly sensitized persons. Loss of fingernails due to persisting allergic contact dermatis in an artificial gel nail designer is rarely reported (Haglmüller *et al.* 1995). The preparation used in the case reported by Haglmüller *et al.* was a one-component

gel based on aliphatic urethaneacrylate, tetraethyleneglycol-diacrylate and hydroxyfunctional methacrylates.

A laboratory technician working in the manufacture of disposable contact lenses developed neurological and gastrointestinal symptoms after working with UV-curable acrylic monomers. The only skin symptom was transient onycholysis of the fingernails (Andersen 1986).

Industrial sealants which polymerize rapidly under anaerobic conditions in the presence of the metals in steel and brass contain sensitizing *dimethacrylates*. These products have immensely useful applications in the locking of screws firmly into position. Allergic contact dermatitis from such sealants affects principally the pulps of the fingers (Cronin 1980a) and can extend as scaly eczema under the free margin of the nails (Condé-Salazar *et al.* 1986). Kanerva *et al.* (2001) have reported on optician's occupational allergic contact dermatitis, paraesthesia and paronychia caused by anaerobic acrylic sealants. Onycholysis has been described in several such patients (Mathias & Maibach 1984; Guerra *et al.* 1993). Using acrylic resin to repair windscreens may produce dermatitis of the fingertips (Pedersen 1997), with positive tests to 2-hydroxy-ethylmethacrylate (HEMA) and methyl methacrylate (MMA). Patients working with dental prostheses should be patch tested with MMA, HEMA, dimethacrylates, epoxy acrylates and urethane acrylates (Kanerva *et al.* 1993).

Dentin bonding systems seem to be stronger sensitizers than MMA. Furthermore, seven of the 11 patients reported by Kanerva *et al.* (1994) developed paraesthesia.

Triple-cured hybrid-glass ionomers contain the same sensitizing acrylics, for example dimethacrylates, as dental composite resins and bonding agents. As they are mixed manually, and acrylics rapidly penetrate protective gloves (Munksgaard 1992), the risk of becoming occupationally sensitized is evident (Kanerva *et al.* 1997c). Thus, no-touch techniques should be used when handling uncured acrylics.

Printing workers sensitized to *photopolymerizable acrylic resin* may show eczematous lesions on the fingertips and around the nail plate, extending to the distal subungual area (Calas *et al.* 1977). Thumb, index and middle fingers of both hands are affected with fissuring and scaling (Goday *et al.* 1997).

'*Caine' local anaesthetics*, especially amethocaine and procaine, cause an allergic contact dermatitis in dental personnel particularly on the pulps of the first three digits, either due to contact with the preparatory topical preparation or with the liquid to be injected. *Propanidid* can produce a similar pattern in anaesthetists with paronychia, sometimes of both hands (Castelain & Piriou 1980) (Fig. 7.9).

*Cement dermatitis* may be allergic, due to the dichromate content, or may result from alkaline irritation and burns. Dermatitis of the dorsum of the proximal nail fold and koilonychia are frequent (Fig. 7.10). The latter is usually accompanied by distolateral subungual hyperkeratosis lifting the lateral edges of the nail. Painful fissures in the same area are common (Calnan 1960).

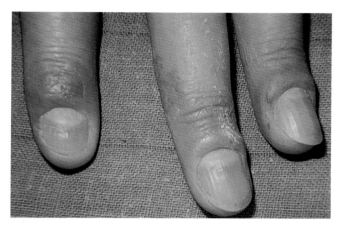

**Fig. 7.9** Propanidid paronychia, usually seen in anaesthetists. (Courtesy of P.Y. Castelain, France.)

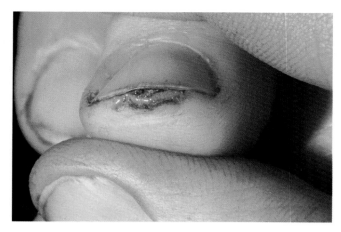

**Fig. 7.11** Codeine sensitization—pharmaceutical industry workers. (Courtesy of C. Romaguera, Spain.)

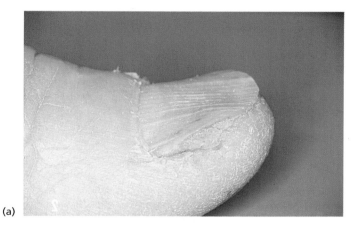

(a)

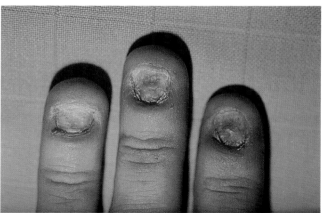

(b)

**Fig. 7.10** (a) Cement dermatitis nail signs with lateral subungual hyperkeratosis. (b) Nail atrophy—cement worker. (Courtesy of J.L. Levy, France.)

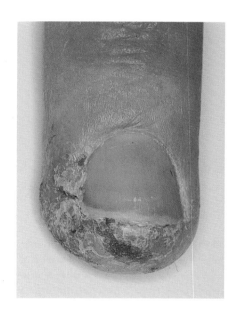

**Fig. 7.12** Epoxy resin 'dermatitis'.

*Codeine* sensitization in pharmaceutical workers has been associated with subungual hyperkeratosis, onycholysis and nail atrophy, as well as dermatitis of the hands, arms and face (Romaguera & Grimalt 1983) (Fig. 7.11).

*Epoxy resin* dermatitis (Bord & Castelain 1966; Brooke & Beck 1999) especially involves the right first two fingertips, producing erosion and crusting or necrotic-appearing lesions (Fowler 1990); the resin oligomer may collect under the free edge of the nail and polymerize slowly as it dries (Fig. 7.12).

*Ethyl-cyanocrylate*-containing adhesive used in nail wrapping, in which linen or silk is glued to the abraded nail and filed down, as well as for attaching preformed plastic nails, can cause a periungual contact dermatitis in manicurists and/or clients (Shelley & Shelley 1988) and in hairstylists attaching pieces of false hair to bald scalps (Tomb *et al.* 1993). It spreads to the eyelids and may appear as patches over the backs of the hands (Fitzgerald *et al.* 1995) simulating small-plaque parapsoriasis (Shelley & Shelley 1984).

Plate makers and those with *food allergy* such as to onions (Fig. 7.13), garlic (Burgess 1952; Burks 1954; Jappe *et al.*

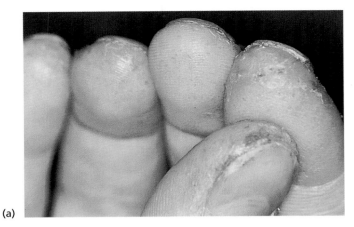

(a)

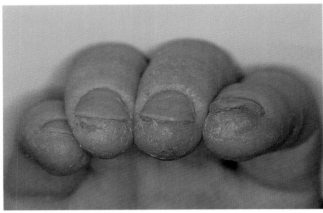

(b)

**Fig. 7.13** (a,b) Nail changes due to contact with onions.

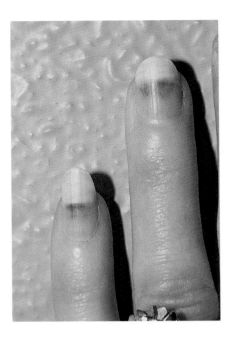

**Fig. 7.14** Nail dystrophy with subungual haemorrhage due to formaldehyde.

1999), tomatoes, etc., may develop finger pulp dermatitis with hyperkeratosis and fissuring, paronychia (Tosti *et al.* 1992) and onycholysis. The nails may also present with several transverse depressions (Bleumink *et al.* 1972). Food handlers who have contact with uncooked food may develop immediate type hypersensitivity in the form of protein contact dermatitis, a variant of contact urticaria (English 1998).

*Formaldehyde* (Fig. 7.14) is responsible for sensitization in many occupational groups, including hospital staff, when an eczema of the fingers with nail dystrophy may result (Cronin 1980b).

*Glutaraldehyde*, the active ingredient in many commonly used cold sterilizing agents, may be responsible for a papulovesicular, scaly, pruritic dermatitis. This was primarily around the fingertips in the case reported by Fowler's (1991); onychodystrophy was also noted.

*Hydroxylamine*, which is both a sensitizer and an irritant, may produce onycholysis and/or paronychia (Pellerat & Chabeau 1976; Goh 1990; Baran 1991). It has been widely used in colour photograph processing, the chemical industry (oximes synthesis), the pharmaceutical industry (bactericide, fungicide, anti-algal) and in the manufacture of rubber and plastic compounds, cosmetics and soap.

*1-Methylquinoxalinium-p-toluene sulfonate* sensitization, from a conditioner applied to offset lithography plates in order to render the image receptive to ink, causes dermatitis of the fingertips and periungual areas, particularly of the index, middle and ring fingers of the right hand (English *et al.* 1986).

Contact sensitivity to a cycloplegic *mydriatic agent* and to its pharmacological components tropicamide and phenylephrine hydrochloride was reported on the finger of a nurse. Her work included the instillation of eyedrops into patients undergoing routine fundoscopic examination. The lesions showed well-demarcated brownish erythema with scaling on the 2nd and 3rd fingers of her left hand. She used these fingers when separating the lids of patients for the instillation of mydriatic drops, some of which leaked on to her hands (Okamoto & Kawai 1991).

Allergic contact dermatitis from *nonoxynol-6*, a non-ionic emulsifier in an industrial waterless hand cleanser, was associated with a transverse dystrophy of the fingernails (Nethercott & Lawrence 1984).

*Propacetamol* is an analgesic and antipyretic medication which may induce fissured fingertip eczema in nurses preparing injections of this drug (Barbaud *et al.* 1997).

*Quaternium-15*, a broad-spectrum bactericidal formaldehyde releaser, was responsible for throbbing pain and tenderness in fingernails which had gradually become thickened and discoloured. Uncommonly seen, it has occurred in hairdressers (Marren *et al.* 1991).

During the summer of 1979 women in Britain using adhesive to attach a brand of plastic artificial nails began to present with onycholysis, subungual hyperkeratosis, atrophy of the nail plate and dermatitis of the periungual skin (Rycroft *et al.* 1980). This was traced to contact sensitization by p-*tertiary*

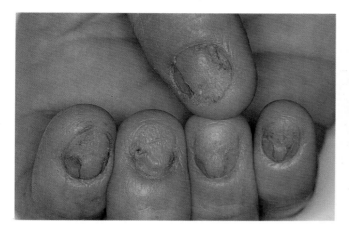

**Fig. 7.15** Dystrophy due to *p*-tertiary butylphenol (PTBP) formaldehyde resin.

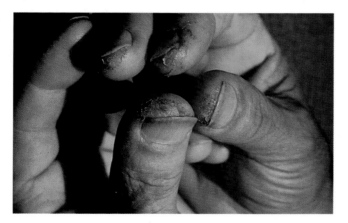

**Fig. 7.16** Fisherman's dystrophy due to escavenitis. (Caused by sea-worm coelomic fluid.) (Courtesy of P. Angelini, Italy.)

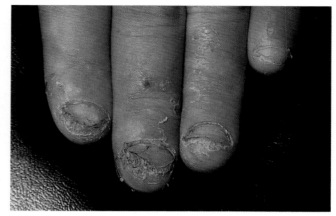

**Fig. 7.17** Severe dermatitis and nail dystrophy due to bryozoans. (Courtesy of C. Audebert, France.)

*Bryozoans* ('moss animals'), invertebrate animals resembling seaweeds, cause contact and photocontact dermatitis with nail involvement, including pitting, paronychia, extensive distal nail dystrophy and subungual hyperkeratosis (Audebert & Lamoureux 1978) (Fig. 7.17).

## Chemical irritants

An irritant patch test reaction is a sharply demarcated erythema with minimal infiltration and with pustules (English 1998).

The nails can be softened and gradually destroyed by prolonged immersion in water containing high concentrations of *alkalis*, *alkaline chlorine-containing compounds* (Coskey 1974) or powerful *detergents* (Fig. 7.18). Irritant reactions appear around and under the nails when the hands come into contact with concentrated enzyme powder. Bleeding ulcerations under the nails may be seen (Göthe *et al.* 1972).

*Aminoethyl ethanolamine*-containing soldering flux in the electronics industry is usually irritant and may sometimes cause allergic contact dermatitis (Goh 1985), beginning periungually, with onycholysis, and spreading down the fingers and patchily onto the backs of the hands.

Permanent wave chemicals (*ammonium thioglycolate*) may cause koilonychia in hairdressers in conjunction with soreness of the distal nail beds, without associated dermatitis (Alanko *et al.* 1997) (Fig. 7.19). Thioglycolates in depilatories (chemical hair removers) are a further domestic cause of acute chemical onycholysis, several fingernails being involved at the same time (Baran 1980).

The application of a solution containing *arsenic*, *copper acetate* and *hydrochloric acid*, used to give a patina to belt-buckles, produced a marked throbbing pain in the distal phalanx of all the fingers of the right hand after 3 days. A green-blue coloration appeared in the nails, in the surrounding tissues and in the pulp, together with an oedema of the affected region (Fig. 7.20). Onycholysis, slight subungual hyperkeratosis and acropulpitis were still evident after 6 months (Balguerie 1990).

*butylphenol (PTBP) formaldehyde resin* in a particular batch of the adhesive (Fig. 7.15). This was a particular problem because the patients using these nails tended to have occupations which brought them into the public eye.

*Thiourea* contained in silver polish may produce contact and photocontact allergy with vesicular eruption of the fingertips and invasion under the fingernails (Dooms-Goossens *et al.* 1988).

*Unsaturated polyester (UP) resin cements* can sensitize car repairers and mould makers, the resulting dermatitis sometimes having an element of subungual hyperkeratosis (Tarvainen *et al.* 1993).

## Biological sensitivity

*Escavenitis* (Montel & Gouyer 1957) (Fig. 7.16). The coelomic fluid of a sea-worm (*Nesreis diversicolor*) used as bait can cause an exudative onychopathy with onycholysis of the first three fingers of the right hand in fishermen.

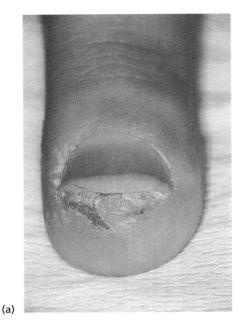

(a)

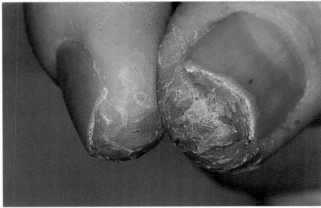

(b)

**Fig. 7.18** (a,b) Subungual and fingertip inflammatory eruption due to powerful detergents.

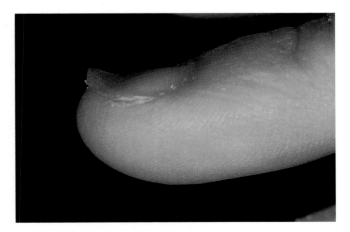

**Fig. 7.19** Koilonychia in a hairdresser (thioglycolate). (Courtesy of L. Kanerva, Finland.)

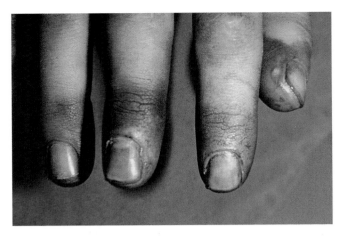

**Fig. 7.20** Discoloration of the digits and nails with oedematous changes, due to solution used to give patina to belt-buckles. (Courtesy of X. Balguerie, France.)

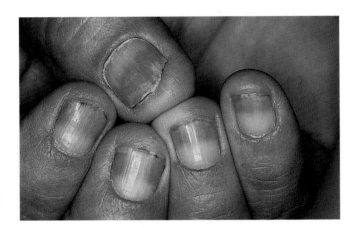

**Fig. 7.21** Nail discoloration and onycholysis due to 5% dinitroorthocresol.

The weed killers *diquat* and *paraquat* can also soften and discolour the nail plate, leading to nail loss (Botella *et al.* 1985). This can happen either from contact with the chemicals in concentrated form (Samman & Johnston 1969) or following gross contamination with diluted solutions (Hearn & Keir 1971). Similar changes have been described in a man using *5% dinitro-orthocresol* (Fig. 7.21), without further recommended dilution, for spraying fruit trees (Baran 1974). *Dinobuton* handlers may present with yellow nails and hair (Wahlberg 1974) (Fig. 7.22).

Enzyme detergents were found to cause acute onychia and onycholysis in housewives (Hodgson & Mayon-White 1971); symptoms appeared after 2 weeks of using an enzyme detergent for approximately an hour each day without gloves. Patch tests with 1% and 2% aqueous solutions of the detergent were negative.

Prolonged occupational contact with *formaldehyde* solutions can cause softening and brown discoloration of the nail plate (Schwartz *et al.* 1957b). Formalin (37–50% solution of

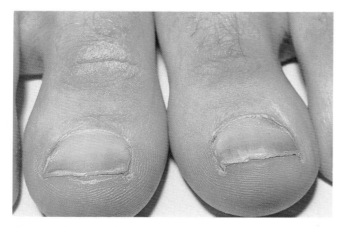

**Fig. 7.22** Yellow nails in a dinobuton handler. (Courtesy of J.E. Wahlberg, Sweden.)

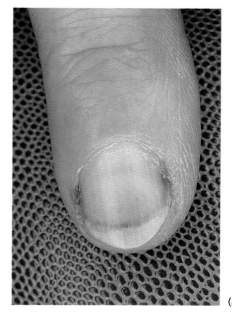
(a)

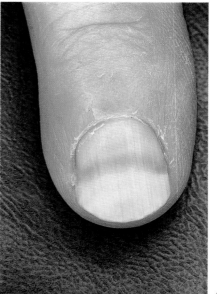
(b)

formaldehyde in water) is widely used industrially. It can be used as a preservative, a tanning agent and to augment the water resistance of paper.

*Gold potassium cyanide* is responsible for a purplish-brown discoloration and onycholysis of the nails among electroplaters and electronics workers (Budden & Wilkinson 1978).

*Hydrofluoric acid* especially damages the subungual tissues, which are a common portal of entry for this highly destructive chemical (Fig. 7.23). The acid readily diffuses through minute holes in rubber gloves. Frequently the burn is unrecognized until up to 24 h later when excruciating pain begins; severe progressive tissue destruction results from the unique properties of the fluoride ion. The subungual tissues are especially susceptible to its destructive effect (Sebastian 1994) and specific treatment with a topical 2% calcium gluconate preparation is indicated (MacKinnon 1986; Julie *et al.* 1988), or, even better, intra-arterial injection with a bolus of calcium (14 mg/kg) followed by prophylactic nail avulsion and continuous topical calcium gluconate therapy for 4–6 days (Sebastian 1994). Hydrofluoric acid is widely used in the semiconductor industry but can be a component of rust-removing agents (Shewmake & Anderson 1979; Baran 1980; Pedersen 1980). It is used, considerably diluted, to remove rust stains from fabrics prior to laundering and dry cleaning. It is also used in the manufacture of plastics, germicides, dyes, tanning solutions, solvents and fire-proofing materials; the glazing of pottery; photography; metal electropolishing; graphite processing; cleaning brick, stone, iron and steel; and in the brewing of beer to control fermentation and to cleanse rubber pipes.

*Organic solvents* (Fig. 7.24) and *motor oils* (Fig. 7.25) also soften the nail plate.

*Oxalic acid*, which is used in bleaching animal and vegetable materials, can cause redness and swelling of the fingertips

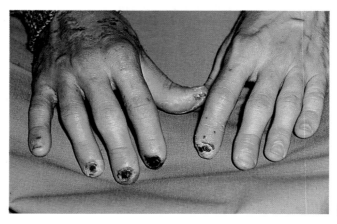
(c)

**Fig. 7.23** (right) (a,b) Terminal subungual hyperkeratosis and onycholysis due to hydrofluoric acid. (c) Necrosis of the distal digits (courtesy of G. Sebastian, Germany).

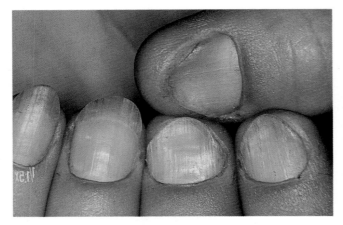

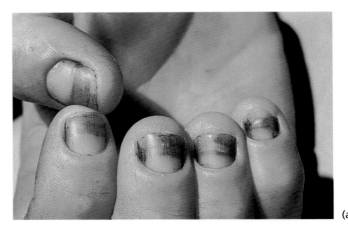

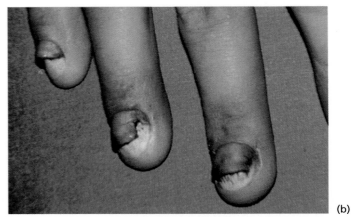

**Fig. 7.24** Nail signs (1st, 2nd and 3rd fingers) due to oven cleaning foam.

together with a bluish discoloration and brittleness of the nails (Schwartz *et al.* 1957a).

## Bacterial infections

*Abrasions and lacerations* can cause problems. Even trivial breaks of the periungual skin may lead to more serious conditions such as *cellulitis, erysipelas* and *septicaemia.* The usual microorganisms are coagulase-positive staphylococci and various streptococci.

*Pseudomonas* infection results in the cosmetically distressing green nail syndrome. Health care personnel with green nails may be a source of nosocomial infections (Greenberg 1975).

*Paronychial infections* are common and usually caused by a mixture of pathogenic organisms. Kitchen employees, agricultural workers and pianists are particularly liable to develop this condition. Acute paronychia is frequently seen in meat handlers and streptoccal paronychia has been reported in workers in a chicken factory (Barnham & Kerby 1984).

Inoculation through the periungual tissues of the spores of *Clostridium tetani,* which are widespread in soil, may lead to a full-blown *tetanus* infection.

*Erysipeloid,* fish handler's disease, is a bacterial infection (Fig. 7.26). The causative organism, *Erysipelothrix rhusiopathiae,* infests salt-water fish, shellfish, meat and poultry. Therefore at-risk occupations include fishermen, butchers and poultry dressers. Breaks in the periungual area provide a portal of entry, although it can penetrate intact skin (English 1998). Erysipeloid is a mild subacute cellulitis that resembles erysipelas. It presents as a painful, purplish papule, with a slowly spreading, dusky erythema as the centre clears, and with lymphadenitis which may be associated with paronychia. Septicaemia may occur.

Erysipeloid resolves spontaneously or with antibiotic therapy (penicillin).

Erysipeloid must be differentiated from 'seal finger', which occurs in aquarium workers and veterinarians following

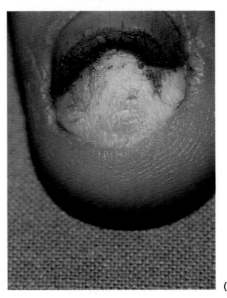

**Fig. 7.25** (a) Motor mechanic's fingers after prolonged handling of oil. (b,c) Onycholysis and subungual thickening due to mineral oils.

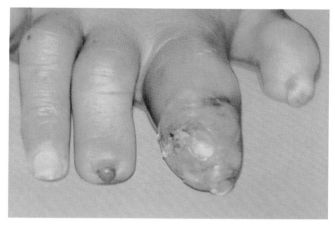

**Fig. 7.26** Leishmaniasis mimicking erysipeloid, usually seen in meat or fish handlers. (Courtesy of A. Zahaff, Tunisia.)

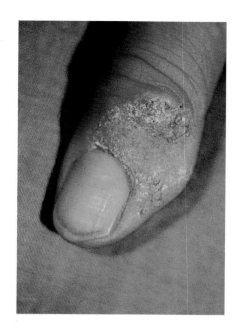

**Fig. 7.28** Verrucous TB—reinoculation type (prosector's wart).

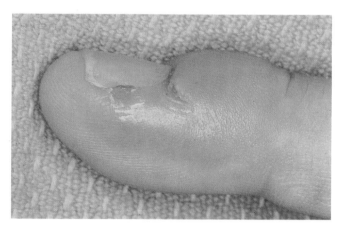

**Fig. 7.27** TB infection—primary (prosector's paronychia). (Courtesy of D. Geoette, USA.)

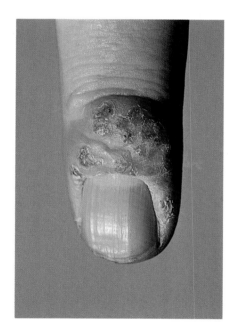

**Fig. 7.29** Swimming pool granuloma (*Mycobacterium marinum* infection).

trauma associated with working with seals. Zahaff *et al.* (1987) has described a case of leishmaniasis mimicking erysipeloid.

The *prosector's paronychia* is a primary inoculation infection with *Mycobacterium tuberculosis* (Fig. 7.27). The prosector's wart (tuberculosis verrucosa cutis, verrucosa necrogenica) signifies a reinoculation of cutaneous tuberculosis (Fig. 7.28) more often than a primary inoculation infection. Infection usually occurs at an autopsy on a tuberculotic cadaver and it may occasionally be seen in pathologists, morgue attendants and other hospital personnel (Jetton & Coker 1969; O'Donnell *et al.* 1971; Goette *et al.* 1978; Hooker *et al.* 1979). Penetrating trauma is necessary for the initiation of the infection because the tubercle bacillus cannot traverse the normal skin barrier. Such primary inoculation tuberculosis is associated with a negative tuberculin test prior to infection, cf. reinoculation cutaneous tuberculosis; the differential diagnosis includes chancriform conditions of deep fungal or bacterial origin (Hoyt 1981).

*Mycobacterium marinum infection* (*swimming pool granuloma*) gives rise to a slightly tender papule that develops at the proximal nail fold, which becomes pustular and drains: the latter ceases within a week but the papule persists, gradually increasing in size (Fig. 7.29). The dorsal surface of the distal phalanx of the finger appears erythematous and verrucous (Horn 1981). The differential diagnosis includes atypical mycobacterial infection, sporotrichosis and tuberculosis verrucosa cutis.

Frequently, swimming pool granuloma is a self-limited infection which may last for several months. Small lesions may be satisfactorily excised (Pettit 1982). However, if the infectious material is not completely eradicated, relapse can be expected. Tetracyline in doses ranging from 1 to 2 g/day (or minocycline,

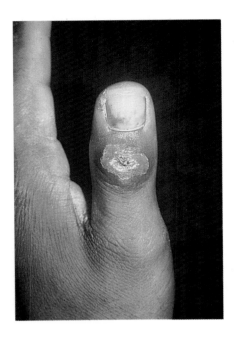

**Fig. 7.30** Tularaemia—inoculation lesion. (Courtesy of R. Arenas, Mexico DF.)

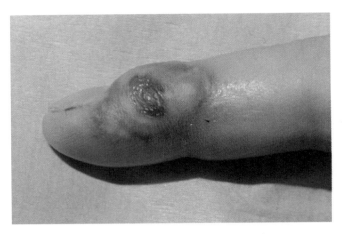

**Fig. 7.31** Orf virus infection. (Courtesy of J.L. Verret, Angers, France.)

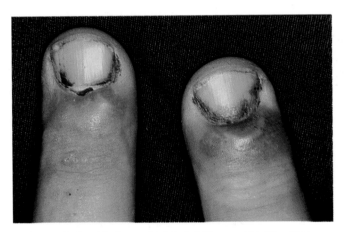

**Fig. 7.32** Milker's nodules (paravaccinia infection). (Courtesy of R.K. Scher, USA.)

100 mg bid) should be considered the treatment of choice in swimming pool granuloma.

*Tularaemia* results from infection with the coccobacillus *Pasteurella tularensis*. Infection around the nail may be transmitted to humans by direct contact with infected wildlife (rabbits are the principal reservoirs of tularaemia in nature). However, most infections are due to contact with animal carcasses (Lewis 1982). Ulceroglandular tularaemia (Fig. 7.30), the most common form, consists of a primary papule which becomes ulcerated, suppurative and granulomatous at the site of inoculation, with regional lymphadenitis (bubonic tularemia). Over half the patients with any cutaneous ulcers present with multiple lesions, including shallow erosions into the subungual tissues (Young *et al.* 1969). Streptomycin is generally the drug of choice, but chloramphenicol, gentamicin and tetracycline are also used in the treatment of tularaemia.

Primary *syphilis* may be acquired occupationally, for example by doctors.

## Viral infections

The *orf* virus infects sheep, goats and even reindeer in and around the mouth and can be transmitted to man. The lesion in the human is most commonly on the dorsum of the right index finger (Amichai *et al.* 1993) (Fig. 7.31), and it can take on a target-like appearance. Spontaneous healing occurs, leaving a small scar (Arnaud *et al.* 1986). Examination of an aspirate by electron microscopy confirms the diagnosis. The lesion resolves spontaneously within 6 weeks (Gill *et al.* 1990).

*Milker's nodules* is a clinically similar viral infection (Fig. 7.32) caused by a paravaccinia virus and afflicts mostly agricultural workers and veterinarians. Viral cultures permit differenti-

ation from orf. This condition passes through the same clinical sequence as orf, in appearance and timing, and heals spontaneously in 21–70 days without scarring (Marriot 1982).

Orf and milker's nodule infection have distinctive histopathological features, and viral changes may frequently be found (Groves *et al.* 1991).

In 'farmyard pox' Shelley and Shelley (1983) recommend a less conservative attitude, suggesting its complete removal by epidermal subsection using a Gillette 'Super blue' blade. Curettage followed by cautery was carried out in cases reported from North Jutland (Hansen *et al.* 1996).

*Herpes simplex* infection is an occupational hazard of dentists (Rames *et al.* 1984), nurses (Kanaar 1967), surgeons and anaesthetists (Rosato *et al.* 1970), and pathologists (Haedicke *et al.* 1989). The eruption may resemble pyogenic paronychia to some extent, but the presence of several closely grouped vesicles on an erythematous base should suggest the diagnosis (Jones 1985). Two or more fingers may be involved at the same time.

*Viral warts* are more common in butchers (Jablonska *et al.* 1987; Aloi *et al.* 1988; Keef *et al.* 1994). Zerboni *et al.* (1994)

**Table 7.1** Individuals at risk of fungal infections.

Athletes
Dustmen
Employees of indoor swimming pools
Excavation workers
Mine workers
Rubber industry workers
Sewer workers
Soldiers
Steel and furnace workers
Wood cutters
Wood pulp workers

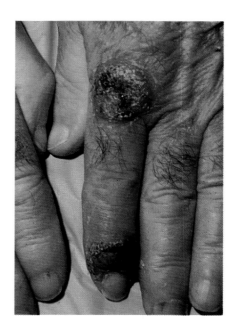

**Fig. 7.33** Blastomycosis —primary lesion in a pathologist. (Courtesy of D. Sweeny, USA.)

have studied the prevalence of warts among the employees of a butchery: 29.7% in the butchers themselves, 11.8% in the meat packers and 2.7% in the office staff. Viral warts are also common in poultry handlers (Moragon *et al.* 1987), poultry processing workers (Stehr-Green *et al.* 1993) and fish handlers (Rüdlinger *et al.* 1989), in whom many of the lesions are periungual or subungual.

## Fungal infections

Fungal infection of the nails and periungual region are common occupational problems (Table 7.1), particularly *candidiasis*. Those with occupations requiring the hands to be wet or exposed to detergents for prolonged periods, such as dishwashers in restaurants, are prone to candidal paronychia and onycholysis. *Candida* infections are also often seen in poultry and fish handlers.

Dermatophytic toenail infections are known to occur with increased prevalence in coal miners and colleagues who work in hot humid environments and who share washing facilities. Infection with *Trichophyton rubrum* often involves both feet and only one hand. Either the dominant or the other hand may be involved (Gellin 1972). A useful diagnostic feature of fungal nail involvement is the sparing of one or more nails, as opposed to psoriatic nail involvement where all the nails tend to be affected.

Alkiewicz and Sowinski (1967) noted two cases of *Trichophyton* infection of the fingernails, a cashier and a teacher; their occupations required moistening of the tips of the fingers continually with a wet sponge. Fungal infections of the toenails have been reported in 6.5–27% of miners (Götz & Hantschke 1965; Tappeiner & Male 1966) often associated with *Scytalidium dimidiatum* and *Scytalidium hyalinum* (Gugnani & Oyeka 1989). Onychomycosis and keratomycosis were caused by *Alternaria* spp. in a wood-pulp worker on chronic steroid therapy (Arrese *et al.* 1996).

Primary cutaneous *blastomycosis* (Fig. 7.33) can be an occupational hazard to pathologists (Larson *et al.* 1983). A reddish-purple furuncle of the distal part of the finger presents

2 weeks after accidental inoculation into a deep cut in the same area.

## Systemic conditions

Besides chemical percutaneous absorption, which may be responsible for methaemoglobinaemia, systemic conditions, such as neurological and gastrointestinal symptoms related to patch tests with UV curable acrylic monomers (Andersen 1986) and even death (Ford *et al.* 1978), may be due to chemical absorption by the inhalation route. After exposure to cobalt and tungsten (Desoille *et al.* 1962), asbestos (Petry 1966), talc, beryllium and silica (Kern 1990), pneumoconiotic lung diseases can produce clubbing. In a dental technician exposed to silica, Erasmus syndrome was associated with necrosis of the digits (Caux *et al.* 1991).

Pseudo-clubbing with acroosteolysis may develop after occupational exposure to excessive levels of vinyl chloride monomer which is responsible for systemic sclerosis (Markowitz *et al.* 1972).

Systemic sclerosis may also be caused by epoxy resin vapour, trichlorethylene, trichlorethane and silica (Rustin *et al.* 1989).

Davies *et al.* (1990) reported on a cutaneous haemangioendothelioma developed on a toe nail bed of a patient who had worked with polyvinyl chloride.

Sclerodactyly with nail fold capillary changes, Raynaud's phenomenon and acroosteolysis (Bachurzewska & Borucka 1986; Flindt-Hansen & Isager 1987) may also result from exposure to vibrations (Nagata *et al.* 1993).

Lupus erythematosus-like erythema and periungual telangiectasia among coffee plantation workers has been reported (Narahari *et al.* 1990).

## Principal nail dystrophies associated with their occupational origin

Tables 7.2 to 7.9 demonstrate the principal nail dystrophies found in occupational nail disorders, but there are few correlations between clinical patterns and aetiology (English 1998).

**Table 7.2** Individuals at risk of nail fragility syndrome resulting from repeated microtrauma. This syndrome leads to a gradual destruction of the nail plate (Ronchese 1962a,b, 1969), which becomes brittle and atrophic. Nail fragility may occur in isolation or be associated with paronychia and/or onycholysis (see parentheses for other presenting features ).

Bean shellers and potato peelers (paronychia)
Butchers
Cement workers
Chemists and laboratory workers (paronychia)
Dentists (onycholysis, subungual hyperkeratosis, dermatitis)
Engravers (paronychia)
Etchers (paronychia)
File makers
Glaziers (paronychia)
Hat cleaners (paronychia)
Nurses
Optical glass handlers
Packers
Painters (paronychia)
Photographers (paronychia, discoloration)
Plasterers (corroded nails)
Porcelain workers (serrated nails)
Pottery workers
Radio workers (paronychia and nail loss)
Rope workers
Shoe makers (onycholysis and paronychia)
Shoe shiners
Silk weavers (Ronchese 1955)
Wet work (paronychia)
Wood workers (paronychia and stains)
Workers exposed to microwave radiation (onycholysis)
Workers handling small instruments
Workers lifting repeatedly heavy plastic bags (Schubert et al. 1977)

**Table 7.3** Toenail dystrophy resulting from repeated microtrauma.

Dancers (exostosis) (Sebastian 1977)
Rickshaw pullers (koilonychia) (Bentley-Philips & Bayles 1971)
Miners (onychomycosis) (Gugnani & Oyeka 1989)
Sportsmen (haematoma, nail shedding)
    Athletes
    Joggers
    Walking
    Squash players
    Soccer players
    Tennis players

**Table 7.4** Paronychia.

Agricultural workers
Animal origin (bristles, sea urchin, oyster shell)
Automotive workers (sulfuric acid exposure from batteries)
Bakers and pastry cooks
Barbers and hairdressers (onycholysis) (Stone 1975)
Bartenders
Bean shellers
Book binders (paste)
Bricklayers (limes, cement, mortar)
Builders and carpenters (including glass fibre)
Button makers
Cement workers
Chemists and laboratory workers
Chicken factory workers
Cooks
Cosmetic workers
Dentists (Kanerva et al. 1997d)
Dinitro-salicylic acid (Fregert & Trulson 1980)
Dyers (aniline dyes, producing stains and necrosis)
Engravers (brittle nail)
Etchers, glass etchers (brittle nail)
Fishermen
Fishmongers
Florists and gardeners (onycholysis) (hyacinth, daffodil and narcissus bulbs, tulip fingers)
Glaziers (brittle nail)
Groundskeepers
Harpists
Housewives/husbands and house cleaners
Janitorial and domestic workers
Manicurists (artificial nails)
Meat handlers
Mechanics
Milkers (onycholysis from bristle)
Oil-rig workers
Painters
Photographic developers (brittle nail,discoloration)
Pianists
Physicians, dentists, nurses
Potato peelers
Prosector's paronychia
Radio workers (methanol, causing pigmentation and nail loss)
Salt plant workers (ulcers)
Shoe workers (brittle nails)
Swimming pool granuloma
Tanners (whitlow)
Textile workers (threads of fabric)
Violinists (nail dystrophy)
Wood workers (brittle nails, stains)
Wool workers (wool thread).

**Table 7.5** Alterations in colour of the nail plate .

| Sign | Workers affected |
| --- | --- |
| Leuconychia | Arsenic workers |
| | Butchers (Fig. 7.34) |
| | Key punchers (Honda *et al.* 1976) |
| | Salt plant workers and contact with salted intestines (Ferreira-Marques 1939; Frenk & Leu 1966) (see Fig. 7.34) |
| | Weedkillers (paraquat) (Dobbelaere & Bouffioux 1974; Botella *et al.* 1985) |
| | Workers manufacturing thallium rodenticides |
| | Fly tyer's finger (apparent leuconychia) (Mac Aulay 1990) |
| Blue | Anodizers (aluminium) |
| | Local argyria (Bergfeld & McMahon 1987; Sarsfield 1992) |
| | Car mechanics (oxalic acid in radiators) |
| | Cyanosis from methaemoglobinaemia or sulfhaemoglobinaemia |
| | Dye makers |
| | Electroplaters |
| | Gold platers |
| | Metal cleaners, metal patina solution |
| | Ink makers |
| | Paint removers |
| | Photographers |
| | Rust removers |
| | Silver workers (presenting generalized argyria) (Bleehen *et al.* 1981) |
| | Textile workers |
| Brown/black | Cigar makers |
| | Cobblers |
| | Coffee bean workers |
| | Cooks and bakers (burnt sugar) |
| | Electric bulb cleaners (hydrochloric acid) |
| | Gunsmith |
| | Hairdressers (Fig. 7.35) |
| | Photographers |
| | Roadway pavers |
| | Shoe-shiners |
| | Vintners (red wine) |
| | Walnut pickers (pecans) (Fig. 7.36) |
| | Woodworkers (ebony, mahogany) (Harris & Rosen 1989) |
| | Woodworkers (varnish) |
| Green (usually caused by *Pseudomonas* infection) | Bartenders |
| | Dish-washers |
| | Electricians |
| | Fruit handlers |
| | Laundry workers |
| | Metallurgists |
| | Restaurant workers |
| | Sugar factory workers |
| Yellow | Epoxy system handlers: metaphenylenediamine and 4,4'-methylenedianiline (Cohen 1985) (Fig. 7.37) |
| | Flower handlers |
| | Pesticide workers: diquat (Samman & Johnston 1969; Clark & Hurst 1970), paraquat (Samman & Johnston 1969; Hearn & Keir 1971), dinitro-orthocresol (Baran 1974), dinobuton (Wahlberg 1974) |
| | Workers handling chromium salts |
| | Workers handling dyestuffs: dinitro-salicylic acid (Fregert & Trulson 1980), dinitrobenzene, dinitrotoluene and trinitrotoluene |

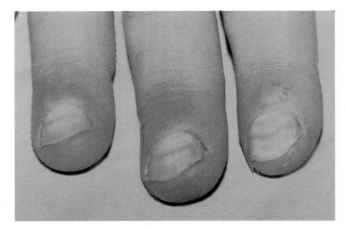

**Fig. 7.34** Butcher's leuconychia. (Courtesy of F. Leu, Switzerland.)

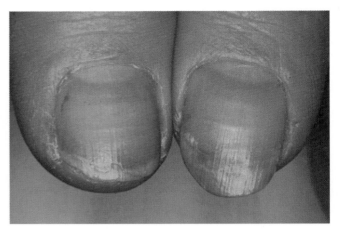

**Fig. 7.37** Yellow staining in a handler of epoxy resin system chemicals. (Courtesy of S.R. Cohen, USA.)

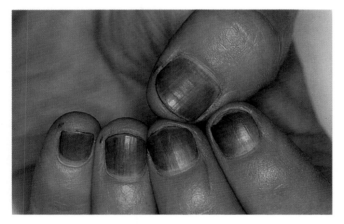

**Fig. 7.35** Brown discoloration of nails due to dye (in a hairdresser).

**Table 7.6** Koilonychia.

Car mechanics (Dawber 1974)
Chimney sweeps
Coil winders (Smith *et al.* 1980)
Glass workers
Hairdressers (thioglycolates) (Alanko *et al.* 1997)
Mushroom growers (Schubert *et al.* 1977)
Oil burner repairers (Meyer-Hamme & Quadripur 1983)
Organic chemists (organic solvents) (Ancona-Alayon 1975)
Rickshaw pullers (feet) (Bentley-Phillips & Bayles 1971)
Slaughterhouse workers (Forck & Kästner 1967)

*Note*: after a while, nail changes may become irreversible (Pedersen 1982).

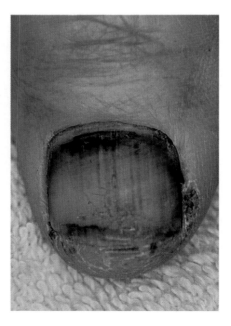

**Fig. 7.36** Colour changes (walnut picker). (Courtesy of S. Salasche, USA.)

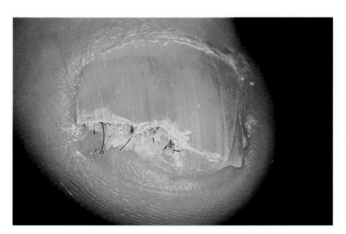

**Fig. 7.38** Onycholysis and subungual thickening associated with subungual hairs in a hairdresser.

**Table 7.7** Onycholysis. Occupational onycholysis may be associated with acute trauma (metal) or repeated microtrauma, but most frequently it is due to chemical irritants or sensitizers as described in the text. In addition, there are infective causes, which tend to be limited to medical personnel (herpes) (Louis & Silva 1979) and occupations which entail prolonged soaking of the hands (*Candida* and *Pseudomonas*); there are also traumatic causes.

Repeated minor injuries (Ronchese 1962a; Forck & Kästner 1967; Somov *et al.* 1976; Menné *et al.* 1985)
 Cropping
 De-stalking mushrooms
 Milking
 Nut cracking
 Poultry plucking
 Scraping
 Separating meat from bone
 Shell casing

Introduction of foreign bodies (they may also produce paronychial infection)

After acute trauma or repeated microtrauma
 Animal origin (see Table 7.4)

Metal, glass, fibre glass (Rogaïlin *et al.* 1975), plastic

Splinters of hair (Hogan 1988; de Berker *et al.* 1994; Buendia-Eisman *et al.* 1997; Haddad *et al.* 1999) (Fig. 7.38)

Plants
 Thorn, splinter, hyacinth and narcissus bulbs raphide cells with crystal of calcium oxalate (Hjorth & Wilkinson 1968; Julian & Bowers 1997)

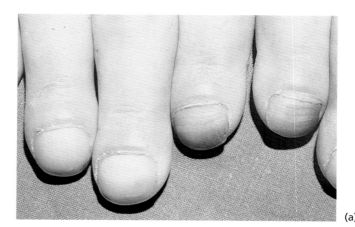

(a)

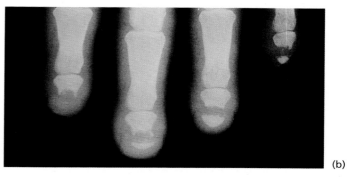

(b)

**Fig. 7.39** (a) Pseudo-clubbing due to occupational acroosteolysis. (Courtesy G. Moulin, France.) (b) Occupational acroosteolysis—X-ray changes in terminal phalanges.

**Tables 7.8** Clubbing and pseudo-clubbing.

| Clinical sign | Exposure to: |
|---|---|
| Clubbing (resulting from pneumoconiotic lung diseases) | Asbestos (Petry 1966) |
| | Talc |
| | Beryllium (Kern 1990) |
| | Silica |
| | Cobalt (Desoille *et al.* 1962) |
| | Tungsten (Desoille *et al.* 1962) |
| Pseudo-clubbing (systemic sclerosis with acroosteolysis) (Fig. 7.39) | Vinyl chloride monomer (Rustin *et al.* 1989) |
| Cutaneous haemangioendothelioma | Polyvinyl chloride (Davies *et al.* 1990) |
| Collagen diseases Systemic sclerosis | Vinyl chloride monomer Epoxy resin (vapours) Trichlorethylene, trichlorethane Silica (Rustin *et al.* 1989) |
| Sclerodactyly associated with nail fold capillary changes, Raynaud's phenomenon, acroosteolysis) (Bachurzewska & Borucka 1986; Flindt-Hansen & Isager 1987) | Vibrations (Nagata *et al.* 1993) |
| Lupus eythematosus-like erythema and periungual telangiectasia | Coffee (in plantation workers) (Narahari *et al.* 1990) |

**Tables 7.9** Distal bone anomaly.

| | |
|---|---|
| Fracture of the distal phalanx | Acute injury |
| Subungual exostosis | Dancers (Sebastian 1977) |
| Acroosteolysis | Guitar players (Baran & Tosti 1993) |
| Pseudo-clubbing with | Vinyl chloride monomer |
| acroosteolysis (Fig. 7.39) | (Markowitz et al. 1972) |
| Sclerodactyly with acroosteolysis | Exposure to vibrations (Nagata et al. 1993) |
| Necrosis of the digits | Erasmus syndrome (Caux et al. 1991) |

## Dyschromia of the nail

Nail dyschromia indicates an abnormality in colour of the fabric and/or surface of the nail plate and/or subungual tissue.

Abnormalities of colour depend on the transparency of the nail, its attachment to the underlying tissue and the character of the latter.

*Examination of the abnormal nails* should be carried out with the fingers completely relaxed and not pressed against any surface. Then, the fingertips should be blanched to see if the pigmented abnormality is grossly altered; this may help to differentiate between discoloration of the nail plate itself and discoloration of the vascular nail bed. If the abnormality lies in the latter it usually disappears.

Further information may be gleaned by transillumination of the nail. The modifications observed are differentiated readily from the diffuse homogeneous reddish glow of the normal nail plate (Goldman 1962). If the discoloration is in the subungual soft tissues, its exact position can more easily be identified.

When discoloration results from *abnormalities at the nail plate–nail bed attachment*, leading to onycholysis and/or subungual hyperkeratosis, the history of the condition will help in diagnosis. Chemicals, wet occupation, trauma or infection may be implicated. Thus the history of the condition may, for example, confirm the traumatic origin of a haematoma. However, the possibility of malignant melanoma following trauma to a nail as a coincidental or causal event should be kept in mind (Roberts 1984).

When the *discoloration is confined to the nail plate*, in patients whose nails are in contact with occupationally derived agents, or with the topical application of therapeutic agents, neither fingertip pressure producing blanching nor the pen-torch placed against the pulp will alter the pigmentation. The discoloration often follows the shape of the proximal nail fold. It can be removed by scraping the nail plate or cleaning it with a solvent such as acetone.

To determine if the colour is within the nail plate, a piece of nail should be cut off and examined while immersed in water. When specimens are allowed to dry, their true colour may be obscured by the scattering of the transmitted light (Baden 1987).

When the pigmentation involves all the digits, it results from the *systemic absorption of a chemical*:

1 When the route of systemic absorption is oral, the discoloration is more likely to correspond to the shape of the lunula. Transverse leuconychia might occur, for example, in thallium poisoning.
2 When systemic absorption of a chemical through the lung or the skin produces dyschromia, there are two possibilities (Kern 1990):

(a) Disappearance of the pigmentation on the nail bed blanching test means that the pigment originates from the blood vessels. Methaemoglobinaemia, as an example, manifests as a bluish discoloration of the terminal digits and should be looked for in an otherwise asymptomatic worker, i.e. following exposure to aromatic nitro and amino compounds that can penetrate all glove materials. The colour disappears within 16 h of leaving work, in contrast to sulfhaemoglobinaemia, which presents with the same distal discoloration as an early warning sign of intoxication, but which disappears only with the normal life span of the red blood cell, i.e. 4 months (Kern 1990). Deaths from asphyxia among fishermen have been reported (Ford *et al.* 1978). The workers had previously been involved in dipping shrimps into a sodium bisulfite solution used routinely to control 'black spots', a discoloration associated with decay. A fungicide, zinc ethylene bisdithiocarbamate, was also responsible for sulfhaemoglobinemia and acute haemolytic anaemia in a patient with glucose-6-phosphate dehydrogenase deficiency and hypocatalasaemia (Pinkhas *et al.* 1963).

(b) If the pigmentation is not altered on the nail bed blanching test, but it is obliterated by the pen-torch pressed against the pulp, then the *pigment is deposited in the nail bed tissue*, as observed in the blue nails of silver refinery workers (Bleehen *et al.* 1981).

However, the distinction between oral absorption and systemic absorption of the chemical through the lung or the skin is not clear cut. For example, occupational exposure to polychlorinated biphenyls (PCBs) is usually through direct contact, but inhalation and ingestion may also be operative in some cases. Discoloration of the nails appeared in 2.5% of PCB-exposed capacitor manufacturing workers (Fischbein *et al.* 1979).

## Non-occupational nail hazards

There are few direct hazards to the nails that are not occupational and these very largely consist of cosmetic applications to the nails. Nail preparations rarely damage the nails themselves. When they do, their effect is usually quickly perceived and the product either radically altered or withdrawn from the market.

The principles of diagnosis of these rare non-occupational but exogenous nail disorders are the same as those for occupational nail disorders outlined under 'Diagnosis of occupational nail disorders' above. Besides the cosmetic hazards that are specified in this section, there are several conditions described above that can sometimes also arise non-occupationally from

**Tables 7.10** General guidance on glove materials.*

| Material | Protective against | Additional notes |
|---|---|---|
| Natural rubber | Soaps and detergents, water-soluble irritants, dilute acids and alkalis | Not good for organic, solvents, strong acids and alkalis, many other organic compounds |
| Butyl rubber | Aldehydes, most amines, amides, ketones, formaldehyde resins, epoxy resins, most acrylates, isocyanates | |
| Chloroprene | Soaps and detergents, dilute acids and alkalis, certain amines and esters, most alcohols, vegetable oils | Not good for aldehydes, ketones, nitro- and halogenated compounds |
| Fluorocarbon | Organic solvents, particularly halogenated and aromatic hydrocarbons | Cost 30–40 times as much as natural rubber |
| Nitrile rubber | Organic acids, certain alcohols, amines, ethers, peroxides, inorganic alkalis, vegetable oils | Also protect against organophosphorus compounds to some extent |
| Styrene-butadiene rubber | | Hypoallergenic surgical gloves only |
| Polyethylene | Mainly for food handlers and medical personnel | Chemical resistance dependent on seams |
| Polyvinyl alcohol | Several organic solvents, most esters | Not resistant to water or aqueous solutions |
| Polyvinyl chloride | Soaps and detergents, oils, metalworking fluids, dilute acids and alkalis, vegetable oils | Not good for most organic solvents |

* Actual protection depends on glove thickness, manufacturing quality, chemical concentration, duration of contact, environmental temperature and humidity, etc.

leisure pursuits e.g. 'do-it-yourself' activities and housework. These are not repeated here. Allergic contact dermatitis from acrylic sculptured nails has been included earlier because of its occurrence in manicurists as well as in their clients. Permanent loss of fingernails due to allergic reaction to an acrylic nail preparation seems unique (Fisher 1989). The use of cyanoacrylate nail glue preparations may produce allergic reactions in the nail plate and paronychial area, which may be prolonged with resultant marked dystrophy of the nails (Shelley & Shelley 1988), and even partial loss that may eventually prove permanent (Fisher 1987).

## Cosmetic physical hazards

See Chapter 8.

## Cosmetic chemical sensitizers or irritants

See Chapter 8.

## Discoloration of the nail plate

See Chapter 8.

## Nail protection at work

Gloves are the best form of such protection, but only if they are considered safe to wear and if they are made of material appro-

priate to the agent against which protection is required. Neither natural rubber nor polyvinyl chloride (PVC) gloves, for example, are a good protection against organic solvents. Further general guidance is given in Table 7.10. Expert detailed advice is now available (Mellström 1985; Forsberg & Keith 1989).

## Nail cosmetic hazards at work

Can it definitively be proved that artificial nails or even nail varnish present absolutely no risk of spreading bacteria?

In 1982 Nava, a researcher, noted that polished nails pose no infection problem as long as they are manicured and have no chips or cracks. A statement confirmed by Baumgardner *et al.* (1993): nail polish worn on short, healthy nails does not appear to be associated with increased microbial counts on the fingernails. This contradicts, however, a previous statement that nail polish and rings make hands difficult to decontaminate (Bennet & Brachman 1979) and 'recommended practices preclude artificial nails' (Ricards 1985): it has been shown that chipped fingernail polish or fingernail polish worn longer than 4 days fosters increased numbers of bacteria on the fingernails of operating room nurses after surgical hand scrubs (Wynd *et al.* 1994).

After handwashing, there were higher numbers of colony-forming units of gram-negative rods cultured from the fingertips of nurses with artificial nails than from those of nurses with natural nails. Because of the number of nosocomial infections caused by gram-negative rods, health care workers who wear artificial nails should consider the potential risk of increased carriage of gram-negative rods (Pottinger *et al.* 1989). Certain genera of bacteria, for example *Serratia*, *Acinetobacter* and *Pseudomonas*, were recovered only from nurses with artificial nails.

Anecdotal reports from North America have also suggested that nurses who wear acrylic fingernails may become colonized or infected by *Candida* and, thus, become a possible risk to susceptible patients. This possibility remains to be established in clinical practice, though there are theoretical reasons for concern, notably the capacity of *Candida* to adhere to acrylic surfaces, as recognized in denture stomatitis (Symonds *et al.* 1993).

Three case reports of *Pseudomonas* corneal ulcers following injury to the eye with artificial nails have been published (Parker *et al.* 1989). If transmission occurs on one individual, there is no reason why it cannot occur from one person to another (Senay 1991).

The Association of Operating Room Nurses (AORN) recommends that artificial nails are not worn by operating room personnel, citing reports of fungal and bacterial infections. In addition, concerns have also been raised by others that the use of artificial fingernails and nail polish may discourage vigorous handwashing (Larson & Lusk 1985). Therefore, many hospitals have adopted AORN's guidelines, and some have extended them beyond the operating room, for example in prohibiting nurses who work in the neonatal intensive care and labour and delivery units from wearing artificial nails (Hill 1998).

Some food processing plants have also banned artificial nails and nail polish, because they cannot let anything fall into the 'food stream'. A number of occupations and companies now have policies regarding the maintenance and appearance of their employees' nails.

## References

Agahian, B., Lee, J., Nelson, J. *et al.* (1990) Arsenic levels in fingernails as a biological indicator of exposure to arsenic. *American Industrial Hygiene Association Journal* **51**, 646–651.

Alanko, K., Kanerva, L., Estlander, T. *et al.* (1997) Hairdresser's koilonychia. *American Journal of Contact Dermatitis* **8**, 177–178.

Alkiewicz, J. & Sowinski, W. (1967) Die Trichophytie der Fingernägel als berufliches problem. *Mycosen* **10**, 463.

Aloi, F.G., Molinero, A., Passera, A. *et al.* (1988) Viral warts in butchers. Clinical and statistical study. *Giornale Italiano di Dermatologia e Venereologia* **123**, 341–344.

Amichai, B., Grunwald, M.H., Abraham, A. *et al.* (1993) Tense bullous lesions on fingers. *Archives of Dermatology* **129**, 1043–1048.

Ancona-Alayón, A. (1975) Occupational koilonychia from organic solvents. *Contact Dermatitis* **1**, 367–369.

Andersen, K.E. (1986) Systemic symptoms related to patch test with UV curable acrylic monomers. *Contact Dermatitis* **14**, 180.

Arnaud, J.P., Bernard, P., Souyri, N. *et al.* (1986) Human orf disease localized in the hand. A study of eight cases. *Annales de Chirurgie de la Main* **5**, 129–132.

Arrese, J., Pierard-Franchimont, C. & Pierard, G.E. (1996) Onychomycosis and keratomycosis caused by *Alternaria* sp. A bipolar opportunistic infection in a wood-pulp worker on chronic steroid therapy. *American Journal of Dermatology* **18**, 611–613.

Audebert, C. & Lamoureux, P. (1978) Eczema professionnel du marin pêcheur par contact de bryozoaires en baie de Seine. *Annales de Dermatologie et de Vénéréologie* **105**, 187–192.

Bachurzewska, B. & Borucka, I. (1986) Gefässläsionen bei Einsenbahnnarbeiterinnen die mit Epoxidharzen in Berührung kommen. *Dermatosen* **34**, 77–79.

Baden, H.P. (1987) *Diseases of the Hair and Nails*, p. 21. Year Book Medical Publishers, Chicago.

Bajaj, A.K., Pasricha, J.S., Gupta, S.C. *et al.* (1996) *Tabernaemontana coronaria* causing fingertip dermatitis. *Contact Dermatitis* **35**, 104–105.

Balguerie, X. (1990) Arsénicisme cutané aigu. *Nouvelle Dermatologie* **9**, 340–345.

Baran, R. (1974) Nail damage caused by weed killers and insecticides. *Archives of Dermatology* **110**, 467.

Baran, R. (1978) Pigmentations of the nails (chromonychia). *Journal of Dermatologic Surgery and Oncology* **4**, 250–254.

Baran, R. (1980) Acute onycholysis from rust-removing agents. *Archives of Dermatology* **116**, 382–383.

Baran, R. (1991) Onycholysis from hydroxylamine. *Contact Dermatitis* **24**, 158.

Baran, R. & Bureau, H. (1981) Surgical treatment of recalcitrant chronic paronychias of the fingers. *Journal of Dermatologic Surgery and Oncology* **7**, 106–107.

Baran, R. & Schibli, H. (1990) Permanent paresthesia to sculptured nails. A distressing problem. *Dermatologic Clinics* **8**, 139–141.

Baran, R. & Tosti, A. (1993) Occupational acroosteolysis in a guitar player. *Annales de Dermatologie et de Vénéréologie* **73**, 64–65.

Barbaud, A., Reichert-Penetrat, S., Tréchot, P. *et al.* (1997) Occupational contact dermatitis to propacetamol. *Dermatology* **195**, 329–331.

Barnham, M. & Kerby, J. (1984) A profile of skin sepsis in meat handlers. *Journal of Infection* **9**, 43–50.

Baumgardner, C.A., Maragos, C.S., Walz, J.A. *et al.* (1993) Effects of nail polish on microbial growth of fingernails. *AORN Journal* **58**, 84–88.

Bennet, J.V. & Brachman, P.S. (eds) (1979) *Hospital Infections*, pp. 88–89. Little, Brown & Co., Boston.

Bentley-Phillips, B. & Bayles, M.A.H. (1971) Occupational koilonychia of the toe nails. *British Journal of Dermatology* **85**, 140–144.

Bergfeld, W.F. & McMahon, J.T. (1987) Cutaneous metalloid hyperpigmentation. In: *Advances in Dermatology*, Vol. 1 (eds J.P. Callen, M.V. Dahl, L.E. Golitz & S.J. Stegman), pp. 123–124. Year Book, Chicago.

de Berker, D., Dawber, R. & Wojnarowska, F. (1994) Subungual hair implantation in hairdressers. *British Journal of Dermatology* **130**, 400–401.

Bleehen, S.S., Gould, D.J., Harrington, C.I. *et al.* (1981) Occupational argyria: light and electron microscopic studies and X-ray microanalysis. *British Journal of Dermatology* **104**, 19–26.

Bleumink, E., Doeglas, H.M.G., Klokke, A.H. *et al.* (1972) Allergic contact dermatitis to garlic. *British Journal of Dermatology* **87**, 6–9.

Bord, A. & Castelain, P.Y. (1966) Les dermatoses professionnelles dans l'industrie aéronautique. *Bulletin de la Societé Française de Dermatologie et de Syphiligraphie* **73**, 396–401.

Botella, R., Sastre, A. & Castells, A. (1985) Contact dermatitis to paraquat. *Contact Dermatitis* **13**, 123–124.

Boyle, J.C., Smith, N.J. & Burke, F.D. (1988) Vibration white finger. *Hand Surgery* **13B**, 171–175.

Brodkin, R.H. & Bleiberg, J. (1973) Cutaneous microwave injury. A report of two cases. *Acta Dermato-Venereologica* **53**, 50–52.

Brooke, R.C. & Beck, M.H. (1999) Occupational allergic contact dermatitis from epoxy resin used to restore window frames. *Contact Dermatitis* **41**, 227–228.

Brooke, R. & Coulson, I. (1998) Toast-makers' fingers. *Contact Dermatitis* **39**, 86.

Brun, R. (1978) Contact dermatitis to orange-wood in a manacurist. *Contact Dermatitis* **4**, 315.

Bruynzeel, D.P. (1986) Allergic contact dermatitis to hydrangea. *Contact Dermatitis* **14**, 128.

Bruynzeel, D.P. (1997) Bulb dermatitis. Dermatological problems in the flower bulb industries. *Contact Dermatitis* **37**, 70–77.

Budden, M.G. & Wilkinson, D.S. (1978) Skin and nail lesions from gold potassium cyanide. *Contact Dermatitis* **4**, 172–173.

Buendia-Eisman, A., Serrano-Ortega, S. & Ortega del Olmo, R.M. (1997) Hair fragments as a subungual foreign body in a hairdresser. *European Journal of Dermatology* **7**, 517–518.

Burgess, J.F. (1952) Occupational dermatitis due to onion and garlic. *Canadian Medical Asssociation Journal* **66**, 275.

Burks, J.W. Jr (1954) Classic aspects of onion and garlic dermatitis in housewives. *Annals of Allergy* September–October 592–596.

Calas, E., Castelain, P.Y., Raulot Lapointe, H. *et al.* (1977) Allergic contact dermatitis to a photopolymerizable resin used in printing. *Contact Dermatitis* **3**, 186–194.

Calnan, C.D. (1960) Cement dermatitis. *Journal of Occupational Medicine* **2**, 15.

Castelain, P.-Y. & Piriou, A. (1980) Contact dermatitis due to propanidid in an anesthetist. *Contact Dermatitis* **6**, 360.

Caux, F., Chosidow, O., De Cremoux, H. *et al.* (1991) Le prothésiste dentaire, un sujet à risque de syndrome d'Erasmus. *Annales de Dermatologie et de Vénéréologie* **118**, 301–304.

Clark, D.G. & Hurst, E.W. (1970) The toxicity of diquat. *British Journal of Industrial Medicine* **27**, 51–55.

Cohen, S.R. (1985) Yellow staining caused by 4,4'-methylenedianiline exposure. *Archives of Dermatology* **121**, 1022–1027.

Condé-Salazar, L., Guimaraens, D. & Romero, L.V. (1986) Occupational allergic contact dermatitis from anaerobic acrylic sealants. *Contact Dermatitis* **18**, 129–132.

Coskey, R.J. (1974) Onycholysis from sodium hypochlorite. *Archives of Dermatology* **109**, 96.

Cronin, E. (1980a) *Contact Dermatitis*, p. 586. Churchill Livingstone, Edinburgh.

Cronin, E. (1980b) *Contact Dermatitis*, p. 792. Churchill Livingstone, Edinburgh.

Davies, M.F.P., Curtis, M. & Howat, J.M.T. (1990) Cutaneous hemangioendothelioma: possible link with chronic exposure to vinyl chloride. *British Journal of Industrial Medicine* **47**, 65–67.

Dawber, R. (1974) Occupational koilonychia. *British Journal of Dermatology* **91** (Suppl. 10), 11.

De Dulanto, F. & Camacho, F. (1979) Radiodermatitis. *Acta Dermato-Sifilitica* **70**, 67–94.

Derrick, E. & Darley, C. (1997) Contact dermatitis to nasturtium. *British Journal of Dermatology* **136**, 20–291.

Desoille, H., Brouet, G., Assouly, M. *et al.* (1962) Fibrose pulmonaire diffuse chez un sujet exposé aux poussières de cobalt et de carbure de tungstène. *Archives des Maladies Professionnelles* **23**, 570–578.

Dobbelaere, F. & Bouffioux, J. (1974) Leuconychie en bandes due au paraquat. *Archives Belges de Dermatologie* **30**, 283–384.

Dolma, T., Norboo, T., Yayha, M. *et al.* (1990) Seasonal koilonychia in Ladakh. *Contact Dermatitis* **22**, 78–80.

Dooms-Goossens, A., Dubusschère, K., Morren, M. *et al.* (1988) Silver polish: another source of contact dermatitis reactions to thiourea. *Contact Dermatitis* **19**, 133–135.

Ekenvall, L. (1987) Clinical assessment of suspected damage from hand-held vibrating tools. *Scandinavian Journal of Work, Environment and Health* **13**, 271–274.

English, J.S.C. (1998) *Occupational Dermatology*. Manson Publishing, London.

English, J.S.C., White, I.R. & Rycroft, R.J.G. (1986) Sensitization by 1-methylquinoxalinium-*p*-sulfonate. *Contact Dermatitis* **14**, 261–262.

Fairbairn, J.F., Juergeas, J.L. & Spittell, J.A. (1972) *Peripheral Vascular Disease*, 4th edn, p. 428. Philadelphia, Saunders.

Ferreira-Marques, J. (1939) Une forme particulière de leuconychia, la leuconychie en large bande longitudinale (stigmate professionnel). *Annals of Dermatology* **10**, 688–691.

Finlay, A.Y. & Ryan, T.J. (1996) Disability and handicap in dermatology. *International Journal of Dermatology* **35**, 305–311.

Fischbein, A., Wolf, M.S., Lilis, R. *et al.* (1979) Clinical findings among PCB-exposed capacitor manufacturing workers. *Annals of the New York Academy of Sciences* **320**, 703–715.

Fisher, A.A. (1987) Allergic reactions to cyanoacrylate 'Crazy glue' nail preparations. *Cutis* **40**, 475–476.

Fisher, A.A. (1989) Permanent loss of fingernails due to allergic reaction to an acrylic nail preparation: a sixteen-year follow-up study. *Cutis* **43**, 404–406.

Fisher, A.A. & Baran, R. (1992) Occupational nail disorders with a reference to Koebner's phenomenon. *American Journal of Contact Dermatitis* **3**, 16–23.

Fitzgerald, D.A. & English, J.S.C. (1994) Widespread contact dermatitis from sculptured nails. *Contact Dermatitis* **30**, 117.

Fitzgerald, D.A., Bhaggoe, R. & English, J.S.C. (1995) Contact sensitivity to cyanocrylate nail-adhesive with dermatitis at remote sites. *Contact Dermatitis* **32**, 175–176.

Flindt-Hansen, H. & Isager, H. (1987) Scleroderma after occupational exposure to trichlorethylene and trichlorethane. *Acta Dermato-Venereologica* **67**, 263–264.

Forck, G. & Kästner, H. (1967) Charakteristische onycholysis traumatica bei Fleissbandarbeiter in Geflügelschlachterei. *Hautarzt* **18**, 85–87.

Ford, R., Shkor, J., Akman, W.V. *et al.* (1978) Deaths from asphyxia among Fisherman. *Morbidity and Mortality Weekly Report* **27**, 309–315.

Forsberg, K. & Keith, L.H. (1989) *Chemical Protective Clothing Performance Index Book*. Wiley, New York.

Fowler, J.F. (1990) Occupational dermatitis of the fingertips. *American Journal of Contact Dermatitis* **1**, 210–211.

Fowler, J.F. (1991) Fingertip eczema in a dental worker. *American Journal of Contact Dermatitis* **2**, 76–77.

Freeman, S. & Rosen, R.H. (1990) Friction as a cause of irritant contact dermatitis. *American Journal of Contact Dermatitis* **1**, 165–170.

Freeman, S., Lee, M.-S. & Gudmundsen, K. (1995) Adverse contact reactions to sculptured acrylic nails: four case reports and a literature review. *Contact Dermatitis* **33**, 381–385.

Fregert, S. & Trulson, L. (1980) Yellow stained skin from dinitrosalicylic acid. *Contact Dermatitis* 6, 362.

Frenk, E. & Leu, F. (1966) Leukonychie durch beruflichen Kontakt mit gesalzenen Därmen. *Hautarzt* 17, 233–235.

Fulghum, D.D. (1972) Allergic contact onycholysis due to poison ivy oleoresin. *Contact Dermatitis Newsletter* 11, 266.

Gallaghar, R.G., Zavon, M. & Doyle, H.N. (1955) Radioactive contamination in a radium therapy clinic. *Publications Health Report* 70, 617–624.

Gellin, G.A. (1972) *Occupational Diseases*, p. 78. American Medical Association, Chicago.

Gette, M.T. & Marks, J.E. (1990) Tulip fingers. *Archives of Dermatology* 126, 203–205.

Gibbs, R.C. (1973) Tennis toe. *Archives of Dermatology* 107, 918.

Gill, M.J., Arlette, J., Buchan, K.A. *et al.* (1990) Human orf. *Archives of Dermatology* 126, 356–358.

Goday, J.J., Yanguas, I., Aguirre, A. *et al.* (1997) Occupational contact dermatitis from a photopolymerising printing plate. *Journal of the European Academy of Dermatology and Venereology* 9, 78–93.

Goette, D.K., Jacobson, K.W. & Doty, R.D. (1978) Primary inoculation tuberculosis of the skin. Prosector's paronychia. *Archives of Dermatology* 114, 567.

Goh, C.L. (1985) Occupational dermatitis from soldering flux among workers in the electronic industry. *Contact Dermatitis* 13, 85–90.

Goh, C.L. (1990) Allergic contact dermatitis and onycholysis from hydroxylamine sulphate in colour developer. *Contact Dermatitis* 22, 109.

Goldman, L. (1962) Transillumination of the fingertip as aid in examination of nail changes. *Archives of Dermatology* 85, 644.

Goodwin, P. (1976) Onycholysis due to acrylic nail applications. *Clinical and Experimental Dermatology* 1, 191.

Göthe, C.J., Nilzen, A., Holmgren, A. *et al.* (1972) Medical problems in the detergent industry caused by proteolytic enzymes from bacillus subtilis. *Acta Allergica* 27, 63.

Götz, H. & Hantschke, D. (1965) Einblicke in die Epidemiologie der Dermatomykosen im Kohlenbergbau. *Hautarzt* 16, 543.

Greenberg, J.H. (1975) Green fingernails: a possible pathway of nosocomial pseudomonas infection. *Military Medicine* 145, 356.

Groves, R.W., Wilson-Jones, E. & MacDonald, D.M. (1991) Haman orf and milkers' nodules: a clinicopathologic study. *Journal of the American Academy of Dermatology* 25, 706–711.

Guerra, L., Vincenzi, C., Peluso, A.M. & Tosti, A. (1993) Prevalence and sources of occupational contact sensitization to acrylates in Italy. *Contact Dermatitis* 28, 101–103.

Gugnani, H.C. & Oyeka, C.A. (1989) Foot infections due to *Hendersonula toruloidea* and *Scytalidium hyalinum* in coal miners. *Journal of Medical and Veterinary Mycology* 27, 169–179.

Haddad, V. Jr, Facouri, C.N. & Lima Dillon, N. (1999) Fragmento capilares provocando paroniquia e onicolise em barbeiros/cabeleiros: uma dermatose ocupacional. *Anais da Brasileira Dermatology* 74, 155–156.

Haedicke, G.J., Grossman, J.A.I. & Fisher, A.E. (1989) Herpetic whitlow of the digits. *Journal of Hand Surgery* 14B, 443–446.

Haglmüller, T., Hemmer, W., Kusak, I. *et al.* (1995) Loss of fingernails due to persistant allergic contact dermatitis in an artificial nail designer. *Journal of Allergy and Clinical Immunology* 95, 250.

Hansen, S.K., Mertz, H., Krogdahl, A. *et al.* (1996) Milker's nodule. A report of 15 cases in the county of north Jutland. *Acta Dermato-Venereologica* 76, 88.

Harris, A.O. & Rosen, T. (1989) Nail discoloration due to mahogany. *Cutis* 43, 55–56.

Harvell, J. & Maibach, H.I. (1992) Skin disease among musicians. *Medical Problems in the Performing Arts* 7, 114–120.

Hausen, B.M. (1982) Airborne contact dermatitis caused by tulip bulbs. *Journal of the American Academy of Dermatology* 7, 500–503.

Head, S. (1984) Victualler's thumb nail—a condition of subungual osmotrauma. *Journal of the Royal College of General Practitioners* 34, 118.

Hearn, C.E.D. & Keir, W. (1971) Nail damage in spray operators exposed to paraquat. *British Journal of Industrial Medicine* 28, 399.

Heidenheim, M. & Jemec, G.B.E. (1991) Side effects of cryotherapy. *Journal of the American Academy of Dermatology* 24, 653.

Hill, S. (1998) Outlawed nails. *Nails Magazine* 8, 56–61.

Hjorth, N. & Wilkinson, D.S. (1968) Contact dermatitis IV. Tulip fingers, hyacinth itch and lily rash. *British Journal of Dermatology* 80, 696–698.

Hodgson, G. & Mayon-White, R.T. (1971) Acute onychia and onycholysis due to an enzyme detergent. *British Medical Journal* 3, 352.

Hogan, D.J. (1988) Subungual trichogranuloma in a hairdresser. *Cutis* 42, 105–106.

Honda, M., Hattori, S., Koyama, L. *et al.* (1976) Leukonychia striae. *Archives of Dermatology* 112, 1147.

Hooker, R.P., Eberts, T.J. & Strickland, J.A. (1979) Primary inoculation tuberculosis. *Journal of Hand Surgery* 4, 270.

Horn, M.S. (1981) *Mycobacterium marinum* infection. *Journal of the Association of Military Dermatology* 7 (2), 25.

Hoyt, E.M. (1981) Primary inoculation tuberculosis. Report of a case. *Journal of the American Medical Association* 245, 1556.

Jablonska, S., Obalek, S., Favre, M. *et al.* (1987) The morphology of butcher's warts as related to papillomo-virus types. *Archives of Dermatological Research* 279, 566–572.

Jappe, U., Bonnekoh, B., Hausen, B.M. & Gollnick, H. (1999) Garlic-related dermatoses: case report and review of the literature. *American Journal of Contact Dermatitis* 10, 37–39.

Jetton, R.L. & Coker, W.L. (1969) Tuberculosis verrucosa cutis (prosector's wart). *Archives of Dermatology* 100, 380.

Jillson (1979) The Frisbee nail. *Journal of the American Academy of Dermatology* 1, 163.

Jones, J.G. (1985) Herpetic whitlow: an infectious occupational hazard. *Journal of Occupational Medicine* 27, 725–728.

Julian, C.G. & Bowers, P.W. (1997) The nature and distribution of daffodil pickers' rash. *Contact Dermatitis* 37, 259–262.

Julie, R., Barbier, F., Lambert, J. *et al.* (1988) Brûlures par acide fluorhydrique. A propos d'une série de 32 cas. *Semaine des Hôpitaux de Paris* 64, 31–39.

Kanaar, P. (1967) Primary herpes simplex infection of fingers in nurses. *Dermatologica* 134, 346.

Kanerva, L., Estland, T., Jolanki, R. *et al.* (1993) Occupational allergic contact dermatitis caused by exposure to acrylate during work with dental prostheses. *Contact Dermatitis* 28, 268–275.

Kanerva, L., Henricks-Eckerman, M.-L., Estlander, T. *et al.* (1994) Occupational allergic contact dermatitis and composition of acrylates in dentin bonding systems. *Journal of the European Academy of Dermatology and Venereology* 3, 157–168.

Kanerva, L., Lauerma, A., Estlander, T. *et al.* (1996) Occupational allergic contact dermatitis caused by photobonded sculptured nails and a review of (meth)acrylates in nail cosmetics. *American Journal of Contact Dermatitis* 7, 109–115.

Kanerva, L., Henriks-Ekerman, M.-L., Jolanki, R. et al. (1997a) Plastics/acrylics: material safety data sheets need to be improved. Clinical Dermatology 15, 533–546.

Kanerva, L., Jolanki, R. & Estlander, T. (1997b) 10 years of patch testing with the (meth) acrylate series. Contact Dermatitis 37, 255–258.

Kanerva, L., Estlander, T. & Jolanki, R. (1997c) Occupational allergic contact dermatitis caused by acrylic tri-cure glass ionomer. Contact Dermatitis 37, 49–50.

Kanerva, L., Henricks-Eckerman, M.-L., Estlander, T. et al. (1997d) Dentist's occupational allergic paronychia and contact dermatitis caused by acrylics. European Journal of Dermatology 7, 177–180.

Kanerva, L., Mikola, H., Enricks-Eckerman, M.-L. et al. (1998) Fingertip paresthesia and occupational allergic contact dermatitis caused by acrylics in a dental nurse. Contact Dermatitis 38, 114–116.

Kanerva, L., Estlander, T. & Jolanki, R. (2001) Optician's occupational allergic contact dermatitis, paraesthesia and paronychia caused by anaerobic acrylic sealants. Contact Dermatitis 41, 117–119.

Keef, M., Al Ghamdi, A., Coggon, D. et al. (1994) Cutaneous warts in butchers. British Journal of Dermatology 130, 9–14.

Kern, D.G. (1990) Occupational disease. In: Nails, Therapy, Diagnosis, Surgery (ed. D. Scher), pp. 224–243. W.B. Saunders, Philadelphia.

Kulcsár, S. (1966) Deformity of the finger nails caused by vibrations. A case report. Berufsdermatosen 14, 244.

Larson, D.M., Eckman, M.R., Albert, R.L. et al. (1983) Primary cutaneous (inoculation) blastomycosis: an occupational hazard to pathologists. American Journal of Clinical Pathology 79, 253–255.

Larson, E. & Lusk, E. (1985) Evaluating handwashing technique. Journal of Advances in Nursing 10, 547–522.

Lewis, J.E. (1982) Suppurative inflammatory eruption occurring in septicemic tularemia. Cutis 30, 92.

Long, P.I. (1958) Subungual hermorrhage in pan washer. Journal of the American Medical Association 168, 1226.

Louis, D.S. & Silva, J. Jr (1979) Herpetic whitlow infections of the digits. Journal of Hand Surgery 4, 90.

MacAulay, J.C. (1990) Fly tyer's finger. Canadian Journal of Dermatology 2, 67.

MacKinnon, M.A. (1986) Treatment of hydrofluoric acid burns. Journal of Occupational Medicine 22, 804.

Markowitz, S.S., MacDonald, C.J. & Fethiere, W. (1972) Occupational acroosteolysis. Archives of Dermatology 106, 219–233.

Marks, J.G., Bishop, M.E. & Willis, W.F. (1979) Allergic contact dermatitis to sculptured nails. Archives of Dermatology 115, 100.

Marren, P., De Berker, D., Dawber, R.P.R. et al. (1991) Occupational contact dermatitis due to quaternium-15 presenting as nail dystrophy. Contact Dermatitis 25, 253–254.

Marriot, W. (1982) Some viral disease: orf and Milker's nodule: tropical dermatology syllabus. In: XVI Congressus Internationalis Dermatologiae, Tokyo.

Mathias, C.G. & Maibach, H.I. (1984) Allergic contact dermatitis from anaerobic acrylic sealants. Archives of Dermatology 120, 1202–1205.

Mellström, G. (1985) Protective effect of gloves—compiled in a data base. Contact Dermatitis 13, 162–165.

Menné, T., Roed-Petersen, J. & Hjorth, N. (1985) Pressure onycholysis in slaughterhouse workers. Acta Dermatoven 65 (Suppl. 120), 88–89.

Messite, J., Troisi, F.M. & Kleinfeld, M. (1957) Radiological hazards due to X-radiation in veterinarians. Archives of Industrial Health 16, 48–51.

Meyer-Hamme, S. & Quadripur, S.A. (1983) Berufsbedingte Koilonychie. Hautarzt 34, 577–579.

Montel, M.L. & Gouyer, E. (1957) L'Escavenite. Bulletin de la Société Française de Dermatologie et de Syphiligraphie 64, 672.

Moragon, M., Ibañez, M.D., San Juan, L. et al. (1987) L'incidence des verrues vulgaires chez les travailleurs d'abattoirs industriels de volaille de la province de Valence. Archives des Maladies Professionnelles 48, 41–43.

Munksgaard, E.C. (1992) Permeability of protective gloves to (di) methacrylates in resinous dental materials. Scandinavian Journal of Dental Research 100, 189–192.

Murdoch, D. (1993) Koilonychia in Sherpas. British Journal of Dermatology 128, 594–595.

Mürer, A.J.L., Poulsen, O.M., Roed-Petersen, J. et al. (1995) Skin problems among Danish dental technicians. Contact Dermatitis 33, 42–47.

Nagata, C., Yoshida, H., Mirbod, S.M. et al. (1993) Cutaneous signs (Raynaud's phenomenon, sclerodactylia and edema of the hands) and hand-arm vibration exposure. International Archives of Occupational and Environmental Health 64, 587–591.

Narahari, S.R., Skinivas, C.R. & Kelkar, S.K. (1990) L.E.-like erythema and periungual telangiectasia among coffee plantation workers. Contact Dermatitis 22, 296–297.

Nava, S. (1982) Removing rings when washing hands necessary in family-centered OB ward. Hospital Infection Control 9, 168.

Nethercott, J.R. & Lawrence, M.J. (1984) Allergic contact dermatitis due to nonylphenol ethoxylate. Contact Dermatitis 10, 235–239.

O'Donnell, T.F., Jurgenson, P.F. & Weyerich, N.F. (1971) An occupational hazard, tuberculous paronychia. Archives of Surgery 103, 757.

Okamoto, H. & Kawai, S. (1991) Allergic contact sensitivity to mydriatic agents on a nurse's fingers. Cutis 47, 357–358.

Parker, A.V., Cohen, E.J. & Arentsen, J.J. (1989) Pseudomonas corneal ulcers after artificial fingernail injuries. American Journal of Ophthalmology 107, 548–549.

Pedersen, N.B. (1980) Edema of fingers from hydrogen fluoride containing aluminium blancher. Contact Dermatitis 6, 41.

Pedersen, N.B. (1982) Persistent occupational koilonychia. Contact Dermatitis 8, 134.

Pedersen, N.B. (1997) Allergic contact dermatitis from acrylic resin repair of windscreens. Contact Dermatitis 39, 99.

Pellerat, M. & Chabeau, G. (1976) Hydroxylamine et dermatoses professionnelles. Bulletin de la Société Française de Dermatologie et de Syphiligraphie 83, 238–239.

Peters, K., Gammelgaard, B. & Menne, T. (1991) Nickel concentrations in fingernails as a measure of occupational exposure to nickel. Contact Dermatitis 25, 237–241.

Petry, H. (1966) Uhrglasnägel und Trommelschlegelfinger bei Asbestose. International Archiv der Gewebepathologie und Gewebehygiene 22, 55–59.

Pettit, J.H.S. (1982) Skin tuberculosis and mycobacterial ulcers. Tropical dermatology Syllabus. In: XVI Congressus Internationalis Dermatologicae, Tokyo.

Pinkhas, J., Djaldetti, M., Joshua, H. et al. (1963) Sulfhemoglobinemia and acute Hemolytic anemia with Heinzbodies following contact with a fungicide—Zinc Ethylene Bisdithiocarbamate in a subject with glucose—6—phosphate dehydrogenase deficiency and hypocatalasemia. *Blood* **21**, 484–494.

Pottinger, J., Burns, S. & Manske, C. (1989) Bacterial carriage by artificial versus natural nails *American Journal of Infection Control* **17**, 340–344.

Rames, S., Folkmar, T. & Roed-Petersen, B. (1984) Herpes simplex as a possible occupational disease in dentists of the county of Aarhus, Denmark. *Acta Dermato-Venereologica* **64**, 163–165.

Ricards, J. (1985) Recommended practices preclude artificial nails. *AORN Journal* **42**, 793.

Roberts, A.H.N. (1984) Subungual melanoma following a single injury. *Journal of Hand Surgery* **9B**, 328–330.

Rogaïlin, V.I., Selisski, G.D. & Zakharov, G.A. (1975) Clinical characteristics of skin disease in production of glass fibre. *Sovetskaia Meditsina* **9**, 154.

Romaguera, C. & Grimalt, F. (1983) Dermatitis de contacto profesional por codeina. *Boletin Inform GEIDC* **5**, 21–23.

Ronchese, F. (1953) Occupational nail marks, true and false. *Indian Journal of Medical Surgery* **22**, 45–48.

Ronchese, F. (1955) Peculiar silk weavers' nails. A new type of artefacts. *Archives of Dermatology* **71**, 525–526.

Ronchese, F. (1962a) Nail defect and occupational trauma. *Archives of Dermatology* **85**, 404.

Ronchese, F. (1962b) *Nails: Injuries and Disease in Traumatic Medicine and Surgery for the Attorney*, Vol. 6, pp. 626–639. Butterworth, Washington.

Ronchese, F. (1969) Occupational nails. *Cutis* **5**, 164–165.

Rosato, F.E., Rosato, E.F. & Plotkin, S.A. (1970) Herpetic paronychia, an occupational hazard of medical personnel. *New England Journal of Medicine* **283**, 804–805.

Rosenthal, E.A. (1983) Treatment of finger tip and nail bed injuries. *Orthopedic Clinics of North America* **14**, 675–697.

Rosenzweig, R. & Scher, R.K. (1993) Nail cosmetics: adverse reactions. *American Journal of Contact Dermatitis* **4**, 71–77.

Rüdlinger, R., Bunney, M.H., Grab, R. et al. (1989) Warts in fish handlers. *British Journal of Dermatology* **120**, 375–381.

Rustemeyer, T. & Frosch, P.J. (1996) Occupational skin diseases in dental laboratory technicians (1). Clinical pictures and causative factors. *Contact Dermatitis* **34**, 125–133.

Rustin, M.H.A., Bull, H.A., Ziegler, V. et al. (1989) Silica exposure and silica-associated systemic sclerosis. *British Journal of Dermatology* **121** (Suppl. 34), 29–30.

Ryan, A.M. & Goldsmith, L.A. (1995) Golfer's nails. *Archives of Dermatology* **131**, 857–858.

Rycroft, R.J.G. (1977) Contact dermatitis from acrylic compounds. *British Journal of Dermatology* **96**, 685–687.

Rycroft, R.J.G. & Calnan, C.D. (1981) Alstroemeria dermatitis. *Contact Dermatitis* **7**, 284.

Rycroft, R.J.G., Wilkinson, J.D., Holmes, R. et al. (1980) Contact sensitization to *p*-tertiary butylphenol (PTBP) resin in plastic nail adhesive. *Contact Dermatitis* **5**, 441–445.

Samman, P.D. & Johnston, E.N.M. (1969) Nail damage associated with handling of paraquat and diquat. *British Medical Journal* **1**, 818–819.

Sarsfield, P., White, T.E. & Theaker, J.M. (1992) Silverworker's finger: an unusual occupational hazard mimicking a melanocytic lesion. *Histopathology* **20**, 73–75.

Scher, R.K. (1988) Occupational nail disorders. *Dermatologic Clinics* **6**, 2733.

Schubert, B., Minard, J.J., Baran, R. et al. (1977) Onychopathie des champignonnistes. *Annales de Dermatologie et de Vénéréologie* **104**, 627–630.

Schwartz, L., Tulipan, L. & Birmingham, D.J. (1957a) *Occupational Disease of the Skin*, 3rd edn, pp. 242, 760. Henry Kimpton, London.

Schwartz, L., Tulipan, L. & Birmingham, D.J. (1957b) *Occupational Disease of the Skin*, 3rd edn, pp. 759–760. Henry Kimpton, London.

Sebastian, G. (1977) Subungual Exostose der Grosszche, Berufsstigma bei Tänzern. *Dermatologische Monatsschrift* **163**, 998–1000.

Sebastian, G. (1994) Praxisrelevante Therapie emfehlungen bei Flussäure verätzungen. *Hautarzt* **45**, 453–459.

Senay, H. (1991) Acrylic nails and transmission of infection. *Canadian Journal of Infection Control* **6**, 52.

Shelley, D.E. & Shelley, W.B. (1984) Chronic dermatitis simulating small-plaque parapsoriasis due to cyanoacrylate adhesive used in fingernails. *Journal of the American Medical Association* **252**, 2455–2456.

Shelley, D.E. & Shelley, W.B. (1988) Nail dystrophy and periungual dermatitis due to cyanoacrylate glue sensitivity. *Journal of the American Academy of Dermatology* **19**, 574–575.

Shelley, W.B. & Shelley, E.D. (1983) Surgical treatment of farmyard pox. *Cutis* **31**, 191–192.

Shelley, W.B. & Shelley, D.E. (1995) Portrait of a practice 'Judo' nails. *Cutis* **56**, 91–92.

Shewmake, S.W. & Anderson, B.G. (1979) Hydrofluoric acid burns. *Archives of Dermatology* **115**, 593–596.

Smith, S.J., Yoder, F.W. & Knox, D.W. (1980) Occupational koilonychia. *Archives of Dermatology* **116**, 861.

Somov, B.A., Lipets, M.E., Ivanov, V.V. et al. (1976) Occupational onycholysis. *Vestnik Dermatologii i Venereologii* **2**, 51–55.

Stehr-Green, P.A., Hewer, P., Meekin, G.E. et al. (1993) The aetiology and risk factors for warts among poultry processing workers. *International Journal of Epidemiology* **22**, 294–298.

Stone, O.J. (1975) Chronic paronychia in which hair has a foreign body. *International Journal of Dermatology* **14**, 661–663.

Symonds, J.M. & O'Dell, C.A. (1993) Letters to the editor. *Journal of Hospital Infection* **23**, 243–244.

Tappeiner, J. & Male, O. (1966) Nagelveränderungen durch Schimmelpilze. *Dermatology International* **5**, 145.

Tarvainen, K., Jolanki, R. & Estlander, T. (1993) Occupational contact allergy to unsaturated polyester resin cements. *Contact Dermatitis* **28**, 220–224.

Taylor, W. (1982) Vibration white finger in the workplace. *Journal of the Society of Occupational Medicine* **32**, 159–166.

Tomb, R.R., Lepoittevin, J.P., Durepaire, F. et al. (1993) Ectopic contact dermatitis from ethyl cyanoacrylate instant adhesives. *Contact Dermatitis* **28**, 206–208.

Tosti, A., Guerra, L., Morelli, R. et al. (1992) Role of foods in the pathogenesis of chronic paronychia. *Journal of the American Academy of Dermatology* **27**, 706–710.

Veccherini-Blineau, M.F. & Guiheneuc, P. (1988) Syndrome digital des vibrations et syndrome du canal carpien: deux entités électrophysiologiques différentes ? *Neurophysiologie Clinique* **18**, 541–548.

Wahlberg, J.E. (1974) Yellow staining of hair and nails and contact sensitivity to dinobuton. *Contact Dermatitis Newsletter* **16**, 481.

Washburn, B. (1962) Frostbite: what is it. How to prevent it. Emergency treatment. *New England Journal of Medicine* **266**, 974–989.

Wynd, C.A., Samstag, D.E. & Lapp, A.M. (1994) Bacterial carriage on the fingernails of OR nurses *AORN Journal* **60**, 796–805.

Young, L.S., Bicknell, D.S., Archer, B.G. *et al.* (1969) Tularemia epidemic: Vermont 1968. Forty-seven cases linked to contact with muskrats. *New England Journal of Medicine* 280, 1253.

Yu Hsin-Su, Yao Tsing-Hua, Tseng Ho-Ming *et al.* (1988) Vibration syndrome with special reference to the effects of temperature on vibration-induced white finger. *Journal of Dermatology* 15, 466–472.

Zahaff, A., Sevestre, H., Fraitag, S. *et al.* (1987) Leishmaniose cutanée dans le sud (ouest tunisien). *Nouvelle Dermatologie* 6, 551–555.

Zerboni, R., Tarantini, G., Muratori, S. *et al.* (1994) Virus warts in a meat-processing factory. *Dermatosen in Beruf und Umwelt* 12, 237–240.

# CHAPTER 8

# Cosmetics: the care and adornment of the nail

**E. Brauer & R. Baran**

In this chapter attention is directed to the care and adornment of normal nail-free disease or obvious genetic defect though variations in physical characteristics such as colour, nail thickness, contour, flexibility and surface smoothness are considered.

The human nail, chemically similar to horn and hoof, is not essential for the survival of *Homo sapiens*, but it has many important functions that are crucial for the efficient use of the hands and the feet (Chapter 1). The nail is a prime source for the transmission of organisms, both macroscopic and microscopic, toxins, irritants and allergens. Maintaining nail cleanliness is essential to many aspects of health.

The nail is also a locus of critical importance (Figs 8.1 & 8.2). For many, cleanliness does not achieve aesthetic satisfaction. A multitude of products, implements and procedures are now on sale to fulfil the quest of those seeking nails (and therefore fingertips) with enhanced attractiveness (Figs 8.3 & 8.4). While the cosmetic industry encourages and caters to the trappings of nail care and adornment, the motivation is probably innate; nail beautification was an established practice in societies long past (Barnett & Scher 1992); the long fingernail, often accentuated by gold and jewelled fingertip extenders, was indicative of high rank and station in society.

The principle is the same today, only style and intensity has changed. The appearance of the nail remains the major distinguishing feature of the hands of the labourer, male or female.

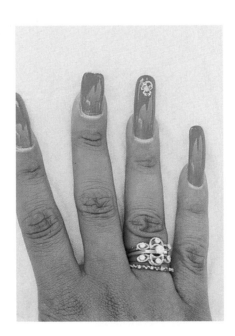

**Fig. 8.1** Long artificial painted nails; cf. Fig. 8.2.

Basic nail grooming is a universal practice; nail adornment is not limited to, only more obvious in, the female. Attractive fingertips, in conjunction with many other grooming characteristics, contribute to an elevation in personnal appraisal—improvement in confidence and self-image. The physician is

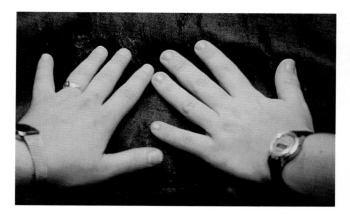

**Fig. 8.2** Short 'stubby' nails; cf. Fig. 8.1—less attractive.

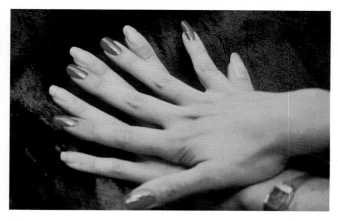

**Fig. 8.4** Showing the aesthetic difference between long red nails and uncoloured ones, same individual.

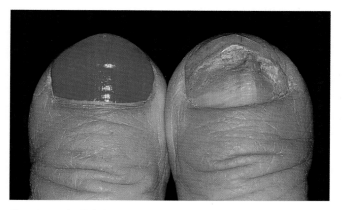

**Fig. 8.3** Varnish adds little in cosmetic improvement to a broad, short fingernail.

well advised to recognize this means for achieving a psychological 'lift' in his/her patients. The great benefit achieved dwarfs to insignificance the small risk of adverse reaction. A thorough discussion of the principles of good nail hygiene and cosmetic usage follows, including descriptions of products and implements (Figs 8.5–8.7) (Brauer 1969; Baran 1982).

The purist might easily discuss nail care as requiring only soap, water, and perhaps a brush. The same can be said for the maintenance of any hard surface, even a kitchen floor. One easily recognizes that abrasives, solvents, waxes, stains, varnishes, paints and floor coverings (which do not exhaust the catalogue of items in daily use) not only create a clean, sanitary deck, but also an attractive one as well. The nail, whose exposure to environmental insult is greater, is a vital surface that reproduces

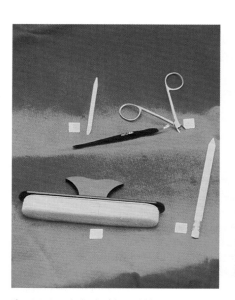

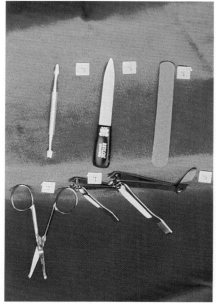

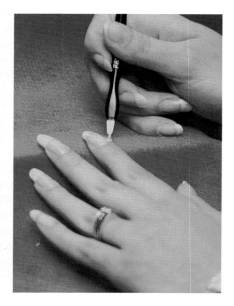

**Figs 8.5–8.7** The 'tools of the trade' for nail apparatus manicure (see Table 8.1).

**Table 8.1**  Items for nail care (Figs 8.5–8.7).

| Item | Description |
| --- | --- |
| Clippers | Slightly curved, jaw-like blades operated by a spring mechanism for severing the free edge |
| Scissors | Slightly curved blades for cutting soft, thin, flexible nail plates. Note: blunted ends of blades to minimize injury to soft tissue |
| Emery board | A flat disposable 'paper-board' wand, coated with powdered emery to shape as well as file down length or smoothen sharp, rough portions of the free edge of the nail |
| Nail file | An elongated board made of wood or foam covered with abrasives that vary in grit depending on the intended use. The grit is the determination of how many abrasive particles there are per cubic centimetre. Low-grit boards (60–120 grits) are for quickly removing a layer of a articicial nails. Medium-grit boards (120–180) are for smoothing and shaping both artificial and natural nails |
| Blocks | These are similar to files, but usually take the form of a larger, rectangular foam block that fits comfortably into the hand. Files and blocks are the most widely used types of abrasives |
| Metal particle file | Fine metallic particles are electroplated on a metal wand; this lasts indefinitely and has the delicacy, speed and efficiency of the emery board |
| Acrylic nippers | They are designed specifically to chip back the acrylic at the base of the nail in preparation for a fill |
| Cobalt steel fibreglass shear | These are fine, but strong, scissors that bear up well against fibreglass while maintaining a sharp cutting edge |
| Cuticle pusher | A polished, metallic probe with various shaped ends for separating the cuticle edge from the nail plate and loosening cuticle remnants. The probe has rounded edges to minimize injury to soft tissue |
| Orange stick | A reed-like wooden or flexible pencil-shaped plastic implement that is used as the cuticle pusher above. It is less likely to cause injury to the nail fold. It was originally fabricated from orange wood |
| Cuticle trimmer | Tiny clipper-jawed scissors for cutting frayed cuticle. Recently, a curette-like V-shaped blade, mounted in a plastic handle, has been introduced to efficiently shave down this tissue |
| Nail buffer | Chamois or similar fabric, usually padded and mounted on a convenient holding device for polishing the nail plate. It is used in conjunction with mild pumice-type abrasive creams or waxes to produce a high lustre to the nail surface |
| Nail whitener | This is a pencil-like device with a white clay (kaolin) core that is used to deposit colour on the undersurface of the free edge of the nail |
| Disinfectant container | This should be large enough to hold a disinfecting solution in which items to be sanitized are immersed |

Pedicures demand a special set of implements due to the size and thickness of toenails. A typical toenail cutter works with a squeeze grip action.

itself, imperfections included, every few months. With its delicate biological system it cannot be expected to be served by fewer agents if cleanliness, beauty and personal taste are to be satisfied. Table 8.1 lists, with a brief description, the major items in general use for nail care.

## The art of nail care

The manner in which each of the items in Tables 8.1 and 8.2 is used and the sequence for performing the professional manicure in a beauty salon follows. An individual at home will usually shorten or omit completely selected steps to conform to constraints of time and dexterity. The physician, familiarizing him/herself with the procedure, will gain insight into the use and abuse which occasionally may lead to ungual and periungual problems.

An attractive fingernail is oval in shape, but there are three other basic nail shapes: round, rectangular and pointed. Length creates the impression of thin, tapered and graceful fingers. Excessive length, however, interferes with the efficiency of the hand's performance (Fig. 8.8).

### Manicure routine (Fig. 8.9)

1  Old nail enamel or buffer waxes and oils are thoroughly removed with a cottonwool ball saturated with nail enamel remover.
2  The nails are shaped with a file or emery board in preference to clipping. The latter tends to cause a shearing action on the nail plate that promotes fracturing.
3  The tissues of the fingertips are then softened by soaking them in a bath of warm, soapy water for several minutes; the cuticular edge is then gently and bluntly retracted from the nail plate. The best and safest way to achieve this is by covering the nail with a soft fabric. The manicurist then grasps the patron's fingertip between her thumb and index finger. The operator then pushes her thumb in a proximal direction exerting gentle pressure on the cuticular rim that surrounds the nail. The

**Table 8.2** Toiletries and cosmetics.

| | |
|---|---|
| Nail enamel solvents | Solvents of acetone and/or ethyl acetate or similar compounds that quickly soften and solubilize nail enamel, oils and waxes for quick and easy cleansing |
| Cuticle and nail creams and lotions | Oil-in-water emulsion preparations to aid in softening keratin of nail plate and contiguous skin. This is achieved initially by the addition of water, and subsequently by the reduction in evaporation into the environment of the tissues' inherent moisture |
| Cuticle removers | These are lotions or gels containing approximately 0.4% sodium or potassium hydroxide. They are applied to the proximal edge of the nail plate in the vicinity of the cuticlar ridge. Their purpose is to 'digest' the remnants of cuticle that adhere to the nail plate as it grows outward. The lotion is left in place for approximately 10 min and then washed off. These products are not meant to remove the fibrous cuticular ridge |
| Base coats, top coats and nail enamel | These three products have similar basic formulas. They consist of a film former, such as nitrocellulose, a thermoplastic resin for gloss and adhesion (e.g. toluenesulfonamide/formaldehyde*) and a plasticizer (e.g. dibutyl phthalate) for flexibility; these are incorporated in an acetate and ketone solvent. (A nail enamel differs only in containing pigments and suspending agents to achieve colour.) The quantities of the basic ingredients vary with desired product performance. For example, with a base coat good adhesion or bonding to the nail plate and the superimposed nail enamel is accentuated at the price of gloss; with a top coat, which is applied over the nail enamel, the gloss factor is dominant |
| Film drying accelerant | Mineral oil is sprayed or brushed over freshly applied enamel to give fast protection from minor environmental insults while the enamel sets |
| Sanitation | This can use physical agents (ultraviolet rays, moist and dry heat) or chemicals (alcohol, quaternary compounds, etc.). It is preferable to use the dry heat temperature for 10 s in the electric glass bead sterilizer that reaches 475°F (245°C) |

* New analytical technology reveals that this resin may contain a trace of formaldehyde (Nater *et al.* 1985).

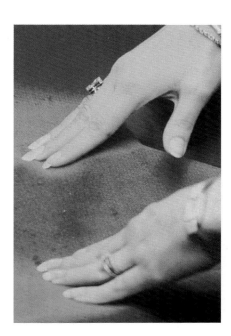

**Fig. 8.8** The 'lever' effect of long nails may lead to onycholysis. Excessively long nails may interfere with the subtle functions of the hands.

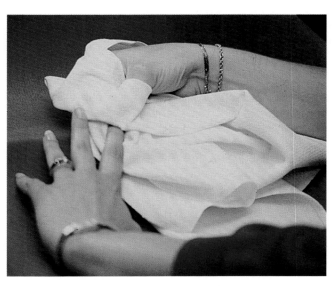

**Fig. 8.9** Manicure routine.

tension created on the fibrous band gradually causes it to thin while more of the proximal nail is exposed to create an oval shape. This desired appearance will only be achieved after a number of treatments of this type, over several weeks. The novice tries to accomplish this rapidly by pressure with the 'cuticle-pusher'; this may damage the softened nail matrix resulting in a nail with multiple transverse ridges.

4 As necessary, cuticle remover is then applied to the exposed new nail growth. After several minutes it is rinsed off thoroughly with water. Any remnants of cuticle adhering to the

plate can be gently rubbed away with an orange stick or similar wand to create a smooth, even surface.

5 Any ragged edges are then trimmed from the cuticle. No attempt is made to eliminate this fibrous band, which creates a thin, attractive, framed edge to the proximal nail.

6 The nail plate should be cleansed again with nail enamel remover. It may now be polished with the application of wax and suitably buffed or coated with nail enamel.

7 Nail enamel provides gloss and colour in a broad spectrum of shades. Two or three coats are necessary for an even, attractive finish with five polish options: full coverage, free edge, hairline tip, slim line or free wall, halfmoon unpolished. A nail base coat applied before the nail enamel will increase bonding of the enamel to the plate and reduce the tendency for some shades of nail enamel to stain the nail plate. (See 'Discoloration of the nail' below). The application of a top coat product to the dried enamel will increase gloss and enhance wear characteristics.

These details mainly relate to fingernails. Toenails require similar care for cleanliness. However, toenail plates should be clipped and filed to achieve almost a square or slightly oval free edge carried just beyond the toe, in order not to interfere with the pressure of footwear, and to avoid the ingrown nail. Adornment is usually less vigorous, especially when self-administered due to difficulty in access. It is easier to groom toenails if a firm, pencil-thick roll of cottonwool is placed between the digits.

## Special products and procedures
(Baran & Schoon 1998a,b)

### Nail mending kits (Fig. 8.10)

Cultivated nails of pleasing, matched length demand an investment of time, care and devotion. The reward is aesthetic satisfaction and considerable pride; damage to such a prized possession is of significant concern. Fracture to the free edge can be splinted by the application of mending papers that are saturated with clear, thickened basic nail enamel substance. When dry, conventional nail enamel may be applied with reasonably good cosmetic effect so that the damaged plate can be protected until normal growth permits filing to the length and shape desired. Quick, efficient nail mending kits are available. These consist of transparent plastic film strips that are applied to the nail fracture with a cyanoacrylate glue. Even a totally severed nail plate tip can be mended by this method. Since application is made to a non-viable portion of the nail, the possibility of an allergic reaction is minimized. However, this substance requires much care and skill in its use. It dries rapidly and firmly. Fingers, even eyelids, have been bound together by this substance, requiring medical attention for resolution.

### Nail hardeners (Figs 8.11–8.13)

Fragile, or very flexible nail plates pose difficulties to those desiring long tapered nails. Regular application of 5–10%

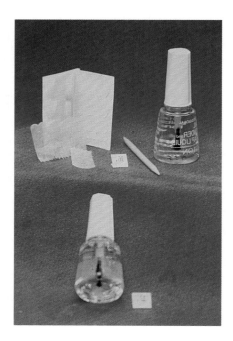

**Fig. 8.10** Nail mending kit.

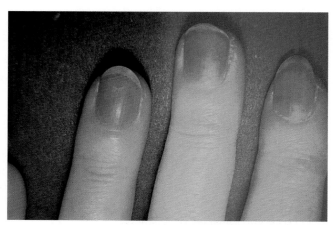

**Fig. 8.11** Reactions to nail hardeners. Subungual haemorrhage due to formaldehyde. (Courtesy of P. Lazar, USA.)

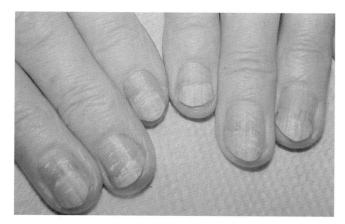

**Fig. 8.12** Reactions to nail hardeners—onycholysis. (Courtesy of P. Lazar, USA.)

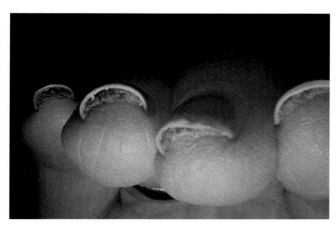

**Fig. 8.13** Reactions to nail hardeners—subungual hyperkeratosis. (Courtesy of P. Lazar, USA.)

aqueous formalin will stiffen the nails but lower flexibility and increased strength will result in an imbalance called brittleness. Moreover, local irritation, allergic dermatitis, pain, onycholysis, subungual hyperkeratosis and even subungual haemorrhage have been reported (Lazar 1966). In addition prolonged use of formaldehyde causes the nail to become split, dry and brittle.

For approximately 20 years the United States Food and Drug Administration has restricted the marketing of such commercial products. Formaldehyde is also prohibited in Japan. In the European Common Market, products containing formaldehyde must state this clearly on the label. They may be dispensed on prescription. Because of the ability of nail enamel films to protect, splint and modestly fortify the nail plate itself, products with minor modifications in quality and quantity of the resin are now offered as 'hardeners'. These contain no formaldehyde other than a trace which may result from the chemical reaction to create the basic resin. The United States Food and Drug Administration permits a formaldehyde concentration of 0.2% or less, which is far too low to have any hardening benefit. In fact the property that people really want is toughness, which is a favourable balance between strength and flexibility (Schoon 1996). Formaldehyde is merely the chemical moiety upon which the resin is formed. Mitchell (1981) has reported a non-inflammatory onycholysis from formaldehyde-containing nail hardener.

### Nail wrapping

Nail wrapping is performed in salons; each operator has her own technique and product mix. Essentially, the free edge of each nail is splinted with layers of a fibrous substance, such as cottonwool, paper, silk, linen, plastic film or fibre glass and affixed with cyanoacrylate glue. After drying the edge is fashioned to suit, and the nail is coated with enamel. Fibre glass has become very popular. Most fibre glass systems consist of three basic elements: resin or adhesive, fibre glass mesh, and an activator or catalyst hastening the resin (cyanoacrylate) polymerization.

Depending on the skill and quality of workmanship, the procedure may require as much as 2 h to perform. The reinforced, durable, free edge resists wear and tear and permits growth of a long nail. Fresh nail enamel is applied after several days and the entire procedure repeated every 2 weeks. The previous wrappings are easily removed with nail enamel remover. Care must be taken to keep the edge of the nail coated with nail enamel to prevent snagging as it wears.

Contact sensitization to cyanoacrylate adhesive may result in severe onychodystrophy (Guin *et al.* 1998; Kanerva & Estlander 1999; Higashi *et al.* 2000) and dermatitis at remote sites (Fitzgerald *et al.* 1995).

### Sculptured nails (Figs 8.14–8.17)

This procedure is performed in salons. A plastic 'nail' is constructed upon the natural nail or nail substance of each fingertip. A metallized paperboard template is placed upon the natural nail surface to frame the 'nail' to be. Liquid-and-powder systems are based on methacrylates. The powder is a polymer which contains the initiator and other additives. A fresh acrylic mixture of ethyl methacrylate (or related moieties) monomer and polyethyl polymer powder is moulded within the template so that a plastic 'nail' of desired thickness and length is created. When hardened, the template is removed. The prosthesis is filed to shape and the surface polished. Nail enamel is then applied. It is cosmetically elegant and exceedingly durable. Depending on the skill and quality of workmanship, several hours are required to complete a very costly procedure which must be refurbished every few weeks to fill in the surface defect apparent at the lunula as the new growth becomes evident. The bonding created is profound. The removal of sculpured nails requires acetone. Some chemicals may be dangerous. One specific solvent, identified as

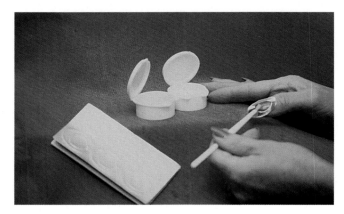

**Fig. 8.14** Nail sculpturing.

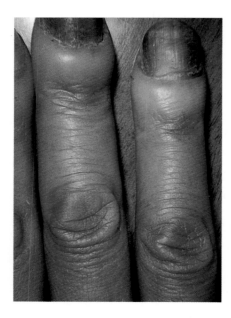

**Fig. 8.15** Nail sculpturing, side effects and complications (see text)—paronychia. (Courtesy of A. Fisher, USA.)

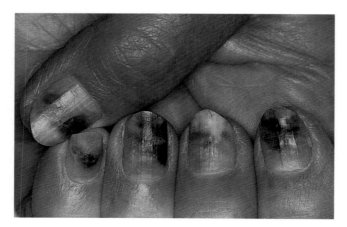

**Fig. 8.16** Nail sculpturing, side effects and complications.

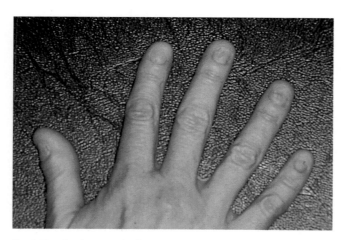

**Fig. 8.17** Nail sculpturing, side-effects and complications. Permanent anonychia.

acetonitrile, liberates inorganic cyanide when metabolized (Turchen *et al.* 1991; Rainey & Roberts 1993). Paediatric cyanide deaths following ingestion have been reported (Caravati & Litovitz 1988). Nitroethane poisoning from artificial nail remover has led to cyanosis and 39% methaemoglobinaemia (Hornfeldt & Rab 1994). Methaemoglobinaemia has also been reported from the ingestion of artificial nail solution (Kao *et al.* 1997).

Removal, if necessary, can be a painful surgical event. Allergic contact-type inflammation of ungual and periungual areas, infection, foreign body reactions, haemorrhage and severe pain have been reported, secondary nail dystrophy is not unusual (Marks *et al.* 1979). Fisher (1980, 1989) described a single case of persistent paraesthaesia and anonychia from the procedure 16 years previously. Since these publications new cases of paraesthaesia have been reported (Freeman *et al.* 1995; Kanerva *et al.* 1998). Baran and Schibli (1990) then Fisher and Baran (1991) observed a case of permanent paraesthaesia without anonychia and without sensitization to the acrylic monomer. Many individuals however, happily tolerate the method regularly over many years.

There are different types of acrylic giving the technician more choice in treating clients (hard acrylic, acrylic with high UV absorbency and a clearer acrylic). Homopolymers made from ethyl monomer are more flexible. Homopolymers made from methyl monomer are harder and stronger. In general copolymers blend the best of both monomers (Schoon 1996).

The new odourless products contain hydroxy ethyl methacrylate. They require proper ventilation just as much as traditional products.

Koppula *et al.* (1995) found that several acrylates are useful as screening patch test allergens.

### Premixed acrylic gels (UV light-cured gels)

These products are very similar to two-part, monomer-and-polymer systems. The initiator, catalyst and oligomers can be combined together into a single product that is supplied premixed and easy to use. Initiators are activated by powerful UV lights (Schoon 1996).

Coloured gels may be recommended to clients who do not change polish colour often.

To improve the adhesion between the natural nail and the artificial nail, a substance called 'primer' may be needed. There are two types of primer: acid primer (acrylic acids) and non-acid primer or non-etching primer (without methacrylic acid). Artificial nail primers containing methacrylic acid represent a corrosive hazard to young children and have been associated with severe injuries (Woolf & Shaw 1998).

Primer should be used when recommended by the manufacturer. Any formula which uses only ethyl, methyl (outlawed in the USA) or isobutyl methacrylate has a low affinity for the natural nail. By contrast, cyanoacrylates form extremely strong bonds and require no primers.

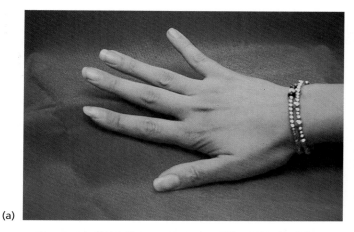

(a)

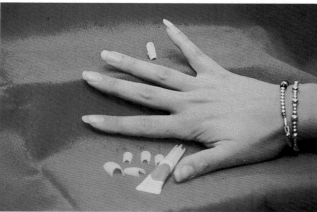

(b)

**Fig. 8.18** (a,b) Preformed artificial nails.

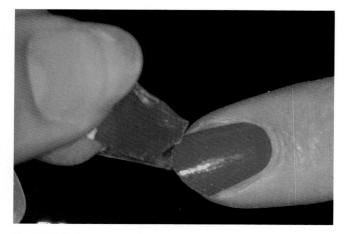

**Fig. 8.19** Self-adherent plastic nails, press-on type.

### Preformed artificial nails (Fig. 8.18)

Preformed, plastic prosthetic full nails may be used as temporary natural overlays, not worn for longer than 48 h each time they are used. They are more often used as permanent nail tip extensions cemented in place with various types of glues, especially ethyl cyanoacrylate adhesive with its accompanying hazard (Fisher 1987; Shelley & Shelley 1988). The cosmetic effect is good (Figs 8.18 & 8.19). Significant improvement has been made in adhesives for cosmetic use. The setting time has been slowed down while removal with ordinary nail enamel removers is now possible. Most nail technicians now use acrylic tips associated with overlays.

### 'Press-on' nail colour

Self-adherent various sized, nail-shaped, coloured plastic films are affixed to the nail plate to duplicate a nail enamel effect (Fig. 8.19). Although the cosmetic benefit is achieved quite quickly and easily, the wear is poor and its use not popular (Calnan 1958).

### Removal of nail coatings

The most commonly used solvent for the removal of nail products is acetone. Warming the solvent with great care can cut product removal time in half. However, most gels are difficult to remove because they are highly cross-linked and resistant to many solvents. Therefore gel enhancements should be removed slowly with a medium-grit file (not drill), leaving a very thin layer of product, then soak in warm product remover. Once softened, scrape the remaining product away with a wooden pusher stick (Schoon 1996).

## Nail care and adornment in medical practice

### Benefits

#### General

A clean, well-groomed nail is important to one's health and self esteem. Nail adornment is a common practice among fashion-conscious individuals who are devoted to projecting attractiveness and social status. It is a mistake for the physician to view a patient's complaint of unattractive nails as too trivial for medical consideration. Many of the products and procedures previously described will help overcome cosmetic defects.

#### Specific

The habit of *nail biting and cuticle picking* may be discouraged by a regimen of nail care, particularly with added colour.

*Dystrophic, atrophic, absent or diseased nails*, particularly where only a few are involved, can be improved cosmetically with one of the procedures previously described (Figs 8.20 & 8.21). Due to the severity of adverse reactions with the 'permanently' adhering sculptured nail, caution should be exercised in its recommendation.

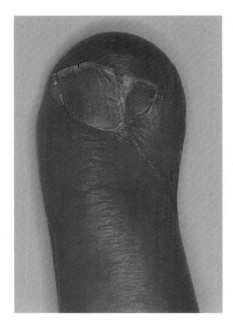

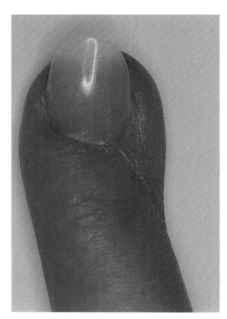

**Fig. 8.20** Dystrophic nail.

**Fig. 8.21** After a nail prosthesis has been applied (cf. Fig. 8.20).

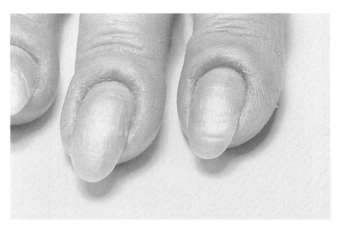

**Fig. 8.22** Paronychia due to overzealous manicuring. (Courtesy of R. Staughton, UK.)

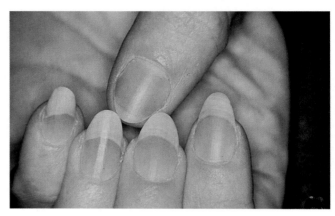

**Fig. 8.23** Discoloration of the nails due to nail enamels.

## Adverse effects (see also Chapter 7)

### Paronychia (Fig. 8.22)

This occasionally appears when poor manicuring skill causes skin penetration by sharp and pointed implements (Roberge *et al.* 1999).

### Ridging

Transverse ridging of nail plates, as well as transverse leukony-

chia, may result from overzealous use of manicure tools in the vicinity of the lunula, particularly in association with the use of cuticle removers.

### Discoloration of the nail (Fig. 8.23)

Deeper shades of red and brown nail enamel may cause mild staining of nail keratin (Calnan 1967). This phenomenon occurs in only a few users and is without satisfactory explanation. Nail staining begins near the cuticle, extends to the top of the nail, and becomes progressively darker from base to tip. With the leaching out of the varnish, the dyes (D & C Red no. 6, 7 and 34; FD & C yellow no. 5 Lake) generally penetrate into the nail too deeply to be removed.

This poses a cosmetic problem only if the user elects not to continue with a coloured nail enamel. The staining is significantly, or completely, avoided by the application of a base coat prior to the use of the offending nail enamel.

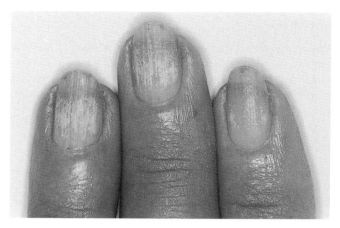

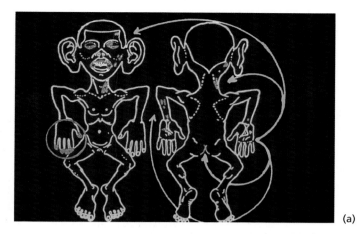

(a)

Fig. 8.24 'Granulation' of the nail plate due to multiple layers of enamel.

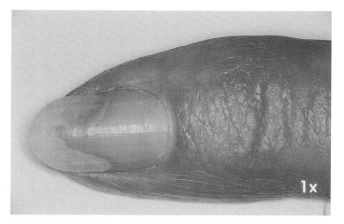

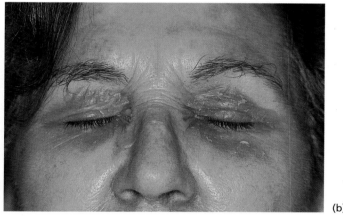

(b)

Fig. 8.26 (a,b) Sites of origin and transfer of allergens. (After C. Bonu, Italy.)

Fig. 8.25 Onycholysis due to nail cosmetic procedures—patch testing is required to find the cause, but here the nail plate–nail bed separation was due to overzealous cleaning with an orange stick (sculptured onycholysis).

### Granulation of nail keratin (Fig. 8.24)

Granulation is occasionally observed in individuals who apply fresh coats of enamel on top of old, worn enamel, for several weeks in succession. It results in superficial friability (Baran 1985). It may be avoided by following a 5–7-day nail care schedule as described previously.

### Onycholysis (Fig. 8.25)

Impervious coatings, such as cemented, preformed artificial nails, sculptured nails or similar films may cause spontaneous, uncomplicated separation of the natural plate from its bed due to the interference with normal vapour exchange (Guin & Wilson 1999).

Nail enamels and related products reduce, but do not eliminate, the vapour exchange from nail bed to the environment. Although nail enamels have been mentioned in association with onycholysis, considering the extensive worldwide use, the cause-and-effect relationship must be most unusual.

Significant attention to nail care often yields longer nails. Onycholysis of the distal portion of the fingertip may be caused by the increased leverage created by the length of nail beyond the fingertip (Fig. 8.8).

### Contact dermatitis (allergic) (Figs 8.26 & 8.27)

Conventional nail care and nail enamel products are rarely associated with local (fingertips) allergic eczematous-type contact reactions (Liden *et al.* 1993). A patchy eruption on distant sites, such as eyelids, neck and deltoid areas, even the genitals, may appear due to contact with fingers. Besides ectopic dermatitis, allergic airborne contact dermatitis should be suspected when the lesions involving the face, neck and ears are symmetrical. The allergen in nail enamels is usually the thermoplastic resin. Diagnostic patch testing with nail enamel should be performed without occlusive covering, or with dry enamel films to avoid false-positive reactions from solvent. Interestingly ectopic contact dermatitis from henna used to dye nails has been reported (Etienne *et al.* 1997).

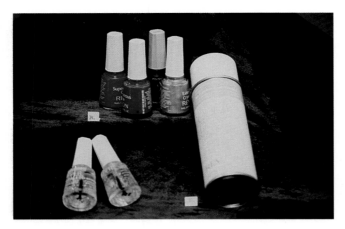

**Fig. 8.27** Some of the agents causing type IV hypersensitivity.

## Overall risk

Precise figures are not available for the number of adverse reactions related to the use of cosmetics in general, and certainly none for nail care products in particular. However, by reviewing data collected from several souces, a reasonable estimate can be made.

### *North American Contact Dermatitis Group*

In a 64-month interval between 1977 and 1983, 12 dermatologists representing various geographical areas of the USA studied 713 patients with cosmetic dermatitis. Of this number, 55, or 8%, had adverse reactions to the entire category of nail preparation.

## Summary

No matter how one reviews and analyses the figures from all sources, the incidence of untoward reactions related to the use of cosmetics by the general population is very small (approximately 2 per million units sold). Nail care products as a subgroup probably account for under 10% of cosmetic reactions. The rare injury of any significance is caused by the acrylate resins where the monomer and polymer are mixed on the fingertip to create the sculptured nail. These are products of low volume use which are not marketed, presently, by any of the large well-known cosmetic manufacturers.

Typical of cosmetics, nail care products are fashion orientated. Short-lived fads have not been considered in this discussion because they would lack pertinence. Likewise, this chapter is not meant to be an historical review of past irrelevant literature. For example, nail care products with ingredient compositions that are no longer available commercially have been omitted. Regrettably, current dermatological literature continues to cite nail enamel base coats as singularly responsible for adverse reactions when the product formula in question has not been marketed for more than 50 years.

There are many products, implements and devices for maintaining clean well-groomed nails to satisfy individual needs. These benefits are obtained with small risk. The physician can and should be well versed in the nail care and adornment that aid patients in achieving an improved positive self-image.

The recommendation to a patient to use a product labelled 'hypoallergenic' is naive, as it is used in the cosmetic industry purely for promotion. Dermatologically, it is without any merit. It serves only to mislead the practitioner and confuse the patient. There are almost as many patients who react to products labelled 'hypoallergenic' as to any other; for example, tosylamide/formaldehyde resin has been responsible for desquamative gingivitis (Staines *et al*. 1998).

All reputable manufacturers are committed to market products with as low a sensitizing potential as possible. A patient with an allergic sensivity to substance R can benefit only if the product is free of substance R. If substance W is substituted for it, the product can hardly be hypoallergenic to another patient with an allergic sensivity to substance W. Frequently, so-called hypoallergenic products are identical in ingredient content to products not so labelled. The physician may wish to subject a particular patient to an extensive, time-consuming battery of skin patch tests to identify the offending substance and then seek a product free of it. However, initially, the patient is pragmatically better served by being asked to change the type of the product (e.g. from cream to lotion or powder form), or the brand name or manufacturer.

In the case of nail enamel resins, there are several different types used in manufacture so switching brands to present a different resin is a reasonable approach. In countries that require ingredient disclosure on the label, product differences may be readily identified; allergen identification by means of detailed skin patch test work-up may be worthwhile. When the practice proves successful, the new product, though tolerated, still cannot be called hypoallergenic. The patient may eventually become allergic to another substance in the new product.

Haemorrhage, paronychia and foreign-body reactions have been associated with unusual contact-type reactions. (See 'Sculptured nails' above.)

## References

Baran, R. (1982) Pathology induced by the application of cosmetics to the nail. In: *Principles of Cosmetics for the Dermatologist* (eds P. Frost & S. Horwitz), p. 181. Mosby, St Louis.

Baran, R. (1985) Cosmetics and the fingernails—old and new facts. In: *Society of Cosmetic Scientists Symposium on Recent Advances in Skin Biology in Relation to Cosmetics*, Paper 14, 11–12 November.

Baran, R. & Schibli, H. (1990) Permanent paresthesia to sculptured nail. A distressing problem. *Dermatologic Clinics* 8, 139–141.

Baran, R. & Schoon, D.D. (1998a) Cosmetology of normal nails. In: *Textbook of Cosmetic Dermatology* (eds R. Baran & H. Maiback), 2nd edn. Martin Dunitz, London.

Baran, R. & Schoon, D.D. (1998b) Cosmetics for abnormal and pathological nails. In: *Textbook of Cosmetic Dermatology* (eds R. Baran & H. Maiback), 2nd edn. Martin Dunitz, London.

Barnett, J.M. & Scher, R.K. (1992) Nail cosmetics. *International Journal of Dermatology* 31, 675–681.

Brauer, E.W. (1969) *Your Skin and Hair. A Basic Guide to Care and Beauty.* MacMillan, New York.

Calnan, C.D. (1958) Onychia from synthetic nail coverage. *Transactions of the St John Hospital Dermatology Society* 41, 66–68.

Calnan, C.D. (1967) Reactions to artificial colouring materials. *Journal of the Society of Cosmetic Chemistry* 18, 215–223.

Caravati, E.M. & Litovitz, T.L. (1988) Pediatric cyanide intoxication and death from an acetonitrile-containing cosmetic. *Journal of the American Medical Association* 260, 3470–3473.

Etienne, A., Piletta, P., Hauser, C. *et al.* (1997) Ectopic contact dermatitis from Henna. *Contact Dermatitis* 37, 183.

Fisher, A.A. (1980) Permanent loss of finger nails from sensitization and reaction to acrylic in a preparation designed to make artificial nails. *Journal of Dermatologic Surgery and Oncology* 6, 70–71.

Fisher, A.A. (1987) Allergic reactions to cyanoacrylate 'Krazy glue' nail preparations. *Cutis* 40, 475–476.

Fisher, A.A. (1989) Permanent loss of finger nails due to allergic reaction to an acrylic nail preparation. A sixteen-year follow-up study. *Cutis* 43, 404–406.

Fisher, A.A. & Baran, R. (1991) Adverse reactions to acrylate sculptured nails with particular reference to prolonged paresthesia. *American Journal of Contact Dermatitis* 2, 38–42.

Fitzgerald, D.A., Bhaggoe, R. & English, J.S.C. (1995) Contact sensitivity to cyanoacrylate nail adhesive with dermatitis at remote sites. *Contact Dermatitis* 32, 175–176.

Freeman, S., Lee, M.S. & Gudmunsen, K. (1995) Adverse contact reactions to sculptured acrylic nails: 4 case reports and a literature review. *Contact Dermatitis* 33, 381–385.

Guin, J.D. & Wilson, P. (1999) Onycholysis from nail lacquer: a complication of enamel enhancement? *American Journal of Contact Dermatitis* 10, 34–36.

Guin, J.D., Baas, K. & Nelson-Adsokan, P. (1998) Contact senistization to cyanoacrylate adhesive as a cause of severe onychodystrophy. *International Journal of Dermatology* 37, 31–36.

Higashi, N., Kume, A. *et al.* (2000) Two cases of allergic contact dermatitis from nail cosmetics. *Environmental Dermatology* 7, 79–83.

Hornfeldt, C.S. & Rab, W.H. (1994) Nitroethane poisoning from an artificial nail remover. *Journal of Toxicology and Clinical Toxicology* 32, 321–324.

Kanerva, L., Mikola, H., Enricks-Eckerman, M.L. *et al.* (1998) Fingertip paresthesia and occupational allergic contact dermatitis caused by acrylics in a dental nurse. *Contact Dermatitis* 38, 114–116.

Kanerva, L. & Estlander, L. (1999) Allergic onycholysis and paronychia caused by cyanoacrylate nail glue, but not by photobonded methacrylate nails. *European Journal of Dermatology* 9, 223–225.

Kao, L., Leiking, J.B., Crockett, M. *et al.* (1997) Methemoglobinemia from artificial fingernail solution. *Journal of the American Medical Association* 278, 549–550.

Koppula, S.V., Fellman, J.H. & Storrs, F.J. (1995) Screening allergens for acrylate dermatitis associated with artificial nails. *American Journal of Contact Dermatitis* 6, 78–85.

Lazar, P. (1966) Reactions to nail hardeners. *Archives of Dermatology* 94, 446–448.

Liden, C., Berg, M., Färm, G. & Wrangsjo, K. (1993) Nail varnish allergy with far-reaching consequences. *British Journal of Dermatology* 128, 57–62.

Marks, J.G., Bishop, M.E. & Willis, W.F. (1979) Allergic contact dermatitis to sculptured nails. *Archives of Dermatology* 115, 100.

Mitchell, J.C. (1981) Non-inflammatory onycholysis from formaldehyde-containing nail hardener. *Contact Dermatitis* 7, 173.

Nater, J.P., de Groot, A.C. & Miem, D.H. (1985) *Unwanted Effects of Cosmetics and Drugs Used in Dermatology,* 2nd edn, pp. 337–342. Excerpta Medica. Amsterdam.

North American Contact Dermatitis Group (1982) *Prospective Study of Cosmetics Reactions: 1977–1980,* Vol. 6, pp. 909–917.

Rainey, P.M. & Roberts, W.L. (1993) Diagnosis and misdiagnosis of poisoning with cyanide precursor acetonitrile: nail polish remover or nail glue remover? *American Journal of Emergency Medicine* 11, 104–108.

Roberge, R.J., Weinsteine, D. & Thimons, M.M. (1999) Perionychial infections associated with sculptured nails. *American Journal of Emergency Medicine* 17, 581–582.

Schoon, D.D. (1996) *Nail Structure and Products Chemistry.* Milady Publishing, Albany, NY.

Shelley, E.D. & Shelley, W.D. (1988) Nail dystrophy and periungual dermatitis due to acrylate glue sensitivity. *Journal of the American Academy of Dermatology* 19, 574–575.

Staines, K.S., Felix, D.H. & Forsyth, A. (1998) Desquamating gingivitis, sole manifestation of tosylamide/formaldehyde resin allergy. *Contact Dermatitis* 39, 10.

Turchen, S.G., Monaguerra, A.S. & Whitney, C. (1991) Severe cyanide poisoning from the ingestion of an acetonitrile containing cosmetic. *American Journal of Emergency Medicine* 9, 264–267.

Woolf, A. & Shaw, J. (1998) Childhood injuries from artificial nail primer cosmetic products. *Archives of Pediatric and Adolescent Medicine* 152, 41–46.

# Hereditary and congenital nail disorders

**L. Juhlin & R. Baran**

## Introduction

Many of the defects of the nails are accompanied by developmental changes in other organs, such as skin, teeth, brain and bones. The many abnormalities of the nails described here are often of minor importance when making a diagnosis. Of greater interest are apparently isolated nail defects, since they may help in the diagnosis of hidden syndromes or more generalized disease. In categorizing these disorders the nail has been placed in the 'centre' but disorders have also been grouped according to the most obvious symptoms. Such a practical division aims to aid the physician observing nail changes as a help to diagnosis.

In view of the large number of unique and rare syndromes with nail involvement, we have resolved much of this chapter into comprehensive tables stressing the nail apparatus changes and major associated abnormalities. The MIM (Mendelian Inheritance in Man) numbers have been added when available (McKusick 1998). Autosomal entries initiated before 20 May 1994 have numbers 100050–195002 and 200100–280000. Later appearing autosomal entries are numbered 600000–601922. X-linked disorders are numbers 300000–315000, Y-linked 400000–490000 and mitochondrial entries numbers 502000–598500. An asterisk indicates that an entry describes a distinct gene or phenotype. An absence of the sign preceding the number indicates that the distinctness of the phenotype or the characterization of the gene in the human is not established. The sign # means that the phenotype is caused by mutation in a gene also represented by other entries.

### Reference

McKusick, V.A. (1998) *Mendelian Inheritance in Man. A Catalogue of Human Genes and Genetic Disorders*, 12th edn, Vols I–III. Johns Hopkins University Press, Baltimore.

## Nail embryology

The human nail apparatus begins to develop during the 9th week of intrauterine life; nail plate growth is evident by 14 weeks and may be complete by 20 weeks (Chapter 1). Nail defects occurring during this period are called embryopathies and those appearing later are the fetopathies. The embryopathies are often hereditary whereas the fetopathies as a rule are caused by vascular or mechanical factors. Some hereditary defects do not become apparent until later in life, mainly because they are due to increased susceptibility to infections or secondary damage. Telfer *et al.* (1988) classified the congenital and hereditary nail dystrophies according to whether the defects occurred in the nail matrix, the nail field or the nail bed. A defect in the nail matrix is the most common cause of abnormal nails. The matrix can have an abnormal position, size or quality. The nail field is the area in which the entire nail unit (nail matrix and nail bed) develops. Proliferation of the nail bed will produce a thickened nail which, as in pachyonychia congenita, is not evident until early childhood.

## Reference

Telfer, N.R., Barth, J.H. & Dawber, R.P.R. (1988) Congenital and hereditary nail dystrophies—an embryological approach to classification. *Clinical and Experimental Dermatology* **13**, 160–163.

## Anonychia

Total absence of all nails from birth is rare (Solammadevi 1981). Often there are rudimentary nails on some fingers or toes (MIM 107000); therefore, there is frequently only a quantitative difference between anonychia and hyponychia and they often occur together (Timerman *et al.* 1969). The first two cases with anonychia were described in 1842 by the physician to the King of Saxony, Dr F.A. Amman; Cockayne (1933) reviewed some of the earlier cases.

Isolated anonychia (Fig. 9.1) without other symptoms can be inherited as a dominant, recessive or sporadic abnormality (see Salamon 1966; Mahloudji & Amidi 1971; Hopsu-Havu & Jansén *et al.* 1973; MIM *206800). Cockayne (1933) and Strandskov (1939) described families with absent thumbnails from birth (MIM 188200). If an X-ray is undertaken an underlying bone abnormality is generally found (Baran & Juhlin 1986). There will be no nail if the distal phalanx is lacking; when the latter is hypoplastic the nails may be absent, dystrophic or normal. Often anonychia is combined with other symptoms (Nevin *et al.* 1982, 1995) (Fig. 9.2) such as broad, small hands, due to various skeletal anomalies such as loss of phalanges (MIM 106990, *106995) or isolated fingers and toes (ectrodactyly) (MIM 106900), syndactyly (Figs 9.3 & 9.4) or polydactyly (Salamon 1966; Lawrence 1969; Rahbari *et al.*

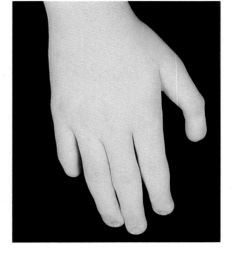

**Fig. 9.2** Anonychia/hyponychia in DOOR syndrome. (Courtesy of Professor Nevin, Belfast.)

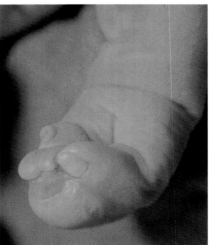

**Fig. 9.3** Syndactyly.

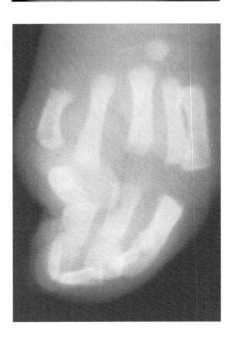

**Fig. 9.4** Syndactyly— X-ray changes in digits of patient in Fig. 9.3.

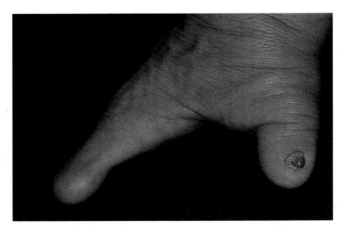

**Fig. 9.1** Anonychia/hyponychia.

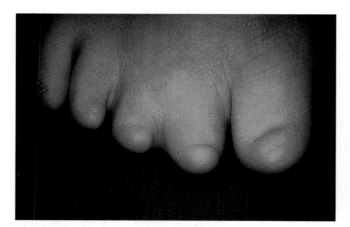

**Fig. 9.5** Anonychia—pseudo-amputee appearance.

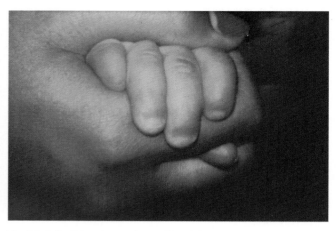

**Fig. 9.6** Coffin–Siris syndrome—absence of the 5th fingernail. (Courtesy of Professor Schinzel, Switzerland.)

1975; Kurgan *et al.* 1976; Cooks *et al.* 1985; Kumar & Levick 1986; Ortonne *et al.* 1986; Hatzis & Soulacos 1994; Wood 1996). In the brachydactyly variant called apical dystrophy by MacArthur and McCullough (1932) or banana fingers, the four ulnar digits barely project beyond the thumb and the fingers look amputated and have no nails (Fig. 9.5). Absence of nails on the ring fingers and rudimentary nails on other fingers with brachydactyly in six generations was reported by Schott (1978). Families with total anonychia and microcephaly with normal intelligence have also been described (Teebi & Kaurah 1996).

## Anonychia with other symptoms

Anonychia can occur with retarded development of the teeth (Baisch 1931). Freire-Maia and Pinheiro (1979) described recessive total anonychia with a dominant dental anomaly and aplasia or hypoplasia of the upper lateral incisors, spaced teeth and lack of some molars. Loss of toenails and bradydactyly with dental changes was reported by Tennstedt *et al.* (1985). Congenital absence of three toenails with linear skin atrophy, scaring alopecia and scar-like lesions of the tongue was reported by Sequeiros and Sack (1985). Absence or hypoplasia of nails on thumbs and halluces can, together with gingival fibromatosis (MIM *135500), be diagnostic features for Zimmerman–Laband syndrome (Chodriker *et al.* 1986; Robertson *et al.* 1998). Anonychia can be combined with deafness, onychoosteodystrophy and mental retardation (Fig. 9.2) (DOOR syndrome) (Table 9.3). These patients have an inborn metabolic error with an increase of 2-oxyglutamate in plasma and urine (Patton *et al.* 1987). Pfeiffer (1982) reported the otoonychoperoneal syndrome with absence of nails on thumbs, index fingers and big toes with dysplastic ears and hypoplasia of the fibula (MIM 259780).

Anonychia is described in the rare glossopalatine ankylosis syndrome in which the mouth is abnormal, the tongue being attached to the temporomandibular joint (Gorlin *et al.* 1976). Absence of nails on thumbs and great toe due to absence of epi-

physical centres and poor modelling of the distal phalanges was reported as a possible new autosomal disorder by Lynch *et al.* (1997). The patients also had bulbous nasal tip, long philtrum kinosogenic choreoathetosis and developmental delay. A family with dominant anonychia with bizarre flexural pigmentation (MIM 106750) and hair abnormalities was reported by Verbov (1975). Anonychia has also been described in the dyscephalic-mandibulo-oculofacial syndrome (MIM 234100) of Hallerman–Streiff–Francois with bird-like faces (Guérineau & Plassart 1965; Cohen 1991) and craniofrontal nasal dysplasia (Table 9.6). Familial absence of the 5th fingernails (Fig. 9.6) in combination with mental retardation, coarse faces with full lips and scalp hypotrichosis (MIM 135900) were first described by Coffin and Siris (1970). Carey and Hall (1978) and Haspeslagh *et al.* (1984) have reviewed the literature and described new cases. Hypoglycaemia in the syndrome was reported by Imaizumi *et al.* (1995) and data on cognitive development was presented by Swillen *et al.* (1995). This disorder belongs to the group of epidermal dysplasias which often have other abnormalities as described in Table 9.2. In the popliteal pterygium syndrome (Klein's syndrome) the nails are missing on the 5th toe (MIM *119500). The patients also have pterygium and fissures on the 1st toe with syndactyly (Klein 1962; Soekarman *et al.* 1995). In congenital onychodysplasia of the index finger (COIF) or Kikuchi syndrome the nail on the index finger can be missing (see page 399 and Table 9.6). Lack of thumbnails can occur in the nail–patella syndrome.

## Nail–patella syndrome or hereditary osteo-onychodysplasia (MIM *161200)

This was described by Chatelain (1820) and Little (1897) (cited in Raman & Haslock 1983). Early diagnosis of the nail–patella syndrome or hereditary osteo-onychodysplasia (HOOD) can be made by examining the nails, which give clues to the possibility of other organs being involved.

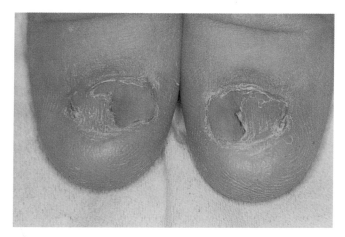

**Fig. 9.7** Nail–patella syndrome—hypoplastic thumbnails.

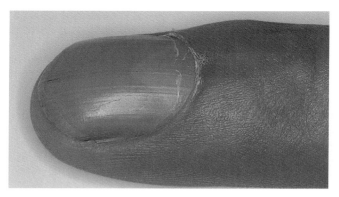

**Fig. 9.8** Nail–patella syndrome—triangular, pointed lunula.

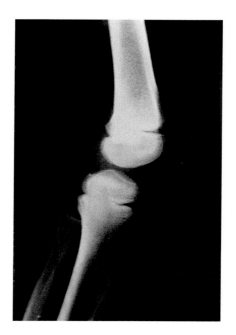

**Fig. 9.9** Nail–patella syndrome—X-ray to show aplastic patellae.

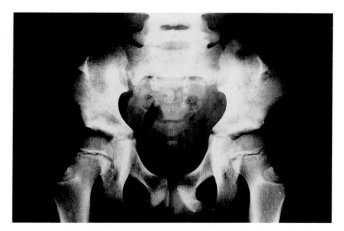

**Fig. 9.10** Nail–patella syndrome—X-ray showing bilateral posterior iliac horns.

## Nails (Fig. 9.7)

The nail changes are most pronounced on the ulnar side of the thumbs and decrease towards the 5th finger. The toenails are rarely affected. The nails, especially on the thumbs, might be absent or short, narrow, spoon shaped, soft and/or fragile. The lunula can be triangular or V shaped (Fig. 9.8), which is almost pathognomonic for the condition (Norton & Mescon 1968; Daniel *et al.* 1980).

## Bones

The patella is aplastic or luxated in 90% of patients (Fig. 9.9). Pain in the knee or gait problems after exercise often bring the patient to the doctor. The changes can result in early osteoarthritis. The radius head is small which can cause limitation in elbow motion or subluxation of radius. Bilateral posterior iliac horns are pathognomic (Fig. 9.10). Other bone changes can be seen, such as scapular hypoplasia, scoliosis, genu valgum and hypoplastic lateral humerus epicondyle.

## Kidney

Renal involvement is seen in 42% of the cases with various degrees of dysfunction (Carbonara & Albert 1964; Croock *et al.* 1987). It has recently been described as the only manifestation of the syndrome (Dombros & Katz 1982; Salcedo 1984; Gubler *et al.* 1990). The presence of collagen-like fibrils in the glomerular basement membrane as revealed by electron microscopy is diagnostic (Morita *et al.* 1973). The renal symptoms are usually first discovered in adults as asymptomatic proteinuria. The end result can be a nephrotic-like picture which can result in renal failure.

## Eye

Heterochromia of the iris with hyperpigmentation of the papillary margin are also helpful diagnostic signs. In addition microcornea and glaucoma have been reported.

## Other signs

Webs on fingers and pterygia in the popliteal or antecubital areas can occur. (Rizzo *et al.* 1993). Other features described are cutis laxa and palmoplantar hyperhidrosis (Peckman & Bergfeld 1980).

## Genetics

The syndrome is autosomal dominant and the gene is located on the long arm of the 9th chromosome (Westerveld *et al.* 1976). The locus is linked to that of the ABO group (Renwick & Lawler 1955). Ferguson-Smith *et al.* (1976) assigned the linkage group to 9q34. McIntosh *et al.* (1997) and Eyaid *et al.* (1998) further positioned the nail–patella syndrome interval between DqS60 and AKI.

## References

Baisch, A. (1931) Anonychia congenita, kombiniert mit Polydactylie und verzögertem abnormen Zalindurchbruch. *Deutsche Zeitschrift für Chirurgie* 232, 450.

Baran, R. & Juhlin, L. (1986) Bone dependent nail formation. *British Journal of Dermatology* 114, 371–375.

Carbonara, P. & Albert, M. (1964) Hereditary osteoonychodysplasia (HOOD). *American Journal of the Medical Sciences* 248, 139.

Carey, J.C. & Hall, B.D. (1978) The Coffin–Siris syndrome. Five new cases including two siblings. *American Journal of Diseases of Children* 132, 667.

Chodriker, B.N., Chudley, A.E., Toffler, M.A. & Reed, M.H. (1986) Brief clinical report: Zimmerman–Laband syndrome and profound mental retardation. *American Journal of Medical Genetics* 25, 543.

Cockayne, E.A. (1933) Abnormalities of the nails. *Inherited Abnormalities of Skin and its Appendages*, p. 265, Oxford University Press, London.

Coffin, G.S. & Siris, E. (1970) Mental retardation with absent fifth fingernail and terminal phalanx. *American Journal of Diseases of Children* 119, 433.

Cohen, M.M. Jr (1991) Hallerman–Streiff syndrome: a review. *American Journal of Medical Genetics* 41, 488.

Cooks, R., Hertz, M., Katznelson, M. & Goodman, R.M. (1985) A new nail dysplasia syndrome with onychonychia and absence and/or hypoplasia of distal phalanges. *Clinical Genetics* 27, 85.

Croock, A.D., Kahaleh, M.B. & Powers, J.M. (1987) Vasculitis and renal disease in nail–patella syndrome: case report and literature review. *Annals of the Rheumatic Diseases* 46, 562.

Daniel, C.R., Osment, L.S. & Noojin, R.O. (1980) Triangular lunulae. *Archives of Dermatology* 116, 448.

Dombros, N. & Katz, A. (1982) Nail patella-like renal lesions in the absence of skeletal abnormalities. *American Journal of Kidney Diseases* 1, 237.

Eyaid, W.M., Clough, M.V., Root, H. *et al.* (1998) Physical mapping of the nail patella syndrome interval at 9q34: ordering of STSs and ESTs. *Human Genetics* 103, 525.

Ferguson-Smith, M.A., Aitken, D.A., Turleau, C. & de Grouchy, J. (1976) Localization of the human ABO : Np-1 : AK-1 linkage group by regional assignment of AK-1–9q34. *Human Genetics* 34, 35.

Freire-Maia, N. & Pinheiro, M. (1979) Recessive anonychia totalis and dominant aplasia (or hypoplasia) of upper lateral incisors in the same kindred. *Journal of Medical Genetics* 16, 45.

Gorlin, R.J., Pindborg, J.J. & Cohen, M.M. (1976) *Syndromes of the Head and Neck*, 2nd edn. McGraw-Hill, New York.

Gubler, M.C., Dommersures, J.P., Furioli, J. *et al.* (1990) Syndrome de 'nail–patella' sans atteinte extrarenale. Une nouvelle nephropathie hereditaire glomerulaire. *Annales de Pediatrie (Paris)* 37, 78.

Guerinéau, P. & Plassart, H. (1965) Syndrome dyscéphalique de Francois a propos d'un nourrison de race maure. *Archives Françaises de Pediatrie (Paris)* 22, 882.

Haspeslagh, M., Fryns, J.P. & van den Berghe, H. (1984) The Coffin–Siris syndrome: report of a family and further delineation. *Clinical Genetics* 26, 374.

Hatzis, J. & Soulacos, P.N. (1994) Anonychia of all toes with absence of phalangeal bones. *Australian Journal of Dermatology* 35, 83.

Hopsu-Havu, V.K. & Jansén, C.T. (1973) Anonychia congenita. *Archives of Dermatology* 107, 752.

Imaizumi, K., Nakamura, M., Masuno, M., Makita, Y. & Kuroki, Y. (1995) Hypoglycemia in Coffin–Siris syndrome. *Journal of Medical Genetics* 59, 49.

Klein, D. (1962) Cheilo-palatoschizis avec fistules de la levre inférieure associé a une syndactylie, une onychodysplasie particuliere, un pterygion poplité unilatéeral et des pieds varus équins. *Journal de Genetique Humaine* 11, 65.

Kumar, D. & Levick, R.K. (1986) Autosomal dominant onychodystrophy and anonychia with type B brachydactyly and ectrodactyly. *Clinical Genetics* 30, 219.

Kurgan, A., Hirsch, M. & Williams, F.J. (1976) Aplasia of toe phalanges and nails. *Israeli Journal of Medical Sciences* 12, 570.

Lawrence, R. (1969) Absence of phalanges and toenails. *Medical Radiography and Photography* 45, 46.

Lynch, S.A., Gardner-Medwin, D., Burn, J. & Bushby, K.M.D. (1997) Absent nails, kinesogenic choreoathetosis, epilepsy and developmental delay—a new autosomal dominant disorder? *Clinical Dysmorphology* 6, 133.

MacArthur, J.W. & McCullough, F. (1932) Apical dystrophy, an inherited defect of hands and feet. *Human Biology* 4, 179.

McIntosh, I., Clough, M.V., Schaffer, A., Puffenberger, E.G. *et al.* (1997) Fine mapping of the nail–patella locus at 9q34. *American Journal of Human Genetics* 60, 133–142.

McKusick, V.A. (1998) *Mendelian Inheritance in Man. A Catalogue of Human Genes and Genetic Disorders*, 12th edn, Vols I–III. The Johns Hopkins University Press, Baltimore.

Mahloudji, M. & Amidi, M. (1971) Simple anonychia. Further evidence for autosomal recessive inheritance. *Journal of Medical Genetics* 8, 478.

Morita, T., Laughlin, O., Kawano, K. & Kimmelstiel, P. (1973) Nail–patella syndrome. *Archives of Internal Medicine* 131, 271.

Nevin, N.C., Thomas, P.S., Calvert, J. & Reid, M. (1982) Deafness, onycho-osteodystrophy, mental retardation (DOOR) syndrome. *American Journal of Medical Genetics* 13, 325.

Nevin, N.C., Thomas, P.C., Eedy, D.J. & Shepherd, C. (1995) Anonychia and absence/hypoplasia of distal phalanges (Cooks syndrome): report of a second family. *Journal of Medical Genetics* 32, 638.

Norton, L.A. & Mescon, H. (1968) Nail–patella–elbow syndrome. *Archives of Dermatology* 98, 372.

Ortonne, J.-P., Juhlin, L. & Lacour, J.-P. (1986) Anonychia with ectrodactyly of one foot. *International Journal of Dermatology* 25, 188.

Patton, M.A., Krywawych, S., Winter, R.M., Brenton, D.P. & Baraitser, M. (1987) DOOR syndrome (deafness, onycho-osteo-dystrophy and mental retardation). Elevated plasma and urinary 2-oxyglutamate in three unrelated patients. *American Journal of Medical Genetics* **26**, 207.

Peckman, K.J. & Bergfeld, W.F. (1980) Palmo-plantar hyperhidrosis occurring in a kindred with nail–patella syndrome. *Journal of the American Academy of Dermatology* **3**, 627.

Pfeiffer, R.A. (1982) The oto-onycho–peroneal syndrome. A probably new genetic entity. *European Journal of Paediatrics* **138**, 217.

Rahbari, H., Heath, L. & Chapel, T. (1975) Anonychia with ectro-dactyly. *Archives of Dermatology* **111**, 1482.

Raman, D. & Haslock, I. (1983) The nail–patella syndrome—a report of two cases and a literature review. *British Journal of Rheumatology* **22**, 41.

Renwick, J.H. & Lawler, S.D. (1955) Genetic linkage between the ABO and nail–patella loci. *Annals of Human Genetics* **19**, 312.

Rizzo, R., Pavone, L., Micali, G. & Hall, J.G. (1993) Familial bilateral antecubital pterygia with severe renal involvement in nail–patella syndrome. *Clinical Genetics* **44**, 1.

Robertson, S.P., Lipp, H. & Bankier, A. (1998) Zimmermann–Laband syndrome in an adult. Long term follow-up of a patient with vascular and cardiac complications. *American Journal of Medical Genetics* **78**, 160.

Salamon, T. (1966) Erbkrankheiten der Nägel. In: *Handbuch der Haut- und Geschlechtkrankbeiten Erganzungswerk*, Vol. 7, p. 409. Springer, Berlin.

Salcedo, J.R. (1984) An autosomal recessive disorder with glomerular basement membrane abnormalities similar to those seen in the nail patella syndrome: report of a kindred. *American Journal of Medical Genetics* **19**, 579.

Schott, G.D. (1978) Hereditary brachydactyly with nail dysplasia. *Journal of Medical Genetics* **15**, 119.

Sequeiros, J. & Sack, G.H. Jr (1985) Linear skin atrophy, scaring alopecia. *American Journal of Medical Genetics* **17**, 579.

Soekarman, D., Cobben, J.M., Vogels, A., Spauwen, P.H. & Fryns, J.-P. (1995) Variable expression of the popliteal pterygium syndrome in two 3-generation families. *Clinical Genetics* **47**, 169.

Solammadevi, S.V. (1981) Simple anonychia. *Southern Medical Journal* **74**, 1555–1557.

Strandskov, H.H. (1939) Inheritance of absence of thumb nails. *Journal of Heredity* **30**, 53.

Swillen, A., Glorieux, N., Peeters, M. & Fryns, J.-P. (1995) The Coffin–Siris syndrome: data on mental development, language, behaviour and social skills in children. *Clinical Genetics* **48**, 177.

Teebi, A.S. & Kaurah, P. (1996) Total anonychia congenita and micro-cephaly with normal intelligence: a new autosomal recessive syndrome? *American Journal of Medical Genetics* **66**, 257.

Tennstedt, D., Lachapelle, J.-M. & Baran, R. (1985) Brachydactylie avec anonychia. *Annales de Dermatologie et de Vénéréologie* **112**, 901.

Timerman, L., Museteanu, C. & Simionescu, N.N. (1969) Dominant anonychia onychodystrophy. *Journal of Medical Genetics* **6**, 105.

Verbov, J. (1975) Anonychia with bizarre flexural pigmentation. An autosomal dominant dermatosis. *British Journal of Dermatology* **92**, 469–474.

Westerveld, A., Jongsma, A.P.M., Meera Khan, P., Van Someren, H. & Bootsma, D. (1976) Assignment of the AK : Np : ABO linkage group to human chromosome 9. *Proceedings of the National Academy of Sciences of the United States of America* **73**, 895–899.

Wood, V.E. (1996) Absence of nails with absent distal phalanges. *Journal of Hand Surgery* **21B** (3), 403.

## Hereditary ectodermal dysplasias

The term hereditary ectodermal dysplasia (HED) was intro-duced by Weech (1929). It is used to cover a heterogeneous group of primary epidermal disorders where at least one of the follow-ing signs occur: hypotrichosis, hypodontia, onychodysplasia and anhidrosis, plus at least one sign affecting other structures of epidermal origin as classified by Freire-Maia (1977) and Freire-Maia and Pinheiro 1988). Solomon and Kcuer (1980) prefer to exclude diseases which are progressive. The list of HED now includes over 90 different conditions. Whether there is a reduction in sweating in certain areas has in many cases not been fully tested, which makes this part of the classification weak (Berg *et al.* 1990). We therefore prefer to list skin changes instead of hidrotic changes. Additional ectodermal tissues which can be involved are ears, lens of eyes, anterior pituitary gland, central nervous system and adrenal medulla. Other embryolo-gical germ layers may also be involved, but when they dominate and when epidermal changes are secondary they are not con-sidered as HED.

Tables 9.1–9.3 list the combinations and features where the nails are involved. Since thickening of the soles and palms is an easily recognized sign, those with keratoderma palmoplantar have been grouped together (Table 9.1). The various types of keratoderma palmoplantar have been reviewed by Stevens *et al.* (1996). Here we have only included those with nail changes. The nail changes in other ectodermal dysplasias with changes of teeth and hair or skin are listed in Table 9.2 and those where the teeth are normal in Table 9.3. Four important conditions listed in Tables 9.1–9.3 will be further described.

### Hypohidrotic ectodermal dysplasia (Fig. 9.11)

Charles Darwin (1875) first described a Hindu family with ectodermal dysplasia of X-linked type; today this is called Christ–Siemens–Touraine syndrome (Reed *et al.* 1970; Norval *et al.* 1988; Sybert 1989). A more rare autosomal recessive type was first described by Passarge *et al.* (1966) and Passarge and Fried (1977). The prominent features are the typical facies suggestive of congenital syphilis, often with a depressed nasal bridge (saddleback nose), large and conspicuous nostrils, high cheek bones and a narrow lower face. The eyebrows are scanty and the eyes slant upwards. The lips can be thick and the buccal commissures have radiating furrows. Sebaceous gland hyperplasia and telangiectases are often seen on the cheeks. The hair of the scalp and body is thin and sparse. There is hypodontia, reduced sweating and decreased function of the lacrimal ducts. The nails can be normal, fragile, dystrophic or absent at birth (Fig. 9.11). A combination with hypothy-roidism and ciliary dyskinesia was described by Pabst *et al.*

**Table 9.1** Hereditary ectodermal dysplasia (ED) with keratoderma palmoplantare and nail changes.

| Condition | Inheritance MIM No. | Nails | Hair | Skin with palmoplantar hyperkeratosis+ | Teeth | Ear | Eye | Other findings |
|---|---|---|---|---|---|---|---|---|
| Cardio-facio-cutaneous syndrome (Reynolds et al. 1986; Borradori & Blanchet-Bardon 1993; Manoukian et al. 1996; Leichtman 1996; Neri & Zollino 1996) | AD? 115150 | Thin koilonychia dysplastic | Sparse, thin scalp, eyelashes, eyebrows | Ichtyosiform or follicular hyperkeratosis | Normal or dysplastic | Angulated. Prominent helices | Palpebral fissures | Congenital heart defects. Cranial vault. Depressed bridge of nose. Variant of Noonan syndrome? |
| Dermatopathia pigmentosa reticularis (Rycroft et al. 1977; Heimer et al. 1992) | AD 125595 | Longitudinal ridging and lamellar splitting | Sparse scalp, eyebrows, axilla | Reticulate hyperpigmentation since early age often on the trunk. Adermato glyphia. | Normal | – | Corneal changes | Acral bullae giving contractures |
| Dyskeratosis congenita, Zinsser–Engman–Cole syndrome (Connor & Teague 1981; Kalb et al. 1986; Caux et al. 1996) (p. 389) | XLR 30500 | Short, atrophic after late childhood, most prominent on fingers where often they are lost | Normal or scarring alopecia | Mainly palmar hyperkeratosis. Hyperhidrosis of palms and soles. Reticulated hyperpigmentation of neck, face and chest | Sometimes malformed | Deafness | Blepharitis with loss of cilia. Leucoplakia on conjunctive. Lacrimal duct obstruction | Acrocyanosis. Aplastic anaemia. Pancytopenia. Oral lesions and leukoplakia. Immunological abnormalities. Testicular atrophy. Avascular necrosis of femur |
| Scoggins' type (1971) | AD 127550 | Short, atrophic after late childhood, most prominent on fingers where are lost | Normal or scarring alopecia | Mainly palmar hyperkeratosis. Hyperhidrosis of palms and soles. Reticulated hyperpigmentation of neck, face and chest | Sometimes malformed | Deafness | Blepharitis with loss of cilia. Leukoplakia on conjunctive. Lacrimal duct obstruction | Acrocyanosis. Aplastic anaemia. Pancytopenia. Oral lesions and leukoplakia. Immunological abnormalities. Testicular atrophy. Avascular necrosis of femur |
| ED–AOHD syndrome (Freire-Maia et al. 1977) | AD – | Onychodysplasia: thick, dark and deformed toenails | Alopecia or fair thin hair | Hypohidrosis. Hyperkeratosis of knees and elbows. Dermatoglyphics abnormal | Normal | Neural deafness | Photophobia, hyperopia | Palpebral slanting, EEG abnormal, retarded bone age. Unusual face, prominent nose |
| Ectrodactyly-clefting (EEC) syndrome. (Cockayne 1936; Ogur & Yüksel 1988; Rollnick & Hoo 1988; Buss et al. 1995; Maas et al. 1996) | AD 129900 | Deformed, thin, brittle, striated: pitted and terminated irregular (Fig. 9.8) | Wiry, hypopigmented | Fair, hypopigmented, scaly skin with comedo-naevus (Leibowitz & Jenkins 1984) | Dysplasia. Partial anodentia. Caries | | Blue sclera. Photophobia. Absence of lacrimal puncta. Tearing. Blepharitis. Meibom's glands deficient. Corneal scarring. Blindness | Cleft lip + palate. Short stature. Ectrodactyly + syndactyly. Claw-shaped hands. Genital and urinary tract abnormalities. Growth hormone deficiency (Knudtzon & Aarskog 1987). Responsible gene in the region 7q11.2–q21.3 (Qumsiey 1992) |
| Epidermolysis bullosa simplex with hyperpigmentation, palmoplantar keratosis (Fischer & Gedde-Dahl 1979; Boss et al. 1981) | AD #131960 | Terminal onycholysis, 'peaked' lunula | Normal | Speckled hyperpigmentation. Blistering tendency of hands and feet in infancy. Punctate keratosis of palms and soles | Normal | – | – | Mutation VI domain of keratin 5 (Irvine et al. 1997). Same as Kindler syndrome? (see this table) |

| Disorder (references) | Inheritance / MIM | Nails | Hair | Skin | Teeth | Ears | Eyes | Other features / genetics |
|---|---|---|---|---|---|---|---|---|
| Focal dermal hypoplasia. Goltz and Gorlin syndrome (Goltz et al. 1970; Malfait et al. 1989; Moore & Mallory 1989; Pujol et al. 1992; Kore-Eda et al. 1995) | XLD *305600 | Thin, spoon-shaped. Can be absent in 50%. No lunula | Sparse in focal areas of scalp and publis | Focal thin skin with herniation of fat. Linear hypo- and hyperpigmentation. Papillomas | Normal | – | Multiple severe anomalies | Small stature. Asymmetrical face. Cranial, spinal and bone anomalies. Cleft lip and palate. Papillomas of mucous membranes. Urinary abnormality. Gene region Xp 22.31 |
| Hidrotic ED (Clouston 1929; Wilkey & Stevenson 1945; Freire-Maia & Pinheiro 1984; Ando et al. 1988; Hassed et al. 1996) | AD 129500 | Thick on toes or dystrophic. Grow slowly. Change more marked with age. Onycholysis, pits ridges. Often small and conical. Paronychia. Hyperkeratotic nail bed looks like thickened nails (Figs 9.12–9.14) | In 50% sparse, short and thin. Eyebrows and eyelashes often absent | Normal sweat. Hyperpigmentation especially over joints. Clubbing of fingers | Normal but occasionally hypodontia and natal teeth | Deafness in some. Mutation 13q11–q12 (Kelsell et al. 1997) | Occasionally strabism and cataracts | Gene mapped to chromosome 13q (Kibar et al. 1996) |
| Hyperpigmentation, hypotrichosis and dystrophy of nails. NFJ syndrome (Sparrow et al. 1976; Itin et al. 1993) | AD *161000 | Distal thickening, subungual hyperkeratosis, onycholysis | Normal | Symmetrical hyperpigmentation most marked on neck and in axillae, fading after puberty. Hypohydrosis. Hypoplastic dermatoglyphic pattern. Punctate keratosis on palms and soles | Enamel defects. Early loss | – | – | Malalignment of great toenails common |
| Hystrix-like keratosis (Schulz-Kiesow et al. 1996) | AD | Markedly thick with distal dystrophy | Normal | Localized hyperkeratosis on pressure area of soles. Spiny keratosis trunk, arm, legs | Normal | – | – | Long fingers. Hyperextensible joints |
| Keratoderma palmoplantare Thost-Unna (Kuster & Becker 1992) | AD 14190 | Thick | Normal | Hyperhidrosis of palms and soles | Normal | – | – | Gene mapped to 17q11–q21.2 Keartin 9 gene site of mutation (Rothnagel et al. 1995; Kobayashi et al. 1998 for ref.) |
| Keratoderma palmoplantare progressiva (type Meleda) (Salamon 1982; Protonotarios et al. 1986; Lestringant et al. 1997; Bouadjar et al. 2000) | AR 248300 | Onychogryphosis koilonychia, short subungual hyperkeratosis; proximal part of nail pink, distal pale | Normal or woolly hair (Tosti et al. 1994) | Hyperhidrosis of palms and soles. Erythema of face and sacral region. Keratosis of elbows and knees | Normal | – | – | Cardiomegaly. Mental retardation may occur. Increased risk for cardiomyopathy when woolly hair (Carvajal-Huert 1998) |
| Keratoderma palmoplantare and alopecia (Stevanovic 1959) | AD 104100 | Dystrophic nail plate. Proximal parts hyperkeratotic and brittle | Scanty hair. Eyebrows and eyelashes absent | Otherwise normal | Normal | – | – | – |

(continued p. 378)

**Table 9.1** (cont'd)

| Condition | Inheritance MIM No. | Nails | Hair | Skin with palmoplantar hyperkeratosis+ | Teeth | Ear | Eye | Other findings |
|---|---|---|---|---|---|---|---|---|
| Keratoderma palmoplantare with periodontosis (Papillon & Lefevre 1924; Gorlin et al. 1964; Haneke 1979; Nazzaro et al. 1988; Hart et al. 1998) | AR 245000 | Punctate depressions. Occasionally spoon-shaped or thick | Normal or sparse after 25 years | Hyperhidrosis of palms and soles. Erythema of face and sacral region. Hyperkeratosis of elbows, knees and Achilles area. Pyogenic infections | Periodontitis. Premature loss of teeth. Bleeding of gingiva | Deafness (Thorel 1964) | – | Calcification of the dura common. Acroosteolysis. Pyogenic infections (Bergman & Friedman-Birnbaum 1988). Locus on 11q14–q21 (Hart et al. 1998 for ref.) |
| Keratoderma palmoplantare with periodontosis and onychogryphosis (Puliyel & Sridharan Iyer 1986) | AR 245010 | Onrychogryphosis of thumbs and big toe | Normal | Hyperkeratosis after extending on to dorsum of hands and feet and on extensor area of arms and legs | Periodontosis | – | – | Pes planus. arachnodactyly, acroosteolysis. Linked to cytokeratin genes on chromosomes 12 and 17 (Hart et al. 1997) |
| Keratoderma palmoplantare with papulosa Buschke–Fischer (Shirren & Dinger 1965; Stevens et al. 1996) | AD 148600 | Subungual hyperkeratosis, onychogryphosis, longitudinal furrows | Normal | Papuloverrucoid palmoplantar lesions after puberty and progressively increasing. Hyperhidrosis of palms and soles may occur as well as hyperkeratosis over knees | Normal | – | – | Gene clusters on 12q and 17q (Kelsell et al. 1997) |
| Keratoderma with leuconychia totalis (Crosti et al. 1983; Basran et al. 1995) | AD? | Leuconychia totalis | Coiled with furrows. Trichorrhexis nodosa | Follicular hyperkeratosis | Transversal furrows of incisors | Deafness | – | – |
| Keratoderma palmoplantare with leuconychia and deafness (Schwann 1963; Bart & Pumphrey 1967; Ramer et al. 1994) | AD *149200 | Leuconychia on thumbs and big toes. Longitudinal white spots on other nails. Frequently koilonychia | Normal | Hyperkeratotic areas knuckle pads on the dorsal side of the fingers and toes | Normal | Deafness since birth | – | Dupuytren's contracture |
| Keratoderma palmoplantare mutilans with deafness (Vohwinkel 1929; Bhatia et al. 1989) | AD #124500 | Pseudo-ainhum | Alopecia | Polygonal papules on knees, elbows, backs of hands and feet and ichthyosiform dermatitis | Normal | Deafness high tones | – | Insertional mutation in loricrin at chromosome 1q21 (Armstrong et al. 1998) |
| Keratoderma palmoplantare with atrophic fibrosis of the extremities (Huriez et al. 1969; de Berker & Kavanagh 1993; Delaporte 1995) | AD 181600 | Hypoplastic with fracture of free edge. Longitudinal ridging, koilonychia and complete aplasia. Transverse and increased longitudinal curvature | Retroauricular alopecia | Since birth palmoplantar hyperkeratosis and scleroderma-like atrophy of tips of fingers and toes and over finger joints. Risk for squamous cell carcinoma. Hypohidrosis | Microdontia | – | – | Increased risk of intestinal cancer |

| Disorder | Inheritance/OMIM | Nails | Hair | Skin | Teeth | Hearing | Eyes | Other |
|---|---|---|---|---|---|---|---|---|
| Keratoderma palmoplantare and clubbing of nails (Bureau et al. 1959; Barraud-Klenovsek et al. 1997) | – | Thick, with clubbing, watch glass like | Normal | Increased sweating especially on extremities. Recidivating leg ulcers | Normal | – | – | Tall massive body but small head. Hypertrophy of long bones. Decreased bone density with thin cortex. Distal phalanges enlarged |
| Keratoderma palmoplantare and neuropathy (Tolmie et al. 1988b) | AD 148360 | Dystrophic nails at birth or early childhood with painful longitudinal cracks | Normal | Focal hyperkeratosis on palms and soles | Not mentioned | – | – | Motor and sensory neuropathy |
| Keratoderma palmoplantare and gingiva (Raphael et al. 1968; Gorlin et al. 1976) | AD 148730 | Sub- and periungual hyperkeratosis | Normal | Changes marked on friction areas. Appear at age 5 on fingers. Later on toes | Normal | – | – | Gingival hyperplasia |
| Keratoderma with widespread scale-crust formation (McGrath 1999) | AR | Thick dystrophic | Short Sparse | Initial pink skin with blisters of soles, perioral erythema, erosions. General skin fragility with scales and crusts. Later palmoplantar keratosis. Painful walking | Normal | Normal | – | Fail to sweat Plakophilin 1 mutation |
| Keratoderma palmoplantare with cystic eyelids, hypodontia and hypotrichosis (Schöpf et al. 1971; Font et al. 1986; Happle & Rampen 1987; Nordin et al. 1988; Craigen et al. 1997) | AR *224750 | Fragile with longitudinal and oblique furrows | Sparse on vertex | – | Hypodontia | – | Cyst on upper and lower eyelids. Senile cataract | Squamous cell carcinoma on a finger in one patient |
| Keratosis, ichthyosis and deafness (KID syndrome) (Senter et al. 1978; Skinner et al. 1981; Langer et al. 1990; McGrae 1990) | AR 242150 | Thick white nails most marked on fingers | Hypotrichosis. Eyebrows and eyelashes absent | Erythrokeratoderma on knees and palms. Pitted type of hyperkeratosis. Plaques on central portion of face. Hypohidrosis | Normal or abnormal | Neurosensory deafness | Vascularization of cornea; keratitis | Tight heel cords may occur. Fungal infections common |
| Lamellar ichthyosis (ichthyosiform erythroderma) (Rand & Baden 1983; Hoeger et al. 1998) | AR 242100 | Thick-striated subungual hyperkeratosis. Can be normal or absent | Normal | Ichthyosis on erythemic skin. Hyperhidrosis of soles and palms | Normal | – | Ectropion. Corneal dystrophies. Photophobia | Cardiomyopathy. Occasionally small stature and mental retardation (BIDS syndrome) |
| Odontoonychodermal dysplasia (Fadhil et al. 1983; Arnold et al. 1995) | AR 257980 | Dystrophic | Dry, sparse, thin | Hyperhidrosis | Hypodontia. Peg-shaped incisors | – | – | Mild mental deficiency |
| Olmsted's syndrome (Poulin et al. 1984; Atherton et al. 1990) | AD? – | Thick, transversal, rigid. Subungual hyperkeratosis | Alopecia or hypohidrosis | Keratotic plaques around body orifices and in groins. Linear keratosis of flexor surfaces, later mutilating contractions of fingers. Anhidrosis. Constricting bands on fingers | Premolar can be lacking | Audiogram abnormal for higher frequencies | – | Leukokeratosis. Hyperlaxity of joints. Atresia of distal phalanges |

(continued p. 380)

**Table 9.1** (cont'd)

| Condition | Inheritance MIM No. | Nails | Hair | Skin with palmoplantar hyperkeratosis+ | Teeth | Ear | Eye | Other findings |
|---|---|---|---|---|---|---|---|---|
| Pachyonychia congenita (Jadassohn & Lewandowsky 1906; Thomas et al. 1984) (see also p. 388) | AD 167200 | Yellow or brown at age 3–5 months, followed by thickening of nail bed. Paronychia common. Onycholysis | Normal | Hyperhidrosis palmoplantare often with bullae. Follicular hyperkeratosis with hyperpigmentation Leukokeratosis of tongue | Natal teeth caries or normal | Deafness | Cataract and corneal dyskeratosis | Short stature. Mental retardation. Hoarseness |
| Pachyonychia congenita (Jackson & Lawler 1951; Clementi et al. 1986) | AD 167210 | Thick subungual hyperkeratosis at early age | Dry, kinky, sometimes alopecia | Palmar and plantar hyperhidrosis. Follicular keratosis | Teeth present at birth | – | – | Epidermal cysts. Sebocystomatoses |
| Pachyonychia congenita with amyloidosis and hyperpigmentation (Buckly & Cassuto 1962; Tidman et al. 1987) | AD – | Thick and discoloured in infancy but improving in adulthood | Normal | Diffuse rippled and macular. Hyperpigmentation of neck, axilla, trunk, thighs and popliteal fossa. Fading when adult. Amyloid deposits in papillary dermis of hyperpigmented areas | Normal | Normal | Normal | – |
| Pachyonychia congenita with leuconychia (Haber & Rose 1986) | AR 260131 | Proximal leuconychia with obliteration of lunula after age 12. Mild onycholysis of toes with slight elevation of nail plate | – | Bulla on plantar surface. Punctate keratoderma. Hyperkeratotic papules on dorsa of toes and fingers. Angular cheilitis | Normal | Normal | Normal | – |
| Poikiloderm bullous Kindler's syndrome (Kindler 1954; Forman et al. 1989, Hovnanian et al. 1989), see also epidermolysis bullosa in this table | AR *173650 | Dystrophic | Normal | Poikiloderma gradually appearing with cutaneous atrophy and reticulated pigmentation. Friction blisters in infancy. Hyperkeratosis of palms and soles, often mild | | – | – | Photosensitivity in childhood. Gingival fragility. Leukokeratosis. Webbing of digits. Ainhum-like constrictions. Urethral and oesophageal stenoses |
| Poikiloderma acrokeratotic. Weary syndrome (Weary et al. 1971; Larregue et al. 1981) | AD *173650 | Dystrophi (Fig. 9.15) | Normal | Vesiculopustules hands and feet. Dermatitis. Reticulated pigmentation without telangiectasia or severe atrophy. Spares the head. Keratotic papules of dorsal hands, feet ellbows and knees. Sometimes also on palms and soles | Poor dentition can occur | | | |

Inheritances are indicated as follows: AD, autosomal dominant; AR, autosomal recessive; XLR, sex-linked, recessive; XLD dominant transmission; AW, autosomal semidominant.

**Table 9.2** Ectodermal dysplasias with nail and teeth changes: hair and skin often involved.

| Condition | Inheritance | Nails | Hair | Skin | Teeth | Ear | Eye | Other findings |
|---|---|---|---|---|---|---|---|---|
| AEC syndrome (Hay & Wells 1976; Schwayder et al. 1986; Seres-Santamaria 1993) | AD 106260 | Absent or dystrophic | Partial or complete loss | Dry. Partial anhidrosis, often thick palms and soles. Hidrocystoma (Brilon & Rütten 1993) | Widely spaced | Auricular deformities common | Ankyloblepharon. Lacrimal duct atresia | Cleft lip and palate. Syndactyly, supernumerary nipples. Adhesions between jaws can occur |
| ADULT syndrome (Propping & Zerres 1993) | AD 103285 | Concave dysplastic | Thin | Excessive freckling | Hypodontia. Loss of teeth | – | Obstruction of lacrimal duct | Ectrodactyly |
| ANOTHER syndrome (see p. 388) (Pike et al. 1986) | AR | Ridged, fragile, brittle | Thin, sparse | Dry. Hypohidrosis. Speckled brown pigmentation | Hypodontia. Conical teeth | Conductive hearing deficit. Otitis media | Ciliary dyskinesia | Respiratory tract infection. Infantile hypothyroidism. Absent breast tissue |
| Acrorenal ectodermal dysplasia (AREDYLD) syndrome (Pinheiro et al. 1983; Breslau-Siderius et al. 1992) | AR? 207780 | Transverse and longitudinal grooves of fingernails | Hypotrichosis. Slow growing | Reduced sweating | Hypodontia. Anodontia | – | – | Lipotrophic diabetes and hypomastia. Unusual face |
| Chondroectodermal dysplasia (Ellis & van Creveld 1940; Christan et al. 1980) | AR *225500 | Dystrophic koilonychia. Brittle. No need to be cut | Sparse, thin, brittle and hypochromic | Normal | Natal teeth in 25%. Hypodontia. Oligodontia. Conically crowned | – | – | Broad nose. Short limbs. Polydactyly. Fusion of bones. Respiratory difficulties and heart defects common. Gene located on chromosome 4 p16 (Polymeropoulus et al. 1996) |
| Chondroectodermal dysplasia (Curry & Hall 1979; Schapiro et al. 1984) | AD – | As above + nails splitting | Normal | Normal | As above | – | – | As above |
| Coffin–Siris syndrome (Coffin & Siris 1970; Carey & Hall 1978; Lucaya et al. 1981; Patel et al. 1987; Braun-Quintin et al. 1996) | AD 135900 | 5th fingernail and toenails hypoplastic or absent, other nails sometimes hypoplastic (Fig. 9.3) | Sparse on scalp, eyebrows and lashes. Hirsutism of limbs, forehead and back | Dermatoglyphic changes | Delayed eruption. Microdontia | – | – | Thick lips. Low nasal bridge. Microcephaly. Psychomotor and growth retardation. Absence or hypoplasia of distal phalanges especially of finger 5 and toe 5. Patellae dysplasia. Respiratory infections |
| Congenital hypoparathyroidism (Moshkowitz et al. 1969; Braverman 1981) | – | Distal half brittle. Irregular grooves. Onychorrhexia. Leuconychia | Normal | Normal | Malocclusion caries. Loss of enamel | – | Cataract | Hypoparathyroidism. Epilepsy |

(continued p. 382)

**Table 9.2** (cont'd)

| Condition | Inheritance | Nails | Hair | Skin | Teeth | Ear | Eye | Other findings |
|---|---|---|---|---|---|---|---|---|
| Dentooculocutaneous syndrome (Ackerman et al. 1973) | AR 200970 | Horizontal ridging with distal onychoschizia | Scanty, no beard | Indurated and hyperpigmented over finger joints | Taurodont, pyramidal or fused molar roots | – | Juvenile glaucoma. Ectropion lower lids | Upper lip lacking. Cupid bow. Philtrum thick and wide. Syndactyly. Clinodactyly |
| Ectodermal dysplasia with distinctive facial appearance, alopecia and polydactyly | – 129540 | Rounded, especially index fingers | Very few hairs on scalp and body | Normal | Thin enamal. Pitted teeth | – | Eccentric pupils | Wide nasal bridge, flat philtrum. Chromosomes normal. No consanguinity |
| Fried's tooth and nail syndrome (Fried 1977) | AR – | Thin on finger. On toes also small and concave | Fine, short and scanty eyebrows | Normal | Hypodontia peg-shaped | – | – | Prominent lip and chin. Cleft lip, brachial cyst on the neck |
| Hay–Wells syndrome; see AEC syndrome | | | | | | | | |
| Hypohidrotic ED. Christ Siemens–Touraine-syndrome (Pinheiro et al. 1981; Sybert 1989) (p. 375) | XR 305100 | Often normal, may be dystrophic | Thin, sparse on scalp and body | Thin, dry shiny. No or decreased sweating. Dermoglyphic changes | Delayed eruption. Hypodontia. Peg shaped, conical | Hearing loss may occur | – | Saddle-shaped nose. Small nostrils. Oral dryness causes hoarseness. Genetic location Xq12–q13 (Zonana et al. 1988). Mutation (Kere et al. 1996) |
| Hypohidrotic ED (Marshall 1958; Passarge et al. 1966; Gorlin et al. 1970) | AR *224900 | Small, concave koilonychia | Thin and sparse | Mild hypohidrosis | Adontia or normal teeth | Hearing loss may occur | Cataract myopia | As above |
| Hypohidrotic ED with multiple anomalies (Rapp & Hodgkin 1968; Schroeder & Sybert 1987; O'Donnell & James 1992; Kantaputra et al. 1998) | AD *129400 | Small, disfigured with distal soft tissue. Subungual keratosis | On scalp sparse, short, slow growing, wiry or pili torti. Sparse eyelashes, eyebrows and body hair | Mild palmoplantar keratosis. One or more café au lait spots. Keratoderma or normal | Slow development. Hypodontia conically shaped. Caries | – | Aplasia of lacrimal punctate | Absence lingual frenelum. Short stature + cleft lip and palate. Hypospadias. Syndactyly |
| Hypoplastic-enamel-onycholysis-hypohidrosis syndrome (Witkop et al. 1975) | AD *104570 | Onycholysis. Thin koilonychia. Subungual keratosis | Normal | Hypohydrosis. Seborrhoeic dermatitis of scalp | Hypoplastic hypocalified enamel. Partial anodontia | – | – | – |
| Lacrimo-auriculodento-digital (LADD) syndrome (Hollister et al. 1973; Francannet et al. 1994) | AD 149730 | Ectopic nails. Large thumbnail | Normal | Normal | Enamel poor. Peg-shaped incisors. Darkening of teeth | Hearing loss. Cup-shaped ears | Aplasia of lacrimal punctata. Eye infections | Digital and radial malformations. Kidney anomalies can occur. Prenatal ultrasonography for diagnosis |
| Nail, tooth, ear syndrome (Robinson et al. 1962). See also DOOR syndrome, Table 9.3 | AD 124480 | Hypoplastic and dysplastic with furrows and cracks | Normal | Chloride increased in sweat | Partial anodontia coniform | Sensory deafness | – | Syndactyly. Polydactyly may occur |

| Syndrome | Inheritance / MIM | Nails | Hair | Skin | Teeth | Ears | Eyes | Other |
|---|---|---|---|---|---|---|---|---|
| Oculo-dento-digital (ODD or ODOD) syndrome (O'Rourk & Bravos 1969; Traboulsi et al. 1986; Norton et al. 1995) | AD or AR *164200; AR 257850 rare | Dysplastic; fusion of nails and phalanges between 4th and 5th fingers | Hypotrichosis | Normal | Microdontia. Hypodontia. Conical incisive. Enamel hypoplasia | Unilateral deformity of external ear | Microphthalmia. Ectropia. Nystagmus. Iris atrophy | Small alae nasi. Anteversion of nostrils. Microstomia, micrognathia. Polydactyly, syndactyly, hypophalangy. AD locus 6q22–q24 (Gladwin et al. 1997) |
| Oculo-tricho-dysplasia (OTD) syndrome (de Cecatto Lima et al. 1988) | AR 257960 | Fragile, brittle | Hypohidrosis | Normal | Small, widely spaced | – | – | Retinitis pigmentosa |
| Odonto-trichomelic hypohidrotic ED (Cat et al. 1972; Pavone et al. 1989) | AR 273400 | Hypoplastic nails and no nail on some fingers | Hypotrichosis | Thin, dry, shiny | Hypodontia | Auricles abnormal | – | Protruding lips, enlarged nose, hypoplastic nipples and areola. Tetramelic reductions Oligophreny. Metabolic defects. ECG abnormalities. Retarded growth |
| Odontomicronychial dysplasia (Pinheiro et al. 1996) | AR 601319 | Slow growing, short, thin | Normal | Normal | Precocious eruption of primary and secondary teeth with short roots | – | – | – |
| Odontoonyco dysplasia with alopecia (Pinheiro et al. 1985; Zirbel et al. 1995) | AR – | Fragile and brittle with a subungual corneal layer | Almost total alopecia. Absent axillary and pubic hair. Abnormal dermatoglyphics | Hypohidrosis | Micro- and hypodentia. Widely spaced teeth with hypolastic enamel | – | Blepharitis | Syndactyly. Irregular arreata mammae. Photophobia |
| Odonto-trichungual digital palmar syndrome (Mendoza & Valiente 1997) | AD | Dystrophic. Absent great toe | Straw like | Interdigital folds. Transverse palmar creases | Natal teeth | – | – | Hypoplasia of distal phalanges and metacarpal bones |
| Popliteal pterygium syndrome (Gorlin et al. 1976; Escobar & Weaver 1978; Brun et al. 1994; Soekarman et al. 1995) | AD *119500 | Absent or dystrophic longitudinal stria. Brittle. Subungual hyperkeratosis | Hypotrichosis. No eyebrows or eyelashes. Fair and depigmented | Hypoludrosis. Cutaneous folds on limbs | Microdontia. Conical | Hypoplasia on earlobes | Black iris | Hare lip. Supernumary nipples. Right thumb lacking. Alteration of genitalia. Popliteal and perianal pterygia |
| Salamon syndrome (Salamon et al. 1967) | AR 278200 | Dystrophic | Woolly hair. Sparse, dry lustreless. Pili torn. Trichorhexis nodosa | Normal | Hypodontia. Microdontia | – | Chronic blepharoconjunctivitis. Punctate keratitis. Atrophia retina. Trichiasis palpebra | Piriform nose. Slight osteoporosis of arms and legs |
| Tooth and nail syndrome (Witkop et al. 1975; Kinch et al. 1983; Chitty et al. 1996) | AD *189500 | Small and spoon shaped. Slow growth in children. Longitudinal ridging | Fine and brittle | Dry. Wrinkles in face | Hypodontia. Cone shaped. Widely spaced | Big ears | – | Everted lips |

(continued p. 384)

**Table 9.2** (cont'd)

| Condition | Inheritance | Nails | Hair | Skin | Teeth | Ear | Eye | Other findings |
|---|---|---|---|---|---|---|---|---|
| Variant of previous (Ellis & Dawber 1980) | AD – | As previous. Nail fold thick | Fine and brittle | Reduced palmar sweat duct potency | As previous | Big ears | – | Mental retardation |
| Tricho-dento-osseous (TDO) syndrome. Enamel hypoplasia and curly hair (Robinson et al. 1966; Lichtenstein et al. 1972; Seow 1993) | AD *190320 | Flat, thick, malformed, striated. Break off easily | Thick with short curls. Dry and rough | Normal | Small pitted, widely spaced. Caries. Hypoplastic enamel | – | – | Sclerosteosis especially of the skull. Gene locus 17q21 DLX3 gene deletion mutation (Price et al. 1998) |
| Tricho-odonto-onycho dermal (TOOD) syndrome (Tsakalakos et al. 1986) | AD? 129510 | Dystrophic nails, some absent | Hypotrichosis | Dry, atrophic, poikiloderma-like spots. Palmar keratosis | Delayed eruption. Hypodontia. Enamel hypoplasia. Abnormal shape. Supernumerary teeth | Nerve deafness | – | Microstomia. Thin lips. Linear hypoplastic tip of nose. Eyelids, or perioral hyperpigmentation. Absent nipple. Phalangeal changes |
| Tricho-odonto-onychial dysplasia (Pinheiro et al. 1983; Mégarbané 1998) | AR 275450 | Thin, concave digits 1–3. Toenail dystrophic | Thin and dry | Normal sweating. Dry skin | Widely spaced first teeth. Most permanent teeth absent except conical incisors | – | – | Probably subtype of Frieds or Witkops type (in this table) |
| Tricho-rhino-phalangeal syndrome I (TRP I) (Giedion 1967; Parizel et al. 1987; Carrington et al. 1994) | AD 190350 and AR 275500 | Thin, short with stria. Flattened thumbnail. Koilonychia | Sparse, blond fine and slow growing. Eyebrows laterally sparse | Normal | Supernumerary, peg shaped | – | – | Prominent lip and chin. Pear-shaped nose. Short fingers. Brachial cyst on the neck. Cleft lip seen. High arched palate. Deletion 8q24.12 (Ludecke et al. 1995) |
| Tricho-rhino-phalangeal syndrome II (TRP II) (Langer et al. 1984; Sánchez et al. 1985; Bühler et al. 1987) | AR #150230 | Thin, short with stria. Flattened thumbnail. Koilonychia | Sparse, blond fine and slow growing. Eyebrows laterally sparse | Normal | Supernumerary, peg shaped | – | – | As above + multiple exostosis. Deletion 5 Mb |
| Triphalangy of thumbs and toes (Qazi & Smithwick 1970). Could be same as DOOR syndrome (Table 9.1) | AR *220500? | Hypoplastic | Normal | Dermatoglyphic abnormalities | Widely spaced. Poorly formed | – | – | Three phalanges in both thumbs and big toes. Hypoplasia of distal phalanges |
| Xeroderma, talipes and enamel defect (XTE) syndrome | AD – | Small, malformed | Dry, slow growing. No lower lashes | Hypohidrosis | Yellow enamel | – | Photophobic | Clubfoot. Oligophrenia |

Inheritances are indicated as follows: AD, autosomal dominant; AR, autosomal recessive; XR, sex-linked recessive.

**Table 9.3** Ectodermal dysplasia with hair and/or skin changes but without dental changes.

| Condition | Inheritance | Nails | Hair | Skin | Teeth | Ear | Eye | Other findings |
|---|---|---|---|---|---|---|---|---|
| Aplasia cutis congenita. See focal dermal hypoplasia | | | | | | | | |
| Aplasia cutis with dystrophic nails (Harari et al. 1976; Evers et al. 1995) | AD 107600 | Short thin grey nail plate. Longitudinal stria. Some onychogryphostis | Normal | Aplasia cutis of scalp and/or trunk | Normal | – | – | – |
| Apical dysplasia of fingers (Dodinval 1972) | AD | Transverse depressions | Normal | Epidermal dysplastic ridges. Fingerpads hypoplastic with painful chaps | Normal | – | – | – |
| Atrichia with nail dystrophy (Vogt et al. 1988) | AR | Distal parts dystrophic and brittle | Alopecia. A few pigmented short hairs on scalp. Eyebrows and lashes sparse | Normal | Normal | – | – | Moderate retardation with delayed speaking. Abnormal facies with depressed nasal bridge, hypertelorism and long philtrums |
| BIDS, IBIDS and PIBIDS syndromes; see trichothiodystrophy | | | | | | | | |
| CHANDS syndrome curly hair, ankyloblepharon, nail dysplasias (Baughman 1971; Toriello et al. 1979) | AR 214350 | Small, hypoplastic | Curly | Normal | Normal | – | Ankyloblepharon | Ataxia |
| Chondrodysplasia punctata (Happle 1979; O'Brien 1990; Gobello et al. 1995) | XD 302960 | Flattened and split into layers (Fig. 9.9) | Circumscribed alopecia. Trichorrhexis nodosa. Sparse lashes and eyebrows | First year transient. Ichthyosiform hyperkeratosis. Athrophoderma. Pseudopelade. Pigmentary changes | Normal | Dysplastic auricles described | Cataract common. Epicanthus. Nystagmus and hazy cornea also described | Short stature. Flat nose bridge and peculiar shape of face. Malformation of limbs and vertebral column. Locus at Xp22.3. Sulfatase deficiency (Franco et al. 1995) |
| Chondrodysplasia punctata (Sheffield et al. 1976; Curry 1979) | XR *302950 | Mild dystrophy | Eyebrows sparse | Slight ichthyosiform | – | – | – | Hypoplasia, distal phalanges. Short stature. Depressed tip of nose. Mental retardations |
| DOOR syndrome (Feinmesser & Zelig 1961; Walbaum 1970; Cantwell 1975; Qazi & Nangia 1984; Patton et al. 1987; Lin et al. 1993) | AR *220500 | Onychodythstrophy since birth. Nails do not grow | Normal or alopecia | Abnormal dermatoglyphics. Spiny hyperkeratosis | Normal | Deafness | – | Osteodystrophy. Mental retardation, seizures. Increase of 2-oxyglutarate |
| ED with onychogryphosis (Freire-Maia et al. 1975) | – | Severe onychogryphosis | Eyebrows lacking, scarce eyelashes | Dry. Hypohidrosis. Follicular hyperkeratosis, hyper and hypochromic spots | Normal | – | Nuclear cataract | Psychomotor and growth retardation. Frontal bossing. Depressed bridge of the nose |

(continued p. 386)

**Table 9.3** (cont'd)

| Condition | Inheritance | Nails | Hair | Skin | Teeth | Ear | Eye | Other findings |
|---|---|---|---|---|---|---|---|---|
| ED with abnormal papillar ridging (Basan 1965; Reed & Schreiner 1983) | AD *129200 | Transverse overcurvature, irregular, atrophic with central fissures and ridging | Normal | Papillar ridging lacking. Abnormal furrows of hands | Normal | – | – | – |
| Focal dermal hypoplasia. Goltz and Gorlin syndrome (Goltz et al. 1970; Sybert 1985; Moore & Mallory 1989; Goltz 1992; Bellosta et al. 1996) | XLD *305600 | Thin, spoon shaped. Can be absent in 50% | Sparse in focal areas of scalp and pubis | Focal thin skin with herniation of fat. Papilloma, telangiectasis. Linear hypo- and hyperpigmentation. Keratotic lesions in palms and soles in 11%. Epidermolysis bullosa (Jones et al. 1992) | Normal or enamel defects | – | Multiple severe anomalies | Small stature. Asymmetrical face. Cranial, spinal and bone anomalies. Cleft lip and palate. Striated pattern of long bones (Larrègue & Duterque 1975) |
| Hair–nail dysplasia (Pinheiro & Freire-Maia 1992) | AD | Short, fragile, spoon shaped | Thin, fragile, slow growing, sparse | Normal | Normal | Normal | – | – |
| Hair–nail dysplasia (Barbareschi et al. 1997) | AD | Micronychia onychorexis. Triangular nail plate. | Hypotrichosis temporal eyebrows. Folliculitis decalvans neck | Normal | Normal | – | – | |
| Hair and nail dysplasia (Christianson & Fourie 1996) | AD 601375 | Dystrophic and thick. Distal half not attached to nail bed | Thin, sparse, short on scalp. Eyebrows, exilla, pubic absent. Eyelashes short and sparse | Normal | Normal | – | – | |
| Hyper- and hypopigmentation with dystrophic nails (Moon-Adams & Slatkin 1955) | AD | Thin, brittle with longitudinal furrows | Normal | Symmetrical pigmentation and hyperkeratosis of non-exposed skin with areas of hypopigmentation | Normal | – | – | Probably same as dermopathia pigmentosa reticularis (see above). Table 9.1 |
| Ichthyosis follicularis with alopecia (Rothe et al. 1990) | AD | Onychodystrophy and paronychia | Total alopecia | Follicular hyperkeratosis. Hyperkeratosis of extensive aspect of hands, knees and elbows. Perineal plaques | Normal | Hearing defect | Photophobia | Angular cheilitis |
| Ichthyosis follicularis–alopecia–photophobia IFAP syndrome (Martino et al. 1992) | XR? | Dystrophic hyperconvex | Atrichia | Erythematous follicular ichthyosis hypohidrosis | Normal or enamel dysplasia | Large ears | Myopia. Corneal dystrophy | Vertebral defects. Short stature. Megacolon. Renal anomalies. Brain atrophy |
| Onychotrichodysplasia with neutropenia (Cantú et al. 1975; Hernandez et al. 1979; Verhage et al. 1987; Dalapiccola et al. 1994) | AR 258360 | Hypoplastic. Onychorrhexis. Koilonychia | Trichorrhexis. Dry, short curly, sparse | Mild keratosis follicularis. Thick, wrinkled palms and soles with pustules | Normal | – | Conjunctivitis. Ectropion | No or mild mental retardation. Neutropenia and repeated infections. Sulfur deficient hairs (Itin & Pittelkow 1990) |

| Disorder | Inheritance | Number | Nails | Hair | Skin | Teeth | | Eyes | General features |
|---|---|---|---|---|---|---|---|---|---|
| Pili torti and onychodysplasia (Calzavara-Pinton et al. 1991) | AR | | Dystrophic of distal part | Scalp, beard, pubic and axillary hair broken at 1–10 mm length. Eyebrows, eyelashes and body hair absent | Normal | Normal | Normal | Normal | Facial dysmorphism with long philthrum |
| Retinal angiomas with hair and nail defects (Tolmie et al. 1988a) | AR | | Dysplastic | Sparse | Normal | Normal | Normal | Strabismus. Retinal angioma | Intracranial calcification |
| Thumb deformity and alopecia (Winter et al. 1988) | AD 188150 | | – | Alopecia | Hyper- and depigmentation in the groin | Single upper. Incisor in some patients | – | – | Short stature. Mental retardation (Chiba & Miura 1979). Hypoplastic thumbs |
| Tricho-oculo-dermal vertebral syndrome (Alves et al. 1981; Stratton et al. 1993; Gorlin 1997) | AR (601701) | | Thin and brittle fingernails. Toes wide and short with paronychia | Hypotrichosis. Dry and rough | Dry. Fissures. Infections. Hyperkeratotic spots, especially on soles. Scaling. Skin webbing of fingers. Dermoglyphic changes | Normal | – | Bilateral nuclear cataract. Narrow palperal fissures. Entropion | Wide nasal bridge and hypoplasia of nasal alae. Micrognathia. Enlarged interphalangeal joints. Germ valga. Kyphoscolios is. Spina bifida oculta |
| Trichothiodystrophy, BIDS syndrome (Jackson et al. 1974) Sabin's syndrome (Itin & Pittelkow 1990) (p. 390) | AR *234050 | | Break easily. Do not grow long | Brittle, short, trichoschizis, trichorrhexis nodosa in some | Normal or dry | Normal or carious | Normal | Punctate cataracts | Intellectual, impairment common. Decreased fertility. Short stature common. Poor motor coordination |
| Trichothiodystrophy (TTD). IBDS or Tay syndrome (Jorizzo et al. 1982; Blomquist et al. 1991 for ref.) | AR #601675 | | Brittle and dystrophic or thick, convex curvature subungual hyperkeratosis | Brittle, short, trichoschizis, trichorrhexis nodosa in some | Collodion baby. Ichthyosis form erythroderma (photosensitivity in 50%). Lack of subcutaneous fat | Normal | Normal | Punctate cataracts. Nystagmus | Intellectual impairment common. Decreased fertility. Short stature common Poor motor coordination. Hypogonadism. Recurrent infections |
| Trichothiodystrophy with PIB(D)S syndrome (van Neste et al. 1980, 1988; Rebora & Crovato, 1987; Klejer et al. 1994) | AR #278730 | | Hypoplastic or dystrophic with spotted leuconychia and lamellar splitting | Brittle, short, trichoschizis, trichorrhexis nodosa in some | Normal at birth. Later xerosis or non-congenital ichthyosis vulgaris. Xeroderma pigmentosum. Photosensitivity | – | Neurosensory loss | Nystagmus, myopia, retinal dystrophia can occur | Intellectual impairment. Short stature. Smiling outgoing personality Photosensitivity |
| Trichothiodystrophy with transient immunodeficiency (Baden & Katz 1988) | – | | Short with horizontal splitting. Thin and often spoon shaped | Short, sparse or uneven length | Normal | Normal | Normal | Normal | Transient immunodeficiency in one patient, otherwise healthy |
| Trichothiodystrophy with neutropenia (see onychotrichodysplasia with neutropenia) | 258360 | | | | | | | | |

Inheritances are indicated as follows: AD, autosomal dominant; AR, autosomal recessive; XLD, sex-linked dominant transmission; XR, sex-linked recessive.

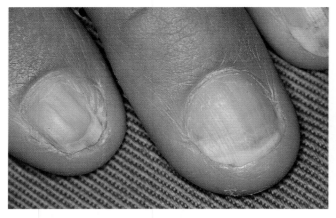

**Fig. 9.11** Hypohidrotic ectodermal dysplasia—nail dystrophy.

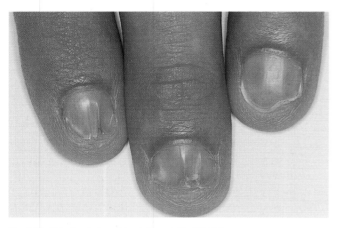

**Fig. 9.12** Hidrotic ectodermal dysplasia—small 'nail fields'.

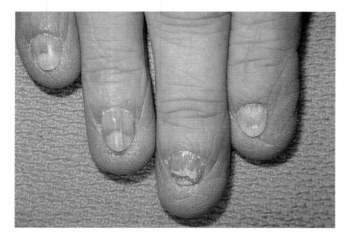

**Fig. 9.13** Hidrotic ectodermal dysplasia—small 'nail fields' with short, overcurved nails. (Courtesy of L. Norton, USA.)

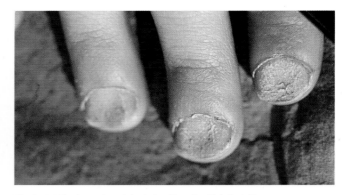

**Fig. 9.14** Hidrotic ectodermal dysplasia—thin nails with koilonychia.

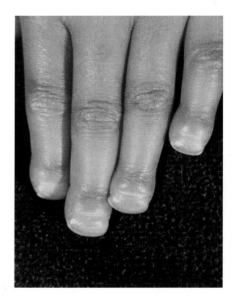

**Fig. 9.15** Poikiloderma acrokeratotic. Weary syndrome. (Courtesy of M. Fazio, Italy.) (See Table 9.1.)

(1981). Other syndromes are described where cleft lip and palate dominate the picture—Rapp–Hodgkin syndrome, or ankyloblepharon-ectodermal-cleft (AEC) syndrome and ectrodactyly ectodermal clefting (EEC) syndrome. Genitourin-ary anomalies can also occur with this syndrome (Freire-Maia & Pinheiro 1984; Schwayder *et al.* 1986; Schroeder & Sybert 1987; Rollnick & Hoo 1988). Pike *et al.* (1986), Morris *et al.* (1987) and Pinheiro *et al.* (1989b) called this condition ANOTHER syndrome (alopecia, nail dystrophy, ophthalmic complications, thyroid dysfunction, hypohidrosis, ephelides and enteropathy, and respiratory tract infections). A woman with manifestations of Rapp–Hodgkin syndrome had a malformed newborn son with EEC syndrome and also ankyloblepharon as in the AEC syndrome (Moerman & Fryns 1996). The authors suggested the syndrome could be the same disorder.

## Pachyonychia congenita

This is a hereditary ectodermal dysplasia with thickening of the nails and subungeal hyperkeratosis appearing within the first 6 months of life but late onset has also been reported (Paller *et al.* 1991; Iraci *et al.* 1993) (Figs 9.16 & 9.17). There is also abnormal keratinization of skin and mucosa membranes.

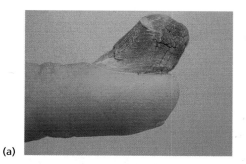

(a)

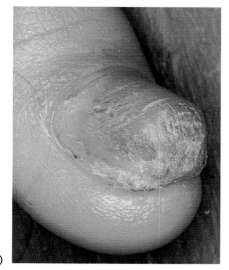

(b)

**Fig. 9.16** (a,b) Pachyonychia congenita.

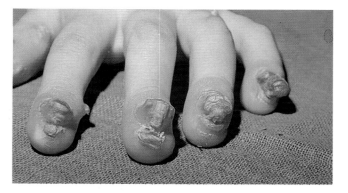

**Fig. 9.17** Pachyonychia congenita.

The nail changes with keratosis of the palms and soles were mentioned in the literature from the 17th and 18th century (Bondesson 1993) and well described in a thesis by the Danish physician Musaeus (1716). Colcott-Fox (1897), Müller (1904) and Garrick-Wilson (1905) reported the condition. The following year Jadassohn and Lewandowsky described the full syndrome in two siblings. Feinstein *et al.* (1988) classified pachonychia congenita into four clinical types with increasing symptoms. In some cases only the nails are affected. (Chang *et al.* 1994; Pryce & Verbov 1994).

Type I is most common (56%). On all fingers and toes the nails become yellow-brown usually within months after birth and show subungual hyperkeratosis with elevation of the nail plates. The nails become progressively thicker with wedge-shaped nails. Families with onset of the symptoms in the 2nd to 4th decade have also been described and may be a genetically distinct subtype (Paller *et al.* 1991; Iraci *et al.* 1993; Lucker & Steijlen 1995; Mouaci-Midoun *et al.* 1996). The patients also have palmoplantar hyperkeratosis, follicular hyperkeratosis of the body and oral leukokeratoses.

Type II (25%) has clinical findings as in type I, but also bullae and hyperhidrosis of palms and soles, early dentition and steatocystoma multiplex.

Type III occurs in 12% of the patients and has in addition angular cheilosis, corneal dyskeratosis and cataracts. Type IV (7%) has these features plus laryngeal lesions, hoarseness, mental retardation and hair anomalies. This grouping is likely to be changed in the future with increasing information about the genetic background.

The inheritance is usually autosomal dominant, although an autosomal recessive has been described (Table 9.1) In the Jadassohn–Lewandowsky type (PC-1) there are mutations in keratin 16 or its expression partner keratin 6a (Bowden *et al.* 1995; McLean *et al.* 1995). In the Jackson–Lawler type (PC-2) similar genetic lesions have been established in keratin 17 (McLean *et al.* 1995). Mutations in K16 have also been identified in patients with palmoplantar keratoderma (Shamsheer *et al.* 1995) and K17 mutations were found in patients with steatocytoma multiplex (Smith *et al.* 1997). Covello *et al.* (1998) also demonstrated that K17 mutations underlie both PC-2 and steatocytoma multiplex and that alternate phenotypes can arise from these genetic lesions.

The differential diagnosis can be epidermolysis bullosa, onychogryphosis, psoriasis and oral thrush, but the presence of thick wedge-shaped, pinched-up or claw-like nails with yellowish-brown pigmentation together with other symptoms rarely offers any diagnostic problems.

Treatment with retinoids has been tried with, as a rule, only moderate improvement of skin and nail lesions, but positive results have also been reported (Hoting & Wassilew 1985). Distal avulsion with nail bed scarification and matrix destruction is needed to prevent the growth of nails. Areas of ulceration should be observed for possible skin malignancy (Su *et al.* 1990).

## Dyskeratosis congenita (Zinsser–Engman–Cole syndrome)

Here one finds short and atrophic fingernails appearing after late childhood. The nail can initially be thin, concave with longitudinal ridging and pterygium (Burkhardt *et al.* 1994) and the changes may progress to loss of nails (Fig. 9.18). At the same time crops of vesicles appear in the mouth, which ulcerate and leave an atrophic mucosa. There is palmar hyperkeratosis and hyperhidrosis and almost always a reticulated hyperpigmentation of the face, neck and chest. The complete syndrome is not apparent until the 2nd or 3rd decade of life (Connor &

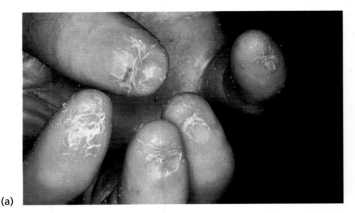

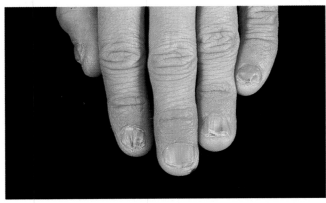

**Fig. 9.18** (a,b) Dyskeratosis congenita. ((a) courtesy of S. Aractingi, France; (b) courtesy of U. Blume-Peytaki, Germany.)

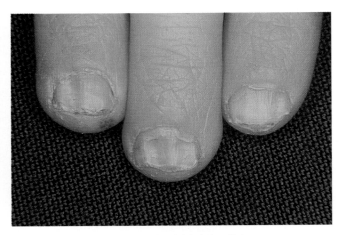

**Fig. 9.19** Trichothiodystrophy (thin nails and slight koilonychia).

Teague 1981; Kalb *et al.* 1986; Ogden *et al.* 1988). Continuous lacrimation due to atresia of the lacrimal duct and thickened fissured mucosal leukoplakia are common not only in the mouth but also in the oesophagus, anus, urethra and vagina. There is a high risk of developing early malignancy in these lesions and frequent biopsies are often needed. Dental caries and early loss of teeth are seen. The eye manifestations are epiphora, fundus changes, blepharitis and loss of eyelashes. The ear manifestations include transparent tympanic membrane, meatal atresia and malformations of the middle ear. Intracranial calcification and increased fragility of bones have been reported. Abnormal immunology with haematopoietic disorders occur in 50% of patients in the 2nd and 3rd decades and may be the presenting changes. The manifestations include anaemia, bone marrow hypoplasia, thrombocytopenia and pancytopenia (Dodd *et al.* 1985). Testicular atrophy is common.

The inheritance is X-linked recessive and the gene has been assigned to Xq28 by linkage of DNA markers (Connor *et al.* 1986). Knight *et al.* (1996) further fine mapped the locus on Xq28. Highly skewed X inactivation was seen in leucocytes, fibroblasts and mucosa (Devriendt *et al.* 1997). The disease should therefore be a good candidate for gene therapy (Dokal 1996).

## Trichothiodystrophy

Patients with trichothiodystrophy (TTD) have brittle hair and nails due to low cystine-rich matrix proteins (Price *et al.* 1980). In addition the patients frequently have nail dysplasia, splitting and koilonychia (Fig. 9.19). In one type called Tay syndrome or IBDS (ichthyotic, brittle hair, decreased fertility, short stature Table 9.3) the skin is ichthyotic and the nails can also be thick with subungual hyperkeratosis (Jorizzo *et al.* 1982). The palms and soles could be thickened and fissured, but keratodermia was not mentioned in the review of 95 cases by Itin and Pittelkow (1991).

Cell fusion experiments have shown that all except three of the TTD cells strains have a repair deficiency with the same complementation group as that in xeroderma pigmentosum group D, where the defect involves the *ERCC2* gene (Stefanini *et al.* 1993). This form is referred to as TTD 1. In the three exceptional cases the excision-repair defect was complemented in all xeroderma pigmentosum groups and this form was called TTD 2. A third complementation group was reported in 3 sibs by Weeda *et al.* (1997) with a mutation in the *ERCC3/XPB* gene. The clinical description of the condition was as that described in TTD with congenital ichthyosis.

The clinical features of the TTD with PIBI (D)S (photosensitivity ichthyosis, brittle hair, intellectual impairment, decreased fertility, short stature) are similar and repair studies of one patient showed reduced repair synthesis and the patient was assigned to xeroderma pigmentosum group D (Kleijer *et al.* 1994). Therefore PIBI(D)S syndrome is probably a variant of the IBDS syndrome.

A different trichothiodystrophy is the hair–brain syndrome or BIDS syndrome where the skin is normal (Jackson *et al.* 1974). The Sabinas brittle hair syndrome (Arbisser *et al.* 1976) and the trichorexis nodosa with mental defect (Pollitt *et al.* 1968) may be identical. Minor dental abnormalities such as caries were mentioned in 10% of the cases (Table 9.3). Itin and Pittelkow (1991) described sulphur-deficient hair in a patient who also had neutropenia. Such a syndrome has earlier been described (but not examined for sulphur) as onychotrichodysplasia with neutropenia (Table 9.3) by Cantú *et al.* (1975), Hernandez *et al.* (1979) and Verhage *et al.* (1987). It is possible therefore that the family of trichothiodystrophies will increase in the future as more cases are examined for sulfur content.

## References

Ackerman, J.L., Ackerman, A.L. & Ackerman, A.B. (1973) A new dental ocular and cutaneous syndrome. *International Journal of Dermatology* **12**, 285.

Alves, A.F.P., dos Santos, P.A.B., Castelo-Branco-Neto, E. & Freire-Maia, N. (1981) Brief clinical report: an autosomal recessive ectodermal dysplasia syndrome of hypotrichosis, onychodysplasia, hyperkeratosis, kyphoscoliosis, cataract, and other manifestations. *American Journal of Medical Genetics* **10**, 213.

Ando, Y., Tanaka, T., Horiguchi, Y., Ikai, K. & Tomono, H. (1988) Hidrotic ectodermal dysplasia: a clinical and ultrastructural observation. *Dermatologica* **176**, 205.

Arbisser, A.I., Scott, C.I. Jr & Howell, R.R. (1976) A syndrome manifested by brittle hair with morphologic and biochemical abnormalities, developmental delay and normal stature. *Birth Defects* **12**, 219.

Armstrong, D.K.B., McKenna, K.E. & Hughes, A.E. (1998) A novel insertional mutation in loricrin in Vohwinkel's keratoderma. *Journal of Investigative Dermatology* **111**, 702.

Arnold, W.P., Merkx, M.A.W. & Steijlen, P.M. (1995) Variant of odontoonychodermal dysplasia? *American Journal of Medical Genetics* **59**, 242.

Atherton, D.J., Sutton, C. & Jones, B.M. (1990) Mutilating palmoplantar keratoderma with periorificial keratotic plaques (Olmsted's syndrome). *British Journal of Dermatology* **122**, 245.

Baden, H.P. & Katz, A. (1988) Trichothiodystrophy without retardation: one patient exhibiting transient combined immunodeficiency syndrome. *Pediatric Dermatology* **5**, 257.

Barbareschi, M., Cambiaghi, S., Crupi, A.C. & Tadini, G. (1997) Family with 'pure' hair–nail ectodermal dysplasia. *American Journal of Medical Genetics* **72**, 91.

Barraud-Klenovsek, M.M., Lübbe, J. & Burg, G. (1997) Primary digital clubbing associated with palmoplantar keratoderma. *Dermatology* **194**, 302.

Bart, R.S. & Pumphrey, R.E. (1967) Knuckle pads, leukonychia and deafness. A dominantly inherited syndrome. *New England Journal of Medicine* **276**, 202.

Basan, M. (1965) Ektodermale Dysplasie. Fehlendes Papillarmuster Nagelveraenderungen und Vierfingerfurche. *Archiv für klinische und experimentelle Dermatologie* **222**, 546.

Basran, F., Yilmaz, E., Alpsoy, E. & Yilmas, G. (1995) Keratoderma, hypotrichosis and leukonychia totalis: a new syndrome? *British Journal of Dermatology* **133**, 636.

Baughman, F.A. Jr (1971) CHANDS: the curly hair ankyloblepharon–nail dysplasia syndrome. *Birth Defects* **7**, 100.

Bellosta, M., Trespolli, D., Ghiselli, E., Capra, E. & Scappaticci, S. (1996) Focal dermal hypoplasia: report of a family with 7 affected women in 3 generations. *European Journal of Dermatology* **6**, 499.

Berg, D., Weingold, D.H., Abson, K.G. & Olsen, E.A. (1990) Sweating in ectodemal dysplasia syndromes. *Archives of Dermatology* **126**, 1075.

Bergman, R. & Friedman-Birnbaum, R. (1988) Papillon–Lefevre syndrome: a study of the long-term clinical course of recurrent pyogenic infections and the effects of etretinate treatment. *British Journal of Dermatology* **119**, 731.

de Berker, D. & Kavanagh, G. (1993) Distinctive nail changes in scleroatrophy of Huriez. *British Journal of Dermatology* **129** (Suppl. 42), 36.

Bhatia, K.K., Chaudhary, S. & Palima U.S. &Mehrotra, G.C. (1989) Keratoma hereditaria mutilans (Vohwinkel's disease) with congenital alopecia universalis (atrichia congenita). *Journal of Dermatology* **16**, 231.

Blomquist, H.K., Bäck, O., Fagerlund, B., Holmgren, G. & Steckén-Blicks, C. (1991) Tay or IBDS syndrome. *Acta Paediatrica Scandinavica* **80**, 1241.

Bondesson, J. (1993) Pachonychia congenita. A historical note. *American Journal of Dermatopathology* **15**, 594.

Borradori, L. & Blanchet-Bardon, C. (1993) Skin manifestations of cardio-facio–cutaneous syndrome. *Journal of the American Academy of Dermatology* **28**, 815.

Boss, J.M., Matthews, C.N.A., Peachey, R.D.G. & Summerly, R. (1981) Speckled hyperpigmentation, palmo-plantar punctate keratoses and childhood blistering: a clinical triad, with variable associations. A report of two families. *British Journal of Dermatology* **105**, 579.

Bouadjar, B., Benmazouzia, S., Prudhomme, J.F. *et al.* (2000) Clinical and genetic studies of 3 large, consanguineous Algerian families with Mal de Meleda. *Archives of Dermatology* **136**, 1247–1252.

Bowden, P.E., Haley, J.L., Kansky, A., Rothnogel, J.A., Jones, D.O. & Turner, R.J. (1995) Mutation of a type II keratin gene (K6a) in pachyonychia congenita. *Nature Genetics* **10**, 363.

Braun-Quintin, C., Kapferer, L. & Kotzot, D. (1996) Variant of Coffin–Siris syndrome or previously undescribed syndrome. *American Journal of Medical Genetics* **84**, 568.

Braverman, I.M. (1981) *Skin Signs of Systemic Disease*, 2nd edn, p. 640. W.B. Saunders, Philadelphia.

Breslau-Siderius, E.J., Toonstra, J., Baart, J.A., Koppeschaar, H.P.F., Maassen, J.A. & Beemer, F.A. (1992) Ectodermal dysplasia, lipoatrophy, diabetes mellitus and amastia: a second case of the AREDYLD syndrome. *American Journal of Medical Genetics* **44**, 374.

Brilon, C. & Rütten, C. (1993) Hay–Wells-Syndrome mit multiplen ekkrinen Hidrozystomen. *Aktuelle Dermatologie* **19**, 86.

Brun, M.-F., Delcampe, P., Retout, A., Bachy, B. & Peron, J.-M. (1994) Syndromes des ptérygions poplités. *Revue de Stomatologie et de Chirurgie Maxillo-Faciale* **95**, 343.

Buckly, W.R. & Cassuto, J. (1962) Pachyonychia congenita. *Archives of Dermatology* **85**, 397.

Bühler, E.M., Bühler, U.K., Beutier, C. & Fessler, R. (1987) A final word on the trichorhino–phalangeal syndromes. *Clinical Genetics* **31**, 273.

Bureau, Y., Barrière, H. & Thomas, M. (1959) Hippocratisme digital congénital avec hyperkératose palmo-plantaire et troubles osseux. *Annales de Dermatologie et de Vénéréologie* **86**, 611.

Burkhardt, D., Schirren, C.G., Schuffenhauer, S., Ullman, S. & Schirren, H. (1994) Dyskeratosis congenita bei monozygoten Zwillingen. *Hautarzt* **45**, 249.

Buss, P.W., Hughes, H.E. & Clarke, A. (1995) Twenty-four cases of the EEC syndrome: clinical presentation and management. *Journal of Medical Genetics* **32**, 716.

Calzavara-Pinton, P., Carlino, A., Benetti, A. & de Panfilis, G. (1991) Pili torti and onychodysplasia. Report of a previously undescribed hidrotic ectodermal dysplasia. *Dermatologica* **182**, 184.

Cantú, J.M., Arias, J., Foncerada, M. et al. (1975) Syndrome of onycho-trichodysplasia with chronic neutropenia in an infant from consanguineous parents. Birth Defects: Original Article Series XI, 2.63.

Cantwell, R.J. (1975) Congenital sensori-neural deafness associated with onycho-osteo-dystrophy and mental retardation (DOOR syndrome). Humangenetik 26, 261.

Carey, J.C. & Hall, B.D. (1978) The Coffin–Siris syndrome. Five new cases including two siblings. American Journal of Diseases of Children 132, 667.

Carrington, P.R., Chen, H. & Altick, J.A. (1994) Trichorhinophalangeal syndrome, type I. Journal of the American Academy of Dermatology 31, 331.

Carvajal-Huerta, L. (1998) Epidermolytic palmoplantar keratoderma with woolly hair and dilated cardiomyopathy. Journal of the American Academy of Dermatology 39, 418.

Cat, L., Costa, O. & Freire-Maia, N. (1972) Odontotrichomelic hypohidrotic dysplasia. A clinical reappraisal. Human Heredity 22, 91.

Caux, F., Aractingi, S., Sawaf, M.H., Ouhayoun, J.-P., Dubertret, L. & Gluckman, E. (1996) Dyskeratosis congenita. European Journal of Dermatology 6, 332.

de Cecatto Lima, L., Pinheiro, M. & Freire-Maia, N. (1988) Oculotricho-dysplasia (OTD): a new probably autosomal recessive condition. Journal of Medical Genetics 25, 430.

Chang, A., Lucker, G.P.H., van de Kerkhof, P.C.M. & Steijlen, P.M. (1994) Pachonychia congenita in the absence of other syndrome abnormalities. Journal of the American Academy of Dermatology 30, 1017.

Chiba, A. & Miura, T. (1979) A family with hypotrichosis associated with congenital hypoplasia of the thumb. Japanese Journal of Genetics 24, 111.

Chitty, L.S., Dennis, N. & Baraitser, M. (1996) Hidrotic ectodermal dysplasia of hair, teeth and nails: case reports and review. Journal of Medical Genetics 33, 707.

Christan, J.C., Dexter, R.N., Palmer, C.G. & Muller, J. (1980) A family with three recessive traits and homozygosity for a long 9gh+ chromosome segment. American Journal of Medical Genetics 6, 301.

Christianson, A.L. & Fourie, S. (1996) Family with autosomal dominant hidrotic ectodermal dysplasia: a previously unrecognised syndrome? American Journal of Medical Genetics 63, 549.

Clementi, M., Cardin de Stefani, E., Dei Rossi, C., Avventi, V. & Tenconi, R. (1986) Pachyonychia congenita Jackson–Lawler type: a distinct malformation syndrome. British Journal of Dermatology 114, 367.

Clouston, H.R. (1929) A hereditary ectodermal dystrophy. Canadian Medical Association Journal 21, 10.

Cockayne, E.A. (1936) Cleft palate-lip, hare lip, dacrocystitis, and cleft hand and foot. Biometrika 28, 60.

Coffin, G.S. & Siris, E. (1970) Mental retardation with absent fifth fingernail and terminal phalanx. American Journal of Diseases of Children 119, 433.

Colcott-Fox, T. (1897) Symmetrical hyperkeratosis of the nail beds of the hands and feet and other areas chiefly on the palms and soles. Clinical Society Transactions (London) 30, 242.

Connor, J.M. & Teague, R.H. (1981) Dyskeratosis congenita. Report of a large kindred. British Journal of Dermatology 105, 321.

Connor, J.M., Gatherer, D., Gray, F.C., Pirrit, A. & Affara, N.A. (1986) Assignment of the gene for dyskeratosis congenita to Xq28. Human Genetics 72, 348.

Covello, S.P., Smith, F.J.D., Sillevis Smitt, J.H. et al. (1998) Keratin 17 mutations cause either steatocystoma multiplex or pachonychia conconita type 2. British Journal of Dermatology 139, 475.

Craigen, W.J., Levy, M.L. & Lewis, R.A. (1997) Schöpt–Schulz–Pasaige syndrome with an unusual pattern of inheritance. American Journal of Medical Genetics 71, 186.

Crosti, C., Sala, R., Bertani, E., Gasparini, G. & Menni, S. (1983) Leuconychie totale et dysplasie ectodermique. Observation de deux cas. Annales de Dermatologie et de Vénéréologie 110, 617.

Curry, C. (1979) Personal communication. McKusick, V. M. Mendelian Inheritance in Man, 12th edn, p. 3276, 1998.

Curry, C.J.R. & Hall, B.P. (1979) Polydactyly, conical teeth, nail dysplasia, and short limbs: a new autosomal dominant malformation syndrome. Journal of Bone and Joint Surgery 53B, 101.

Dalapiccola, B., Mingarelli, R. & Obregon, G. (1994) Onychotrichodysplasia and chronic neutropenia and mild mental retardation: delineation of the syndrome. Clinical Genetics 15, 147.

Darwin, C. (1875) The Variation of Animals and Plants Under Domestication, p. 319, 2nd edn. John Murray Publishers, London.

Delaporte, E., N'Guyen-Mailfer, C., Janin, A. et al. (1995) Keratoderma with scleroatrophy of the extremities or sclerotylosis (Huriez syndrome): a reappraisal. British Journal of Dermatology 133, 409.

Devriendt, K., Matthijs, G., Legius, E. et al. (1997) Skewed X-chromosome inactivation in female carriers of dyskeratosis congenita. American Journal of Human Genetics 60, 581.

Dodd, H.J., Devereux, S. & Sarkany, J. (1985) Dyskeratosis congenita with pancytopenia. Clinical and Experimental Dermatology 10, 73.

Dodinval, P. (1972) The dysplasia of epidermal ridges revisited. Evidence of an apical dysplasia of the fingers. Humangenetik 15, 20.

Dokal, I. (1996) Dyskeratosis congenita: an inherited bone marrow failure syndrome. British Journal of Haematology 92, 775.

Ellis, J. & Dawber, R.P.R. (1980) Ectodermal dysplasia syndrome: a family study. Clinical and Experimental Dermatology 5, 295.

Ellis, R.W.B. & van Creveld, S. (1940) A syndrome characterized by ectodermal dysplasia, polydactyly, chondro-dysplasia and congenital morbus cordis: report of three cases. Archives of Disease in Childhood 15, 65.

Escobar, V. & Weaver, D.D. (1978) The facio-genito-popliteal syndrome. Birth Defect: Original Article Series XIV (6B), 185.

Evers, M.E.J.W., Steijlen, P.M. & Hamel, B.C.J. (1995) Aplasia cutis ongenita and associated disorders: an update. Clinical Genetics 47, 295.

Fadhil, M., Ghabra, T.A., Deeb, M. & Der Kaloustian, V.M. (1983) Odontoonychodermal dysplasia: a previously apparantly undescribed ectodermal dysplasia. American Journal of Medical Genetics 14, 335.

Feinmesser, M. & Zelig, S. (1961) Congenital deafness associated with onychodystrophy. Archives of Otolaryngology 74, 507.

Feinstein, A., Friedman, J. & Schewach-Millet, M.S. (1988) Pachyonychia congenita. Journal of the American Academy of Dermatology 19, 705.

Font, R.L., Seabury Stone, M., Schanzer, M.C. & Lewis, R.A. (1986) Apocrine hidrocystomas of the lids, hypodontia, palmar-plantar hyperkeratosis, and onychodystrophy—a new variant of ectodermal dysplasia. Archives of Ophthalmology 104, 1811.

Forman, A.B., Prendiville, J.S., Esterly, N.B. et al. (1989) Kindler syndrome: report of two cases and review of the literature. Pediatric Dermatology 6, 91.

Francannet, C., Vanlieferinghen, P., Dechelotte, P., Urbain, M.F.,

Campagne, D. & Malpuech, G. (1994) LADD syndrome in five members of a three-generation family and prenatal diagnosis. *Genetics Counselling* **5**, 85.

Franco, B., Meroni, G., Parenti, G. *et al.* (1995) A cluster of sulphatase genes on Xp22.3: mutations in chondrodysplasia punctata (CD PX) and implications for warfarin embryopathy. *Cell* **81**, 15.

Freire-Maia, N. (1977) Ectodermal dysplasias revisited. *Acta Geneticae Medicae et Gemellologiae (Roma)* **26**, 121.

Freire-Maia, N., Cat, I. & Rapone Gaidzinsky, R. (1977) An ectodermal dysplasia syndrome of alopecia, onychodysplasia, hypohidrosis, hyperkeratosis, deafness and other manifestations. *Human Heredity* **27**, 127.

Freire-Maia, N. & Pinheiro, M. (1984) *Ectodermal Dysplasias, A Clinical and Genetic Study*. Alan R. Liss, New York.

Freire-Maia, N. & Pinheiro, M. (1988) Ectodermal dysplasias—some recollections and a classifications. *Birth Defects: Original Article Series* **24**, 3.

Freire-Maia, N., Fortes, V.A., Pereira, L.C., Opitz, J.M., Marcallo, F.A. & Cavalli, I.J. (1975) A syndrome of hypohidrotic ectodermal dysplasia with normal teeth, peculiar facies, pigmentary disturbances, psychomotor and growth retardation, bilateral nuclear cataract, and other signs. *Journal of Medical Genetics* **12**, 308.

Fried, K. (1977) Autosomal recessive hydrotic ectodermal dysplasia. *Journal of Medical Genetics* **14**, 137.

Gamborg Nielsen, P. (1983) Mutilating palmo-plantar keratoderma. *Acta Dermato-Venereologica* **63**, 365.

Garrick-Wilson, A. (1905) Three cases of hereditary hyperkeratosis of the nail bed. *British Journal of Dermatology* **17**, 13.

Giedion, A. (1967) Cone-shaped epiphyses of the hands and their diagnostic value: the tricho-rhino-phalangeal syndrome. *Annals of Radiology (Paris)* **10**, 322.

Gladwin, A., Donnai, D., Metcalfe, K. *et al.* (1997) Localization of a gene for oculodentodigital syndrome to human chromosome 6q22–q24. *Human Molecular Genetics* **6**, 123.

Gobello, T., Mazzanti, C., Fileccia, P. *et al.* (1995) X-linked dominant chondrodysplasia punctata (Happle syndrome) with uncommon symmetrical shortening of the tubular bones. *Dermatology* **191**, 323.

Goltz, R.W. (1992) Focal dermal hypoplasia syndrome: an up-date [editorial]. *Archives of Dermatology* **128**, 1108.

Goltz, R.W., Henderson, R.R., Hitch, J.M. & Ott, J.E. (1970) Focal dermal hypoplasia syndrome. *Archives of Dermatology* **101**, 1.

Gorlin, R.J. (1997) Personal comments, p. 3158. In: *Mendelian Inheritance in Man 1998* (ed. V.A. McKusick), 12th edn. Johns Hopkins University Press.

Gorlin, R.J., Sedano, H. & Anderson, V.E. (1964) The syndrome of palmar-plantar hyperkeratosis and premature periodontal destruction of the teeth. *Journal of Pediatrics* **65**, 895.

Gorlin, R.J., Old, T. & Anderson, V.A. (1970) Hypohidrotic ectodermal dysplasia in females: a critical analysis and argument for genetic heterogeneity. *Zeitschrift für Kinderheilkd* **108**, 1.

Gorlin, R.J., Pindborg, J.J. & Cohen, M.M. (1976) *Syndromes of the Head and Neck*, 2nd edn. McGraw-Hill, New York.

Haber, R.M. & Rose, T.H. (1986) Autosomal recessive pachyonychia congenita. *Archives of Dermatology* **122**, 919.

Haneke, E. (1979) The Papillon–Lefèvre syndrome: keratosis palmoplantaris with periodontopathy. *Human Genetics* **51**, 1.

Happle, R. (1979) X-linked dominant chondrodysplasia punctata. *Humangenetik* **53**, 65.

Happle, R. & Rampen, F.H.J. (1987) Multiple eyelid hidrocystoma syndrome: a new cancer syndrome? In: *Proceedings of the 17th World Congress on Dermatology (Berlin). Clinical Dermatology* (eds D.S. Wilkinson, J.M. Mascaro & C.E. Orfanos), p. 290. Schattawer, Stuttgart.

Harari, Z., Pasmanik, A., Dvoretzky, I., Schewach-Millet, M. & Fischer, B.K. (1976) Aplasia cutis congenita with dystrophic nail changes. *Dermatologica* **153**, 363.

Hart, T.C., Stabholz, A., Meyle, J., Shapira, L. *et al.* (1997) Genetic studies with severe periodontis and palmoplantar hyperkeratosis. *Journal of Periodontal Research* **32**, 81.

Hart, T.C., Bowden, D.W., Ghaffar, K.A. *et al.* (1998) Sublocalization of the Papillon–Lefevre syndrome locus 11q14–21. *American Journal of Human Genetics* **79**, 134.

Hassed, S.J., Kincannon, J.M. & Arnold, G.L. (1996) Clouston syndrome: an ectodermal dysplasia without significant dental findings. *American Journal of Human Genetics* **61**, 274.

Hay, R.J. & Wells, R.S. (1976) The syndrome of ankyloblepharon, ectodermal defects and cleft lip and palate: an autosomal dominant condition. *British Journal of Dermatology* **94**, 277.

Heimer, W.L., Brauner, G. & James, W.D. (1992) Dermatopathia pigmentosa reticularis: a report of a family demonstrating autosomal dominant inheritance. *Journal of the American Academy of Dermatology* **26**, 298.

Hernandez, A., Olivares, F. & Cantu, J.M. (1979) Autosomal recessive onychotrichodysplasia, chronic neutropenia and mild mental retardation. *Clinical Genetics* **15**, 147.

Hoeger, P.H., Adwani, S.S., Whitehead, B.F., Finley, A.Y. & Harper, J.J. (1998) Ichtyosiform erythroderma and cardiomyopathy: report of two cases and review of the literature. *British Journal of Dermatology* **139**, 1055.

Hollister, D.W., Klein, S.N., de Jager, H.J., Lachman, R.S. & Rimoin, D.L. (1973) The lacrimo-auriculo-dento-digital syndrome. *Journal of Pediatrics* **83**, 438.

Hoting, E. & Wassilew, S.W. (1985) Systemische Retinoidtherapie mit Etretinat bei Pachyonychia congenita. *Hautarzt* **36**, 526.

Hovnanian, A., Blanchet-Bardon, C. & de Prost, Y. (1989) Poikiloderma of Theresa Kindler: report of a case with ultrastructural study, and review of the literature. *Pediatric Dermatology* **6**, 82.

Huriez, C.L., Deminati, M., Agache, R., Delmas-Marsalet, Y. & Mennecier, M. (1969) Génodermatose scléro-atrophiante et kéeratodermique des extrémitées. *Annales de Dermatologie et de Syphiligraphie* **6**, 135.

Iraci, S., Bianchi, L., Gatti, S., Carozzo, A.M., Bettini, D. & Nini, G. (1993) Pachynychia congenita with late onset of nail dystrophy—a new clinical entity? *Clinical and Experimental Dermatology* **18**, 478.

Irvine, A.D., McKenna, K.E., Jenkinson, H. & Hughes, A.E. (1997) A mutation in the VI domain of keratin 5 causes epidermolysis bullosa simplex with mottled pigmentation. *Journal of Investigative Dermatology* **108**, 809.

Itin, P.H. & Pittelkow, M.R. (1990) Trichothiodystrophy: review of sulfur-deficient brittle hair syndromes and association with the ectodermal dysplasias. *Journal of the American Academy of Dermatology* **22**, 705.

Itin, P.H. & Pittelkow, M.R. (1991) Trichothiodystrophy with chronic neutropenia and mild mental retardation. *Archives of Dermatology* **24**, 356.

Itin, P.H., Lautenschlager, S., Meyer, R., Mevorah, B. & Rufli, T.

(1993) Natural history of the Naegeli–Franceschetti–Jadassohn syndrome and futher definition of its clinical manifestations. *Journal of the American Academy of Dermatology* **28**, 742.

Jackson, A.D.M. & Lawler, S.D. (1951) Pachyonychia congenita: a report of six cases in one family. *Annals of Eugenics (London)* **16**, 141.

Jackson, C.E., Eiss, L. & Watson, J.H.L. (1974) Brittle hair with short stature; intellectual impairment and decreased fertility: an autosomal recessive syndrome in an Amish kindred. *Pediatrics* **54**, 201.

Jadassohn, J. & Lewandowsky, F. (1906) Pachyonychia congenita. *Ikonographical Dermatology* **1**, 29.

Jones, E.M., Hersch, J.H. & Yusk, J.W. (1992) Aplasia cutis congenita, cleft palate, epidermolysis bullosa, and ectrodactyly. A new syndrome? *Pediatric Dermatology* **9**, 293.

Jorizzo, J.L., Atherton, D.J., Crounse, R.G. & Wells, R.S. (1982) Ichthyosis, brittle hair, impaired intelligence, decreased fertility and short stature (I.B.D.S. syndrome). *British Journal of Dermatology* **106**, 705.

Kalb, R.E., Grossman, M.E. & Hutt, C. (1986) Avascular necrosis of bone in dyskeratosis congenita. *American Journal of Medicine* **80**, 511.

Kantaputra, P.N., Pruksachatkunakorn, C. & Vanittanakom, P. (1998) Rapp–Hodgkin syndrome with palmoplantar keratoderma, glossy tongue, congenital absence of lingual frenelum and of sublingual caruncles. *American Journal of Medical Genetics* **79**, 343.

Kelsell, D.P., Dunlop, J., Stevens, H.P. *et al.* (1997) Connexin 26 mutations in hereditary non-syndromic sensorineural deafness. *Nature* **387**, 80.

Kere, J., Srivastava, A.K., Montonen, O. *et al.* (1996) X-linked anhidrotic (hypohidrotic) ectodermal dysplasia is caused by mutation in a novel transmembrane protein. *Nature Genetics* **13**, 409.

Kibar, Z., Der Kaloustian, V.M., Brais, B. *et al.* (1996) The gene responsible for Clouston hidrotic ectodermal dysplasia maps to the pericentromeric region of chromosome 13q. *Human Molecular Genetics* **5**, 543.

Kindler, T. (1954) Congenital poikilodermia with traumatic bullae formation and progressive cutaneous atrophy. *British Journal of Dermatology* **66**, 104.

Kleijer, W.J., Beemer, F.A. & Boom, B.W. (1994) Intermittent hair loss in a child with PIBI(D)S syndrome and trichothiodystrophy with defective DNA repair xeroderma pigmentosum group D. *American Journal of Medical Genetics* **52**, 227.

Knight, S.W., Vulliamy, T., Forni, G.L., Oscier, D., Mason, P.J. & Dokal, I. (1996) Fine mapping of the dyskeratosis locus in Xq28. *Journal of Medical Genetics* **33**, 993.

Knudtzon, J. & Aarskog, D. (1987) Growth hormone deficiency associated with the ectrodactyly–ectodermal dysplasia–clefting syndrome and isolated absent septum pellucidum. *Pediatrics* **79**, 410.

Kobyashi, S., Tanaka, T., Matsuyoshi, N. & Imamura, S. (1996) Keratin 9 point mutation in the pedigree of epidermolytic hereditary palmoplantar keratoderma perturbs keratin intermediate filament network formation. *FEBS Letters* **386**, 149.

Kore-Eda, S., Yoneda, K., Ohtani, T., Tachibana, T., Furukawa, F. & Imamura, S. (1995) Focal dermal hypoplasia (Goltz syndrome) associated with multiple giant papillomas. *British Journal of Dermatology* **133**, 997.

Kuster, W. & Becker, A. (1992) Indication for the identity of palmoplantar keratoderma type Unna–Thost with type Vorner, Thost's family revisted 110 years later. *Acta Dermato-Venereologica* **72**, 120.

Langer, K., Konrad, K. & Wolff, K. (1990) Keratitis, ichthyosis and deafness (KID)—syndrome: report of three cases and a review of the literature. *British Journal of Dermatology* **122**, 689.

Langer, L.O., Krassikoff, N., Laxova, R. *et al.* (1984) The trichorhinophalangeal syndrome with exostoses (or Langer–Gideon syndrome): four additional patients without mental retardation and review of the literature. *American Journal of Medical Genetics* **19**, 81.

Larregue, M. & Duterque, M. (1975) Striated osteopathy in focal dermal hypoplasia. *Archives of Dermatology* **111**, 1365.

Larregue, M., Prigent, F., Lorette, G., Canuel, C. & Ramdenee, P. (1981) Acrokeratose poikilodermique bulleuse et hereditaire de Weary–Kindler. *Annales de Dermatologie et de Vénéréologie* **108**, 69.

Leibowitz, M.R. & Jenkins, T. (1984) A newly recognized feature of ectrodactyly, ectodermal dysplasia, clefting (EEC) syndrome: comedone naevus. *Dermatologica* **169**, 80.

Leichtman, L.G. (1996) Are cardio-facio-cutaneous syndrome and Noonan syndrome distinct? A case of CFC offspring of a mother with Noonan syndrome. *Clinical Dysmorphology* **5**, 61.

Lestringant, G.G., Frossard, P.M., Adeghate, E. & Qayed, K.I. (1997) Mal de Meleda: a report of four cases from the United Arab Emirates. *Pediatric Dermatology* **14**, 186.

Levan, N.E. (1961) Congenital defect of thumbnails. *Archives of Dermatology* **83**, 938.

Lichtenstein, J., Warson, R. & Jorgenson, R. (1972) The trichodento-osseous (TDO) syndrome. *American Journal of Human Genetics* **24**, 569.

Lin, H.J., Kakkis, E.D., Ereson, D.J. & Lachman, R.S. (1993) DOOR syndrome (deafness, onycho-osteodystrophy and mental retardation): a new patient and delineation of neurologic variability among recessive cases. *American Journal of Medical Genetics* **47**, 534.

Lucaya, J., Garcia-Conesa, J.A., Bosch-Banyeras, J.M. & Pons-Peadejordi, G. (1981) The Coffin–Siris syndrome. A report of four cases and review of the literature. *Pediatric Radiology* **11**, 35.

Lucker, G.P.H. & Steijlen, P.M. (1995) Pachonychia congenita tarda. *Clinical and Experimental Dermatology* **20**, 226.

Maas, S.M., de Jong, T.P.V.M., Buss, P. & Hennekam, R.C.M. (1996) EEC syndrome and genitourinary anomalies: an up-date. *American Journal of Medical Genetics* **63**, 472.

Malfait, Y., Decroix, J., Vandaele, R. & Bourlond, A. (1989) Un nouveau cas de syndrome de Goltz. *Annales de Dermatologie et de Vénéréologie* **116**, 715.

Manoukian, S., Lalatta, F., Selicorni, A., Tadini, G., Cavalli, R. & Neri, G. (1996) Cardio-facio-cutaneous (CFC) syndrome: report of an adult without mental retardation. *American Journal of Medical Genetics* **63**, 382.

Marshall, D. (1958) Ectodermal dysplasia. Report of a kindred with ocular abnormalities and hearing defect. *American Journal of Ophthalmology* **45**, 143.

Martino, R., D'Eufemia, P., Pergola, M.S. *et al.* (1992) Child with manifestations of dermotrichic syndrome and ichthyosis follicularis-alopecia-photophobia (IFAP) syndrome. *American Journal of Medical Genetics* **44**, 233.

McGrae, J.D. (1990) Keratitis, ichthyosis, and deafness (KID) syndrome. *International Journal of Dermatology* **29**, 89.

McGrath, J.A. (1999) A novel genodermatosis caused by mutations in plakophilin 1, A structural component of desmosomes. *Journal of Dermatology* **26**, 764–769.

McLean, W.H.I., Rugg, E.L., Lunny, D.P. *et al.* (1995) Keratin 16 and keratin 17 mutations cause pachonychia congenita. *Nature Genetics* 9, 273.

Mégarbané, A., Noujeim, Z., Fabre, M. & Der Kaloustian, V.M. (1998) New form of hidrotic ectodermal dysplasia in a Lebanese family. *American Journal of Medical Genetics* 75, 196.

Mendoza, H.R. & Valiente, M.D. (1997) A newly recognized autosomal dominant ectodermal dysplasia syndrome: the odonto-tricho-ungual-digital-palmar syndrome. *American Journal of Medical Genetics* 71, 144.

Moerman, P. & Fryns, J.-P. (1996) Ectodermal dysplasia, Rapp–Hodgkin type in a mother and severe ectrodactyly–ectodermal clefting syndrome (EEC) in her child. *American Journal of Medical Genetics* 63, 479.

Moon-Adams, D. & Slatkin, M.H. (1955) Familial pigmentation with dystrophy of the nails. *Archives of Dermatology* 71, 591.

Moore, D.J. & Mallory, S.B. (1989) Goltz syndrome. *Pediatric Dermatology* 6, 251.

Morris, C.A., Carey, J.C. & Demsey, S.A. (1987) Another case. *Proceedings of the Greenwood Genetics Center* 6, 145.

Moshkowitz, A., Abrahamov, A. & Pisanti, S. (1969) Congenital hypoparathyroidism simulating epilepsy, with other symptoms and dental signs of intra-uterine hypocalcemia. *Pediatrics* 44, 401.

Mouaci-Midoun, N., Cambiaghi, S. & Abimelec, P. (1996) Pachonychia congenita tarda. *Journal of the American Academy of Dermatology* 35, 334.

Müller, C. (1904) On the causes of congenital onychogryphosis. *München Medicine Wochenschrift* 49, 2180.

Murdoch-Kinch, C.A., Miles, A.D. & Poon, C.-K. (1993) Hypodontia and nail dysplasia syndrome. *Oral Surgery Oral Medicine Oral Pathology* 75, 403.

Musaeus, C. (1716) *Dissertatio inauguralis medica de unguibus montrosis.* J.S. Martin, Copenhagen.

Nazzaro, V., Blanchet-Bardon, C., Mimoz, C., Revuz, J. & Puissant, A. (1988) Papillon–Lefèvre syndrome. Ultrastructural study and successful treatment with acitretin. *Archives of Dermatology* 124, 533.

Neri, G. & Zollino, M. (1996) More on the Noonan–CFC. controversy [editorial]. *American Journal of Medical Genetics* 65, 100.

van Neste, D., Miller, X. & Bohnert, E. (1988) Trichothiodystrophie. *Aktuelle Dermatologie* 14, 191.

van Neste, D., Thomas, P. & Desmons, F. (1980) Trichoschisis, photosensibilité. Retard staturopondéral. Nouveau syndrome congénital. *Annales de Dermatologie et de Vénéréologie* 107, 718.

Nordin, H., Månsson, T. & Svensson, A. (1988) Familial occurrence of eccrine tumours in a family with ectodermal dysplasia. *Annales de Dermatologie et de Vénéréologie* 68, 523.

Norton, K.K., Carey, J.C. & Gutmann, D.H. (1995) Oculodental dysplasia with cerebral white matter abnormalities in a two-generation family. *American Journal of Medical Genetics* 57, 458.

Norval, L., van Wyk, C.W., Basson, N.J. & Coldrey, J. (1988) Hypohidrotic ectodermal dysplasia: a genealogic, stereomicroscope, and scanning electron microscope study. *Pediatric Dermatology* 5, 159.

O'Brien, T.J. (1990) Chondrodysplasia punctata (Conradi disease). *International Journal of Dermatology* 29, 472.

O'Donnell, B.P. & James, W.D. (1992) Rapp–Hodgkin ectodermal dysplasia. *Journal of the American Academy of Dermatology* 27, 323.

O'Rourk, T.R. & Bravos, A. (1969) An oculo-dento-digital dysplasia. *Birth Defects* 5, 226.

Ogden, G.R., Connor, E. & Chisholm, D.M. (1988) Dyskeratosis congenita: report of a case and review literature. *Oral Surgery Oral Medicine Oral Pathology* 65, 586.

Ogur, G. & Yüksel, M. (1988) Association of syndactyly, ectodermal dysplasia, and cleft lip and palate: report of two sibs from Turkey. *Journal of Medical Genetics* 25, 37.

Pabst, H.F., Groth, O. & McCoy, E.E. (1981) Hypohidrotic ectodermal dysplasia with hypothyroidism. *Journal of Pediatrics* 98, 223.

Paller, A.S., Moore, J.A. & Scher, R. (1991) Pachyonychia congenita tarda. A late onset form of pachyonychia congenita. *Archives of Dermatology* 127, 701.

Papillon, P. & Lefevre, P. (1924) Deux cas de kératodermie plamaire et plantaire symétrique familiale (maladie de Méléeda) chez le frère et la soeur: coexistence dans les 2 cas d'altérations dentaires graves. *Bulletin de la Societé Française de Dermatologie et de Syphiligraphie* 31, 82.

Parizel, P.M., Dumon, J., Vossen, P., Rigaux, A. & De Scheppes, A.M. (1987) The trichorhino-phalangeal syndrome revisited. *European Journal of Radiology* 7, 154.

Passarge, E. & Fried, E. (1977) Autosomal recessive hypohidrotic ectodermal dysplasia with subclinical manifestations in the heterozygote. In: *Birth Defects* (ed. D. Bersma), pp. 95–100. Williams & Wilkins, Baltimore.

Passarge, E., Nuzum, L.T. & Schubert, W.K. (1966) Anhidrotic ectodermal dysplasia as autosomal recessive trait in an inherited kindred. *Humangenetik* 3, 181.

Patel, Z.M., Mulye, V.R., Raghavan, K. & Shah, S.B. (1987) Translocation in Coffin–Sirris syndrome. *Indian Pediatrics* 24, 435.

Patrizi, A., Di Lernia, V. & Patrone, P. (1992) Palmoplantar keratoderma with sclerodactyly (Huriez syndrome). *Journal of the American Academy of Dermatology* 26, 855.

Patton, M.A., Krywawych, S., Winter, R.M., Brenton, D.P. & Baraitser, M. (1987) DOOR syndrome (deafness, onycho-osteodystrophy, and mental retardation): elevated plasma and urinary 2-oxoglutarate in three unrelated patients. *American Journal of Medical Genetics* 26, 207.

Pavone, L., Rizzo, R., Tine, A., Micali, G., Sorge, G. & Neri, G. (1989) A case of the Freire–Maia odontotrichomelic syndrome: nosology with EEC syndrome. *American Journal of Medical Genetics* 33, 190.

Pike, M.G., Baraitser, M., Dinwiddie, R. & Atherton, D.J. (1986) A distinctive type of hypohidrotic ectodermal dysplasia featuring hypothyroidism. *Journal of Pediatrics* 108, 109.

Pinheiro, M. & Freire-Maia, N. (1992) Hair–nail dysplasia—a new pure autosomal dominant ectodermal dysplasia. *Clinical Genetics* 41, 296.

Pinheiro, M., Ideriha, M.T., Chautard-Freire-Maia, E.A. *et al.* (1981) Christ–Siemens–Touraine syndrome. Investigations on two large Brazilian kindreds with a new estimate of the manifestation rate among carriers. *Human Genetics* 57, 428.

Pinheiro, M., Freire-Maia, N. & Roth, A.J. (1983a) Trichoodonto-onychial dysplasia—a new meso-ectodermal dysplasia. *American Journal of Medical Genetics* 15, 67.

Pinheiro, M., Freire-Maia, N., Chautard-Freire-Maia, E.A., Araujo, L.M.B. & Libermar, B. (1983b) A syndrome combining an acrorenal field defect, ectodermal dysplasia, lipoatrophic diabetes and other manifestations. *American Journal of Medical Genetics* 16, 29–33.

Pinheiro, M., Freire-Maia, N. & Gollop, T.R. (1985) Odonto-onychodysplasia with alopecia: a new pure ectodermal dysplasia with probable autosomal recessive inheritance. *American Journal of Medical Genetics* **20**, 197.

Pinheiro, M., José Penna, F. & Freire-Maia, N. (1989) Two other cases of another syndrome? Family report and update. *Clinical Genetics* **35**, 237.

Pinheiro, M., Gomes-de-Sá-Filho, F.P. & Freire-Maia, N. (1990) New cases of dermoodontodysplasia? *American Journal of Medical Genetics* **36**, 161.

Pinheiro, M., Snel, A.I. & Freire-Maia, N. (1996) Odontomicronychial ectodermal dysplasia. *Journal of Medical Genetics* **33**, 230.

Pollitt, R.J., Jenner, F.A. & Davies, M. (1968) Sibs with mental and physical retardation and trichorrhexis nodosa with abnormal amino acid composition of the hair. *Archives of Disease in Childhood* **43**, 211.

Polymeropoulus, M.H., Ide, S.E., Wright, M. *et al.* (1996) The gene for the Ellis–van Creveld syndrome is located on chromosome 4p16. *Genomics* **35**, 1.

Poulin, Y., Perry, H.O. & Muller, S.A. (1984) Olmsted syndrome congenital palmplantar and periorifacial keratoderma. *Journal of the American Academy of Dermatology* **10**, 600.

Price, J.A., Wright, J.T., Kula, K., Bowden, D.W. & Hart, T.C. (1998) A common DLX3 gene mutation is responsible for tricho-dento-osseous syndrome in Virginia and North Carolina Families. *Journal of Medical Genetics* **35**, 825.

Price, V.H., Odom, R.B., Ward, W.H. & Jones, F.T. (1980) Trichothiodystrophy. *Archives of Dermatology* **116**, 1375.

Propping, P. & Zerres, K. (1993) ADULT syndrome: an autosomal-dominant disorder with pigment anomalies, ectrodactyly, nail dysplasia, and hypodontia. *American Journal of Medical Genetics* **45**, 642.

Protonotarios, N., Tsatsopoulou, A., Patsourakos, P. *et al.* (1986) Cardiac abnormalities in familial palmplantar keratosis. *British Heart Journal* **56**, 321.

Pryce, D.W. & Verbov, J.L. (1994) A family with pachyonychia congenita affecting the nails only. *Clinical and Experimental Dermatology* **20**, 226.

Pujol, R.M., Casanova, J.M., Pérez, M., Matias-Guiu, X., Planagumà, M. & de Moragas, J.M. (1992) Focal dermal hypoplasia (Goltz syndrome). Report of two cases with minor cutaneous and extracutaneous manifestations. *Pediatric Dermatology* **9**, 112.

Puliyel, J.M. & Sridharan Iyer, K.S. (1986) A syndrome of keratosis palmo-plantaris congenita, pes planus, onychogryphosis, periodontosis, arachnodactyly and a peculiar acroosteolysis. *British Journal of Dermatology* **115**, 243.

Qazi, Q.H. & Nangia, B.S. (1984) Abnormal distal phalanges and nails; deafness, mental retardation; and seizure disorder: a new familiar syndrome. *Journal of Pediatrics* **104**, 391.

Qazi, Q.H. & Smithwick, E.M. (1970) Triphalangy of thumbs and great toes. *American Journal of Diseases of Children* **120**, 255.

Qumsiyeh, M.B. (1992) EEC syndrome (ectrodactyly, ectodermal dysplasia and cleft lip/palate is on 7p11.2–q21.3. *Clinical Genetics* **42**, 101.

Ramer, J.C., Vasily, D.B. & Ladda, R.L. (1994) Familial leuconychia, knuckle pads, keratosis palmoplantaris: an additional family with Bart–Pumphrey syndrome. *Journal of Medical Genetics* **31**, 68.

Rand, R.E. & Baden, H.P. (1983) The ichthyosis—a review. *Journal of the American Academy of Dermatology* **8**, 285.

Raphael, A.L., Baer, P.N. & Lee, W.B. (1968) Hyperkeratosis of gingival and plantar surfaces. *Periodontics* **6**, 118.

Rapp, R.S. & Hodgkin, W.E. (1968) Anhidrotic ectodermal dysplasia: autosomal dominant inheritance with palate and lip anomalies. *Journal of Medical Genetics* **5**, 269.

Rebora, A. & Crovato, F. (1987) PIBI(D)S syndrome—trichothiodystrophy with xeroderma pigmentosurn (group D) mutation. *Journal of the American Academy of Dermatology* **16**, 940.

Reed, W.B., Lopez, A. & Landing, B. (1970) Clinical spectrum of anhidrotic ectodermal dysplasia. *Archives of Dermatology* **102**, 134.

Reed, T. & Schreiner, R.L. (1983) Absence of dermal ridge patterns: genetic heterogeneity. *American Journal of Medical Genetics* **16**, 81.

Reynolds, J.F., Neri, G., Herrmann, J.P. *et al.* (1986) New multiple congenital anomalies/mental retardation syndrome with cardio-facio-cutaneous involvement—the CFC syndrome. *American Journal of Medical Genetics* **25**, 413.

Robinson, G.C., Miller, J.R. & Bensimon, J.R. (1962) Familial ectodermal dysplasia with sensori-neural deafness and other anomalies. *Pediatrics* **30**, 797.

Robinson, G.C., Miller, J.R. & Worth, H.M. (1966) Hereditary enamel hypoplasia: its association with characteristic hair structure. *Pediatrics* **37**, 498.

Rollnick, B.R. & Hoo, J.J. (1988) Genitourinary anomalies are a competent manifestation in the ectodermal dysplasia, ectrodactyly, cleft lip/palate (EEC) syndrome. *American Journal of Medical Genetics* **29**, 131.

Rothe, M.J., Weiss, D.S., Dubner, B.H., Weitzner, J.M., Lucky, A.W. & Schachner, L. (1990) Ichthyosis follicularis in two girls: an autosomal dominant disorder. *Pediatric Dermatology* **7**, 287.

Rothnagel, J.A., Wojcik, S., Liefer, K.M. *et al.* (1995) Mutations in the 1A domain of keratin 9 in patients with epidermolytic palmoplantar keratoderma. *Journal of Investigative Dermatology* **104**, 430.

Rycroft, R.J., Calnan, C.D. & Allenby, C.F. (1977) Dermatopathia pigmentosa reticularis. *Clinical and Experimental Dermatology* **2**, 37.

Salamon, T. (1982) Nagelveränderungen bei des krankheit von Mijet. *Zeitschrift für Hautkrankheiten* **57**, 1496.

Salamon, T., Cubela, V., Bogdanovic, B., Lazovic, O. & Bulatovic, N. (1967) Uber ein Geschwisterpaar mit einer eigenartigen ektodermalen Dysplasie. *Archives of Clinical and Experimental Dermatology* **230**, 60.

Sánchez, J.M., Laberta, J.D., de Negrotti, T.C. & Migliorini, A.M. (1985) Complex translocation in a boy with trichorhinophalangeal syndrome. *Journal of Medical Genetics* **22**, 314.

Schapiro, S.D., Jorgenson, R.J. & Salinas, C.F. (1984) Brief clinical report: Curry–Hall syndrome. *American Journal of Medical Genetics* **17**, 579.

Schöpf, E., Schultz, H. & Passarge, E. (1971) Syndrome of cystic eyelids, palmo-plantar keratosis. Hypodontia and hypotrichosis as a possible autosomal recessive trait. *Birth Defects: Original Article Series* **VII (8)**, 219.

Schroeder, H.W. & Sybert, V.P. (1987) Rapp–Hodgkin ectodermal dysplasia. *Journal of Pediatrics* **110**, 72.

Schulz-Kiesow, M., Metze, D. & Traupe, H. (1996) Hystrix-like keratosis with nail and joint involvement: a new genodermatosis? *Dermatology* **192**, 321.

Schwann, J. (1963) Keratosis palmaris et plantaris cum surditate congenita et leuconychia totali ungium. *Dermatologica* **126**, 335.

Schwayder, T.A., Lane, A.T. & Miller, M.E. (1986) Hay–Wells syndrome. *Pediatric Dermatology* **3**, 399.

Scoggins, R.B., Prescott, K.J., Asher, G.H., Blaylock, W.K. & Bright, R.W. (1971) Dyskeratosis congenita with Fanconi-type anemia: investigations of immunologic and other defects. *Clinical Research* **19**, 409.

Senter, T.P., Jones, K.L., Sahati, N. & Nyham, W.L. (1978) Atypical ichthyosiform erythroderma and congenital neurosensory deafness. A distinct syndrome. *Journal of Pediatrics* **92**, 68.

Seow, K. (1993) Trichodentoosseous (TDO) syndrome: case report and literature review. *Pediatric Dentistry* **15**, 355.

Seres-Santamaria, A., Arimany, J.L. & Muniz, F. (1993) Two sibs with cleft palate, ankyloblepharon, alveolar synechiae, and ectodermal defects: a new recessive syndrome? *Journal of Medical Genetics* **30**, 793.

Shamsheer, M.K., Navscaria, H.A., Stevens, H.P. *et al.* (1995) Novel mutations in keratin-1b gene underly focal non-epidermolytic palmoplantar keratoderma. (NEPPK) in 2 families. *Human Molecular Genetics* **4**, 1875.

Sheffield, L.J., Danks, D.M., Mayne, V. & Hutchinson, L.A. (1976) Chondrodysplasia punctata—23 cases of a mild and relatively common variety. *Journal of Pediatrics* **89**, 916.

Shirren, V. & Dinger, R. (1965) Untersuchungen bei keratosis palmo-plantaris papulosa. *Archives of Clinical and Experimental Dermatology* **221**, 481.

Skinner, B.A., Greist, M.C. & Norins, A.L. (1981) Keratitis, ichthyosis and deafness (KID) syndrome. *Archives of Dermatology* **117**, 285.

Smith, F.J.D., Corden, L.D., Rugg, E.L. *et al.* (1997) Missense mutations in keratin 17 cause either pachyonychia congenita type 2 or a phenotype resembling steatocystoma multiplex. *Journal of Investigative Dermatology* **108**, 220.

Soekarman, D., Cobben, J.M., Vogels, A., Spauwen, P.H. & Fryns, J.P. (1995) Variable expression of the popliteal pterygium syndrome in two 3-generation families. *Clinical Genetics* **47**, 169.

Solomon, L.M. & Kcuer, E.J. (1980) The ectodermal dysplasias. Problems of classification and some newer syndromes. *Archives of Dermatology* **116**, 1295.

Sparrow, G.D., Samman, P.D. & Wells, R.S. (1976) Hyperpigmentation and hypohidrosis. *Clinical and Experimental Dermatology* **1**, 127.

Stefanini, M., Vermeulen, W., Weeda, G. *et al.* (1993) A new nucleotide-excision-repair gene associated with the disorder trichothio-dystrophy. *American Journal of Human Genetics* **53**, 817.

Stevanovic, D.V. (1959) Alopecia congenita. *Acta Geneticae Medicae et Gemellologiae (Roma)* **9**, 127.

Stevens, H.P., Kelsell, D.P., Bryant, S.P. *et al.* (1996) Linkage of an American pedigree with palmoplantar keratoderma and malignancy (palmoplantar dysplasia type III) to 17q24. *Archives of Dermatology* **132**, 640.

Stratton, R.F., Jorgensen, R.J. & Krause, I.C. (1993) Possible second case of tricho-oculo-dermo-vertebral (alves) syndrome. *American Journal of Medical Genetics* **46**, 313.

Su, W.P.D., Chun, S.I., Hammond, D.E. & Gordon, H. (1990) Pachyonychia congenita: a clinical study of 12 cases and review of the literature. *Pediatric Dermatology* **7**, 33.

Sybert, V.P. (1985) Aplasia cutis congenita: a report of 12 new families and review of the literature. *Pediatric Dermatology* **3**, 1.

Sybert, V.P. (1989) Hypohidrotic ectodermal dysplasia: argument against an autosomal recessive form clinically indistinguishable from X-linked hypohidrotic ectodermal dysplasia (Christ–Siemens–Touraine syndrome). *Pediatric Dermatology* **6**, 76.

Thomas, D.R., Jorizzo, J.L., Brysk, M.M., Tschen, J.A., Miller, J. & Tschen, E.H. (1984) Pachyonychia congenita. *Archives of Dermatology* **120**, 1475.

Thorel, F.M. (1964) Un cas de maladie de Méléda, variété Papillin-Lefèvre avec surdité. *Bulletin de la Société Française de Dermatologie et de Syphiligraphie* **71**, 707.

Tidman, M.J., Wells, R.S. & MacDonald, D.M. (1987) Pachyonychia congenita with cutaneous amyloidosis and hyperpigmentation—a distinct variant. *Journal of the American Academy of Dermatology* **16**, 935.

Tolmie, J.L., Browne, B.H., McGettrick, P.M. & Stephenson, J.B.P. (1988a) A familial syndrome with coats' reaction retina angiomas, hair and nail defects and intracranial calcification. *Eye* **2**, 297.

Tolmie, J.L., Wilcox, D.E., McWilliam, R., Assindi, A. & Stephenson, J.P.B. (1988b) Palmoplantar keratoderma; nail dystrophy, and hereditary motor and sensory neuropathy: an autosomal dominant trait. *Journal of Medical Genetics* **25**, 754.

Toriello, H.V., Lindstrom, J.A., Waterman, D.F. & Baugham, F.A. (1979) Reevaluation of CHANDS. *Journal of Medical Genetics* **16**, 316.

Tosti, A., Miscali, C., Piraccini, B., Barbaraschi, M. & Ferretti, R.M. (1994) Woolly hair, palmoplantar keratoderma and cardiac abnormalities: report of a family. *Archives of Dermatology* **130**, 522.

Traboulsi, E.I., Faris, B.M. & Kaloustian, V.M. (1986) Persistant hyperplastic primary vitreous and recessive oculodentoosseous dysplasia. *American Journal of Medical Genetics* **24**, 95.

Tsakalakos, N., Jordaan, F.H., Taaljaard, J.J. & Hough, S.F. (1986) A previously undescribed ectodermal dysplasia of the tricho-odonto-onychial subgroup in a family. *Archives of Dermatology* **122**, 1047.

Verhage, J., Habbema, L., Vrensen, G.F.J., Roord, J.J. & Bleeker-Wagemakers, E.H. (1987) A patient with onychotrichodysplasia, neutropenia and normal intelligence. *Clinical Genetics* **31**, 374.

Vogt, B.R., Traupe, H. & Hamm, H. (1988) Congenital atrichia with nail dystrophy, abnormal facies, and retarded psychomotor development in two siblings: a new autosomal recessive syndrome? *Pediatric Dermatology* **5**, 236.

Vohwinkel, K.H. (1929) Keratoma hereditarium mutilans. *Archives of Dermatology* **158**, 354.

Walbaum, R., Fontaine, G., Lienhardt, J. & Piquet, J.J. (1970) Surdite familiale avec osteo-onycho-dysplasie. *Journal de Genetique Humaine* **18**, 101.

Weary, P.E., Manley, W.F. Jr & Graham, G.F. (1971) Hereditary acrokeratotic poikiloderma. *Archives of Dermatology* **103**, 409.

Weech, A.A. (1929) Hereditary ectodermal dysplasia (congenital ectodermal defect). A report of two cases. *American Journal of Diseases of Children* **37**, 766.

Weeda, G., Eveno, E., Donker, I. *et al.* (1997) A mutation in the XPB/ERCC3 DNA repair transcription gene, associated with trichothiodystrophy. *American Journal of Human Genetics* **60**, 320.

Wilkey, W.D. & Stevenson, G.H. (1945) A family with inherited ectodermal dystrophy. *Canadian Medical Association Journal* **53**, 226.

Wilson, W.G., Greer, K.E., Martof, A.B., McIlhenny, J. & Hatter, D.L. (1989) 'New' ectodermal dysplasia syndrome with distinctive facial appearance and preaxial polydactyly of feet. *American Journal of Medical Genetics* **34**, 227.

Winter, R.M., MacDermott, K.D. & Hill, F.J. (1988) Sparse hair, short stature, hypoplastic thumbs, single upper central incisor and abnormal skin pigmentation: a possible 'new' form of ectodermal dysplasia. *American Journal of Medical Genetics* **29**, 209.

Witkop, C.J., Brearly, L.J. & Gentry, W.D. (1975) Hypoplastic enamel, onycholysis and hypohidrosis inherited as an autosomal dominant trait. *Oral Surgery* **39**, 71.

Zirbel, G.M., Ruttum, M.S., Post, A.C. & Esterly, N.B. (1995) Odonto-onychodermal dysplasia. *British Journal of Dermatology* **133**, 797.

Zonana, J., Clarke, A., Sarfarazi, M. *et al.* (1988) X-linked hypohidrotic ectodermal dysplasia: localization within the region Xq11–21.1 by linkage analysis and implications for carrier detection and prenatal diagnosis. *American Journal of Human Genetics* **43**, 75.

## Disease loci and chromosome anomalies

Chromosomal localization has now been established for several genetic traits. Mapping of important disease loci has increased rapidly during the last years. As the specific genes and their products are discovered for particular disorders, disease names no longer appear in the individual chromosome tables. Syndromes with chromosome anomalies usually have mental deficiency and dysmorphic changes as the main features together with multiple defects (McKusick 1998). The nails are often convex or hypoplastic from birth. The Noonan or male Turner's syndrome (MIM *163950) has a 45X chromosomal abberation. The patients have small stature and lymphoedema of the hands and feet (Fig. 9.20). The short and wide nails show koilonychia and are sometimes missing. Same as cardio-facio-cutaneous syndrome (Table 9.1) (Ward *et al.* 1994).

### References

McKusick, V.A. (1998) *Mendelian Inheritance in Man. A Catalogue of Human Genes and Genetic Disorders*, 12th Edn, Vol. II. Johns Hopkins University Press, Baltimore.

Ward, K.A., Moss, C. & McKeown, C. (1994) The cardio-facio-cutaneous syndrome: a manifestation of the Noonan syndrome? *British Journal of Dermatology* **131**, 270.

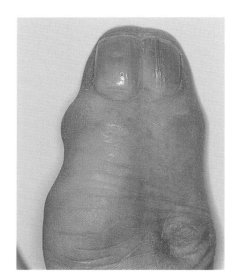

**Fig. 9.21** Fused digits and nails.

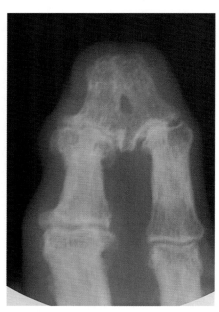

**Fig. 9.22** X-ray of digits in Fig. 9.21—only terminal phalanges are fused.

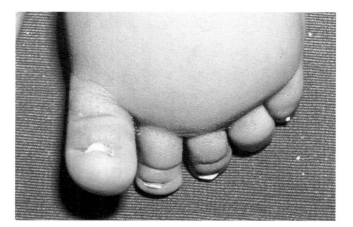

**Fig. 9.20** Turner's syndrome (Table 9.5). Narrow hypoplastic nails associated with limb lymphoedema. (Courtesy of L. Tamayo, Mexico DF.)

## Nail change in syndromes with predominant skeletal anomalies

In patients with bradydactyly, syndactyly, zygodactyly and polydactyly the nails are sometimes malformed or absent. When the distal phalanges are involved the nails are often longitudinally convex and/or broad (Figs 9.21 & 9.22). Skeletal changes are also found in syndromes with ectodermal dysplasia (Tables 9.1 & 9.2) and with chromosomal anomalies.

### Hypoplastic or atrophic nails with skeletal anomalies

These disorders are listed in Table 9.4. In particular, congenital onychodysplasia of the index fingers (COIF), also termed Kikuchi syndrome, will be discussed (Figs 9.23–9.26). Baran

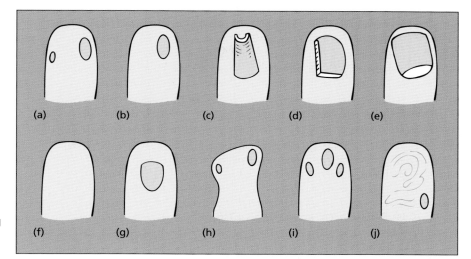

**Fig. 9.23** Types of micronychia and other dystrophies seen particularly in congenital onychodystrophy of the index fingers (COIF). (a) Polyonychia in COIF; (b) micronychia in COIF; (c) 'rolled' micronychia in COIF; (d) hemionychogryphosis in COIF; (e) malalignment in COIF; (f) anonychia in COIF; (g) usual micronychia; (h) polyonychia in syndactyly; (i) polyonychia in congenital skin disease; (j) onychoheterotopia (Ohya's type). (After Baran 1980; Kikuchi 1991; Millman & Strier 1982.)

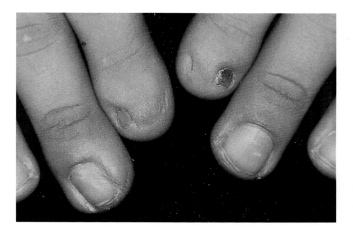

**Fig. 9.24** Kikuchi (COIF) syndrome—see Fig. 9.23; classical involvement of the index fingers.

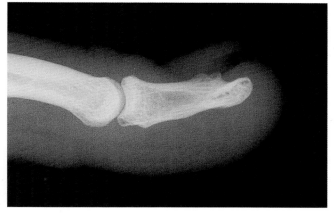

**Fig. 9.26** COIF syndrome—X-ray showing Y-shaped bifurcation of the distal phalanx.

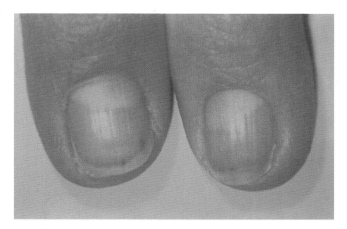

**Fig. 9.25** COIF syndrome—asymmetrical lunula leading to hemionychogryphosis.

(1980) suggested that it was congenital and characterized by a variety of nail deformities affecting one or both index fingers (Fig. 9.23) and by bone abnormalities, such as a Y-shaped bifurcation of the distal phalanx, visible on lateral X-ray pictures (Fig. 9.26). Such a bone abnormality may occur under both normal and abnormal nails. The defects are mainly seen on the radial side of the index fingers. Kikuchi *et al.* (1981) related this to the smaller calibre of the artery on the radial side. Micronychia is the commonest clinical manifestation. The so-called 'rolled micronychia' is a rare variant. Anonychia, hemionychogryphosis or simple malalignment are also less frequent presentations. A deformed lunula was described by Baran and Stroud (1984). Millman and Strier (1982), in an extensive article, described nine members of one family who suffered from the COIF syndrome; the clinical spectrum was broadened to include autosomal dominant inheritance. This syndrome was described in identical twins (Kameyoshi *et al.* 1998). Kikuchi (1991) described a case where both thumbnails also were involved. He thought that it could be related to an

**Table 9.4** Atrophic or hypoplastic nails with skeletal anomalies.

| Disease | Inheritance | Nails | Other symptoms |
|---|---|---|---|
| Acrogeria. Gottron syndrome (Grüneberg 1960; de Groot et al. 1980) | 201200 | Atrophic nails | Thin skin with senile changes limited to distal extremities |
| Brachydactyly with absence of middle phalanges and hypoplastic nails (Bass 1968; Cuevas-Sosa & Garcia-Segur 1971; Schott 1978) | AD *112900 | Hypoplasia or absence of several nails | Brachydactyly. Duplicated phalanges of thumbs. Sometimes syndactyly |
| Brachymorphism-onychodysplasia-dysphalangism (BOD) syndrome (Verloes et al. 1993) | AD? 113477 | Hypoplasia or absent | Hypoplasia distal phalanges. Facial dysmorphism, short stature |
| CHARGE association (Meinecke et al. 1989) 14q22–q24.3 duplication (North et al. 1995) | AR 214800 | Hypoplastic | Colomboma, heart anomaly, choanal atresia. Retardation. Genital and ear anomalies |
| Chondrodysplasia type Grebe (Hattab et al. 1996) | AR *200700 | Short dysplastic on bud-like fingertips | Asymmetrical dysplasia of long bones, prominent forehead, hypodontia, hearing loss |
| COIF syndrome (see below) | | | |
| Congenital hemidysplasia with ichthyosiform erythroderma and limb defects. CHILD syndrome (Happle et al. 1980; Christiansen et al. 1984; von Schlenzka et al. 1989; Hashimoto et al. 1995) | XD 308050 | Dystrophic on affected side | Mainly in females. Postzygotic mutation (Happle et al. 1996) |
| Cleidocranial dysostosis with micrognathia, absent thumbs and distal aphangia (Yunis & Varon 1980; Rabe et al. 1996) | AD *216340 | Hypoplastic or absent. Short fingertips and toes | |
| Craniofrontonasal dysplasia (Grutzner & Gorlin 1988; Orlow 1992; Saavedra et al. 1996) | XD 304110 | Longitudinally grooved nails, heminychia or anonychia | Hypertelorism, broad nasal root, syndactyly craniosynostosis. Curly hair |
| Frontometaphyseal dysplasia (Gorlin & Cohen 1969; Glass & Rosenbaum 1995) | AD *305620 | Short nails | Marked supraorbital bony ridge. Skeletal alteration. Deafness. Missing teeth |
| Fryns syndrome (Fryns 1987; Van Hove et al. 1995) | AR *229850 | Hypoplastic and small | Characteristic facies with broad nasal bridge, cleft palate, distal digital hypoplasia and urogenital and neurological anomalies |
| Hairy elbows syndrome (Beighton 1970; Edwards et al. 1994) | AR 139600 | Short | Hypertrichosis of elbows. Short stature. Facial asymmetry |
| Incontinentia pigmenti, Bloch-Sulzberger syndrome (Carney & Carney 1970; El-Benhawi & George 1988; Dolan et al. 1992; Sybert 1994) | XD *308310 Xq28 Male, lethal *308300 Xq1121 Sporadic | Dystrophic. In 7% koilonychia. At 15 years subungual tender tumours which clear spontaneously (Hartman 1966; Pinol Aguade et al. 1973; Mascaro et al. 1985) | Vesicular, verrucous and swirling pattern of pigmented macular lesions. Later hypopigmented. Anomalies of eyes (30–50%), nervous system (30%), teeth (65%), skeleton (13%), alopecia (40%) |

| Syndrome | Inheritance | OMIM | Nail changes | Other features |
|---|---|---|---|---|
| Kikuchi COIF syndrome, congenital onychodysplasia of the index fingers (Brunzlow et al. 1987; Millman & Strier 1982; Bittar et al. 1988; Youn et al. 1996) | AD | – | Anonychia, micronychia or polyonychia of index finger (Figs 9.4–9.6) | |
| Lethal syndrome with cloudy cornea, diaphragmatic and distal defects (Fryns et al. 1979; Young et al. 1986) | AR | *229800 | Small, hypoplastic | Stillborn or dead shortly after birth. Coarse face, small eyes, cleft palate, hypoplasia of lungs; diaphragm and distal bone deformation |
| Osteo-onychodysplasia. Nail–patella syndrome (Pye-Smith 1893; Gibbs et al. 1964). See page 372 | AD | *161200 | Short, narrow, fragile, changes most pronounced on the thumb where the nails might be missing. Sometimes koilonychia. Toes rarely affected. Pterygium. Lunula missing or V-shaped (Fig. 9.2) | Patella absent 92%. Radius head small. Iliac crest exocytosis. Eyes and kidney abnormalities as well as other changes occasionally. Linked to ABO blood group. Locus localized on chromosome |
| Pallister-Hall syndrome (Verloes et al. 1995) | AD | | Hypoplastic | Hypothalamin hamartoblastoma. Facial dysmorphism cleft epiglottis and bony anomalies |
| Poikiloderma congenita. Rothmund–Thomson syndrome (Silver 1966; Vennos et al. 1992) | AR | *268400 | Nails small; thin and dystrophic in 25% | Short phalanges. Small stature. Saddle nose. Frontal bossing. Photosensitive cataracts. Skin of cheeks red and swollen about the 3rd month of age, then on extensor surface of extremities. Later atrophy, pigmentation and telangiectasia |
| Pre- and postnatal growth retardation, mental retardation and acral limb deficiences (Cartwright et al. 1991) | – | – | Small, hyperconvex and poorly keratinized | Facial dysmorphism |
| Progeria. Hutchinson–Gilford syndrome (De Busk 1972; Jimbow et al. 1988; Badame 1989; Brown et al. 1990; Erdem et al. 1994) | AR | 176670 | Thin, yellow, atrophic | Dwarfism, pseudosenility. Small face giving a hydrocephalic appearance. Bird face. Narrow chest, other bone deformations. Arteriosclerosis. Atrophic skin. Gene on chromosome 1 |
| Rüdiger syndrome (Rüdiger et al. 1970) | AR | 268650 | Hypoplastic | Somatic retardation, small fingers, ureteral stenosis, cleft palate, coarse facies Death within 1st year of life |
| Weaver syndrome (Fitch 1980; Dumic et al. 1993) | AD | 277590 | Thin, deep set nails | Unusual facies. Increased weight, height and bifrontal diameter. Hypertonia. Prominent fingerpads. Hoarse voice |
| Werner syndrome (Epstein et al. 1966; Yu et al. 1997) | AR | *277700 | Atrophic nails | Short stature, premature greying and baldness. Juvenile cataracts. Hypogonadism, diabetes, calcification of blood vessels, osteoporosis. Atrophic skin. Wasting of musculature. Loss of WRN gene product |
| Williams elfin facies syndrome (Jones & Smith 1975; Perez Jurado et al. 1996; Dutly & Schinzel 1996 for ref.) | AD | #194050 | Short, deep set or brittle | Coarse facies, depressed nasal bridge, hoarse voice, aortic stenosis, growth deficiency and mental retardation. Deletion of elastin, ELN locus chromosome 7q11.23 |

Inheritances are indicated as follows: AD, autosomal dominant; AR, autosomal recessive; XD, sex-linked dominant.

abnormal handgrip in fetal life. Kitamaya and Tsukada (1983) prefer the term congenital onychodysplasia because it is not only located on the index finger. They assumed that it is due to ischaemic damage in embryonic life. Kikuchi's syndrome has also been reported with anomaly of the great toe (Koizumi *et al.* 1998). Isolated congenital onychodysplasia of the toenails has been observed (Biedermann *et al.* 1995; Herzberger & Runne 1998).

## References

Badame, A.J. (1989) Progeria. *Archives of Dermatology* **125**, 540.

Baran, R. (1980) Syndrome d'Iso et Kikuchi. *Annales de Dermatologie et de Vénéréologie* **107**, 431.

Baran, R. & Stroud, J.D. (1984) Congenital onychodysplasia of the index finger (Iso and Kikuchi syndrome). *Archives of Dermatology* **120**, 243.

Bass, H.N. (1968) Familial absence of middle phalanges with nail dysplasia: a new syndrome. *Pediatrics* **42**, 318.

Beighton, P.H. (1970) Familial hypertrichosis cubiti: hairy elbows syndrome. *Journal of Medical Genetics* **7**, 158.

Biedermann, T., Schirren, C.G., Schirren, H. *et al.* (1995) Kongenitale Onychodysplasie (Iso–Kikuchi syndrome). *Hautarzt* **46**, 53–56.

Bittar, E.O., Parra, C.A., de Prieto, G.L., Briggs, E. & Baeza, O.O. (1988) Kongenitale ischämische Onychodystrophie (Iso–Kikuchi-Syndrom) und chronischer Lupus erythematodes. *Hautarzt* **39**, 750.

Brown, W.T., Abenur, J., Goonewardena, P. *et al.* (1990) Hutchinson–Gilford progeria syndrome, clinical, chromosomal and metabolic abnormalities [abstract]. *American Journal of Human Genetics* **47** (Suppl.), A50.

Brunzlow, H., Lorck, D. & Neumann, J. (1987) Beitrag zum Iso–Kikuchi-Syndrom Kongenitale Onychodysplasie. *Radiologia Diagnostica (Berlin)* **6**, 773.

Carney, R.G. & Carney, G. Jr (1970) Incontinentia pigmenti. *Archives of Dermatology* **102**, 157.

Cartwright, J., Nelson, M. & Fryns, F.P. (1991) Pre- and postnatal growth retardation–severe mental retardation–acral limb deficiences with poorly keratinized nails. *Genetics Counselling* **2**, 147.

Christiansen, J.V., Petersen, H.O. & Søgaard, H. (1984) The CHILD-syndrome—congential hemidysplasia with ichthyosiform erythroderma and limb defects. A case report. *Acta Dermato-Venereologica* **64**, 165.

Cuevas-Sosa, A. & Garcia-Segur, F. (1971) Brachydactyly with absence of middle phalanges and hypoplastic nails. A new herediatry syndrome. *Journal of Bone and Joint Surgery* **53B**, 101.

De Busk, F.L. (1972) The Hutchinson–Gilford progeria syndrome. *Journal of Pediatrics* **80**, 697.

Dolan, O.M., Bingham, E.A. & Corbett, J.R. (1992) Incontinentia pigmenti. *British Journal of Dermatology* **127** (Suppl. 40), 54.

Dumic, M., Vukovic, J., Cvitkovic, M. & Medica, I. (1993) Twins and their mildly affected mother with Weaver syndrome. *Clinical Genetics* **44**, 338.

Dutly, F. & Schinzel, A. (1996) Unequal interchromosomal rearrangements may result in elastin gene deletions causing the Williams–Beuren syndrome. *Human Molecular Genetics* **5**, 1893.

Edwards, M.J., Crawford, A.E., Jammu, V. & Wise, G. (1994) Hypotrichosis 'cubiti'. *American Journal of Medical Genetics* **26**, 382.

El-Benhawi, M.O. & George, W.M. (1988) Incontinentia pigmenti: a review. *Cutis* **41**, 259.

Epstein, C.J., Martin, G.M., Schultz, A.L. & Motulsky, A.G. (1966) Werner's syndrome. Review of its symptomatology, natural history, pathology features, genetics and relationships to natural aging process. *Medicine (Baltimore)* **45**, 177.

Fitch, N. (1980) The syndromes of Marshall and Weaver. *Journal of Medical Genetics* **17**, 174.

Fryns, J.P. (1987) Fryns syndrome: a variable MCA syndrome with diaphragmatic defects, coarse face, and distal limb hypoplasia. *Journal of Medical Genetics* **24**, 271.

Fryns, J.P., Moerman, R., Goddeeris, P., Bossuyt, C. & van den Berghe, H. (1979) A new lethal syndrome with cloudy corneae, diaphragmatic defects and distal limbs deformities. *Human Genetics* **50**, 65.

Gibbs, R., Berczellar, P.H. & Hyman, A.B. (1964) Nail–patella–elbow syndrome. *Archives of Dermatology* **89**, 196.

Glass, R.B.J. & Rosenbaum, K.N. (1995) Frontometaphyseal dysplasia: neonatal radiographic diagnosis. *American Journal of Medical Genetics* **57**, 1.

Gorlin, R.J. & Cohen, M.M. Jr (1969) Frontometaphyseal dysplasia: a new syndrome. *American Journal of Diseases of Children* **118**, 487.

de Groot, W.P., Tafelkruyer, J. & Woerdeman, M.J. (1980) Familial acrogeria (Gottron). *British Journal of Dermatology* **103**, 213.

Grüneberg, T. (1960) Die Akrogerie (Gottron). *Archives of Clinical and Experimental Dermatology* **210**, 409.

Grutzner, E. & Gorlin, R.J. (1988) Craniofrontonasal dysplasia: phenotypic expression in females and males and genetic considerations. *Oral Surgery Oral Medicine Oral Pathology* **65**, 436.

Happle, R., Koch, H. & Lenz, W. (1980) The CHILD-syndrome. Congenital hemidysplasia with ichthyosiform erythroderma and limb defects. *European Journal of Pediatrics* **134**, 27.

Happle, R., Effendy, I., Megahed, M., Orlov, S.J. & Kuster, W. (1996) CHILD syndrome in a boy. *American Journal of Medical Genetics* **62**, 192.

Hartman, D.L. (1966) Incontinentia pigmenti associated with subungual tumour. *Archives of Dermatology* **94**, 632.

Hashimoto, K., Topper, S., Sharata, H. & Edwards, M. (1995) Child syndrome: analysis of abnormal keratinization and ultrastructure. *Pediatric Dermatology* **12**, 116.

Hattab, F.N., Al-Khateeb, T. & Mansour, M. (1996) Oral manifestations of severe short limb dwarfism resembling Grebe chondrodysplasia. *Oral Surgery Oral Medicine Oral Pathology* **81**, 550.

Herzberger, G. & Runne, U. (1998) Isolierte Kongenitale anonychie der Zehennägel D2–D4 beidseits (Iso–Kikuchi Syndrom). *Zeitschrift für Hautkrankheiten* **73**, 550.

Jimbow, K., Kobayashi, H., Ishii, M., Oyanagi, A. & Ooshima, A. (1988) Scar and keloid-like lesions in progeria. An electron-microscopic and immunohistochemical study. *Archives of Dermatology* **124**, 1261.

Jones, K. & Smith, D.W. (1975) The Williams elfin facies syndrome: a new perspective. *Journal of Pediatrics* **86**, 718.

Kameyoshi, Y., Iwazaki, Y., Hide, M. & Yamamoto, S. (1998) Congenital onychodysplasia of the index finger in identical twins. *British Journal of Dermatology* **139**, 1120.

Kikuchi, I. (1991) Congenital onychodysplasia of the index fingers: a case involving the thumbnails. *Seminars in Dermatology* **10**, 7.

Kikuchi, I., Ishii, Y., Idemori, M. & Ogata, K. (1981) Congenital onychodysplasia of the index fingers. *Journal of Dermatology* **8**, 51.

Kitamaya, Y. & Tsukada, S. (1983) Congenital onychodysplasia: report of 11 cases. *Archives of Dermatology* **119**, 8.

Koizumi, H., Tomoyori, T. & Ohkawaza, A. (1998) Congenital onychodysplasia of the index fingers with anomaly of the great toe. *Acta Dermato-Venereologica* **76**, 322–323.

Mascaro, J.M., Palou, J. & Vives, P. (1985) Painful subungual keratotic tumors in incontinentia pigmenti. *Journal of the American Academy of Dermatology* **13**, 913.

Meinecke, P., Pole, A. & Schmiegelow, P. (1989) Limb anomalies in the CHARGE association. *Journal of Medical Genetics* **26**, 202.

Millman, A.J. & Strier, R.P. (1982) Congenital onychodysplasia of the index fingers. *Journal of the American Academy of Dermatology* **7**, 57.

North, K.N., Wu, B.L., Cao, B.N., Whiteman, D.A.H. & Korf, B.R. (1995) CHARGE association in a child with *de novo* inverted duplication (14) (q22–q24.3). *American Journal of Medical Genetics* **26**, 202.

Orlow, S.J. (1992) Cutaneous findings in craniofacial malformation syndromes. *Archives of Dermatology* **128**, 1379.

Perez Jurado, L.A., Peoples, R., Kaplan, P., Hamel, B.C.J. & Francke, U. (1996) Molecular definition of the chromosome 7 deletion: Williams syndrome and parent-of-origin effects on growth. *American Journal of Human Genetics* **59**, 781.

Pinol Aguade, J., Mascaro, J.M., Herrero, C. & Castel, T. (1973) Tumeurs sous-unguéales dyskératosiques douloureuses et spontanément résolutives. Les rapports avec l'Incontinentia Pigmenti. *Annales de Dermatologie et de Syphiligraphie* **100**, 159.

Pye-Smith, R.J. (1893) Notes on a family presenting in most of its members certain deformities of the joints of both limbs. *Medicine Press* **34**, 504.

Rabe, H., Brune, T., Rossi, R. *et al.* (1996) Yunis–Varon syndrome. *Clinical Dysmorphology* **5**, 217.

Rüdiger, R.A., Haase, W. & Passarge, E. (1970) Association of ectrodactyly, ectodermal dysplasia and cleft lip-palate. *American Journal of Diseases of Children* **120**, 160.

Saavedra, D., Richieri-Costa, A., Guion-Almeida, M.L. & Cohen, M.M. Jr (1996) Craniofrontonasal syndrome: study of 41 patients. *American Journal of Medical Genetics* **61**, 147.

von Schlenzka, K., Gehre, M., Neumann, H.-J. & Sochor, H. (1989) CHILD-Syndrome—kasuistischer Beitreag zur Kenntnis dieser seltenen Genodermatose. *Dermatologische Monatsschrift* **175**, 100.

Schott, G.D. (1978) Hereditary brachydactyly with nail dysplasia. *Journal of Medical Genetics* **15**, 119.

Silver, H.K. (1966) Rothmund–Thomson syndrome: an oculocutaneous disorder. *American Journal of Diseases of Children* **111**, 182.

Sybert, V.P. (1994) Incontinentia pigmenti nomenclature [letter]. *American Journal of Human Genetics*. **55**, 209.

Van Hove, J.L.K., Spiridigliozzi, G.A., Heinz, R., McConkie-Rosell, A., Iafolla, K. & Kahler, S.G. (1995) Fryns syndrome: survivors and neurologic outcome. *American Journal of Medical Genetics* **59**, 334.

Vennos, E.M., Collins, M. & James, W.D. (1992) Rothmund–Thomson syndrome: review of the world literature. *Journal of the American Academy of Dermatology* **27**, 750.

Verloes, A., Bonneau, D., Guidi, O. *et al.* (1993) Brachymorphism-onychodysplasia-dysphalangism syndrome. *Journal of Medical Genetics* **30**, 158.

Youn, S.H., Kwon, O.S., Park, K.C. *et al.* (1996) Congenital onychodysplasia of the index fingers. Iso–Kikuchi syndrome. A case involving the second toenail. *Clinical and Experimental Dermatology* **21**, 457–458.

Young, I.D., Simpson, K. & Winter, R.M. (1986) A case of Fryns syndrome. *Journal of Medical Genetics* **23**, 82.

Yu, C.-E., Oshima, J., Wijsman, E.M. *et al.* (1997) Werner's syndrome collaborative group: mutations in the concensus helicase domains of the Werner syndrome gene. *American Journal of Human Genetics* **60**, 330.

Yunis, E. & Varon, H. (1980) Cleidocranial dysostosis, severe micrognathism, bilateral abscence of thumbs and 1st metatarsal bone, and distal aphalangia: a new genetic syndrome. *American Journal of Diseases of Children* **134**, 649.

## Hyperonychia, hyperplastic thick nails

Large nails are seen in patients with macrodactylia due to epidermal naevus, gigantism and various connective tissue syndromes (Greenberg *et al.* 1987). Thick nails are common in patients with various types of keratoderma (Table 9.1) and in ichthyosiform dermatitis (Table 9.2). Schulze (1966), Burg (1975) and Bazex *et al.* (1990) described families with thick and hard nails with partial onycholysis (MIM 164800) but without other anomalies (Fig. 9.27). Thick nails that split into double layers (matrix doubling syndrome) on the fingers and toes was reported by Vigh & Pinter 1973. The patients also showed oculomotor paresis, debility and external ear aplasia. Three cases of nail bed hyperkeratosis where the base is normal, the surface smooth but the distal part of the nail is raised up from the nail bed by a dark friable horny mass, were described by Garrick Wilson and Cantab (1905). A special form is pachonychia, i.e. thickening of the nail bed with elevation of the nail plate, which occurs in pachonychia congenita (page 388). Pachyonychia on the toes was found in patients having a rare syndrome with severe mental retardation and unusual facies together with large ears; this is associated with a stable ring group G chromosome (Dubowitz *et al.* 1971).

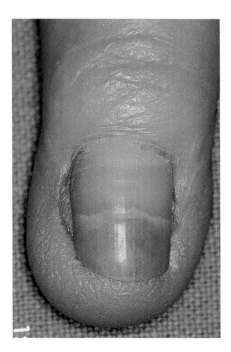

**Fig. 9.27** Congenital 'onycholysis'.

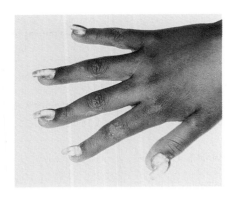

**Fig. 9.28** Congenital onychogryphosis.

Onychogryphosis (Fig. 9.28) can occur with autosomal dominant inheritance, but usually appears first in early childhood (Heller 1927; Clement 1928; Orel 1928; Videbaeck 1948; Lubach 1982). It can also be seen with other ectodermal malformations (Tables 9.1 & 9.2).

## References

Bazex, J., Baran, R., Monbrun, F., Griforieff-Larrue, N. & Marguery, M.C. (1990) Hereditary distal onycholysis—a case report. *Clinical and Experimental Dermatology* **15**, 146.

Burg, G. (1975) Onycholysis partialis hereditaria cum scleronychia. *Hautarzt* **26**, 386.

Clement, L.S. (1928) A claw-fingered family. The inheritance of nail mutation in man. *Journal of Heredity* **19**, 529.

Dubowitz, V., Cooke, P., Colver, D. & Harris, F. (1971) Mental retardation, unusual facies and abnormal nails associated with a group G ring chromosome. *Journal of Medical Genetics* **8**, 195.

Garrick Wilson, A. & Cantab, M.B. (1905) Three cases of hereditary hyperkeratosis of the nail bed. *British Journal of Dermatology* **17**, 13.

Greenberg, G.M., Pess, G.M. & May, J.W. (1987) Macrodactyly and the epidermal nevus syndrome. *Journal of Hand Surgery* **12**, 730.

Heller, J. (1927) Die Krankheiten der Nägel. In: *Handbuch der Haut und Geschlechtskrankheiten*, Bd VIII/2 (ed. J.J. Jadassohn), pp. 1–423. Springer, Berlin.

Lubach, D. (1982) Erbliche Onychogryposis. *Hautarzt* **33**, 331.

Orel, H. (1928) Über eine Familie mit erblicher Onychogryposis. *Archives of Rassenbiology* **20**, 169.

Schulze, H.D. (1966) Hereditary Onycholysis partialis mit Skleronychie. *Dermatologische Wochenschrift* **30**, 766.

Videbaeck, A. (1948) Hereditary onychogryphosis. *Annals of Eugenics (London)* **14**, 139.

Vigh, G. & Pinter, L. (1973) Nagelmatrix-Verdoppelungssyndrom. *Zeitschrift für Haut und Geschlechtskrankheiten* **48**, 125.

Youn, S.H., Kwon, O.S., Park, K.C., Youn, J.I. & Chung, J.H. (1996) Congenital dysplasia of the index fingers—Iso–Kikuchi syndrome. *Clinical and Experimental Dermatology* **21**, 457–458.

## Clubbing, acropachy, hippocratic nails (*119900)

Here the nails are thick and curved. Most common are the acquired forms seen in association with pulmonary and other systemic diseases. A hereditary form of clubbing without any other symptoms has been reviewed by Fischer *et al.* (1964). It has a gradual onset from puberty. The cause of the clubbing is unknown and it is usually not evident before early childhood. Clubbing can also be seen as a part of various syndromes, which are listed in Table 9.5.

## References

Andrén, L., Dymling, J.F., Hogeman, K.E. & Wendeberg, B. (1962) Osteoporosis acroosteolytica: a syndrome of osteoporosis, acro-osteolysis and open sutures of the skull. *Acta Chirurgica Scandinavica* **12**, 496.

Barrière, H., Liton, R. & Bureau, B. (1977) Kératose liqénoide striée: Forme congenitale. *Annales de Dermatologie et de Vénéréologie* **104**, 767.

Bureau, Y., Barrière, H. & Thomas, M. (1959) Hippocratisme digital congénital avec hyperkératose palmo-plantaire et trobules osseux. *Annales de Dermatologie et de Vénéréologie* **86**, 611.

Cheney, W.D. (1965) Acro-osteolysis. *American Journal of Roentgenology* **94**, 595.

Christian, C.D., McLoughlin, T.G., Cathcart, E.S. & Eisenberg, M.M. (1964) Peutz–Jegher's syndrome associated with functioning ovarian tumor. *Journal of the American Medical Association* **190**, 935.

David, T.J. & Burwood, R.L. (1972) The nature and inheritance of Kirner's deformity. *Journal of Medical Genetics* **9**, 430.

Dore, D.D., MacEwen, G.D. & Boulos, M.I. (1987) Cleidocranial dysostosis and syringomyelia: review of the literature and case report. *Clinical Orthopedics* **214**, 229.

Elias, A.N., Pinals, R.S., Andersson, C.H., Gould, L.V. & Streeten, D.H.P. (1978) Hereditary osteodysplasia with acro-osteolysis (the Hajdu–Cheney syndrome). *American Journal of Medicine* **65**, 627.

Erdem, N., Günes, A.T., Avci, O. & Osma, E. (1994) A case of Hutchinson–Gilford progeria syndrome mimicking scleredema in early infancy. *Dermatology* **188**, 318.

Fazio, M., Lisi, S., Amantea, A., Maini, A. *et al.* (1995) Poikilodermie sclérosante héréditaire de Weary. *Annales de Dermatologie et de Vénéréologie* **122**, 618.

Fischer, D.R., Singer, D.H. & Feldman, S.M. (1964) Clubbing, a review with emphasis on hereditary acropachy. *Medicine* **43**, 459.

Fryburg, J.S. & Sidhu-Malik, N. (1995) Long-term follow-up of cutaneous changes in siblings with mandibuloacral dysplasia who were originally considered to have hereditary sclerosing poikiloderma. *Journal of the American Academy of Dermatology* **33**, 900.

Fryns, J.-P., Stinckens, C. & Feenestra, L. (1997) Vocal cord paralysis and cystic kidney disease in Hajdu–Cheney syndrome. *Clinical Genetics* **51**, 271.

Gelb, B.D., Shi, G.-P., Chapman, H.A. & Desnick, R.J. (1996) Pycnodysostosis, a lysosomal disease caused by cathepsin K deficiency. *Science* **273**, 1236.

Greer, K.E., Weary, P.E., Nagy, R. & Robinow, M. (1978) Hereditary sclerosing poikiloderma. *International Journal of Dermatology* **17**, 316.

Hemminki, A., Tomlinson, I., Markie, D. *et al.* (1997) Localization of a susceptibility locus for Peutz–Jeghers syndrome to 19p using comparative genomic hybridization and targeted linkage analysis. *Nature Genetics* **15**, 87.

Kirner, J. (1927) Doppelseitige Verkrümmungen des Kleinfingerendglides als selbständiges Krankheitsbild. *Fortschritte Röntgenologie* **36**, 804.

**Table 9.5** Hereditary forms of clubbed fingernails.

| Disease | Inheritance | Comments |
|---|---|---|
| Acroosteolysis with osteoporosis (Andrén et al. 1962; Cheney 1965; Elias et al. 1978; Udell et al. 1986; Fryns et al. 1997) | AD *102500 | Increased curvature of nails with pitting. Broad distal phalanges with two ossicies. Increase of bitemporal diameter of the skull and flattening of the vertex. Osteoporosis of the mandible. Mast cell increase. Cystic kidneys. Vocal cord paralysis |
| Cartilage–hair hypoplasia, (McKusick et al. 1965; Polmat & Pierce 1986) | AR 250250 | Short fingers, especially of terminal phalanges. Short stature and thin sparse hair. Impaired cell function |
| Cleidocranial dysostosis (Lacroux et al. 1965; Dore et al. 1987; Mundlos et al. 1997) | AD #119600 | Aplasia of clavicles, delayed ossification of fontanelles, typical facies, coxa vara, abnormal terminal phalanges. Multiple associated anomalies. Micronychia. Syringomyelia. Gene assigned to 6p21 in 1.5-MG region |
| Dystelephalangy (Kirner 1927; David & Burwood 1972) | AD *128000 | Distal phalange of digit V is curved. Sometimes with absence of middle finger |
| Hereditary clubbing of digits (Fischer et al. 1964) | AD *119900 | Gradual onset puberty. More common in males |
| Ichthyosiform dermatosis with linear keratotic flexural papules and sclerosing palmoplantar keratodermia (Barrière et al. 1977; Pujol et al. 1989) | AR | Increased curvature of the nail plate and clubbing of nails. Pseudohainum of fingers. Dental abnormalities |
| Keratoderma palmoplantare and clubbing of nails (Bureau et al. 1959; Barraud-Klenovsek et al. 1995) | | See Table 9.1. Recidivating leg ulcers. Small head. Bone changes with enlarged distal phalanges |
| Mandibuloacral dysplasia (Young et al. 1971; Fryburg & Sidhu-Malik 1995; Toriello 1995) | AR *248370 | As above + mandibular hypoplasia. Crowding of teeth, short stature, alopecia prominent eyes, fat deposit over abdomen |
| Nodular erythema with digital changes. Nakajo syndrome (Kitano et al. 1985) | AR 256040 | Nodular erythema. Long and thick fingers. Joint mobility restricted. Loss of adipose tissue of the upper part of body. Large eyes, nose, lips and ears |
| Oto-onycho-peroneal syndrome (Pfeiffer 1982) | AR 259780 | Enlarged fingertips, dysmorphic cranofacial features, hypoplasia of fibula, contractures of hip, knee and ankle joints |
| Pachydermoperiostosis (Pramatarov et al. 1988; Singh & Menon 1995) | AD 167100 | Thickening and furrowing of face and scalp. Clubbing of digits and periosteal new bone, formation starting about puberty |
| Peutz–Jeghers–Touraine syndrome (Christian et al. 1964; Valero & Sherf 1965; Wilson et al. 1986; Hemminki et al. 1997) | AD *175200 | Pigmented macule and intestinal polyps. Ovarian and testicular tumours also reported. Black nails (see Table 9.7). Defect in single locus on 19p |
| Pycnodysostosis (Maroteaux & Lamy 1965; Andren et al. 1962; Gelb et al. 1996) | AR #265800 *601105 | Stubby digits simulating clubbing. Short, brittle nails. Dystrophy. Dwarfism, sclerotic bones which easily fracture. Basic defect in cathepsin K-gene |
| Sclerosing poikiloderma (Weary et al. 1969; Greer et al. 1978; Fazio et al. 1995) | AD? 173700 | Clubbing of fingernails: generalized poikiloderma increased in flexural areas and extensor area of elbows and knees. Sclerosis of palms and soles. Linear and reticulated hyperkeratotic and sclerotic bands in axilla antecubital on popliteal fossa |

Inheritances are indicated as follows: AD, autosomal dominant; AR, autosomal recessive.

Kitano, Y., Matsunaga, E., Morimoto, T., Okada, N. & Sano, S. (1985) A syndrome with nodular erythema, elongated and thickened fingers, and emaciation. *Archives of Dermatology* **121**, 1053.

Lacroux, R., Delahaya, R.P. & Laynaud, S. (1965) Dystrophies unguéales et macrocheilite dans la dysostose cleido-cranienne. *Bulletin de la Societé Française de Dermatologie et de Syphiligraphie* **72**, 366.

McKusick, V.A., Elridge, R., Hostetler, J.A., Egeland, J.A. & Ruangwit, U. (1965) Dwarfism in the Amish II. Cartilage–hair hypoplasia. *Bulletin of the Johns Hopkins Hospital* **116**, 285.

Maroteaux, P. & Lamy, M. (1965) The malady of Tolouse-Lautrec. *Journal of the American Medical Association* **191**, 715.

Mundlos, S., Otto, F., Mundlos, C. et al. (1997) Mutations involving the transcription factor CB FA1 cause cleidocranial dysplasia. *Cell* **89**, 773.

Pfeiffer, R.A. (1982) The oto-onycho–peroneal syndrome. A probably new genetic entity. *European Journal of Pediatrics* **138**, 317.

Polmat, S.H. & Pierce, G.F. (1986) Cartilage hair hypoplasia: immunological aspects and their clinical implications. *Clinical Immunology and Immunopathology* **40**, 87.

Pramatarov, K., Daskarev, L., Schurliev, L. & Tonev, S. (1988) Pachy-dermoperiostose (Touraine–Solente–Golé-syndrome). *Zeitschrift für Hautkrankheiten* **63**, 55.

Pujol, R.M., Moreno, A., Alomar, A. & de Moragas, J.M. (1989) Congenital ichthyosiform dermatosis with linear keratotis flexural papules and sclerosing palmoplantar keratoderma. *Archives of Dermatology* **125**, 103.

Singh, G.R. & Menon, P.S.N. (1995) Pachydermoperiostosis in a 13-year-old boy presenting as an acromegaly-like syndrome. *Journal of Pediatric Endocrinology and Metabolism* **8**, 51.

Toriello, H.V. (1995) Mandibulo-acral dysplasia: heterogenicity versus variability. *Clinical Dysmorphology* **4**, 12.

Udell, J., Schumacher, H.R. Jr, Kaplan, F. & Fallon, M.D. (1986) Idiopathic familial acroosteolysis: histomorphometric study of bone and literature review of the Haidu–Cheney syndrome. *Arthritis and Rheumatism* **29**, 1032.

Valero, A. & Sherf, K. (1965) Pigmented nails in Peutz–Jeghers syndrome. *American Journal of Gastroenterology* **43**, 56.

Verloes, A., David, A., Ngo, L. & Bottani, A. (1995) Stringent delineation of Pallister–Hall syndrome in two long surviving patients: importance of radiological anomalies of the hands. *Journal of Medical Genetics* **32**, 605.

Weary, P.E., Hsu, Y.T., Richardson, D.R., Caravati, C.M. & Wood, B.T. (1969) Hereditary sclerosing poikiloderma: report of two families with an unusual and distinctive genodermatosis. *Archives of Dermatology* **100**, 413.

Wilson, D.M., Pitts, W.C., Hintz, R.L. & Rosenfeld, R.G. (1986) Testicular tumors with Peutz–Jeghers syndrome. *Cancer* **57**, 2238.

Young, L.W., Radebaugh, J.F., Rubin, P. *et al.* (1971) A new syndrome manifested by mandibular hypoplasia, acroosteolysis, stiff joints and cutaneous atrophy (mandibuloacral dysplasia) in two unrelated boys. *Birth Defects* **7**, 291.

Yunis, E. & Varon, H. (1980) Cleidocranial dysostosis, severe micrognathism, bilateral absence of thumbs and first metatarsal bone, and distal aphalangia: a new genetic syndrome. *American Journal of Diseases of Children* **134**, 649.

## Broad nails and pseudoclubbing

When the terminal phalanx is short or dysmorphic, the nail is sometimes curved which is termed pseudoclubbing. In other cases the nail appears only broad and short. Stub thumb (brachydactyly type D, 'murderer's thumb') is a rather common genetic disorder without any other defects. The overlying nail is often called 'racquet nail' (Chapter 2). It is also seen in connection with the various syndromes listed in Table 9.6.

## References

Apert, E. (1906) De l'acrocéphalosyndactylie. *Bulletin of the Society of Medicine (Paris)* **23**, 1310.

Barsky, A.J. (1967) Macrodactyly. *Journal of Bone and Joint Surgery* **49A**, 1255.

Berry, A.C. (1987) Rubinstein–Taybi syndrome. *Journal of Medical Genetics* **24**, 562.

Biggs, P.J., Wooster, R., Ford, D. *et al.* (1995) Familial cylindromatosis (turban tumor syndrome) gene localised to chromosome 16q2–q13: evidence for its role as a tumor suppressor gene. *Nature Genetics* **11**, 41.

Butler, M.G., Hall, B.D., Maclean, R.N. & Lozzio, C.B. (1987) Do some patients with Seckel syndrome have haematological problems and/or chromosome breakage? *American Journal of Medical Genetics* **27**, 645.

Camarasa, J.G. & Moreno, A. (1987) Juvenile hyaline fibromatosis. *Journal of the American Academy of Dermatology* **16**, 881.

Fitch, N. (1982) Albright's hereditary osteodystrophy: a review. *American Journal of Medical Genetics* **11**, 11.

Gorlin, R.J., Pindborg, J.J. & Cohen, M.M. (1976) *Syndromes of the Head and Neck*, 2nd edn. McGraw Hill, New York.

Greither, A. & Rehrmann, A. (1980) Spiegler-Karzinome mit assoziierten Symptomen. Ein neues Syndrom? *Dermatologica* **160**, 361.

Herranz, P., Borbujo, J., Martínez, W., Vidaurrózaga, C., Diaz, R. & Casado, M. (1994) Rubenstein–Taybi syndrome with piebaldism. *Clinical and Experimental Dermatology* **19**, 170.

Keipert, J.A., Fitzgerald, M.G. & Danks, D.M. (1973) A new syndrome of broad terminal phalanges and facial abnormalities. *Australian Pediatric Journal* **9**, 10.

Kunze, J. & Kaufmann, H.J. (1985) Greig cephalopolysyndactyly syndrome. Report of a sporadic case. *Helvetica Paediatrica Acta* **40**, 489.

Larsen, L.J., Schottstaedt, E.R. & Bost, F.C. (1950) Multiple congenital dislocations associated with characteristic facial abnormality. *Journal of Pediatrics* **37**, 574.

Le Merrer, M., Girot, R., Parent, P., Cormier-Daire, V. & Maroteaux, P. (1995) Acral dysostosis dyserythropoiesis syndrome. *European Journal of Pediatrics* **154**, 384.

Leri, A. (1921) Une maladie congénitale et héréditarire: la pléonostéose familiale. *Bulletin of the Society of Medicine (Paris)* **45**, 1228.

Levine, M.A., Madi, W.S. & O'Brian, S.J. (1991) Mapping of the gene encoding the alpha subunit of the stimulatory G protein of adenyl cyclase (GNAS) to 20q13.2–q13.3 in humans by *in vitro* hybridization. *Genomics* **11**, 478.

McKusick, V.A. (1998) *Mendelian Inheritance in Man*, 12th edn. Johns Hopkins University Press, Baltimore.

Maroteaux, P. & Malamut, G. (1968) L'acrodysostose. *Presse Medicale* **76**, 2189.

Marques, M.N.T. (1980) Larsen's syndrome: clinical and genetic aspects. *Journal de Genetique Humaine* **28**, 83.

Pazzaglia, U.E. & Beluffi, G. (1986) Oto-palato-digital syndrome in four generations of a large family. *Clinical Genetics* **30**, 338.

Pfeiffer, R.A. (1964) Dominant erbliche Akrocephalosyndaktylie. *Zeitschrift für Kinderheilkund* **90**, 300.

Puretic, S., Puretic, B., Fiser-Herman, M. & Adamcic, M. (1962) A unique form of mesenchymal dysplasia. *British Journal of Dermatology* **74**, 8.

Rasmussen, S.A. & Frias, J.L. (1988) Mild expression of the Pfeiffer syndrome. *Clinical Genetics* **33**, 5.

Robinow, M., Pfeiffer, R.A., Gorlin, R.J. *et al.* (1971) Acrodysostosis: a syndrome of peripheral dysostosis, nasal hypoplasia, and mental retardation. *American Journal of Diseases of Children* **121**, 195.

Rubenstein, J.H. & Taybi, H. (1963) Broad thumbs and toes and facial abnormalities. *American Journal of Diseases of Children* **105**, 588.

Seckel, H.P.G. (1960) *Bird-headed Dwarfs: Studies in Developmental Anthropology including Human Proportion.* Charles C. Thomas, Springfield, IL.

Taine, L., Goizet, C., Wen, Z.Q. *et al.* (1998) Submicroscopic deletion

**Table 9.6** Hereditary forms of broad nails and some also with pseudoclubbing.

| Disease | Inheritance | Comments |
| --- | --- | --- |
| Acrocephalosyndactyly (Apert 1906; Pfeiffer 1964; Rasmussen & Frias 1988) | AD 101200 101400 101600 | Craniosynostosis. Syndactyly. Ankylosis and other skeletal deformities |
| Acrodysostosis (Maroteaux & Malamut 1968; Robinow et al. 1971) | AD 180700 *101800 | Fingernails short, broad and oval in shape. Short fingers. Nasal and midface hypoplasia. Mental retardation. Growth failure. Pigmented naevi. Combination with congenital dyserythropoetic anemia reported. (Le Merrer et al. 1995) |
| Dwarfism-brachydactyly syndrome (Tonoki et al. 1990) | XL 223610? | Nails broad, deformed and hypoplastic. Mental retardation. Multiple anomalies |
| Greig cephalopolysyndactyly syndrome (Kunze & Kaufmann 1985) | AD #175700 | Hexdactyly, syndactyly craniofacial abnormalities. Nails small; broad and dystrophic |
| Larsen's syndrome (Larsen et al. 1950; Marques 1980; Tsang et al. 1986) | AR *245400 AD *150250 | Stub thumbs, cylindrical fingers, flattened peculiar facies, widespread eyes. Multiple dislocations, short metacarpals |
| Mandibuloacral dysplasia (Zina et al. 1981; Tenconi et al. 1986) | AR *248370 | Club-shaped terminal phalanges. Mandibular hypoplasia, delayed cranial closure. Dysplastic clavicles. Atrophy of skin over hands and feet. Alopecia |
| Megalodactyly (Barsky 1967) | AD 155500 | One or two fingers markedly enlarged |
| Bird-headed dwarfism (Seckel 1960; Butler et al. 1987) | AR 210600 | Low birth weight with adult head circumference. Mental retardation. Beak-like protrusion of nose. Multiple osseous anomalies. Clubbing of fingers |
| Nasodigitoacoustic syndrome (Keipert et al. 1973; Gorlin et al. 1976) | AR 255980 | Facial abnormalities. Broad distal phalanges. Deafness |
| Cranio-otopalatodigital syndrome (Taybi 1962; Pazzaglia & Beluffi 1986) | XR or AR *311300 type 304120 | Broad, short nails of thumbs and big toes. Mental retardation. Prominent occiput. Hypoplasia of facial bones. Cloven palate. Conductive deafness |
| Pleonosteosis (Léri 1921) | *151200 | Short stature. Spade-like hand with thick palmar pads. Massive knobby thumbs. Short flexed fingers. Limited joint motion with contractures |
| Pseudohypoparathyroidism, Albright hereditary osteodystrophy (Gorlin et al. 1976; Fitch 1982; Levine et al. 1991; McKusick 1998) | XD, AR, AD #103580 *139320 203330 300800 | Short stature. Round face. Depressed nasal bridge. Short metacarpals. Mental retardation. Cataracts in 25%. Enamel hypoplasia. Calcification of skin. Mutation in GNAS1 gene located on chromosome 20q13.2–q13.3. Genetics unclear |
| Puretic syndrome juvenile hyaline fibromatosis (Puretic et al. 1962; Camarasa & Moreno 1987) | AR *228600 | Subcutaneous tumours causing deformities of face and skull. Osteolysis of peripheral phalanges. Stunted growth. Contracture of joints. Multiple subcutaneous nodes, atrophic sclerodermic skin. Gingival fibromatosis |
| Rubinstein-Taybi syndrome (Rubinstein & Taybi 1963; Berry 1987; Taine et al. 1998) | AR #180849 | Broad thumb and great toes. High palate, short stature, mental retardation, peculiar facies, keloid formation. Deletion chromoscome 16p 13.3. One case combined with piebaldism (Herranz et al. 1994) |
| Spiegler tumours and racquet nails (Tsambaos et al. 1979; Greither & Rehrmann 1980; Biggs et al. 1995) | ? *132700 | Brachydactyly. Turban tumours with gene localized to chromosome 16q12–q13 |
| Stub thumb with racquet nail (Zaun et al. 1987) | AD *113200 | No other defects |

Inheritances are indicated as follows: AD, autosomal dominant; AR, autosomal recessive; XL, sex-linked transmission; XD, sex-linked dominant; XR, sex-linked recessive.

of chromosome 16p13.3 in patients with Rubenstein–Taybi syndrome. *American Journal of Medical Genetics* **78**, 267.

Taybi, H. (1962) Generalized skeletal dysplasia with multiple anomalies. A note on Pyle's disease. *American Journal of Roentgenology* **88**, 450.

Tenconi, R., Miotti, E., Miotti, A. *et al.* (1986) Another Italian family with mandibuloacral dysplasia: why does it seem more frequent in Italy? *American Journal of Medical Genetics* **24**, 357.

Tonoki, H., Kishino, T. & Niikawa, N. (1990) A new syndrome of dwarfism, brachydactyly, nail dysplasia, and mental retardation in sibs. *American Journal of Medical Genetics* **36**, 89.

Tsambaos, D., Greither, A. & Orfanos, C.E. (1979) Multiple malignant Spiegler tumors with brachydactyly and racket-nails. *Journal of Cutaneous Pathology* **6**, 31.

Tsang, M.C.K., Ling, J.Y.K., King, N.M. & Chow, S.K. (1986) Oral and craniofacial morphology of a patient with Larsen syndrome. *Journal of Craniofacial Genetics and Developmental Biology* **6**, 357.

Zaun, R., Payeur, M. & Stenger, D. (1987) Brachyonychie unterschiedlichen Typs bei Mutter und Tochter. *Hautarzt* **38**, 104.

Zina, A.M., Cravario, A. & Bundino, S. (1981) Familial mandibuloacral dysplasia. *British Journal of Dermatology* **105**, 719.

## Isolated congenital nail dysplasia

Hamm *et al.* (2000) have described a new autosomal condition, clinically very close to restricted nail lichen planus. Histology abnormalities include prominent granular layer of the nail matrix and epithelial strands, and buds extending from the nail bed.

### Reference

Hamm, H., Karl, S. & Bröcker, E.B. (2000) Isolated congenital nail dysplasia: a new autosomal dominant condition. *Archives of Dermatology* **136**, 1239–1243.

## Koilonychia—spoon nails (MIM *149300)

In koilonychia the contour is concave instead of convex. Acquired forms are often associated with anaemia, thyroid dysfunction or trauma. Familial koilonychia without other defects is rare, but the cases reported suggest autosomal dominant transmission (Bumpers & Bishop 1980; Almagor & Haim 1981; Crosby & Petersen 1989). Koilonychia with dominantly inherited leuconychia was described by de Graciansky and Boule (1961) and Baran and Achten (1969), and with leuconychia, keratoderma palmoplantare, knuckle pads and deafness by Bart and Pumphrey (1967). Koilonychia is also seen with keratoderma palmoplantare progressiva (type Meleda; Table 9.1); some other ectodermal dysplasias (Tables 9.2 & 9.3); monilethrix (Walzer 1930; Lewis 1942); onychogryphosis (Curtis & Netherton 1939); the nail–patella syndrome (page 372); incontinentia pigmenti (Table 9.6); trichoepithelioma multiplex (Cramers 1981); and in a syndrome with abnormally

long eyelashes (Zaun *et al.* 1984). In trichomegaly koilonychia has otherwise not been reported (Gray 1944).

### References

Almagor, G. & Haim, S. (1981) Familial koilonychia. *Dermatologica* **162**, 400.

Baran, R. & Achten, G. (1969) Les associations congénitales de koilonychie et de leuconychie totale. *Archives Belges Dermatologique* **25**, 13.

Bart, R.S. & Pumphrey, R.E. (1967) Knuckle pads, leukonychia and deafness. A dominantly inherited syndrome. *New England Journal of Medicine* **276**, 202.

Bumpers, R.D. & Bishop, M.E. (1980) Familial koilonychia. *Archives of Dermatology* **116**, 845.

Cramers, M. (1981) Trichoepithelioma multiplex and dystrophia unguis congenita. A new syndrome? *Acta Dermato-Venereologica* **61**, 364.

Crosby, D.L. & Petersen, M.J. (1989) Familial koilonychia. *Cutis* **44**, 209.

Curtis, G.H. & Netherton, F.W. (1939) Congenital koilonychia and onychogryphosis. *Archives of Dermatology* **40**, 839.

de Graciansky, P. & Boule, S. (1961) Association de koilonychie et de leuconychie transmises en dominance. *Bulletin de la Societé Française de Dermatologie et de Syphiligraphie* **68**, 15.

Gray, H. (1944) Trichomegaly or movie lashes. *Stanford Medical Bulletin* **2**, 157.

Lewis, G.M. (1942) Monilethrix, koilonychia. *Archives of Dermatology* **45**, 209.

Walzer, A. (1930) Monilethrix and koilonychia. *Archives of Dermatology* **21**, 1054.

Zaun, H., Stenger, D., Zabransky, S. & Zankl, M. (1984) Das Syndrom der langen Wimpern ('Trichomegaliesyndrom', Oliver–McFarlane). *Hautarzt* **35**, 162.

## Curved nail of the 4th toe (MIM 219070)

Plantarly curved nail deformity of the 4th toe with hypoplasia of the bone and soft tissue of the distal phalange was described by Iwasawa *et al.* (1991). Eight cases were reported by Higashi *et al.* (1999) without other anomalies of the extremities.

### References

Higashi, M., Kume, A., Taganogushi, T. *et al.* (1999) Congenital curved nail of the fourth toe. *Journal of Pediatric Dermatology* **18**, 99–101.

Iwasawa, M., Hirose, T. & Matsao, K. (1991) Congenital curved nail of the fourth toe. *Plastic and Reconstructive Surgery* **87**, 553.

## Overcurvature of the nails

This is an excessive transverse curvature of one or more nails giving the effect of an ingrowing toenail, often causing considerable discomfort (Chapman 1973; Samman 1978). In hidrotic ectodermal dysplasia (Table 9.1) the nails are conical with distal ingrowing and increased convexity. They often fail to reach the end of the digit, appear small and may have onycholysis and/or spontaneous shedding. Circumferential nails (Table 9.10) also have an excessive curvature (Chavda & Crosby *et al.* 1993).

## References

Chapman, R.S. (1973) Overcurvature of the nails. An inherited disorder. *British Journal of Dermatology* **89**, 317.

Chavda, D.V. & Crosby, L.A. (1993) Circumferential toenail. *Foot and Ankle* **14**, 111.

Samman, P.D. (1978) Great toenail dystrophy. *Clinical and Experimental Dermatology* **3**, 81.

## Ectopic nails, onychoheterotopia (Figs 9.29–9.31)

After trauma to the nail matrix a portion of it can produce a nail outside the nail fold. A normal looking congenital ectopic nail on the palmar aspect of the thumb was described by Ohya (1931, cited in Kikuchi *et al.* 1978).

Kalisman and Kleinert (1983) and Allieu *et al.* (1985) reported a boy with circumferential nail growth over all sides of the small finger. Alves *et al.* (1999) reported the same anomaly on a left ring finger. Congenital claw-like fingers and toes were seen in two siblings (Egawa 1977).

Ectopic calcaneal nail (Kopera *et al.* 1996) has been reported in a patient whose sister, father and father's brother had the same lesion in the same location.

In Kuniyuki's case (1998) the right 5th finger and the left 4th finger presented with hard keratotic papules on the thin tip

associated with a Y-shaped bifurcation on the distal phalanx of the former and an M-shaped depressed deformity in the phalanx of the latter.

Ida *et al.* (1997) reported a case of congenital ectopic nails on bilateral little fingers presenting as hyperkeratinized elevations on the tip of the palmar side below the nails and close to the free edge. X-ray showed a depression on the tip of the distal phalanx.

A similar case was associated with Pierre Robin syndrome (Roger *et al.* 1986). Circumferential toenails have also been described (Chavda & Crosby *et al.* 1993). A fingernail and

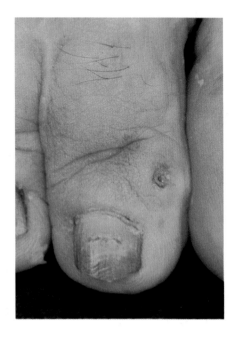

**Fig. 9.29** Ectopic nail. (Courtesy of K. Aoki, Japan.)

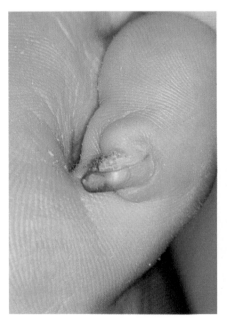

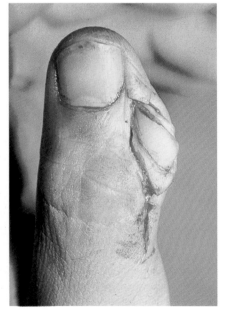

**Fig. 9.30** Ectopic nail. (a) On the palmar aspect of the thumb. (Courtesy of E. Grosshans, France.) (b) In the process of removal. (Courtesy of P. Maksène, France.)

(a)　　　　　　　　　(b)

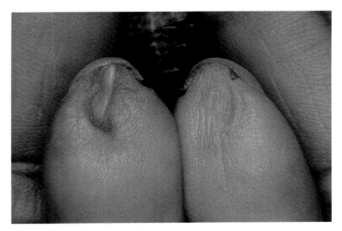

**Fig. 9.31** Ectopic nail on the palmar surface of the fingertip. (Courtesy of Lindsay, USA.)

dorsal skin on the palmar surface with a normal nail on the dorsal surface was reported by Keret and Ger (1987). Two patients with congenital ectopic palmar nails of the little finger were associated with absent flexion in the finger (Rider 1992). In other reported cases the nails have been abnormally shaped (Kikuchi *et al.* 1978, 1984; Miura 1978; Aoki & Suzuki 1984; Yamasaki *et al.* 1984; Markinson *et al.* 1988; Kuniyuki 1996; Tomita *et al.* 1997; Kamibayashi *et al.* 1998). They all appeared on the palmar (Fig. 9.31) or dorsal side 1 cm from the normal nail. Kinoshita *et al.* (1993) reported a clam-like deformity of the little finger expressing the unusual appearance of the nail wrapping around the fingertip (probably close to the circumferential nail). Ectopic nails should be differentiated from rudimentary polydactyly (Baden *et al.* 1976; Chung *et al.* 1994), from COIF (Millman & Strier 1982) and from the nail matrix doubling syndrome of Vigh and Pinter (1973), with thick nails, oculomotor paresis, debility and aplasia of the external ear. A boy with a double nail on the right 5th finger and an ectopic nail on the left has also been described (Muraoka *et al.* 1996).

## References

Allieu, Y., Benichou, M., Tessier, J. & Baldet, P. (1985) L'ongle annulaire, une malformation congénitale exceptionnelle de la main. *Annales de Chirurgie Plastique et Esthétique* **30**, 217.

Alves, G.F., Poon, E., John, J. *et al.* (1999) Circumferential fingernail. *British Journal of Dermatology* **140**, 960–962.

Aoki, K. & Suzuki, H. (1984) The morphology and hardness of the nail in 2 cases of congenital onychoheterotopia. *British Journal of Dermatology* **110**, 717–723.

Baden, H.P., Alper, J.C. & Lee, L.D. (1976) Rudimentary polydactyly presenting as a claw. *Archives of Dermatology* **112**, 1006.

Chavda, A.V. & Crosby, L.A. (1993) Circumferential toenail. *Foot and Ankle* **14**, 111.

Chung, J., Nam, I.W., Ahu, S.K., Lee, S.H., Kim, J.G. & Sung, Y.O. (1994) Rudimentary polydactyly. *Journal of Dermatology* **21**, 54.

Egawa, T. (1977) Congenital claw-like fingers and toes. Case report of two siblings. *Plastic and Reconstructive Surgery* **59**, 569–574.

Ida, N., Fukuya, Y., Yoshitana, K. *et al.* (1997) A case of congenital ectopic nails on bilateral little finger. *Journal of Dermatology* **24**, 38–42.

Kalisman, M. & Kleinert, H.E. (1983) A circumferential fingernail. Fingernail on the palmar aspect on the finger. *Journal of Hand Surgery* **8**, 58.

Kamibayashi, Y., Abe, S., Fujita, T. *et al.* (1998) Congenital ectopic nail with bone deformity. *British Journal of Plastic Surgery* **51**, 321–323.

Keret, D. & Ger, E. (1987) Double fingernails on the small fingers. *Journal of Hand Surgery* **12A**, 608.

Kikuchi, L., Ono, T. & Ogata, K. (1978) Ectopic nail. *Plastic and Reconstructive Surgery* **61**, 781.

Kikuchi, L., Ogata, K. & Idemori, M. (1984) Vertically growing ectopic nail. Nature's experiment on nail growth direction. *Journal of the American Academy of Dermatology* **10**, 114.

Kinoshita, Y., Kojima, T. & Ushida, M. (1993) Clam nail deformity of the little finger. *Plastic and Reconstructive Surgery* **91**, 158.

Kopera, D., Soyer, H.P. & Kerl, H. (1996) Ectopic calcaneal nail. *Journal of the American Academy of Dermatology* **35**, 484–485.

Kuniyuki, S. (1996) Congenital ectopic nails of the fingers associated with bone deformities. *Acta Dermato-Venereologica* **76**, 322–323.

Markinson, B., Brenner, A.R. & McGrath, M. (1988) Congenital ectopic nail. A case study. *Journal of the American Podiatric Medical Association* **78**, 318.

Millman, A.J. & Strier, R.P. (1982) Congenital onychodysplasia of the index fingers. *Journal of the American Academy of Dermatology* **7**, 57.

Miura, T. (1978) Two families with congenital nail anomalies: nail formation in ectopic areas. *Journal of Hand Surgery* **3**, 348.

Muraoka, M., Yoshioka, N. & Hyodo, T. (1996) A case of double fingernail and ectopic fingernail. *Annals of Plastic Surgery* **36**, 201–205.

Rider, M.A. (1992) Congenital palmar nail syndrome. *Journal of Hand Surgery* **17B**, 371.

Roger, H., Souteyrand, P., Collin, J.P., Vanneuville, G. & Teinturier, P. (1986) Onychohétérotopie avec polyonychie associée a un syndrome de Pierre Robin: a propos d'une nouvelle observation. *Annales de Dermatologie et de Vénéréologie* **113**, 235.

Tomita, K., Inoue, K., Ichikawa, H. *et al.* (1997) Congenital ectopic nails. *Plastic and Reconstructive Surgery* **100**, 1497–1499.

Vigh, G. & Pinter, L. (1973) Nagelmatrix-Verdoppelungssyndrom. *Zeitschrift für Haut und Geschlechtskrankheiten* **48**, 125.

Yamasaki, R., Yamasaki, M., Kokoroishi, T. & Jidoi, J. (1984) Ectopic nail associated with bone deformity. *Journal of Dermatology* **11**, 295.

## Congenital malformations caused by drugs or infections

Hydantoin (phenytoin) taken during pregnancy (MIM 132810) is known to cause malformations, including hypoplasia of nail and fingers, a broad short nose, ocular hypertelorism, ptosis, strabismus and ear and mouth abnormalities (Sabry & Farag 1996). Cleft lip, ventricular septal defects and psychomotor retardation can also occur (Silverman *et al.* 1988). Trimethadione, paramethadione and valproic acid can produce similar multiple defects (Gorlin *et al.* 1976; Rosen & Lightner 1978;

Jäger-Roman *et al.* 1986). After valproic acid the nails were long and hyperconvex. After carbamazepine only hypoplastic nail changes were reported which normalized after some months (Niesen & Fröscher 1985). After phenobarbitone hypoplasia of nails and phalanges was observed (Thakker *et al.* 1991). Hyperpigmentation of several fingernails after hydantoin has also been described (Johnson & Goldsmith 1981; Verdeguer *et al.* 1988). It can be distal with detachment of the nail plate, diffuse or occur as dark longitudinal streaks.

Anticoagulant therapy with warfarin during the 1st trimester of pregnancy may give hypoplasia of nasal bones and the terminal phalanges together with stippled epiphyses: the fingernails are small and malformed. The syndrome has many features in common with the dominant type of chondrodysplasia punctata (Pettifor & Benson 1975). Malformations in infants of chronically alcoholic women are common and include growth deficiency, bone, eye and cardiac anomalies as well as hirsutism and nail hypoplasia (Crain *et al.* 1983). Taylor *et al.* (1988) reported koilonychia, transverse growth, hyperpigmentation and thinning of nails in children born after maternal poisoning with polychlorinated biphenyls (PCB) in rice oil.

Congenital cutaneous candidiasis is uncommon and can involve only the nails (Arbegast *et al.* 1990). In congenital acquired immune deficiency syndrome (AIDS) the nails appear yellow (Chernosky & Finley 1985; Daniel 1986).

## References

Arbegast, K.D., Lamberty, L.F., Koh, J.K. *et al.* (1990) Congenital candidiasis limited to the nail plates. *Pediatric Dermatology* 7, 310.

Chernosky, M.E. & Finley, V.K. (1985) Yellow nail syndrome in patients with acquired immunodeficiency disease. *Journal of the American Academy of Dermatology* 13, 731.

Crain, L.S., Fitsmaurice, N.E. & Mondry, C. (1983) Nail dysplasia and fetal alcohol syndrome. *American Journal of Diseases of Children* 137, 1069.

Daniel, C.R. III (1986) Yellow nail syndrome and acquired immunodeficiency disease. *Journal of the American Academy of Dermatology* 14, 844.

Gorlin, R.J., Pindborg, J.J. & Cohen, M.M. (1976) *Syndromes of the Head and Neck*, 2nd edn. McGraw-Hill, New York.

Jäger-Roman, E., Deichl, A., Jakob, S. *et al.* (1986) Fetal growth, major malformations, and minor anomalies in infants born to women receiving valproic acid. *Journal of Paediatrics* 108, 997.

Johnson, R.B. & Goldsmith, L.A. (1981) Dilantin digital effects. *Journal of the American Academy of Dermatology* 5, 191.

Niesen, M. & Fröscher, W. (1985) Finger- and toenail hypoplasia after carbamazepine monotherapy in late pregnancy. *Neuropediatrics* 16, 167–168.

Pettifor, J.M. & Benson, R. (1975) Congenital malformations associated with the administration of oral anticoagulants during pregnancy. *Journal of Pediatrics* 86, 459.

Rosen, R.C. & Lightner, E.S. (1978) Phenotypic malformations in association with maternal trimethadione therapy. *Journal of Pediatrics* 92, 240.

Sabry, M.A. & Farag, T.I. (1996) Hand anomalies in fetal–hydantoin syndrome: from nail/phalangeal hypoplasia to unilateral acheiria. *American Journal of Medical Genetics* 62, 410.

Silverman, A.K., Fairley, J. & Wong, R.C. (1988) Cutaneous and immunologic reactions to phenytoin. *Journal of the American Academy of Dermatology* 18, 721.

Taylor, J.S., Rogan, W.J. & Cwi, J. (1988) Congenital Yucheng-dermatological findings. In: *Proceedings of the American Dermatological Association*, p. 30.

Thakker, J.C., Kothari, S.S., Deshmu, K.L. *et al.* (1991) Hypoplasia of nails and phalanges: a teratogenic manifestation of phenobarbitone. *Indian Pediatrics* 28, 73.

Verdeguer, J.M., Ramon, D., Moragon, M. *et al.* (1988) Onychopathy in a patient with fetal hydantoin syndrome. *Pediatric Dermatology* 5, 56.

## Nail discoloration

Discoloration of nails is common. Abnormal colour due to external factors staining the nail have been reviewed by Daniel (1985) and the influence of drugs and systemic disorders has recently been discussed (Daniel 1990). Leuconychias and their classification have been reviewed by Grossman and Scher (1990). The conditions with congenital and/or hereditary discoloration are listed in Table 9.7 according to colour changes. Several of them are combined with other abnormalities and are therefore also mentioned elsewhere.

## References

Albright, S.D. & Wheeler, C.I. (1964) Leukonychia. Total and partial leukonychia in a single family with a review of the literature. *Archives of Dermatology* 90, 392.

Baran, R. & Achten, G. (1969) Les associations congénitales de koilonychie et de leuconychie totale. *Archives Belges Dermatologique* 25, 13.

Bart, B.J., Gorlin, R.J., Anderson, E.V. & Lynch, E.W. (1966) Congenital localized absence of skin and associated abnormalities resembling epidermolysis bullosa. *Archives of Dermatology* 93, 296.

Bart, R.S. & Pumphrey, R.E. (1967) Knuckle pads, leukonychia and deafness. A dominantly inherited syndrome. *New England Journal of Medicine* 176, 202.

Bearn, A. & McKusick, V.A. (1958) Azure lunulae: an unusual change in the fingernails in two patients with hepatolenticular degeneration (Wilson's disease). *Journal of the American Medical Association* 166, 903.

Buskshell, L.L. & Gorlin, R.J. (1975) Leukonychia totalis, multiple sebacous cysts, renal calculi. *Archives of Dermatology* 111, 899.

Carmel, R. (1985) Hair and fingernail changes in acquired and congenital pernicious anemia. *Archives of Internal Medicine* 145, 484.

Caron, G.A. (1962) Familial congenital pigmented naevi of the nails. *Lancet* i, 508.

Chevrant-Breton, J., Simon, M., Bourel, M. & Ferrand, B. (1977) Cutaneous manifestations of idiopathic hemochromatosis. *Archives of Dermatology* 113, 161.

Christensen, K. & Manthrope, R. (1983) Alkaptonuria and ochronosis: a survey and 5 cases. *Human Heredity* 33, 140.

**Table 9.7** Conditions with congenital and/or hereditary discoloration of nails listed according to colour changes.

| Disease | Colour of nail | Inheritance | Comments and references |
|---|---|---|---|
| Keratitis, ichthyosis and deafness | White, thick | AR 242150 | See Table 9.1, KID syndrome |
| Keratoderma palmoplantare with atrophic fibrosis of extremities | White | AD 181600 | (Huriez et al. 1969) |
| Leopard syndrome | White with koilonychia | AD *151100 | Lentigines, electrocardiographic changes, ocular hypertelorism, pulmonary stenosis, abnormalities of genitalia, retarded growth, deafness (Selmanowitz et al. 1971; Voron et al. 1976) |
| Leuconychia totalis | Milky or porcelain | AD *151600 | (Albright & Wheeler 1964; Kates et al. 1986; Grossman & Scher 1990; Stevens et al. 1998) |
| Leuconychia totalis + epiphyseal dysplasia (Lowry–Wood) syndrome | Milky | AR *226960 | Also nystagmus, hypoplasia of corpus callosum, microcephaly (Yamamoto et al. 1995) |
| Leuconychia subtotalis | Milky or porcelain | AD *151600 | Pink area (2–4 mm), distal to white area (Juhlin 1963) |
| Leuconychia striatus | Milky or porcelain | AD | Longitudinal or transverse band (Sibley 1922; Higashi 1971; Mahler et al. 1987) |
| Leuconychia striatus + eruptive milia | Milky or porcelain | | (Schimpf & Pons 1974) |
| Leuconychia + koilonychia | Milky or porcelain | AD | (de Graciansky & Boule 1961; Baran & Achten 1969) |
| Leuconychia + koilonychia + deafness + knuckle pads + keratoderma palmoplantare | Milky or porcelain | AD *149200 | (Bart & Pumphrey 1967; Crosti et al. 1983) |
| Leuconychia + multiple sebaceous cysts + renal calculi, (FLOTCH syndrome) | Milky or porcelain | AD | (Bushkell & Gorlin 1975; Friedel et al. 1986) |
| Leuconychia + onychorhexis + hypoparathyroidism + dental changes + cataract | Milky or porcelain | AR | (Moshkowitz et al. 1969) |
| Leuconychia duodenal ulcer and gallstones | Milky or porcelain | ? | (Ingegno & Yatto 1982) |
| Leuconychia + pili torti | White | | (Giustina et al. 1985) |
| Acrokeratosis verruciformis (Hopf's disease) | White in early years. Brown with ridging and subungual hyperkeratosis in later life | AD *101900 | Verrucous or lichenoid papules on the dorsa of hands and fingers. Palms and soles may be involved as translucent punctae (Niedelman & McKusick 1962; Herndon & Wilson 1966; Schueller 1972) |
| Haemochromatosis | White, grey or brownish | AD *235200 | Koilonychia in 50%. Periungual area brown (Chevrant-Breton et al. 1977; Kalk 1957) |
| Familial amyloidosis with polyneuropathy | Yellow | | More marked on distal toenails (Hendricks 1980) |
| Incontinentia pigmenti | Slightly yellow | AD | See Table 9.6 |
| Macular amyloidosis with familial nail dystrophy | Yellow-brown | AD | Resolution of nail changes during 3rd or 4th decade (Shaw et al. 1983) |
| Aplasia cutis with dystrophic nails | Grey-yellow, brown periungual skin | AD | (Bart et al. 1966) |
| Pachyonychia congenita | Yellow or brown | AD | See Table 9.5 |
| Progeria | Yellow, atrophic | AR 176670 | See Table 9.5 |
| Yellow nail syndrome congenital | Yellow | AD 153300 | Family history of lymphoedema (Marks & Ellis 1970). See Table 9.9 |

*(continued)*

**Table 9.7** (cont'd)

| Disease | Colour of nail | Inheritance | Comments and references |
|---|---|---|---|
| Acrodermatitis enteropathica | Brownish | *201100 | (Kamatani et al. 1978) |
| Acanthosis nigricans | Grey-brown | AD 100600 | (Magid et al. 1987) |
| Darier's disease | Brown, red or white | AD *124200 | Usually as longitudinal white and red streaks. Subungeal, V-shaped keratoses (Ronchese 1965; Zaias & Ackerman 1973). Gene localized between D12S234 and DS12S129 (Wakem et al. 1996) |
| Congenital phenytoin effect | Brown, red and white | 132810 | – |
| Congenital pigmented naevi of the nails | Brown, sometimes as longitudinal band | AD *162900 | (Caron 1962; Coskey 1983) |
| Epidermal naevus | Dark | | – |
| Hereditary ectodermal dysplasia syndromes | Dark, brown | | See Table 9.1 |
| Congenital porphyria (Günther's) | Brown | AR *263700 | Possible mutilation of hands and feet. Koilonychia |
| Porphyria cutanea tarda | Yellow-brown. Pigmentation in bands. Photoonycholysis | AR 176100 | Usually distal. Absence of lunula, early koilonychia (Puissant et al. 1971) |
| Erythropoietic protoporphyria | Grey-blue-brown, opaque. Can be red in Wood's light. Photoonycholysis (white). Absence of lunula | AR *177000 | (Redeker & Berke 1962; Thivolet et al. 1968; Marsden & Dawber 1977) |
| Alkaptonuria (Ochronosis) | Grey blue | AR *203500 | Appears in adults (Teller & Winkler 1973) with alkaptonuria (Christensen & Manthrope 1983). Gene 3q13.3–q21 (Schmidt et al. 1997) |
| Angioma | Bluish-red nail bed | – | – |
| Facioscapulohumoral muscular dystrophy (Coat's syndrome) | Bluish-red nail bed with telangiectasia | AR *158900 | Telangiectasia of face, conjunctiva, retina. Deafness, muscle weakness. Mental retardation (Small 1968). Gene on 4q35 (van Deutekom et al. 1996) |
| Congenital heart disease | Red-bluish lunula | AD #121000 | Clubbing. Deletion of chromosome 22 (Wilson et al. 1992) |
| Hepatolenticular degeneration, Wilson's disease | Azure lunula | AR *277900 | (Bearn & McKusick 1958) |
| Telangiectasia, hereditary benign | Blue lunula and nail bed | AD *187260 | Blue lips and nipples, telangiectasia of chest, elbows and dorsum of hands. Varicosities of lower legs (Ryan & Wells 1971; Mills & Dicken 1979) |
| Hereditary haemorrhagic teleangiectasia (Rendu–Olser–Weber syndrome) | Blue fine blood vessels (Fig. 9.11) | AD #187300 | Telangiectasia of face, conjunctiva, fingers, mucosa of nasopharynx, gastrointestinal tract and bladder (Gorlin & Sedano 1978; Graft 1983) |
| Klippel–Trénaunay syndrome | Bluish | AD 149000 | Large haemangioma with hypertrophy of bones and soft tissue (Samuel & Spitz 1995) |
| Nigraemia. Haemoglobin M disease | Blue cyanotic | AD *141800 | Cyanosis of face. No clubbing. Brown haemoglobin M band on electrophoresis (Shibata et al. 1967) |
| Pernicious anaemia | Blue | AD or AR 170900 261000 | Hair changes (Carmel 1985; Noppakun & Swasdikul 1986) |
| Peutz–Jeghers–Touraine syndrome | Black | AD *175200 | Longitudinal bands; unusual clubbing (Valero & Sherf 1965). See Table 9.5 |

Inheritances are indicated as follows: AD, autosomal dominant; AR, autosomal recessive.

Coskey, R. (1983) Congenital subugual naevus. *Journal of the American Academy of Dermatology* 9, 747.

Crosti, C., Sala, E., Bertani, E., Gasparini, G. & Menni, S. (1983) Leuconychie totale et dysplasie ectodermique. Observation de deux cas. *Annales de Dermatologie et de Vénéréologie* 110, 617.

Daniel, C.R. III (1985) Nail pigmentation abnormalities. *Dermatologic Clinics* 3, 431.

Daniel, C.R. III (1990) Pigmentation abnormaties. In: *Nails: Therapy, Diagnosis, Surgery* (eds R.K. Scher & C.R. Daniel), p. 153. W.B. Saunders, Philadelphia.

Friedel, J., Heid, E. & Grosshans, E. (1986) Le Syndrome 'Flotch', Survenue Familiale d'une LeucOnychie totale, de kystes Trichilemmaux et d'une dystrophie Ciliaire à Hérédité autosomique dominante. *Annales de Dermatologie et de Vénéréologie* 113, 549.

Giustina, T.A., Woo, T.X., Campbell, J.P. & Ellis, C.N. (1985) Association of pili torti and leukonychia. *Cutis* 35, 533.

Gorlin, R.J. & Sedano, H.O. (1978) Hereditary hemorrhagic telangiectasia. The Rendu–Weber–Osler syndrome. *Journal of Dermatologic Surgery and Oncology* 4, 864.

de Graciansky, P. & Boule, S. (1961) Association de koilonychie et de leuconychie transmises en dominance. *Bulletin de la Societé Française de Dermatologie et de Syphiligraphie* 68, 15.

Graft, G.E. (1983) A review of hereditary hemorrhagic telangiectasia. *Journal of the American Osteopathic Association* 82, 412.

Grossman, M. & Scher, R.K. (1990) Leukonychia. Review and classification. *International Journal of Dermatology* 29, 535.

Hendricks, A.A. (1980) Yellow lunulae with fluorescence after tetracycline therapy. *Archives of Dermatology* 116, 438.

Herndon, J.H. & Wilson, J.D. (1966) Acrokeratosis verruciformis (Hopf) and Darier's disease. *Archives of Dermatology* 93, 305.

Higashi, N. (1971) Leukonychia striata longitudinalis. *Archives of Dermatology* 104, 142.

Huriez, C., Deminati, M., Agache, R., Delmas-Marsalet, Y. & Mennecier, M. (1969) Génodermatose scléro-atrophiante et kératodermique des extrémités. *Annales de Dermatologie et de Syphiligraphie* 96, 135.

Ingegno, A.D. & Yatto, R.P. (1982) Hereditary white nails (leuconychia totalis), duodenal ulcer and gallstones: genetic implications. *New York State Journal of Medicine* 82, 1797.

Juhlin, L. (1963) Hereditary leuconychia. *Acta Dermato-Venereologica* 43, 136.

Kalk, H.O. (1957) Über Hautzeichen bei Leberkrankheiten. *Deutsche Medizinische Wochenschrift* 38, 1637.

Kamatani, M., Rai, A., Hen, H. et al. (1978) Yellow nail syndrome associated with mental retardation in two siblings. *British Journal of Dermatology* 99, 329.

Kates, S.L., Harris, G.D. & Nagle, D.J. (1986) Leukonychia totalis. *Journal of Hand Surgery* 11B, 465.

Magid, M., Esterly, N.B., Prendiville, J. & Fujisaki, C. (1987) The yellow nail syndrome in an 8-year-old girl. *Pediatric Dermatology* 4, 90.

Mahler, R.H., Gerstein, W. & Watters, K. (1987) Congenital leukonychia striata. *Cutis* 39, 453.

Marks, R. & Ellis, J.P. (1970) Yellow nails. A report of six cases. *Archives of Dermatology* 102, 619.

Marsden, R.A. & Dawber, R.P.R. (1977) Erythropoietic protoporphyria with onycholysis. *Proceedings of the Royal Society of Medicine* 70, 252.

Mills, J.L. & Dicken, C.H. (1979) Hereditary acrolabial telangiectasia. *Archives of Dermatology* 115, 474.

Moshkowitz, A., Abrahamov, A. & Pisanti, S. (1969) Congenital hypoparathyroidism simulating epilepsy, with other symptoms and dental signs of intra-uterine hypocalcemia. *Pediatrics* 44, 401.

Niedelman, M.L. & McKusick, V. (1962) Acrokeratosis verruciformis (Hopf). *Archives of Dermatology* 86, 779.

Noppakun, N. & Swasdikul, D. (1986) Reversible hyperpigmentation of skin and nails with white hair due to vitamin $B_{12}$ deficiency. *Archives of Dermatology* 122, 896.

Puissant, A., David, V., Lachiver, D. & Aitken, G. (1971) Formes cliniques atypiques de la porphyrie cutanée tardive. *Bollettino dell Istituto Dermatologico San Gallicano* 7, 19.

Redeker, A. & Berke, M. (1962) Erythropoietic protoporphyria with eczema solare. *Archives of Dermatology* 86, 569.

Reilly, P.J. & Nostrant, T.T. (1984) Clinical manifestations of hereditary hemorrhagic telangiectasia. *American Journal of Gastroenterology* 79, 363.

Ronchese, F. (1965) The nail in Darier's disease. *Archives of Dermatology* 91, 617.

Ryan, T.J. & Wells, R.S. (1971) Hereditary benign telangiectasia. *Transactions of the St John's Hospital Dermatologic Society* 57, 148.

Samuel, M. & Spitz, L. (1995) Klippel–Trenaunay syndrome: clinical features, complications and management in children. *British Journal of Surgery* 82, 757.

Schimpf, A. & Pons, F. (1974) Multiple eruptive Millien und striäre leukonychia. *Zeitschrift für Hautkrankheiten* 49, 207.

Schmidt, S.R., Gehrig, A., Koehler, M.R., Schmid, M., Muller, C.R. & Kress, W. (1997) Cloning of the homogentisate 1,2-dioxygenase gene, the key enzyme of alkaptonuria in mouse. *Mammalian Genome* 8, 168.

Schueller, W.A. (1972) Acrokeratosis verruciformis of Hopf. *Archives of Dermatology* 106, 81.

Selmanowitz, V.J., Orentreich, N. & Felsenstein, J.M. (1971) Lentiginous profusa syndrome (multiple lentigines syndrome). *Archives of Dermatology* 104, 393.

Shaw, M., Jurecka, W., Black, M.M. & Kurwa, A. (1983) Macular amyloidosis associated with familial nail dystrophy. *Clinical and Experimental Dermatology* 8, 363.

Shibata, S., Miyagi, T., Iuchi, L., Ohba, Y. & Yamamoto, K. (1967) Hemoglobin Ms of the Japanese. *Bulletin of the Yamaguchi Medical School* 14, 141.

Sibley, K. (1922) Leukonychia striata. *British Journal of Dermatology and Syphilis* 34, 238.

Small, R.G. (1968) Coat's disease and muscular dystrophy. *Transactions of the American Academy of Ophthalmology* 72, 225.

Stevens, K.R., Leis, P.F., Peters, S., Baer, S. & Orengo, I. (1998) Congenital leukonychia. *Journal of the American Academy of Dermatology* 39, 509.

Teller, H. & Winkler, K. (1973) Zur Klinik und Histopathologie der endogenen Ochronose. *Hautartz* 12, 537.

Thivolet, J., Freycon, J., Perrot, H., Gaubaud, P. & Beyvin, A.J. (1968) Protoporphyrie érythropoietique. *Bulletin de la Societé Française de Dermatologie et de Syphiligraphie* 75, 829.

Valero, A. & Sherf, K. (1965) Pigmented nails in Peutz–Jeghers syndrome. *American Journal of Gastroenterology* 43, 56.

Van Deutekom, J.C.T., Lemmers, R.J.L.F., Grewal, P.K. et al. (1996) Identification of the first gene (FRG1) from the FSDH region on human chromosome 4q35. *Human Molecular Genetics* 5, 581.

Voron, D.A., Hatfield, H.H. & Kalkhoff, R.X. (1976) Multiple lentigines syndrome. Case report and review of literature. *American Journal of Medicine* 60, 446.

Wakem, P., Ikeda, S., Haake, A. *et al.* (1996) Localization of the Darier disease gene to a 2-cM portion of 12q23–24.1. *Journal of Investigative Dermatology* 106, 365.

Wilson, D.I., Goodship, J.A., Burn, J., Cross, I.E. & Scambler, P.J. (1992) Deletions within chromosome 22q11 in familial congenital heart disease. *Lancet* 340, 573.

Yamamoto, T., Tohyama, J., Koeda, T., Maegaki, Y. & Takahashi, Y. (1995) Multiple epiphyseal dysplasia with small head, congenital nystagmus, hypoplasia of corpus callosum, and leukonychia totalis: a variant of Lowry–Wood syndrome? *American Journal of Medical Genetics* 56, 6.

Zaias, N. & Ackerman, B. (1973) The nail in Darier–White disease. *Archives of Dermatology* 107, 193.

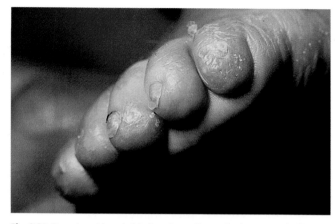

**Fig. 9.34** Recessive epidermolysis bullosa dystrophica—nails of an 11-month-old female. (Courtesy of I. Anton-Lambrecht, Germany.)

## Epidermolysis bullosa (Figs 9.32–9.42)

The various forms of epidermolysis bullosa and their nail changes which might help in diagnosis are listed in Table 9.8.

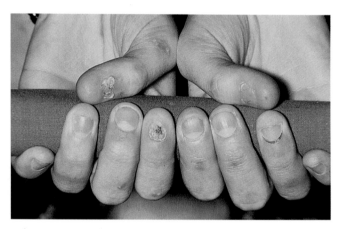

**Fig. 9.32** Recessive epidermolysis bullosa dystrophica (Hallopeau–Siemens). Twenty-four-year-old female—some nails normal, some dystrophic, some absent.

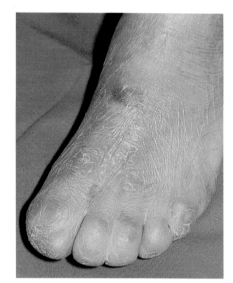

**Fig. 9.35** Recessive epidermolysis bullosa dystrophica—11-month-old male with complete loss of nails. (Courtesy of I. Anton-Lambrecht, Germany.)

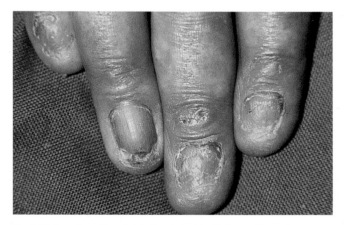

**Fig. 9.33** Recessive epidermolysis bullosa dystraphica (Hallopeau–Siemens). Forty-two-year-old male—severe nail dystrophy; mutilating epidermolysis bullosa with widespread blistering.

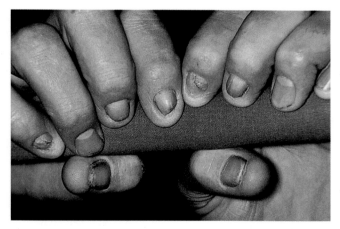

**Fig. 9.36** Dominant epidermolysis bullosa dystrophica (Cockayne–Touraine)—36-year-old male with nail dystrophy and blisters limited to the hands and feet. (Courtesy of I. Anton-Lambrecht, Germany.)

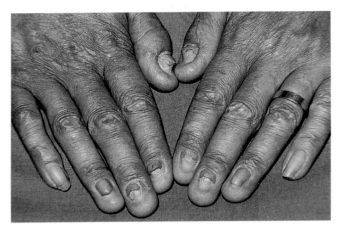

**Fig. 9.37** Dominant epidermolysis bullosa dystrophica, albulopapuloid (Pasini)—41-year-old male with thickened, short and brittle nails. (Courtesy of I. Anton-Lambrecht, Germany.)

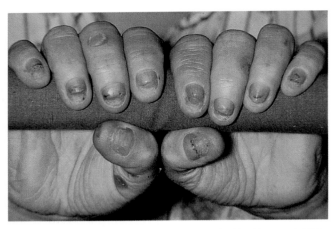

**Fig. 9.40** Epidermolysis bullosa atrophicans mitis, generalized (Hashimoto *et al*. 1976) —42-year-old female with thickened, raised nails with early onychogryphosis. (Courtesy of I. Anton-Lambrecht, Germany.)

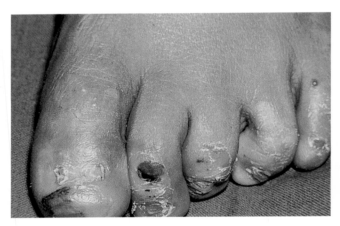

**Fig. 9.38** Dominant epidermolysis bullosa dystrophica, albulopapuloid (Pasini)—5-year-old daughter of patient in Fig. 9.37; toe blisters and nail dystrophy. (Courtesy of I. Anton-Lambrecht, Germany.)

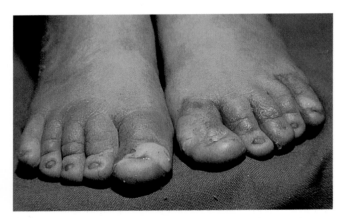

**Fig. 9.41** Epidermolysis bullosa atrophicans mitis, generalized (Hashimoto *et al*. 1976)—5-year-old male with severe toenail dystrophy and generalized blistering. (Courtesy of I. Anton-Lambrecht, Germany.)

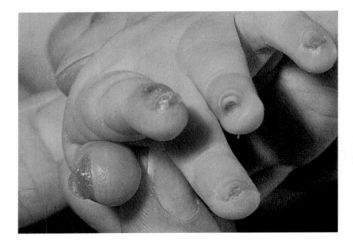

**Fig. 9.39** Epidermolysis bullosa atrophicans gravis, generalized (Herlitz)—4-week-old male with heaped-up nails and subungual granulation tissue (Voigtländer *et al*. 1979). (Courtesy of I. Anton-Lambrecht, Germany.)

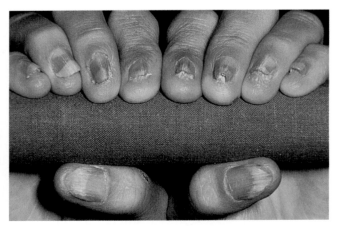

**Fig. 9.42** Epidermolysis bullosa atrophicans, localized (Hashimoto *et al*. 1976)—27-year-old female with raised, dome-shaped, partly onychogryphotic nails. (Courtesy of I. Anton-Lambrecht, Germany.)

A slight modification of the classification recommended by a consensus group on epidermolysis bullosa has been used here (Fine *et al.* 1991a). Different types of epidermolysis can arise from missense mutations in the same codon and can contribute far more to the clinical severity than previously thought (Shemanko *et al.* 1998). The different subtypes of epidermolysis bullosa could therefore be gradations of clinical severity rather than distinct genetic diseases. This area of research has expanded markedly in recent years, and the references given in Table 9.8 can only serve as a guide to further references. The nail changes in epidermolysis bullosa have been reviewed by Bruckner-Tuderman *et al.* in 1995. Epidermolysis bullosa with congenital skin defects described as a new syndrome by Bart *et al.* (1966) was excluded in our 2nd edition because it was regarded as damage caused *in utero* which can occur in most types of epidermolysis bullosa (Wojnarowska *et al.* 1983; Bedane *et al.* 1990). Investigations of the original kindred and their descendants by Zelickson *et al.* (1995) showed persistance of blistering into adult life with atrophic scarring. The gene was mapped to 3p near the site of the gene encoding type VII collagen. Christiano *et al.* (1996a) demonstrated the mutation in the *COL 7AI* gene. Bart's syndrome seems therefore to be a variant of dystrophic epidermolysis bullosa where it now has been added.

## References

Altomare, G.F., Polenghi, M., Pigatto, P.D. *et al.* (1990) Dystrophic epidermolysis bullosa inversa: a case report. *Dermatologica* **181**, 145.

**Table 9.8** Nails in patients with epidermolysis bullosa. (Modified after Fine *et al.* 1991.)

| Type of disease | Nails | Inheritance | Comments |
|---|---|---|---|
| INTRAEPIDERMAL | | | |
| *EB simplex localized* | | | |
| Hands and feet (Weber Cokayne type) EB simplex (Müller *et al.* 1998) | Normal. Rarely dystrophic | AD #131800 | Mainly palmoplantar with callus. Mutation in keratin 5 or 14 gene (McKenna *et al.* 1992) |
| With anodontia (Kallin's syndrome) (Gamborg Nielsen & Sjölund 1985) | Thick or curved | AR #601001? | Alopecia, blisters mainly on hands and feet. No teeth |
| *EB simplex, generalized* | | | |
| Koebner type (Galligan *et al.* 1998) | Usually normal | AD #131900 | Lesions on hands and feet. Mutation in keratin 5 gene |
| Herpetiformis (Dowling-Meara Buchbinder *et al.* 1986; McGrath *et al.* 1992; Letai *et al.* 1993) | Loss of nails with regeneration. End result dystrophic or normal nails | AD #131760 | Herpetiform groups of bloody blister since birth. Keratodermia. Mutation in keratin 5 or 14 gene. |
| EBS with mottled pigmentation (Fischer & Gedde-Dahl 1979; Bruckner-Tuderman *et al.* 1989). Can overlap with Dowling-Meara | Peculiar curving. Partially dystrophic | AD #131960 | Pigmentation neck, abdomen. Variant with punctate keratoderma (Medenica-Mojsilovic *et al.* 1986). Transition in keratin V (Irvine *et al.* 1997) |
| Ogna variant (Gedde-Dahl 1971) | Onychogryphosis of big toe in adulthood | AD *131950 | Haemorrhagic blisters. Localized to 8q24 |
| Superficialis (Fine *et al.* 1989) | Often dystrophic | AD | Subcorneal blisters |
| With neuromuscular disease (Salih *et al.* 1985; Niemi *et al.* 1988; Gache *et al.* 1996; Smith *et al.* 1996) | Can be dystrophic | AR #226670 | Scarring alopecia. Mysthenica gravis. Genetic defect in plectin in the 8q24.13-qter region |
| Macular (Mendes da Costa) (van der Valk 1908; Lungarotti *et al.* 1994; Wijker *et al.* 1995) | Dysmorphic | XR *302000 | No hairs, hyper and depigmentation, microcephaly. Short fingers. Lethal to males. Gene in the Xq27.3-qter region |
| JUNCTIONAL | | | |
| *Junctional localized* | | | |
| Inversa (Gedde-Dahl *et al.* 1994) | Dystrophic or absent sometimes heaped up. Easily shed | AR *226450 | Teeth dystrophic. Locus EBR2A assigned to 1q31 |

(continued p. 418)

Lichtenwald, D.J., Hanna, W., Sauder, D.N., Jakubovic, H.R. & Rosenthal, D. (1990) Pretibial epidermolysis bullosa: report of a case. *Journal of the American Academy of Dermatology* 22, 346.

Lin, A.N., Smith, L.T. & Fine, J.-D. (1995) Dystrophic epidermolysis bullosa inversa: report of two cases with further correlation between electron microscopic and immunofluorescence studies. *Journal of the American Academy of Dermatology* 33, 361.

Lungarotti, M.S., Martello, C., Barboni, G., Mezzetti, D., Mariotti, G. & Calabro, A. (1994) X-linked retardation, microcephaly, and growth delay associated with hereditary bullous dystrophy macular type: report of a second family. *American Journal of Medical Genetics* 51, 598.

McGrath, J.A., Ishida-Yamamoto, A., Tidman, M.J., Heagerty, A.H.M., Schofield, O.M.V. & Eady, R.A.J. (1992) Epidermolysis bullosa simplex (Dowling–Meara): a clinicopathological review. *British Journal of Dermatology* 126, 421.

McGrath, J.A., Gatalica, B., Christiano, A.M. *et al.* (1995) Mutations in the 180-kD bullous pemphigoid antigen (BPAG2), a hemidesmosomal transmembrane collagen (COL7A1) in generalized atrophic benign epidermolysis bullosa. *Nature Genetics* 11, 83.

McGrath, J.A., Kivirikko, S., Ciatti, S., Moss, C., Christiano, A.M. & Uitto, J. (1996) A recurrent homozygous nonsense mutation within the LAMA3 gene as a cause of Herlitz junctional epidermolysis bullosa in patients of Pakistan ancestry evidence for a founder effect. *Journal of Investigative Dermatology* 106, 781.

McKenna, K.E., Hughes, A.E., Bingham, E.A. & Nevin, N.C. (1992) Linkage of epidermolysis bullosa simplex to keratin gene loci. *Journal of Medical Genetics* 29, 568.

Medenica-Mojsilovic, L., Fenske, N.A. & Espinoza, C.G. (1986) Epidermolysis bullosa herpetiformis with mottled pigmentation and an unusual punctate keratoderma. *Archives of Dermatology* 122, 900.

Mellerio, J.E., Salas-Alanis, J.C., Talamantes, M.L. *et al.* (1998) A recurrent glycine substitution mutation, G2043R, in the type VII collagen gene (COL7A1) in dominant dystrophic epidermolysis bullosa. *British Journal of Dermatology* 139, 730.

Mendes da Costa, S. & Van der Valk, J.W. (1908) Typus maculatus der bullosen hereditaren Dystrophie. *Archives of Dermatology and Syphilis* 91, 1.

Müller, F.P., Küster, W., Bruckner-Tuderman, L. & Korge, B.P. (1998) Novel K5 and K14 mutations in German patients with the Weber–Cockayne variant of epidermolysis bullosa simplex. *Journal of Investigative Dermatology* 111, 900.

Nakar, S., Ingber, A., Kremer, I. *et al.* (1992) Late-onset junctional epidermolysis bullosa and mental retardation: a distinct autosomal recessive syndrome. *American Journal of Medical Genetics* 43, 776.

Niemi, K.-M., Sommer, F.L., Kero, M. *et al.* (1988) Epidermolysis bullosa simplex associated with muscular dystrophy with recessive inheritance. *Archives of Dermatology* 124, 551.

Priestley, G.C., Tidman, M.J., Weiss, J.B. & Eady, R.A.J. (1990) *Epidermolysis Bullosa: A Comprehensive Review of Classification, Management and Laboratory Studies.* DEBRA, Crowthorne, Berkshire.

Ramelet, A.A. & Boillat, C. (1985) Epidermolyse bulleuse dystrophique albupapuloide autosomique recessive. *Dermatologica* 171, 397.

Salih, M.A.M., Lake, B.D., El Hag, M.A. *et al.* (1985) Lethal epidermolytic epidermolysis bullosa: a new autosomal recessive type of epidermolysis bullosa. *British Journal of Dermatology* 113, 135.

Schurig, B., Krieg, T., Landthaler, M. & Braun-Falco, O. (1987) Epidermolysis bullosa hereditaria dystrophica (Hallopeau–Siemens). *Hautarzt* 38, 619.

Shemanko, C.S., Mellerio, J.E., Tidman, M.J., Lane, B.E. & Eady. R.A.J. (1998) Severe palmo-plantar hyperkeratosis in Dowling–Meara epidermolysis bullosa simplex caused by a mutation in the keratin 14 gene (*KRT14*). *Journal of Investigative Dermatology* 111, 893.

Smith, F.J.D., Eady, R.A.J., Leigh, I.M. *et al.* (1996) Plectin deficiency results in muscular dystrophy with epidermolysis bullosa. *Nature Genetics* 13, 450.

Smith, F.J.D., Maingi, C., Covello, S.P. *et al.* (1998) Genomic organization and fine mapping of the keratin 2e gene (*KRT2E*): K2e V1 domain polymorphism and novel mutations in ichthyosis bullosa of Siemens. *Journal of Investigative Dermatology* 111, 817.

Takizawa, Y., Shimizu, H., Pulkkinen, L. *et al.* (1998) Novel mutations in the LAMB3 gene shared by two Japanese unrelated families with Herlitz junctional epidermolysis bullosa, and their application for prenatal testing. *Journal of Investigative Dermatology* 110, 174.

Terracina, M., Posteraro, P., Schubert, M. *et al.* (1998) Compound heterozygosity for a recessive glycine substitution and a splice site mutation in the COL7A1 gene causes an epidermolysis bullosa. *Journal of Investigative Dermatology* 111, 744.

Wijker, M., Ligtenberg, M.J.L., Schoute, F. *et al.* (1995) The gene for hereditary bullous dystrophy, X-linked macular type, maps to the Xq27.3-qter region. *American Journal of Human Genetics* 56, 1096.

Wojnarowska, F.T., Eady, R.A.J. & Wells, R.S. (1983) Dystrophic epidermolysis bullosa presenting with congenital absence of skin: report of four cases. *British Journal of Dermatology* 108, 477.

Wright, J.T., Fine, J.-D., Johnson, L.B. & Steinmetz, T.T. (1993) Oral involvement of recessive dystrophic epidermolysis bullosa inversa. *American Journal of Medical Genetics* 47, 1184.

Zelickson, B., Matsumura, K., Kist, D., Epstein, E. & Bart, B.J. (1995) Bart's syndrome. Ultrastructure and genetic linkage. *Archives of Dermatology* 131, 663.

## Secondary nail changes and some miscellaneous nail conditions

Various hereditary disorders with secondary nail changes appear in Table 9.9. In Table 9.10 disorders with non-classified nail involvement are listed.

## References

Ainsworth, J.R., Shabbir, G., Spencer, A.F. & Cockburn, F. (1992) Multisystem disorder of Punjabi children exhibiting spontaneous dermal and submucosal granulation tissue formation: LOGIC syndrome. *Clinical Dysmorphology* 1, 3.

Allieu, Y., Benichou, M., Teissier, J. & Baldet, P. (1985) L'ongle annulaire, une malformation congénitale exceptionnelle de la main. *Annales de Chirurgie Plastique et Esthétique* 30, 217.

Baran, R. & Bureau, H. (1982) Malalignment of the big toenail as a cause of ingrowing toenail in infancy. Pathology and treatment. *British Journal of Dermatology* 107, 33.

Baran, R. & Bureau, H. (1983) Congenital malalignment of the big

**Table 9.9** Hereditary disorders with secondary nail changes.

| Disease | Inheritance MIM | Nails | Comments |
|---|---|---|---|
| Acanthosis nigricans (benign hereditary) (Tasjian & Jarrat 1984) | AD *100600 | Thick, friable, dull, grey or normal | Pigmented, thick skin neck, axilla of inguinal region |
| Acrodermatitis enteropathica | AR *201100 | Periungual eczema, candida infections. Multiple Beau's lines | Alopecia, typical acral skin lesion, enteropathia |
| Aminogenic alopecia deficiency (Shelley & Rawnsley 1965) | AR | Brittle | Argininosuccinic aciduria. Loss of hair |
| Citrullinaemia (Bonafe et al. 1984) | AR *215700 | Clubbed. Red transverse band distally | Trichorrhexis. Cutaneous atrophy. Hyperammoniaemia |
| Congenital loss of pain (Thomson et al. 1980; Rosenberg et al. 1994) | AR #256800 | Brittle | Argininosuccinic synthetase deficiency. Antihidrotic. Mental retardation |
| Diabetes | AR *222100 | *Candida* infection. Thick finger nails and toenails | – |
| Gingival fibromatosis, Zimmerman–Laband syndrome (Laband et al. 1964; Chodirker et al. 1986) | AD *135500 | Small or absent nails of thumb and big toe | Gingival fibroma. Big nose and ears. Hepatosplenomegaly. Distal phalanges short. Sometimes hypertrichosis, mental retardation or ocular changes |
| Hyper-IgE syndrome (Davis et al. 1966; Koch et al. 1992) | AR 147060 | Hyperkeratotic or atrophic nails due to candida infections. Mild clubbing | Defect in polymorphonuclear neutrophil function. Red scaly skin lesions. Cold staphylococcal abscess High IgE levels. Craniosynostosis (Hoger et al. 1985) |
| Hyperuricaemia (Gospos, 1976) | AD 240000 | Thick, split, dystrophic | Mental retardation |
| Lesh–Nyhan syndrome (Gharbi et al. 1989) | XL 308950 | Destroyed | Self-mutilation |
| Lichen planus hereditaria (Copeman et al. 1978; Mahood 1983; Valsecchi et al. 1990) | 151620 | Destroyed | – |
| Lymphoedema with yellow nails (Wells 1966) and mental retardation (Kamatani et al. 1978) | AD 153300 | Thick yellow nails | Congenital lymphoedema with adult onset and respiratory tract infection |
| Multiple cartilaginous exostosis. Diaphyseal aclasis (Krooth et al. 1961; Solomon 1964; Hazen & Smith 1990) | AD 133700 | Non-tender nodules of proximal part of nail fold with elevation and splitting of nail | Retardation of growth of long bones and sarcomatous degeneration reported |
| Neurofibromatosis (Recklinghausen) (Chao 1959; Riccardi & Eichner 1986) | AD *162200 | One or more hypertrophic fingers or toes with dislocation of nails | Multiple neurofibromas, cutaneous pigmentation, central nervous involvement |
| Porokeratosis Mibelli (Scappaticci et al. 1989) | AD *175800 | Thick, ridged or fissured | Centrifugal spreading patches with central atrophy. Chromosome 3p14p12 |
| Pityriasis rubra pilaris | AD *173200 | One or more hypertrophic | – |
| Psoriasis | AD *177900 | Pitting. Onycholysis, hyperkeratosis | |
| Tuberous sclerosis, epiloia, (Bourneville–Pringle) | AD *191100 | Koenen's tumours. Subungual fibroma dislocating nails | Epilepsy, mental retardation. Angiofibroma of face and oral mucosa, intracranial calcification |
| Zimmerman–Laband syndrome (see gingival fibromatosis above) | | | |

Inheritances are indicated as follows: AD, autosomal dominant; AR, autosomal recessive; XD, sex-linked dominant.

**Table 9.10** Various hereditary, familial or congenital disorders with nail involvement.

| Disease | Nails | Inheritance MIM | Comments |
|---|---|---|---|
| Acrorenal ocular syndrome (Halal *et al.* 1984) | Thumbnail hypoplasia | AD 102520 | Renal and ocular anomalies. Ptosis |
| Ainhum, amniotic constriction band (Feingold 1984) | Dysplastic | 103400 | Swelling, brachydactylia or amputations *in utero* |
| Circumferential, curved fingernail. Congenital claw-like fingers and toes (Egawa 1977; Kalisman & Kleinert 1983; Allieu *et al.* 1985; Iwasawa *et al.* 1991) | Nails cover both dorsal and lateral or all sides of one or more fingers | AR 219070 | One case combined with Pierre Robin syndrome |
| Congenital hereditary endothelial dystrophy (CHED) (Stirling *et al.* 1994; Toma *et al.* 1995) | Hypoplastic short on fingers and feet | AD *121700 AR *217700 | Corneal clouding. Gene mapped to chromosome 20 |
| Congenital ingrown toenails (Hendricks 1979) resulting in malalignment of the big toe nail (Baran *et al.* 1979; Baran & Bureau 1982, 1983; Barth *et al.* 1986) | Thick with transverse ridging onycholysis, shedding. Panonychia common. Fibrous tumours of nailfold (Hammerton & Shrank 1988) | ? | Early surgical operation advised. Seen in monozygotic twins |
| Congenital subungual pterygium (Odom *et al.* 1974; Christophers 1975; Dugois *et al.* 1975; Chams-Davatchi 1980; Runne & Orfanos 1981, Nogita *et al.* 1991) | Aberrant hyponychium. Painful fractures of nails may occur | ? | Mainly females |
| Dysplasia of the 5 toenail (Hundeiker 1969) | After age 2 on the 5th toe, longitudinal furrows and distal onycholysis with splitting of nails | AD? | – |
| Epidermodysplasia verruciformis-like dermatoses with nail changes (Salamon *et al.* 1987) | Thick with longitudinal furrows. White, yellow pigmentation. Subungual hyperkeratoses | XD 305350 | Symmetrical flat warts. Hyper- and hypopigmented spots |
| Familial twenty-nail dystrophy (Knöll *et al.* 1989; Commens 1990) | Longitudinal ridging, rough, loss of lustre | AD *161050 | Trachonychia can also be acquired |
| Great toenail dystrophy (Samman 1978) | Affected nails, dystrophic and brownish | – | See congenital malalignment of big toe nail |
| Hypocalcified enamel and dystrophic nails (Takeda *et al.* 1989) | Dysplastic, striated on finger and toes | XR | Hypoplastic enamel on permanent teeth. Patients otherwise normal |
| Idiopathic familial onychomadesis (Mehra *et al.* 2000) | Recurrent onychomadesis | | Multiple digits. Absence of any causal disease and medication |
| Inherited toenail dystrophy (Dawson 1979, 1982) | Said to be identical to Samman's dystrophy | AD | Spontaneous resolution can occur |
| Laryngo-onychocutaneous syndrome (Shabbir *et al.* 1986; Ainsworth *et al.* 1992; Philips *et al.* 1994) | Dystrophic nails sometimes thick | AR 245660 | Hoarseness in early life. Ulcerative pyogenic granuloma-like lesions mainly around mouth and nose. Teeth showed notching and crenations. Lamina lucida defect. Junctional EB? |
| Leprechaunism (Roth *et al.* 1981; Cantani *et al.* 1987; Hone *et al.* 1994) | Hyperconvex | #246200 | Wrinkled loose skin. Decreased subcutaneous fat. Thick lips. Acanthosis nigricans. Hypotrichosis. Hyperinsulinaemia. Mutation in insulin receptor gene |
| Macular amyloidosis with familial nail dystrophy (Shaw *et al.* 1983) | See Table 9.6 | – | – |

*(continued)*

**Table 9.10** (cont'd)

| Disease | Nails | Inheritance MIM | Comments |
|---|---|---|---|
| Osteopoikilosis: Buscke-Ollendorf syndrome (Giro et al. 1992; Colla et al. 1995) | Pitting and 'oil'-spots. Onycholysis (psoriasis?) | AD *166700 | Dermatofibrosis lenticularis yellow papular arms and legs. Radiological features typical |
| Pili torti (Beare) syndrome (Beare 1952) | Onychodysplasia | AD 261900 | Appears after puberty. See also pili torti, page 387 |
| Rud syndrome (Wallach et al. 1987) | Increased lunula on hands. Micronychia on toes | AR or XL 308200 | Congenital ichthyosis and male hypogonadism, epilepsy, mental retardation, retinitis pigmentosa |
| Soft nail disease (Prandi & Caccialanza 1977) | Atrophic short soft nail. Absence of lunula | | A single case |
| Trichoepithelioma multiple and dystrophic nails (Cramers 1981; Harada et al. 1996) | Thumb nails most affected. Koilonychia of index finger | AD? *161606 | Only dystrophic nails in some. Gene mapped to chromosome 9p21. |
| Trichomegaly syndrome (Zaun et al. 1984) | Koilonychia | AD 190330 | Abnormally long eyelashes. Sparse scalp hair, eye disorders and mental retardation can occur (Goldstein & Hurt 1972) |

Inheritance: AD, autosomal dominant; AR, autosomal recessive; XL, sex-linked transmission; XD, sex-linked dominant; XR, sex-linked recessive.

toe-nail as a cause of ingrowing toe-nail in infancy. Pathology and treatment (a study of thirty cases). *Clinical and Experimental Dermatology* 8, 619.

Baran, R., Bureau, H. & Sayag, J. (1979) Congenital malalignment of the big toenail. *Clinical and Experimental Dermatology* 4, 359.

Barth, J.H., Dawber, R.P.R., Ashton, R.E. & Baran, R. (1986) Congenital malalignment of great toenails in 2 sets of monozygotic twins. *Archives of Dermatology* 122, 379.

Beare, J.M. (1952) Congenital defect showing features of pili torti. *British Journal of Dermatology* 64, 566.

Björnberg, A. (1961) Adenoma sebaceum. Review, case reports and discussion of eugenic aspects. *Acta Dermato-Venereologica* 41, 213.

Bonafe, J.L., Pieraggi, M.T., Abravanel, M., Benque, A. & Abravanel, G. (1984) Skin, hair and nail changes in a case of citrullinemia with late manifestation. *Dermatologica* 168, 213.

Cantani, A., Ziruolo, M.G. & Tacconi, M.L. (1987) Un syndrome polydysmorphique rare: Le Lepréchaunisme. *Annals of Genetics* 30, 221.

Chams-Davatchi, C. (1980) Pterygium inversum ungueal. *Annales de Dermatologie et de Vénéréologie* 107, 83.

Chao, D.H.-C. (1959) Congenital neurocutaneous syndromes in childhood. *Journal of Pediatrics* 55, 189.

Chodirker, B.X., Chudley, A.E., Toffler, M.A. & Reed, M.H. (1986) Brief clinical report: Zimmerman–Laband syndrome and profound mental retardation. *American Journal of Medical Genetics* 25, 543.

Christophers, E. (1975) Familiäre subunguale pterygion. *Hautarzt* 26, 543.

Colla, F., Brühlmann, P., Panizzon, P. & Michel, B.A. (1995) Osteopoikilie—Haut und Gelenkmanifestationen. *Zeitschrift für Rheumatologie* 54, 123.

Commens, C.A. (1990) Twenty nail dystrophy in identical twins. *Pediatric Dermatology* 5, 117.

Copeman, P.W.M., Tan, R.S.-H., Timlin, D. & Samman, P.D. (1978) Familial lichen planus. Another disease or a distinct people? *British Journal of Dermatology* 98, 573.

Cramers, M. (1981) Trichoepithelioma multiplex and dystrophia unguis congenita. A new syndrome? *Acta Dermato-Venereologica* 61, 364.

Davis, S.D., Schaller, J. & Wedgwood, R.J. (1966) Job's syndrome. Recurrent 'cold' staphylococcal abscesses. *Lancet* i, 1013.

Dawson, T.A.J. (1979) An inherited nail dystrophy principally affecting the great toenails. *Clinical and Experimental Dermatology* 4, 309.

Dawson, T.A.J. (1982) An inherited nail dystrophy principally affecting the great toenails: further observations. *Clinical and Experimental Dermatology* 7, 455.

Dugois, P., Amblard, P., Martel, C. & Reymond, J.L. (1975) Pterygium inversum unguis familial. *Bulletin de la Societé Française de Dermatologie et de Syphiligraphie* 82, 283.

Egawa, T. (1977) Congenital claw-like fingers and toes. Case report of two siblings. *Plastic and Reconstructive Surgery* 59, 569.

Feingold, M. (1984) Amniotic constriction bands (Streeter dysplasia, ring constrictions). *American Journal of Diseases of Children* 138, 199.

Gharbi, M.-R., Fazaa, B., Ferchiou, A., Mokhtar, I. & Lahmar, M.L. (1989) Le syndrome de Lesch et Nyhan. *Revue Européene de Dermatologie et Maladie Sexuelle Transmissible* 2, 87.

Giro, M.G., Duvic, M., Smith, L.T. et al. (1992) Buschke–Ollendorff syndrome associated with elevated elastin production by affected skin fibroblasts in culture. *Journal of Investigative Dermatology* 99, 129.

Goldstein, J.H. & Hurt, A.E. (1972) Trichomegaly, cataract, and hereditary spherocytosis in two siblings. *American Journal of Ophthalmology* 73, 333.

Gospos, C. (1976) Gicht. Subakute periarticulare knotige Hautgicht der Endphalangen mit Nageldystrophie. *Zeitschrift für Hautkrankheiten* 51, 29.

Halal, F., Homsy, M. & Perreault, G. (1984) Actro-renal–ocular syndrome: autosomal dominant thumb hypoplasia, renal ectopia, and eye defect. *American Journal of Medical Genetics* 17, 753.

Hammerton, M.D. & Shrank, A.B. (1988) Congenital hypertrophy of the lateral nail folds of the hallux. *Pediatric Dermatology* 5, 243.

Harada, H., Hashimoto, K. & Ko, M.S. (1996) The gene for multiple familial trichoepithelioma maps to chromosome 9p21. *Journal of Investigative Dermatology* 107, 41.

Hazen, P.G. & Smith, D.E. (1990) Hereditary multiple exostoses: report of a case presenting with proximal nail fold and nail swelling. *Journal of the American Academy of Dermatology* 22, 132.

Hendricks, W.M. (1979) Congenital ingrown toenails. *Cutis* 24, 393.

Hoger, P.H., Boltshauser, E. & Hitzig, W.H. (1985) Craniosynostosis in hyper IgE syndrome. *European Journal of Pediatrics* 144, 414.

Hone, J., Accili, D., Al-Gazali, L.I., Lestringant, G., Orban, T. & Taylor, S.I. (1994) Homozygosity for a new mutation (ile 19-to-met) in the insulin receptor gene in five sibs with familial insulin resistance. *Journal of Medical Genetics* 31, 715.

Hundeiker, M. (1969) Herditäre Nageldysplasie der 5 Zehe. *Hautarzt* 20, 282.

Iwasawa, M., Hirose, T. & Matsuo, K. (1991) Congenital curved nail of the fourth toe. *Plastic and Reconstructive Surgery* 87, 553.

Kalisman, M. & Kleinert, H.E. (1983) A circumferential fingernail. Fingernail on the palmar aspect of the finger. *Journal of Hand Surgery* 8, 58.

Kamatani, M., Rai, A., Hen, H. *et al.* (1978) Yellow nail syndrome associated with mental retardation in two siblings. *British Journal of Dermatology* 99, 329.

Knöll, R., Ulrich, R. & Schäfer, R. (1989) Autosomal-dominant verebte 20-Nägel-Dystrophie. *Archives of Dermatology* 15, 213.

Koch, P., Wettstein, A., Knauber, J. & Zaun, H. (1992) A new case of Zimmermann–Laband syndrome with atypical retinitis pigmentosa. *Acta Dermato-Venereologica* 72, 376.

Krooth, R.S., Macklin, M.T. & Hilbish, T.F. (1961) Diaphysial aclasis (multiple exostosis) on Guam. *American Journal of Human Genetics* 13, 340.

Laband, P.F., Habib, G. & Humphreys, G.S. (1964) Hereditary gingival fibromatosis. Report of an affected family with associated splenomegaly and skeletal and soft-tissue abnormalities. *Oral Surgery* 17, 339.

Mahood, J.M. (1983) Familial lichen planus. *Archives of Dermatology* 119, 292.

Mehra, A., Murphy, R.J. & Wilson, B.B. (2000) Idiopathic familial onychomadesis. *Journal of the American Academy of Dermatology* 43, 349–350.

Nogita, T., Yamashita, H., Kawashima, M. & Hidano, A. (1991) Pterygium inversum unguis. *Journal of the American Academy of Dermatology* 24, 787.

Odom, R.B., Stein, K.M. & Maibach, H. (1974) Congenital, painful, abberant hyponychium. *Archives of Dermatology* 110, 89.

Philips, R.J., Atherton, D.J., Gibbs, M.L., Strobel, S. & Lake, B.D. (1994) Laryngo-onycho-cutaneous syndrome: an inherited epithelial defect. *Archives of Disease in Childhood* 70, 319.

Prandi, G. & Caccialanza, M. (1977) An unusual congenital nail dystrophy ('soft nail disease'). *Clinical and Experimental Dermatology* 2, 265.

Riccardi, V.M. & Eichner, J.E. (1986) *Neurofibromatosis: Phenotype, Natural History and Pathogenesis*. Johns Hopkins University Press. Baltimore.

Rosenberg, S., Nagahashi Marie, S.K. & Kliemann, S. (1994) Congenital insensitivity to pain with anhidrosis (hereditary, sensory and autonomic neuropathy type IV). *Pediatric Neurology* 11, 50.

Roth, S.I., Schedewie, H.K., Herzberg, V.K., Olefsky, J., Elders, M.J. & Rubinstein, A. (1981) Cutaneous manifestations of leprechaunism. *Archives of Dermatology* 117, 531.

Runne, U. & Orfanos, C.E. (1981) The human nail. *Current Problems in Dermatology* 9, 102.

Salamon, T., Halepovic, E., Berberovic, L. *et al.* (1987) Epidermodysplasia verruciformis-ähnliche Genodermatose mit Veränderungen der Nägel. *Hautarzt* 38, 525.

Samman, P.D. (1978) Great toenail dystrophy. *Clinical and Experimental Dermatology* 3, 81.

Scappaticci, S., Lambiase, S., Orecchia, G. & Fraccaro, M. (1989) Clonal chromosome abnormalities with preferential involvement of chromosome 3 in patients with porokeratosis of Mibelli. *Cancer Genetics and Cytogenetics* 43, 89.

Shabbir, G., Hassan, M. & Kazmi, A. (1986) Laryngo-onychocutaneous syndrome. A study of 22 cases. *Biomedicine* 2, 15.

Shaw, M., Jurecka, W., Black, M.M. & Kurwa, A. (1983) Macular amyloidosis associated with familial nail dystrophy. *Clinical and Experimental Dermatology* 8, 363.

Shelley, W. & Rawnsley, H.M. (1965) Aminogenic alopecia: hair loss associated with argininosuccinic aciduria. *Lancet* ii, 1327.

Solomon, L. (1964) Hereditary multiple exostosis. *American Journal of Human Genetics* 16, 351.

Stirling, R., Pitts, J., Galloway, N.R., Robson, K. & Newbury-Ecob, R. (1994) Congenital hereditary endothelial dystrophy associated with nail hypoplasia. *British Journal of Ophthalmology* 78, 77.

Takeda, Y., Itagaki, M. & Ishibashi, K. (1989) Hypoplastic-hypocalcified enamel of teeth and dysplastic nails: an undescribed ectodermal dysplasia syndrome. *International Journal of Oral and Maxillofacial Surgery* 18, 73.

Tasjian, D. & Jarrattt, M. (1984) Familial acanthosis nigricans. *Archives of Dermatology* 120, 1351.

Thomson, C.C., Park, R.I. & Prescot, G.H. (1980) Oral manifestations of the congenital insensitivity to pain syndrome. *Oral Surgery* 50, 220.

Toma, N.M.G., Ebenezer, N.D., Inglehearn, C.F., Plant, C., Ficker, L.A. & Bhattacharya, S.S. (1995) Linkage of congenital hereditary endothelial dystrophy to chromosome 20. *Human Molecular Genetics* 4, 2395.

Valsecchi, R., Bontempelli, M., di Landro, A., Barcella, A. & Lainelli, T. (1990) Familial lichen planus. *Acta Dermato-Venereologica* 70, 272.

Voigtländer, V., Schnyder, U.W. & Anton-Lamprect, I. (1979) *Dermatologie in Praxis und Klinik*, Band III, p. 2245. Georg Thieme-Verlag, Stuttgart.

Wallach, D., Foldes, G., Cattan, E. & Dulac, O. (1987) Syndrome de Rud. *Annales de Dermatologie et de Vénéréologie* 144, 1462.

Wells, G.C. (1966) Yellow nail syndrome with familial primary hypoplasia of lymphatics, manifest late in life. *Proceedings of the Royal Society of Medicine* 59, 447.

Zaun, H., Stenger, D., Zabransky, S. & Zankl, M. (1984) Das Syndrom der langen Wimpern ('Trichomegaliesyndrom', Oliver-McFarlane). *Hautarzt* 35, 162.

# CHAPTER 10

# Nail surgery and traumatic abnormalities

**E.G. Zook, R. Baran, E. Haneke & R.P.R. Dawber**
**(with the participation of G.J. Brauner)**

This chapter has drawn on the skills of four experts in nail surgery working in different countries in the specialties of dermatological surgery and hand surgery. In order to illustrate how things can be done differently and achieve excellent results we have organized the content in a manner to reflect the differences and common ground between the authors. Elvin Zook's contribution has been placed in *italic letters* so that the perspective of the hand surgeon can throw a different light on the material addressed by the dermatological surgeon.

The surgery of the nail and its associated structures has generated considerable interest during the last decade; a deformed nail has always been a cosmetic handicap but, until recently, the possibilities for surgical correction were limited. The application by the dermatologist of the techniques of plastic surgery and the more refined skills of the specialized hand surgeon have brought fresh optimism to the field. The objectives of surgery are:

1 To facilitate diagnosis: this may entail biopsy.
2 To alleviate pain.
3 To treat infection, which may or may not be directly associated.
4 To correct or prevent anatomical, traumatic, congenital, infectious, parasitic or iatrogenic deformities.
5 To remove local tumours.
6 To ensure the best cosmetic result.

These objectives are interrelated and must be viewed as a therapeutic whole.

## Anatomy

*Detailed anatomy of the perionychium is presented in Chapter 1. The terms for the perionychium vary from specialty to specialty and country to country, so only a brief discussion of anatomy as it will be used in this chapter will be given here.*

*The perionychium consists of the paronychium (surrounding soft tissue) and the nail bed (Lewis 1954). It has been described on numerous occasions (Jones 1941; McCash 1956; Pardo-Castello 1960; Stone & Mullins 1963; Lewin 1965; Barron 1970; Samman 1972; Zaias 1980; Samman 1983; Zook 1985, 1990a). The lateral anatomy in diagrammatic form that will be used in this chapter is shown in Fig. 10.1. The hyponychium is the junction between the distal nail bed and the skin of the fingertip. The proximal nail fits into a dorsal fold called the nail fold. The skin over the nail fold is the nail wall and the thin arched area where the dorsal roof of the nail fold covers the nail is called the eponychium. The lunula is the curved white line just distal to the eponychium. The nail matrix is the tissue that produces material that is incorporated to make up the nail volume.*

*The nail is made of material from three areas in the nail bed. (Jarrett & Spearman 1966; de Berker et al. 1996) (Fig. 10.2). Lewis (1954) attributed approximately 90% of nail production*

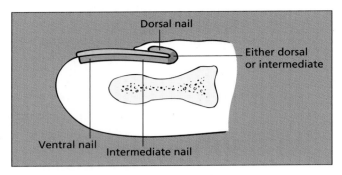

**Fig. 10.2** The three areas of nail production. © E. Zook.

*to the germinal matrix, which lies on the proximal ventral floor of the nail fold in proximity to the periosteum of the distal phalanx. The nail bed from the distal edge of the germinal matrix to the hyponychium is known as the 'sterile matrix' and produces nail cells that adhere the nail to the nail bed as new cells are produced and flow into the nail. The proximal one-half of the dorsal roof of the nail fold produces cells that flow out onto the nail surface and add the shine to the nail. Loss of the eponychium and nail wall will eliminate the shine on the nail and cause roughness of the surface. While Lewis (1954) suggests that all three areas produce nail, Zaias (1980) states only the portion produced by the germinal matrix is true nail.*

*The general terms nail bed, nail matrix or matrix will be used interchangeably in this chapter. References to specific areas of the nail bed or nail matrix will be so stated.*

## Physiology

*During the first 30 days postinjury the nail grows less rapidly then overgrows for 50 days and subsequently grows slower for 14 days. This creates a ridge on all injured nails, which will eventually grow off to leave a flat nail if severity of the injury has not obviated achievement of a normal nail.*

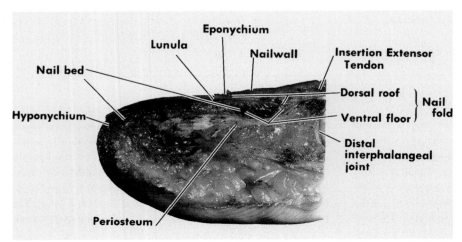

**Fig. 10.1** The anatomy of the perionychium as used in this chapter. © E. Zook.

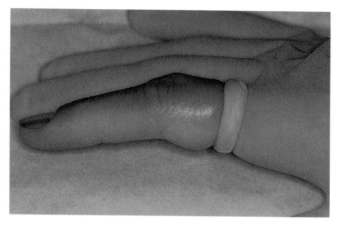

**Fig. 10.3** Aseptic technique using the 'rolled-up' rubber glove finger method.

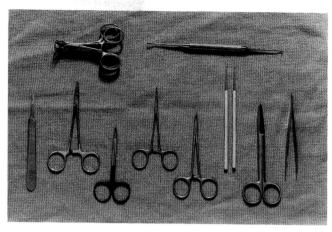

(a)

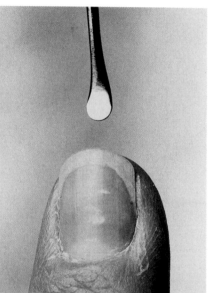

(b)

**Fig. 10.4** (a) The various fine instruments, which make up a pack for nail bed surgery. (b) A Kleinert–Kutz elevator to remove the nail is shown in comparison with the size of the nail. © E. Zook.

## History and patient examination

General examination of the patient should be carried out to exclude peripheral vascular disease, diabetes and blood dyscrasias, collagen disease, peripheral neurological disease, prosthetic cardiac valves, elderly and incapacited patients in poor general health and immunocompromised patients. The concomitant administration of drugs should be noted: these may affect anaesthesia, for example monoaminoxidase inhibitors, β-blockers or phenothiazines; those that prolong bleeding, for example aspirin or anticoagulants; drugs that delay healing, for example systemic or topical steroids, or have toxic effects on nail, for example retinoids. Additionally there may be a history of allergy to lidocaine or carbocaine or parabens (contained in both as a preservative); local anaesthetics may be contraindicated in patients with cardiac disease such as heart block. A knowledge of previous antitetanus immunization is important since tetanus toxoid is advisable when handling the toenail area or in traumatic lesions that come into contact with soil. The affected digit should be inspected with regard to the quality and colour of the surrounding skin and compared to the unaffected contralateral digit. The presence of signs of infection, particularly in association with pyrexia, may modify the site or type of anaesthesia or delay surgery until appropriate systemic antibiotic therapy has had effect.

Xeroradiography, echography, MRI allow evaluation of the phalanx and soft tissue.

## Preoperative measures

The hand is prepared for nail surgery using a surgical scrub with povidone-iodine or alternative disinfectant soap. A sterile surgical glove with the tip of the appropriate finger removed provides an aseptic covering of the patient's hand (Fig. 10.3).

The foot should first be soaked in appropriate antiseptic solutions before surgery is performed on the toenails. If cutting

the nail plate is needed it is wise to soak the digit for about 10 min in water to soften it, thus facilitating nail section. The foot is draped in the usual aseptic manner with sterile towels which are secured with towel clamps.

## Instrumentation

*It is essential that fine instrumentation be available for fingernail surgery. This includes fine curved iris scissors, fine toothed pick-ups, a scalpel with a small blade, skin hooks, needle holder, and the periosteal elevator. I prefer the Kleinert–Kutz elevator, which has a small end, which is ideal for raising the nail from the nail bed and out of the nail fold (Fig. 10.4). The fine toothless needle holder and suture such as 6 or 7-0 chromic*

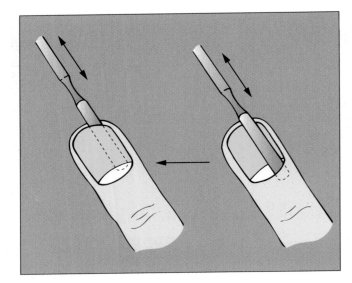

**Fig. 10.5** Nail avulsion with a dental spatula.

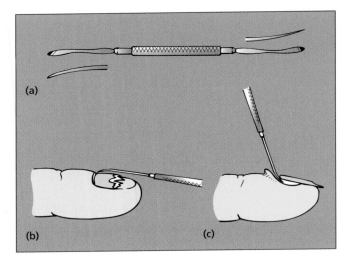

**Fig. 10.6** Cordero's method of nail plate avulsion. (a) Freer septum elevator. (b) The instrument shown is pushed under the proximal nail fold to the far edge of the nail plate and is in the process of freeing it from side to side. (c) The instrument is shown slipped along the natural plane of cleavage between nail plate and bed, thus freeing it entirely.

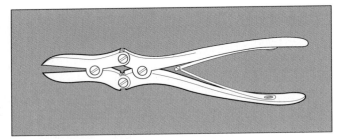

**Fig. 10.7** Double action nail clipper (bone rongeur).

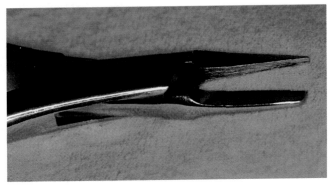

**Fig. 10.8** The English nail splitter.

and 6-0 nylon are essential for accurate approximation and minimal tissue reaction.

In addition dermatologists use nail elevators (Figs 10.5–10.8) (dental spatula or Freer septum elevator), single or double pronged skin hooks (flexible retractors), double action nail clippers (bone rongeur), nail splitting scissors, English nail splitter (the lower blade is unique, with its smooth undersurface that glides atraumatically along the nail bed, while the anvil-like upper surface slides under the nail, the regular scissor's upper blade then cuts through the nail plate), pointed scissors (Gradle scissors), curved iris scissors, small-nosed mosquito haemostats and no. 11 and no. 15 scalpel blades, the chisel-like

number 81 blade of the Beaver system is useful as a nail splitter for thickened or friable nails (Salasche & Peters 1985); disposable punches (2, 3, 3.5, 4, 5 and 6 mm), tourniquet (Penrose drains), Luer–Lock syringe and 30-gauge needle. Sutures are monofilament non-absorbable polypropylene (e.g. Prolene) or 6-0 colourless absorbable threads (e.g. PDS).

The use of a magnifier lens (×3 or ×5) or a microscope facilitates surgery.

## Anaesthesia

*Anaesthesia of the finger is essential for good surgical care of the nail and its problems. If pain occurs during the procedure, it may complicate or hinder the correct treatment of the nail. Various techniques have been described for anaesthetizing the fingertip including injections over the dorsal finger proximal to the nail. I find this injection uncomfortable for the patient and prefer a total finger block (Fig. 10.9). This is done in a variety of ways, which include penetration of the skin on each side of the finger in the area of the digital nerve and injection of local anaesthetic agent. Lignocaine (lidocaine) without adrenaline (epinephrine) has quick action and a low toxicity. Penetrate the skin over the digital nerve at the base of the finger down to the periosteum with a fine (25–30) gauge needle. While withdrawing the needle inject 1 mL of local anaesthetic, then angle 45 degrees volar and inject another 1 mL and then 45 degrees dorsal*

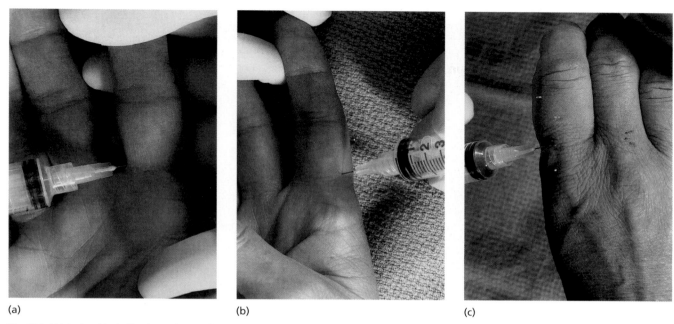

(a)                    (b)                   (c)

**Fig. 10.9** (a) Injection of 3 mL of local anaesthetic in a fanshape on the lateral aspect of the finger. (b) Similar injection on the opposite side of the finger. (c) Injection of a bead of local anaesthetic across the dorsum of the finger. © E. Zook.

*and inject another 1 mL. Do the same bilaterally which uses approximately 6 mL of lignocaine. Then run a bead 1–2 mL of lignocaine beneath the dorsal skin of the proximal phalanx. It is important to give the anaesthetic time to be effective which takes 8–10 min. Bupivacaine may be used either before or after the procedure for prolonged anaesthesia. Onset of anaesthesia takes longer with bupivacaine and the toxicity is higher than lignocaine but in small amounts used for a finger block that is rarely of consequence.*

### Wing block local distal digital anaesthesia
(Salasche & Peters 1985) (Fig. 10.10)

Using a 30 gauge needle, the injection is started 2–3 mm proximal to the junction of the proximal and lateral nail fold. It is continued distally and downward to deaden the lateral digital nerve and its branches. The injection is then carried across the proximal nail fold, to involve the transverse nerve, and finally to the other side of the digit: the lateral and proximal nail folds will be seen to distend and blanch, the anaesthetic solution partially acts as a tourniquet. For distal nail bed operations, a supplementary injection at the tip of the digit is often necessary. Unilateral 'wing' block is used for isolated surgery of the nail border.

Anaesthesia takes effect almost immediately.

### Central local distant digital anaesthesia (Zaias 1990)
(Fig. 10.11)

In children's digits and small toes, a single injection of the anaesthetic into the proximal nail fold area furthur delivers the

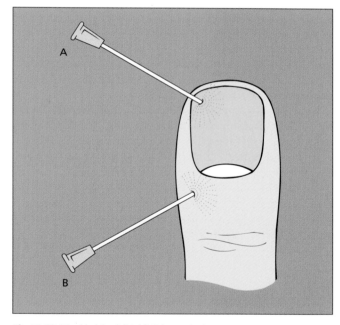

**Fig. 10.10** Wing block local distal digital anaesthesia.

anaesthetic into the dermis of the lunula. The anaesthetic will cover all the matrix and nail bed region. We have obtained good, but inconsistant, results in adults, even in injecting the great toe.

Local distant digital anaesthesia is contraindicated if there is infection in the terminal phalangeal region.

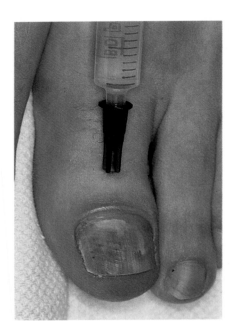

**Fig. 10.11** Central local distal digital anaesthesia.

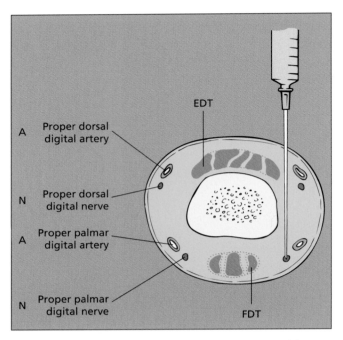

**Fig. 10.13** Digital cross-section showing the various structures present in relation to the nerves to be injected (N); A, artery; EDT, extensor digitorum tendon; FDT, flexor digitorum tendon.

## Metacarpal block (Kleinert 1959) (Figs 10.12–10.15)

A wheal is raised on the dorsum of the hand 2–3 cm proximal to the web. A 30 gauge needle is placed 2–3 cm proximal to the dorsal web and 2 mL of the local anaesthetic agent is infiltrated at the level of the digital nerve which is volar to the deep transverse intermetacarpal ligament. The needle is reinserted on the opposite side of the metacarpal to block the other digital nerve. A small subcutaneous wheal is raised on the dorsum of the hand to block the dorsal sensory branches.

It takes 10–15 min for anaesthesia to develop in digital nerve blocks. Metacarpal blocks and webspace blocks are of use for anaesthetizing the lateral aspect of adjacent digits.

Digital nerve block performed in the web or in the metacarpal area is safer than one performed more distally, because hydrostatic pressure of the injection creates a tourniquet effect.

In addition, digital block anaesthesia may facilitate the extension of a pre-existing infection and carries a risk of spreading it higher up the extremity. Therefore hand surgeons favour general anaesthesia or regional block (if only the distal phalanx is involved).

## Transthecal digital block (Chiu 1990)

Flexor tendon sheath may be used as an avenue for introducing anaesthetics to the core of the digit. Through centrifugal anaesthetic diffusion all four digital nerves are anaesthetized

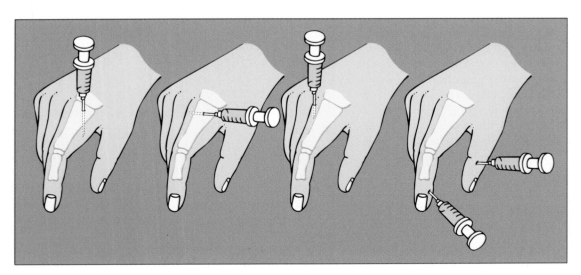

**Fig. 10.12** Diagram to show the various digital sites suggested for adequate anaesthesia of the nail apparatus (see text). (After Petres & Hundeiker.)

rapidly. This technique involves palmar percutaneous injection of 2 mL of lignocaine into the potential space of the flexor tendon sheath at the level of the palmar flexion crease with a 3-mL syringe and a no. 25–27 gauge hypodermic needle.

## Regional anaesthesia (Kleinert 1959; Abadir 1975; Hutton *et al.* 1991)

Regional anaesthesia is indicated for extensive surgery.

### Wrist block (Fig. 10.16)

This is the anaesthesia of choice when treating several fingertips or when there is infection or vascular impairement in the affected digits. This procedure involves truncal infiltration of the median and ulnar nerves.

### Median nerve block at wrist

Locate palmaris longus tendon and flexor carpi radialis by asking the subject to flex the hand against resistance. At the distal crease at the wrist between the two tendons raise a small skin wheel with a 2-cm needle, advance the needle about 8–12 mm. Care should be exercised so that the nerve is not transfixed. Advance the needle slowly to contact the nerve if paraesthesia is desired. When it is elicited withdraw the needle 1–2 mm. Then inject 5–8 mL of suitable anaesthetic.

### Ulnar nerve block

At the proximal crease of the wrist, immediately medial to the ulna, advance a 2-cm needle diagonally pointing posteriorly and cephalad until the medial surface of the ulna is contacted by

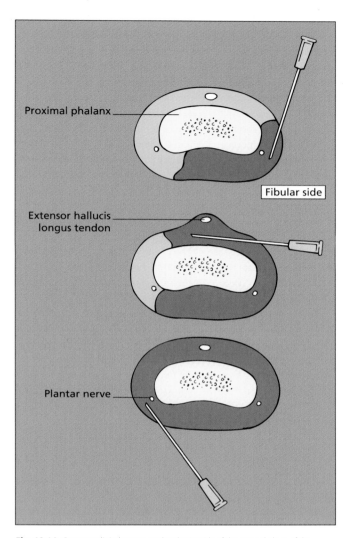

**Fig. 10.14** Great toe digital nerves on the plantar side of the coronal plane of the phalanx—sites of anaesthesia. (After W.R. Ross, USA.)

Proximal phalanx

Fibular side

Extensor hallucis longus tendon

Plantar nerve

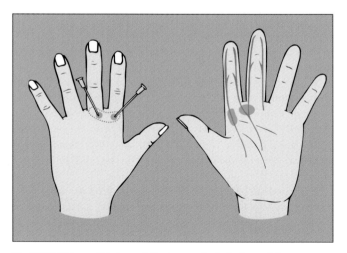

**Fig. 10.15** Metacarpal block—useful for the anaesthesia of adjacent digits.

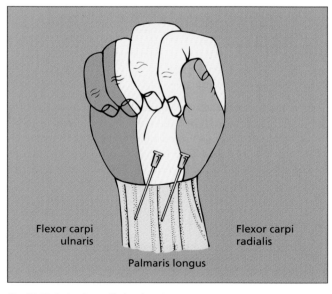

Flexor carpi ulnaris

Flexor carpi radialis

Palmaris longus

**Fig. 10.16** Regional nerve block at the wrist.

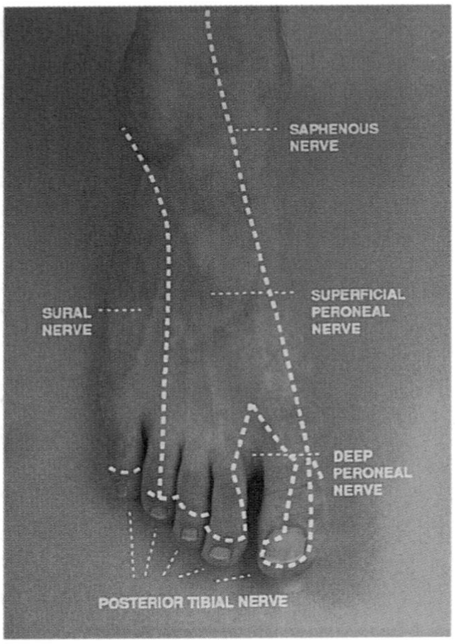

**Fig. 10.17** Nerve supply to the foot.

the advancing needle. Withdraw the needle a few millimetres then readvance in a slightly more medial direction until the tip of the needle is felt tenting the skin of the dorsal surface of the arm by the operator's other hand. Aspirate, to insure absence of blood. Then inject 8–10 mL of any suitable local anaesthetic while withdrawing the needle. The injection site has to traverse the course of the ulnar nerve and its branches. The success rate is almost 100% with this block (Abadir 1975).

### Radial nerve block

In order to inject the radial nerve, the sharp edge of the curve of the lower end of the radius is used as a guide. The anaesthetic is placed subcutaneously in the deep layer of fat, starting at the edge of the radius 5–8 cm above the wrist, where the nerve emerges under the brachioradialis tendon.

Anaesthesia becomes established in 5–15 min.

### Nerve blocks for the toes (Fig. 10.17)

Digital blocks are usually adequate for procedures involving the distal toes. However, in rare, selected cases (nail avulsion of several digits, for example) nerve blocks involving the posterior tibial, deep peroneal, sural or saphenous nerve, or a combination of them should be considered, as indicated by the specific surgical site (Cohen & Roenigk 1991).

### Brachial plexus anaesthesia

This does not seem appropriate for nail surgery.

### Intravenous regional analgesia

This method is now seldom used by hand surgeons: this is induced by lignocaine or bupivacaine. The operative field is exsanguinated either by elevating the limb, or by application of Esmarch bands. It is then excluded from the general circulation by the use of an arterial tourniquet inflated to 30 mmHg above systolic blood pressure. The anaesthetic is then given; in 20 min, this results in an excellent analgesia which lasts for nearly 2 h. Pain may be quite distressing when the anaesthetic wears off. The tourniquet may be removed after 1 h. The analgesia generally persists for a short time, inadequate to ensure haemostasis and satisfactory cutaneous suturing. This mode of anaesthesia requires a minimum of preoperative tests and may be ideal for ambulatory surgery, but is not without hazard, especially with bupivacaine.

Irrespective of the technique used, the following points are relevant:
- Xylocaine 1 or 2% should be given without adrenaline, since the ischaemia lasts too long and may result in gangrene.
- Depending on the site of the injection, it takes 3–10 min for anaesthesia to develop.

*Tourniquets are essential for haemostasis and visualization of the nail bed. After the local block is in effect, a Penrose drain (Fig. 10.18) is wrapped around the finger starting distally and winding proximally overlapping each wrap slightly. At the proximal finger a loop is pulled up from each side and a clamp placed across the Penrose. An alternative is extravasating the blood from the finger with either a Penrose drain or elevation and using the metal tourniquet shown (Fig. 10.19).*

### General anaesthesia

General anaesthesia may be indicated in children, or for psychological or medical reasons in adults.

## Incisions

*Access to the nail fold is best achieved by incisions made radially from the eponychium at its proximal corners (Fig. 10.20). The radial incision allows the eponychium to be reapproximated more accurately with fine nylon sutures and decreases the chance of notching that develops with incisions paralleling the paronychial fold.*

*Access to the bone of the distal phalanx is made through an arc incision just on the skin side of the hyponychium. The nail must be removed from the nail bed if extensive exposure is required. The nail bed may then be raised from the periosteum of the distal phalanx allowing most of the distal phalanx to be exposed. The nail bed is then replaced on the bone and sutured distally.*

*For removal of naevi or small tumours of the nail bed a longitudinal incision in the germinal and/or sterile matrix is preferred. The matrix edges are carefully undermined so the incision can be closed without tension. A transverse incision is more difficult to close without tension and gives a higher incidence of non-adherence of the nail. The longitudinal incision*

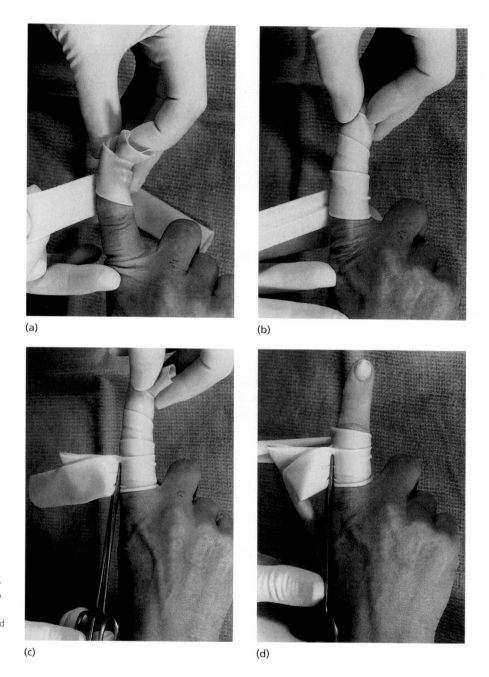

(a)

(b)

(c)

(d)

**Fig. 10.18** (a) Tip of a no. 1 Penrose drain is held free distally and then the finger is wrapped with the Penrose. (b) The wrapping of the finger has been completed. (c) A clamp is placed across the base of the Penrose drain to serve as a tourniquet. (d) The end of the Penrose is pulled to unwind the Penrose and expose the nail bed and perionychium. © E. Zook.

*may sometimes give some ridging or splitting of the nail particularly if it is closed under tension.*

*The distal interphalangeal (DIP) joint is best accessed by a transverse incision over the joint with a perpendicular arm on the lateral aspect of the finger converting the transverse incision to a 'T' if the lesion is on one side, or an 'H' if access to the entire joint is necessary to debride osteophytes.*

## References

Abadir, A. (1975) Use of local anaesthetics in dermatology. *Journal of Dermatologic Surgery* **1**, 68–72.

Barron, J.N. (1970) The structure and function of the skin of the hand. *Hand* **2**, 93–96.

Chiu, D.T.W. (1990) Transthecal digital block: flexor tendon sheath used for anaesthetic infusion. *Journal of Hand Surgery* **15A**, 471–473.

Cohen, S.J. & Roenigk, R.K. (1991) Nerve blocks for cutaneous surgery on the foot. *Journal of Dermatologic Surgery and Oncology* **17**, 527–534.

de Berker, D. & Mawhinney, B. & Sviland, L. (1996) Quantification of regional matrix nail production. *British Journal of Dermatology* **134**, 1083–1086.

Hutton, K.P., Podolsky, A., Roenigk, R.K. *et al.* (1991) Regional anaesthesia of the hand for dermatologic surgery. *Journal of Dermatologic Surgery and Oncology* **17**, 881–888.

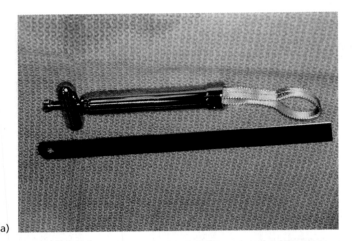

(a)

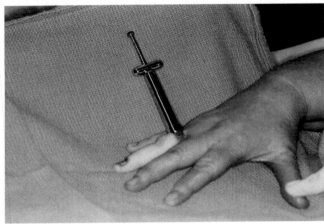

(b)

**Fig. 10.19** (a) A commercially available metal tourniquet, which has a wide metal band, to avoid localized compression of the nerve. (b) Blood extravasated from the finger and the tourniquet applied. © E. Zook.

Jarrett, A. & Spearman, R.I.C. (1966) The histochemistry of the human nail. *Archives of Dermatology* **94**, 652–657.

Jones, F.W. (1941) *The Principles of Anatomy as Seen in the Hand*, 2nd edn. Baillière, Tindall and Cox, London.

Kleinert, H.E. (1959) Fingertip injuries and their management. *American Surgery* **25**, 41–45.

Lewin, K. (1965) The normal finger nail. *British Journal of Dermatology* **77**, 421–430.

Lewis, B.L. (1954) Microscopic studies of fetal and mature nail and surrounding soft tissue. *Archives of Dermatology* **70**, 732–747.

McCash, C.R. (1956) Free nail grafting. *British Journal of Plastic Surgery* **8**, 19–33.

Pardo-Castello, V. (1960) *Disease of the Nail*, 3rd edn. Charles C. Thomas, Springfield, IL.

Salasche, S. & Peters, V.J. (1985) Tips on nail surgery. *Cutis* **35**, 428–438.

Samman, P.D. (1972) *The Nails in Disease*, 2nd edn. Charles C. Thomas, Springfield, IL.

Samman, P.D. (1983) *The Nails in Disease*, 3rd edn. Year Book Medical Publishers, Chicago.

Stone, O.J. & Mullins, J.F. (1963) The distal course of nail matrix hemorrhage. *Archives of Dermatology* **79**, 186–187.

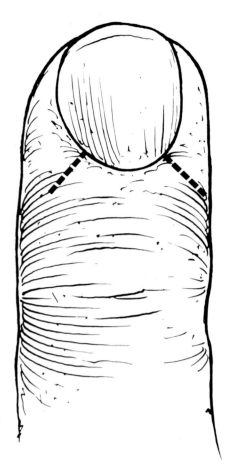

**Fig. 10.20** Incisions to expose the nail fold should be made tangentially from the eponychium as shown. © E. Zook.

Zaias, N. (1980) *The Nail in Health and Disease*. Spectrum Publications, Jamaica, NY.

Zaias, N. (1990) *The Nail in Health and Disease*, 2nd edn. Appleton & Lange, Norwalk, CN.

Zook, E.G. (1985) Nail bed injuries. *Hand Clinics* **1**, 701–716.

Zook, E.G. & Russell, R.C. (1990) Reconstruction of a functional and esthetic nail. *Hand Clinics* **6**, 59–68.

## Dressing

*If the nail is available and of reasonably normal contour, scrape the undersurface with a 15 scalpel blade to remove the adhering fragments of matrix and soak the nail in povidone-iodine solution (Betadine) or other antiseptic solution while performing surgery on the nail bed. After the procedure is completed the nail may be replaced into the nail fold and held there with a 5-0 nylon suture through the hyponychium and the nail. Replacing the nail contours the tissue between the stitches gives better sensation while the new nail is growing out, maintains fracture reduction and is less uncomfortable than an exposed matrix. If the nail is not available, is too deformed, or fragmented a piece of 20/1000th reinforced silicone sheeting will maintain the nail fold open until healing occurs and contour the matrix edges*

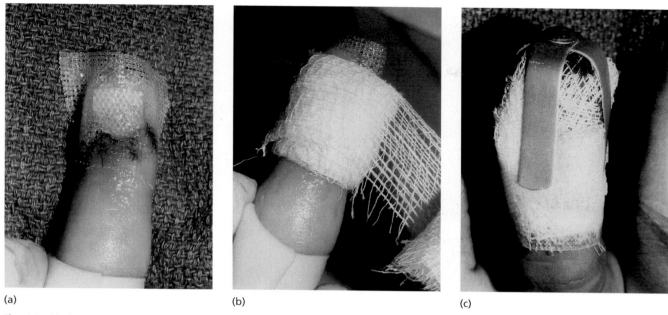

(a)  (b)  (c)

**Fig. 10.21** (a) After repair of the nail bed non-adherent gauze such as adaptic is placed over the nail. (b) An absorbent gauze and Kling to hold it in place is applied. (c) A 4-post splint of either metal or plastic is used to protect the end of the finger. © E. Zook.

*between sutures. Commercially available nails may be used but correct size and shape must be found. If none of the aforementioned is available, a piece of adaptic or other non-adherent gauze may be cut in the shape of the nail and placed into the nail fold and over the matrix. The gauze will adhere and does not need to be sutured. An absorbable gauze is placed over the non-adherent gauze to collect drainage from the nail bed. A 1-inch (2.5 cm) Kling dressing is wrapped to maintain the gauze in place. A metal four-post or plastic cap splint over the dressing prevents bumping and increases the comfort of the patient in the first few weeks while the finger is healing (Fig. 10.21).*

The involved extremity should be elevated during the first 48 h. For toenail surgery the patient should be warned in advance to bring an open-toed shoe, slipper or sandal. The patient has to be kept recumbent. Depending on the type of operation the first dressing should be removed after 24–48 h: any surgical operation of a non-sterile nail area, for example, an ingrowing toenail with oozing granulation tissue or a nail biopsy on a mycotic nail with subungual hyperkeratosis, as well as considerable bleeding, should prompt a change of dressing after 24 h. After removal of the outer layers of the dressing, the extremity is put into lukewarm water with disinfectant soap, for example povidone-iodine soap, until the inner layers of the dressing float off. This ensures an entirely painless procedure. If there is any sign of infection, antiseptic soaks should be commenced once to three times daily (Haneke 1991). If the operation wound does not show any sign of inflammation, the second dressing may be left for 5–7 days.

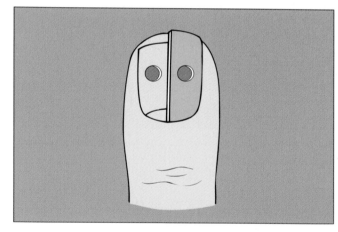

**Fig. 10.22** Biopsy of the nail bed: right half, showing one punch technique without nail plate avulsion; left half, biopsy after partial nail avulsion.

## Reference

Haneke, E. (1991) Operationen am Nagelorgan—Planung, Durchführung, Fehlermöglichkeiten und ihre Vermeidung. *Zeitschrift für Hautkrankheiten* **66** (Suppl. 3), 132–133.

## Biopsy of the nail area (Figs 10.22–10.26, Tables 10.1 & 10.2)

Biopsy of the nail area is almost as simple as at any other site

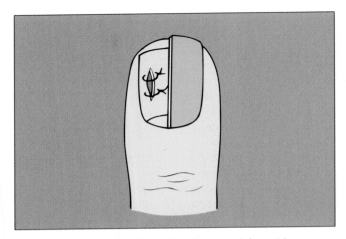

**Fig. 10.23** Biopsy of the nail bed; longitudinal ellipse removed after partial plate avulsion.

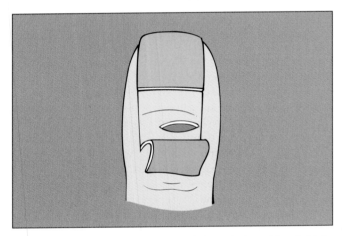

**Fig. 10.24** Crescent or fusiform matrix biopsy: only the proximal part of the nail plate is cut to permit biopsy.

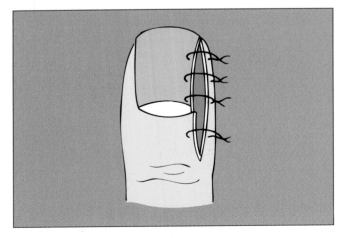

**Fig. 10.25** Longitudinal biopsy on the lateral aspect.

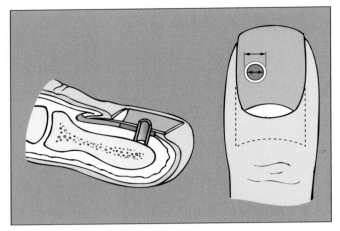

**Fig. 10.26** Diagram showing nail bed biopsy using the double punch technique.

**Table 10.1** Nail biopsies. (From Gonzalvez-Serva 1990, with permission from the author and publisher.)

*According to site*
Matrix
Bed
Combined (proximal fold–matrix bed–hyponychium)
Paronychium
Plate

*According to field preparation*
Without avulsion of plate (translaminar)
With prior avulsion of plate (open)

*Acccording to sampling method*
Punch
Incisional
Shave (trimming):
  (a) Soft tissues
  (b) Nail plate

*According to orientation*
Transverse
Longitudinal

*According to comprehensiveness*
Local (one component of nail unit)
En bloc (several components of nail unit)
A large sample of a single component

and may be a very useful procedure (André & Achten 1987; Kechijian 1987; Rich 1992).

**Why and when?** (Baran & Sayag 1976; Scher & Ackerman 1980)

**1** To demonstrate pathogenicity of fungal organisms in diseased nails (Chapter 5) (Achten 1972; Scher & Ackerman 1980a; Haneke 1985).

**Table 10.2** Clinico-pathological limitations of nail biopsies (from Gonzalvez-Serva 1990, with permission from the author and publisher).

*Regarding inflammatory diseases*

1. Clinical and histological signs of dystrophy (plate abnormality) are shared by several diseases, both inflammatory and otherwise
2. Superimposition of common reactional patterns unrelated to primary aetiology:
    (a) Metaplastic epidermalization (reversing of specialized nail epithelia to 'genetic' epidermoid squamous epithelium)
    (b) Lichen simplex chronicus onychalis (post-traumatic orthokeratotic hyperplasia of nail epithelia)
3. Different histological appearances than homologous cutaneous dermatosis
4. Primary trauma may mimic specific inflammation
5. Microorganisms are difficult to detect or assess as primary agents, i.e. they may represent colonizers

*Regarding solid tumours*

1. Non-specific appearance at clinical examination
2. Different behaviour than cutaneous homologue (e.g. keratoacanthoma)
3. Frequent history of trauma obscures neoplastic nature
4. Associated chronic infection
5. Late diagnosis:
    (a) Lack of radiologic studies
    (b) Reticence to biopsy early in course
    (c) Insufficient tissue sample
    (d) Difficult discrimination between some neoplasms and reactive changes

*Regarding pigmented lesions*

1. Difficult discrimination between pigments: haemosiderin and melanin may look alike
2. Biopsy may reveal pigment but not its source: the matrix should be assessed because melanocytic lesions, malignant melanoma, primarily reside there
3. Not all deposition of melanin is neoplastic. Ephelis-like hyperplasia is the most common cause
4. Not all melanocytic neoplasms are malignant. Dysplastic naevi probably exist in the nail field
5. Criteria for diagnosis of melanoma may be of difficult application. Acral lentiginous melanoma traditionally is considered difficult to diagnose

2 To differentiate between mycotic and psoriatic nail disease (Scher & Ackerman 1980b; Haneke 1991).

3 To aid in the diagnosis of dystrophies limited to the nail apparatus, such as lichen planus, since it would require special treatment to avoid further nail destruction (Zaias 1967; Hanno *et al.* 1986).

4 To establish early diagnosis of malignant subungual and periungual neoplasia or to facilitate the diagnosis of certain benign tumours.

Nail biopsy is not recommended in immunocompromised subjects, diabetes mellitus or peripheral vascular disease.

## How and where?

1 Using scissors or a bone rongeur, it is easy to take specimens that include a piece of the distal plate and the underlying hyponychium. This technique may be adequate for the diagnosis of some mycotic nail infections (Achten 1972).

2 A 3-mm punch biopsy can be restricted to the nail plate. This can be used when there is a possibility that the suspected mycotic pathology is not confined to the distal portion. Soaking in tepid warm water 10 min immediately prior to punching the nail may be helpful.

3 Except for this purpose, it may also be useful to thin the nail by electric grinding before biopsying the nail bed. This facilitates translaminar punch biopsy. When the punch reaches the periosteum, it is withdrawn and fine (Graddle) scissors should be used to release the specimen. Biopsy specimens from the nail matrix or bed are delicate and can be ruined by either crushing the tissue with forceps or shredding it while attempting to separate it from its attachments to the bone below. This can be avoided by securely skewering the specimen with a 30 gauge needle after the specimen has been punched or excised down to the bone. The distal end of the needle is then bent with a haemostat to prevent the specimen from slipping off (Salasche & Peters 1985). Pressure on the nail plate also forces the tissue cylinder up so that it can be cut at its base.

Only direct pressure or oxycel is used for haemostasis (Stone *et al.* 1978). Biopsy sites usually heal satisfactorily. Siegle and Swanson (1982) have developed a two-punch technique for the nail bed. The first and larger punch (6 mm) removes a circular defect in the nail plate, and the second smaller 3–4-mm punch biopsies the nail bed through the nail plate defect created by the first larger punch. The 6-mm nail disc is then put back in its original place. The authors favour this method which overcomes the difficulty to extract within the confines of a 3–4-mm window in the nail plate the fibrous nail bed firmly attached, both to the periosteum and the surrounding nail bed connective tissue (Kechijian 1987). In some cases a small area of onycholysis may be seen.

4 A 3-mm punch biopsy performed into matrix will not produce a noticeable or permanent deformity (Higashi 1970). This is not Zook's opinion: '*I have treated several 3-mm punch biopsies, which resulted in a split nail. Therefore, make the biopsy with a tool as small as possible to make the diagnosis. An incisional biopsy usually will be 1–2 mm in width and 3–4 mm in length. Incisional biopsies should be sutured with fine chromic gut and the nail replaced.*'

## Longitudinal nail bed biopsy (Fig. 10.25)

Sometimes the size of the tissue to be removed necessitates a longitudinal elliptical wedge resection. This is carried out to the bone, the nail plate being fully avulsed, or its longitudinal half partially removed. The wedge biopsy should be long and narrow, parallel with the longitudinal ridges of the rosette nail bed. After the wedge of tissue has been removed, the edges of the ellipse are undermined to facilitate primary closure. Relaxing incisions may be useful at the lateral margins of the nail bed to facilitate primary closure with 6-0 colourless PDS. The indications for this procedure include diagnosis of skin disease, tumours, or unknown lesions.

### Transverse matrix biopsy (Fig. 10.24)

#### Crescent or fusiform matrix biopsy

It is important when performing nail matrix biopsies to maintain the distal curved configuration of the distal lunula. Two small oblique incisions are made on each side of the proximal nail fold; the fold is then retracted in order to expose the matrix area. The proximal third of the plate is dissected and removed, enabling the distal two-thirds of the plate to be retained for the protection of the distal rosette nail bed. The lesion is identified and either part or all of the lesion is removed by a crescent-shaped wedge of tissue with the convex portion of the crescent matching the anterior border of the lunula. The incision is carried down deep to the bone (Fosnaugh 1982). Fusiform biopsy is preferable, as a crescent-shaped biopsy often provides specimens of inadequate width. Using a fine hook, the matrix is then undermined to allow primary suture. Closing is accomplished with interrupted 6-0 PDS sutures. As long as the proximal part of the matrix is not disturbed, transverse biopsy will merely thin the nail plate and will not leave the fissure which may result from a central longitudinal biopsy.

### Nail matrix—nail bed biopsy combined (Fig. 10.25)

1 *Lateral longitudinal biopsy.* The best specimens for histopathological examination are achieved using the lateral longitudinal nail biopsy that includes the proximal nail fold, matrix, nail bed and hyponychium. It could be done at the lateral margin. This method gives as much information as the median longitudinal nail biopsy, but avoids the split-like nail deformity resulting commonly from the latter technique. Beginning in the lateral nail groove, the incisions reach to the bone, parallel for the most part to the lateral margin of the nail plate, including a 3–4-mm nail segment. This ensures that a full thickness fragment of the nail bed and the matrix with its lateral horn is obtained. The most proximal incisions reach the most distal crease of the distal joint and the most distal incisions reach the hyponychium. Slightly curved iris scissors or, better, a surgical blade, are useful for releasing the tissue from the bone. Starting at the tip of the digit one proceeds proximally while maintaining contact with the bony phalanx. Normal sutures are placed on the proximal nail fold and the hyponychium. The lateral nail fold is sutured to the nail plate using back-stitches to provide the reconstruction of the lateral nail fold (Haneke 1984, 1988).

The method of lateral longitudinal biopsy associated with removal of the homologous lateral nail fold (Bennett 1976) is not suitable.

2 In certain cases, it may be necessary to determine the extent of probable malignancy (Siegle & Swanson 1982). If the nail plate is to be part of the biopsy specimen, then only the plate on

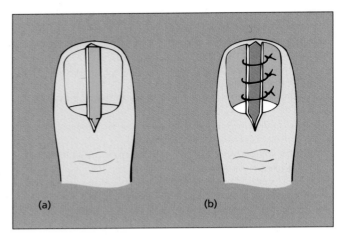

**Fig. 10.27** Nail matrix–nail bed biopsy. (a) The nail plate on either side of the area to be biopsied is removed. (b) Excision of a rectangular block down to bone.

each side of the area to be biopsied should be avulsed (Scher 1980) (Fig. 10.27). However it is quite possible with the scalpel to avulse a rectangular block 3 mm wide down to the bone without avulsing the nail plate on either side of it. This will include the hyponychium, nail bed, nail matrix and proximal nail fold. The surrounding tissues are then undermined and closed, again taking care to ensure good lunular approximation.

### Biopsy of proximal nail fold

Occasionally the proximal nail fold needs to be biopsied. Depending on the purpose, there are three techniques for biopsying this area. When the indications are the same as for routine skin biopsy, a 2-mm punch is advanced down to the nail plate (Stone *et al.* 1978); the plug can then be lifted free. When a punch biopsy is taken, the distal margin of the proximal nail fold should be preserved. For surface biopsy the razor blade technique is ideal (Shelley 1975). Prior to use, each blade is manually broken into two halves by longitudinal bending. The half blade, which is held securely with the fingers and thumb, is kept perfectly flat or bent to the exact arc which conforms to the depth of tissue one desires to remove.

Haemostasis is obtained by a sliding gauze pressure and the application of Monsel's solution (or aluminium chloride) to the resultant dry, non-bleeding field. When more tissue is required, for example in collagen diseases, a crescent-shaped tissue excision, 2–3 mm wide, of the edge of the proximal nail fold is performed. This amount of tissue allows histology, immunohistology and electron microscopy examination to be carried out (Schnitzler *et al.* 1976, 1980). Healing is rapid—by secondary intention. Usually no scarring is visible after 4 weeks, and no nail dystrophy develops.

Treatment of some tumours of the proximal nail fold is possible with the previous techniques. They may be used according to the type and the location of the tumours in the proximal nail fold:

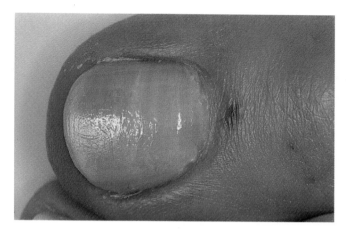

**Fig. 10.28** Crescentic proximal nail fold removal for distal melanocytic naevus: before treatment.

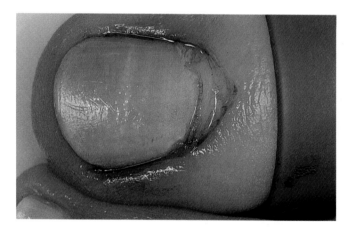

**Fig. 10.29** Crescentic proximal nail fold removal for distal melanocytic naevus: after surgery.

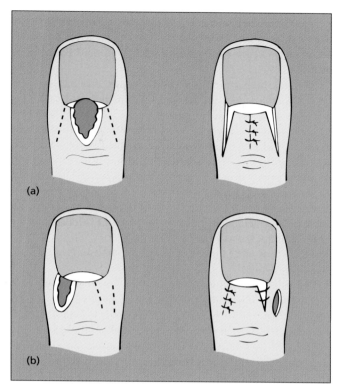

**Fig. 10.30** Method for removal of small lesions from the proximal nail fold.

**1** Some tumours such as myxoid pseudocysts (Salasche 1984), melanocytic naevi and fibrokeratomas (Baran 1986) may be successfully treated by a crescent-shaped piece of proximal nail fold when they are located at its most distal portion. This crescent should not exceed 3–4 mm at its greatest width, to prevent the appearance of a rough nail (Figs 10.28 & 10.29).

**2** Small lesions in the median part of the proximal nail fold may be excised as a wedge. Two lateral incisions are made in the proximal nail fold which is separated from the underlying nail allowing suture of the excisional wound. The narrow secondary defects readily heal by secondary intention (Haneke & Baran 1991) (Fig. 10.30a).

**3** A small lesion in the lateral part of the proximal nail fold may be excised as a wedge. Only one lateral incision is made at the opposite region of the proximal nail fold. To obtain a better healing of the secondary defect which is less narrow than in the previous procedure, the operation may be supplemented by a relaxing incision in the proximal nail fold (Fig. 10.30b).

**4** A dorsal flap can be raised from the proximal nail fold using two dorso-lateral incisions and a horizontal one, proximal to

the cuticle. This permits a clear view of a subcutaneous tumour, or myxoid pseudocyst.

## Longitudinal melanonychia and its biopsy (Baran & Haneke 1984; Baran & Kechijian 1989)

Longitudinal melanonychia (LM) is characterized by a tan, brown or black longitudinal streak within the nail plate. LM results from increased melanin deposition in the nail plate. The presence of blood or chromogens, however, may simulate this disorder. LM invariably poses a diagnostic challenge. The mimics and causes of longitudinal melanonychia are numerous and often impossible to differentiate from one another by history and clinical inspection alone. The diagnosis of subungual melanoma must always be included in the differential diagnosis of LM.

If the cause of LM is not apparent, it should be established by biopsy.

The dangers of an error of judgement by carrying out this procedure are twofold (Sanderson & MacKie 1979):

**1** That the proper treatment of a malignant lesion will be delayed and so allow the disease to disseminate.

**2** That the treatment, correct for a malignant melanoma, will lead to severe, totally unnecessary, cosmetic disability if employed for a benign tumour.

For these reasons, isolated pigmented streaks, involving any portion of the nail apparatus, necessitate biopsy, especially when the thumb or the great toe are involved. The only possible exceptions are in black and oriental patients, in whom it could represent a normal finding, in children when the band remains stable and in Laugier–Hunziker–Baran's syndrome (Baran 1979; Haneke 1991).

No single biopsy method meets the needs of all patients with LM. The following considerations will be helpful in selecting the procedure that is most appropriate:

1 Postoperative dystrophy is less likely to occur with distal matrix biopsies than with biopsies of proximal matrix. However, accordingly, it is important to locate precisely the origin of pigment production so that the most appropriate surgical procedure can be selected.

2 Complete excision of LM is accomplished more easily and with less cosmetic deformity when the band is located in the lateral third of the nail plate.

3 Thin bands of LM are more amenable to complete excision than wide bands.

4 The features outlined later (e.g. presence or absence of Hutchinson's sign, thumb or great toe involvement, patient age, race, lesion history and clinical features) provide information that is helpful in establishing the likelihood of subungual melanoma. In instances where the likelihood of subungual melanoma is high, biopsy should be pursued with less regard for cosmetic appearance and with greater concern for complete extirpation.

5 The appearance and functional integrity of the nail are less crucial in the toes than in the fingers.

6 LM in the finger of a person whose occupation depends on the functional and cosmetic integrity of the hand often presents a formidable challenge.

7 Because LM is more likely to represent subungual melanoma in older patients, biopsy should be performed aggressively.

Fortunately, postoperative appearance and functional nail integrity are less often a critical concern in elderly patients.

8 In general, postoperative appearance is of greater concern in women than in men.

## Biopsy methods

Various surgical approaches are available for nail biopsies in LM. The procedure that is ultimately selected will depend on: (a) the likelihood of subungual melanoma; (b) the need to select a procedure that will minimize the risk of postoperative dystrophy; (c) location (medial or lateral) of the band within the nail plate; (d) band width; and (e) the matrix origin (proximal or distal) of LM. The patient must be fully apprised of the risk of permanent postoperative dystrophy.

### Periungual pigmentation present (Fig. 10.31)

When LM is accompanied by periungual pigmentation, the likelihood of subungual melanoma is high. X-ray studies should be obtained and the patient examined for lymphadenopathy. If the risk of malignancy (according to the criteria outlined later) is great, if there is no history of previous nail surgery, no history of ingestion of photosensitizing medications, and no evidence for a syndrome associated with hyperpigmentation and if there is unequivocal evidence that the pigment is located within (and not beneath) the proximal and/or lateral nail folds, all affected portions of the nail apparatus (proximal and lateral nail folds, nail plate, nail bed, hyponychium, and skin) are removed *en bloc* down to bone, with relative disregard for cosmetic appearance. To ensure complete

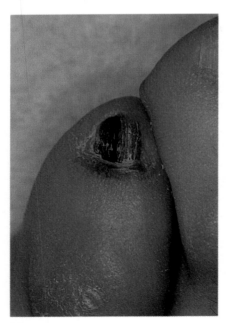

(a)

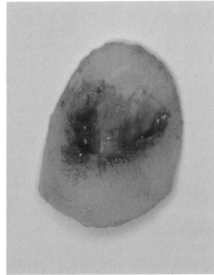

(b)

**Fig. 10.31** (a) Ungual and periungual pigmentation. (b) After surgery asked for by the patient the diagnosis turned out to be 'frictional melanonychia' with pseudo-Hutchinson's sign.

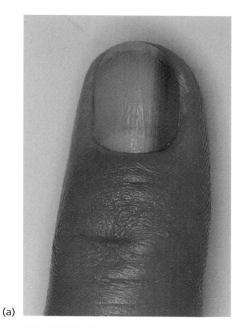

(a)

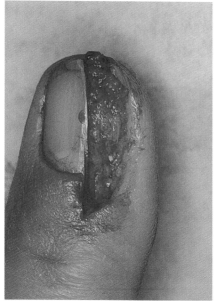

(b)

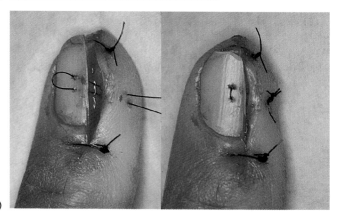

(c)

**Fig. 10.32** (left) (a–c) Lateral longitudinal biopsy for lateral nail pigmentation.

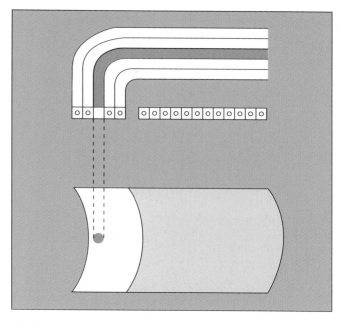

**Fig. 10.33** The site of matrix pigment pathology in relation to the depth of nail plate pigmentation. (After Higashi 1970.)

biopsy and excision, 1 mm of normal tissue is included in the excision. The advantage of this method lies in the completeness of excision. The pathologist is able to study the lesion in its entirety, render a precise diagnosis, and draw salient conclusions regarding prognosis. The conspicuous disadvantage of this approach is the potential for significant postoperative deformity.

### Lateral third of the nail plate involved (Fig. 10.32)

Lateral longitudinal biopsy is the preferred method when LM involves the lateral third of the nail plate. The advantages of this technique include the following: (a) all affected tissue including the matrix, proximal nail fold, cuticle, upper portion of the lateral nail fold adjacent to the proximal nail fold, nail bed and nail plate, are completely removed; (b) the pathologist is able to examine the lesion in its entirety; (c) pigment recurrence or persistence is unlikely; and (d) postoperatively, the patient is left with a good cosmetic result with just a narrowed nail.

### Midportion of the nail plate involved (Figs 10.33–10.35)

When LM lies within the midportion of the nail plate, the potential for postoperative dystrophy may be great and the selection of the optimal biopsy method is difficult.

It is necessary to identify the origin (proximal or distal matrix) of pigmentation in LM. Pigment histologically localized within the dorsal half of the nail plate indicates a proximal

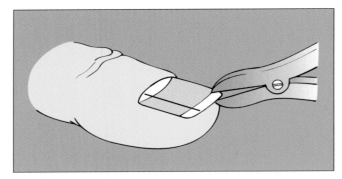

**Fig. 10.34** Nail clipping of the free edge to define the depth of pigment with the nail.

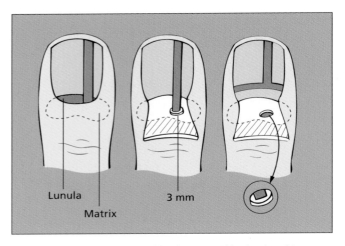

**Fig. 10.36** Sites of biopsy for lesions of less than 3 mm width; taken through intact nail plate.

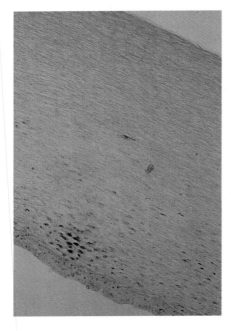

**Fig. 10.35** Nail pigmentation localized within the ventral nail plate (distal matrix production).

matrix origin; pigment localized within the ventral nail plate indicates a distal matrix origin (Fig. 10.33).

The level of pigment within the nail plate is defined microsopically with Fontana–Masson staining of clippings obtained from the free edge of the nail. When a distal matrix origin seems likely, the cuticle can be retracted proximally to confirm the distal origin of LM without reflexion of the proximal nail fold.

**Thin band, less than 3 mm in width** (Higashi 1970; Kopf *et al.* 1984) (Figs 10.36–10.38)

When the band is thin, it represents a low risk for subungual melanoma (e.g. an 8-year-old patient with index nail involvement), and originates in the distal two-thirds of the matrix, a 3-mm punch excision is indicated. Punch excision is performed through the nail plate with direct visualization of the band at its origin.

The origin of the band is exposed by reflecting the proximal nail fold with relaxing incisions, if necessary. With a 3-mm

punch, a circumferential incision is made around the origin of the band; the cylinder of involved tissue is not removed at this time. The next step consists in removal of the proximal (surrounding) third of the nail plate, leaving in place the cylinder of tissue containing the origin of LM. In the absence of the nail plate, the surgeon is able to inspect the surrounding nail matrix and bed with a head magnifier lens to determine whether pigment extends distally of laterally from the punch incision. The cylinder of tissue containing the origin of LM is then removed. Because the surrounding nail plate has been previously detached, the cylinder of tissue is completely accessible and excised with relative ease (Fig. 10.36). The detached nail plate and cylinder of LM are submitted to the pathologist for sectioning through the band. With assistance from the surgeon, the pathologist is able to orientate the specimens properly to ensure optimal sectioning and microscopic interpretation.

Alternatively, a punch biopsy of the LM origin with *en bloc* removal of the nail plate and matrix can be performed without first removing the surrounding nail plate. Another method is to perform a biopsy on the involved matrix after removing the overlying involved nail plate.

The stage method is preferable for the following reasons:
1 If punch excision is conducted without initially removing surrounding nail plate, the biopsy cylinder may be difficult to separate from surrounding tissues. In addition, removal of the proximal third of the nail plate before matrix excision permits direct operative visualization of the underlying nail matrix or bed to verify that the band origin is enclosed within the cylinder of tissue.
2 If the involved nail plate is removed before biopsy, the origin of LM (in the underlying matrix) may be 'lost' when the nail is torn off.
3 Punch excision through affected nail plate and underlying involved matrix ensures that the lesion will be removed *en bloc*, usually with the nail plate attached to the underlying matrix.

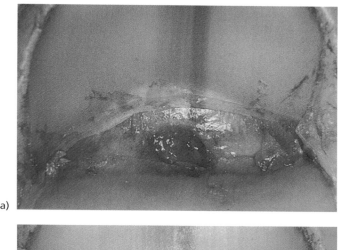

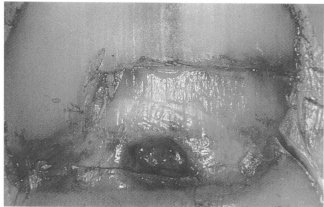

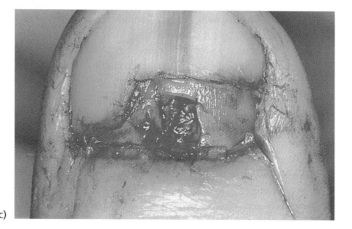

**Fig. 10.37** (a) Punch biopsy through the matrix at the proximal end of a narrow LM band; after biopsy pigment is still seen in front of the biopsy site. (b) Enlargement of the nail window to check the extent of the pigmentation. (c) Removal of the latter.

4 When the origin of LM is completely excised, the likelihood of postoperative pigment recurrence is negligible, and the pathologist is afforded the opportunity to examine the lesion intact and in its entirety. The risk of postoperative dystrophy is minimal because only 3 mm of distal matrix is removed.

Biopsies of a thin band less than 3 mm in width that originate in the proximal one-third of the matrix, can also be performed

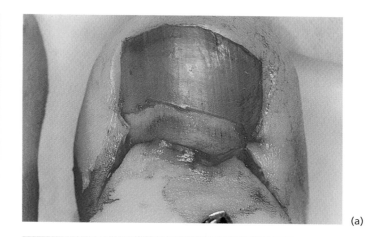

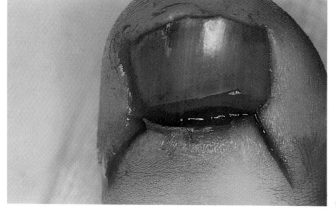

**Fig. 10.38** (a) Pigmentation of the whole nail with distal origin in the matrix; proximal nail removal prior to biopsy. (b) Transverse biopsy of the matrix.

with a 3-mm punch. The proximal nail fold must be reflected completely to ensure full exposure of the band. An attempt may be made to close the (proximal matrix) defect with 6-0 absorbable suture. Because the matrix is fragile and liable to tear easily, it is sufficient to achieve partial approximation rather than to attempt complete closure of the matrix biopsy margins. The risk of postoperative dystrophy is substantial.

### Bands 3–6 mm in width (Figs 10.38 & 10.39)

For bands between 3 and 6 mm wide that involve the distal two-thirds of the matrix, transverse elliptic excision is indicated (Fig. 10.38). Although the potential for postoperative dystrophy is significant, an effort should be made, depending on the clinical circumstances, to excise completely the origin of the band not only to prevent postoperative recurrence of LM but also to ensure that representative tissue is submitted for study. Because the proximal matrix remains intact, a thinned nail plate will regenerate postoperatively.

When 3–6-mm wide bands involve the proximal third of the matrix, the releasing flap method of Schernberg and Amiel (1985) is indicated (Fig. 10.39). This technique enables

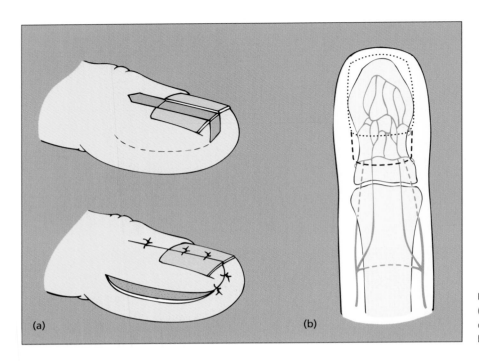

**Fig. 10.39** Proximal third of the matrix is involved. (a) Removal of the band using the releasing flap method of Schernberg and Amiel (1985); the flap is vascularized by branches of the medial phalangeal artery (b).

removal of the proximal portion of the matrix with acceptable postoperative changes in the nail apparatus; the nail plate is diminished in width but is otherwise normal except for slight dystrophy, such as a longitudinal ridge. In this method, the pigmented band is completely excised in a rectangular monoblock comprising involved nail plate, bed, matrix, and proximal nail fold delineated laterally by a curved incision running from the distal end of the monoblock incision to the proximal edge of the matrix. Inferiorly, the nail bed and matrix are separated from the underlying bony phalanx to provide complete mobility. The flap is rotated into position (abutting the incised medial portion of the nail plate, bed, matrix, and proximal nail fold) and closed with 5-0 nylon sutures. The defect in the lateral nail fold is allowed to heal by secondary intention.

### Bands wider than 6 mm (Fig. 10.40)

If the band is wider than 6 mm or if the full thickness of the nail is pigmented, a large portion of the matrix would necessarily be involved. Under these circumstances, the underlying disease process is unlikely to be benign. Depending on the clinical condition, partial longitudinal biopsy, transverse elliptic excision or punch biopsies from selected areas of the matrix can be performed or the entire portion of the involved nail apparatus can be excised *en bloc*.

### Shave excision of the matrix (Haneke 2001) (Fig. 10.40f)

Benign longitudinal melanonychia is usually due to a lentigo or junctional naevus of the matrix. Hence a deep biopsy or excision down to the bone is not necessary for diagnostic and

therapeutic purposes. We have therefore changed our attitude when treating brown streaks in the nail which are not indicative of subungual melanoma.

Under a proximal ring block of the digit, the proximal nail fold is incised at both sides, separated from the underlying nail fold and reflected to allow visualization of the entire length of the brown streak. An elevator is slipped under the proximal end of the nail plate to free it from the matrix and distal nail bed. A transverse section is made over two-thirds of the nail plate at about the level of the lunula margin to permit the proximal nail plate portion to be elevated and the pigmented spot in the matrix to be inspected. Using a no. 15 scalpel, a superficial incision through the matrix epithelium and the papillary dermis is carried out around the melanocyte focus with about 2 mm safety margin. The scalpel is then held parallel to the matrix surface and the entire lesion is removed by cutting horizontally. This leaves a wound area about 1 mm deep.

The specimen is immediately transferred to wet gauze upside down and then stuck to a piece of filter paper which is put into the fixative, thus ensuring a perfectly straight specimen.

The nail plate is laid back on the matrix and fixed to the lateral nail sulcus by a simple stitch. Wound healing was uneventful in all 12 cases operated with this technique thus far. Almost no postoperative nail dystrophy was visible after complete regrowth of the nail. This is probably due to two factors: firstly, the wound is very superficial leaving almost the entire matrix connective tissue intact which allows wound healing to take place very rapidly with re-epithelialization taking place from the wound margins under morphogenetic influence of matrical connective tissue. Secondly, about one-half of the matrix epithelium remains attached to the nail plate during sur-

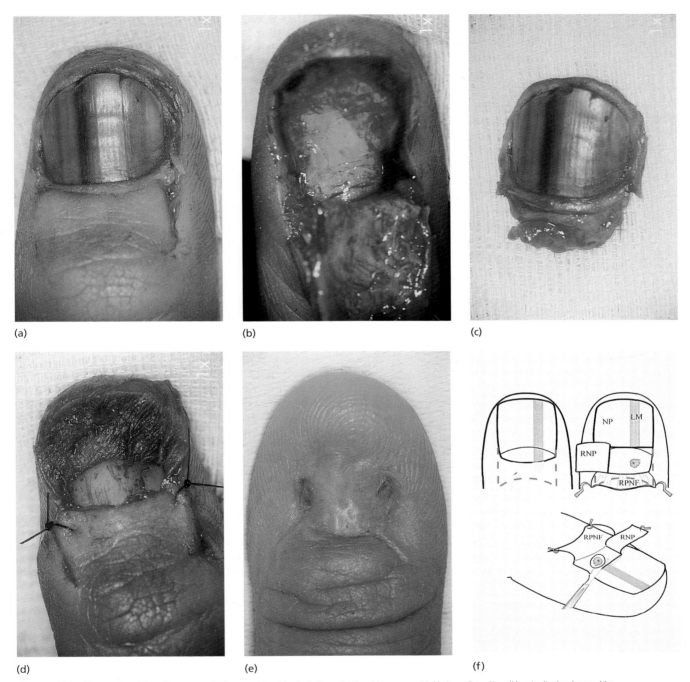

**Fig. 10.40** (a) En bloc excision of the nail apparatus; (b) for appropriate histological examination; (c) in a case with (d,e) very 'broad band' longitudinal melanonychia; (f) shave excision of the matrix.

gical nail detachment from the matrix; this might perhaps act like an epithelial graft.

Histopathological examination of the specimens always revealed junctional naevi or lentigo. However, in case of sub-ungual melanoma, any other more invasive surgical approach may be performed without delay.

## Handling biopsy specimens

Commonly, nail biopsies are difficult to handle. This problem starts with the surgical procedure: artefacts may be produced by tearing and dislocation of the nail plate from the nail bed or by squeezing the tissue.

The portion of the biopsy to be examined should have a straight plane section in order to facilitate tissue orientation in the paraffin block. It is obviously important to ensure that tissue of likely pathological interest is indeed included in the histological section. The longitudinal (lateral) biopsy (Zaias 1967; Baran & Sayag 1976) gives information on the effect of disease on all parts of the nail apparatus. Nail biopsies are difficult to cut. The nail plate is very hard and may be torn from the epithelium. This difficulty can partly be overcome by floating the paraffin block, cut surface down for 1 h in 1% aqueous polysorbate 40 at 4°C after trimming it down to expose the surface at the level of the desired section (Lewin *et al.* 1973).

Entirely flat sections are infrequently obtained. Haematoxylin & eosin (H&E) staining is not always sufficient. Periodic acid–Schiff (PAS) and/or Grocott's stain are recommended if onychomycosis is suspected. Intraepithelial polymorphonuclear leucocytes are more easily identified after PAS staining. Physicochemical alterations in the nail keratin are demonstrated with Giemsa's stain by the abrupt change from red to blue. Masson–Goldner's trichrome stain is particularly valuable in demonstrating keratinization processes.

## Treatment after nail biopsy

After biopsy, a simple dressing with antibiotic tulle gauze, or an antibiotic ointment, is applied for 3–5 days. The dressing should be thick in order to prevent the pain which might be produced by inadvertent minor trauma. Maintaining the hand or foot elevated for 1 or 2 days postoperatively will diminish pain during this period. Analgesics are not usually necessary. The first change of the dressing may be painful, especially when clotted blood causes the gauze to adhere. Soaking the finger in an antiseptic solution, for example 3% hydrogen peroxide, or a mixture of diluted hydrogen peroxide with an antiseptic, greatly facilitates the procedure.

Pulsating pain after the second postoperative day, mainly at night, may be indicative of wound infection and the dressing should be changed. If infection is present, the sutures are removed and the wound is drained. Increasing pain after 3–5 days may be an indication of incipient reflex sympathetic dystrophy (Ingram *et al.* 1987; Haneke 1992).

## References

Achten, G. (1972) Histologie unguéale. *Bollettino dell Istituto Dermatologico San Gallicano* 8, 3.

André, J. & Achten, G. (1987) Techniques de la biopsie de l'ongle. *Annales de Dermatologie et de Vénéréologie* 114, 889–892.

Baran, R. (1979) Longitudinal melanotic streaks as a clue to Laugier–Hunziker syndrome. *Archives of Dermatology* 115, 1448–1449.

Baran, R. (1986) Removal of the proximal nail fold. Why, when, how? *Journal of Dermatologic Surgery and Oncology* 12, 234–236.

Baran, R. & Haneke, E. (1984) Diagnostik und Therapie der streifenförmigen Nagelpigmentierung. *Hautarzt* 35, 359–365.

Baran, R. & Kechijian, P. (1989) Longitudinal melanonychia (melanonychia striata). Diagnosis and management. *Journal of the American Academy of Dermatology* 21, 1165–1175.

Baran, R. & Sayag, J. (1976) Nail biopsy. Why, when, where, how? *Journal of Dermatologic Surgery and Oncology* 2, 322–324.

Bennett, R.G. (1976) Technique of biopsy of nails. *Journal of Dermatologic Surgery and Oncology* 2, 325.

Fosnaugh, R.F. (1982) Surgery of the nail. In: *Skin Surgery* (ed. E. Epstein Jr), p. 981, 5th edn. Charles C. Thomas, Springfield, IL.

Gonzalvez-Serva, A. (1990) The problem-oriented ungual biopsy. *Pathology Review* 2 (1).

Haneke, E. (1984) Segmentale Matrixverschmälerung zur Behandlung des eingewachsenen Zehennagels. *Deutsche Medizinische Wochenschrift* 109, 1451–1453.

Haneke, E. (1985) Nail biopsies in onychomycosis. *Mykosen* 28, 473–480.

Haneke, E. (1988) Exzisions—und Biopsieverfahren. *Zeitschrift für Hautkrankheiten* 63 (Suppl.), 17–19.

Haneke, E. (1991) Laugier-Hunziker-Baran-Syndrom. *Hautarzt* 42, 512–515.

Haneke, E. (1992) Sympathische Reflexdystrophie (Sudeck-Dystrophie) nach Nagelbiopsie. *Zentralblatt für Haut und Geschlechtskrankheiten* 160, 263.

Haneke, E. (2001) Tangential matrix excision for longitudinal melanonychia (in press).

Haneke, E. & Baran, R. (1991) Nails: surgical aspects. In: *Aesthetic Dermatology* (eds L.C. Parish & G.P. Lask), pp. 236–247. McGraw-Hill, New York.

Hanno, R., Mathes, B.M. & Krull, E.A. (1986) Longitudinal nail biopsy in evaluation of acquired nail dystrophies. *Journal of the American Academy of Dermatology* 14, 803–809.

Higashi, N. (1970) On the effects of the matrix and nail bed biopsy on the regeneration of the nail plate (in Japanese). *Hifu* 12, 78–80.

Ingram, G.J., Scher, R.K. & Lally, E.V. (1987) Reflex sympathetic dystrophy following nail biopsy. *Journal of the American Academy of Dermatology* 16, 253–256.

Kechijian, P. (1987) Nail biopsy vignettes. *Cutis* 40, 331–335.

Kopf, A., Albom, M. & Ackerman, A.B. (1984) Biopsy technique for longitudinal streaks of pigmentation in nails. *American Journal of Dermatopathology* 6 (Suppl. 1), 309–312.

Lewin, K., DeWitt, S. & Lawson, R. (1973) Softening techniques for nail biopsies. *Archives of Dermatology* 107, 223–224.

Rich, P. (1992) Nail biopsy: indications and methods. *Journal of Dermatology and Oncology* 18, 673–682.

Salasche, S.J. (1984) Myxoid cysts of the proximal nail fold: a surgical approach. *Journal of Dermatologic Surgery and Oncology* 10, 35–39.

Salasche, S.J. & Peters, V.J. (1985) Tips on nail surgery. *Cutis* 35, 428–438.

Sanderson, K.V. & MacKie, R.M. (1979) Tumours of the skin. In: *Textbook of Dermatology* (eds A. Rook, D.S. Wilkinson & F.J.G. Ebling), p. 2129. Blackwell Scientific Publications, Oxford.

Scher, R.K. & Ackerman, A.B. (1980a) Subtle clues to diagnosis from biopsies of nails. The value of nail biopsy for demonstrating fungi not demonstrable by microbiologic techniques. *American Journal of Dermatopathology* 2, 55.

Scher, R.K. & Ackerman, A.B. (1980b) Subtle clues to diagnosis from biopsies of nails. Histologic differential diagnosis of onychomycosis, psoriasis of the nail unit from cornified cells of the nail bed nail alone. *American Journal of Dermatopathology* 2, 255.

Schernberg, F. & Amiel, M. (1985) Etude anatomo-clinique d'un lambeau unguéal complet. *Annales de Chirurgie Plastique et Esthétique* **30**, 217–131.

Schnitzler, L., Baran, R., Civatte, J. *et al.* (1976) Biopsy of the proximal nail fold in collagen diseases. *Journal of Dermatologic Surgery and Oncology* **2**, 313–315.

Schnitzler, L., Civatte, J., Baran, R. *et al.* (1980) Le repli sus-unguéal normal. *Annales de Dermatologie et de Vénéréologie* **107**, 771–774.

Shelley, W.B. (1975) The razor blade in dermatologic practice. *Cutis* **16**, 843.

Siegle, R.J. & Swanson, N.A. (1982) Nail surgery: a review. *Journal of Dermatologic Surgery and Oncology* **8**, 659–666.

Stone, O.J., Barr, R.J. & Herten, R.J. (1978) Biopsy of the nail area. *Cutis* **21**, 257–260.

Zaias, N. (1967) The longitudinal nail biopsy. *Journal of Investigative Dermatology* **49**, 406–408.

## Electroradiosurgery

Electrosurgery was popular for a long time. It was then forgotten for a while but is now back in vogue because of the appearance of radiosurgery and the new flexible electrodes on the market with a flattened triangular tip for treating ingrowing toenail. The insulated matricectomy electrode (Fig. 10.41) is specially coated for the protection of the upper tissue while destroying underlying cells. Destruction of the lateral horn of the matrix is thus possible without injuring the ventral aspect of the proximal nail fold using the uncoated side down on the matrix (Kerman & Kalmus 1982).

Using an English nail splitter the offending lateral border is separated from the nail, cut and the segment is removed with forceps. After selecting 'partially rectified current' the electrode is applied for a period of 3 s to the matrix area, then the power is shut off, the electrode removed and one waits for 10 s. This procedure is repeated twice when treating a great toe. A 0.125-mL dose of dexamethasone phosphate is instilled into the wound. A layer of antibiotic ointment is applied, followed by a sterile com-pressive dressing (Hettinger *et al.* 1991). Complete matricectomy is also possible using the same technique after total nail avulsion.

Radiosurgery can be used to treat warts. When they are subungual they first require a partial avulsion of the distal or lateral half of the nail plate, depending on their location. Radiocoagulation is done superficially, followed by a careful curettage of the area because of the fragile nature of the tissue in the nail bed. Simple pressure with a dressing made of a double thickness of sterile gauze results in haemostasis. In case of persistent bleeding, slight pressure with a Q-tip soaked in 35% aluminium chloride is usually sufficient.

Pyogenic granulomas can be excised with a cutting loop electrode, providing a specimen for the histologist whilst coagulating the base (Pollack 1991).

### References

Hettinger, D.F., Valinsky, M.S., Nucci, G. *et al.* (1991) Nail matrix-ectomies using radio wave technique. *Journal of the American Podiatric Medical Association* **81**, 317–321.

Kerman, B.C. & Kalmus, A. (1982) Partial matricectomy with elec-trodesiccation for permanent repair of ingrowing nail borders. *Journal of Foot Surgery* **21**, 54–56.

Pollack, S.V. (1991) *Electrosurgery of the Skin.* Churchill Livingstone, New York.

## Microscopically controlled surgery

(Mikhail 1991; Goldminz & Bennett 1992; de Berker *et al.* 1996) (Figs 10.42 & 10.43)

Mohs' chemosurgery originally involved serial excisions of chemically fixed tissue and immediate thorough histological study of each specimen until completely negative sections were obtained. This method is now usually performed without 'intravital' fixation (fresh tissue technique). Proper orientation of the surgical specimen and their correct marking are the crucial points. This requires a map of the original lesion and areas of residual tumour at all stages in the procedure of serial excisions.

This technique leads to complete removal of the malignant tumour without sacrificing large amounts of normal tissue. The resulting defect may then be repaired with free grafts, or pedicle flaps, depending on the size and location of the defect.

### References

de Berker, D., Dahl, M.G.C., Malcom, A.J. *et al.* (1996) Micrographic surgery for subungual squamous cell carcinoma. *British Journal of Plastic Surgery* **49**, 414–419.

Goldminz, D. & Bennett, R.G. (1992) Mohs micrographic surgery of the nail unit. *Journal of Dermatologic Surgery and Oncology* **18**, 721–726.

Mikhail, G.R. (1991) *Mohs Micrographic Surgery.* W.B. Saunders, Philadelphia.

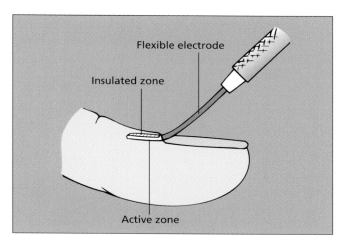

**Fig. 10.41** Matricectomy electrode.

Flexible electrode

Insulated zone

Active zone

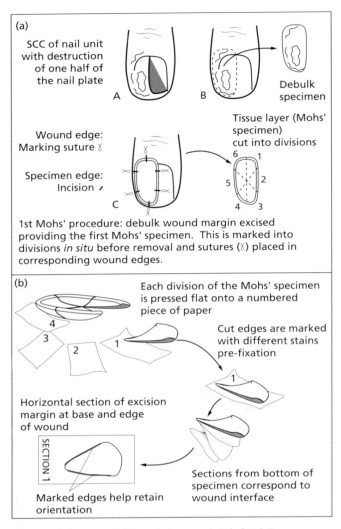

**Fig. 10.42** (a,b) Microscopically controlled surgery—de Berker's technique.

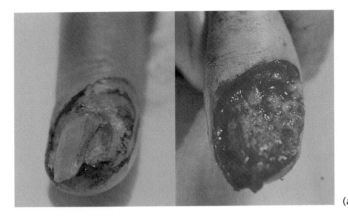

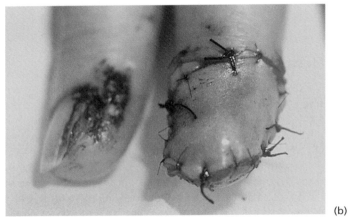

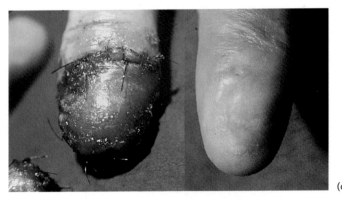

**Fig. 10.43** (a–c) Microscopically controlled surgery for squamous cell carcinoma. (Courtesy of D. Gormley, USA.)

## Non-scalpel techniques (Figs 10.44 & 10.45)

### Cryosurgery in the nail region

The fingertips and nail apparatus are well endowed with sensory nerve endings. Therefore, unless adequate pretreatment analgesia is given, cryosurgery to this area may be relatively painful or resisted by the patient; certainly without such care, repeat treatments for conditions such as warts may be impossible. It should be pointed out that after the initial freeze and thaw, with all but the shortest freeze times, despite the prominent 'burn appearance', pain is considerably less than other methods which cause inflammation, unless the periosteum is frozen. Short freeze times may only induce erythema and blister formation which may be haemorrhagic. Freezing does not damage connective tissue in normal therapeutic doses (Shepherd & Dawber 1984; Dawber *et al.* 1997) and for this reason it has recently been suggested as perhaps better than surgery for

periungual tumours such as myxoid cysts (Dawber *et al.* 1983), particularly those which have discharged and may be difficult to dissect surgically.

Cryosurgery has long been used by dermatologists for periungual warts, because like spontaneous healing, correctly used, scarring should not occur after freezing.

### References

Dawber, R.P.R., Colver, G. & Jackson, A. (1997) *Cutaneous Cryosurgery*, 2nd edn. Martin Dunitz, London.

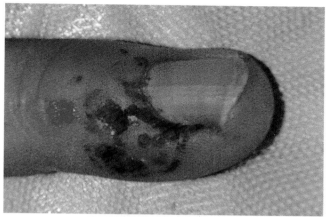

(a)

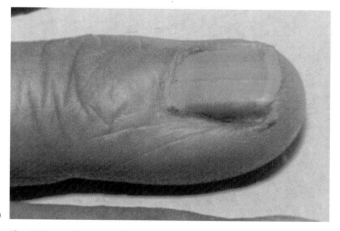

(b)

(c)

**Fig. 10.44** (a–c) Cryosurgery for Bowen's disease. (Courtesy of P. Lauret, France.)

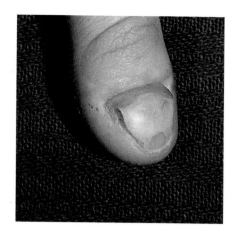

**Fig. 10.45** Onycholysis with leuconychia after cryosurgery for warts. (Courtesy of M. Thuilliez, Belgium.)

Dawber, R.P.R., Sonnex, T., Leonard, J. *et al.* (1983) Myxoid cysts of the finger: treatment by liquid nitrogen spray cryosurgery. *Clinical and Experimental Dermatology* **8**, 153.

Shepherd, J.P. & Dawber, R.P.R. (1984) Wound healing and scarring after cryosurgery. *Cryobiology* **21**, 157–169.

## Laser surgery and the nail unit (by Gary J. Brauner)

LASER is an acronym for Light Amplification by the Stimu-lated Emission of Radiation. The $CO_2$ laser is that laser most utilized for surgery of and around the nail. It produces an intense monochromatic ray of 10 600 nm wavelength, absorbed well in water. When it is absorbed by water-bearing tissue it causes the tissue to heat rapidly and vaporize or carbonize. The handpiece of the $CO_2$ laser has a focusing lens, which can focus a spot to 0.1–0.2 mm when held at one focal length. Although the $CO_2$ laser is frequently used in a focused manner where it emits a power density of perhaps 50 000 $W/cm^2$ and thus haemostatic incisional surgery can be performed, it is generally used in and around the nail in a defocused manner, several focal lengths above the surface of the skin so that one has a spot size of 1 mm or more and a power density of hundreds to thousands of $W/cm^2$. With such a defocused spot, one can haemostatically vaporize away skin cells and 'peel' the skin with extraordinary ability to visualize the tissue.

Why should one use the laser for diseases of the nail? The major virtue of the $CO_2$ laser is increased visualization. Because the laser produces a bloodless wound and one can focus the spot size down to tenths of a millimetre, the laser surgeon can trace abnormal tissue far better than with the smallest curette. Furthermore, because of the haemostasis, one can avoid sacrificing normal surrounding tissue in the attempt to eradicate pathology. Originally, the $CO_2$ laser was utilized with colposcopic magnification. Magnification will also produce more accurate and better results so that the use of magnifying loupes is a necessary adjunct for laser surgery (Pyrcz & Carlson 1990). Such loupes could also be used with cold steel surgery alone to produce better results.

Although haemostasis is a crucial part of visualization and the $CO_2$ laser is a very good instrument for providing it, a simple tourniquet provided by an elastic band or Penrose drain is often necessary in $CO_2$ laser surgery (Borovoy *et al.* 1983; Kaplan *et al.* 1985; Rothermel & Apfelberg 1987; Wright 1989). One might therefore argue that adequate haemostasis might be obtainable with such tourniquets in cold steel surgery as well. One certainly does not need to purchase an expensive $CO_2$ laser to provide postoperative haemostasis when it can be provided with simple application of aluminium chloride or ferric subsulphate solution.

**Table 10.3** Use of carbon dioxide laser for nail disease.

Nail bed
  Subungual haematoma

Nail bed or nail fold tumefactions
  Periungual fibroma
  Pyogenic granuloma
  Mohs' surgery
  Myxoid cyst

Nail plate dystrophy
  Matricectomy total
    Onychogryphosis
    Onychauxis
    Single or double plicature
  Matricectomy partial
    Single plicature

Nail bed ablation
  Pachyonychia congenita

Hyponychial ablation
  Partial or double plicature

Nail fold dystrophy
  Lateral fold ablation
  Hypertrophic lateral nail fold
  Matricectomy, partial

Tinea
  'Waffling' technique
  Nail bed ablation
  Matricectomy, total

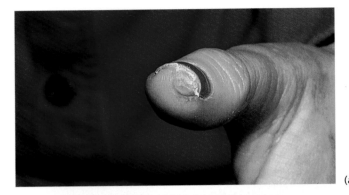

(a)

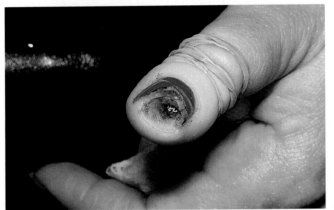

(b)

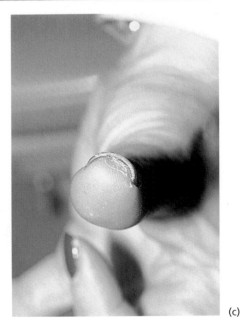

**Fig. 10.46** Subungual fibrokeratoma. (a) Before laser treatment. (b) Immediately after $CO_2$ laser obliteration by vaporization. (c) Minimal residue at 10 weeks.

(c)

Lastly, one can use the laser to burn through the nail plate or to vaporize it. Simple mechanical avulsion may be faster, but is more traumatizing.

Surprisingly, despite extensive and vigorous promotion of laser surgery by podiatrists, there is a paucity of literature concerning the real usefulness of the $CO_2$ laser for ungual and periungual surgery (Bennett 1989).

Table 10.3 indicates uses of the $CO_2$ laser. Subungual haematomas can be treated without the need for local anaesthesia by rapidly penetrating through nail plate with a focused beam. Instead of the nail plate being cut away, it can be vaporized to expose a deeply imbedded subungual splinter for easier extraction (Miller & Brodell 1995), though Epstein (1996) thinks this is unnecessary overuse of laser. One can use the laser as an incisional instrument to excise squamous cell carcinoma in the Mohs' technique or small tumours such as periungual fibromas or pyogenic granulomas (Fig. 10.46). Excisional surgery generally is done at 15–20 W with a focused spot of approximately 1 mm in size and the beam applied in a continuous fashion. A defocused beam will vaporize myxoid cysts around the nail fold.

The main use of the $CO_2$ laser is for subungual and periungual warts (Brauner 1991) (Fig. 10.47). The $CO_2$ laser allows one to carbonize nail plate in pursuit of the subungual or periungual wart, although intraoperative clipping is usually faster. The laser here is operated in a defocused mode with 1–2 mm spot size at 5–10 W output in either intermittent 0.05-s bursts

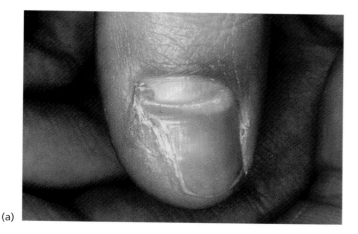

(a)

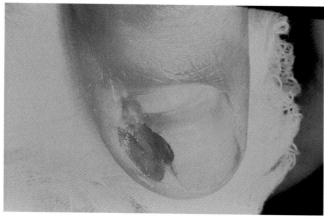

(b)

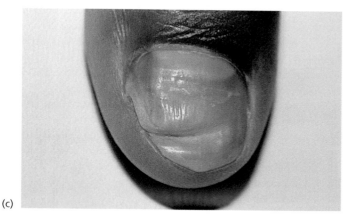

(c)

**Fig. 10.47** Periungual and subungual wart. (a) Before treatment by $CO_2$ laser. (b) Intraoperative, where although apparently free of disease the sulcus shows a small light patch proximally which represents residual wart. (c) After healing

evident dermal papillae, particularly when a tourniquet is also used. One can easily vaporize these remnants but they must be traced well down into the lateral sulci for periungual warts and under the nail plate and onto the nail bed for subungual warts. Caution must be used when approaching the nail matrix lest it be vaporized and produce subsequent nail dystrophy. Healing usually occurs in 3–4 weeks (Apfelberg *et al.* 1984b).

There are times when the nail growth is so distorted that only total ablation of the affected area would produce a cosmetically acceptable result. Onychogryphosis was the first instance in which a laser was employed around the nail (Kaplan *et al.* 1976). Vaporization of the nail bed and matrix to the area overlying the interphalangeal joint was performed after avulsion of the nail. Similar procedures can be used for onychauxis and have also been used by podiatrists for chronic tinea pedis. The technique involves operating the laser at 2–6 W with an irradiance of approximately 60–160 $W/cm^2$ (Kaplan *et al.* 1985; Leshin & Whitaker 1988) with vaporization of the nail matrix after reflection of the proximal nail fold. The vaporization should include both that portion of the nail matrix extending onto the reflection of the nail fold as well as the lunula, and the vaporization must extend to the lateral horns of the nail unit (Siegle & Swanson 1982; Leshin & Whitaker 1988) in order to avoid regrowth of spicules of nail. Although Leshin and Whitaker (1988) found no recurrence after laser surgery, Kaplan *et al.* (1985) had subsequently to use 10% sodium hydroxide, which can be used alone to produce a matricectomy. Rothermel and Apfelberg (1987) performed laser, then curettage and relasering (curettage may also be utilized alone successfully). Wright (1989) noted, with a technique involving lasering proximally, medially and laterally, curetting and relasering, that there was a nail plate recurrence rate of 50% for total matricectomy in 58 nails and 48% for partial matricectomy, whereas his own recurrence rate with more traditional surgical techniques was only 20% for total matricectomy; he concluded that the laser was inferior to traditional surgical podiatric techniques. Siegle and Swanson (1982) cited many published recurrence rates of 0–5% for phenol or cold steel matricectomies. Because of curvature of the finger the lateral horns which are difficult to visualize for accurate lasering, combination therapies of first lasering the nail fold and then applying phenol to run into the lateral horns are now touted as more effective.

Nail bed ablation may be useful palliatively for treatment of nail dystrophies in which the nail bed plays a significant contributing role, such as pachyonychia congenita. Although Thomsen *et al.* (1982) suggest that surgical ablation of the nail fold, not the nail bed, is appropriate in pachyonychia congenita as a totally destructive method, our patients seem to have had a demonstrably better palliative result by treatment of the nail bed alone rather than the nail fold alone with $CO_2$ laser surgery (Fig. 10.48).

Partial matricectomy may be useful for nail plate dystrophies in which one has only a partially plicated nail (partial pincer

or continuous mode (Apfelberg *et al.* 1984a,b; Street & Roenigk 1990; Lim & Goh 1992). As with electrodesiccation, the infected epidermis tends to boil and bubble and usually separates easily from the underlying dermis. The residual charred area then is snipped at the periphery with iris scissors and the roof is avulsed. The typical fish-white appearance or residual wart tissue is easy to demonstrate against the pinker background and

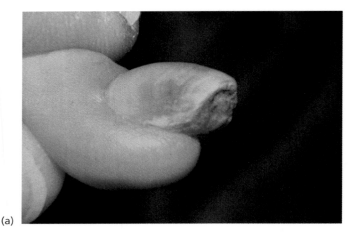

(a)

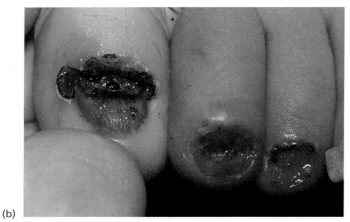

(b)

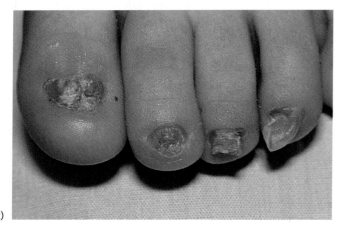

(c)

**Fig. 10.48** Pachyonychia congenita. (a) One digit prior to treatment with marked subungual hyperkeratosis. (b) Immediately postoperative: only the nail fold of the first digit was vaporized. (c) After healing, the nail is most improved where only the nail bed was vigorously vaporized.

nail syndrome). The patient must be forewarned about the narrower resultant nail. In this instance, it is easiest to simply either carbonize the offending portion of the nail, or to incise the entire nail plate longitudinally and then destroy the responsible nail matrix, again remembering to laser into the lateral horn of the nail fold after reflecting the fold.

For a partially plicated nail it is not necessary to destroy the offending portion of the nail plate and its matrix, if the nail dystrophy is not very severe and the pattern is one more of ingrowing into the hyponychium rather than pinching it. One can deliberately produce an atrophic scar of the hyponychium by lasering into the fat and allowing the deformed nail plate to slide over this atrophic area without further discomfort (Fig. 10.49).

The $CO_2$ laser has found wide use in podiatry for treatment of nail fold dystrophy since it is so rapid and haemostatic. In situations where one has uncomfortable or non-cosmetic appearance of the medial and lateral nail folds because of hypertrophy (so-called hypertrophic lips) one can simply laser the offending tissue away and leave the area to heal by secondary intention or tape the remaining normal lateral nail fold to the nail plate, thus closing the wound.

For recurrent nail fold dystrophy produced by onychocryptosis (Morselli & Anselmi 1985; Rothermel & Apfelberg 1987; Leshin & Whitaker 1988; Bennett 1989; Wright 1989; Street & Roenigk 1990) a partial matricectomy can be performed with the above parameters (Fig. 10.50a).

The question of treatment of tinea of the nails is controversial, particularly because the speed of nail ablation may be no faster than simple avulsion. The expense of the use of the laser may well be prohibitive as compared to oral medication such as itraconazole or terbinafine which now need to be taken for only 3 months. (Apfelberg *et al.* 1984a; Rothermel & Apfelberg 1987; Leshin & Whitaker 1988; Wright 1989; Pyrcz & Carlson 1990).

The so-called 'waffling' technique was allegedly developed at the Wenske Institute; small vaporized pits were made in the nail plate as wells which would theoretically hold topical antifungal liquid and allow it to better distribute through the nail plate. Pyrcz and Carlson (1990) note that the treatment was repeated two or three times at 6-week intervals and was allegedly 70% effective in clearing the nail, but this is unsubstantiated by data (Rothermel & Apfelberg 1987; Pyrcz & Carlson 1990). The more standard approach involves either avulsing the nail plate and vaporizing the nail bed or vaporizing both the nail plate and the nail bed. The nail bed is vaporized lightly at approximately 5 W and then curetted. After the wound heals in 2–3 weeks, the area is scrubbed daily and a topical antifungal lotion is applied daily. There is at least an 86% failure rate (Rothermel & Apfelberg 1987) with this technique, though approximately 51% of patients have results where most of the nails remain unaffected by tinea 4 years after treatment (Rothermel & Apfelberg 1987). Carbon dioxide laser ablation of infected nail plates as a sole treatment should be relegated to the bin of past history. Unfortunately, as yet there has been no controlled study to show that laser debulking of diseased nails in combination with the newer short course oral azoles or terbinafine allows for better remission rates or shorter less expensive courses of oral medication. Neev *et al.* (1997) have done preliminary studies on several new ultrashort lasers in the nanosecond and femtosecond pulse-duration range, such as the 2940-nm Er :

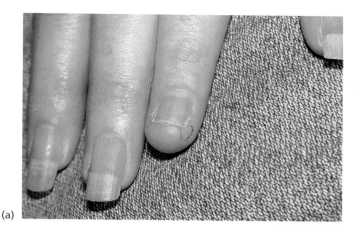

(a)

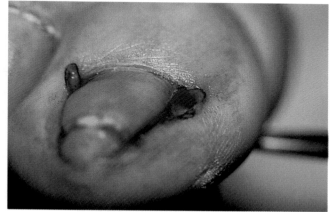

(a)

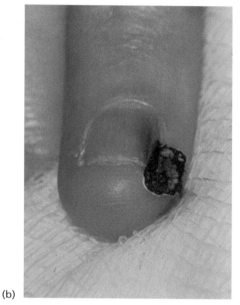

(b)

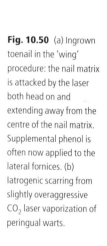

**Fig. 10.50** (a) Ingrown toenail in the 'wing' procedure: the nail matrix is attacked by the laser both head on and extending away from the centre of the nail matrix. Supplemental phenol is often now applied to the lateral fornices. (b) Iatrogenic scarring from slightly overaggressive $CO_2$ laser vaporization of peringual warts.

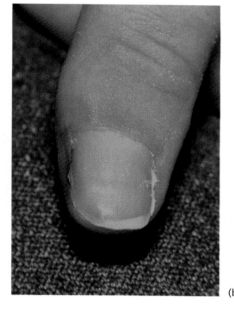

(b)

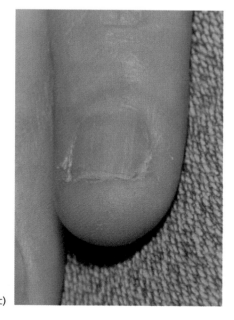

(c)

**Fig. 10.49** Nail dystrophy with finger revision (a). The finger pulp in this instance is deliberately destroyed and made atrophic (b) to allow for proper movement of the plicated nail deformity (c).

YAG, the 2080-nm Ho : YSGG, the 308-nm XeCl excimer and a 1050-nm ultra-ultrashort (femtosecond) laser. Their results suggest that ultrashort lasers may be found effective in thinning the nail plate without its entire removal to allow for better uniform penetration of topical medications, a new variant of the waffle produced by melting and shattering of nail without significant collateral damage.

Although haemostasis and magnification provide for more accurate removal of pathological tissue, it is certainly possible to have undesirable atrophic scarring occur after laser surgery. When scarring has occurred from prior surgical attempts at wart removal, distinction of the infected epidermal tissue from normal dermis becomes extremely difficult and another similar or worse scar will likely be produced. If a huge wart is treated requiring significant destruction, it is possible for subcutaneous tissue to be destroyed resulting not only in epidermal, but dermal and subcutaneous atrophy and dystrophy at the tip of the finger (Fig. 10.50b). When working around the proximal nail fold one must be meticulous in not destroying any matrix lest permanent nail plate dystrophy occur. Here it may be better to undertreat suspicious residual lesions and re-evaluate for further treatment at a later date.

The Er : YAG laser which removes epidermis more precisely and in thinner layers of ablation than the $CO_2$ laser can be used to remove periungual warts without the need for local anaesthesia (Langdon 1998); this laser seems to bear a lesser risk to the operator than electrodesiccation or $CO_2$ laser since wart DNA can not be found in its plume unlike the former two (Garden *et al.* 1988; Gloster & Roenigk 1995; Hughes & Hughes 1998). Human papillomavirus (HPV) has even been found in the $CO_2$ laser plume of subungual squamous cell carcinomas (Ashinoff *et al.* 1991).

The use of non-vaporizing laser treatment for warts was first popularized by Nemeth in 1991 who found that use of the 511-nm green ray of a copper vapour laser was well absorbed by the tan colour (presumably melanin, the 'surrogate target') of wart tissue and led to a high remission rate even in warts recalcitrant to $CO_2$ laser. Wart destruction is evidenced histologically by immunoperoxidase identification of type IV collagen below the 'selectively removed' HPV-containing epidermis. Even when no laser plume is produced, wart remission can be achieved. Remnants of wart virus by polymerase chain reaction (PCR) analysis of ambient room air were not found after such copper vapour laser treatment, unlike 82% of samples of laser plume from $CO_2$ laser-treated wart tissue (Nemeth *et al.* 1992). Others thought the increased vascular pattern in the papillary dermis of warts made them particularly susceptible to green laser light and this accounted better for the copper vapour laser's success. Interruption of perfusion by the coagulative effects of such radiation upon absorption by oxyhaemoglobin makes the wart then infarct.

Following this lead, Tan *et al.* (1993) first used the deeper penetrating and even better absorbed yellow light of the 585 nanometer flashlamp-pumped tunable dye laser (PDL) for wart treatment (Mixter *et al.* 1997). It has been found very effective in treating warts in all locations, even previously resistant warts, by several authors (Kauvar *et al.* 1995), though several (Webster *et al.* 1995; Borovoy *et al.* 1996; Jacobsen *et al.* 1997; Jain & Storwick 1997) report more conservative cure rates of about 70–80% more consistent with other modes of therapy. Some authors refute the effectiveness and persistence of improvement entirely (Huilgol *et al.* 1996). The key to effectiveness seems to be frequent repeat treatments at 2- or 3-week intervals and with multiply stacked bursts of 3–4 bursts at 8–10 $J/cm^2$ after paring the wart hard almost to the point of bleeding.

Geronemus (1992) has reviewed use of green pulsed dye, argon and copper vapour and red Q-switched ruby laser for pigmented lesions in and around the nail where treatment parameters are identical to elsewhere on the skin. Laser is not a reasonable treatment for pigmented nail streaks or hyperpigmentation with Hutchinson's sign. Vascular lesions also have been treated with selective green argon (Fig. 10.51) or copper vapour, yellow pulsed dye or tunable dye and non-

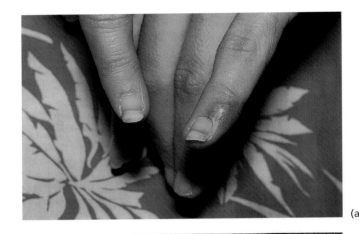

(a)

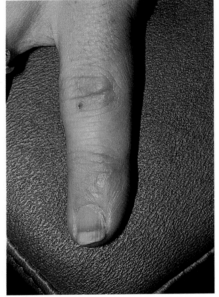

(b)

**Fig. 10.51** Arterial-venous malformation treatment by argon laser. (a) Preoperative. (b) Postoperative—moderate improvement. Lesions thicker than 1 mm are not usually very effectively treated by vascular-lesion lasers.

selective infrared $CO_2$ lasers as in other locations. Congenital portwine stains of the digits are much more resistant to treatment than elsewhere, probably because of higher blood flow interfering with thermocoagulation and more deeply extending vascular malformations.

## References

Apfelberg, D., Maser, M., Lash, H. *et al.* (1984a) Efficacy of the carbon dioxide laser in hand surgery. *Annals of Plastic Surgery* **13**, 320–326.

Apfelberg, D., Rothermel, E., Widtfeld, A. *et al.* (1984b) Preliminary report on the use of carbon dioxide laser in podiatry. *Journal of the American Podiatric Medical Association* **74**, 509–513.

Ashinoff, R., Li, J., Jacobson, M. *et al.* (1991) Detection of human papillomavirus DNA in squamous cell carcinoma of the nail bed and finger determined by polymerase chain reaction. *Archives of Dermatology* **127**, 1813–1818.

Bennett, G. (1989) Laser use in foot surgery. *Foot and Ankle* **10**, 110–114.

Borovoy, M., Fuller, T., Hotz, P. *et al.* (1983) Laser surgery in podiatric medicine. Present and future. *Journal of Foot Surgery* 22, 353–357.

Borovoy, M.A., Borovoy, M., Elson, L. *et al.* (1996) Flashlamp pulsed dye laser (585 nm) treatment of resistant verrucae. *Journal of the American Podiatric Medical Association* 11, 547–550.

Brauner, G. (1991) Treatment of periungual warts [letter; comment]. *Journal of the American Academy of Dermatology* 25, 731.

Epstein, E. (1996) Treatment of subungual splinters [letter]. *Journal of the American Academy of Dermatology* 35, 491.

Garden, J., O'Banion, M., Shelnitz, L. *et al.* (1988) Papillomavirus in the vapor of carbon dioxide, laser-treated verrucae. *Journal of the American Medical Association* 259, 1199–1202.

Geronemus, R. (1992) Laser surgery of the nail unit. *Journal of Dermatological Surgery and Oncology* 18, 735–743.

Gloster, H. & Roenigk, R. (1995) Risk of acquiring human papillomavirus from the plume produced by the carbon dioxide laser in the treatment of warts. *Journal of the American Academy of Dermatology* 32, 436–441.

Hughes, P. & Hughes, A. (1998) Absence of human papillomavirus DNA in the plume of erbium : YAG laser-treated warts. *Journal of the American Academy of Dermatology* 38, 426–428.

Huilgol, S., Barlow, R. & Markey, A. (1996) Failure of pulsed dye laser therapy for resistant verruca. *Clinical and Experimental Dermatology* 21, 93–95.

Jacobsen, E., McGraw, R. & McCagh, S. (1997) Pulsed dye laser efficacy as initial therapy for warts and against recalcitrant verrucae. *Cutis* 59, 206–208.

Jain, A. & Storwick, G. (1997) Effectiveness of the 585 nm flashlamp-pulsed tunable dye laser (PTDL) for treatment of plantar verrucae. *Lasers in Surgery and Medicine* 21, 500–505.

Kaplan, B., D'Angelo, A. & Johnson, C. (1985) The carbon dioxide laser in podiatric medicine. *Clinical Podiatry* 2, 519–522.

Kaplan, B., Labandter, C. & Labandter, H. (1976) Onychogryphosis treated with the $CO_2$ surgical lasers. *British Journal of Plastic Surgery* 29, 102.

Kauvar, A., McDaniel, D. & Geronemus, R. (1995) Pulsed dye laser treatment of warts. *Archives of Family Medicine* 4, 1035–1040.

Langdon, R. (1998) Erbium : YAG laser enables complete ablation of periungual verrucae without the need for injected anesthetics [letter]. *Dermatological Surgery* 24, 157–158.

Leshin, B. & Whitaker, D. (1988) Carbon dioxide laser matricectomy. *Journal of Dermatologic Surgery and Oncology* 14, 608–611.

Lim, J. & Goh, C. (1992) Carbon dioxide laser treatment of periungual and subungual viral warts. *Australasian Journal of Dermatology* 33, 87–91.

Miller, M. & Brodell, R. (1995) Surgical pearl: treatment of subungual splinters. *Journal of the American Academy of Dermatology* 33, 667–668.

Mixter, R., Carson, L., Walton, B. *et al.* (1997) Treatment of recalcitrant verrucae with both the ultrapulse and $CO_2$ and PLDL pulsed dye lasers [letter]. *Plastic and Reconstructive Surgery* 100, 1612–1613.

Morselli, M. & Anselmi, C. (1985) Use of carbon dioxide laser for the treatment of podiatric lesions. In: *International Congress of Dermatologic Surgery, Rome*, 9 October.

Neev, J., Nelson, J.S., Critelli, M. *et al.* (1997) Ablation of human nail by pulsed lasers. *Lasers in Surgery and Medicine* 21, 186–192.

Nemeth, A., Leonardi, C., Wu, X. *et al.* (1992) Investigation of possible wart virus released during copper vapor treatment of anogenital and body warts. *Lasers in Surgery and Medicine* 4, 70.

Pyrcz, R. & Carlson, B. (1990) Lasers in podiatry and orthopedics. *Medical Clinics of North America* 25, 719–723.

Rothermel, E. & Apfelberg, D. (1987) Carbon dioxide laser use for certain diseases of the toenails. *Clinics in Podiatric Medicine and Surgery* 4, 809–821.

Siegle, R. & Swanson, N. (1982) Nail surgery: a review. *Journal of Dermatologic Surgery and Oncology* 8, 659–666.

Street, M. & Roenigk, R. (1990) Recalcitrant periungual verrucae: the role of carbon dioxide laser vaporization. *Journal of the American Academy of Dermatology* 23, 115–120.

Tan, O., Hurwitz, R. & Stafford, T. (1993) Pulsed dye laser treatment of recalcitrant verrucae: a preliminary report. *Lasers in Surgery and Medicine* 13, 127–137.

Thomsen, R., Zuehlke, R. & Beckman, B. (1982) Pachyonychia congenita—surgical management of the nail changes. *Journal of Dermatologic Surgery and Oncology* 8, 24–28.

Webster, G., Satur, N., Goldman, M. *et al.* (1995) Treatment of recalcitrant warts using the pulsed dye laser. *Cutis* 56, 230–232.

Wright, G. (1989) Laser matricectomy in the toes. *Foot and Ankle* 9, 246–247.

## Nail avulsion

Nail avulsion represents significant trauma to the nail apparatus and must therefore only be performed when indicated.

There are two main methods for nail plate removal:

**1** *Distal nail avulsion* (Fig. 10.5). This classical method, may use: (a) the straight haemostat usually recommended in standard texts of dermatology; or (b) sharp, but non-cutting instruments, such as a dental spatula (Albom 1977), or a Freer septum elevator (Baran 1981); (c) small scissors which open and close gently, working beneath the proximal nail fold and under the nail to remove the nail plate.

We use the Freer instrument which is inserted under the proximal nail fold to the proximal edge of the nail plate (by keeping the blunt curved-up end pointing to the nail plate), with motions from one side of the nail to the other, it is then pushed well under each posterolateral aspect of the proximal nail fold, freeing the nail plate on its dorsal surface. Next, the nail plate–nail bed attachment is freed by proceeding in the same manner, from the distal edge toward the matrix, keeping the blunt curved-up end pointing to the nail plate, thus peeling the nail plate off.

**2** *Proximal nail avulsion* (Cordero 1965; Linares 1967) (Fig. 10.6). This method starts proximally and proceeds distally, by the use of a Freer septum elevator.

The first stage of nail plate avulsion is identical in both techniques, commencing by separating the undersurface of the proximal nail fold from the nail plate, and in the use of a longitudinal, side to side, back and forth motion. During the second stage of surgical avulsion by the proximal to distal technique, the nail elevator is inserted below the proximal edge of the nail plate. It is important to free the posterolateral angle of the nail plate as the attachment is firm at this site. During the third stage, the lifted proximal part of the nail plate is placed on the proximal nail fold, after which the instrument can be slipped easily along

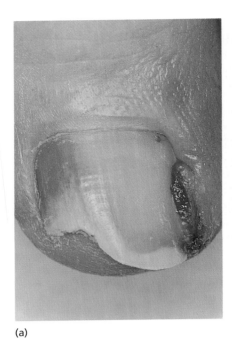

(a)

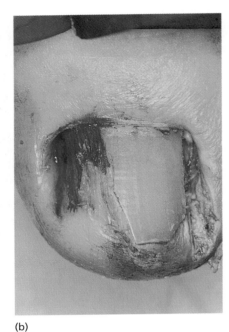

(b)

**Fig. 10.52** (a,b) Partial nail avulsion; before systemic antifungal therapy.

the natural plane of cleavage between nail and bed, allowing the nail plate to be pulled distally. This proximal approach appears to be more valuable when the distal part of the nail has a great deal of subungual hyperkeratosis such as in distal subungual onychomycosis, onychogryphosis, pachyonychia congenita, etc., or when there is no obvious distal fold left.

This technique is feasible because the nail plate, although firmly adherent to the nail bed, has a very loose attachment to the matrix. This explains the histological finding that the epithelium of the nail bed is lining the avulsed nail plate whereas on the part which covers the matrix, there is little matrix epithelium attached to it. Incidental to removing the nail plate, it is imperative that the nail grooves be cleared of subungual debris. This is best accomplished by wiping the nail bed and grooves with gauze wrapped around the end of a 'mosquito-haemostat'. If any remnants adhere, these can be removed with a curette.

After removal of the nail, Zaias (1990) recommends gently pushing the proximal nail fold to ensure an 'open' proximal nail groove and to prevent 'pus' pockets in this groove.

Some signs preclude simple nail avulsion: with malformed nails due to matrix disease, large defects of the nail bed or ingrowing toenails, simply extracting the nail is not curative. Indeed, repeated nail avulsion may cause thickening and overcurvature of the nail plate (Runne 1983). Therefore, it is important to stress that nail avulsion is not a therapy *per se* but enables exposure, then treatment of the subungual structures.

Keratinization of the nail bed following nail avulsion may be avoided by replacing the original nail with a donor 'nail bank transplant'; this will adapt, adhere and function as an autologous nail in a completely satisfactory manner. Preservation of the matrix, the proximal nail fold and the proximal groove is also essential to normal nail regrowth. Whichever method is used, the original nail plate, a 'nail bank transplant' or an artificial nail are helpful for the regeneration of a satisfactory nail.

### Partial nail avulsion (Figs 10.52 & 10.53)

Partial nail avulsion can be more suitable than total avulsion in several circumstances.

Removing the lateral or medial segment of the nail plate should be encouraged in some onychomycoses as enough normal nail is left to counteract the upward forces exerted on the distal soft tissue when walking: this will prevent the appearance of a distal nail wall. The involved portion of the nail is incised from the hyponychium to the proximal nail fold with a nail splitter and the freed nail segment is then avulsed.

In distal subungual onychomycoses with hyperkeratosis, elevation of the nail plate from the nail bed permits the easy removal of the affected portion of the nail with a double action bone rongeur. In such a case a distal edge of the cut portion of the nail plate has only a short distance to grow to reach the distal nail bed, which prevents the slow development of a distal nail wall.

In proximal subungual onychomycosis, removal of the diseased portion of the nail plate is not difficult: the non-adherent lunula region is cut transversely with a nail splitter, by inserting the instrument beneath the lateral edge of the nail plate. The distal portion of the nail is left in place which decreases discomfort.

*Bacterial infection of the nail area* (page 505) and dermatological conditions may benefit from the same techniques. They are also useful when performing some types of nail biopsy.

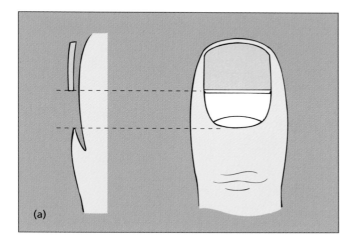

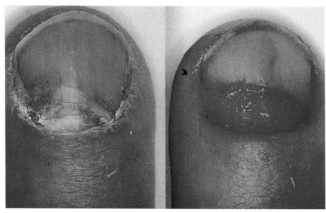

**Fig. 10.53** (a) Avulsion of the proximal portion of the nail plate. (b) Proximal subungual onychomycosis. Removal of the affected proximal portion prior to oral therapy.

## References

Albom, M.J. (1977) Avulsion of a nail plate. *Journal of Dermatologic Surgery and Oncology* **3**, 34–35.

Baran, R. (1981) More on avulsion of nail plate. *Journal of Dermatologic Surgery and Oncology* **7**, 854.

Cordero, C.F.A. (1965) Ablacion ungueal: su uso en la onycomicosis. *Dermatology International* **14**, 21.

Linares, J.L. (1967) Ablacion ungueal. Evaluation terapeutica de la tecnica creada para el Dr FA Cordero. *Dermatologica Revista Mexican* **11**, 161–172.

Runne, U. (1983) Operative Eingriffe an Nagellorgan: Indikationen und Kontraindikationen. *Zeitschrift für Hautkrankheiten* **58**, 324–332.

Zaias, N. (1990) *The Nail in Health and Disease*, 2nd edn. Appleton & Lange, Norwalk, CN.

## Trauma

*Meskinen's law of bureaucracies (1978) states 'there is never time to do it right, but there is always time to do it over' applies to many things in medicine but especially the treatment of nail* bed injuries. *The more adequately the acute injury of the nail bed is treated the fewer reconstructive procedures will be necessary.*

### Treatment of acute injuries

*Ashbell et al. (1967) classified nail bed injuries 30 years ago. Zook et al. (1984) divides the injured nail into: (a) simple lacerations; (b) stellate lacerations; (c) severe crush injuries; and (d) avulsions. Closing a finger in a door is the most common source of perionychial injury, followed by smashing between objects, lacerations from saws and lawn mowers. The age groups most commonly suffering nail bed injuries are children and young adults (age 4–30 years). The long finger is the most frequently injured followed in order by the ring, index, small and thumb. A simple laceration is the most common injury (36%), followed by the stellate laceration (27%), crush (22%), and avulsion (15%) in decreasing frequency. Fifty per cent of injuries of the nail bed also have a fracture of the distal phalanx and/or tuft (Zook et al. 1984, Zook 1985, 1990a).*

*Perionychial injury from a localized object compresses the nail bed between the nail and the bone resulting in a crushing split of the nail bed (Fig. 10.54). When a larger object compresses the nail bed between the nail and the bone a stellate or multiple fragment type injury results (Fig. 10.55).*

### Subungual haematoma

*The nail bed is a very vascular structure and injury to it causes bleeding beneath the nail. This is known as a subungual haematoma and frequently produces very painful throbbing pain. Subungual haematomas that involve less than 50% of the visible nail bed with the paronychium, eponychium and hyponychium intact may be drained by nail perforation to evacuate the haematoma and relieve the pain (Zook 1982a). Perforation is performed by a heated paper clip pressed on the nail surface to burn a hole. Contact with the haematoma will cool the paper clip and avoid injury to the nail bed (Fig. 10.56a) or may also be burned in the nail with an ophthalmic cautery. (Zook 1982b) (Fig. 10.56b). These techniques leave a smooth round hole that will continue to drain for several days. It is essential to clean and scrub the finger and nail prior to making the hole. This decreases the chance of bacteria introduction into the wound leading to infection subungually or osteomyelitis. When more than half of the visible nail is undermined by haematoma or the paronychium, hyponychium, or eponychium is pulled away from the nail, the nail should be removed, the nail bed explored and repaired if necessary. Occasionally there will be no significant laceration of the nail bed but in the vast majority the nail bed requires surgical repair. A recent randomized study has suggested that trephination alone may be adequate for contained subungual haematomas when the nail borders are intact. (Seaberg et al. 1991) These workers, however, agree that if any edge of the nail is dislodged, exploration is indicated.*

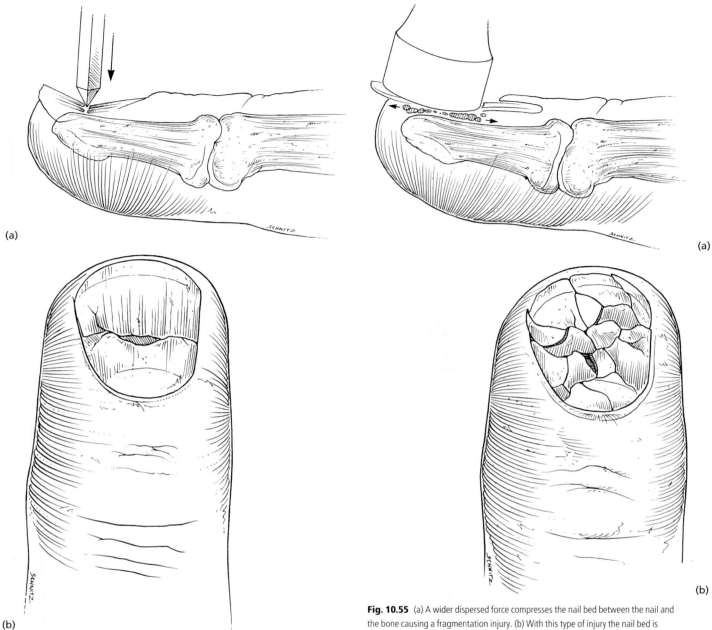

(a)

(b)

**Fig. 10.54** (a) A sharp object striking the nail compresses the nail bed between the nail and the bone causing a crushing laceration. (b) This type of blow may or may not break the nail but gives localized injury to the nail bed. © E. Zook.

(a)

(b)

**Fig. 10.55** (a) A wider dispersed force compresses the nail bed between the nail and the bone causing a fragmentation injury. (b) With this type of injury the nail bed is frequently exploded into many small pieces. © E. Zook.

### Simple laceration

*The most common injury to the nail bed is a simple laceration. (Zook et al. 1984) (Fig. 10.57). The nail is removed following a surgical prep and application of a tourniquet by gently opening and closing iris scissors from distal to proximal. The points of the scissors must be kept against the nail to prevent injury to the matrix. A small periosteal elevator fits the curved undersurface*

*of the nail bed more accurately than a larger tool (Fig. 10.19b) and does less damage to the nail bed (Zook et al. 1985). After the nail is removed it is cleaned of extraneous material from the undersurface and sides by scraping with scalpel blade. The nail is soaked in Betadine solution while the nail bed injury is being repaired. Loupe magnification is advantageous in achieving accurate approximation of the wound edges. Irregularities of the matrix are trimmed only if it is possible to do so without sacrificing significant matrix tissue. If there is question it is best to approximate the irregular wound edges with fine chromic sutures. Replace the nail or silicone sheeting on the nail bed*

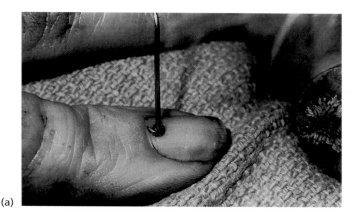

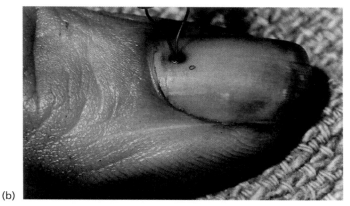

**Fig. 10.56** (a) A heated paper clip is used to perforate the nail and allow drainage of subungual haematoma. (b) A heated ophthalmic cautery will burn a small round hole in the nail and allow continued drainage. © E. Zook.

to mould the irregularities together as accurately as possible and give minimal scarring. One millimetre of undermining of the nail bed from the periosteum will allow slight eversion of the wound edges and more accurate wound approximation. Although 5-0 chromic catgut (Weckesser 1974), and 6-0 plain catgut (Ashbell et al. 1967) have been advocated, I prefer 7-0 chromic on a micropoint spatula double-armed GS-9 ophthalmic needle (Ethicon) (Fig. 10.58). The needle curve allows easy passage through the nail bed and the double needle gives a spare in case one is bent during the repair.

Following repair of the nail bed the nail is retrieved from the antibiotic solution. A hole is drilled through it to allow drainage in an area not over the laceration (Fig. 10.59a–e). Schiller (1957) described replacing the nail into the nail fold. We hold the nail in place with a 5-0 monofilament nylon suture placed through the hyponychium and the free edge of the distal nail. The finger is dressed as previously described and the dressing removed in 5–7 days. The hyponychial suture holding the nail in the fold is removed in 2–3 weeks. The nail remains adherent until pushed off by the new growing nail, which takes 1–2 months.

If the nail is not available the previously described reinforced silicone sheeting may be used as a substitute. We place a 6-0 nylon suture through the nail wall at the proximal nail fold passing through the silastic and then back out to maintain the silicone sheeting in the nail fold (Fig. 10.60) (Zook 1986). This stitch should be removed by 7 days to prevent growth of nail bed cells up the suture track. This nail fold suture is not needed when a stiff nail is available but is with the softer silicone sheet. If the nail or silicone sheet is not available, a nail-shaped piece

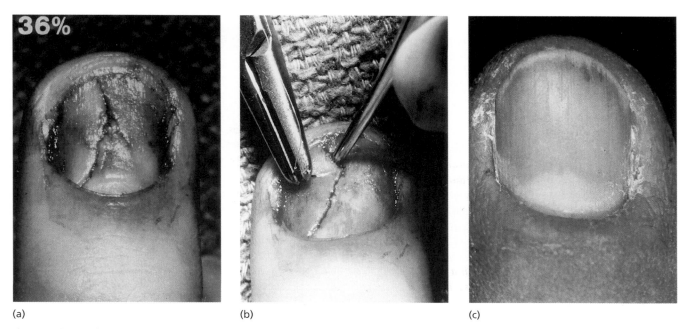

(a)                    (b)                    (c)

**Fig. 10.57** (a) 36% of nail bed injuries are categorized as simple lacerations. (b) Accurate approximation of the nail bed with fine absorbable suture is necessary. (c) One year later a normal nail. © E. Zook.

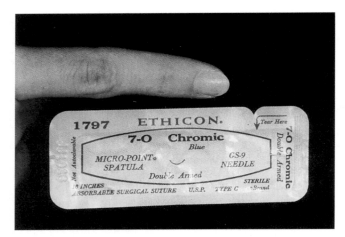

**Fig. 10.58** The suture preferred for repair of the nail bed. © E. Zook.

*of adaptic gauze is placed in the nail fold to maintain patency. After the first dressing change the finger is soaked in warm soapy water for 5–10 min three to four times a day to remove crusts and allow for easier suture removal.*

*When the nail is pulled from the nail fold it is not uncommon for the germinal matrix to remain attached to the nail and be avulsed with the nail. When this occurs the germinal matrix is separated from the nail. The germinal matrix is reapproximated into the nail fold with horizontal mattress sutures on each corner and in the middle (Fig. 10.61). The germinal matrix is accurately repaired with fine sutures. The nail is then replaced into the fold and maintains the fold open so that scarring does not occur from the dorsal roof to the ventral floor.*

*If a laceration involves the dorsal roof and the ventral floor each is repaired with fine chromic sutures with the knots placed in the nail fold rather than in the matrix tissue where they cause inflammation. It is especially important in this case that nail, silicone sheet or gauze be placed in the nail fold to prevent scarring between the dorsal roof and the ventral floor with resultant synechia and nail splitting (Zook 1990b).*

### Stellate lacerations

*Stellate lacerations occur with a more diffuse blow to the nail causing more fragmentation. These are managed in similar fashion to simple lacerations with accurate approximation of all lacerations. Meticulous reapproximation is aided by loupe magnification. Attention should be directed at the nail bed and the undersurface of the nail to retrieve any avulsed fragments of matrix. If found they should be removed from the nail and replaced as grafts. Porcine xenografts have been reported to give good results as a dressing in complicated injuries (Ersek et al. 1985) but are often not readily available.*

### Severe crushing injuries

*A poorer prognosis (Zook et al. 1984) occurs with severe crush-*

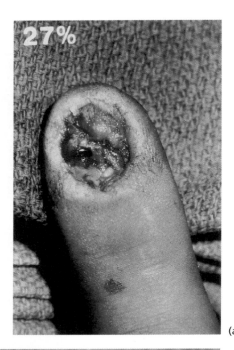

(a)

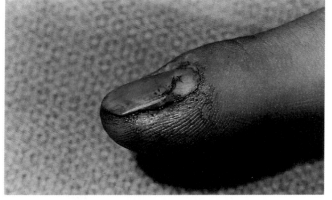

(b)

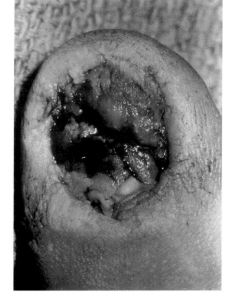

**Fig. 10.59** (a) 27% of nail bed injuries are categorized as stellate lacerations. (b) The proximal nail shown avulsed from the nail fold which is an indication for removal of the nail and exploration of the nail bed. (c) An example of a stellate laceration of the nail bed. (*cont'd*)

(c)

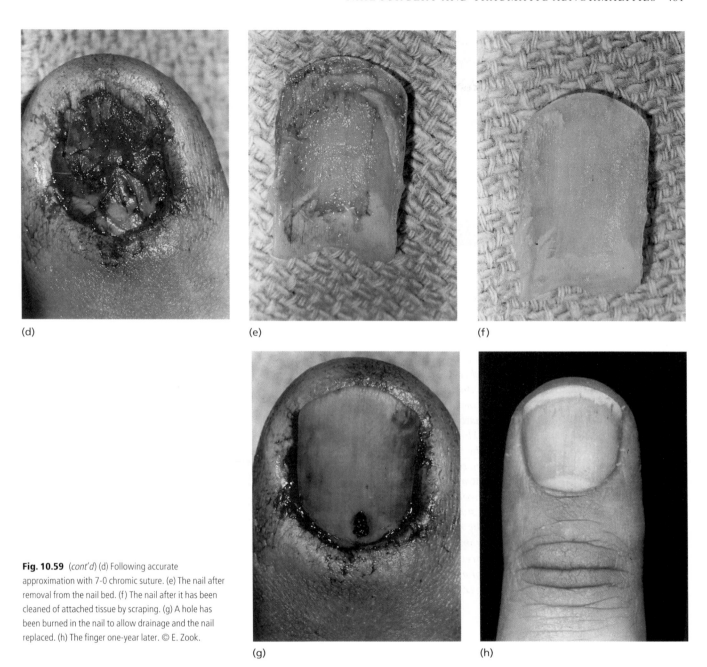

**Fig. 10.59** (cont'd) (d) Following accurate approximation with 7-0 chromic suture. (e) The nail after removal from the nail bed. (f) The nail after it has been cleaned of attached tissue by scraping. (g) A hole has been burned in the nail to allow drainage and the nail replaced. (h) The finger one-year later. © E. Zook.

*ing injuries, which is understandable since they result from greater trauma (Fig. 10.62). All fragments of nail bed should be searched for on the nail and returned and sutured as accurately as possible where they fit on the nail bed. Fragments of nail bed attached by fibres of tissue should be replaced accurately. No portion of sterile or germinal matrix which is available should be discarded but replaced (Zook et al. 1980). The multiple stellate fragments should be approximated as accurately as possible with loupe magnification and nail, silicone sheet or adaptic used to maintain the nail fold open and mould the edges of the wound (Zook 1981).*

### Injuries associated with fractures of the distal phalanx

*Fifty per cent of nail bed injuries have accompanying fracture of the distal phalanx or tuft (Zook et al. 1984). It is essential that accurate approximation of the dorsal cortex be achieved to give normal nail formation. If the fracture is stable, reapplication of the nail will usually hold the fracture reduced and in good position. Bindra (1996) has reported a tension band suture over the nail to provide further stability to the distal phalanx. Displaced and unstable fractures are accurately reduced and fixed with fine longitudinal or crossed K-wires. If a patient is*

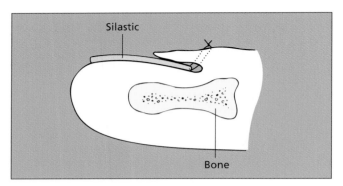

**Fig. 10.60** A nail wall suture used to retain a silastic sheet in the nail fold. © E. Zook.

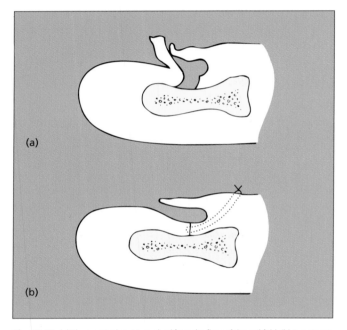

**Fig. 10.61** (a) The germinal matrix avulsed from the floor of the nail fold. (b) A mattress suture through the nail wall used to reapproximate the germinal matrix into the nail fold. © E. Zook.

seen with a displaced fracture in the first several days postinjury the fracture should be reduced and stabilized. The nail bed should be repaired if it has not been. We do not give routine antibiotics for care of nail bed injuries but if there is a delayed treatment we usually administer an appropriate broad-spectrum antibiotic.

### Avulsion of nail matrix

*Avulsion frequently leaves the fragment of nail matrix attached*

**Fig. 10.62** (right) (a) 22% of injuries are classified as severe crushing injuries. (b) After the nail bed is reapproximated as accurately as possible, a piece of 20/1000th silicone sheeting is placed to mould the nail bed and maintain the nail fold open. (c) The patient 1 year later. © E. Zook.

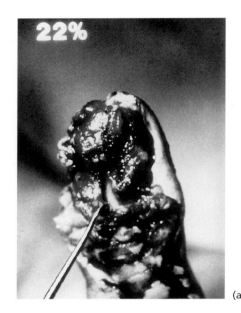

(a)

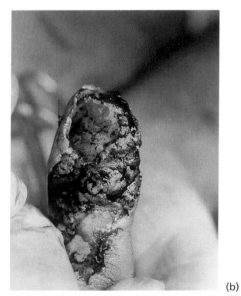

(b)

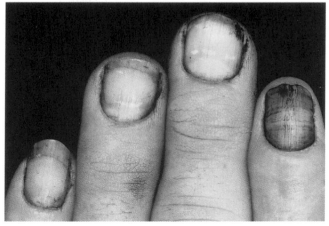

(c)

to the undersurface of the nail. It is important to retrieve the matrix and the nail to return it in its appropriate position on the tip. Schiller (1957) advocated use of the nail since it is the optimum shape and tension to aid inosculation (nourishment) of the nail bed. It is sometimes possible to replace the nail and attached matrix back onto the fingertip in its original position (Fig. 10.63). This may require trimming of the nail so that the edge of the matrix can be seen and approximated accurately. It is frequently necessary with a large avulsed composite fragment to separate the nail from the perionychium to achieve accurate replacement (Fig. 10.64).

A fragment of nail matrix 1 cm in diameter or less will usually live by inosculation and ingrowth of circulation from the periphery even when placed on the bare cortex of the distal phalanx. If the fragment of nail matrix is not available other methods of coverage have been advocated including matrix grafts from other nail beds (Swanker 1947), split thickness skin grafts (Hanrahan 1946; Flatt 1955, 1956; Horner 1966) and reversed dermal grafts. (Ashbell et al. 1967; Clayburgh et al. 1983). However, there has been little success with either of these latter two methods. If an adjacent finger has been amputated and is not replantable, removal of a full thickness matrix graft to replace missing nail matrix is indicated (Fig. 10.65). Harvest of full thickness germinal or sterile matrix from an uninjured finger will leave a significant deformity and is not advised.

Full thickness free nail matrix graft from the toes in acute nail matrix avulsions of the hand has been used by Saita et al. (1983) with excellent results. This unfortunately leaves a deformity of the toenail.

Shepard (1983) published excellent results using split thickness sterile matrix grafts from the adjacent sterile matrix of the injured finger or from a toenail matrix. It has been our experience if there is inadequate, undamaged nail matrix on the injured finger from which to harvest a split matrix graft then a split thickness nail matrix graft will need to be harvested from the large toe to obtain an adequate sized graft (Fig. 10.66a,b). Toes 2 to 5 are as a rule less than one-half the size of a fingernail.

The toenail is removed from the great toe with a periosteal elevator under toe block anaesthesia. A split thickness matrix graft (approximately 8–10/1000 inch thick) is removed from the toe matrix with a surgical blade (Shepard 1990a,b). It is better for the graft to be too thin than too thick to prevent deformity of the toenail. A surgical blade can be used with a back and forth sawing motion to tangentially remove a small fragment (Fig. 10.66c–d). It is impossible to remove a large fragment with this technique due to the curve of the nail bed. If a larger fragment of sterile matrix is needed it is necessary to use the tip of the blade to follow the curve of the matrix (Fig. 10.66e). A pattern of the defect is made with a piece of sterile surgical glove or suture pack. The pattern is placed on the toe matrix (be careful not to turn it over) and outlined to shape and fit. The sterile matrix graft is harvested (Fig. 10.66f)

and sutured in place with fine chromic suture as described earlier (Fig. 10.66h–i). If available the nail is placed over the matrix and into the nail fold.

Split thickness grafts should be taken only from sterile matrix and applied to sterile matrix. If a germinal matrix graft is needed it requires a full thickness germinal matrix graft from a toe. This leaves a toenail deformity and is uncommonly used acutely in the case of trauma. The exception is when there is a non-replantable adjacent finger from which full thickness germinal matrix can be used without resultant deformity. A split thickness sterile matrix graft does not include germinal cells and will not produce nail.

### Delayed matrix repair

If nail bed injuries are seen within 1 week and there is a suspicion of inadequate initial care the nail bed should be explored and repaired. After a week the wound may be so retracted that approximation is impossible (Fig. 10.67). Antibiotics should be used in secondary repairs.

### Tip amputation

Amputation of the fingertip may involve a portion of the nail and matrix. It has been advocated that a skin only amputation be treated with soaks to allow secondary healing. This causes traction on the hyponychium and sometimes gives a significant hook of the nail. With amputation of the skin a split thickness graft from the side of the finger or the hypothenar area of the hand heals the wound and gives less contraction. With simple laceration amputations involving bone, Kutler (1944) flaps (V-Y advancement from bilaterally) or the Atasoy et al. (1970) V-Y flap from the volar aspect of the pad is used to close the finger. If the sterile matrix is pulled over the end of the bone invariably some degree of hooking of the nail will result.

If nail bed distal to the lunula is present, it is best to maintain the sterile and germinal matrix since a short nail is functionally better than no nail. If however only the germinal matrix remains it is best removed to ablate the nail. A short stub of nail usually creates more trouble than benefit. Ablation should be discussed with the patient so they understand what the result will be and the reason for it.

### Reconstruction of the nail bed

As a rule reconstruction of the nail bed following trauma is not as successful as the patient or surgeon desires. Inconsistent results have hindered the process of knowledge development. Every reconstructive procedure on the nail bed must be well thought out using knowledge of anatomy and physiology to achieve the best improvement. In the past the nail matrix has been treated much like the skin which has led to disappointing results and discouragement. Reconstruction can be divided into three areas: germinal matrix, sterile matrix and perionychium.

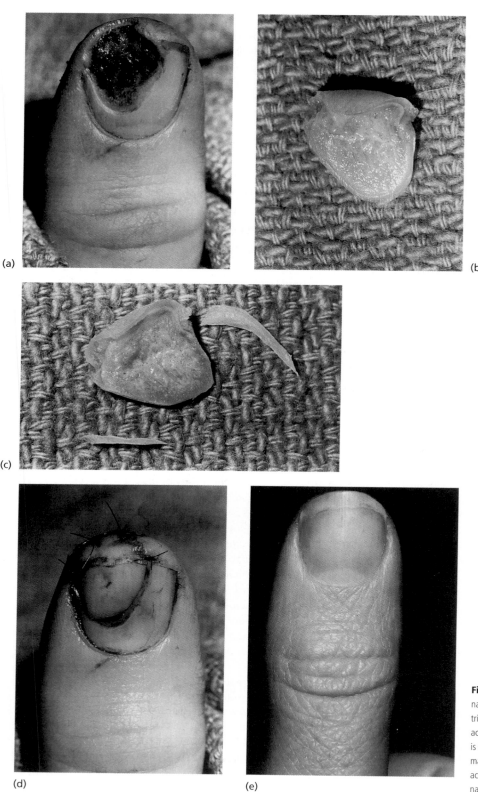

(a)

(b)

(c)

(d)

(e)

**Fig. 10.63** (a) Avulsion of the tip skin, sterile matrix and nail. (b) The undersurface of the fragment. (c) The nail is trimmed from around the edge of the fragment to allow accurate approximation of the edge. (d) The skin of the tip is sutured. The sterile matrix with the nail attached will maintain the size of the nail bed fragment and facilitate accurate approximation. Steri-strips are used to hold the nail in place. (e) One year later. © E. Zook.

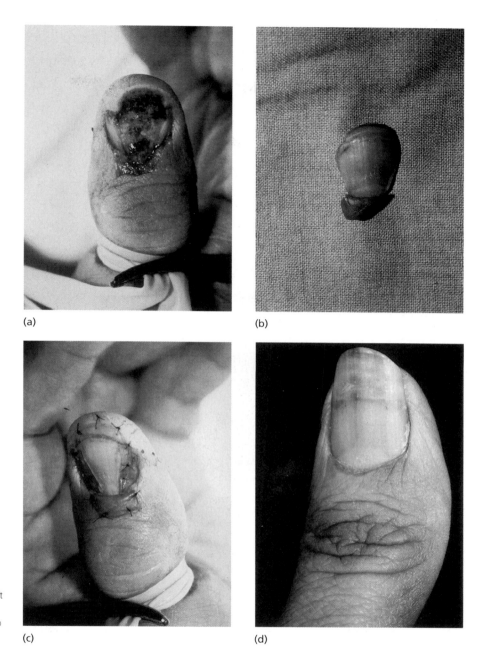

(a)

(b)

(c)

(d)

**Fig. 10.64** (a) Avulsion of the tip, skin, sterile and germinal matrix and dorsal roof of the nail fold. (b) The fragment. (c) The nail is removed and the composite graft accurately replaced. Either the nail or silicone sheeting is used to maintain the nail fold open. (d) One year later. © E. Zook.

## Ridged nail

*Nail ridges are caused by scarring of the nail bed, irregularity of a healed fracture or non-union of the bony tuft. The nail acquires the shape of the nail bed, therefore if the bed is ridged the nail will be ridged (Fig. 10.68). Correction of the ridged nail requires surgical removal of the scar or irregular surface of the distal phalanx which is misshaping the nail bed and causing the ridge. (Ashbell et al. 1967; Tajima 1974).*

*Minor transverse ridges of the nail may be seen following ischaemic periods of the finger or the body such as extended length of tourniquet time, hypoxia from pneumonia, etc. These resolve as the nail grows.*

## Split nail

*A split nail may be caused by ridging of underlying matrix or by a scar in the germinal and/or sterile matrix. Since scar does not produce nail cells, the nail becomes thinner and weaker as it grows distally and is prone to crack and break. If the scar is wide the nail will grow on either side but not in the centre causing a wider split.*

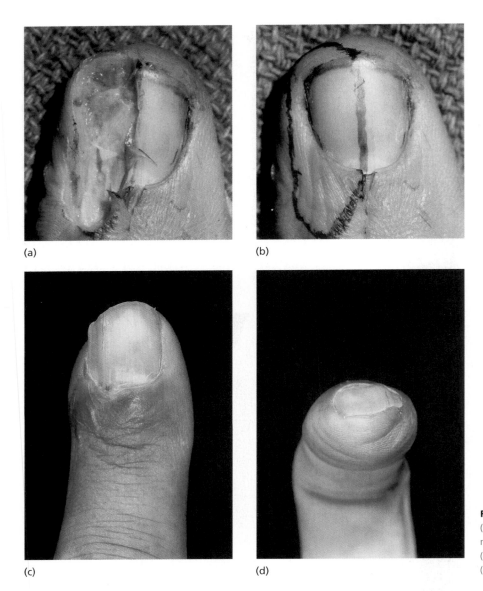

(a)

(b)

(c)

(d)

**Fig. 10.65** (a) Avulsion of one-half of the perionychium. (b) A matched fragment of tissue is removed from a non-replantable finger and grafted onto the injured finger. (c) One-year later growth of the nail is shown. (d) An end-on view. © E. Zook.

*If the scar causing the split involves the sterile matrix it may be treated by resection of a narrow scar and closure of the defect. If the scar is wide enough to cause a split nail it is frequently too wide to close successfully without undue wound tension. (Zook & Russell 1990). We have had reasonable success breaking up longitudinal scars by doing one or two Z-plasties in the sterile matrix making each limb approximately 2 mm long (Fig. 10.69). A split caused by extensive scarring in the sterile matrix, is best treated by scar resection and split thickness sterile matrix graft from an adjacent area of that finger or a toe (Shepard 1990b) (Fig. 10.70).*

*When the split is caused by scar in the germinal matrix no nail is produced in the germinal matrix and the split is complete. Exploration is essential and requires radial incisions from the corners (Fig. 10.20) to expose the germinal matrix. The nail fragments are removed and the nail matrix explored with*

*magnification. Johnson (1971) has advocated incisions in the paronychial fold with advancement of the germinal matrix towards the centre and suturing. I have had little success with this technique and do not use it for reconstruction following trauma. My preference is to transplant germinal matrix from a toenail bed (Fig. 10.71). This graft is harvested somewhat larger than and shaped to fit the defect. Germinal matrix grafts will often require ablation of the toe matrix and nail if the 2nd through 5th are used. If more nail matrix is needed a portion of the large toenail bed is used. In that case one side is usually used so a portion of the nail can be left. (Clark & LeGros-Buxton 1938; Baden 1965). Split thickness grafts of germinal matrix will not produce nail and should never be used.*

*A transverse angled scar in the germinal matrix can cause a horizontal double nail. If the ventral portion is adequate the superficial germinal matrix is excised leaving only the*

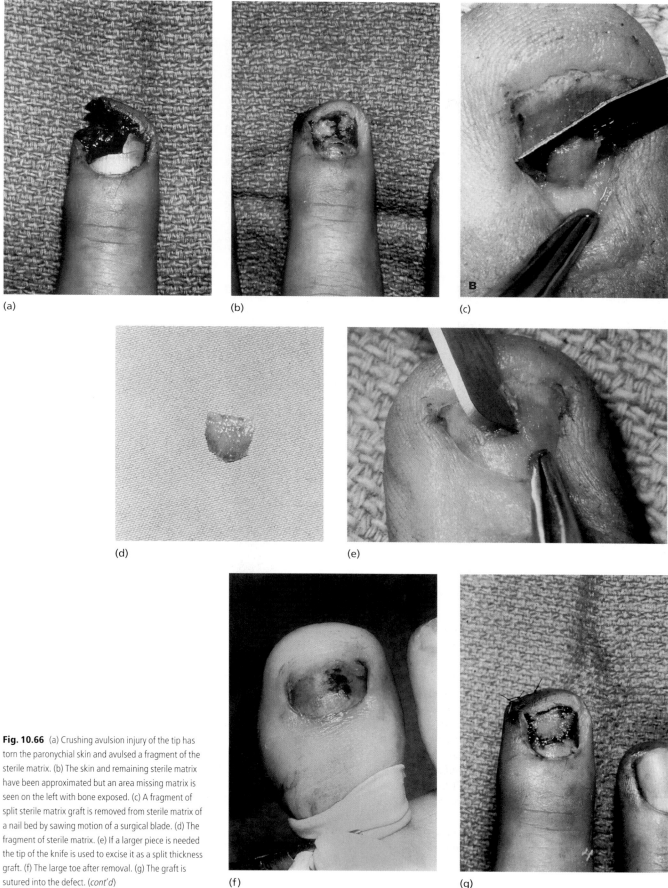

**Fig. 10.66** (a) Crushing avulsion injury of the tip has torn the paronychial skin and avulsed a fragment of the sterile matrix. (b) The skin and remaining sterile matrix have been approximated but an area missing matrix is seen on the left with bone exposed. (c) A fragment of split sterile matrix graft is removed from sterile matrix of a nail bed by sawing motion of a surgical blade. (d) The fragment of sterile matrix. (e) If a larger piece is needed the tip of the knife is used to excise it as a split thickness graft. (f) The large toe after removal. (g) The graft is sutured into the defect. (*cont'd*)

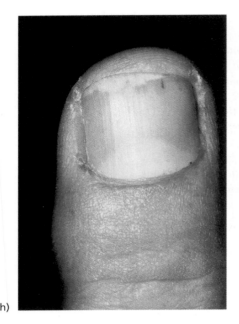

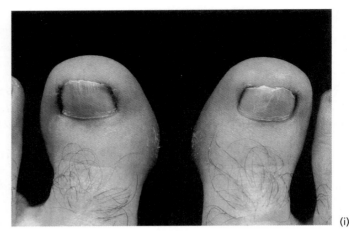

(h)

**Fig. 10.66** (*cont'd*) (h) One year later. (i) The donor toe 1 year later. © E. Zook.

(i)

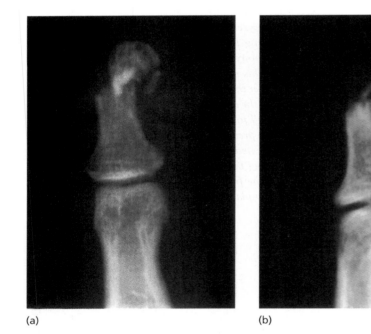

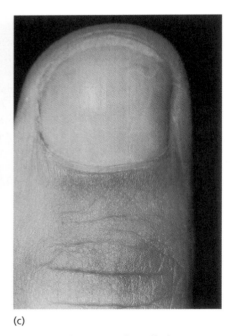

(a)                                          (b)                                          (c)

**Fig. 10.67** (a) A 5-day-old displaced fracture and nail bed injury in the AP view. (b) Volar malalignment of the tuft which requires reduction and pinning as well as nail bed repair. (c) One year following the injury. © E. Zook.

ventral nail (Fig. 10.72). If neither are of adequate volume the intervening scar must be removed to make the nail one again.

### Non-adherence of the nail

*If the non-adherence is distal and unexplained by trauma, removal of the nail and scraping off of the keratinous build-up on the sterile matrix will many times allow the nail to grow normally (Fig. 10.73). This may need to be done on more than one occasion for the nail adherence may improve with each procedure. If scraping does not correct the non-adherence a portion of the abnormal matrix may be replaced with split thickness sterile matrix graft (Fig. 10.74). If the non-adherence is due to scar, the scar is excised and the defect of the scar covered with a split thickness sterile matrix graft from either*

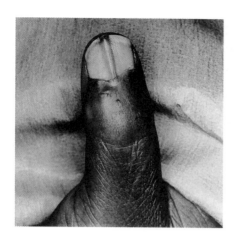

**Fig. 10.68** A ridge in the nail secondary to placement of a longitudinal pin beneath the periosteum of the distal phalanx. © E. Zook.

the adjoining nail or toenail matrix (Fig. 10.75). Again usually if the adjacent nail is not large enough to supply a split thickness graft toes (2nd to 5th) will not be either and the big toe must be used. (Zook et al. 1980).

### Absence of the nail

Absence of a nail may be congenital, secondary to trauma, infection or surgical removal. If toenails are available they may be transferred as a unit to the finger or more successfully may be transferred with microvascular anastomosis (Koshima et al. 1988; Morrison 1990; Pessa et al. 1990; Shibata et al. 1991; Foucher & Sammut 1992; Iwassawa et al. 1992). If toenails are not available, an area of epidermis the shape and size of the corresponding nail on the opposite hand is excised. A split thickness skin graft or full thickness skin graft may be applied to the area and when healed resembles a nail (Fig. 10.76). One can use a split thickness skin graft from the

sterile matrix to simulate the body of the nail and a strip of full thickness skin graft for the lunula and the hyponychium to make these areas white.

Creation of a nail fold with graft has been described into which an artificial nail can be placed. (Buncke & Gonzalez 1962; Barford 1972). However, in my experience although satisfactory initially the fold contracts and after several months has little or no fold left in which to accept the proximal edge of the glued on nail.

Composite grafts from the toe to finger to replace a portion (Fig. 10.77) or an entire fingernail (Fig. 10.78) have the loss of toenail as a consequence.

### Pterygium and eponychial deformities

A pterygium of the eponychium or hyponychium may occur secondary to trauma or congenital absence or collagen vascular diseases such as systemic lupus erythematosus and dermatomyocytis (Caputo et al. 1993). Pterygia of the hyponychium may follow injuries that denervate the fingertip or are secondary to ischaemia. The pad becomes atrophic and the hyponychium is exposed to minor tip traumas. This may be painful and make the finger extremely tender. The hyponychium is detached from the nail by excising the distal 4–5 mm of the sterile matrix (including the hyponychium) and replacing it with split thickness skin graft. This releases the pterygia and allows the nail bed to retract under the protection of the nail (Fig. 10.79).

A pterygium of the eponychium is treated by freeing the dorsal roof of the nail fold from the nail and inserting a silicone sheet beneath it to prevent re-adhesion until the area has healed (Fig. 10.80). The undersurface of the dorsal roof of the nail fold heals releasing the adherence. If that is unsuccessful the dorsal roof may be freed from the nail and a split thickness sterile matrix graft placed on the roof of the nail fold to prevent

**Fig. 10.69** (a) A split in the nail from scar at the junction of the germinal and sterile matrix. (b) One year post revision of the scar and Z-plasty of the sterile matrix. © E. Zook.

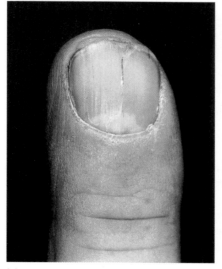
(a)

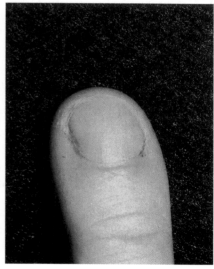
(b)

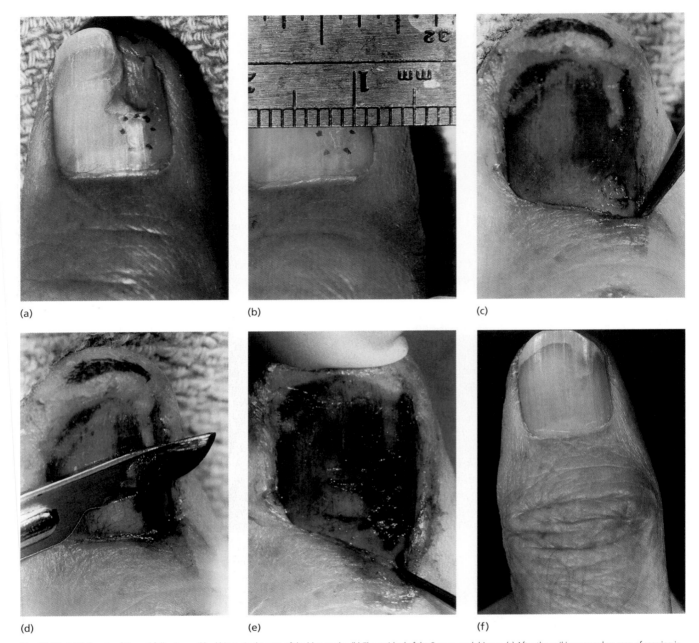

(a)  (b)  (c)

(d)  (e)  (f)

**Fig. 10.70** (a) Deformity of the nail following nail bed biopsy in the area of the blue marks. (b) The residual of the 3-mm punch biopsy. (c) After the nail is removed an area of scarring is seen at the junction of the sterile and germinal matrix. (d) The scarred area is resected and a split thickness sterile matrix graft taken from distally. (e) The split thickness graft is placed over the defect. (f) The patient's nail 1 year later. © E. Zook.

adherence and give improvement in the roughness of the nail (Fig. 10.81). Shephard (1990a) has shown good results with this technique.

A notch in the eponychium may result from trauma or resection of lesions. Baran (1986) has described resection of the lateral edges of the eponychium to create a smooth arc (Fig. 10.82). A notch in the eponychium may be treated with excision and closure, which is not routinely successful, since it

is closed with tension and will frequently pull apart. Several ways to reconstruct the eponychium have been advocated including use of rotation flaps, helical rim of the ear (Rose 1980) or my choice is a free composite eponychial graft from a toe.

The edges of the defect on the eponychium are freshened to allow blood supply and the defect measured (Fig. 10.83). A composite graft of eponychium of a toe (usually the large toe) is used. A fragment of toe eponychium slightly larger than the

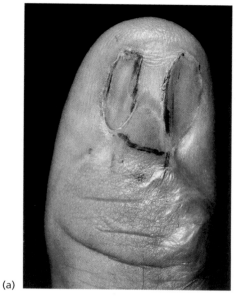

(a)

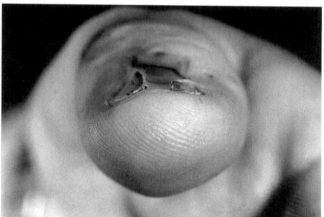

(b)

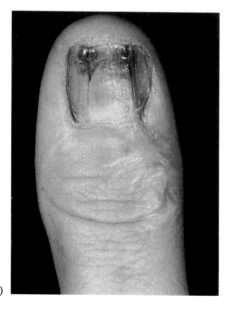

(c)

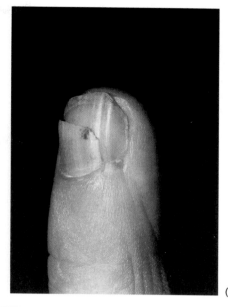

(a)

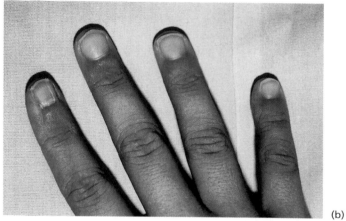

(b)

**Fig. 10.72** (a) A horizontal laceration of the germinal matrix separating the germinal matrix into two portions produces two nails. If the deeper of the two nails is adequate the superficial remnant is resected as in this case. If the inferior nail is not adequate then the scar must be removed from between the two fragments of germinal matrix and reapproximated. (b) The patient's nail 1 year later after removal of the superficial germinal fragment. © E. Zook.

**Fig. 10.71** (a) A wide split of the nail with no nail growing in the centre portion. (b) A distal view showing the two fragments of nail. (c) A germinal and sterile matrix graft from the toe gives regrowth of the nail and is shown 1 year later. © E. Zook.

*defect on the finger is removed. The remaining toe eponychium not used is resected and heals secondarily with little deformity. The composite graft is sutured in place and becomes vascularized from the surrounding tissue (Fig. 10.84).*

*Eponychial deformities secondary to burns are very difficult to correct. A burn of the dorsum of the finger will cause retraction of the eponychium and exposure of the dorsum of the nail with subsequent roughness. (Spauwen et al. 1987). Burns of the hand involving the dorsum of the fingers frequently cause nail deformities. The deformity varies from complete absence of nail to contracture of the dorsal roof with discomfort and roughening of the nail surface. If the nail does not grow several*

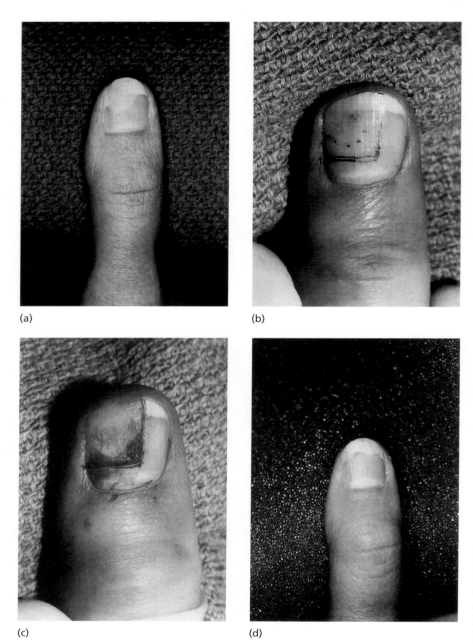

(a)

(b)

(c)

(d)

**Fig. 10.73** (a) Chronic detachment of the nail from the sterile matrix of unknown aetiology, but not secondary to trauma. (b) The area of non-adherence is dotted and the area to be removed is lined. (c) The nail is removed revealing the hyperkeratinous area of non-adherence. This area is scraped down to normal sterile matrix. (d) The nail is seen 1 year later. © E. Zook.

*fingers are usually involved and reconstruction is rarely possible. If it is due to retraction of the dorsal roof and does not involve more than a few fingers, eponychial grafts from the toes will frequently improve the appearance and decrease the symptoms. This is carried out as described earlier for eponychial grafts. Achauer and Welk (1990) have described reconstruction of the dorsal roof of the nail fold by lateral flaps from the fingertips transposed onto the dorsum of the finger to replace the eponychium. Reconstruction of the eponychium has given improved results through the works of several authors. (Hayes 1974; Alsbjorn et al. 1985; Ngim & Soin 1986; Kasai & Ogawa 1989).*

### Cornified nail bed

*It is not uncommon to have a patient complain of non-adherence of the distal portion of the sterile matrix. This is usually caused by either an acute episode of stripping the nail from the hyponychium and distal sterile matrix, followed by the patient attempting to keep dirt from under the nail which causes a chronic problem of nail detachment. The sterile matrix keratinizes and the nail cannot adhere as it grows out. It may also be due to a chronic pulling of the nail from the hyponychium, which occurs in older women when nail growth has slowed. Their fingernails are worn long and the mechanical*

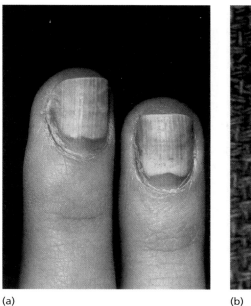
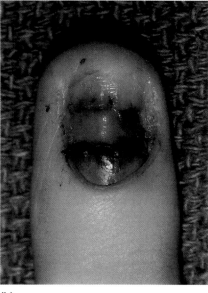
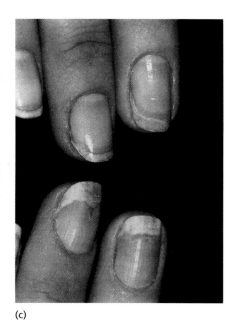

(a)                                    (b)                                    (c)

**Fig. 10.74** (a) Extensive non-adherence of the nail to the sterile matrix of unknown aetiology. (b) The nail is removed and a segment of split thickness sterile matrix graft from the toe is placed distal to the germinal matrix. (c) The patient 1 year later with much improved adherence. © E. Zook.

leverage on the nail causes it to be pulled from the hypony-chium and sterile matrix. Keeping the nail short may allow the nail to readhere to the hyponychial area. If keratinization is the problem, the nail is removed to just proximal to the non-adherence and a scalpel blade is used to scrape the keratin from the sterile matrix. Lubricating creams are applied to allow the nail to grow out and readhere. This may need to be done more than once since the exposed sterile matrix may re-cornify before the nail can cover the most distal portion (Fig. 10.73).

When the germinal matrix has been removed to eliminate nail growth such as frequently has been done for ingrown toenails the keratinization of the sterile matrix is occasionally a problem. The build-up causes roughness, irregularity and sometimes discomfort. The sterile matrix may be excised and replaced with a split thickness skin graft.

## Nail spikes and cysts

Following trauma or attempted removal of nail fragments nail bed may be left and result in nail spikes or cysts. Nail spikes are best treated with complete surgical excision of the fragments of germinal matrix creating the spikes or cysts. Nail cysts are usually slow growing, painful to varying degrees and treated by complete excision of the cyst wall.

## Hyponychium

The hyponychium may become hypertrophic and protrude beyond the tip of the finger and/or nail. It is then frequently tender and painful when pressed or touched. Treatment is excision of the hyponychium and split thickness sterile matrix graft from the adjacent matrix to correct the hypertrophy (Fig. 10.85).

## Hooked nail

Hooked nail occurs with amputation of the fingertip and loss of bony support of the distal nail bed (Fig. 10.86). Pulling the sterile matrix and hyponychium over the bone end also causes hooking. Since nail follows the course of the nail bed the nail hooks distally and volarly. Amputation involving the skin of the tip of the finger has become increasingly treated by secondary healing. This gives a good result for fingertip sensa-tion and coverage but causes some hooking of the nail in most patients.

The symptomatic (painful) hooked nail may be treated by recreating the defect and allowing the sterile matrix to return to the dorsum of the distal phalanx. Following this flap coverage relieves the tension on the nail and usually improves the dis-comfort but does not correct the cosmetic deformity. (Kumar & Satku 1993). To correct a hooked nail completely requires replacement of distal phalanx, fat, skin and nail bed. This can only be done dependably by microvascular replacement of the tissue by transferring from a toe tip (Koshima et al. 1988). Bone grafts onto the distal phalanx with flap coverage as a rule resorb over time and the defect recurs.

A prosthesis rather than a reconstruction can give a good cosmetic result.

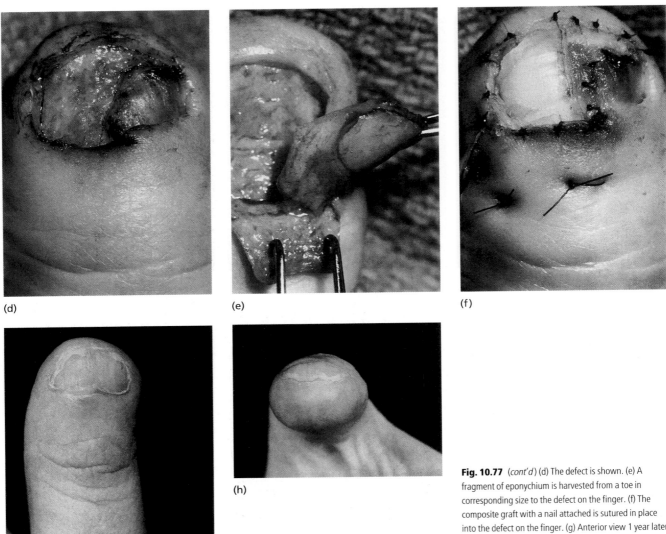

(d)

(e)

(f)

(g)

(h)

**Fig. 10.77** (*cont'd*) (d) The defect is shown. (e) A fragment of eponychium is harvested from a toe in corresponding size to the defect on the finger. (f) The composite graft with a nail attached is sutured in place into the defect on the finger. (g) Anterior view 1 year later showing nail growth. (h) End-on view of the new nail growth. © E. Zook.

They can be plant (thorns, splinter) (Fig. 10.91a,b), animal (urchin, oyster shell) (Haneke *et al.* 1996), metal, plastic or glass, this list being non-exhaustive.

### Patient seen early

Usually the foreign body cannot be seen. Pain, intense when the accident occurred, is at that time moderate, but touching the nail increases the pain. Foreign body must be removed immediately under local anaesthesia with total or partial avulsion of the nail plate. A wet antiseptic dressing must be applied for 2 or 3 days.

### Patient seen later on

Subungual panaritium is the usual reason for the consultation.

Diagnosis is easy because of the yellow colour of the nail bed and the pulsating pain, especially during the night. Removal of the nail plate over the pus and wide drainage of the cavity should be performed if windowing of the nail is not sufficient (Andrus 1980). Usually, antibiotics are not needed and antiseptic dressing applied on the wound. Pain relief is immediately obtained followed by complete recovery within a few days.

Two clinical types deserve special mention.

### Thorns

Thorns of variable origin may induce non-specific inflammatory responses, a suppurative dermatitis with eventual expulsion of the foreign material, or a granuloma with central caseation. In a case of a cactus thorn in the nail bed, a mild inflammatory cell infiltrate with some histiocytes, a few giant

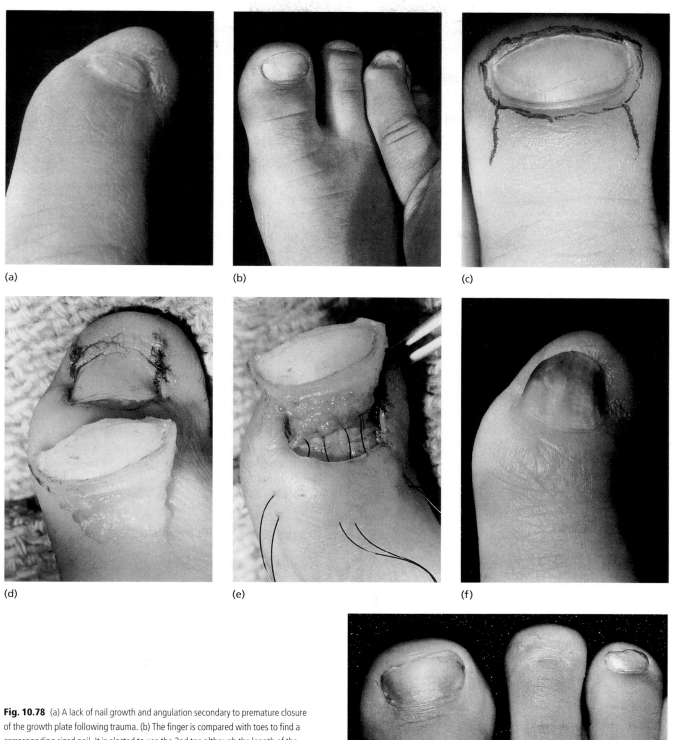

**Fig. 10.78** (a) A lack of nail growth and angulation secondary to premature closure of the growth plate following trauma. (b) The finger is compared with toes to find a corresponding sized nail. It is elected to use the 2nd toe although the length of the 2nd toenail is usually not as long as the finger. (c) The donor toe is marked. (d) The nail, sterile and germinal matrix and hyponychium are excised as a unit and the composite graft transferred to the finger. (e) The composite graft is sutured into the defect and nail fold. (f) One year postgraft finger is seen. Better adherence distally could be attained if the sterile matrix was lengthened with a sterile matrix graft. (g) A 2nd toe postclosure. © E. Zook.

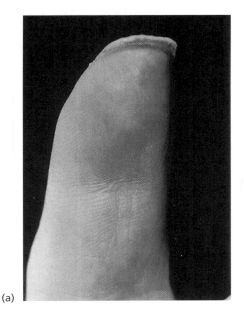

(a)

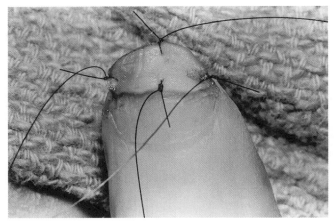

(b)

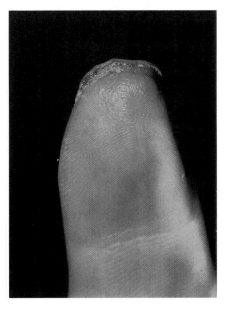

(c)

cells and neutrophils was observed. The foreign body could be identified as a cactus thorn due to its unique structure: On cross-section, it is circular, made up of hexagonal cells with a round central canal and lined by a single layer of flat cells; under polarized light, it is strongly birefringent.

Often the initial injury involving the nail matrix has not been noticed and the patient is examined later on, during the second or third month. There is an uncomfortable, but not really painful, oedema of the whole finger, and its mobility is reduced. This is called 'inoculation synovitis'. Surgical treatment is compulsory, consisting in the removal of the foreign body as well as the oedematous synovial tissue. The colour of the latter is greyish and turbid fluid comes out of it. There is no bacterial infection.

Recovery takes a few days.

A subungual thorn may mimic longitudinal melanonychia (Gotlieb, unpublished).

### Sea urchin granuloma (Fig. 10.91c)

This condition resembles a whitlow. A 35-year-old man with sea urchin granulomas on his left foot including the proximal nail fold and matrix of the 4th toe was seen. The toe was swollen, reddish-blue and tender. The granuloma of the proximal nail fold and matrix had caused a broad split in the nail.

Histopathology showed a thickening of the proximal fold with loss of the cuticle. There was granulomatous inflammation with lymphocytes, histiocytes and large foreign-body-type giant cells some of which had large vacuoles. Remnants of the sea urchin spicules could not be discerned (Haneke *et al.* 1996). Intralesional long-acting steroids are helpful and recovery is seen within 2–3 weeks.

### Delayed post-traumatic deformities

#### Malaligned nail

##### Post-traumatic onycholysis (absence of nail plate–nail bed adhesion)

A functionally stable nail requires at least 5 mm of healthy nail bed distal to the lunula for nail adherence. If the nail grows normally, but fails to adhere to all or part of the nail bed, treatment consists of removing the nail, scraping the epidermis of the nail bed, and covering it immediately with a 'nail bank transplant' or the original nail, if the latter is adequate. In fact, a more satisfactory result can be obtained with resection of the scar which may cause the nail to loosen and its replacement by a split-thickness nail bed graft from either an adjacent area of the nail bed or from a toenail bed (Shepard 1990b).

### References

Achauer, B.M. & Welk, R.A. (1990) One-stage reconstruction of the

**Fig. 10.79** (a) Pterygium of the hyponychium following denervation of the hand and reinnervation which has become painful. (b) The hyponychial area has been excised and a split thickness skin graft placed in the defect to allow the nail bed to detach from the nail. (c) One year later the patient's pain has been relieved. © E. Zook.

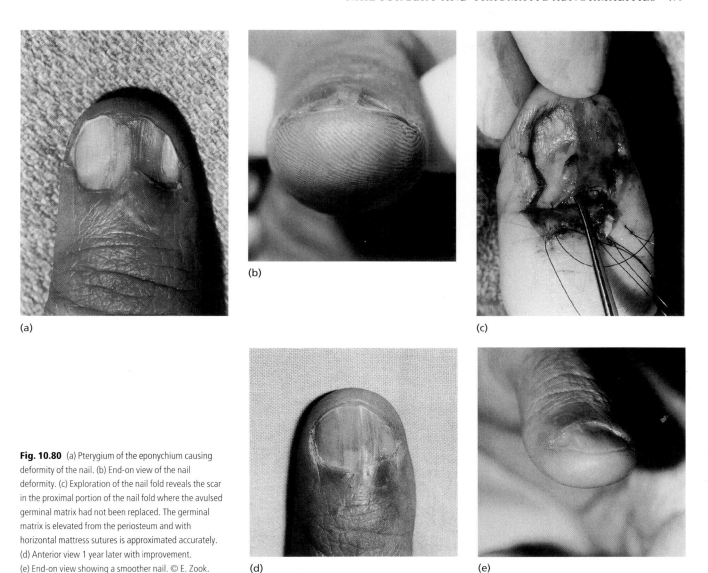

**Fig. 10.80** (a) Pterygium of the eponychium causing deformity of the nail. (b) End-on view of the nail deformity. (c) Exploration of the nail fold reveals the scar in the proximal portion of the nail fold where the avulsed germinal matrix had not been replaced. The germinal matrix is elevated from the periosteum and with horizontal mattress sutures is approximated accurately. (d) Anterior view 1 year later with improvement. (e) End-on view showing a smoother nail. © E. Zook.

postburn nail fold contracture. *Plastic and Reconstructive Surgery* **85**, 937–940.

Alsbjorn, B.F., Metz, P. & Ebbehoj, J. (1985) Nail fold retraction due to burn wound contracture. A surgical procedure. *Burns* **11**, 166–167.

Andrus, C.H. (1980) Instrument and technique for removal of subungual foreign bodies. *American Journal of Surgery* **140**, 588.

Ashbell, T.S., Kleinert, H.E., Putcha, S.M. & Kutz, J.E. (1967) The deformed fingernail, a frequent result of failure to repair nail bed injuries. *Journal of Trauma* **7**, 177–190.

Atasoy, E., Loakimidis, E., Kasdan, M., Kutz, J. & Kleinert, H. (1970) Reconstruction of the amputated fingertip with a triangular volar flap. A new surgical procedure. *Journal of Bone and Joint Surgery* **52A**, 921–926.

Baden, H.P. (1965) Regeneration of the nail. *Archives of Dermatology* **91**, 619–620.

Baran, R. (1986) Removal of the proximal nail fold. Why, when, how? *Journal of Dermatologic Surgery and Oncology* **12**, 234–236.

Barford, B. (1972) Reconstruction of the nail fold. *Hand* **4**, 85–87.

Beasley, R.W. & de Bez, G. (1990) Prosthetic substitution for finger nails. *Hand Clinics* **6**, 105–112.

de Berker, D. & Baran, R. (1998) Acquired malalignment: a complication of lateral longitudinal nail biopsy. *Acta Dermato-Venereologica* **78**, 468–470.

Bindra, R.R. (1996) Management of nail-bed-fracture-lacerations using a tension-band suture. *Journal of Hand Surgery* **21A**, 1111–1113.

Buncke, H.J. & Gonzalez, R.I. (1962) Fingernail reconstruction. *Plastic and Reconstructive Surgery* **30**, 452–461.

Caputo, R., Cappio, F., Rigoni, C. *et al.* (1993) Pterygium inversum unguis. *Archives of Dermatology* **129**, 1307–1309.

Clark, W.E. & LeGros-Buton, L.H.D. (1938) Studies in nail growth. *British Journal of Dermatology* **50**, 221–235.

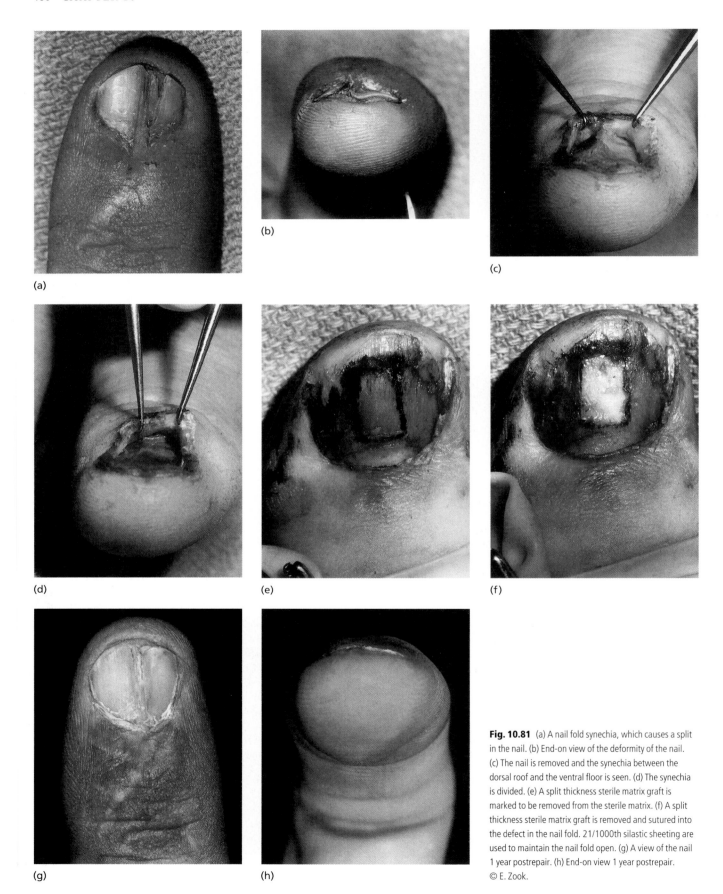

**Fig. 10.81** (a) A nail fold synechia, which causes a split in the nail. (b) End-on view of the deformity of the nail. (c) The nail is removed and the synechia between the dorsal roof and the ventral floor is seen. (d) The synechia is divided. (e) A split thickness sterile matrix graft is marked to be removed from the sterile matrix. (f) A split thickness sterile matrix graft is removed and sutured into the defect in the nail fold. 21/1000th silastic sheeting are used to maintain the nail fold open. (g) A view of the nail 1 year postrepair. (h) End-on view 1 year postrepair. © E. Zook.

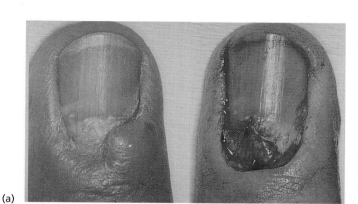

(a)

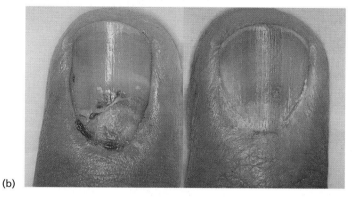

(b)

**Fig. 10.82** (a,b) Procedure to excise jagged proximal nail tissue to give a better cosmetic-result (Baran 1986). © E. Zook.

Clayburgh, R.H., Wood, M.B. & Cooney, W.P. (1983) Nail bed repair and reconstruction by reverse dermal grafts. *Journal of Hand Surgery* **8**, 594–599.

Ersek, R.A., Gadaria, U. & Denton, D.R. (1985) Nail bed avulsions treated with porcine xenografts. *Journal of Hand Surgery* **10A**, 152–153.

Flatt, A.E. (1955) Minor hand injuries. *Journal of Bone and Joint Surgery* **37B**, 117–125.

Flatt, A.E. (1956) Nail-bed injuries. *British Journal of Plastic Surgery* **8**, 34–37.

Foucher, G. & Sammut, D. (1992) Aesthetic improvement of the nail by the 'Illusion' technique in partial toe transfer for thumb reconstruction. *Annals of Plastic Surgery* **28**, 195–199.

Haneke, E., Tosti, A. & Piraccini, B.M. (1996) Sea-urchin granuloma of the nail apparatus. *Dermatology* **192**, 140–142.

Hanrahan, E.M. (1946) The split-thickness skin graft as a covering following removal of a fingernail. *Surgery* **20**, 398–400.

Hayes, C.W. (1974) One-stage nail fold reconstruction. *Hand* **6**, 74–75.

Horner, R.L. & Cohen, B.I. (1966) Injuries to the fingernail. *Rocky Mountain Medical Journal* **63**, 60–62.

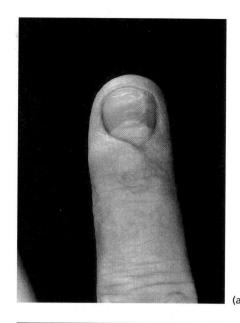

(a)

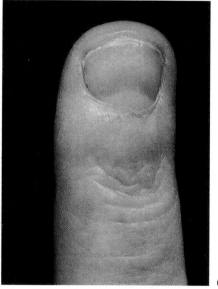

(b)

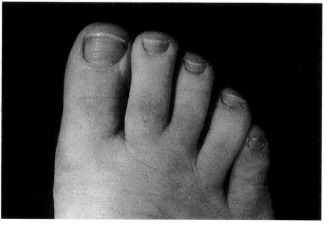

(c)

**Fig. 10.83** (right) (a) Traumatic absence of the dorsal roof of the nail fold causing a notch in the eponychium and roughness of the nail surface. (b) One year posteponychial graft from the 2nd toe with improved surface of the nail and appearance of the eponychium. (c) The 2nd toe donor site 1 year later. © E. Zook.

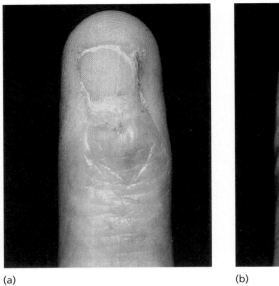

(a)

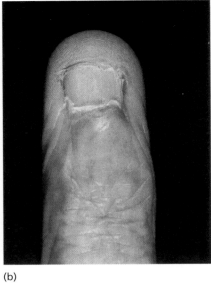

(b)

**Fig. 10.84** (a) Post-laser treatment for eponychial warts which has destroyed the dorsal roof and left a tender, painful proximal nail area. (b) One year posteponychial composite graft from the large toe with relief of pain. © E. Zook.

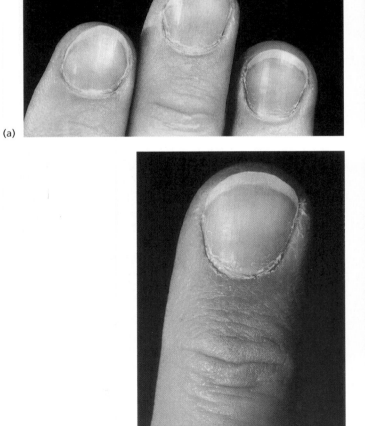

(a)

(c)

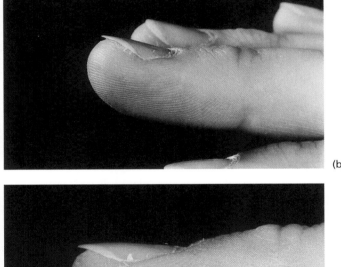

(b)

(d)

**Fig. 10.85** (a) Chronic hypertrophy and avulsion of the hyponychium with painful tip of the long finger. (b) The hypertrophic hyponychium is seen beneath the nail edge. (c) One year later with normal hyponychium and relief of symptoms. (d) Lateral view. © E. Zook.

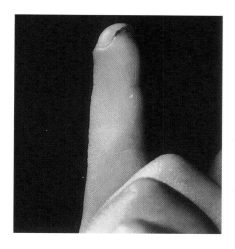

**Fig. 10.86** A painful deformed hooked nail secondary to amputation of tip. © E. Zook.

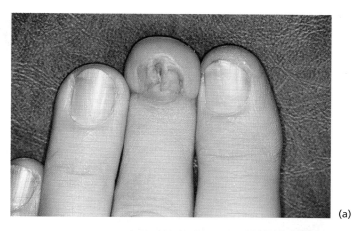

(a)

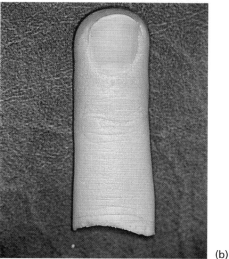

(b)

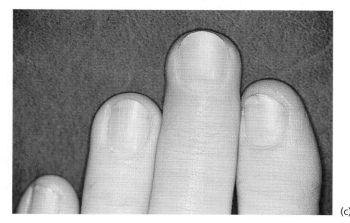

(c)

**Fig. 10.87** (a) Traumatic dystrophy. (b,c) Appropriate digital prosthesis.

Iwassawa, M., Furuta, S., Noguchi, M. & Hirose, T. (1992) Reconstruction of fingertip deformities of the thumb using a venous flap. *Annals of Plastic Surgery* **28**, 187–189.

Johnson, R.K. (1971) Nailplasty. *Plastic and Reconstructive Surgery* **47**, 275–276.

Kasai, K. & Ogawa, Y. (1989) Nailplasty using a distally based ulnar finger dorsum flap. *Aesthetic Plastic Surgery* **13**, 125–128.

Koshima, I., Soeda, S., Takase, T. & Yamasaki, M. (1988) Free vascularized nail grafts. *Journal of Hand Surgery* **13A**, 29–32.

Kumar, V.P. & Satku, K. (1993) Treatment and prevention of 'hook nail' deformity with anatomy correlation. *Journal of Hand Surgery* **18A**, 617–620.

Kutler, W. (1944) A method for repair of fingertip amputation. *Ohio State Medical Journal* **40**, 126.

Morrison, W.A. (1990) Microvascular nail transfer. *Hand Clinics* **6**, 69–76.

Ngim, R.C.K. & Soin, K. (1986) Postburn nail fold retraction: a reconstructive technique. *Journal of Hand Surgery* **11B**, 385–387.

Pessa, J.E., Tsai, T.-M., Li, Y. & Kleinert, H.E. (1990) The repair of nail deformities with the nonvascularized nail bed graft: indications and results. *Journal of Hand Surgery* **15A**, 466–470.

Pillet, J. (1981) The aesthetic hand prosthesis. *Orthopedic Clinics of North America* **12**, 961–969.

Pillet, J. & Didierjean-Pillet, A. (2000) Ungual prostheses. *Journal of Dermatological Treatment* (in press).

Rose, E.H. (1980) Nailplasty utilizing a free composite graft from the helical rim of the ear. *Plastic and Reconstructive Surgery* **66**, 23–29.

Saita, H., Suzuki, Y., Fujino, K. & Tajima, T. (1983) Free nail bed graft for treatment of nail bed injuries of the hand. *Journal of Hand Surgery* **8**, 171–178.

Schiller, C. (1957) Nail replacement in fingertip injuries. *Plastic and Reconstructive Surgery* **19**, 521–530.

Seaberg, D.C., Angelos, W.J. & Paris, P.M. (1991) Treatment of subungual hematomas with nail trephination a prospective study. *American Journal of Emergency Medicine* **9**, 209–210.

Shepard, G.H. (1983) Treatment of nail bed avulsions with split thickness nail bed grafts. *Journal of Hand Surgery* **8**, 49–54.

Shepard, G.H. (1990a) Management of acute nail bed avulsions. *Hand Clinics* **6**, 39–56.

Shepard, G.H. (1990b) Nail grafts for reconstruction. *Hand Clinics* **6**, 79–102.

Shibata, M., Seki, T., Yoshizu, T., Saito, H. & Tajima, T. (1991) Microsurgical toenail transfer to the hand. *Plastic and Reconstructive Surgery* **88**, 102–109.

Spauwen, P.H.M., Brown, I.F., Sauer, E.W. & Klasen, H.J. (1987) Management of fingernail deformities after thermal injury. *Scandinavian Journal of Plastic and Reconstructive Surgery* **21**, 253–255.

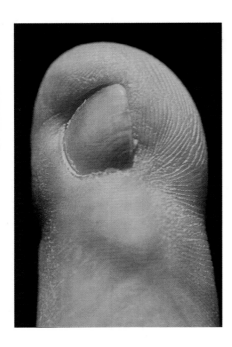

**Fig. 10.88** Traumatic nail malalignment. (Courtesy of G. Cannata, Italy.)

Swanker, W.A. (1947) Reconstructive surgery of the injured nail. *American Journal of Surgery* **74**, 341–345.

Tajima, T. (1974) Treatment of open crushing type of industrial injuries of the hand and forearm: degloving, open circumferential, heat press and nail bed injuries. *Journal of Trauma* **14**, 995–1011.

Weckesser, E.C. (1974) Treatment of hand injuries. In: *Presentation and Restoration of Function*. Year Book Medical Publishers, Chicago.

Zook, E.G. (1981) The perionychium: anatomy, physiology, and care of injuries. *Clinics in Plastic Surgery* **8**, 21–31.

Zook, E.G. (1982a) Fingernail injuries. In: *Difficult Problems in Hand Surgery* (eds J.W. Strickland & J.B. Steichen). CV Mosby, St Louis.

Zook, E.G. (1982b) Injuries of the fingernail. In: *Operative Hand Surgery* (ed. D.P. Green). Churchill Livingstone, New York.

Zook, E.G. (1985) Nail bed injuries. *Hand Clinics* **1**, 701–716.

Zook, E.G. (1986) Complications of the perionychium. *Hand Clinics* **2**, 407–427.

Zook, E.G. (1990a) Anatomy and physiology of the perionychium. *Hand Clinics* **6**, 1–7.

Zook, E.G. (1990b) Discussion of 'Management of acute fingernail injuries'. *Hand Clinics* **6**, 37–38.

Zook, E.G. (1990c) Discussion of 'The etiologies and mechanisms of nail bed injury'. *Hand Clinics* **6**, 21.

Zook, E.G. & Russell, R.C. (1990) Reconstruction of a functional and esthetic nail. *Hand Clinics* **6**, 59–68.

Zook, E.G., Guy, R.J. & Russell, R.C. (1984) A study of nail bed injuries: causes, treatment and prognosis. *Journal of Hand Surgery* **9A**, 247–252.

Zook, E.G., Van Beek, A.L., Russell, R.C. & Beatty, M.E. (1980) Anatomy and physiology of the perionychium: a review of the literature and anatomic study. *Journal of Hand Surgery* **5**, 528–536.

## Chronic trauma of the nail apparatus with podiatric considerations

Dermatologists typically see the nail apparatus in static terms—and frequently give little consideration to the functional aspects of the digit. This is particularly relevant on the toenails for which it is diagnostically and therapeutically mandatory to consider the toe and the foot as a whole and their repetitive movements that may cause nail disease, or aggravate and perpetuate diseases of the nail due to some other primary cause (Dawber *et al.* 1996; Baran *et al.* 1997).

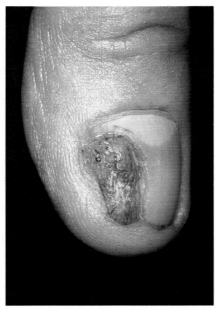

(a)

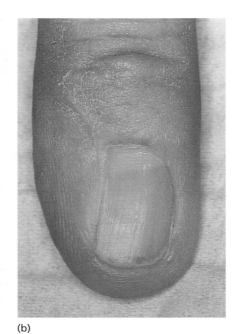

(b)

**Fig. 10.89** (a) Iatrogenic malalignment/squamous cell carcinoma involving the lateral nail bed and distal matrix. (b) Nail deviation following lateral longitudinal excision of the tumour (de Berker & Baran 1998).

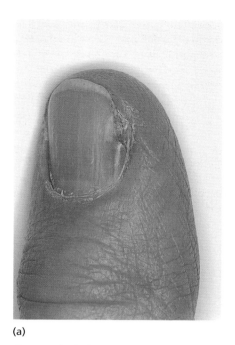
(a)

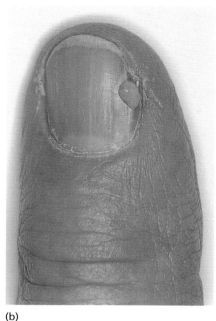
(b)

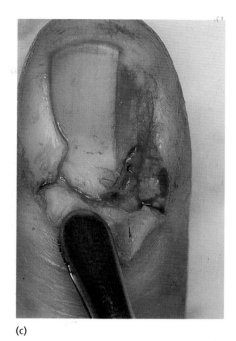
(c)

**Fig. 10.90** (a–c) Subungual thorn and its removal.

Here we mainly consider the toenails and traumatic factors of a more chronic nature—more acute trauma and occupational factors are described elsewhere.

The human foot is a complex structure, made up of 28 bones, including two sesamoid bones, and 40 joints, with 12 extrinsic and 19 intrinsic muscles. The foot has two main functions: to act as a flexible support to the lower limb; and to act as a rigid level to help propulsion during locomotion. Faults in the interrelationship of these structures can cause changes to the surface soft tissues, including nail disorders; such faults may also alter the symptoms and signs of other diseases affecting the foot and nails. The bones and principal joints of the foot are shown in Fig. 10.92; the most important joints in the foot are the ankle, the subtalar joint, the midtarsal joint and the first metatarsophalangeal joint.

## Foot function

When considering toenail problems, it is of great importance to take a full view of the whole foot: common problems often arise as a result of the dynamic functions. When possible external and locomotor precursors of nail disease are considered, the distinct differences between fingernails and toenails need to be taken into account. Being an appendage to the foot, the nail is often contained in footwear for long periods of time and may be subjected to the forces generated during normal movement. Detective work is often needed to highlight causative factors of toenail pathology (Gibbs 1985; Gibbs & Boxer 1989; Wernick & Gibbs et al. 1997). These causes include:

1 Foot function.
2 Foot shape.
3 Footwear.
4 Occupation and other factors.

The human foot has evolved to carry out a specific function —to assist smooth and efficient locomotion. In undertaking this task the foot has developed the ability to alter its structure and its function within a single footstep. To understand this we must briefly look at the normal gait cycle (Fig. 10.92). During normal walking, the first stage (heel strike) begins when the heel comes into contact with the ground. To permit shock absorption the foot must become a flexible unit. It does this by pronation (a triplanar movement occurring mainly at the subtalar and midtarsal joints of the foot). It may be recognized by eversion of the calcaneum, lowering of the arch and slight elongation in the foot length. Subtalar joint pronation unlocks the midtarsal joint so that effectively the foot is flexible to accommodate ground reaction at heel strike. This pronation continues until the whole of the foot is flat to the floor (midstance or full foot). In order for this foot to take full body weight as the opposite foot leaves the ground, it must now become a rigid unit. Once the other limb has passed the plantigrade foot, and undergoes heel strike, the foot begins propulsion—the heel lifts, so body weight is shifted onto the forefoot and the toes. In order to stabilize the foot and balance the whole body forward, the foot becomes supinated. (This is a movement involving the subtalar and midtarsal joints whereby the calcaneum inverts, the arch is raised and the foot is shortened.) This movement effectively locks the foot into rigidity allowing a stable platform for propulsion.

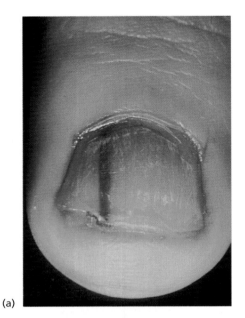

(a)

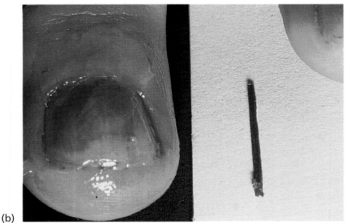

(b)

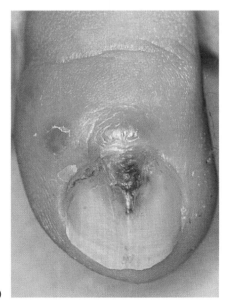

(c)

**Fig. 10.91** (a,b) Subungual thorn mimicking longitudinal melanonychia. (Courtesy of N. Goldfarb, USA.) (c) Sea urchin granuloma involving the proximal nail area (Haneke *et al.* 1996).

Many abnormal foot functions upset this sequence of supination–pronation–resupination. In terms of toenail pathology, these primarily occur around the propulsive phase of the gait cycle. If for any reason the foot has been unable to supinate adequately, there may not be adequate rigidity and propulsion occurs on a 'flexible' foot. So major forces may be dissipated through the forefoot. When repeated many thousands of times a day, this can have adverse effects on the digital area, especially in relation to footwear. If a foot is pronating excessively on propulsion, the foot will elongate (as part pronation) so the distal area will be subject to trauma if the footwear is inadequate in length. Control of the excessive pronation may be obtained by way of prescribed orthoses in footwear.

### Foot shape

Foot shape is also of major importance when considering initiation of toenail disease. Foot shape varies greatly and it is important to remember that foot shape changes with age and the effects of disease. A good example is hallux valgus (Fig. 10.93). At a young age all that may be apparent is slight first metatarsal head enlargement, but within a few years one sees the gradual deviation of the hallux laterally, often under-riding the 2nd toe and forcing it into the upper of a shoe. Such changes in foot shape inevitably affect foot and nail function. Commonly, medial rotation of the toe accompanied by its abduction towards the 2nd toe causes the flesh around the nail edge to roll over the nail plate—a precursor of ingrowing toe nails.

Hallux rigidus is a common condition in which there is a reduction in the normal range of motion at the 1st metatarsophalangeal joint (Fig. 10.94). It is characterized by enlargement of the metatarsal head and general stiffening of the joint; motion is obtained at the nearest functional joint—the interphalangeal joint of the hallux. Over time, this leads to a fixed dorsiflexed distal phalanx; the nail often protrudes dorsally and is open to trauma from footwear and 'stubbing'.

Problems with the lesser digits can also adversely affect the nail apparatus; these may be congenital or acquired. Commonly seen is the foot with the 2nd toe slightly longer than the 1st (Fig. 10.95). This can lead to the longer toe suffering increased trauma from the end of a shoe or stubbing and secondary onychomycosis. Longer toes may suffer trauma in the shoe leading to subungual haematoma and consequent long-term changes in the nail structure. Other types of digital deformities may also predispose to pathology of the nail. Neurological disturbances within the lower limb as a result of diabetes, paresis or other disorders can lead to changes in muscular tone within the leg. Spasticity or atrophy may lead to imbalances between dorsiflexors or plantarflexors of the foot which, in turn, result in digital deformities and nail distortion; the latter will vary in relation to the specific paralysis or orthopaedic change.

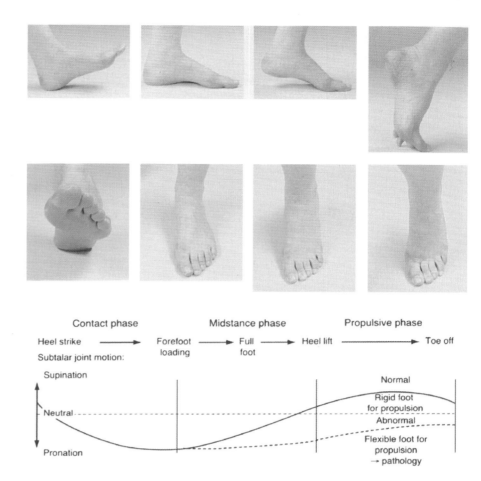

**Fig. 10.92** The normal position of the foot during the normal gait cycle.

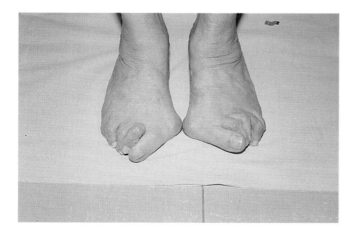

**Fig. 10.93** Hallux abductovalgus—note severe 'crowding' of toes and associated nails.

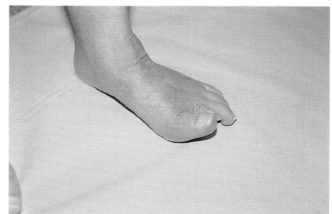

**Fig. 10.94** Hallux rigidus with associated flat foot (pes planus)—the hallux nail ('cock-up' nail) is evidently prone to traumatic influences.

## Footwear (Fig. 10.96)

Footwear is most often overlooked as an aetiological or contributory factor in nail disease (Almeyda 1973; Gibbs 1985; Jackson 1990; Balkin 1993). Patients often state that their shoes feel comfortable: 'it's just my toenail that hurts when I wear them'. Nail pathology from shoes can be due to many factors:
- Poor fitting of footwear.
- Inadequate footwear design or construction.
- Excessive wear to shoes.

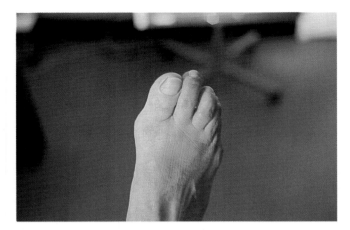

**Fig. 10.95** Longer 2nd toe—this is liable to nail damage.

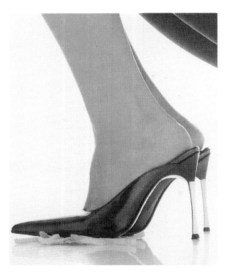

**Fig. 10.96** Very high heels with narrow pointed toe area. These magnificent shoes must not be 'overworn' or toe and toenail problems will accrue!

When looking at shoe fitting, areas of prime importance are:
• Heel height—generally if heels are too high, the foot is forced forward into the toe box with every step, traumatizing the anterior part of the foot, especially around the nail apparatus and apices. The higher the heel, the more damage is likely to occur. It has been the experience of the authors that heel heights greater than 30–35 mm can yield unwanted effects.
• Lack of a suitable fastening—a foot in a shoe without adequate fastening suffers in that the foot freely moves in the shoe and inevitably (as with high heels) it tends to slip forward into the toe box region of the shoe, traumatizing the distal aspect. Laces are, by far, the best method of fastening in a shoe and the higher the laces come up from the front of the shoe the more restraint and support is given to the foot. With patients who, due to arthritic fingers or spine, cannot tie laces, velcro straps make a reasonable substitute.
• Poor toe box design—in order to restrict rubbing and other trauma to the forefoot and nails, a good toe box is a vital feature. Adequate depth and width ensure that no excess pressure

is placed on the digital areas; together with a suitable fastening, this ensures that the foot stays well back from the tip of the shoe and into the heel. In modern shoes, manufacturers still produce types with inadequate width and depth in the toe box area. One can often see the effects of this when toe outlines are visible from the outside of the shoe. When looking at toenail problems it is wise to feel inside the upper of the shoe; one may feel a dent or tear in the inner lining of the shoe corresponding to the affected digit. Other clues can be given by the nail itself. A nail with unusual pigmentation may have acquired this from rubbing on the leather of new shoes. More commonly though, a single toenail with a very 'polished' sheen to it can be the result of continuous rubbing on the soft lining of an upper of a shoe.
• Seams which run over the toe box region of the shoe to give an 'aesthetic touch' can be a cause of problems. Inside the shoe the stitching producing the seam may be readily felt in the shoe upper, impinging on the toe area.
• Shoes which are too long or without a fastening can lead to increased nail trauma as the toes become clawed to maintain ground contact and increase stability. Whether poor fitting shoes are a direct cause of digital deformity continues to be debated.

Specially made shoes for specific foot-cum-toe disorders may be invaluable. For example, the use of half shoes in conjunction with standard diabetic foot care substantially improves outpatient treatment of neuropathic foot/toe ulcers and may be of great help in painful periungual changes.

One can summarize many of these biomechanical factors that induce nail changes briefly (Wernick & Gibbs 1997):
1 *Hallux valgus*—the hallux is shifted and rotated toward the second toe:
   (a) Hypertrophic nail may occur caused by abnormal pressure of the distal nail of the hallux against the shoe.
   (b) Onychocryptosis may develop due to the lateral nail margin of the hallux being pushed against the 2nd toe because of the abducted hallux.
   (c) Subungual haematoma occurs due to the shoe's pressure on the great toe, which overlaps the adjacent toe. Persistent pressure may eventually cause subungual exostosis. Hypertrophic nail usually accompanies or follows haematoma.
2 *Hallux rigidus*—motion is greatly reduced at the 1st metatarsal phalangeal joint, giving excessive motion at the interphalangeal joint of the distal phalanx:
   (a) Hypertrophic nail plate and subungual hyperkeratosis may result from the distal phalanx and nail plate contacting the dorsal and distal surface of the toe box giving recurrent trauma.
   (b) Subungual haematoma and exostosis.
3 *Hammer toes*—the muscles that control the digits are shortened, resulting in a hammer shape of the toes. Subungual hyperkeratosis and hypertrophic lesser nail plate may occur due to the distal phalanx applying pressure to the sole of the shoe.
4 *Overlapping and underlapping toes* result in toes resting on top of or below one another. Hypertrophic nail plate and subungual haematoma occurs from pressure on the nail plate

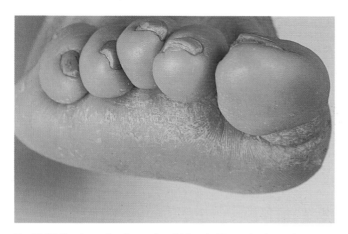

**Fig. 10.97** Hyperkeratotic nails, associated high-arched foot and early stage hammer toes.

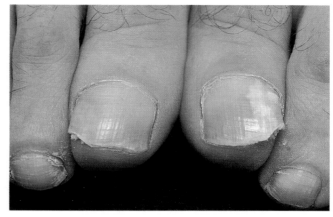

**Fig. 10.98** Primary onycholysis of great toenail 'colonized' by *Scopulariopsis brevicaulis* 'mound growth'.

directly from the toe above or, in the case of any overlapping toe, pressure from the toe box of the shoe.

5 *Rotated toe*—the 5th toe rotates such that the individual walks on the lateral part of the nail plate. Onychoclavus—pressure from the shoe continues to traumatize the nail bed, resulting in hypertrophy and eventual heloma development frequently found in the nail groove. Note: may be associated with hallux valgus.

6 *Shoe-induced change*—the shoe directly causes altered growth of toenails. Onychogryphosis is common; pressure from the shoe encourages abnormal growth of toenails such as tennis toe and pincer nails.

In terms of the changes in toenails potentially due to trauma one can conveniently consider various physical signs seen by the clinician and relate these to factors that may produce them, in contrast to the biomechanical descriptions described above. It is important always to remember that active sports participants (Mortimer & Dawber 1985; Haneke *et al.* 1999) and those with orthopaedic and rheumatological disorders are especially at risk:

1 *Hyperkeratotic nails* (Fig. 10.97). Faults in gait cycle, tight shoe toe box, osteoarthritis; Koebner phenomenon (friction and pressure) in psoriasis (Gibbs & Boxer 1989).

2 *Ingrowing toenail* (*onychocryptosis*, page 494). Broad, short great toenail; men more frequently than women; over-tight footwear.

3 *Primary onycholysis of great toenail* (Fig. 10.98) (Chapter 2). Pressure from adjacent toe—overlapping or cramped toes in narrow toe box (Baran & Badillet 1982).

4 *Onychomycosis* (Fig. 10.99). On the great toenail some degree of trauma in most cases may give a portal of entry for dermatophytes and yeasts (Haneke *et al.* 1999).

5 *Onychogryphosis* (*ram's horn deformity*, Chapter 2). The deformity and its shape is greater with associated hallux abductovalgus.

6 *Acquired pincer and trumpet nails* (page 497). This deformity may cause ingrowing nail and inflammatory hypertrophy

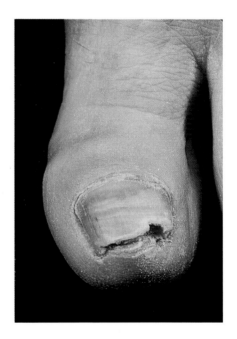

**Fig. 10.99** Hallux rigidus—'raised' nail infected by dermatophyte.

of the lateral nail wall. The pincer nail shape is 'magnified' by natural lateral pressures from adjacent toes and footwear.

7 *Chronic subungual haemorrhage*. Common and often painless in 'stamina' athletes, for example long distance runners (Fig. 10.100). Often leads to subsequent nail shedding or onychomadesis.

8 *Multiple transverse ridges, depressions or white lines* (Baran 1995). More common in the longest toes and nails that are not cut short enough. Hammer toes may generate this sign and also great toenails with hallux rigidus and 'cock-up' toe.

9 *Koilonychia* (Chapter 6). Often seen in rickshaw boys wearing flimsy sandals or with bare feet (Bentley-Phillips & Bayles 1971).

10 *Digital subungual corn* (*heloma; clavus*); (Chapter 3). May be associated with underlying traumatic periosteal thickening.

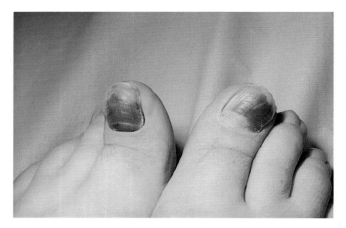

**Fig. 10.100** Bilateral (painless) subungual haemorrhage—common in 'stamina athletes'.

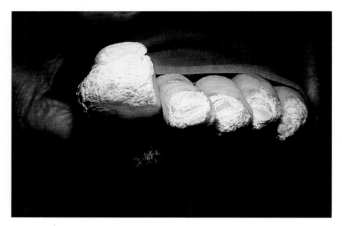

**Fig. 10.102** Psoriasis. Distal subungual thickening—feet have high arches and early hammer toes—?Koebner phenomenon.

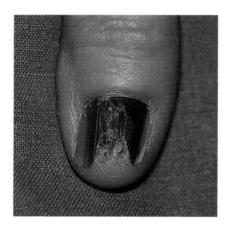

**Fig. 10.101** Malignant melanoma—initially started with acute injury—?cause, ?effect.

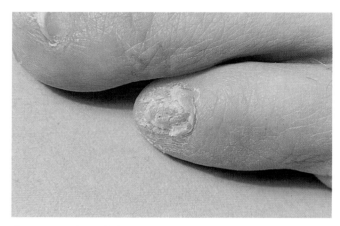

**Fig. 10.103** Viral wart of 5th toenail—the digit is rotated outwards and subject to friction damage and consequent viral colonization.

*End corn* on the tips of toes may distort the nail—more common on hammer toes.

**11** *Longitudinal melanonychia* (Chapter 11). May be due to friction on adjacent footwear; 5th toe involvement may be postinflammatory due to lateral pressure from footwear on lateral rotated toes (Baran 1987).

**12** *Raised, thickened or 'tented' nails* (Chapter 2). May be associated with bony thickening or exostosis; often in footballers or ballet dancers.

Some diseases that are modified by trauma include:

**1** *Congenital malalignment* (page 501). The lateral deviation, thickening and periungual inflammation typically begin when crawling and walking in footwear first occur.

**2** *Melanoma of nail apparatus* (Chapter 11). 50% of cases give a history of initial trauma (Fig. 10.101)—?cause or effect (O'Toole *et al.* 1995).

**3** *Pachyonychia congenita* (Chapter 9). On toenails the changes are made more prominent by friction and pressure.

**4** *Psoriasis* (Chapter 5). Trauma may cause nail shedding in pustular forms: pressure and friction (Fig. 10.102) may give thickening (?Koebner phenomenon). Note: podiatry treatment may be as important as pharmacokinetic treatments!

**5** *Lichen planus* (Chapter 5). Nail apparatus friction and pressure may give erosions.

**6** *Epidermolysis bullosa* (Chapters 3 & 9). All (?) the physical signs in the nail apparatus are mechanobullous (traumatic) except in epidemolysis bullosa acquisita (immunobullous mechanism).

**7** *Subungual and periungual viral warts.* Often occur at sites of minor damage due to friction and pressure (Fig. 10.103).

## References

Almeyda, J. (1973) Platform nails. *British Medical Journal* **1**, 176–177.

Balkin, S.W. (1993) What do women want: comfy shoes—sometimes. *Journal of the American Medical Association* **269**, 215.

Baran, R. (1987) Frictional longitudinal melanonychia. *Dermatologica* **174**, 280–284.

Baran, R. (1995) Transverse leuconychia of toenails due to repeated microtrauma. *British Journal of Dermatology* **133**, 267–269.

Baran, R. & Badillet, G. (1982) Primary onycholysis of the big toenail. *British Journal of Dermatology* 106, 529–534.

Baran, R., Dawber, R.P.R., Tosti, A. & Haneke, E. (1997) Traumatic disorders of the nail. In: *Text Atlas of Nail Disorders*, pp. 169–198. Martin Dunitz, London.

Bentley-Phillips, B. & Bayles, M.A.H. (1971) Occupational koilonychia of the toenails. *British Journal of Dermatology* 85, 140–144.

Dawber, R.P.R., Bristow, I. & Mooney, J. (eds) (1996) The foot. In: *Problems in Podiatry and Dermatology*, pp. 1–35. Martin Dunitz, London.

Gibbs, R.C. (1985) Toenail disease secondary to poorly fitting shoes or abnormal biomechanics. *Cutis* 36, 309–400.

Gibbs, R.C. & Boxer, M.C. (1989) Abnormal biomechanics of feet and their cause of hyperkeratoses. *Journal of the American Academy of Dermatology* 6, 1061–1069.

Haneke, E., Burzykowski, T. & Meuleners, L. (1999) The relationship between sport and mycotic feet. *Journal of European Academy of Dermatology and Venereology* 12 (Suppl. 2), S217–S218.

Jackson, R. (1990) The Chinese foot-binding syndrome. *International Journal of Dermatology* 29, 322.

Mortimer, P.S. & Dawber, R.P.R. (1985) Trauma to the nail unit including sports injuries. *Dermatologic Clinics* 3, 415–420.

O'Toole, E.A., Stephens, R. & Young, M.M. (1995) Subungual melanoma: a relation to direct injury? *Journal of the American Academy of Dermatology* 33, 525–528.

Wernick, J. & Gibbs, R.C. (1997) Pedal biomechanics and toenail disease. In: *Nails: Therapy, Diagnosis, Surgery* (eds R.K. Scher & C.R. Daniel), pp. 301–316, 2nd edn. W.B. Saunders, Philadelphia.

## Miscellaneous nail dystrophies

### Narrowing of the nail

This method has evolved from knowledge obtained over many years using the lateral longitudinal biopsy technique.

Longitudinal matrix narrowing has been found to be useful for the treatment of:
1 Ingrowing toenail.
2 Longitudinal melanonychia involving the lateral third of the nail plate.
3 Longitudinal splitting of the nail at the lateral aspect.
4 Tumours located at the lateral aspect.
5 Racquet thumb.

The so-called wedge excision as depicted in most textbooks of minor surgery is obviously not suited for narrowing the nail: it involves removal of the lateral nail fold (Bennett 1976) and has to include the lateral matrix horns; these, however, are left in most instances.

### Reference

Bennett, R.G. (1976) Technique of biopsy of nails. *Journal of Dermatologic Surgery and Oncology* 2, 325.

### Congenital and/or hereditary nail disorders

Aplastic or dysplastic lesions, produced by restricting amniotic bands, are not amenable to surgery. Tight syndactyly of the Apert type, where the treatment is that of the syndactyly, is beyond the scope of this section.

#### Congenital absence of the nail

Koshima *et al.* (1988) performed free vascularized nail graft utilizing microneurovascular techniques in congenital absence of fingernail.

#### Pachyonychia congenita

Whether the primary site of the pathological process is located in the nail bed (Forsling *et al.* 1973; Shelley 1974), the hyponychium (Kelly & Pinkus 1958) or the matrix (Thomsen *et al.* 1982) is still debatable. A few patients may require excision of the undersurface of the proximal nail fold and the entire subungual tissues in order to achieve permanent total removal of the nail. Full thickness grafting (Cosman *et al.* 1964) or split skin grafting (White & Noon 1977) achieves good results. According to Thomsen *et al.* (1982) the most effective and rapidly performed, and the most acceptable method, lies in vigorous curettage and electrofulguration of the matrix and nail bed. $CO_2$ has been suggested (page 451). Healing proceeds by secondary intention. Phenol cautery may be a useful alternative and can easily be repeated.

#### Racquet thumbs (Fig. 10.104)

A short, broad terminal phalanx of the thumb results in a short and wide nail plate that usually lacks lateral nail folds. The aesthetic appearance may be improved by narrowing the nail plate and creating lateral nail folds.

Lateral–longitudinal nail biopsies are performed on both sides of the thumbnail. The lateral soft aspects of the distal phalanx are dissected from the bone, and back stitches are used to create lateral nail folds. The needle is run into the lateral aspect about 2–3 mm volar to the plane of the nail bed–bone interface, through the nail bed and plate, and back again through the lateral thumb skin, which upon knotting will be elevated, thus forming a lateral nail fold. Nail groove epithelium develops by secondary intention (Haneke 1985).

#### Congenital malalignment of the big toenail
(Baran *et al.* 1979)

See page 502.

### References

Cosman, B., Sysmonds, F.C. & Crikelair, G.F. (1964) Plastic surgery in

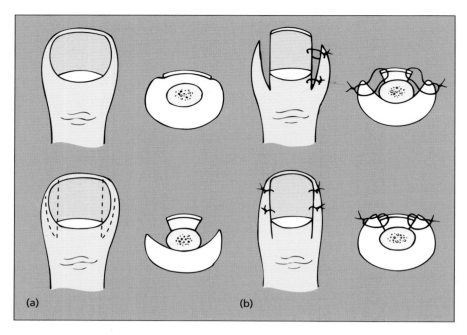

(a)

(b)

**Fig. 10.104** Surgical treatment of racquet thumb. (From Haneke 1985 with permission.)

pachyonychia congenita and other dyskeratoses. *Plastic and Reconstructive Surgery* **33**, 226.

Forsling, B., Nylen, B., Swanbeck, G. *et al.* (1973) Pachyonychia congenita, a histologic and microradiographic study. *Acta Dermato-Venereologica* **53**, 211.

Haneke, E. (1985) Behandlung einiger Nagelfehlbildungen. In: *Fehlbildungen-Navi-Melanome* (eds H.H. Wolff & Schmeller), pp. 71–77. Springer, Berlin.

Kelly, E.W. & Pinkus, H.N. (1958) Report of a case of pachyonychia congenita. *Archives of Dermatology* **77**, 724.

Koshima, I., Soeda, S., Takase, T. *et al.* (1988) Free vascularized nail grafts. *Journal of Hand Surgery* **13A**, 29–32.

Shelley, W.B. (ed.) (1974) Pachyonychia congenita. In: *Consultations in Dermatology*, Vol. II, p. 136. W.B. Saunders, Philadelphia.

Thomsen, R.J., Zuehlke, R.L. & Beckman, B.L. (1982) Pachyonychia congenita. Surgical management of the nail changes. *Journal of Dermatologic Surgery and Oncology* **8**, 24.

White, R.R. & Noon, R.B. (1977) Pachyonychia congenita (Jadassohn–Lewandowki syndrome). Case report. *Plastic and Reconstructive Surgery* **59**, 855.

## Ingrowing toenails

Ingrowing toenail is a common, painful condition, multifactorial in its aetiology, and most frequently seen in young adults. The main factors producing the condition are hereditary, or constitutional, imbalance between the width of the nail plate and that of the nail bed (Haneke 1984, 1986), or overcurvature of the nail plate (Haneke 1992b). Additional factors may be medial rotation of the toe, thinner nails and thicker nail folds (Langford *et al.* 1989). Sweating, convex cutting of the nail, and pointed and/or high-heeled shoes are only participating factors. This is confirmed by the successful results of surgery,

which corrects the discrepancy between the broad nail plate and narrow nail bed, and by the high recurrence rate found with conservative treatment. Disturbed carbohydrate metabolism and constitutional features are common to a group of patients with ingrowing toenails: these include youth with tall stature, hyperhidrosis of hands and feet, the 'unguis incarnatus syndrome' (Steigleder & Stober-Münster 1977); they require special management (Reszler & Mari 1981). There are five major types of ingrowing toenails (Baran 1987):

1 Subcutaneous ingrowing toenail.
2 Hypertrophy of the lateral nail fold.
3 Inward distortion of the nail.
4 Distal nail embedding.
5 Ingrowing toenail in infancy.

### Subcutaneous ingrowing nail (juvenile ingrowing nail)

An ingrowing toenail is created by impingement of the nail plate into the dermal tissue of the lateral nail fold.

It often appears as a result of improper trimming of the nail. A lacerating spicule of the nail margin grows into the soft tissue surrounding the side of the nail, acts as a foreign body and produces irritation and inflammation with pain from perforation of the nail groove epithelium.

In mild cases, separating the offending nail edge from the adjacent soft tissue with a wisp of absorbent cotton coated with collodion gives immediate relief of pain (Fig. 10.105). The collodion which fixes the cotton in place permits bathing (Ilfeld 1991). Treatment for the early stage is conservative.

The foot is soaked daily in lukewarm water with povidone iodine soap or with potassium permanganate (1 : 10 000 dilution).

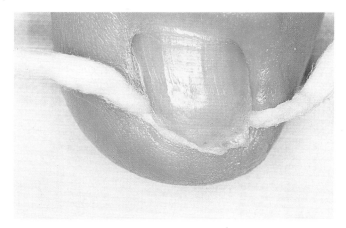

**Fig. 10.105** Ingrowing toenail—separation of ingrowing nail edge from adjacent soft tissue. (Courtesy of G. Cannata, Italy.)

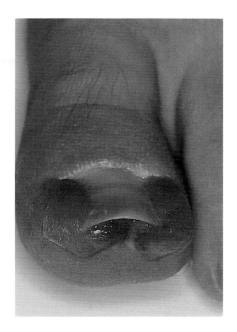

**Fig. 10.106** Ingrowing toenail—excessive bilateral growth of granulation tissue.

To increase pliability of the nail, its centre may be ground down until it is quite thin and the pink nail bed shines through (Maeda *et al.* 1990). Notching a 'V' in the end of the nail may also relieve the pressure at the corners. In fact it is essential to search for and to remove the lateral spike acting as a foreign body under local anaesthesia. Subsequently, a small piece of povidone iodine gauze is forced under the same edge, so that as the nail grows forwards, its lateral margin will not impinge on the soft tissue of the lateral nail fold.

Always cut the nails square, then smooth away sharp corners with an emery board. Conservative management requires a high degree of compliance. Therefore recurrences are frequent because of the mismatch between nail plate width and nail bed width.

### Granulation stage (Fig. 10.106)

The nail groove may be involved along its entire length developing excess granulation tissue. It becomes filled with 'proud flesh' extending under the nail and involving a portion of the nail bed. This together with the swollen lateral nail fold, overlaps the nail plate and since infection is almost always present, pus may exude from the nail groove.

Occasionally steroids covered by a 'Blenderm' tape may control this condition if infection is not prevailing but when the large new mass is covered with surface epithelium, it will require curettage under local anaesthesia. It will enable the 'fish hook' part of the nail to be removed and the acute inflammation of the lateral nail fold to be treated. This may be completed by antibiotic and sublesional injection of steroid suspension. Simple avulsion of the big toenail in the initial management (Murray & Bedi 1975) has so high a recurrence rate that it should not be carried out (Palmer & Jones 1979; Haneke 1986). Moreover, the pulp of the hallux is pushed dorsally during weight bearing and the distal nail groove is obliterated by the development of a distal nail fold (Fig. 10.107) (Fowler

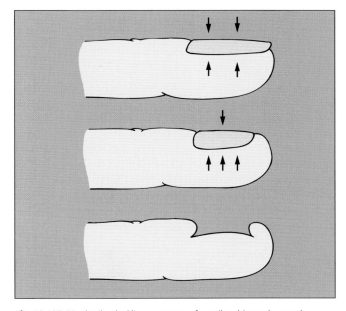

**Fig. 10.107** Distal nail embedding—may occur after nail avulsion and regrowth. (Adapted from Fowler 1958.)

1958). When the newly formed nail advances it becomes embedded in the unsupported pulp which has pressed round the plate distally.

Despite these treatments recurrences are still very frequent and a definitive procedure should usually be undertaken.

### Definitive procedure

Since the nail plate seems too wide for its underlying bed, the logical treatment is aimed at correcting this disparity by the

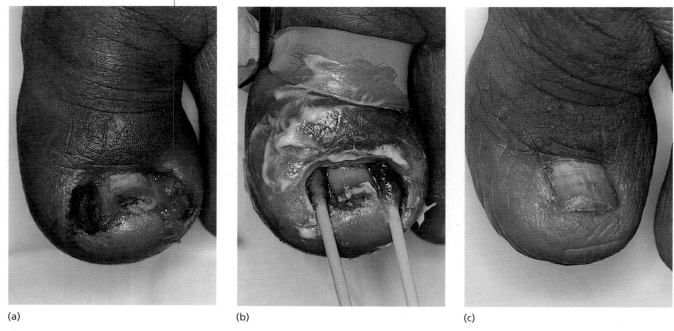

(a)                                (b)                               (c)

**Fig. 10.108** Lateral nail plate excision for recalcitrant ingrowing nail. (a) Before treatment. (b) During phenolic treatment. (c) Late stage many months after healing.

selective matrix excision which permanently narrows the nail. A lateral nail strip is freed from the proximal nail fold, nail bed and matrix with a Freer septum elevator, then cut longitudinally and extracted. This partial nail avulsion may be immediately followed by phenol cauterization—an easy and efficient technique which can be used even when the affected region presents with infection (Dagnall 1976a) (Fig. 10.108).

It is essential to work on a bloodless field, blood inactivating phenol. The haemostasis is accomplished with a tourniquet and the blood carefully cleaned from the space under the proximal nail fold using sterile gauze. The surrounding skin is protected with petroleum jelly and the freshly made solution of liquefied phenol (88%) has to be rubbed vigorously for 3 min in order to achieve complete eradication of the matrix horn epithelium. The cautery is then neutralized with 70% alcohol. Since the nail plate is elevated slightly when the lateral nail strip is cut, the liquefied phenol usually seeps 1–2 mm under the adjacent nail plate, causing lateral onycholysis. This may be partly prevented by rubbing the phenol into the matrix in a rotating motion, moving outward at the nail margin and matrix (Haneke 1984, 1992a).

Postoperative pain is minimal since phenol has a considerable local anaesthetic action. It is also antiseptic. The matrix epithelium is sloughed off and usually exhibits slight oozing for 2–4 weeks. Daily foot baths with povidone-iodine soap will avoid infection and accelerate healing.

The major drawbacks of this procedure are twofold: (a) the length of time required for healing; (b) the prolonged drainage caused by the chemical burn induced by the caustic properties of phenol. Rinaldi *et al.* (1982) have demonstrated that infection may also be a significant cause of the exudation. Poor home care may even be responsible for periostitis (Gilles *et al.* 1986), which may therefore result indirectly from phenol use as well as directly if the procedure is preceded by matricial curettage for example. Using 10% sodium hydroxide (Brown (1981) instead of phenol is an alternative but does not prevent the aforementioned untoward events.

For more skilful surgeons, definitive cure can be obtained by selective lateral matrix excision, which may be performed at the same time or 1 month after the lateral strip of nail has been removed (Fig. 10.109). The remaining granulation tissue is

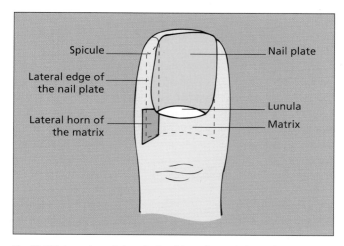

**Fig. 10.109** Ingrowing nail—lateral nail excision and removal of matrix horn.

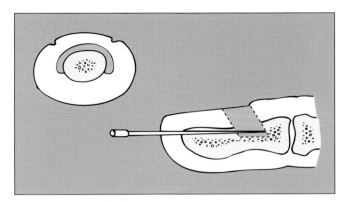

**Fig. 10.110** The number 1 needle is inserted as shown to delineate the limits of the nail matrix. (After R.T. Austin, UK.)

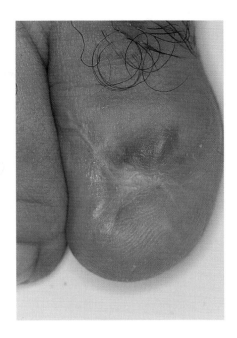

**Fig. 10.111** Terminal Syme operation: a mutilating surgery.

gently curetted, and if infection is severe, oral antibiotic is given and continued for a short time postoperatively. The proximal nail fold is incised obliquely in an angle of about 110 degrees. The incision is opened with fine hooks exhibiting the lateral matrix horn which has to be carefully dissected and excised from the base of the distal phalanx (Haneke 1992a). A no. 1 needle is inserted along the floor of the lateral nail groove until it is arrested by the terminal phalanx (Fig. 10.110). This will serve as a marker for the limits of the matrix (Austin 1970).

The authors do not recommend total ablation of the matrix and nail bed resulting in permanent eradication of the nail organ, which has been advocated in the past (Quenu 1887; Zadik 1950) despite the high rate of recurrence (Murray & Bedi 1975). This procedure is carried out 1 month after nail ablation—the proximal nail fold is reflected after lateral incision exposing the matrix epithelium. Using Austin's technique to determine the most proximo-lateral limits of the matrix, a rectangular block of tissue is excised down to the periosteum, with special attention to the insertion of the extensor tendon beneath the matrix. The block of tissue extends distally, just beyond the edge of the lunular area, proximally almost as far as the joint and laterally until the fatty tissue of the pulp is reached. The proximal nail fold is then replaced and the incisions are closed with steri-strips.

The central flap should be sutured to the remaining distal nail bed only if this can be achieved without tension on the flap. Murray (1979) prefers in many cases to leave the flap free and dress the area with paraffin gauze. If the lateral grooves are deep, the lateral nail folds are excised and the skin edges are sutured to the edges of the nail bed.

### The terminal Syme operation

This procedure is still more radical (Thompson & Terwilliger 1951). It entails the removal of matrix and nail bed with amputation of the distal half of the terminal bone. The ridged skin

of the pulp is then pulled dorsally and sutured over the defect of the former matrix. This operation produces a shortened, bulbous big toe (Murray 1979). This is absolutely unacceptable, both functionally and cosmetically (Fig. 10.111).

These operations are totally inadequate mutilating surgery which only demonstrate the ignorance of surgeons to their patients' needs and complete lack of knowledge of the nail apparatus.

### Hypertrophic lateral nail fold (Fig. 10.112a)

Hypertrophic lateral nail fold usually accompanies longstanding ingrowing nails. The nail, generally, looks normal and the soft tissue appears to be at fault when the lip of the lateral nail fold overgrows the nail plate. Inflammation occurs deep beneath the hypertrophied tissue. Therefore, the treatment consists of narrowing the nail plate by phenol cauterization of the lateral nail horn of the matrix. If the hypertrophic tissue does not regress after 2 months, treatment of the soft tissue is then advised. The authors favour an elliptical wedge of tissue taken from the lateral wall of the toe and its distolateral portion (Fig. 10.112b). This pulls the lateral nail fold away from the offending lateral nail edge.

If lateral nail fold hypertrophy is pronounced its removal has been suggested. In Bose's technique (1971) (Fig. 10.112c) the point of a no. 11 blade is inserted under the lateral nail fold halfway along the nail. Then the nail fold is transfixed, so that the point of the blade emerges at a distance of 5–7 mm from the nail fold. The blade is advanced distally in a straight line, cutting the fold, which exposes the distal half of the side of the nail. This cut fold is steadied with forceps: the direction of the blade is reversed, and the proximal part of the fold is cut in such

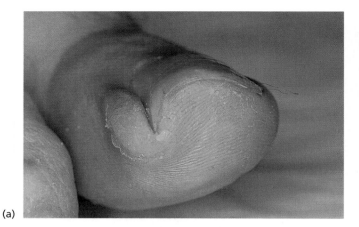

(a)

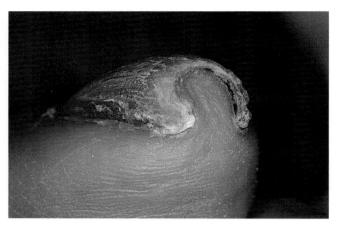

**Fig. 10.113** Pincer nail deformity.

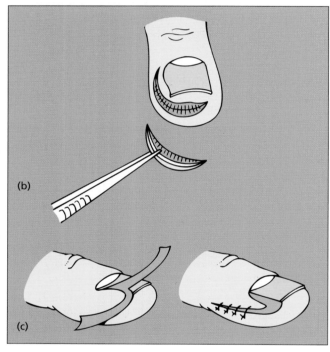

(b)

(c)

**Fig. 10.112** (a) Hypertrophic lateral nail fold. (b) An elliptical wedge of tissue is removed to relieve pressure on the lateral nail fold. (c) A longitudinal wedge, the base of which is at the distal end of the lateral nail fold, is removed and the resultant flap is sutured to the side of the tip of the toe.

### Inward distortion of the nail plate (transverse overcurvature, pincer nail, trumpet nail, unguis constringens, omega nail) (Fig. 10.113)

Pincer nail is a dystrophy characterized by transverse overcurvature that increases along the longitudinal axis of the nail and reaches its greatest extent at the distal part, leading to trumpet nails (Baran 1974) (Fig. 10.114). The edges constrict the nail bed tissue and dig into the lateral grooves. Although pain is not severe in most cases, it may sometimes be excruciating. In patients whose nail plate is involved only at the lateral edge, pain will be felt in the lateral nail groove, simulating an ingrowing toenail. In overcurvature affecting the entire nail, the patients have pain along the lateral nail grooves as well, but on occasion they may develop pain specifically under the midpoint of the distal nail edge, dorsal to the distal phalangeal tuft (Douglas & Krull 1981).

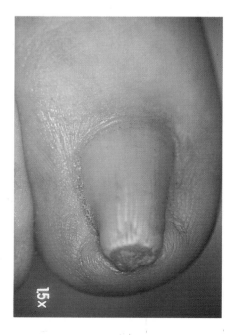

**Fig. 10.114** Trumpet nail.

a way that the slices of tissue so removed thin out gradually. Brisk arterial haemorrhage is arrested with electrocautery. The wound is covered with petroleum jelly gauze and the dressing is changed daily until the wound heels by granulation in approximately 3–4 weeks.

The authors prefer Tweedie and Ranger's procedure (1985) which consists of making a transposition flap of the nail wall. The technique starts as in the previous one but the proximal part of the lateral nail fold is not cut. The flap which is created is then transposed inferiorly and sutured in place with 4/0 nylon sutures. The excess of tissue is cut away.

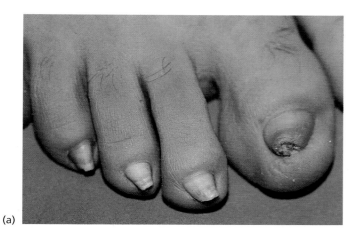

(a)

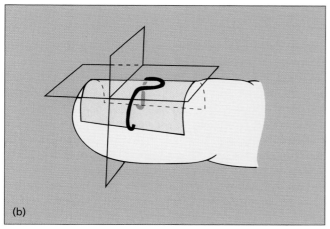

(b)

**Fig. 10.115** (a) Pincer nail deformity with symmetrical involvement of several toes. (b) 'Brace' method to correct the overcurvature of pincer nail.

Two varieties of overcurvature can be distinguished (Haneke 1992b):

1 Asymmetrical involvement of usually only the halluces. The major causes are foot deformities and osteoarthritis.

2 Symmetrical involvement of several toes, usually with a lateral deviation of the long axis of the hallux nails and medial deviation of the lesser toenails (Fig. 10.115a). This is probably genetically determined.

The pincer-nail syndrome (Sorg *et al.* 1989) includes gryphosis of fingernails and toenails in combination with acroosteolytic shortening of the end-phalanx and destructive arthrosis of the terminal joints of the digits. Since deformation of the nail is sometimes accompanied by marked pain, definitive cure may be necessary.

Particularly in the genetic form, X-ray films usually show a wider base of the terminal phalanx, often even exhibiting lateral osteophytes. Hyperostosis is also frequently seen on the dorsal tuft of the terminal phalanx, due to traction from heaped-up nail bed which is firmly attached to the bone by collagen fibres (Haneke 1992b).

Pathogenesis of pincer nail is described in Chapter 2. Acquired pincer nails may be due to a number of different dermatoses of which psoriasis is the most frequent. Tumour of the nail apparatus such as exostosis or implantation cyst (Baran & Broutart 1988) may lead to pincer nails, a condition reversible after treatment of the cause.

Tinea ungium due to *Trichophyton rubrum*, affecting equally the great toe nail and thumb nail, has been responsible for pincer nails (Higashi 1990), which gradually return to normal after systemic antifungal treatment.

Pincer nail deformity may be produced after placement of an arteriovenous fistula (AVF) in the foream (Hwang *et al.* 1999). The nail changes are then restricted to the index and little fingers. This potential and longlasting adverse effect of circulatory disturbance and/or venous hypertension from AVF for haemodialysis is relatively common and should be recognized as a specific sign of circulatory disturbance caused by the AVF.

Pincer nails have been reported after some β-blockers such as practolol and acebutolol (Greiner *et al.* 1998). Transverse overcurvature of the nails is reversible after discontinuation of the drug.

Pronounced pincer nails have developed in association with a metastasizing adenocarcinoma of the sigmoid colon. They have been considered as a marker of gastrointestinal malignancy (Jemec & Thomsen 1997).

Acquired pincer nail deformity in an infant with Kawasaki's disease affected all digits of the hands and to a lesser extent, the toes. Given the absence of pain, the nails were left undisturbed and the overcurvature spontaneously resolved as the nails grew out (Vanderhooft & Vanderhooft 1999).

But the most frequent cause of acquired pincer nails is deformity in the foot with deviation of the phalanges, probably as a result of ill-fitting shoes (Baran *et al.* 1996), and acquired pincer nails of the fingers are commonly seen in degenerative osteoarthritis of the distal interphalangeal joints.

### Conservative management

#### Clipping
Clipping down the lateral edge of the inward distorted nail plate as proximally as is comfortable may be facilitated by emollients such as 3% salicylic acid in petrolatum. This is applied to the nail edge for 2–3 days before the procedure is undertaken.

#### Grooving
For the treatment of early cases, grooving of the nail plate, with a burr extending forwards from the area of the lunula and terminating at the free edge, may be of some help. A central single groove or a series of grooves running parallel to each other should be cut. The latter are cut covering the whole of the dorsal surface of the nail plate. If the nail is greatly thickened, grinding down the thickness may diminish the pressure. This

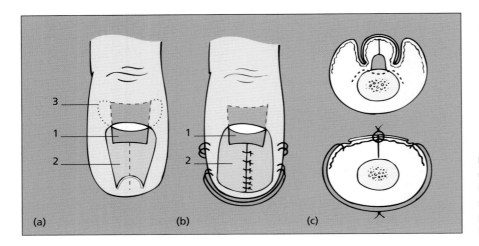

**Fig. 10.116** (a) 1, Nail plate after narrowing and removal of distal two-thirds; 2, nail bed; 3, matrix horn. Removal of lateral matrix horns, bilateral nail strip removal and flattening and spreading of remaining nail plate on previously separated nail bed (b,c). The enclosed hyperostosis is removed with a bone rongeur (c).

procedure may alleviate the pain; however it increases the overcurvature.

*Orthonyx (nail brace technique)* (Dagnall 1976b) (Fig. 10.115b)

Orthonyx is the term coined by Fraser (1967) to describe the field of mechanical correction. This method is based on maintaining tension in the nail plate. The lateral nail grooves are cleaned in order to clear the space under the sides of the nail for the wire. A brace is constructed to fit the curved plate exactly; then, at one selected point, a minute 'adjustment' (a slight bend) is made to the brace and it is fitted to the plate. The nail plate is weaker than the stainless steel wire and the nail will conform to the shape of the brace. Gradually, a series of 'adjustments' are made and almost imperceptibly the curvature decreases. The nail plate will be flattened painlessly within a period of 6 months (Farnsworth 1972). This technique has been successfully employed in overcurvature of fingernails associated with arthritis of the distal joint (R. Baran, unpublished data), but was followed by recurrence within a few weeks in other cases (E. Haneke, unpublished).

Unfortunately, pathogenesis of overcurvature explains why neither nail brace technique nor repeated nail avulsion will cure definitely the condition. Instead some patients report even that nail avulsion exacerbated their difficulties.

Under local anaesthesia, Higashi *et al.* (2000) cut off the digital lateral corners of the nail. Then transverse overcurvature is corrected with the sculptured nail, a procedure repeated at 2- or 3-month intervals with success.

### Surgical treatment

Surgery cannot remove the lateral osteophytes to restore a normal matrix shape, but we have seen good results just with phenol cautery on the matrix horns (Cannata, unpublished data), even on fingernails.

In Haneke's technique (Fig. 10.116) (Haneke 1984) the lateral matrix horns are treated as described above (for subcutaneous ingrowing toenails), then the distal two-thirds of the nail are carefully removed. A longitudinal median incision of the nail bed is carried down to the bone. While doing this, one can usually feel the dorsal traction osteophyte. The entire nail bed is dissected from the phalanx and the dorsal tuft removed with a bone rongeur. The nail bed is spread and sutured with 6-0 PDS atraumatic stitches and kept spread by using reversed tie-over sutures that pull the lateral nail folds apart. To prevent the sutures from cutting through the lateral nail folds, small rubber tubes are placed into the lateral grooves and the threads are laid over them. These stiches are left for 18–21 days to allow the nail bed to adhere in the restored form (Baran & Haneke 1987; Haneke & Baran 1991; Haneke 1992b).

*In Zook's technique, successful treatment of pincer nail involves removing the tubed nail to visualize the nail bed. The paronychium is freed from the periosteum of the distal phalanx through an incision on the tip at the distal end of the paronychium. Fine scissors are used to free the paronychium from the periosteum proximally to beyond the nail fold allowing the nail bed to flatten. A strip of dermis of adequate volume (at least 1 cm in width) is then pulled beneath the paronychium to flatten the nail bed. It is important to not only flatten the sterile matrix but also flatten the lateral portions of the germinal matrix. We have had uniformly good results with this in relief of pain and improvement of appearance (Fig. 10.117) (Brown et al. 2000).*

### Distal nail embedding (Fig. 10.107)

Particularly in the great toe a distal wall may develop after nail avulsion or nail shedding following tennis toe for example. The nail in its normal position counteracts the forces that are exerted during walking. Due to lack of counter pressure, the plantar portion of the hallux pulp becomes distorted dorsally

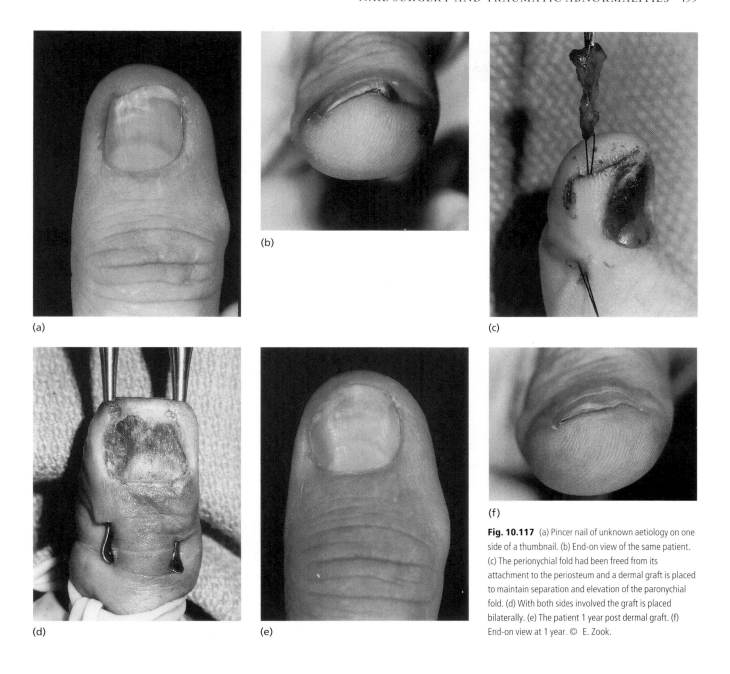

**Fig. 10.117** (a) Pincer nail of unknown aetiology on one side of a thumbnail. (b) End-on view of the same patient. (c) The perionychial fold had been freed from its attachment to the periosteum and a dermal graft is placed to maintain separation and elevation of the paronychial fold. (d) With both sides involved the graft is placed bilaterally. (e) The patient 1 year post dermal graft. (f) End-on view at 1 year. © E. Zook.

when the foot rolls up and the body weight presses on the tip of the big toe during walking. The terminal phalanx looks shorter and the distal wall interferes with the growth of the newly formed nail plate.

When the distal wall cannot be reversed by massaging back in a distal–plantar direction, the anchoring of an acrylic sculptured nail on the stump nail may enable it to overgrow the heaped up distal tissue (Fig. 10.118).

If this procedure is not effective, a crescent-shaped wedge excision becomes necessary (Fig. 10.119). A fish-mouth incision is carried parallel to the distal groove around the tip of the toe,

starting and ending 3–5 mm proximal to the end of the lateral nail fold. A second incision is then done to yield a wedge of 4–8 mm at its greatest width and has to be dissected from the bone (Howard 1893; Greco *et al.* 1973; Dubois 1974; Murray & Robb 1981). The defect is closed with 3–0 nylon, and the stitches are removed 10–14 days later.

### Ingrowing toenail in infancy (see also Chapter 3)

There are five kinds of ingrowing toenail in infancy before age 6 (Baran & Kechijian 1989).

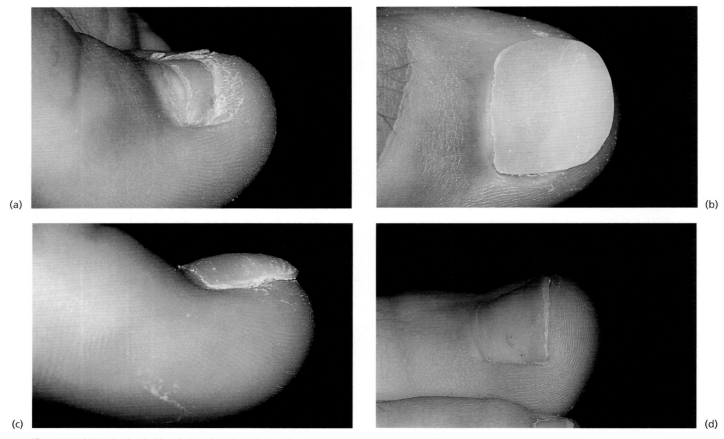

**Fig. 10.118** (a) Distal nail embedding. (b,c) Acrylic sculptured nail anchored into the embedded nail plate. (d) After cure.

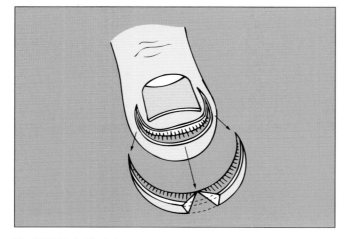

**Fig. 10.119** Dubois' technique.

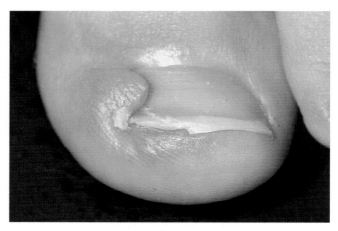

**Fig. 10.120** Congenital hypertrophic lip of the great toe. (Courtesy of J. Civatte, France.)

### *Congenital hypertrophic lip of the hallux* (Fig. 10.120)

In constrast to the hypertrophic lateral nail fold observed in adults, the congenital hypertrophic lip of the hallux disappears spontaneously after several months (Rufli *et al.* 1992) (Chapter 3).

### *Distal toenail embedding with normally directed nail* (Fig. 10.121)

Conservative management is the rule (page 497). In those rare cases where permanent improvement has not been obtained by 1 year of age, a circular soft tissue resection should be performed in an identical manner as in adults.

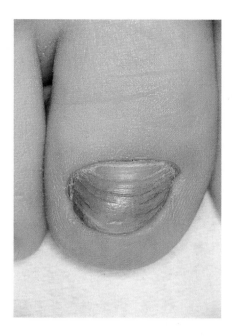

**Fig. 10.121** Distal toenail embedding with normally directed nail.

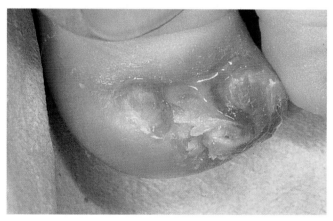

**Fig. 10.122** Distal and lateral ingrowing toenail. (Courtesy of A. Petit, France.)

### *Distolateral nail embedding* (Fig. 10.122)

### *Congenital malalignment of the big toenail* (Baran *et al.* 1979; Baran & Bureau 1983) (Fig. 10.123)

Should an operation be decided in this misrecognized condition (Chapter 3), a crescent wedge-shaped resection must be carried back proximal to and below the nail bed and nail matrix. The crescent has to be larger on the medial than on the lateral aspect. A small, triangular area is also excised at the start of the lateral incision line, thereby enabling the whole nail apparatus to be swung over the resected area so that it can be realigned and then sutured. When the nail deviation is medial instead of lateral, in contrast to the usual type, the crescent has to be larger on the lateral aspect than on the medial one, and a small triangular area is also excised at the start of the medial incision line, thereby enabling the whole nail apparatus to be swung over the resected area, in order that it can be realigned and then sutured (Baran & Bureau 1983).

### *Congenital pincer nails* (Chapman 1973)

## References

Austin, R.T. (1970) A method of excision of the germinal matrix. *Proceedings of the Royal Society of Medicine* **63**, 757–758.

Baran, R. (1974) Pincer and trumpet nails. *Archives of Dermatology* **110**, 639.

Baran, R. (1987) L'ongle incarné. *Annales de Dermatologie et de Vénéréologie* **114**, 1597–1604.

Baran, R. (1989) The treament of ingrowing toenails in infancy. *Journal of Dermatological Treatment* **1**, 55–57.

Baran, R. & Broutart, J.C. (1988) Epidermoid cyst of the thumb presenting as a pincer nail. *Journal of the American Academy of Dermatology* **19**, 143–144.

Baran, R. & Bureau, H. (1983) Congenital malalignment of the big toe-nail as a cause of ingrowing toe-nail in infancy. Pathology and treatment (a study of 30 cases). *Clinical and Experimental Dermatology* **8**, 619–623.

Baran, R. & Haneke, E. (1987) Surgery of the nail. In: *Skin Surgery* (eds E. Epstein & E. Epstein Jr), pp. 534–547. W.B. Saunders, Philadelphia.

Baran, R., Bureau, H. & Sayag, J. (1979) Congenital malalignment of the big toenail. *Clinical and Experimental Dermatology* **4**, 359–360.

Baran, R., Dawber, R.P.R., Tosti, A. & Haneke, E. (1996) *A Text Atlas of Nail Disorders*, p. 29. Martin Dunitz, London.

Bose, B. (1971) A technique for excision of nail fold for ingrowing toenail. *Surgery, Gynecology and Obstetrics* **132**, 511–512.

Brown, F.C. (1981) Chemocautery for ingrown toenails. *Journal of Dermatologic Surgery and Oncology* **7**, 331–333.

Brown, R.E., Zook, E.G. & Williams, J. (2000) Correction of pincer nail deformity using dermal grafting. *Plastic and Reproductive Surgery* **105**, 1658–1661.

Chapman, R.S. (1973) Overcurvature of the nails: an inherited disorder. *British Journal of Dermatology* **89**, 317–318.

Dagnall, J.C. (1976a) The history, development and current status of nail matrix phenolization. *Chiropodist* **36**, 315–324.

Dagnall, J.C. (1976b) The development of nail treatments. *British Journal of Chiropody* **41**, 165.

Douglas, M.C. & Krull, E.A. (1981) Diseases of the nails. In: *Conn's Current Therapy*, p. 712. W.B. Saunders, Philadelphia.

Dubois, J.Ph. (1974) Un traitement de l'ongle incarné. *Nouvelle Presse Medicale* **3**, 1938.

Farnsworth, F.C. (1972) A treatment for convoluted nails. *Journal of the American Podiatric Association* **62**, 110.

Fowler, A.W. (1958) Excision of the germinal matrix: a unified treatment for toenail and onychogryphosis. *British Journal of Surgery* **45**, 382.

Fraser, A.R. (1967) Orthonyx: theory and practice. *British Journal of Chiropody* **32**, 229.

Gilles, G.A., Dennis, K.J. & Harkless, L.B. (1986) Periostitis associated with phenol matricectomies. *Journal of the American Podiatric Association* **76**, 469–472.

Greco, J., Kiniffo, H.V., Chanterelle, A. *et al.* (1973) L'attaque des

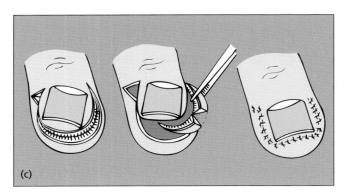

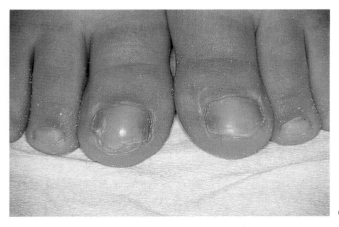

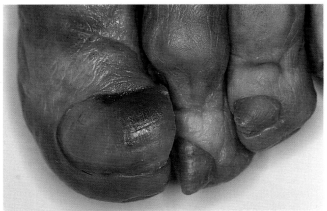

**Fig. 10.123** Congenital malalignment of the great toenail: (a) before treatment; (b) after surgery, using procedure in (c). (d) Congenital malalignment in adulthood.

parties molles, secret de la cure chirurgicale de l'ongle incarné. Un point de technique. *Annales de Chirurgie Plastique* **18**, 363–366.

Greiner, D., Schöfer, H. & Milbradt, R. (1998) Reversible transverse overcurvature of the nails (pincer nails) after treatment with a β-blocker. *Journal of the American Academy of Dermatology* **39**, 486–487.

Haneke, E. (1978) Chirurgische Behandlung des Unguis incarnatus. In: *Operative Dermatologie* (ed. K. Salfed), pp. 185–188. Springer, Berlin.

Haneke, E. (1984) Segmentale Matrixverschmälerung zur Behandlung des eingewachsenen Zehennagels. *Deutsche Medizinische Wochenschrift* **109**, 1451–1453.

Haneke, E. (1986) Surgical treatment of ingrown toenails. *Cutis* **37**, 251–256.

Haneke, E. (1992a) Pathogenese-orientierte Behandlung eingewachsener Zehennägel und des angeborenen Nagelschiefstandes bei Kindern. In: *Fortschritte der operativen Dermatologie 7: Onkologische Dermatologie, neue Aspekte, altersbedingte Besonderheiten* (eds G. Burg, A.A. Hartmann & B. Konz), pp. 243–245. Springer, Berlin.

Haneke, E. (1992b) Etiopathogénie et traitement de l'hypercourbure transversale de l'ongle du gros orteil. *J Med Esth Chir Dermatol* **19**, 123–127.

Haneke, E. & Baran, R. (1991) Nails: surgical aspects. In: *Aesthetic Dermatology* (eds L.C. Parish & G.P. Lask), pp. 236–247. McGraw-Hill, New York.

Higashi, N. (1990) Pincer nail due to tinea unguium. *Hifu* **32**, 40–44.

Higashi, N., Kume, A., Taniguchi, T. *et al.* (2000) Conservative treatment of overcurvature nail with sculptured nail method. *Skin Research* **42**, 437–444.

Howard, W.R. (1893) Ingrown toenail; its surgical treatment. *New York Medical Journal* 579.

Hwang, S.M., Lee, S.H. & Ahn, S.K. (1999) Pincer nail deformity and pseudo-Kaposi's sarcoma: complications of an artificial arteriovenous fistula for haemodialysis. *British Journal of Dermatology* **141**, 1129–1132.

Ilfeld, F.W. (1991) Ingrown toenail treated with cotton collodion insert. *Foot and Ankle* **11**, 312–313.

Jemec, G.B.E. & Thomsen, K. (1997) Pincer nail and alopecia as markers of gastrointestinal malignancy. *Journal of Dermatology* **24**, 479–481.

Langford, D.T., Burke, C. & Robertson, K. (1989) Risk factors in onychocryptosis. *British Journal of Surgery* **76**, 45–48.

Maeda, N., Mizuno, N.M. & Ichikawa, K. (1990) Nail abrasion: a new treatment for ingrown toenails. *Journal of Dermatology* **17**, 746–749.

Murray, W.R. (1979) Onychocryptosis. Principles of non-operative and operative care. *Clinical Orthopedics and Related Research* **142**, 96–102.

Murray, W.R. & Bedi, B.S. (1975) The surgical management of ingrowing toenail. *British Journal of Surgery* **62**, 409–412.

Murray, W.R. & Robb, J.E. (1981) Soft-tissue resection for ingrowing toenails. *Journal of Dermatologic Surgery and Oncology* **7**, 157–158.

Palmer, B.V. & Jones, A. (1979) Ingrowing toenails: the results of treatment. *British Journal of Surgery* **66**, 575–576.

Quenu, M. (1887) Des limites de la matrice de l'ongle. Applications au traitement de l'ongle incarné. *Bulletin de la Societé de Chirurgie Paris* **13**, 252.

Reszler, M. & Mari, B. (1981) Beitrag zum Unguis incarnatus-Syndrom. *Zeitschrift für Hautkrankheiten* **56**, 172–174.

Rinaldi, R., Sabia, M. & Gross, J. (1982) The treatment and prevention of infection in phenol alcohol matricectomies. *Journal of the American Podiatric Association* **72**, 453–457.

Rufli, T., Von Schulthess, A. & Itin, P. (1992) Congenital hypertrophy of the lateral nail folds of the hallux. *Dermatology* **184**, 296–297.

Sorg, M., Krüger, K. & Schattenkirchner, M. (1989) Das Pincer Nail Syndrom—eine seltene Differentialdiagnose des Fingerendgelenks mit Nagelbefall. *Zeitschrift für Rheumatologie* **48**, 204–206.

Steigleder, G.K. & Stober-Münster, J. (1977) Das Syndrom des eingewachsenen Nagel. *Zeitschrift für Hautkrankheiten* **52**, 1225–1229.

Thompson, C. & Terwilliger, C. (1951) The terminal Syme operation for ingrown toenail. *Surgical Clinics of North America* **31**, 575.

Tweedie, J.H. & Ranger, I. (1985) A simple procedure with nail preservation for ingrowing toenails. *Archives of Emergency Medicine* **2**, 149–154.

Vanderhooft, S.L. & Vanderhooft, J.E. (1999) Pincer nail deformity after Kawasaki's disease. *Journal of the American Academy of Dermatology* **41**, 341–342.

Zadik, F.R. (1950) Obliteration of the nail bed of the great toe without shortening the terminal phalanx. *Journal of Bone and Joint Surgery* **32B**, 66.

## Complications in nail surgery (Haneke & Baran 1993)

Proper examination of the patient before performing nail surgery and thorough technique may help one to avoid the commonest complications and enable one to rule out high risk patients (page 426).

For more elaborate techniques than nail avulsion or punch biopsy an exsanguinating tourniquet can be made with a surgical glove. The rubber on the tip of the finger to be operated on is cut across and the glove is rolled down the finger.

If bleeding persists a Penrose drain is secured with a haemostat. The tourniquet can be kept in place for no more than 15 min, otherwise there is a risk of gangrene. Therefore it has to be released for some minutes every 15 min. Hydropneumatic tourniquets are much less traumatizing than rubber strings.

Postoperatively bleeding may be extensive, particularly after the release of the tourniquet. However, because the vessels involved are small, the bleeding can usually be controlled by direct pressure. Oxidized cellulose (oxycel, surgicel, gelfoam) and a dab of aluminium chloride (35%) solution, may be applied for additional surety of haemostasis.

### Pain

There are considerable individual variations in the pain threshold. Preoperative sedation is helpful in most patients undergoing nail surgery. Atarax (hydroxyzime) may be given: 25 mg in the previous evening and repeated 2 h prior to the operation.

Peroperatively pain is due to poor anaesthesia.

Postoperatively (page 434):

1 Dressing must be padded to avoid injury and sealed with papertape, anchored in longitudinal pattern.

2 The extremity should be elevated to reduce oedema, which is frequent, and pain which is decreased when the arm is put in a sling. The foot has to be elevated to 30 degrees and the patient kept recumbent for 48 h.

3 Pain may be significant, and therefore analgesia with paracetamol (acetaminophen) with codeine should be available, mainly for special techniques such as cryosurgery.

The addition of marcaine or ropivacaine at the completion of the surgery is advisable, and may be mixed with 0.4 mL dexamethasone in the original anaesthesia site, if there is no infection (Salasche & Peters 1985).

### Infection

Pre-operatively strict aseptic procedures are similar to those used when performing any cutaneous surgery with local application of antiseptic solutions. The use of a sterile surgical glove, with the appropriate digit removed, will provide an aseptic covering for the rest of the patient's hand. Infection should be controlled since the consequences of extensive digital cellulitis may be severe.

Tetanus toxoid for lesions of the toes should be discussed and advised especially in farmers, for example, as well as the use of prophylactic antibiotics for surgical patients with prosthetic cardiac valves or compromised circulation.

Postoperative infection can happen where infection was latent and not suspected prior to the operation. When infection is present, the organism should be cultured and treated immediately with antibiotics and antiseptic soaks. Postoperative infection has significant morbidity in the distal phalanx including whitlow, compartmental cellulitis and lymphangitis and osteomyelitis.

### Necrosis

Even without overt infection, necrosis may be seen when sutures are too tight and not removed in time.

## Recurrences

They will depend on the nature of the original lesions.

## Permanent residual defects

They may lead to unsightly scarring.

*Matrix involvement*: crushing injuries leave many small pieces of subungual tissue. If these fragments are not incorporated into the repair, some may grow independently and cause nail horns or spicules that must be removed.

For operations involving the lunula border it is cosmetically important to maintain the curvilinear configuration of the distal lunula which plays an important role in shaping the free edge of the nail plate.

Nail deformities have occurred from drilling the nail plate for the release of subungual haematoma and from rough or careless removal of the nail to expose the bed. Nail deformities may also occur from the use of vicryl sutures in nail bed repair. These sutures, if too large, dissolve too slowly and are still present during the new nail growth. This can produce an area of onycholysis and ridging in the nail (Guy 1990).

## Unpredictable complications

*Acquired malalignment complications* may follow a lateral longitudinal nail biopsy (Baran & Haneke 1998; de Berker & Baran 1998).

Two cases of *reflex sympathetic dystrophy* have been reported even following a correct biopsy of the nail bed (Ingram *et al.* 1987; Haneke 1992). The appearance of an epidermoid implantation cyst in an operation scar is another unfortunate example (Baran & Bureau 1988; Nakajima *et al.* 1990). Implantation cyst is not uncommon as a complication of surgery for ingrowing toenails.

Self-resolving deformation of the nail following elastic band traction is unusual in the postoperative management of flexor tendon injuries (Hoddinot & Matthews 1989).

Ingrowing of a big toenail recurring several months after a successful toe-to-thumb transfer should recommend an awareness of the possible complication and treatment of the nail before the transfer (Sadr & Schenck 1982).

## References

Baran, R. & Bureau, H. (1988) Two post-operative epidermoid cysts following realignment of the hallux nail. *British Journal of Dermatology* **119**, 245–247.

Baran, R. & Haneke, E. (1998) Etiology and treatment of nail malalignment. *Dermatologic Surgery* **24**, 719–721.

de Berker, D. & Baran, R. (1998) Acquired malalignment: a complication of lateral longitudinal nail biopsy. *Acta Dermato-Venereologica* **78**, 468–470.

Guy, R.J. (1990) The etiologies and mechanisms of nail bed injuries. The perionychium. *Hand Clinics* **6**, 9–20.

Haneke, E. (1992) Sympathische Reflexdystrophie (Sudeck-Dystrophie) nach Nagelbiopsie. *Zentralblatt für Haut und Geschlechtskrankheiten* **160**, 263.

Haneke, E. & Baran, R. (1993) Nail surgery. In: *Complications in Dermatologic Surgery* (ed. M. Harahap), pp. 84–91. Springer, Berlin.

Hoddinot, C. & Matthews, J.P. (1989) Deformation of the nail following elastic band traction—a case report. *Journal of Hand Surgery* **14B**, 23–24.

Ingram, G.J., Scher, R.K. & Lally, E.V. (1987) Reflex sympathetic dystrophy following nail biopsy. *Journal of the American Academy of Dermatology* **16**, 253–256.

Nakajima, T., Yoshimura, Y. & Yoneda, K. (1990) Open treatment with drainage for ingrowing toenail. *Surgery Gynecology Obstetrics* **170**, 223–224.

Sadr, B. & Schenck, R.R. (1982) Ingrowing nail of a transplanted toe. *Hand* **14**, 337–338.

Salasche, S.J. & Peters, V.J. (1985) Tips on nail surgery. *Cutis* **35**, 428–438.

## Infection

The first stage in treatment of hand infection is accurate and prompt diagnosis (Haussman & Lisser 1992). Radiographs are required to identify foreign bodies, bone lesions, associated fractures and gas formation.

Infection of the nail folds is sometimes superficial (Fig. 10.124a). More often, it is represented by inflammation, swelling and abscess formation. It can be either acute or chronic.

### Bacterial infections

*Acute paronychia is commonly caused by a bacterial infection which gains access to the perionychium at the site of a hangnail. Staphylococcus aureus is the most common bacterium involved (McGinley et al. 1988). If the paronychia is above the nail it is treated by soaking and teasing of the paronychium away from the nail to allow the abscess to drain. However if the abscess has progressed beneath the nail a few millimetres of the lateral nail must be removed to allow adequate drainage (Fig. 10.125). The lateral portion of the nail should be undermined from the eponychium and the nail bed prior to its removal. It is not necessary to make an incision in the eponychium to achieve adequate drainage. An incision in the eponychium in the presence of infection may result in a deformed eponychium. If the abscess becomes a 'runaround' (involves both the paronychium and the dorsal nail fold) the nail should be removed in its entirety to allow drainage. If this abscess has been longstanding it may compromise the germinal matrix by pressure and the nail may not regrow. If the abscess is in the nail fold just the proximal portion of the nail that is involved can be*

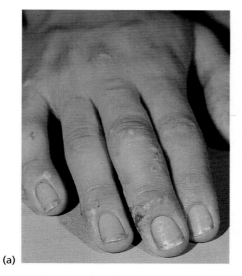

(a)

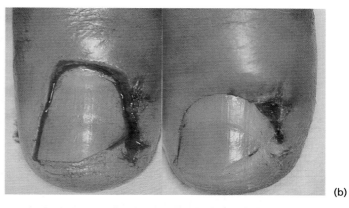

(b)

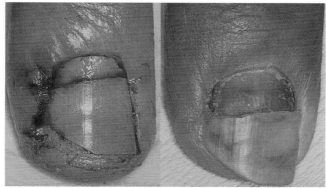

(c)

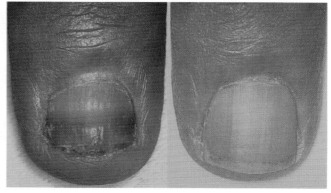

(d)

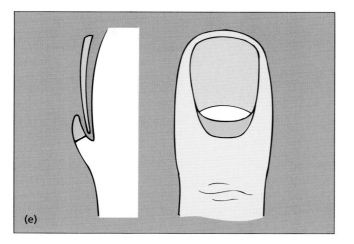

(e)

**Fig. 10.124** (a) Impetigo on the dorsum of some fingers. (b) Chronic paronychia with acute flares. Excision of the proximal nail fold. (c) Avulsion of the proximal nail plate. (d) Good healing. (e) Diagram showing the proximal nail fold removal.

removed leaving the nail over sterile matrix intact which is less uncomfortable.

## Chronic paronychia

*Chronic paronychia involves colonization of the dorsal roof,* soft tissue by a mixed gram-negative and fungal involvement. This may go on for weeks or months before the patient is seen with recurrence episodes of inflammation, which improves with antimicrobial treatment but then recurs. Treatment is an arc (quarter moon) shaped excision of the dorsal roof proximal to the nail fold. The defect heals secondarily with soaks and

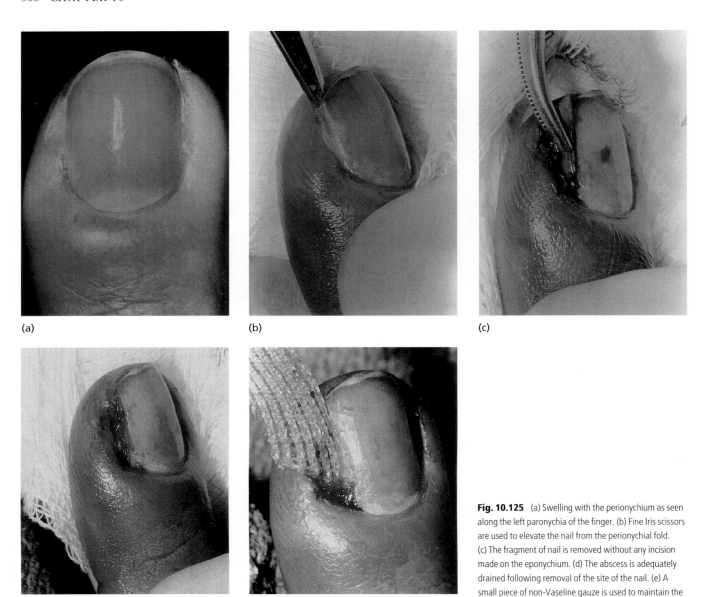

(a)

(b)

(c)

(d)

(e)

**Fig. 10.125** (a) Swelling with the perionychium as seen along the left paronychia of the finger. (b) Fine Iris scissors are used to elevate the nail from the perionychial fold. (c) The fragment of nail is removed without any incision made on the eponychium. (d) The abscess is adequately drained following removal of the site of the nail. (e) A small piece of non-Vaseline gauze is used to maintain the perionychium open. © E. Zook.

*dressing changes. (Keyser & Eaton 1976; Keyser et al. 1990; Bednar & Lane 1991) (Fig. 10.126).*

Baran and Bureau (1981) have described a technique derived from Keyser–Eaton's crescentic marsupialization. A Freer septum elevator is inserted into the proximal nail groove under the proximal nail fold to protect the matrix and extensor tendon. A no. 15 Bard-Parker blade or number 67 Beaver blade is used to excise en bloc a crescent-shaped full thickness skin, 4 mm at its greatest width, which extends from one lateral nail fold to the other. This includes the swollen portion of the proximal nail fold, with the septum elevator moved according to the tip of the scalpel to prevent the matrix from being inadvertently cut. A bevel incision prevents the excision of the nail-producing tissues of the proximal nail fold, responsible for the normal

shine of the nail plate (Fig. 10.124b–d). Subsequently the area is dressed with an antibiotic preparation. Complete healing, by secondary intention, and restoration of the proximal nail fold, with its adherent cuticle, will take place in less than 2 months. The nail fold is generally retracted a few millimetres compared with the original one. In patients who experience repeated acute painful flares associated with chronic paronychia, removal of the base of the nail plate is useful (Baran 1981).

## Subungual infection

### Pyogenic granuloma

*Pyogenic granuloma is a chronic inflammatory process that is*

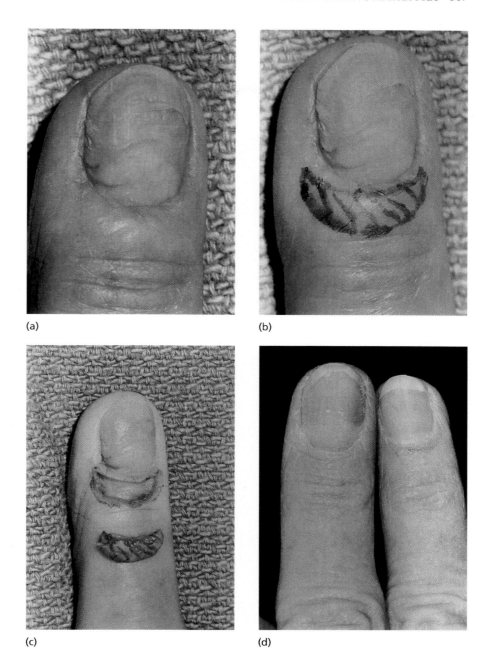

(a)

(b)

(c)

(d)

**Fig. 10.126** (a) A chronic paronychia of 3 years' duration which is painful and unsightly. (b) The area of nail wall to be excised to lower the fungal count. (c) The fragment of nail wall had been removed. (d) The nail is slightly lengthened with more lunula showing but the surface of the nail is much better and the symptoms are relieved. © E. Zook.

*frequently caused by perforation of the nail by over-zealous manicuring or may result from unknown causes. This is a globe of red tissue, which bleeds easily (Fig. 10.127). I treat these with frequent applications of silver nitrate. The differential diagnosis is squamous cell carcinoma which should be considered if these are chronic and non-healing.*

In subungual infection (Figs 10.128 & 10.129) probing will determine the most painful area and provide an indication for the site of fenestration of the nail plate. A U-shaped piece of the distal nail plate is excised in the region loosened by the pus and debridement of the affected nail bed area carried out. The yellow colour due to the subungual pus will sometimes serve as a guide for partial nail avulsion. Soaking the finger in antiseptic solutions, such as chlorhexidine, twice daily and dressing with wet compresses usually result in rapid healing.

**Granulomatous purulent nail bed inflammation ('lectitis purulenta et granulomatosa')** (Runne *et al.* 1978; Eichmann & Baran 1998) (Fig. 10.130)

The nail bed of all the fingers may be affected by lenticular polycyclic macules surrounded by a yellowish area. They are seen through the normal nail plate. After nail avulsion, the nail bed presents with large masses of granulomatous tissue with

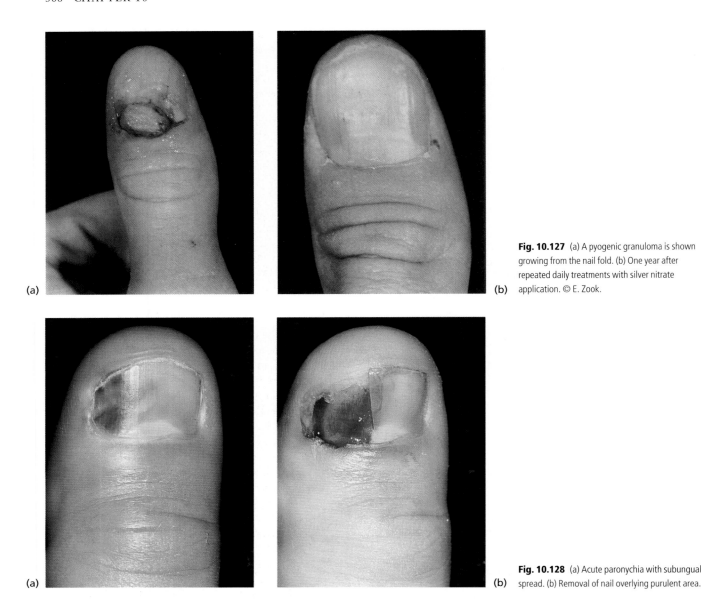

(a)

(b)

**Fig. 10.127** (a) A pyogenic granuloma is shown growing from the nail fold. (b) One year after repeated daily treatments with silver nitrate application. © E. Zook.

(a)

(b)

**Fig. 10.128** (a) Acute paronychia with subungual spread. (b) Removal of nail overlying purulent area.

heavy acanthosis, huge parakeratosis and subcorneal bleeding. There is prominent polymorphonuclear leucocyte inflammation with proliferation of blood vessels. The condition results in permanent sequelae such as onycholysis and thickening of the nail.

Purulent inflammation of the hallux nail bed probably secondary to repeated minor trauma from hiking shoes was observed in a 68-year-old man. The nail covered a grossly enlarged terminal phalanx. It was discoloured and floated on a lake of pus in the nail bed. It could easily be removed, exposing large masses of granulation tissue on the nail bed, lateral sulci and nail walls. Biopsies taken from the nail bed and lateral nail wall showed a very dense, diffuse inflammatory cell infiltrate composed of granulocytes, lymphocytes and abundant eosinophils sometimes giving the appearance of eosinophil abscess formation; eosinophil degranulation then led to intensely

eosinophilic hyalin collagen fibres. The nail bed epithelium was partly lacking or spongiotic. Healing after nail avulsion was uneventful (Haneke, unpublished).

The successful treatment, in a recent case, by local corticoid therapy after a 15-year history (Eichmann & Baran 1998) suggests that lectitis purulenta et granulomatosa is a chronic granulomatous response to repeated minor trauma and could represent a major variant of pyogenic granuloma often observed in the nail bed of the hallux.

## References

Baran, R. (1981) Nail growth direction revisited. (Why do nails grow out instead of up?) *Journal of the American Academy of Dermatology* 4, 78–82.

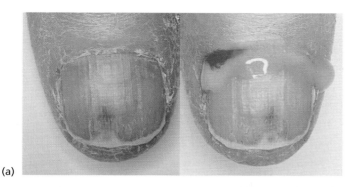

(a)

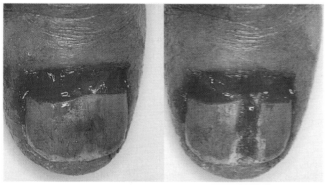

(b)

**Fig. 10.129** (a) Subungual infection. (b) Parts of nail avulsed for the removal of the pus and drainage.

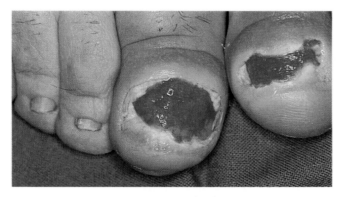

**Fig. 10.130** Granulomatous purulent nail bed inflammation. (Courtesy of J. Bazex, France.)

Baran, R. & Bureau, H. (1981) Surgical treatment of recalcitrant chronic paronychia of fingers. *Journal of Dermatologic Surgery and Oncology* **7**, 106–107.

Bednar, M.S. & Lane, L.B. (1991) Eponychial marsupialization and nail removal for surgical treatment of chronic paronychia. *Journal of Hand Surgery* **16A**, 314–317.

Eichmann, A. & Baran, R. (1998) Lectitis purulenta et granulomatosa. *Dermatology* **196**, 352–353.

Haussman, M.R. & Lisser, S.P. (1992) Hand infections. *Orthopedic Clinics of North America* **23**, 171–185.

Keyser, J.J. & Eaton, R.G. (1976) Surgical cure of chronic paronychia by eponychial marsupialization. *Plastic and Reconstructive Surgery* **58**, 66–70.

Keyser, J.J., Littler, J.W. & Eaton, R.G. (1990) Surgical treatment of infections and lesions of the perionychium. *Hand Clinics* **6**, 137–153.

McGinley, K.J., Larson, E.L. & Leyden, J.J. (1988) Composition and density of microflora in the subungual space of the hand. *Journal of Clinical Microbiology* **26**, 950–953.

Runne, U., Goertz, E. & Weese, A. (1978) Lectitis purulenta et granulomatosa. *Zeitschrift für Hautkrankheiten* **53**, 625.

## The management of diabetic and high risk patients
(Patterson & Hunter 1989)

There are several conditions which put a patient in the high risk group. These and their associated problems include:
• Diabetes mellitus with neuropathy: increased incidence of infection and gangrene.
• Peripheral vascular disease: gangrene.
• Diseases of the nervous system—motor and sensory impairment: infection, gangrene.
• Steroid therapy: infection.
• Anticoagulant therapy: bleeding.
• Prosthetic cardiac valve: infection of the prosthesis.

The toenails should be cut after bathing, when the nails are soft. They should be cut straight across and not too short. It is unwise to use a sharp instrument to clean the subungual area of the free edge of the nail.

If infection is not promptly controlled, it may, within a very short period of time, proceed to rapidly advancing cellulitis, invasion of bony tissue, gangrene and amputation.

Infection must be treated aggressively and antibiotic therapy should be started empirically, without awaiting the bacteriology report. Penicillinase-resistant penicillin, erythromycin or clindamycin should be prescribed.

Prophylactic antibiotic cover for surgical patients with prosthetic cardiac valves or compromised circulation is the rule and may be considered appropriate if blood-sugar control is not optimal (Middleton & Webb 1992). Partial or total nail avulsion with chemical (liquefied phenol BP) ablation of the nail matrix is the most common and least traumatic procedure.

Minimum use of adhesive padding and strapping as well as avoidance of constricting dressing and appliances are recommended.

## References

Middleton, A. & Webb, F. (1992) Toenail surgery for diabetic patients. *Diabetic Medicine* **9**, 680–684.

Patterson, R.S. & Hunter, A.M. (1989) The management of diabetic and other high risk patients. In: *Common Foot Disorders* (eds D. Neale & I.M. Adams), pp. 137–149, 3rd edn. Churchill Livingstone, Edinburgh.

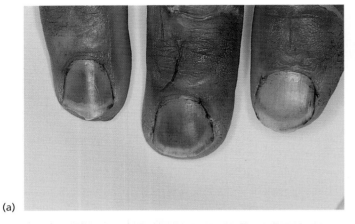

(a)

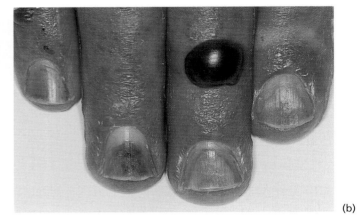

(b)

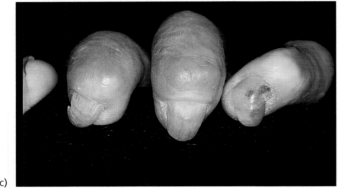

(c)

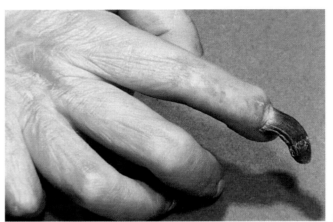

(d)

## Burns (Fig. 10.131)

The nail involvement relates to the severity of the burn and the final result depends on this and other factors such as the site and the depth of the dermal structures involved, the presence of infection, the possibility of keloid formation and the promptness of treatment.

The signs produced will vary with the degree of the burn; with slight thermal injury, the nail plate turns a brownish-yellow hue (Jeune & Ortonne 1979); nail bed involvement may result in transient or permanent onycholysis and a burn of the matrix will lead to loss of the nail, which will be replaced by a dystrophic brownish nail. The extent of the dystrophy reflects the degree of matrix destruction. Involvement of the proximal nail fold and its following synechiae are among the most severe sequelae and are very difficult to correct. However, Barfod's technique (1972) or better procedures derived from this technique (Achauer 1990) (page 472) may give acceptable results. On the other hand early excision-grafting in severe cases of burning will produce better results.

## References

Achauer, B.M. (1990) One-stage reconstruction of the postburn nail fold contracture. *Plastic and Reconstructive Surgery* 85, 937–941.

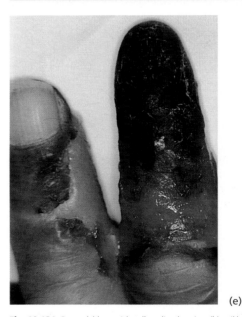

(e)

**Fig. 10.131** Burns: (a) brownish-yellow discoloration; (b) nail bed involvement with onycholysis (may be permanent); (c) scarring with nail and joint dystrophy; (d) black nail due to Hiroshima bomb blast (courtesy of Mr Takahashi, President of the Hiroshima Peace Memorial Museum); (e) acute inflammatory changes which lead to severe nail apparatus scarring (courtesy of A. Tosti, Italy).

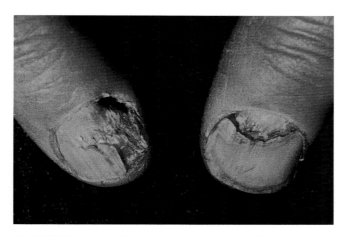

**Fig. 10.132** Hydrofluoric acid burns involving the nail apparatus. (Courtesy of P. Samman.)

Barfod, B. (1972) Reconstruction of the nail fold. *Hand* **4**, 85.

Jeune, R. & Ortonne, J.P. (1979) Chromonychia following thermal injury. *Acta Dermato-Venereologica* **59**, 91.

## Chemical burns

The damage produced by chemical burns is dependent on the concentration of the irritant and its duration of action. Unlike thermal or electric burns, the destruction will continue after the source of the irritant is removed as long as there is residual, active chemical at the site.

In most cases the burn should be irrigated immediately with copious amounts of water. Solid particles, such as lime, bleaching powder, cement or phosphorous should be removed first, preferably with a brush, as water may cause the particles to adhere.

Alkali burns are commonly caused by sodium or potassium hydroxide (lyes) or calcium oxide (lime). These agents are found in many drain cleaners and paint removers. The affected site should be irrigated with water for at least 15 min and the alkali then neutralized with vinegar as emergency remedies in the home (Milner 1982).

Acids produce varying and often characteristic skin discoloration. Hydrofluoric acid burns (Fig. 10.132) should be treated by immersion in lukewarm water until all the surface acid is removed. After irrigation, the burn should be covered with an ointment consisting of one part magnesium oxide and two parts glycerine which precipitates the fluorine as magnesium fluoride. Hydrofluoric acid may continue to penetrate beneath the surface until it is neutralized by bone; many authorities recommend that the inflamed tissue should be infiltrated with 10% solution of calcium gluconate. In fact, the specific treatment consists of intra-arterial infusion of calcium gluconate (Lheureux *et al.* 1991) (Chapter 7).

After the burn has been cleaned and dried, it should be covered with fine mesh gauze soaked in saline. Bulky, dry, sterile dressings are laid over this and held in place by an elastic dressing overall. The burn area should be elevated to prevent oedema, which hinders healing.

Burns are particularly vulnerable to *Clostridium tetanus*. Even in the case of minor burns, the immune status should be checked and the appropriate tetanus prophylaxis instituted.

### References

Lheureux, P., Goldschmidt, D., Hossey, D. *et al.* (1991) Brûlures digitales par l'acide fluorhydrique. *Réanimation Soins Intensive Médicinal Urgence* **7**, 227–230.

Milner, J.E. (1982) The office treatment of minor chemical skin burns. *Cutis* **29**, 285.

## The painful nail

### Diagnosis

Pain is a non-specific symptom of many nail conditions: trauma, infection, tumour, etc. It is often the cause for consulting a physician for an alteration of the nail apparatus or distal phalanx that otherwise was neglected by the patient and/or his physician.

The unique anatomical relations of the nail plate as a firm cover, the nail bed dermis as a very tough fibrous structure, the terminal phalanx as a sensory structure receiving about 60% of the axons of the digital nerves, all are responsible for the sometimes excruciating pain that an otherwise bland alteration would cause.

Diagnosis requires an accurate detailed history:
- Onset: sudden, slow, insidious, unnoticed.
- Course: continuous, repeated, day and/or night.
- Nature: continuous, lancinating, throbbing, nagging, dull, sharp.
- Intensity.
- Response to physical alteration: intensification or relief on raising the corresponding extremity, on cold or heat, on applying a tourniquet.
- Response to specific drugs.

### Exploration

The clinical examination will focus on the nail, the periungual soft and the distal phalanx as well as the entire digit and compare it with its contralateral homologue to be inspected for size, shape, circumference, colour and temperature. The nail has to be examined in a relaxed state, under forced extension and flexion as well as with pressing the fingertips against a hard base; this gives more information about possible differences of blood circulation. A magnifier lens is often of great help.

The next step is careful palpation of the nail region, probing of the nail plate and perionychium, comparison of the consistency of the periungual tissue.

Swellings may be examined using diascopy (glass spatulum pressed on the lesion will make the lesion's proper colour appear) and diaphanoscopy (a light held against the swollen part will make the lesion shine if it is cystic and filled with a clear fluid); again probing is mandatory to locate the point of maximum pain.

Epi-illumination microscopy particularly aids in the clinical diagnosis of pigmented lesions under and around the nail; specifically, dense minute bleedings of the digital tip which tend to get eliminated transepidermally can easily be distinguished from melanin pigmentation.

X-ray investigation is compulsory if pain after a single trauma or inflammation does not subside in due course. We have found xerography with magnification to be of particular value since it permits both the evaluation of the bone and gives outlines of the nail plate and soft tissues.

Magnetic resonance tomography recently proved to be useful for the diagnosis and exact localization of glomus tumours, as did arteriography.

Biopsy is often mandatory and the ultimate tool to make an exact diagnosis.

A number of highly sophisticated techniques, such as MRI and high-frequency ultrasound, are available for research purposes and may, under certain circumstances, be useful for the examination of a painful nail.

## Differential diagnosis

This symptom is so unspecific, subjective, inconstant and not reliable—a feature of many nail conditions. Some patients complain of irresistible pain even in normally painless conditions, some are extremely indolent and pretend not to feel pain.

For the sake of clarity, a few hints to possible differential diagnoses are given according to clinical features and pathology (Tables 10.4 & 10.5).

Whenever the nail apparatus is painful the possible mechanism should be considered. Oedema due to infection, other inflammations or trauma cause pain which is usually alleviated by raising the affected extremity as high as possible. Infection is commonly associated with pulsating pain. Intensifying pain over several days despite surgical intervention of an acute subungual felon may suggest osteitis of the terminal phalanx. Differential diagnosis of periungual pyogenic infection is erysipeloid. Chronic candidal paronychia is characterized by episodic acute flares during which some pain may occur. Herpetic whitlow must be considered, particularly when lymphangitis accompanies the lesions from their beginning and appears to be extraordinarily intense and painful. Ingrown nails are frequent in adolescents and mainly occur on the great toe; whenever a seemingly normal nail on a digit other than the

big toe grows a tumour of the lateral nail groove or wall has to be considered. However, malignant tumours may also develop on the great toe and mimic painful ingrown toenail.

All space-occupying processes such as rapidly growing

**Table 10.4** Some conditions of the nail apparatus which characteristically cause pain.

*Trauma*
Cold injury especially on re-warming
Splinters
Squeezing, crush injuries
Tennis toe, ski-boot toe, sports person's toe

*Inflammation*
Acroosteolysis
Acute osteomyelitis
Cosmetic reactions (prosthetic nails, formaldehyde, etc.)
Herpetic whitlow
Ingrowing toenail
Paronychia (acute and flares in chronic paronychia)
Prosector's wart
Raynaud's phenomenon
Sarcoidosis
Subungual whitlow, subcutaneous abscess

*Tumours of bone or with bone reaction*
Aneurysmal bone cyst
Cirsoid angioma
Enchondroma
Epidermoid cyst
Fibroma
Keratoacanthoma
Leiomyoma, epithelioid leiomyosarcoma
Lipoma
Metastasis to the fingertip
Onychophosis
Osteoid osteoma
Osteoma, exostoses
Secondary infection of slowly growing tumours
Squamous cell carcinoma, basal cell carcinoma
Subungual enchondroma
Subungual corn
Subungual exostosis
Subungual glomus tumour
Subungual neurofibroma
Subungual osteochondroma
Subungual sarcoma, epithelioid sarcoma, chondrosarcoma
Subungual tumour in incontinentia pigmenti
Subungual wart
Synovioma (when it penetrates the distal bony phalanx)

*Non-osseous tumours*
Basal cell carcinoma
Bowen's disease
Cirsoid angioma
Corn
Fibroma
Leimyoma; epithelioid leiomyosarcoma
Lipoma
Melanoma (rarely painful)
Neurofibroma (NFI)
Neuroma (secondary to forgotten trauma)
Onychophosis
Radiodermatitis (acute)

**Table 10.5** Clinical signs in some types of painful nail (Mathes & Hartwig 1993).

| Lesion | Key symptoms and examination |
| --- | --- |
| *Clinically normal appearing nail* | |
| Cold injury | Color of digit, pain on rewarming |
| Enchondroma | X-ray, biopsy |
| Gout | Pain attacks, tophi on fingertip, uric acid determination |
| Neuroma | Biopsy |
| Osteoid osteoma | Nagging pain, poorly localized, more intense at night; X-ray |
| Osteoma | X-ray |
| Raynaud's phenomenon | History of Raynaud's attacks and digiti mortui |
| Some chemical burns | Contact with alkali, caustic substances |
| Subungual glomus tumour | Excruciating pain radiating into arm and triggered by cold, mechanical shock, probing. Pain alleviated after applying a tourniquet |
| | |
| *Visible nail changes, trauma, inflammation* | |
| Acute paronychia | Inspection |
| Dermatomyositis | Inspection, nail fold capillary microscopy |
| Different types of hereditary epidermolysis bullosa | History |
| Hammer blow, crush injury | Personal history |
| Herpetic whitlow | Tzanck test |
| Iatrogenic nails (retinoids, ciclosporine, indinavir, lamivudine, β-blockers) | Inspection, history |
| Ingrowing toenail | Inspection, probing |
| Occlusive vascular disease | Decreased pulses and blood pressure on the affected extremity |
| Pincer nail (Mathes & Hartwig 1993; Baran 1974) | Inspection |
| Pterygium unguis inversum | Inspection |
| Pulpitis sicca and periungual dermatitis | Inspection, history of recurrences |
| Splinter | Inspection, history |
| Subungual cracks | Mainly during cold season |
| Subungual felon | Inspection, bacterial culture |
| Subungual haematoma | Inspection |
| Systemic lupus erythematosus | Inspection, autoimmune phenomena |
| | |
| *Visible nail changes, tumours* | |
| Aneurysmal bone cyst | Bulbous enlargment of phalanx, X-ray |
| Angioleiomyoma | Biopsy |
| Epidermoid cyst | Inspection, history, X-ray |
| Exostosis | Bone-hard tumour, X-ray |
| Glomus tumour (Sheils et al. 1972) | Probing |
| Keratoacanthoma | Inspection, dermatopathology |
| Leiomyoma | Biopsy |
| Maffucci's syndrome | X-ray, history |
| Osteochondroma | Bone-hard tumour, X-ray |
| Pyogenic granuloma | Inspection, biopsy |
| Subungual warts | Inspection (cut away overlying nail plate) |
| Ungual fibrokeratoma | Inspection |

tumours can be painful. Keratoacanthom is a typical example: it elicits pain in contrast to the slow-growing subungual squamous cell (epidermoid) carcinoma. Most other benign tumours and pseudo-tumorous lesions such as dorsal myxoid pseudocysts usually remain asymptomatic.

The best known subungual lesion is the glomus tumour. It is an inherently painful tumour and may cause spontaneous, sometimes pulsating pain which often is precipitated by slight trauma or cold. The pain characteristically radiates up to the shoulder. Application of a tourniquet will relieve the pain. The tumour often seen through the nail plate is a reddish-violaceous spot of 3–10 mm in diameter. A reddish stripe may appear in the nail and be a slight longitudinal elevation in the nail plate. Probing allows further localization of the tumour. Approximately half of the glomus tumours cause a depression in the distal phalanx visible on X-ray films.

## Treatment

Any therapy requires an exact diagnosis. Nail avulsion must never be done without a suspected diagnosis or even as a substitute for treatment: although the nail plate usually obscures the clinical picture it may give invaluable hints as to the history of the disease, its exact localization, etc.

Treatment options for painful nail lesions are summarized in Table 10.2.

## References

Baran, R. (1974) Pincer and trumpet nails. *Archives of Dermatology* **110**, 639.

Mathes, U. & Hartwig, R. (1993) Der empfindliche Nagel. *Zeitschrift für Hautkrankheiten* **68**, 351–358.

Sheils, W.C., Becton, J.L. & Christian, J.D. (1972) Subungual glomus tumor: a cause of pain beneath the finger nail. *Journal of the Medical Association of Georgia* **64**, 268–270.

# CHAPTER 11

# Tumours of the nail apparatus and adjacent tissues

**R. Baran, E. Haneke, J.-L. Drapé & E.G. Zook (with the participation of J.F. Kreusch)**

Glomangiosarcoma

Malignant haemangioendothelioma (haemangiosarcoma, haemangioendothelioma)

Neuroendocrine tumour

*Merkel cell tumour*

Tumours of peripheral nerves

*Neuroma*

*So-called rudimentary supernumerary digits*

*Neurofibroma*

*Systematized multiple fibrillar neuromas*

*Plexiform 'Pacinian' neuroma*

*Glioma, neurilemmoma, schwannoma*

*Granular cell tumour*

*Malignant granular cell tumour*

*Perineurioma*

Osteocartilaginous tumours

*Benign tumours*

Exostosis

Osteochondroma

Multiple exostoses syndrome (diaphysial aclasis)

Soft tissue chondroma

Enchondroma

Enchondromatosis (Ollier's chondrodysplasia)

Maffucci's syndrome (enchondromatosis, or chondrodysplasia with multiple soft tissue haemangiomas)

Osteoid osteoma

Giant cell tumour of the bone

Solitary bone cyst

*Malignant tumours*

Chondrosarcoma

Synovial tumours

*Giant cell tumour (benign synovioma, benign xanthomatous giant cell tumours, villo-nodular pigmented synovitis)*

Lipomatous and myxomatous tumours

*Lipoma*

*Myxoma*

Sarcomas

*Phalangeal sarcoma*

*Epithelioid sarcoma*

*Xanthomatous giant cell sarcoma*

*Glomangiosarcoma*

*Epithelioid leiomyosarcoma*

*Fibrosarcoma*

*Chondrosarcoma*

*Haemangiosarcoma (haemangioendothelioma)*

*Epithelioid angiosarcoma*

*Ewing's sarcoma*

**Pseudotumours**

Myxoid pseudocysts of the digits

Pretibial myxoedema

Primary osteoma cutis

Subungual calcifications

Cutaneous calculi

Oxalate granuloma

Foreign body granuloma (Chapter 10)

Gout (Chapter 6)

**Histiocytic, lymphomatous and metastatic processes**

Histiocytic processes

*Xanthoma*

*Verruciform xanthoma*

*Juvenile xanthogranuloma*

*Multicentric reticulohistiocytosis (Chapter 6)*

Lymphoma (Chapter 6)

Metastases

**Melanocytic lesions**

Subungual melanocytic lesions

Longitudinal melanonychia

Benign melanocytic hyperplasia—focal melanocyte activation

Lentigo simplex and melanocytic naevus

Atypical melanocytic hyperplasia and nail melanoma

Blue naevus

Pseudo-Recklinghausen intradermal naevi

Histopathology of subungual melanoma

Metastasis

Prognosis of subungual melanoma

Nail melanoma in childhood

Nail melanoma in deeply pigmented races

Nail melanoma in transplant recipients

Incident light microscopy of pigmented nail disorders

Spontaneous regression of melanocytic lesions

*Longitudinal melanonychia*

*Melanoma of the nail apparatus*

---

In the original sense of the term, a tumour is a circumscribed swelling which may be due to an increase in cells, acellular tissue components, or both. This term therefore comprises many more lesions than just true neoplasms; however, since the true nature of a tumour often requires a histopathological examination and the differentiation between pseudotumours, degenerative and reactive tumours and 'true' neoplasms is often somewhat arbitrary we will deal in this chapter with most lesions clinically appearing as a 'tumour'. As in Chapter 10, Elvin Zook's contribution has been placed in *italic letters*; Jean-Luc Drapé's contribution is indicated by *italic letters* with a vertical bar in the outer margin.

The clinical differential diagnosis of many tumours in the nail area is difficult. Their common growth pattern may be altered due to anatomical reasons. The nail plate both covers the lesions and may influence the pattern of invasion. Inadvertent, often minor trauma causes the first symptoms so that the diagnosis may be further delayed, and many neoplasms may cause bulbous enlargement of the finger tips with nail clubbing due to bone splaying associated with pressure beneath the nail bed (Guy 1990). Most benign tumours cause nail deformation due to chronic pressure on the matrix. Tumours involving the proximal nail fold can cause pressure from above and produce longitudinal grooving or fissuring of the nail. Some tumours—soft or hard—may occur under the matrix, exerting pressure upward thus causing ridging, overcurvature or even anonychia. Onycholysis may result when they are located beneath or in the nail bed.

Neoplasia of the nail area may be benign, benign but aggressive resulting in nail destruction, or malignant. Since recurrences often occur even in benign tumours and many physicians, as well as pathologists, are not familiar with the particular features of nail tumours, unnecessary amputations have not infrequently been described and sometimes even been recommended as the 'treatment of choice'.

Nail deformation most often denotes benign pathology because this reflects slow growth, while partial or total nail destruction may denote malignancy.

A history of trauma, associated infection, concealment beneath the nail, modifications of tumour behaviour produced by the specialized nail anatomy and variations in pigmentation are all factors which may mislead the diagnostician (Préaux 1978; Salasche & Garland 1985).

## References

Guy, R.J. (1990) The etiologies and mechanisms of nail bed injuries. *Hand Clinics* 6, 9–19.

Préaux, J. (1978) Les tumeurs de la région unguéale des doigts. Problèmes diagnostiques. *Cutis (France)* 2, 481–492.

Salasche, S.J. & Garland, L.D. (1985) Tumors of the nail. *Dermatologic Clinics* 3, 501–519.

## Epithelial tumours

### Benign

**Warts** (Figs 11.1 & 11.2)

Common warts are caused by human papilloma viruses of different DNA types. They are benign, weakly contagious, fibroepithelial tumours with a rough keratotic surface. Most frequently, they are located on the lateral aspect of the proximal nail fold. Subungual warts initially affect the hyponychium, growing slowly toward the nail bed and finally elevating the nail plate which is not often affected although surface

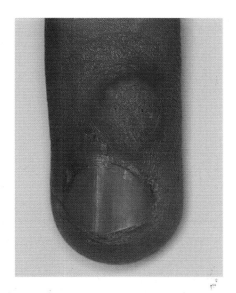

**Fig. 11.1** Wart on the proximal nail fold— pressure has caused a depression on the nail plate.

ridging may occur, but loss of the nail is exceptional. Global nail dystrophy of all 20 nails was a very unusual presentation of HPV infection (type 57) of the nail bed and the matrix in an otherwise immunocompetent patient (McCown *et al.* 1999).

Usually periungual warts are asymptomatic though fissuring may cause pain. Tender periungual nodules are infrequent (Holland *et al.* 1992). Longitudinal grooving is rare. Subungual warts are painful and may mimic a glomus tumour.

Biting, picking and tearing of the nail and nail walls are common habits in subjects with periungual warts. This type of trauma is probably responsible for the spread of the warts and their resistance to treatment.

Bone erosion from verruca vulgaris has been observed (Shapiro *et al.* 1961; Gardner & Acker 1973; Plewig *et al.* 1973; Shah *et al.* 1976; Kumar *et al.* 1980). However, some of these cases may have been keratoacanthomas since the latter as well as epidermoid carcinoma and verruca vulgaris are sometimes indistinguishable from clinical signs alone.

Histopathology of subungual and periungual warts is similar to that of common warts found elsewere. Cytopathogenic effects are not as marked as in plantar warts. An inflammatory infiltrate may be present when the wart has been traumatised repeatedly. Histological examination may be necessary to differentiate extensive periungual warts from verrucous Bowen's disease.

Periungual warts, particularly when located on the hyponychium, may be inconspicuous presenting only a slightly thickened skin-coloured area which swells and after immersion in water, turns white more rapidly than the surrounding skin. Histopathology is then needed to make the diagnosis. It shows considerable thickening of the epidermis, vacuolisation of the granular layer and a loose basket-weave like horny layer (E. Haneke, unpublished observation)

Tuberculosis cutis verrucosa (butcher's nodule, prosector's warts) may occasionally pose difficulties of differential diagnosis, but it is very rare around the nail. Haneke (1983) has

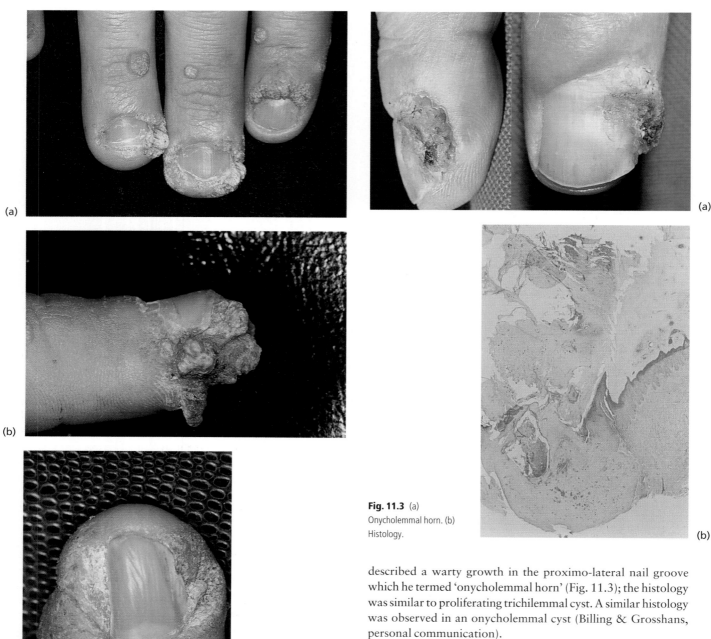

**Fig. 11.2** (a) Multiple periungual warts—more common in nail biters and cuticle/lateral wall pickers. (b) Multiple warts distorting the nail apparatus most frequently seen in immunosuppressed individuals. (c) Periungual warts narrowing the nail plate.

**Fig. 11.3** (a) Onycholemmal horn. (b) Histology.

described a warty growth in the proximo-lateral nail groove which he termed 'onycholemmal horn' (Fig. 11.3); the histology was similar to proliferating trichilemmal cyst. A similar histology was observed in an onycholemmal cyst (Billing & Grosshans, personal communication).

When *mucinous syringometaplasia* involves the distal nail bed, clinical resemblance to warts is striking. Biopsy reveals a focal invagination of the epidermis lined by squamous epithelium, with one or several eccrine ducts leading into the invagination. The eccrine duct epithelium contains mucin-laden goblet cells, and there is mucinous syringometaplasia of the underlying eccrine coils (Scully & Assad 1984).

Differential diagnosis includes onychophosis affecting a lateral fold of the toenails, subungual filamentous tumour, subungual vegetations of amyloidosis subungual corn (heloma), verrucous epidermal naevus, inflammatory linear verrucous epidermal naevus (ILVEN) and multicentric reticulohistiocytosis. With long standing warty lesions, especially in persons over

40 years of age, Bowen's disease must always be considered and a biopsy taken.

Treatment of periungual warts is often frustrating. They have a natural life span of about 4–5 years, but duration may exceed the patience of the patient or physician (Shelley 1972). X-ray and radium treatment have become obsolete. Samman (1979) recommends saturated monochloroacetic acid. It is applied sparingly, allowed to dry and then covered with 40% salicylic acid plaster cut to the size of the wart and held in place with adhesive tape for 2–3 days. After 1–2 weeks most of the wart can be removed and this procedure has to be repeated. This may sometimes become painful when most of the overlying horny layer has been removed (Haneke 1982). Subungual warts are treated similarly, after cutting away the overlying part of the nail plate. Hand or foot baths, as hot as tolerable and performed twice daily, are valuable supportive measures. Due to the vasoconstrictive action of nicotine, smoking will delay healing.

Silver nitrate is known to be an effective cauterizing agent. A comparative study showed the application of silver nitrate by a pencil to be significantly more efficacious than black ink (Yazar & Basaran 1994).

Recalcitrant warts may respond to squaric acid dibutylester (Lee & Mallory 1999) or 2% diphenylcyclopropenone (diphencyprone), an obligate sensitizer which has replaced 2% dinitrochlorobenzene that is mutagenic for salmonella in the Ames test and therefore can no longer be recommended (Wiesner-Menzel & Happle 1984; Orrecchia et al. 1988). Some authors recommend the use of cantharidin (0.007%); 'Cantharone' is applied to the lesions and covered by a plastic tape for 24 hours. The resultant blister roof is removed and the remaining wart re-treated at 2-week intervals, three to four times if necessary. Recently, imiquimod was used successfully in widespread HPV 42 periungual warts in a patient with AIDS (Hengge et al. 1999). Tkach (1989) suggested a trick when using cantharidin for warts in order to avoid blister formation which he believed to cause spreading of the wart, a similar complication occurring with liquid nitrogen. After applying cantharidin, the wart is covered with paper tape. The patient is given an alcohol sponge and instructed to wipe off the cantharidin in 2 h. If there is not enough reaction, the cantharidin is left on progressively longer with subsequent visits. For children Cantharon™ is diluted 1 : 1000 with a 1 : 1 mixture of isopropyl alcohol and acetone and may be left on the skin longer.

5-fluorouracil has been used for treating periungual warts, especially under occlusion. Onychodystrophy (Tanenbaum 1971) and painful onycholysis may appear (Goettmann & Bélaïch 1995).

Shumer and O'Keefe (1983) strongly recommend bleomycin for recalcitrant warts. It is given intralesionally 1 mg per 10 mL at two week intervals. Munn et al. (1996) used bleomycin 1 mg/mL which was dropped on the wart and pricked into the lesion by multiple rapid stabs with a Monolet™ needle. Van der Velden et al. (1997) recommended treatment with increasing concentrations of bleomycin using the Van der

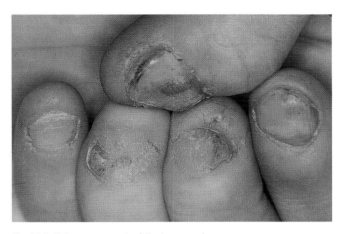

**Fig. 11.4** Nail apparatus scarring following overzealous cryosurgery.

Velden Derma-injector which is a modified tattooing machine. Transitory (Baran 1985a) or permanent (Miller 1984; Urbina-Gonzales 1986) nail dystrophy following intralesional injections of bleomycin for periungual warts has been reported. Vasospastic effects such as permanent Raynaud's phenomenon from intralesional therapy may happen even when using a reduced dose (Epstein 1991).

With a multiple puncture technique under local anaesthesia with a bifurcated vaccination needle to introduce bleomycin sulfate (1 µg/mL) sterile saline solution) into warts, Shelley and Shelley (1991) obtained elimination of 92% of a random series of 258 warts after a single treatment.

Imiquimod used for genital warts may well be in the future one of the best local treatments despite its cost.

Surgical treatment should be avoided if possible. Liquid nitrogen is often used, causing blistering with the blister roof containing the epidermal wart component if the treatment succeeds (Kuflik 1984). However, when treating the proximal nail fold freezing must not be prolonged since one may easily damage the matrix which may result in circumscribed leuconychia or even nail dystrophy. Though scarring is rare, permanent onychoatrophy with pterygium formation has been reported (Baran 1985b) (Fig. 11.4). Particular side effects of cryosurgery include secondary bacterial infection (rare); Beau's lines, onychomadesis, nail loss and pain due to subungual oedema, which is often worse in the very young and very old. Many side effects are avoidable if the freeze times used are carefully controlled, and prophylactic analgesic and subsequent anti-inflammatory treatment is provided.

Oral aspirin 600 mg three times daily, beginning 2 h before and for 3 days after treatment, is helpful. Pre-treatment application of clobetasol propionate (Kersey 1988), beneath an occlusive tape, such as Blenderm, reduces the inflammatory response to the freeze. Massages with this steroid may be continued twice daily for three days.

Destruction using curettage and electrodesiccation may produce considerable scarring. Recently infrared coagulation, argon and $CO_2$ laser treatments, have been used with some success, but permanent nail dystrophy is possible after ablation of periungual warts (Olbright *et al.* 1987; Street & Roenigk 1990). Pulsed-dye laser has also been used successfully for recalcitrant warts with an excellent side effect profile (Ross *et al.* 1999).

Many lay and medical people have 'tricks' for attempting to cure warts. A suggested treatment is 'wrapping' with micropore for example followed 2 weeks later by the careful application of liquefied phenol and then a drop of nitric acid to the lesion. The fuming and spluttering that occurs look efficacious and the wart turns brown (Litt 1978).

Cimetidine, thought to be an immunomodulator, has been disappointing in the treatment of recalcitrant periungual warts (Bauman *et al.* 1996; Yilmaz *et al.* 1996) despite some positive anecdotal reports (Zepeda del Villar 1994).

Since the incubation period of human warts may be up to several months, consistent follow-up, even after seemingly successful therapy, is necessary to allow early treatment of new warts. Wart treatment can only be considered successful when all warts have completely disappeared; reduction in size or number alone is a treatment failure.

## References

Baran, R. (1985a) Brachytelephalangie révélée à l'occasion de dystrophies unguéales induites par cryothérapie. *Annales de Dermatologie et de Vénéréologie* **112**, 365–367.

Baran, R. (1985b) Onychodystrophie induite par injection intralésionnelle de bléomycine pour verrue périunguéale. *Annales de Dermatologie et de Vénéréologie* **112**, 463–464.

Bauman, C., Francis, J.S., Vanderhooft, S. & Sybert, V.P. (1996) Cimetidine therapy for multiple viral warts in children. *Journal of the American Academy of Dermatology* **35**, 271–272.

Epstein, E. (1991) Intralesional bleomycin and Raynaud's phenom-enon. *Journal of the American Academy of Dermatology* **24**, 785–786.

Gardner, L.W. & Acker, D.W. (1973) Bone destruction of a distal phalanx caused by periungual warts. *Archives of Dermatology* **107**, 275–276.

Goettmann, S. & Bélaïch, S. Onycholyse polydactylique sévère au cours d'un traitement des verrues. *Annals of Dermatology* **122S**, 111.

Haneke, E. (1982) Differential diagnose und Therapie von Schwielen, Hühneraugen und Plantarwarzen. *Zeitschrift für Hautkrankheiten* **57**, 263–272.

Haneke, E. (1983) Onycholemmal horn. *Dermatologica* **167**, 155–158.

Hengge, U.R., Esser, S., Schultewolter, T. *et al.* (1999) Self-administered topical 5% imiquimod for the treatment of common warts and mollusca contagiosa. In: *5th Congress German–Japanese Society of Dermatology, Marburg, Book of Abstracts*, p. 18.

Holland, T.T., Weber, C.B. & James, W.D. (1992) Tender periungual nodules. *Archives of Dermatology* **128**, 105–110.

Kersey, P.J.W. (1988) The cold injury response. Natural history and modification by clobetasol propionate in human subjects. Presented at the British Dermatological Surgery Group at the BAD Meeting, London.

Kuflik, E. (1984) Cryosurgical treatment of periungual warts. *Journal of Dermatologic Surgery and Oncology* **10**, 673–676.

Kumar, B., Sharma, S.C. & Kaur, S. (1980) Phalangeal erosions with subungual warts. *Indian Journal of Dermatology and Venereology* **46**, 166–168.

Lee, A.N. & Mallory, S.B. (1999) Contact immunotherapy with squaric acid dibutylester for the treatment of recalcitrant warts. *Journal of the American Academy of Dermatology* **41**, 595–599.

Litt, J.Z. (1978) Don't excise—exorcise. Treatment for subungual and periungual warts. *Cutis* **22**, 327–333.

McCown, H., Thiers, B., Cook, J. *et al.* (1999) Global nail dystrophy associated with HPV type 57 infection. *British Journal of Dermatology* **141**, 731–735.

Miller, R.A.W. (1984) Nail dystrophy following intralesional injections of bleomycin for a periungual wart. *Archives of Dermatology* **120**, 963–964.

Munn, S.E., Higgins, E., Marshall, M. & Clement, M. (1996) A new method of intralesional bleomycin therapy in the treatment of recalcitrant warts. *British Journal of Dermatology* **135**, 969–971.

Olbright, S.M., Stern, R.S., Tang, S.V. *et al.* (1987) Complications of cutaneous laser surgery, a survey. *Archives of Dermatology* **123**, 345–349.

Orrechia, G., Douville, H., Santagostino, L. *et al.* (1988) Treatment of multiple relapsing warts with diphencyprone. *Dermatologica* **177**, 225–231.

Plewig, G., Christophers, E. & Braun-Falco, O. (1973) Mutilierende subunguale Warzen: Abheilung durch Methortrexat. *Hautarzt* **24**, 338–341.

Ross, B.S., Levine, V.J., Nehal, K. *et al.* (1999) Pulsed dye laser treatment for warts: an update. *Dermatologic Surgery* **25**, 277–380.

Samman, P.D. (1979) The nails. In: *Textbook of Dermatology*, 3rd edn (eds A. Rook, D.S. Wilkinson, & F.J.G. Ebling), pp. 1838–1844. Blackwell Scientific Publications, Oxford.

Scully, C. & Assad, A. (1984) Mucinous syringometaplasia. *Journal of the American Academy of Dermatology* **11**, 503–508.

Shah, S.S., Kothari, U.R., Dhoshi, H.V., Bhat, A.C. & Bhalodia, G.C. (1976) Erosion of phalanx by subungual wart. *Indian Journal of Dermatology, Venereology and Leprosy* **42**, 185–186.

Shapiro, L., Flushing, N.Y. & Stoller, N.M. (1961) Erosion of phalanges by subungual warts, report of a case. *Journal of the American Medical Association* **176**, 379.

Shelley, W.B. (1972) *Consultations in Dermatology*, p. 13. W.B. Saunders, Philadelphia.

Shelley, W.B. & Shelley, E.D. (1991) Intralesional bleomycin sulfate therapy for warts: a novel bifurcated needle puncture technique. *Archives of Dermatology* **127**, 234–236.

Shumer, S.M. & O'Keefe, E.J. (1983) Bleomycin in the treatment of recalcitrant warts. *Journal of the American Academy of Dermatology* **9**, 91–96.

Street, M.L. & Roenigk, R.K. (1990) Recalcitrant periungual verrucae: the role of carbon dioxide laser vaporization. *Journal of the American Academy of Dermatology* **23**, 115–120.

Tanenbaum, M.H. (1971) Onychodystrophy after topically applied fluorouracil for warts. *Archives of Dermatology* **103**, 225–226.

Tkach, J.R. (1989) Finding and inventing alternative therapies. How I do it. *Dermatologic Clinics* **7**, 1–18.

Urbina-Gonzales, F., Cristobal-Gil, M. & Aguilar Martinez, A. (1986) Cutaneous toxicity of intralesional bleomycin administration in the treatment of periungual warts. *Archives of Dermatology* **122**, 974–975.

Van der Velden, E.M., Ijsselmuiden, O.E., Drost, B.H. *et al.* (1997) Dermatography with bleomycin as a new treatment for verrucae vulgares. *International Journal of Dermatology* **36**, 145–150.

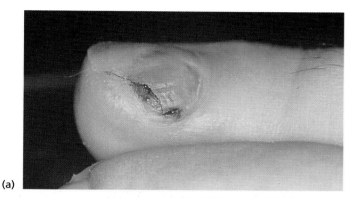

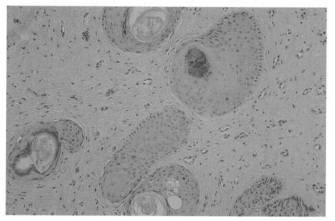

**Fig. 11.5** (a) Syringoma—involvement of the lateral nail bed. (Courtesy of V. Blatière, Montpellier, France.) (b) Syringoma—histology.

Wiesner-Menzel, L. & Happle, R. (1984) Rückbildung von Plantarwarzen nach Behandlung mit Diphencyprone. *Zeitschrift für Hautkrankheiten* **59**, 1080–1083.

Yazar, S. & Basaran, E. (1994) Efficacy of silver nitrate pencils in the treatment of common warts. *Journal of Dermatology* **21**, 329–333.

Yilmaz, E., Alpsoy, E. & Basaran, E. (1996) Cimetidine therapy for warts: a placebo-controlled, double-blind study. *Journal of the American Academy of Dermatology* **34**, 1005–1007.

Zepeda del Villar, J.M. (1994) Cimetidina en el tratamiento de verrugas vulgares. *Dermatologic Reviews of Mexico* **38**, 202–203.

## Syringoma

Syringoma has been reported in the great toe nail bed of a 40-year-old woman presenting with subungual hyperkeratosis and onycholysis following trauma resulting in subungual haematoma. After partial nail avulsion a tumour was discovered, adjacent to the lateral nail fold. Histology showed small tumour islands with duct lumina (Blatière *et al.* 1999) (Fig. 11.5).

## Reference

Blatière, V., Baran, R., Barnéon, G. & Perrin, C. (1999) A syringoma of the big toenail. *Journal of the European Academy of Dermatology and Venereology* **12** (Suppl. 2), S128.

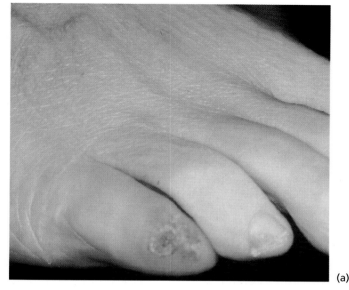

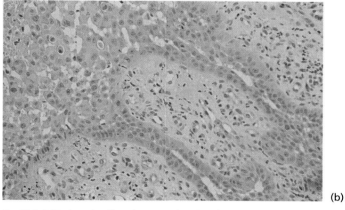

**Fig. 11.6** (a) Eccrine syringofibroadenoma involving the 5th toenail apparatus. (b) Histology of case in (a). (Courtesy of J. Mascaro-Barcelona, Spain.)

## Eccrine syringofibroadenoma (Fig. 11.6)

Clear cell syringofibroadenoma of Mascaró (1963) may present as a keratotic tumour of the nail bed. The first case was found in a man aged 61 and located in the fifth right toenail (Iranzo *et al.* 1999), the second case (Fouilloux *et al.* 2001) was observed in the left ring finger nail in a 71-year-old woman suffering from pain in her finger, occasionally radiating to the wrist and intensifying with pressure. Clinically a 2-mm-wide band ending with horny splinters was seen. Partial nail avulsion displayed keratotic filaments and red granulation tissue. The lesion was successfully removed by curettage. Histology showed anastomosing thin epithelial strands extending from the epithelium of the nail bed into the dermis. The spaces between the strands were filled with fibrovascular stroma. On the superficial level the stroma had a mucoid appearance. The anastomosing cords were made up of cells that were small, cuboidal with a round deeply basophilic nuclueus and scant cytoplasm. Several foci within the tumour showed nests of cells with abundant clear cytoplasm. In places, they formed duct-like structures with amorphous contents. The clear cells stained positively both with colloidal iron and alcian blue.

Periungual involvement of the great toe was shown in one of three cases of familial eccrine syringofibroadenomatosis. The skin appeared fissured and hyperkeratotic (Chen *et al.* 1998).

It is not clear whether solitary eccrine syringofibroadenoma is a true adnexal tumour or a reactive lesion (French 1997).

Eccrine syringofibroadenomatosis may involve the periungual tissues in association with multiple congenital abnormalities (Bell & Guérin 2000).

## References

Bell, H.K. & Guérin, D.M. (2000) Eccrine syringofibroadenomatosis in association with multiple congenital abnormalities. A new inherited syndrome. In: *Poster Abstract Book. AAD 58th meeting, March 10–15, 2000*, poster 137.

Chen, S., Palay, D. & Templeton, S.F. (1998) Familial eccrine syringofibroadenomatosis with associated ophthalmologic abnormalities. *Journal of the American Academy of Dermatology* **39**, 356–358.

Fouilloux, B., Dutoit, M., Cambazard, F. & Perrin, C. (2001) Clear cell syringofibroadenoma (of Mascaró) of the nail. *British Journal of Dermatology* **144**, 625–627.

French, L.E. (1997) Reactive eccrine syringofibroadenoma: an emerging subtype. *Dermatology* **195**, 309–310.

Iranzo, P., Fouilloux, B., Palou, J. *et al.* (1999) Tumor sudoríparo del aparato ungueal? Siringofibroadenoma? Poster, Barcelona.

Mascaró, J.M. (1963) Considérations sur les tumeurs fibroépithéliales: le syringofibradénome eccrine. *Annales de Dermatologie et de Syphiligraphie* **9**, 143–153.

## Eccrine poroma (Fig. 11.7)

Eccrine poroma is a benign proliferation most common on the non-hairy parts of the foot. This tumour reaches 1–3 cm in diameter, is always single, pink, soft and grows slowly. Typically, it is superficial, often protruding or sessile, but occasionally, it may project into the dermis. It may invade the nail bed and elevate the plate (Zaias 1990). When surrounding the nail, the distal phalanx appears enlarged and the nail destroyed (Arenas 1987). Two subungual eccrine poromas in female patients were described by Goettmann *et al.* (1995). The primary diagnosis was pyogenic granuloma since the lesions were pedunculated and one tended to bleed easily. Differential diagnosis includes pyogenic granuloma, amelanotic melanoma, wart, histiocytoma, and carcinoma. Eccrine angiomatous hamartoma (Gabrielsen *et al.* 1991) presents as a painful tumour under the nail (Sammartin *et al.* 1992; Haneke 1993) or on the dorsal aspect of the distal phalanx, the latter led to its amputation (Gabrielsen *et al.* 1991).

Treatment consists of surgical excision of the tumour.

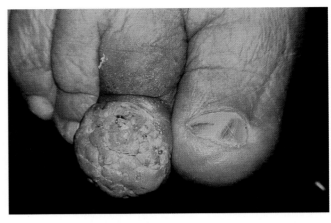

(a)

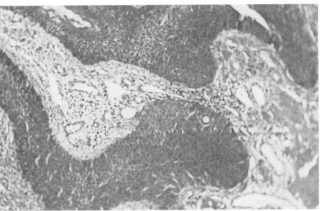

(b)

**Fig. 11.7** (a) Eccrine poroma. (Courtesy of R. Arenas, Mexico DF.) (b) Eccrine poroma—histology. (Courtesy of S. Goettmann-Bonvallot, Paris.)

## References

Arenas, R. (1987) *Dermatología, Atlas, Diagnostico y Tratamiento*, pp. 539–540. McGraw Hill, Mexico.

Gabrielsen, T.O., Elgjo, K. & Sommerschild, H. (1991) Eccrine angiomatous hamartoma of the finger leading to amputation. *Clinical and Experimental Dermatology* **16**, 44–45.

Goettmann, S., Marinho, E., Grossin, M. & Bélaich, S. (1995) Porome eccrine sous-unguéal. A propos de deux observations. *Annales de Dermatologie et de Vénéréologie* **122** (Suppl. 1), S147–S148.

Haneke, E. (1993) Neuro-arterio-syringeal hamartoma in subungual location. In: *14th Congress of the International Society of Dermatological Surgery, Sevilla, 1–4 October 1993, Book of Abstracts*, p. 85.

Sammartin, O., Botella, R., Alegre, V. *et al.* (1992) Congenital eccrine angiomatous harmatoma. *American Journal of Dermatopathology* **14**, 161–164.

Zaias, N. (1990) *The Nail in Health and Disease*, p. 120. Appleton & Lange, Norwalk, CN.

## Porokeratotic eccrine and dermal duct naevus

See p. 531.

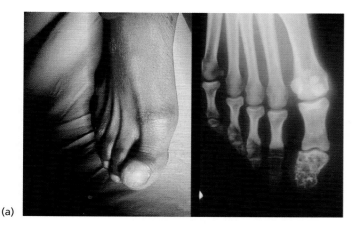

(a)

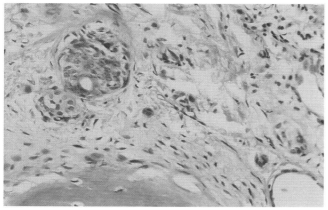

(b)

**Fig. 11.8** (a) Chondroid syringoma. (Courtesy of C.A. Barreto.) (b) Histology of case in (a).

## Chondroid syringoma (Fig. 11.8)

The case of a 25-year-old black woman with a deformed right hallux was reported by Barreto *et al.* (1994). X-ray examination revealed lytic changes in the distal phalanx with reduced technetium uptake on bone scan. The amputation specimen showed a chondroid syringoma of the subungual tissue penetrating and permeating the underlying bone.

Histology revealed an appendageal tumour containing nests of small cuboidal cells and myxoid stroma.

## Reference

Barreto, C.A., Lipton, M.N., Smith, H.B. & Potter, G.K. (1994) Intraosseous chondroid syringoma of the hallux. *Journal of the American Academy of Dermatology* 30, 374–378.

## Distal digital keratoacanthoma (Fig. 11.9)

Subungual and periungual keratoacanthomas (KA) may occur as solitary or multiple tumours. It is a rare benign, but rapidly growing, seemingly aggressive tumour usually situated below the edge of the nail plate or in the most distal portion of the nail bed. Multiple subungual KAs without KAs on other sites are exceptional (Haneke 1991). Many cases have been reported in the literature (Ronchese 1970; Stoll 1980; Cramer 1981; Keeney *et al.* 1988); however, the diagnosis was not definitely confirmed in all cases (Stoll 1980) since many lesions were inadequately biopsied and others persisted for more than 1 year. We have followed 12 patients (Baran & Goettmann 1998). The distal phalanx of the toe was affected in three cases. Spontaneous resolution occurred in one patient. One other recurred after surgery.

Keratoacanthoma is said to arise from hair follicle epithelium, but there are no hair follicles in the subungual and periungual regions; this may be seen as a hint to the close relationship between hair follicle and nail apparatus and explains why some cases may be interpreted as oncholemmal cysts (E. Grosshans, personal communication) (Fig. 11.10).

The lesion may start as a small and painful keratotic nodule visible beneath the free edge, growing rapidly to a one to two centimetre lesion within 4–8 weeks. Its typical gross appearance, as a dome-shaped nodule with a central plug of horny material filling the crater, is not often seen subungually although histology of an adequate biopsy specimen will clearly show the characteristic pattern (Table 11.1). Less frequently the tumour grows out from under the proximal nail fold, which becomes inflamed, and may cover or surround it with a cushion of swollen tissue (Gonzales-Ensenat *et al.* 1988). Spontaneous regression is rare in this area (Van Vloten 1991). The tumour soon erodes the bone and this may be demonstrated radiologically as a fairly well-defined crescent-shaped lytic defect of tuft adjacent to the overlying nail bed (Lovett *et al.* 1995; Haneke *et al.* 1998). Reconstitution of the bony defect can be expected (Levy *et al.* 1985; Pellegrini & Tompkins 1986).

*Magnetic resonance imaging (MRI) may help depict a deep infiltrating lesion of the distal nail bed. MRI is superior to X-ray in detection of an erosion of the distal phalanx. Images show a large nodule with an homogeneous signal (intermediate signal on T1-weighted images and high signal on T2-weighted images). Intravenous injection of gadolinium provides strong peripheral enhancement. A central area of low signal indicates a central plug of horny material filling the crater (Fig. 11.11). The limits may be ill-defined by oedema in the surrounding tissues.*

A case of multiple familial keratoacanthoma (Hilker & Winterscheidt 1987) showed no tendency toward spontaneous involution in contrast to the case of Mittal *et al.* (1984) associated with polyarthritis. Multiple keratoacanthomas may appear in patients on cyclosporin (Guillot *et al.* 1990) and suramin (Kobayashi *et al.* 1996). Histologically perineural invasion in keratoacanthoma may be a risk factor for recurrence (Wagner *et al.* 1987).

Whether trauma (Ronchese 1970) or exposure to steel wool (Fisher 1990) plays a role in the evolution of subungual keratoacanthoma remains uncertain.

Diagnosis of distal digital keratoacanthoma depends on the rapid growth, with bone erosion and characteristic histology.

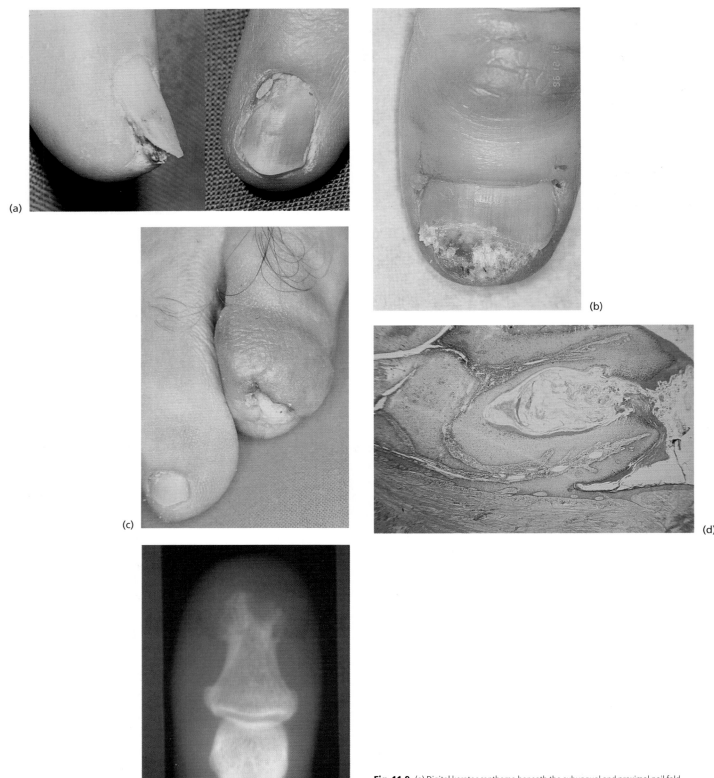

**Fig. 11.9** (a) Digital keratoacanthoma beneath the subungual and proximal nail fold. (b) Distal digital keratoacanthoma involving hyponychium and distal nail bed. (c) Distal digital keratoacanthoma affecting the ventral aspect. (d) Typical histology. (e) Crescent-shaped lytic defect of the tuft. (Courtesy of J. Mascaro, Spain.)

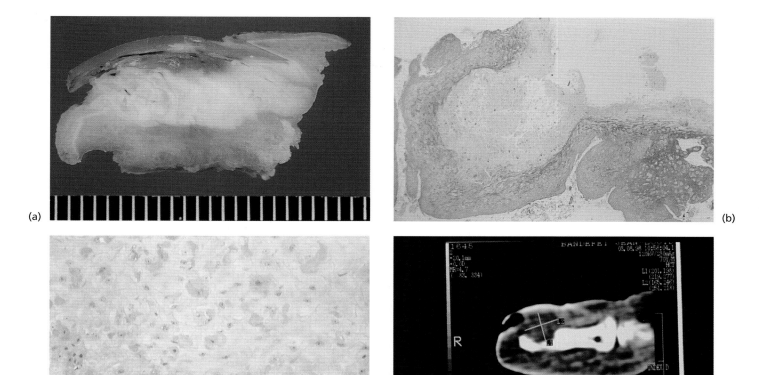

**Fig. 11.10** (a) Proliferating onycholemmal cyst after surgery. (b, c) Histology of case in (a). (d) MRI of case in (a). (Courtesy of Billing & Grosshans, Strasbourg.) (d) MRI shows a large lytic lesion beneath the nail.

**Table 11.1** Difference between keratoacanthoma (KA) on the skin and under the nails. (Adapted from Stoll 1980.)

| | KA on skin | Subungual KA |
| --- | --- | --- |
| Growth direction | More horizontal | More vertical |
| Infiltrate | Many neutrophils and eosinophils | Less neutrophils and eosinophils, no fibrosis at base |
| Bone erosion | Usually none | Rapid |
| Duration | 9–12 months | Longer if not treated |
| Spontaneous regression | Frequent | Infrequent |
| Symptoms | No pain | Pain |

Its clinical differentiation from squamous cell carcinoma is nevertheless difficult (Table 11.2) (Shapiro & Baraf 1970; Bräuninger & Hoede 1986).

Histopathology of subungual keratoacanthoma differs slightly from that of the skin. In this particular location, the tumour is more narrow but deeply infiltrating. It shows a marked shoulder with an epidermal lip, a central crater filled with keratin and the tumour cells are large, pale and often develop keratohyalin granules. This feature corresponds with filaggrin expression as revealed by immunohistochemistry. However, neither involucrin, cytokeratin and filaggrin expression nor staining for the lectin peanut agglutinin (PNA) allow differentiation of keratoacanthoma from subungual squamous cell carcinoma. Their staining is too variable. An antibody directed against transforming growth factor (TGF-α) was shown to give different staining patterns in keratoacanthoma and squamous cell carcinoma (Ho *et al.* 1991), but further studies are needed to establish its discriminating value. Demonstration of markers such as p53, PCNA and Ki1 gives a more peripheral staining in KA than in squamous cell carcinoma, but this again is not a safe differential diagnostic feature (Schulze & Haneke, unpublished data).

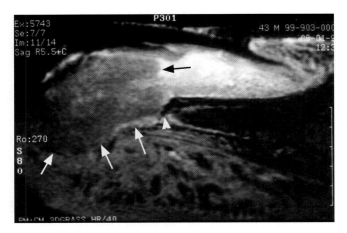

**Fig. 11.11** Keratoacanthoma (arrows). MR sagittal gradient echo image after injection of gadolinium. Note the osteolysis of the distal phalanx (arrowhead).

**Table 11.2** Differentiation between subungual keratoacanthoma and squamous cell carcinoma (adapted from Norton 1980).

|  | Subungual KA | Subungual carcinoma |
| --- | --- | --- |
| Sex | M > F | M > F |
| Age (year) | 35–65 | 60–80 |
| Incidence | Very rare | Relatively common |
| Growth rate | Rapid | Slow |
| Duration of symptoms | Short | Long |
| History of trauma | Rarely | Sometimes |
| Tumour mass | Always present | Often not present |
| Bone invasion | Early | Late |
| Radiography | Bone erosion | Late bone destruction |
| Mutiple tumours | Common | Rare |

### Treatment of keratoacanthoma

Management of subungual KA ranges from conservative local excision to amputation, but aggressive ablative surgery as the initial intervention for this benign condition has probably occurred due to either misdiagnosis or misinterpretation of the nature of the pathology.

The treatment of choice is removal of the entire tumour with histological control of the resection margins. The patient should then be followed for an adequate period of time to rule out a recurrence since subungual keratoacanthoma has been reported to recur as late as 22 months (Scarini *et al.* 1983). Mohs' micrographic surgery may be used as has been advocated by Moreno-Gimenez *et al.* (1987). Pellegrini and Tompkins (1986) reviewed 18 cases reported in the literature revealing that 86% of the lesions treated by curettage were cured by eventual conservative amputation; this is strong evidence that curettage is not the adequate therapy for subungual KA. Further curettage or amputations of the distal phalanx, according to the amount of bone destruction and function ought then not to be necessary for a recurrence (Patel & Desai 1989).

Retinoids may be beneficial in keratoacanthoma (Yoshikawa *et al.* 1985), sometimes combined with surgical removal (Voigtländer & Baum 1990). Eruptive keratoacanthomas have responded to oral etretinate 1 mg/kg/day with complete resolution. Recurrence can occur after cessation of treatment, requiring maintenance therapy (10 mg on alternate days), however, this mode of treatment is more effective as prophylaxis in multiple keratoacanthoma. 5-Fluorouracil has also been used either injected into the lesion, or applied as a 20% ointment three times daily for 3–4 weeks (Bennet *et al.* 1985). Intralesional bleomycin may be tried in the distal nail area (Sayama & Tagami 1983), as well as methotrexate (Melton *et al.* 1991).

### References

Baran, R. & Goettmann, S. (1998) Distal digital keratoanthoma: a report of 12 cases and review of the literature. *British Journal of Dermatology* **139**, 512–515.

Bennet, R., Epstein, E. & Goette, D. (1985) Current management of keratoacanthoma using 5-FU. *Cutis* **36**, 218–236.

Bräuninger, W. & Hoede, N. (1986) Subunguales Keratoakanthom. *Hautarzt* **37**, 270–273.

Cramer, S.F. (1981) Subungual keratoacanthoma. A benign bone-eroding neoplasm of the distal phalanx. *American Journal of Clinical Pathology* **75**, 425–429.

Fisher, A.A. (1990) Subungual keratoacanthoma: possible relationship with exposure to steel wool. *Cutis* **46**, 26–28.

Gonzales-Ensenat, A., Vilalta, A. & Torras, H. (1988) Keratoacanthome péri et sous-unguéal. *Annales de Dermatologie et de Vénéréologie* **115**, 329–331.

Guillot, B., Fesneau, H., Mourad, G. *et al.* (1990) Kerato-acanthomes multiples sous ciclosporine. *Presse Medical* **19**, 1286.

Haneke, E. (1991) Multiple subungual keratoacanthomas. In: *XII International Congress of Dermatologic Surgery Munich*. *Zentralblatt für Haut- und Geschlechtskrankheiten* **159**, 337–338.

Haneke, E., Mainusch, O. & Hilker, O. (1998) Subunguale Tumoren: Keratoakanthom, Neurofibrom, Nagelbett-Melanom. *Zeitschrift für Dermatologie* **184**, 86–102.

Hilker, O. & Winterscheidt, M. (1987) Familiäre multiple Keratoakanthome. *Zeitschrift für Hautkrankheiten* **62**, 284–289.

Ho, T., Horn, T. & Finzi, E. (1991) Transforming growth factor α expression helps to distinguish keratoacanthomas from squamous cell carcinomas. *Archives of Dermatology* **127**, 1167–1171.

Keeney, G.L., Banks, P.M. & Linscheid, R.L. (1988) Subungual keratoacanthoma. Report of a case and review of the literature. *Archives of Dermatology* **124**, 1074–1076.

Kobayashi, K., Pezen, D.S. & Vogelzang, N.J. (1996) Keratoacanthomas and skin neoplasms associated with suramin therapy. *Archives of Dermatology* **132**, 96–98.

Levy, D.W., Bonakdarpour, A., Putong, P.B. *et al.* (1985) Subungual keratoacanthoma. *Skeletal Radiology* **13**, 287–290.

Lovett, J.A., Haines, T.A. & Bentz, M.L. (1995) Subungual keratoacanthoma masquerading as a chronic paronychia. *Plastic Surgery* **38**, 84–87.

Melton, J.L., Nelson, B.R., Stough, D.B. *et al.* (1991) Treatment of keratoacanthomas with intralesional methotrexate. *Journal of the American Academy of Dermatology* **25**, 1017–1023.

Mittal, R., Mittal, R.L., Chopra, A. *et al.* (1984) Polyarthritis with atypical keratotic nodular dermatosis or polyarthritis with multiple keratoacanthoma. *Dermatologica* **169**, 199–202.

Moreno-Gimenez, J.C., Lerma Puerta, E., Sanchez Conejo-Mir, J. *et al.* (1987) Queratoacantoma subungual. *Acta Dermato-Sifilitica* **78**, 561–564.

Patel, M.R. & Desai, S.S. (1989) Subungual keratoacanthoma in the hand. *Journal of Hand Surgery* **14A**, 139–142.

Pellegrini, V.D. & Tompkins, A. (1986) Management of subungual keratoacanthoma. *Journal of Hand Surgery* **11A**, 718–724.

Ronchese, F. (1970) Subungual keratoacanthoma. *Chronic Dermatology* **1**, 3–4.

Sayama, S. & Tagami, H. (1983) Treatment of keratoacanthoma with intralesional bleomycin. *British Journal of Dermatology* **109**, 449–452.

Scarini, P., Ghigi, G., Bertarelli, C. *et al.* (1983) Subungual keratoacanthoma. A variant of verrucous squamous cell carcinoma of the skin. *Applied Pathology* **1**, 339–342.

Shapiro, L. & Baraf, C.S. (1970) Subungual epidermoid carcinoma and keratoacanthoma. *Cancer* **25**, 141–152.

Stoll, D.M. (1980) Subungual keratoacanthoma. *American Journal of Dermatopathology* **2**, 265–271.

Van Vloten, W. (1991) Subungual keratoacanthoma. Case presented at the Annual Meeting of the Collegium Dermato-Pathologicum Unna-Darier, Graz, Austria.

Voigtländer, V. & Baum, C. (1990) Destruierendes subunguales Keratoakanthom: Erhaltung der Endphalanx durch kombinierte operative und medikamentöse Therapie. *Zeitschrift für Hautkrankheiten* **66** (Suppl. 3), 110–111.

Wagner, R.F., Cottel, W.I. & Smoller, B.K. (1987) Perineural invasion associated with recurrent sporadic multiple self-healing squamous carcinomas. *Archives of Dermatology* **123**, 1275–1276.

Yoshikawa, K., Hirano, S. & Kato, T. (1985) A case of eruptive keratoacanthoma treated by oral etretinate. *British Journal of Dermatology* **112**, 579–583.

## Distal digital incontinentia pigmenti tumours (Fig. 11.12)

Incontinentia pigmenti (IP), or Bloch-Sulzberger syndrome, is a multi-organ disease with an X-linked dominant inheritance which affects females and usually is lethal in males. Independent sporadic cases resembling X-autosomal translocations involving the same X-chromosome breakpoint have been reported but recent DNA probes have failed to confirm this localisation (Harris *et al.* 1988).

There are three clinical stages of skin changes: a linear erythemato-vesiculous and bullous reaction which is present at birth is followed by a second stage of verrucous lesions which gradually disappear. The third stage is characterized by a splashed or whorled pigmentation in a pattern which follows Blaschko's lines.

From 15 to 30 years of age, painful subungual keratotic tumours (Piñol-Aguadé *et al.* 1973; Mascaró *et al.* 1985; Simmons *et al.* 1986; Adeniran *et al.* 1993) or warty periungual tumours (Moss & Ince 1987) can appear as a manifestation of IP. It is usually the fingers which are involved; but warty brownish growths arranged linearly along the great toes have been observed (El-Benhawi & George 1988). The keratotic sub-

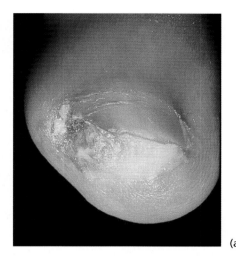

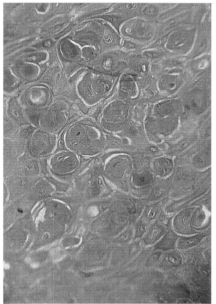

**Fig. 11.12** (a) Subungual incontinentia pigmenti tumour. (b) Dyskeratotic cells of case in (a). (Courtesy of J. Mascaro, Spain.)

ungual mass produces dystrophy or simple onycholysis of the nail which is displaced from its bed. Erythema and swelling of the finger tip are found at the border of the lesion. The tumour may be localized only on the proximal subungual area leading to the destruction of a portion of the nail plate, or the fold with tender swellings which are smooth proximally and warty distally (Moss & Ince 1987). The tumours destroy the distal bony phalanx. They may disappear spontaneously after several months leaving a 2 mm scar on the pulp just under the free edge of the nail at the site of a warty lesion (Moss & Ince 1987). Hartman and Danville (1976) reported the case of a 30-year-old woman with painful subungual tumours from the age of 20 years. The keratotic lesions resulted in nail dystrophy and scalloped bone deformities of the terminal phalanges of the fingers. Regression followed pregnancy on two occasions. Eight fingernails and one toenail were affected over a 20-year period in a female who developed her first lesion at 16 years of age (Hermanns & Piérard 1986).

Histological examination of the tumours shows a verrucous or pseudoepitheliomatous hyperplasia of the epidermis with hyperkeratosis and hypergranulosis where dyskeratotic cells are found at all levels thus resembling the second stage of IP development. Differential diagnoses include warts, epidermoid cysts, subungual fibromas, squamous cell carcinoma and above all keratoacanthoma which is clinically and histologically indistinguishable (Baran & Goettmann 1998). Despite possible self healing, the patient asks for treatment because of the intense pain (Nurse 1979) and disability. Management by desiccation and curettage or surgical excision are usually successful but permanent nail atrophy may occur. A course of systemic retinoids should be considered despite possible recurrence (Bessems et al. 1988). Malvehy et al. (1998) gave 1 mg etretinate /kg bodyweight and produced a rapid response with resolution of pain and marked reduction of the lesion including improvement of the bony alterations and nail deformity.

## References

Adeniran, A., Townsend, P.L.G. & Peachey, R.D.G. (1993) Incontinentia pigmenti (Bloch–Sulzberger syndrome) manifesting as painful periungual and subungual tumours. *Journal of Hand Surgery* **18B**, 667–669

Baran, R. & Goettmann, S. (1998) Distal digital keratoacanthoma: a report of 12 cases and a review of the literature. *British Journal of Dermatology* **139**, 512–515.

Bessems, P.J.M., Jagtman, B.A. & Van de Staak, W. (1988) Progressive, persistent, hyperkeratotic lesions in incontinentia pigmenti. *Archives of Dermatology* **124**, 29–30.

El-Benhawi, M.O. & George, W.M. (1988) Incontinentia pigmenti. A review. *Cutis* **41**, 259–262.

Hartman, D.L. & Danville, P.A. (1976) Incontinentia pigmenti associated with subungual tumours. *Archives of Dermatology* **112**, 535–542.

Harris, A., Shelley, L., Haan, E. et al. (1988) The gene for incontinentia pigmenti: failure of linkage studies using DNA probes to confirm cytogenetic localization. *Clinical Genetics* **34**, 1–6.

Hermanns, J.F. & Piérard, G.E. (1986) Onychodystrophie hypertrophique de l'incontinentia pigmenti. *Nouvelle Dermatologie* **5**, 421.

Malvehy, J., Palou, J. & Mascaró, J.M. (1998) Painful subungual tumour in incontinentia pigmenti. Response to treatment with etretinate. *British Journal of Dermatology* **138**, 554–555.

Mascaró, J.M., Palou, J. & Vives, P. (1985) Painful subungual keratotic tumors in incontinentia pigmenti. *Journal of the American Academy of Dermatology* **13**, 913–918.

Moss, C. & Ince, P. (1987) Anhidrotic and achromians lesions in incontinentia pigmenti. *British Journal of Dermatology* **116**, 839–849.

Nurse, D.S. (1979) Help-wanted: incontinentia pigmenti. *Schoch Letter* **29**, 3.

Piñol-Aguadé, J.P., Mascaró, J.M., Herrero, C. & Castel, T. (1973) Tumeurs sous-unguéales dyskératosiques douloureuses et spontanément résolutives: ses rapports avec l'incontinentia pigmenti. *Annales de Dermatologie et de Syphiligraphie* **100**, 159–168.

Simmons, D.A., Kegel, M.F., Scher, R.K. et al. (1986) Subungual tumors in incontinentia pigmenti. *Archives of Dermatology* **122**, 1431–1434.

## Subungual papilloma

Subungual papillomas were briefly reviewed by Heller (1927) who stressed that papilloma is only a descriptive term and does not define a single entity. The history and morphology appears to vary in almost every case. Subungual papillomatosis may be seen in systemic amyloidosis.

## Reference

Heller, J. (1927) Die Krankheiten der Nägel. In: *Handbuch der Haut und Geschlechtskrankheiten*, pp. 150–172. Bd VIII/2 (ed. J. Jadassohn). Spezielle Dermatologie, S.

## Subungual linear keratotic melanonychia
(Baran & Perrin 1999) (Fig. 11.13)

Longitudinal melanonychia displaying features of keratininzed acanthoma is described in two patients. In both cases, a pigmented band consisting of a subungual keratinized epithelial ridge originates in the nail bed. The origin of the pigment is linked to its synthesis within the acanthoma of the nail bed. Interestingly, these lesions are reminiscent of pigmented seborrhoeic keratoses.

## Reference

Baran, R. & Perrin, C. (1999) Linear melanonychia due to subungual keratosis of the nail bed: a report of two cases. *British Journal of Dermatology* **140**, 730–733.

## Localized multinucleate distal subungual keratosis
(Baran & Perrin 1995) (Fig. 11.14)

Distal subungual keratosis with occasional dyskeratotic cells is a small horny lesion originating from the hyponychium region, resembling a form fruste of distal subungual fibrokeratoma. It may be followed clinically and histologically as far as the lunula and is well demonstrated by MRI. This condition belongs to the group of onychopapillomas of the nail bed.

## Reference

Baran, R. & Perrin, C. (1995) Localised multinucleate distal subungual keratosis. *British Journal of Dermatology* **133**, 77–82.

## Onychopapilloma of the nail bed (associated with longitudinal erythronychia) (Baran & Perrin 2000)
(Figs 11.15 & 11.16)

We have biopsied longitudinal erythronychia in 16 subjects

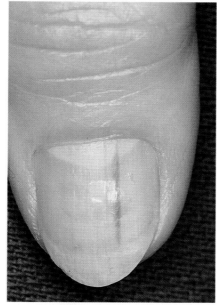

(a)

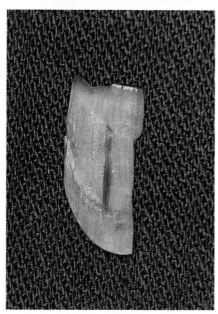

(b)

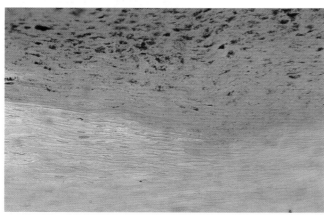

(c)

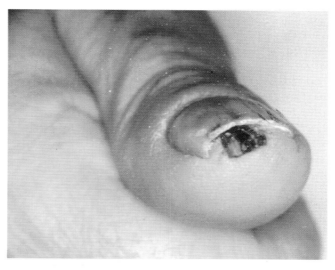

**Fig. 11.14** Distal subungual keratotis with multinucleation. (Courtesy of A. Villaneva, Valencia, Spain.)

showing an onychopapilloma in 14 cases and SCC in the remaining two. Shared clinical features in addition to erythronychia (or sometimes an interrupted line made up of splinter haemorrhages) were typically a longitudinal marked ridge of the nail bed expanded at the distal nail bed as subungual keratosis and associated localised onycholysis. In all cases of 'onychopapilloma' nail bed acanthosis and papillomatosis was evident, and was combined with a keratogenous zone identical to the nail matrix. In addition, we found multinucleate giant cells in four onychopapillomas. In two cases, dysplasia amounting to squamous cell carcinoma *in situ* was found in the absence of any other diagnosis or as a part of Darier's disease. We have therefore suggested that the term 'localized, distal, subungual keratosis with multinucleate cells' should be replaced by 'onychopapilloma' (nail producing papilloma). The presentation of SCC in this pattern has not been previously reported.

### Reference

Baran, R. & Perrin, C. (2000) Longitudinal erythronychia with distal subungual keratosis. Onychopapilloma of the nail bed and Bowen's disease. *British Journal of Dermatology* **143**, 132–135.

**Subungual warty dyskeratoma** (Higashi 1990; Baran & Perrin 1997) (Fig. 11.17)

Longitudinal erythronychia was the presenting sign of Higashi's patient (1990).

A longitudinal reddish ridge was seen in the left third finger nail of a 73-year-old man. Originating in the lunula, it was

**Fig. 11.13** (left) (a) Subungual linear keratotic melanonychia. (b) Ventral aspect of the avulsed portion of the nail plate. (c) Histology of the keratotic lesion.

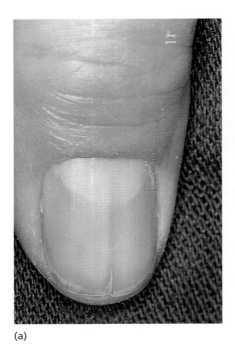

(a)

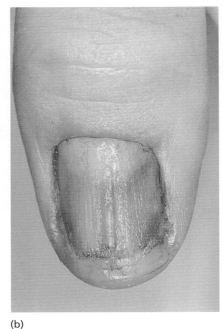

(b)

**Fig. 11.15** (a) Longitudinal erythronychia with onychopapilloma of the nail bed. (b) After nail avulsion the linear subungual papilloma is visible.

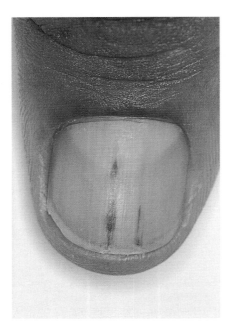

**Fig. 11.16** Double interrupted longitudinal lines made up of splinter haemorrhages with double subungual papilloma.

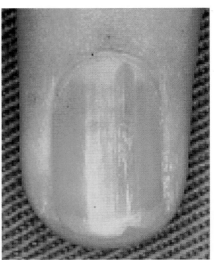

(a)

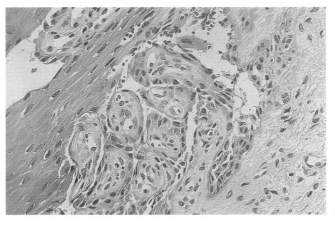

(b)

bordered by splinter haemorrhages and eventually caused a red line. The nail plate was slightly fissured at its free margin. Nail avulsion revealed a longitudinal ridge in the nail bed. Histology showed nail bed papillomatosis with long thin digitations penetrating the underlying connective tissue almost horizontally. Numerous multinucleate cells were seen. A crateriform impres-

**Fig. 11.17** (right) (a) Longitudinal erythronychia caused by warty dyskeratoma. (b) Histology in the hyponychium area. (Courtesy of N. Higashi, Osaka, Japan.)

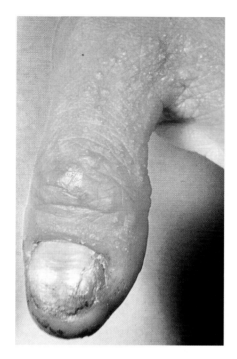

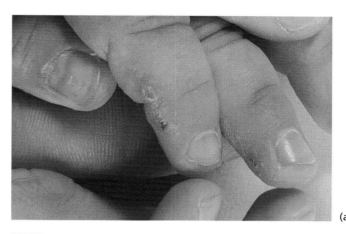

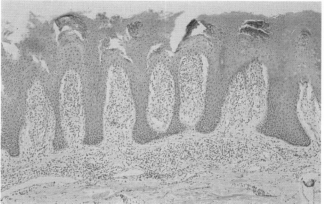

**Fig. 11.18** Verrucous epidermal naevus.

**Fig. 11.19** (a) Inflammatory linear verrucous naevus (ILVEN). (Courtesy of A.J. Landwehr.) (b) ILVEN-marked dermal chronic inflammatory changes.

sion existed at the hyponychium with epithelial digitations containing dyskeratotic cells, corps ronds and grains as well as suprabasal acantholysis (Baran & Perrin 1997). Almost identical lesions, but not as focal as in this case, can be seen in dyskeratosis follicularis of Darier.

## References

Baran, R. & Perrin, C. (1997) Focal subungual warty dyskeratoma. *Dermatology* **195**, 278–280.

Higashi, N. (1990) Focal acantholytic dyskeratosis. *Hifu* **32**, 507–510.

## Verrucous epidermal naevus (Fig. 11.18)

Involvement of the distal phalanx and nails by verrucous epidermal naevi is rare. They may be congenital or late onset lesions. The history and linear arrangement usually enable easy differentiation from extensive warts.

Verrucous epidermal naevi are as a rule asymptomatic, except for examples when they impinge upon the proximal nail fold, where they may cause recurrent paronychia and distort the nail (Atherton 1998).

Involvement of the nail bed causes ridging, splitting, discoloration or dystrophy. Any linear verrucous epidermal naevus whether with or without granular degeneration (epidermolytic hyperkeratosis) may affect the nail.

Differential diagnosis includes lichen striatus and inflammatory linear verrucous epidermal naevus (Fig. 11.19).

Histopathology shows papillomatosis with hyperkeratosis giving a wart-like appearance. However, HPV-characteristic cytopathic effects are lacking. In the matrix and nail bed, the typical epithelium is no longer discernible and the verrucous naevus does not produce a normal nail plate.

A clinically similar aspect was seen in a 3-year-old girl with a *porokeratotic eccrine duct naevus* affecting the periungual skin of her fifth right toe (Vicente *et al.* 1998).

## References

Atherton, D.J. (1998) Naevi and other developmental defects. In: *Textbook of Dermatology*, 6th edn (eds R.H. Champion, J.L. Burton, D.A. Burns & S.M. Breathnach), pp. 523–526. Blackwell Science, Oxford.

Vicente, M.A., Baselga, E., Garcia-Puig, R. *et al.* (1998) Porokeratotic eccrine duct and hair follicle nevus. A familial case with systematized involvement. *Annales de Dermatologie et de Vénéréologie* **125** (Suppl. 1), S176.

## Keratin cysts (Figs 11.20–11.23)

Implantation epidermoid cyst (synonyms: keratin, squamous epithelial or traumatic cysts).

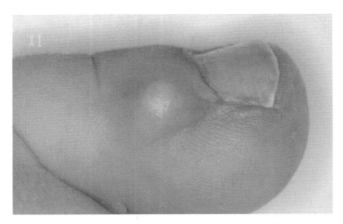

**Fig. 11.20** Postoperative implantation cyst in the posterolateral nail fold.

Epidermoid cysts in the tip of the digits are usually secondary to heavy or penetrating trauma, with implantation of epidermis into subcutaneous tissue or even into the bone; the trauma may have been long ago (even decades) or may not always be remembered. Post-operative epidermoid cysts may occur in the proximity of scars and often follow surgery for ingrown toenail (Baran & Bureau 1989; Challier *et al.* 1996). Persisting discomfort after surgery of the foot may warrant investigation by X-ray or MRI since an intraosseous epidermal inclusion cyst can be a late complication or an underlying condition (Berghs & Feyen 1998).

The distal phalanx gradually enlarges and clubbing becomes evident. Tenderness or pain are of late onset, result from compression of the bone and may eventually result in a fracture.

Shooting pain was described in one case, where there was soft tissue involvement alone (Yung & Estes 1980). Acquired pincer nail is an unusual presentation (Baran & Broutard 1989).

Differential diagnosis comprises virtually all lesions, both reactive and neoplastic, that can cause swelling of the terminal phalanx (Kasdan *et al.* 1991).

Phalangeal intraosseous epidermoid cysts occur twice as frequently in men as in women and the left hand is more often affected than the right (Lerner & Southwick 1986). Pain and swelling of the terminal phalanx are the most frequent clinical signs. The lesion appears as a round, osteolytic zone embedded in the bone, without trabeculae and sclerosis (cf. enchondroma) or as a marginal defect of the cortical substance of bone (Drewes *et al.* 1985; Challier *et al.* 1996). The clinical and radiological differential diagnosis may be very difficult (Schajowicz *et al.* 1970). Rarely, the cyst may contain a penetrating foreign body (Samlaska & Hansen 1992).

*Early in the disease, the bone erosion is absent or subtle and not visible on radiographs. MRI shows a regular mass with homogeneous or slightly heterogeneous content and intermediate signal on T1- and T2-weighted images. A heterogeneous enhancement is noted after injection of gadolinium (Fig. 11.24). The thin epidermal layer is depicted as a regular rim with a high signal identical to that of normal epidermis. Bone erosions, even when subtle, are easily detected on axial images. The area of an old penetrating injury may be marked by dark artefacts on gradient echo images.*

*Inclusion cysts of the distal phalanx are the result of epithelium becoming buried in the bone following trauma. The epithelial cells continue to regenerate creating a cyst in the bone. As the cyst expands first medullary and cortical bone are eroded*

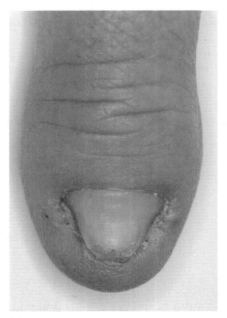

(a)

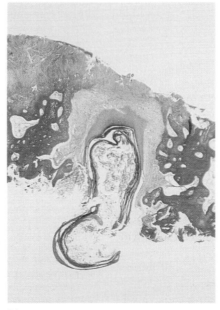

(b)

**Fig. 11.21** (a) Pincer nail deformity due to epidermoid cyst. (b) Intraosseous epidermoid cyst—histological changes.

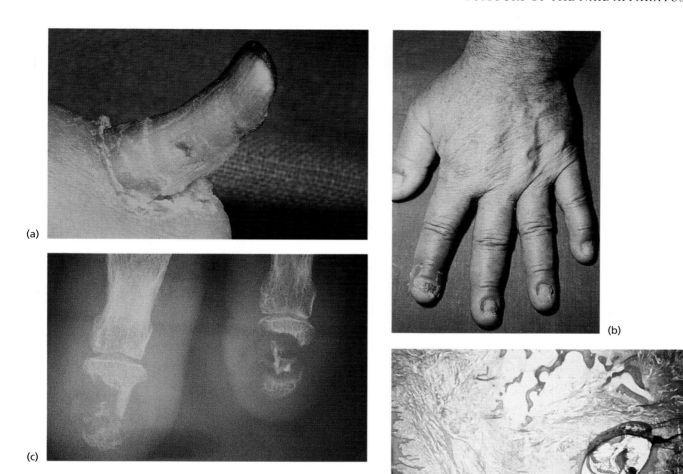

**Fig. 11.22** (a) Psoriatic nail horn. (b) After steroid treatment using dermo-jet. (c) X-ray showing distal bone destruction. (d) Histology demonstrating implantation cysts. (Courtesy of J. Mascaro, Spain.)

*creating a change of the dorsal surface of the distal phalanx and a resultant deformity of the nail bed and nail. Treatment is curettage of cyst and its lining allowing the defect to fill on its own or if it is large, medullary bone graft to fill the defect and give support to the nail bed.*

*Depending on the location of the cyst the surgical approach may be through a lateral incision or, as in the one shown, a fish-mouth incision around the tip of the finger laying the nail and matrix back to treat the cyst (Fig. 11.25).*

Histopathology shows a simple epidermoid cyst filled with orthokeratin and lined by a thin epidermis. However, if remnants of matrix epithelium were displaced into the subcutaneous tissue, the cyst may also contain areas exactly resembling 'tricholemmal' cyst epithelium (matrix cyst), but usually these cysts contain both epidermoid and onycholemmal lining

parts (Haneke 1983). These matrix or onycholemmal cysts are usually seen after inadequate wedge excision for ingrown toenails.

## References

Baran, R. & Broutard, J.C. (1989) Epidermoid cyst of the thumb presenting as a pincer nail. *Journal of the American Academy of Dermatology* **19**, 143–144.

Baran, R. & Bureau, H. (1989) Two post-operative epidermoid cysts following realignment of the hallux nail. *British Journal of Dermatology* **119**, 245–247.

Berghs, B. & Feyen, J. (1998) Intraosseous epidermal inclusion cyst following surgery for ingrowing toenail. *Foot* **8**, 138–140.

Challier, L., Binet, O., Baran, R., Levy, A., Beltzer-Garelly, E. & Revol, M. (1996) Kystes épidermoides d'implantation intra-osseuse de la

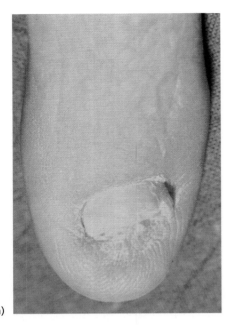

(a)

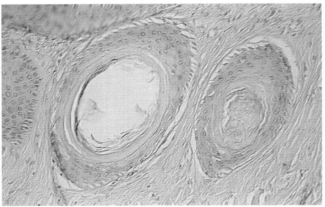

(b)

**Fig. 11.23** (a) Subungual epidermoid inclusion with distal dystrophic nail. (b) Histology of case in (a). Nail bed epithelial hyperplasia and dermal epidermoid. (Courtesy of P.A. Fanti & A. Tosti, Bologna, Italy.)

phalange distale des deux gros orteils. *Annales de Dermatologie et de Vénéréologie* **123**, 203–204.

Drewes, J., Günther, D. & Nolden, H.H. (1985) Intraossäre Epiderm-iszysten der Finger und Zehen. *Aktuelle Chirurgie* **20**, 171–177.

Haneke, E. (1983) Onycholemmal horn. *Dermatologica* **167**, 155–158.

Kasdan, M.L., Stutts, J.T., Kassan, M.A. & Clanton, J.N. (1991) Sebaceous gland carcinoma of the finger. *Journal of Hand Surgery* **16A**, 870–872.

Lerner, M.R. & Southwick, W.O. (1968) Keratin cysts in phalangeal bones. *Journal of Bone and Joint Surgery* **50A**, 365–372.

Samlaska, C.P. & Hansen, M.F. (1992) Intraosseous epidermoid cysts. *Journal of the American Academy of Dermatology* **27**, 454–455.

Schajowicz, F., Aiello, C.A. & Slullitel, I. (1970) Cystic and pseudo-cystic lesions of the terminal phalanx with special reference to epidermoid cyst. *Clinical Orthopedics and Related Research* **68**, 84–92.

Yung, W. & Estes, S.A. (1980) Subungual epidermal cyst. *Journal of the American Academy of Dermatology* **3**, 599–601.

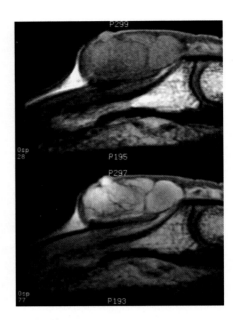

**Fig. 11.24** Epidermoid cyst of the posterior nail fold. Sagittal spin echo T1-weighted image before (top) and after injection of gadolinium (bottom).

### Subungual epidermoid inclusions

Multiple subungual epidermoid inclusions (epidermal buds; Zaias 1990) develop from the ridges of the nail bed epithelium. Although their lining is histologically identical with subungual epidermoid cysts, they usually remain microscopic. Exceptionally they become large enough to produce symptoms, such as swelling of the nail bed. Trauma is a possible cause in some instances (Samman 1959). They occur especially with finger clubbing but also without associated dystrophy (Lewin 1969).

In addition to the two main varieties, eight cases of a new type of subungual epidermoid inclusion have been reported (Fanti & Tosti 1989) (Fig. 11.23a). The most striking clinical features are subungual hyperkeratosis associated with shortened and dystrophic nail plates. Onycholysis was observed in one case. A history of trauma is frequent, but the condition is symp-tomless. In all cases, biopsy shows marked hyperplasia of the nail bed and epidermoid cysts in the dermis (Fig. 11.23b). Ony-chomycosis and psoriasis are the main differential diagnosis.

### References

Fanti, P.A. & Tosti, A. (1989) Subungual epidermoid inclusions: report of 8 cases. *Dermatologica* **17**, 209–212.

Lewin, K. (1969) Subungual epidermoid inclusion. *British Journal of Dermatology* **81**, 671–675.

Samman, P.D. (1959) The human toenail, its genesis and blood supply. *British Journal of Dermatology* **71**, 296–302.

Zaias, N. (1990) *The Nail in Health and Disease*, p. 218. Appleton & Lange, Norwalk, CN.

### Fibroepithelial tumours

Fibrokeratomas (see p. 550).
    Invaginated fibrokeratoma (see p. 552).

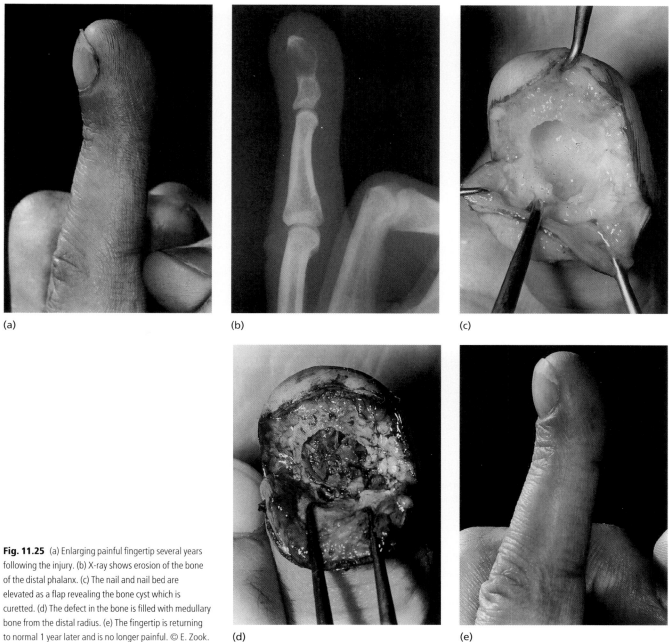

(a)

(b)

(c)

(d)

(e)

**Fig. 11.25** (a) Enlarging painful fingertip several years following the injury. (b) X-ray shows erosion of the bone of the distal phalanx. (c) The nail and nail bed are elevated as a flap revealing the bone cyst which is curetted. (d) The defect in the bone is filled with medullary bone from the distal radius. (e) The fingertip is returning to normal 1 year later and is no longer painful. © E. Zook.

## Onychomatricoma (Fig. 11.26)

Onychomatricoma was recently identified as an uncommon tumour specific to the nail apparatus (Baran & Kint 1991, 1992). Finger nails are much more often involved than toenails (Juillard *et al.* 1994). More than 20 cases have now been identified (Haneke & Fränken 1995; Duhard *et al.* 1996; Perrin *et al.* 1998; Raison-Peyron *et al.* 1998; Van Holder *et al.* 1999; Fraga *et al.* 2001). Only one patient was black (Tosti *et al.* 2000).

Four main clinical signs are striking enough to either make the diagnosis or at least to arouse suspicion of this condition:
1 A yellow longitudinal band of variable width, leaving a single or double portion of normal pink nail, either side.
2 Splinter haemorrhages may be seen in the yellow area involving the proximal nail region in a characteristic manner. Longitudinal ridging is prominent in the affected nail (Fig. 11.27).
3 A tendency toward transverse overcurvature of the affected nail portion which is more pronounced as the yellow colour is more extensive.

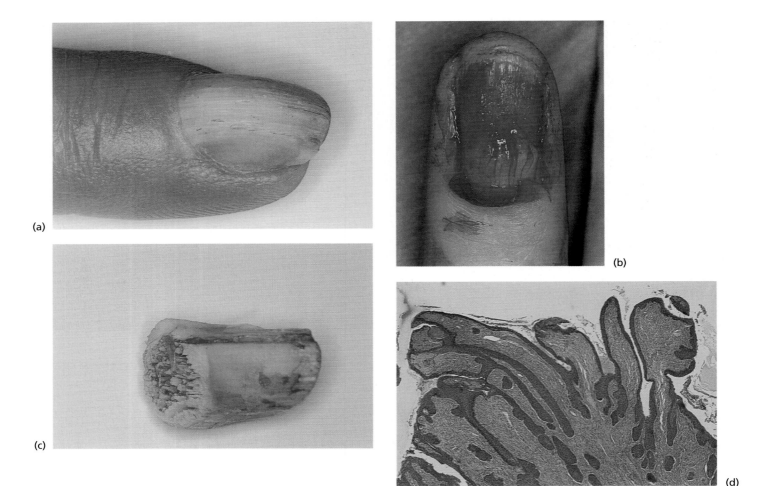

**Fig. 11.26** (a) Onychomatricoma of long duration. Yellow hue of the nail plate. (b) Emerging nail tumour visible after nail avulsion. (c) Nail plate undersurface showing in its proximal portion the holes storing the filamentous digitations. (d) Fibroepithelial proliferations with lobules surrounded by normal basal cells.

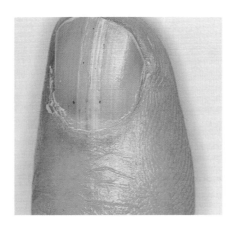

**Fig. 11.27** Onychomatricoma (recent) presenting as a longitudinal xanthonychia.

4 Nail avulsion exposes a villous tumour emerging from the matrix while the nail appears as a thickened funnel, storing filamentous digitations of matrix fitting into the holes of the proximal nail extremity. The villous projections in the nail plate can be so pronounced that nail cutting may produce bleeding (Raison-Peyron *et al.* 1998). However, in some cases the clinical presentation may be confusing: the longitudinal melanonychia may hide the yellow hue and the proximal nail fold may be swollen at its junction with the lateral nail fold. This swelling gives the affected nail the texture of a cutaneous horn. In some cases, this horn is completely separated from the nail plate. Histological examination establishes the diagnosis (Perrin *et al.* 1998). In three cases, the tumour was associated with onychomycosis (Fayol *et al.* 2000).

*MR images are typical (Goettmann* et al. *1994). The sagittal images highlight the tumoral core in the matrix area and the invagination of the lesion into the funnel-shaped nail plate. The centre shows a low signal on all images with a peripheral rim with a signal identical to that of normal epidermis (Fig. 11.28). The distal filamentous extensions present a higher signal on T2-weighted images due to a mucoid stroma with high water content. Axial slices accurately show the holes in the substance of the nail plate, filled with the filamentous extensions.*

Onychomatricoma can also be defined on histological grounds (Perrin *et al.* 1998). This fibroepithelial tumour consists of two anatomical zones, three histological criteria are used for each one. The proximal zone is located beneath the proximal nail

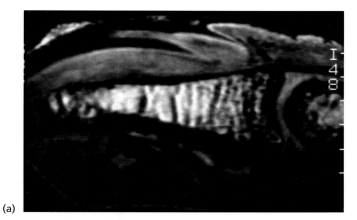

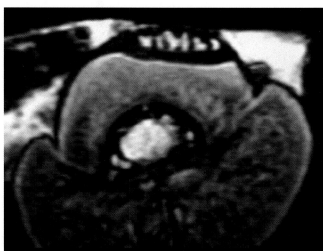

**Fig. 11.28** Onychomatricoma. Sagittal (a) and axial (b) gradient echo MR images.

fold with a proximal border starting at the root of the nail and a distal border corresponding to the cuticle. It is characterized by: (a) deep epithelial invaginations filled with a thick V-shaped keratogenous zone; (b) a thickened nail plate without cavitation but with an undulating inferior border ending in ungual spurs; (c) a fibrillar stroma clearly demarcated from the undersurface.

The distal zone corresponds to the lunula and is characterized by multiple 'glove finger' digitation lined with: (a) matrix epithelium oriented around antero-oblique connective tissue axes; (b) perforation of the nail plate by mutiple cavities that, generally at the distal edge of the lunula, lose their epithelial digitations and become filled with serous fluid; (c) the connective tissue stroma of the digitations extends deeply into the dermis and is not demarcated from healthy tissue.

The loose and vascular stroma of these epithelial digitations explains the proximal splinter haemorrhages seen clinically. The yellow colour of the nail plate from lunula to hyponychium is caused by thickening of the nail as a result of the keratogenous layers surrounding these digitations.

Two histological differential diagnoses can be discussed (Perrin *et al.* 1998):

1 In the longitudinal sections the structure is reminiscent of a fibrokeratoma. However, a diagnosis of fibrokeratoma of the nail matrix can be excluded on the basis of the multiplicity of fibroepithelial digitations, absence of a horny corn, and at the distal border of the thickned nail plate, the presence of cavitation filled with serous fluid.

2 The stroma of the lunular segment of the onychomatricoma can suggest a fibroma. However, the latter can be ruled out on the basis of the hyperplastic and onychogenic nature of the epithelium. Histologically, an ungual fibroma compresses and thins the matrix epithelium which results clinically in thinning of the nail plate in the form of a longitudinal groove.

Immunohistochemistry using the proliferation marker Ki-67 (MIB-1) showed only a low proliferation rate (Haneke & Fränken 1995).

Examination by electron microscopy (Kint *et al.* 1997) shows basal cells in the proximal zone of the onychomatricoma with various features: some being lacunar while others have only a limited cytoplasmic rim containing mitochondria and tonofilamants. In the parakeratotic cell columns, the cells elongate and homogenized tonofilaments appear. Around the lacunae the cells are poorly differentiated and their cytoplasm is granular. It can be concluded that the basal cells have a decreased number of tonofilaments and desmosomes and that their evolution is not uniform. The tumour may be considered as the result of disturbed differentiation of nail matrix cells. Whether it is a true benign neoplasm or a reactive proliferation is not yet clear.

## References

Baran, R. & Kint, A. (1991) Surgical treatment of a filamentous tufted tumour in the matrix of a funnel-shaped nail—a new entity. *Zentralblatt für Haut- und Geschlechtskrankheiten* **159**, 337.

Baran, R. & Kint, A. (1992) Onychomatrixoma. Filamentous tufted tumour in the matrix of a funnel-shaped nail: a new entity. *British Journal of Dermatology* **126**, 510–515.

Duhard, E., Baptiste, C. & Monegier du Sorbier, C. (1996) Onychomatricome: deux nouveaux cas. *Nouvelles Dermatologie* **15**, 461.

Fayol, J., Baran, R., Perrin, C. *et al.* (2000) Onychomatricoma with misleading features. *Acta Dermato-Venereologica* **80**, 370–372.

Fraga, G.R., Patterson, J.W. & McHargue, C.A. (2001) Onychomatricoma: report of a case and its comparison with fibrokeratoma of the nailbed. *American Journal of Dermatopathology* **23**, 36–40.

Goettmann, S., Drapé, J.L., Baran, R., Perrin, C., Haneke, E. & Bélaïch, S. (1994) Onychomatricome: 3 nouveaux cas, intérêt de la résonance magnétique nucléaire. *Annales de Dermatologie et de Vénéréologie* **121**, S145.

Haneke, E. & Fränken, J. (1995) Onychomatricoma. *Dermatologic Surgery* **21**, 984–987.

Juillard, J., Michaud, T. & Schubert, B. (1994) Onychomatricome. In: *1er Symposium International d'Onychologie, Paris, Book of Abstracts*, p. 51.

Kint, A., Baran, R. & Geerts, M.L. (1997) The onychomatricoma: an electron microscopic study. *Journal of Cutaneous Pathology* **24**, 183–188.

Perrin, C., Goettmann, S. & Baran, R. (1998) Onychomatricoma: clinical and histopathologic findings in 12 cases. *Journal of the American Academy of Dermatology* **39**, 560–564.

Raison-Peyron, N., Alirezai, M., Meunier, L., Barnéon, G. & Meynadier, J. (1998) Onychomatricoma: an unusual cause of nail bleeding. *Clinical and Experimental Dermatology* **23**, 138.

Tosti, A., Piraccini, B.M., Calderoni, O. *et al.* (2000) Onychomatricoma: report of three cases including the first recognized in a coloured man. *European Journal of Dermatology* **10**, 604–606.

Van Holder, C., Dumontier, C. & Abimelec, P. (1999) Onychomatricoma. *Journal of Hand Surgery* **24B**, 120–121.

## Premalignant lesions

### Actinic keratosis and arsenical keratosis

Actinic keratoses are the most common precancerous lesion of the skin. Although the nail provides only partial protection of the nail bed from solar damage, as judged by the occurrence of subungual keratoacanthoma and squamous cell carcinoma (Norton 1980), actinic keratoses seem to be exceptionally rare in the subungual area. They usually present as cutaneous 'horns' on the proximal nail fold. Since, however, only about one-third of cutaneous horns overlie actinic keratoses, each lesion must be biopsied or completely excised. Common warts, Bowen's disease, squamous cell carcinoma, chronic radiodermatitis, arsenical keratoses and keratoacanthoma may also give rise to cutaneous horns.

Arsenical keratoses are due to a high content of arsenic in water or wine, or to iatrogenic arsenic ingestion. Microscopically, they cannot definitely be differentiated from other types of keratoses such as actinic keratoses, however, they lack the actinic elastosis associated with an actinic keratosis. Keratotic papules and plaques develop on the periungual skin or nail bed. The latter may also become diffusely hyperkeratotic. Nail dystrophy subsequently develops. All patients with signs of chronic arsenical poisoning must be carefully examined and followed-up, since arsenic has a high carcinogenic potential for various organs.

### Reference

Norton, L.A. (1980) Nail disorders. *Journal of the American Academy of Dermatology* **2**, 451–467.

### Radiodermatitis (Figs 11.29–11.32)

Acute radiodermatitis results from gross overdosages, accidental or therapeutic. Marked painful oedema with erythema and vesiculation develop and a peculiar bluish pigmentation of the nails is commonly noted (Epstein 1962). In more severe instances, the nails may be shed, permanently or temporarily (Gallaghar *et al.* 1955) or may become deformed.

Acute necrosis of the fingertip, nail apparatus and the distal phalanx can occur from massive radiation overdose. Chronic

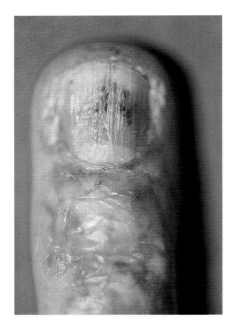

**Fig. 11.29** Radiodermatitis—chronic changes many years after X-irradiation for psoriasis.

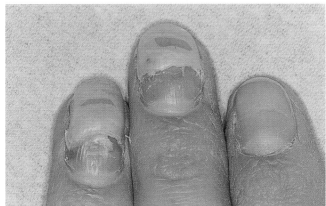

**Fig. 11.30** Acute radiodermatitis—progressive nail shedding.

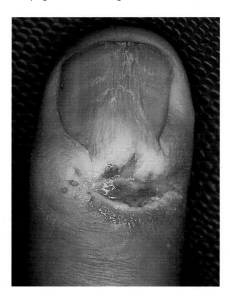

**Fig. 11.31** Ulceration (benign), pterygium formation and nail plate dystrophy. Late changes of X-irradiations.

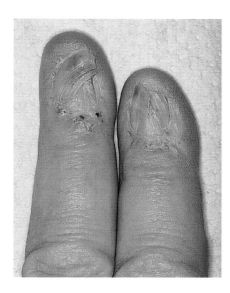

**Fig. 11.32** X-irradiation-induced scarring and nail plate distortion. (Courtesy of B. Richert, Liège, Belgium.)

effects have been seen after the treatment of eczema, psoriasis, onychomycosis, warts and in health care workers before the institution of proper precautions (Guy 1990).

Chronic radiodermatitis (Messite *et al.* 1957) can be caused by ionizing radiation which may lead to skin cancer up to 30 years after exposure. The earliest signs are longitudinal ridging and brittleness. Later, the surrounding skin appears sclerotic and atrophic with telangiectasia and hyperkeratosis. Ulceration may occur and is slow or impossible to cure. The nail plate becomes dull and slightly opaque with a brownish hue. A hyperkeratotic black mass of the distal nail bed due to increased dermal capillaries in a sclerotic connective tissue has been found to be associated with pseudoclubbing (Richert & de la Brassine 1993). Involved nails become variably thickened or distorted with splitting of the distal edges. The nail bed may develop fine, red longitudinal striations which proceed into punctate charcoal patches. A verrucous lesion appearing on the hyponychium or adjacent nail bed may herald malignant degeneration. Hyperkeratosis of the nail bed elevates the nail and causes pain. It may be associated with onycholysis and leuconychia (von Zons 1997). Paronychia-like flares are the rule. Occupational radiodermatitis from Iridium-192 exposure was reported from Spain (Condé-Salazar *et al.* 1986). After an acute episode, an asymptomatic period of several months may follow before the typical picture of chronic radiodermatitis appears. Similar lesions also occurred after exposure to radioactivity from the nuclear plant explosion at Chernobyl.

Treatment depends on the size and location of the keratotic lesions. For small nail bed lesions, curettage may be efficient after a U-shaped piece of the distal nail has been removed. En-bloc excision of the nail apparatus with healing by secondary intention (de Dulanto & Camacho 1979), or Mohs' fresh tissue technique which spares the normal surrounding tissue are treatments of choice. The defect can be covered with a free graft or a flap (Lagrot & Greco 1978), or left to heal by secondary intention.

## References

Condé-Salazar, L., Guimaraens, D. & Romero, L.V. (1986) Occupational radiodermatitis from Ir-192 exposure. *Contact Dermatitis* **15**, 202–204.

de Dulanto, F. & Camacho, F. (1979) Radiodermatitis. *Acta Dermato-Sifilitica* **70**, 67–94.

Epstein, E. (1962) *Radiodermatitis*, p. 50. Charles Thomas, Springfield, IL.

Gallaghar, R.G., Zavon, M. & Doyle, H.N. (1955) Radioactive contamination in a radium therapy clinic. *Public Health Reports* **70**, 617–624.

Guy, R.J. (1990) The etiologies and mechanisms of nail bed injuries. *Hand Clinics* **6**, 9–20.

Lagrot, F. & Greco, J. (1978) Les lésions des ongles dans les radiodermites chroniques des mains. *Cutis* **2**, 507–528.

Messite, J., Troisi, F.M. & Kleinfeld, M. (1957) Radiological hazards due to X-radiation in veterinarians. *Archives of Industrial Health* **16**, 48–51.

Richert, B. & de la Brassine, M. (1993) Subungual chronic radiodermatitis. *Dermatology* **186**, 290–293.

von Zons, P.J. (1997) Radiodermatitis nach Strahlentherapie von Fingerwarzen. *Zeitschrift für Dermatologie* **183**, 190–191.

## Malignant epithelial tumours

When dealing with malignant nail tumours four features should always be taken into account:
- variation in nail colour;
- nail plate deformity;
- partial or total disappearance of the nail plate;
- periungual soft tissue abnormality.

### Epidermoid carcinoma of the nail apparatus

#### Bowen's disease and squamous cell carcinoma
(Figs 11.33–11.43)

Bowen's disease is a non-aggressive malignant condition (the first recognized example of carcinoma *in situ*) which has gained interest for several reasons: (a) the increasing awareness of its frequency with recent reports in the literature; (b) the identification of new clinical patterns such as longitudinal melanonychia (Baran & Simon 1988); (c) our experience indicates that Bowen's disease of the finger nail structures should always be regarded as a potentially polydactylous process with the passage of time (Strong 1983; Baran & Gormley 1987; Delaporte *et al.* 1992; Goodman *et al.* 1995); (d) finally the now proven link with HPV 16, 34 and 35 which sheds new light on the aetiology of this type of cancer (Theunis *et al.* 1999).

Bowen's disease of the nail apparatus is a distinctive type of squamous cell carcinoma that differs from other variants. However, some authors prefer to avoid the use of the term Bowen's disease for *in situ* epidermoid carcinoma occurring beneath the nail plate, because: (a) it is not always easy to

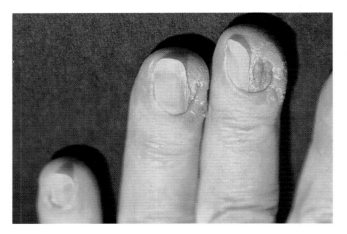

**Fig. 11.33** Epidermoid carcinoma—Bowen's disease (two digits affected). (Courtesy of D. Gormely, Los Angeles, USA.)

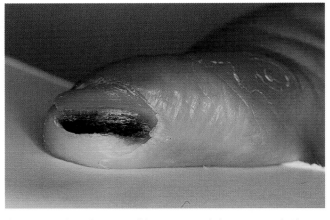

**Fig. 11.36** Epidermoid carcinoma of the matrix. Bowen's disease associated with longitudinal melanonychia.

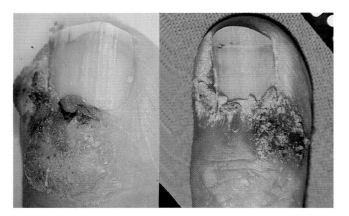

**Fig. 11.34** Epidermoid carcinoma *in situ*, periungual warty proliferations.

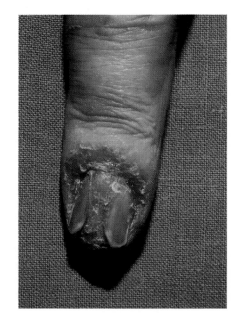

**Fig. 11.37** Epidermoid carcinoma *in situ*. Marked inflammatory changes.

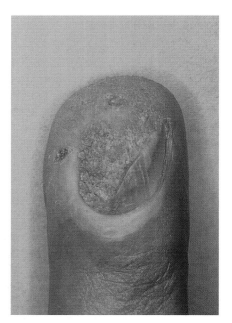

**Fig. 11.35** Epidermoid carcinoma *in situ*. Whitish cuticle area and nail dystrophy. (Courtesy of N. Zaias, Miami, USA.)

separate invasive from *in-situ* carcinoma; (b) it cannot be over-emphasized that a biopsy specimen showing Bowen's disease does not exclude the possibility of invasive carcinoma in other areas of the lesions (Mikhail 1984; Goodman *et al.* 1995).

The malignant process may develop in the epithelium of the periungual area as well as in the subungual tissues. Periungual involvement includes: hyperkeratotic or papillomatous or fibrokeratoma-like growth (Haneke 1991) which may be in subungual location (Baran & Perrin 1994); erosions, scaling and fissuring of the nail folds; whitish cuticle (Zaias 1990); periungual swelling from deep tumour proliferation, with erythema caused by inflammation due to infection; fissure or ulceration of the lateral nail groove, sometimes crusted with granulation-like tissue beneath the scab.

Subungual involvement was consistent in the 12 cases of Guitart *et al.* (1990). It may present with onycholysis and clip-

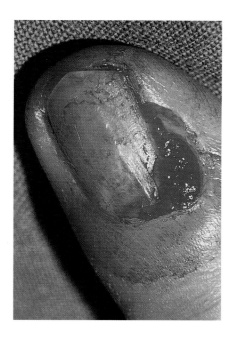

**Fig. 11.38** Epidermoid carcinoma *in situ*. Lateral ulcerated variety. (Courtesy of G. Moulin, Lyon, France.)

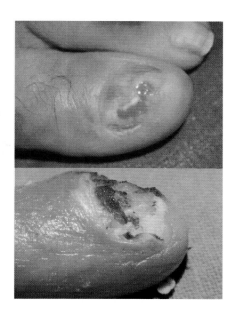

**Fig. 11.41** Epidermoid carcinoma ulceration and bleeding.

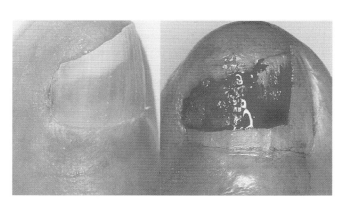

**Fig. 11.39** Pseudo-Hutchinson's sign in Bowen's disease with polydactylic involvement.

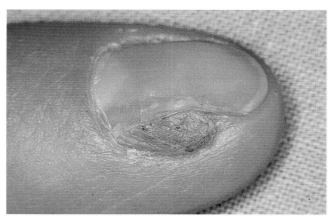

**Fig. 11.42** Epidermoid carcinoma mimicking acquired periungual fibrokeratoma.

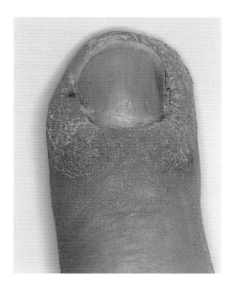

**Fig. 11.40** Epidermoid carcinoma *in situ* with periungual warty lesions, and longitudinal melanonychia along the lateral edge of the nail plate.

ping away of the non-adherent portion of the nail plate shows hyperkeratosis or oozing ulceration of the nail bed. Appearance of longitudinal melanonychia, with classical pattern of the band (Saijo *et al.* 1990; Lemont & Haas 1994) or irregular appearance (Baran & Simon 1988; Baran & Eichmann 1993; Sass *et al.* 1998), is a recent finding. We have also seen longitudinal erythronychia in two cases of subungual Bowen's disease (Baran & Perrin 2000). The nail plate may become dystrophic, ingrown, or there may be partial or total nail loss which shows that the malignant process has developed in the nail matrix. Localized pain may be noted, for example, when the patient uses a keyboard.

The presence of ulceration, bleeding or nodule formation indicates that the carcinoma has become invasive (Mikhail 1984). Bone involvement is seen in less than 20% of the patients (Long & Espinella 1978; Salasche & Garland 1985). Metastases have been reported in patients with hereditary ecto-

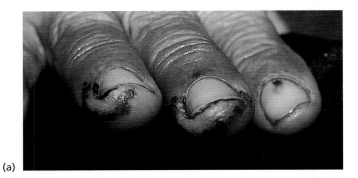

(a)

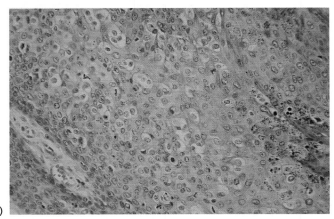

(b)

**Fig. 11.43** (a) Bowen's disease with pseudo-Hutchinson sign. (Courtesy of J. Domingez-Cherit, Mexico DF.) (b) Bowen's disease—histology.

dermal dysplasia (Campell & Keokarn 1966; Mauro *et al.* 1972) and also in patients without ectodermal dysplasia (Fromer 1970; Morule & Adamthwaite 1984; Lai *et al.* 1996; Canovas *et al.* 1998).

The key to diagnosis is the histological examination. The picture is identical with that of Bowen's disease of other skin areas (Haneke *et al.* 1997). The most important feature is the intact basement membrane.

Bowen's disease has been reported in individuals between the ages of 19 and 90, the incidence being highest in the 50–69 year range. The tumour grows slowly and the duration of signs and symptoms from onset to the time of diagnosis has varied from several months to 30 years (Holgado *et al.* 2000). The diagnostic biopsy is often delayed because of the patient's reluctance, technical difficulties, or because the physician has failed to suspect the disease. The digits of the hand are significantly more frequently affected than the toes (Lewis & Mendicino 1994; Uezato *et al.* 1999), and the thumbs are the most common site.

The neoplastic process most commonly originates in the nail folds or nail grooves and may thus clinically mimic warts, infections and other chronic inflammatory conditions.

### Differential diagnosis
The lesions are often mistaken for chronic inflammatory conditions including bacterial infections (Bizzle 1992) as well as

pyogenic granuloma, verruca vulgaris, subungual exostosis, malignant melanoma, glomus tumour and subungual keratoacanthoma, and even acquired ungual fibrokeratoma (Haneke 1991; Baran & Perrin 1994).

The aetiology of subungual epidermoid carcinoma remains unclear. Arsenic cannot be excluded in old psoriatic patients, for example. Trauma, infection and chronic paronychia (Failla 1996; Saccone & Rayan 1993), but above all, exposure to X-ray (physicians, dentists, patients) have been cited as aetiological factors. This may be followed by radiodermatitis (de Dulanto & Camacho 1979) which is with discovery of HPV-infection, the most common factor for the development of squamous cell carcinoma (Guitart *et al.* 1990). HPV-16, 34 (Kawashima *et al.* 1986) and 35 (Rüdlinger *et al.* 1989) have been detected in *in-situ* and invasive epidermoid carcinoma. HPV genome was found in 8 out of 10 periungual lesions by dot-blot analysis of frozen tissue and 6 of them were related to HPV 16 (Moy *et al.* 1989). Using the polymerase chain reaction to detect human papillomavirus in formalin-fixed, paraffin-embedded specimens of periungual squamous cell carcinoma, Ashinoff *et al.* (1991) found that 5 of the 7 periungual lesions contained HPV 16. *In-situ* hybridization failed to identify HPV in any of these patient's tumours. Up to now, more than 24 cases of ungual Bowen's disease proved to be associated with HPV 16 (Delaporte *et al.* 1992; De Dobbeleer *et al.* 1993; Sau *et al.* 1994, Tosti *et al.* 1994; Kapranos *et al.* 1996; Forslund *et al.* 1997; Mitsuishi *et al.* 1997; Sass *et al.* 1998).

This finding prompts one to speculate whether genital-digital transmission of the virus occurs. In Rüdlinger's *et al.* case (1989), Bowen's disease of the nail apparatus and the bowenoid papulosis of the anogenital area revealed an identical HPV 35 infection. As the patient suffered from long-lasting pruritus of the anogenital area, scratching may have resulted in autoinoculation. Similarly, HPV 16 genome from digital Bowen's disease of two women was identical with HPV DNA from archival samples of their genital dysplasia (Forslund *et al.* 1997). However, in the case of Bowen's disease reported by Ostrow *et al.* (1989), the HPV 16 DNA was discovered in a solitary subungual warty lesion and the integration of the HPV 16 DNA appears (so far) to be closely associated with the progression of a premalignant lesion to a malignant one. Cytophotometric analysis of a case of bilateral subungual Bowen's disease with HPV 16 suggested a lack of HPV 16 genome integration into the host DNA of squamous cell carcinoma (Kapranos *et al.* 1996). There is no reason to assume that benign viral warts undergo malignant transformation.

### Treatment
The need for complete removal of the lesion cannot be overemphasized:

**1** The best treatment is Mohs' micrographic surgery allowing adequate excision with maximal preservation of normal tissue and function (Mikhail 1984; Masini & Tulli 1994; de Berker *et al.* 1996; Kuschner & Lane 1997). This can be performed with routine instrumentation (Fig. 11.44) as well as with the $CO_2$ laser in a focused beam incisional mode, which avoids bleeding and ensures minimal post-operative discomfort for the patient.

2 Excisional surgery may be used in some cases or for complete removal of the nail apparatus, with healing by secondary intention, grafting, or repair with a bridge flap (Haneke *et al.* 1997).

3 Electrosurgery is a therapeutic alternative in a very few selected cases.

4 Liquid nitrogen may give good results in experienced hands. Both electrosurgery and liquid nitrogen do not allow adequate histological control of tumour margins. There has been some success using photodynamic therapy with 5-aminolaevulinic acid.

5 Bone involvement requires amputation of the distal phalanx.

*A perionychial squamous cell carcinoma without bone involvement requires complete removal with margins of one-half to one centimeter and usually requires coverage with a skin graft. If there is bony involvement or extensive soft tissue involvement, amputation of the distal interphalangeal joint or more proximally should be considered. Lymph node dissection is indicated if papable lymph nodes do not disappear within 3–4 weeks after amputation or excision as many lymph node enlargements are due to chronic inflammation (Shapiro & Baraf 1970).*

## References

Ashinoff, R., Junli, J., Jacobson, M. *et al.* (1991) Detection of HPV DNA in squamous cell carcinoma of the nail bed and finger determined by polymerase chain reaction. *Archives of Dermatology* **127**, 1813–1818.

Baran, R. & Eichmann, A. (1993) Longitudinal melanonychia associated with Bowen disease. *Dermatology* **18**, 159–160.

Baran, R. & Gormley, D. (1987) Polydactylous Bowen's disease of the nail. *Journal of the American Academy of Dermatology* **17**, 201–204.

Baran, R. & Perrin, C. (1994) Pseudo-fibrokeratoma of the nail apparatus: a new clue for Bowen disease. *Archives of Dermatology* **74**, 449–450.

Baran, R. & Perrin, C. (2000) Longitudinal erythronychia with distal subungual keratosis: onychopapilloma of the nail bed and Bowen's disease. *British Journal of Dermatology* **143**, 132–135.

Baran, R. & Simon, C. (1988) Longitudinal melanonychia: a symptom of Bowen's disease. *Journal of the American Academy of Dermatology* **18**, 1359–1360.

de Berker, D.A.R., Dahl, M.G.C., Malcolm, A.J. & Lawrence, C.M. (1996) Micrographic surgery for subungual squamous cell carcinoma. *British Journal of Plastic Surgery* **49**, 414–419.

Bizzle, P.G. (1992) Subungual squamous cell carcinoma of the thumb masked by infection. *Orthopedics* **15**, 1350–1352.

Campbell, J. & Keokarn, T. (1966) Squamous-cell carcinoma of the nail bed in epidermal dysplasia. *Journal of Bone and Joint Surgery* **48A**, 92–99.

Canovas, F., Dereure, O. & Bonnel, F. (1998) A propos d'un cas de carcinome épidermoide du lit unguéal avec métastase intraneurale du nerf médian. *Annales de Chirurgie de la Main* **17**, 232–235.

Delaporte, E., Breuillard, F., Piette, F. *et al.* (1992) Papillomavirus humain type 16 dans une maladie de Bowen péri-unguéale multifocale. In: *20e Congrés de l'Association de Dermatologie et Syphiligraphie de Langue Française (Montréal), 8–11 June 1992*, pp. 121–122.

De Dobbeleer, G., André, J., Laporte, M. *et al.* (1993) Human papillomavirus type 6/11 and 16 in periungual squamous carcinoma *in situ*. *European Journal of Dermatology* **3**, 12–14.

de Dulanto, F. & Camacho, F. (1979) Radiodermatitis. *Acta Dermato-Sifilitica* **70**, 67–94.

Failla, J.M. (1996) Subungual lipoma, squamous carcinoma of the nail bed, and secondary chronic infection. *Journal of Hand Surgery* **21A**, 512–514.

Forslund, O., Nordin, P., Andersson, K., Stenquist, B. & Hansson, B.G. (1997) DNA analysis indicates patient-specific human papillomavirus type 16 strains in Bowen's disease of fingers and in archival samples from genital dysplasia. *British Journal of Dermatology* **136**, 678–682.

Fromer, J.L. (1970) Carcinoma of the nail bed: discussion. *Archives of Dermatology* **101**, 66–67.

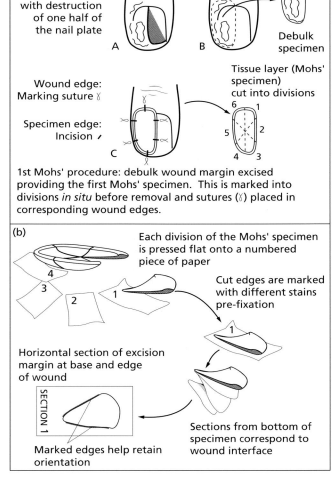

(a)

SCC of nail unit with destruction of one half of the nail plate

A    B    Debulk specimen

Wound edge: Marking suture ɣ

Specimen edge: Incision ⁄

Tissue layer (Mohs' specimen) cut into divisions

6  1
5     2
4  3

C

1st Mohs' procedure: debulk wound margin excised providing the first Mohs' specimen. This is marked into divisions *in situ* before removal and sutures (ɣ) placed in corresponding wound edges.

(b)

4
3    2    1

Each division of the Mohs' specimen is pressed flat onto a numbered piece of paper

Cut edges are marked with different stains pre-fixation

1

Horizontal section of excision margin at base and edge of wound

SECTION 1

Marked edges help retain orientation

1

Sections from bottom of specimen correspond to wound interface

**Fig. 11.44** (a) Mohs' technique used for epidermoid carcinoma. (Courtesy of D. de Berker, UK.) (b) Mohs' technique. (Courtesy of D. de Berker, UK.)

Goodman, G., Mason, G. & O'Brien, T. (1995) Polydactylous Bowen's disease of the nail bed. *Australasian Journal of Dermatology* **36**, 164–165.

Guitart, J., Bergfeld, W.F., Tuthull, R.J. *et al.* (1990) Squamous cell carcinoma of the nail bed: a clinicopathological study of 12 cases. *British Journal of Dermatology* **123**, 215–222.

Haneke, E. (1991) Epidermoid carcinoma (Bowen's disease) of the nail simulating acquired ungual fibrokeratoma. *Skin Cancer* **6**, 217–221.

Haneke, E., Bragadini, L.A. & Mainusch, O. (1997) Enfermedad de Bowen de células claras del aparato ungular. *Acta Terapie Dermatologie* **20**, 311–313.

Holgado, R.D., Ward, S.C. & Suryaprasad, S.G. (2000) Squamous cell carcinoma of the hallux. *Journal of the American Podiatric Association* **90**, 309–312.

Kapranos, N., Aronis, E., Braziotis, A., Tsambaos, D. & Berger, H. (1996) HPV-16-assoziierter Morbus Bowen des Nagelbetts und der Periungual-Region beider Daumen. *Zeitschrift für Hautkrankheiten* **71**, 48–50.

Kawashima, M., Jablonska, S., Favre, M. *et al.* (1986) Characterization of a new type of human papillomavirus found in a lesion of Bowen's disease of the skin. *Journal of Virology* **57**, 688–692.

Kuschner, S.H. & Lane, C.S. (1997) Squamous cell carcinoma of the perionychium. *Bulletin of the Hospital for Joint Disease* **56**, 111–112.

Lai, C.-S., Lin, S.-D., Tsai, C.-W. & Chou, C.-K. (1996) Squamous cell carcinoma of the nail bed. *Cutis* **57**, 341–345.

Lemont, H. & Haas, R. (1994) Subungual pigmented Bowen's disease in a nineteen-year-old black female. *Journal of the American Podiatric Medical Association* **84**, 39–40.

Lewis, J. & Mendicino, R.W. (1994) Squamous cell carcinoma of the great toe. *Journal of Foot and Ankle Surgery* **33**, 482–485.

Long, P.I. & Espinella, J.L. (1978) Squamous cell carcinoma of the nail bed. *Journal of the American Medical Association* **239**, 2154–2155.

Masini, C. & Tulli, A. (1994) Squamous cell carcinoma of the periungual region. Treatment by Mohs surgery. *Giornale Italiano di Dermatologia e Venereologia* **129**, 189–192.

Mauro, J.A., Maslyn, R. & Stein, A.A. (1972) Squamous-cell carcinoma of nail bed in hereditary ectodermal dysplasia. *New York State Journal of Medicine* **72**, 1065–1066.

Mikhail, G. (1984) Subungual epidermoid carcinoma. *Journal of the American Academy of Dermatology* **11**, 291–298.

Mitsuishi, T., Sata, T., Matsukura, T. *et al.* (1997) The presence of mucosal HPV in Bowen's disease of the hands. *Cancer* **79**, 1911–1917.

Morule, A. & Adamthwaite, D.N. (1984) Squamous carcinoma of the nail bed. A case report. *South African Medical Journal* **65**, 63–64.

Moy, R.L., Eliezri, Y., Nuovo, G.J., Zitelli, J.A., Bennett, R.G. & Silverstein, S. (1989) Human papillomavirus Type 16 DNA in periungual squamous cell carcinomas. *Journal of the American Medical Association* **261**, 2669–2673.

Ostrow, R.S., Shaver, M.A., Turnquist, S. *et al.* (1989) Human papillomavirus-16 DNA in a cutaneous invasive cancer. *Archives of Dermatology* **125**, 666–669.

Rüdlinger, R., Grob, R., Yu, Y.X. & Schnyder, U.W. (1989) Human papillomavirus-35 positive bowenoid papulosis of the anogenital area and concurrent with bowenoid dysplasia of the periungual area. *Archives of Dermatology* **125**, 655–659.

Saccone, P.G. & Rayan, G.M. (1993) Subungual malignant degenera-tion following chronic perionychial infection. *Orthopedic Reviews* **5**, 623–626.

Saijo, S., Kato, T. & Tagami, H. (1990) Pigmented nail streak associated with Bowen's disease of the nail matrix. *Dermatologica* **181**, 156–158.

Salasche, S.S. & Garland, L.D. (1985) Tumours of the nail. *Dermatologic Clinics* **3**, 501–519.

Sass, U., André, J., Stene, J.J. *et al.* (1998) Longitudinal melanonychia revealing an intraepidermal carcinoma of the nail apparatus: detection of integrated HPV-16 DNA. *Journal of the American Academy of Dermatology* **39**, 490–493.

Sau, P., McMarlin, S.L., Sperling, L.C. & Katz, R. (1994) Bowen's disease of the nail bed and periungual area. A clinicopathologic analysis of seven cases. *Archives of Dermatology* **130**, 204–209.

Shapiro, L. & Baraf, C.S. (1970) Subungual epidermoid carcinoma and keratoacanthoma. *Cancer* **25**, 141–152.

Strong, M.L. (1983) Bowen's disease in multiple nail beds. Case report. *Journal of Hand Surgery* **8**, 329–330.

Theunis, A., André, J. & Noel, J.C. (1999) Evaluation of the role of genital HPV in the pathogenesis of ungual squamous carcinoma. *Dermatology* **198**, 206–208.

Tosti, A., La Placa, A., Fanti, P.A. *et al.* (1994) Human papillomavirus type 16-associated periungual squamous cell carcinoma in a patient with acquired immunodeficiency syndrome. *Acta Dermato-Venereologica* **74**, 478–479.

Uezato, H., Hagiwara, K., Ramuzi, S.T. *et al.* (1999) Detection of human papilloma virus type 56 in extragenital Bowen's disease. *Acta Dermato-Venereologica* **79**, 311–313.

Zaias, N. (1990) *The Nail in Health and Disease*, 2nd edn. Appleton & Lange. Norwalk, CN.

### *Epithelioma cuniculatum* (Figs 11.45 & 11.46)

Epithelioma (carcinoma) cuniculatum is a rare, slow growing, but locally destructive, low-grade cancer of squamous cell

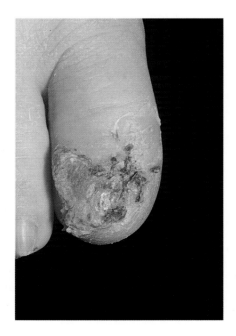

**Fig. 11.45** Verrucous carcinoma. (Courtesy of J. Van Geertruyden, Belgium.)

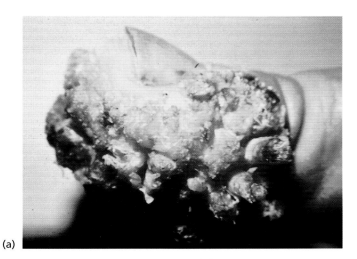

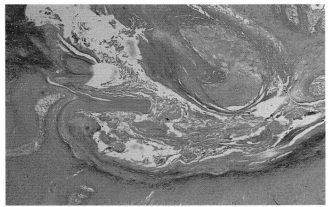

**Fig. 11.46** (a) Verrucous carcinoma. (Courtesy of L. Jaimovich, Buenos Aires, Argentina.) (b) Histology of case in (a).

The radiograph of most of the patients shows erosion or disappearance of the distal third of the phalanx.

Carcinoma cuniculatum is a rare variant of verrucous carcinoma characterized by a system of epithelium-lined tunnels in the tumour. Cellular atypia is usually mild and the lesion may be misdiagnosed as pseudoepitheliomatous hyperplasia. Histology shows a proliferation of epithelial cell complexes with squamous differentiation, formation of fistulae filled with keratinous debris, and a pushing border rather than frank invasion. Mitoses are rare as are dyskeratoses. Usually, there is a marked focal hypergranulosis.

Immunohistochemistry using antibodies to different cytokeratins, involucrin and filaggrin as well as lectin histochemistry with peanut agglutinin only reflect the high degree of differentiation (Haneke & Baran 1990). Filaggrin is present where keratohyalin can be seen in H & E stained section and involucrin is also expressed by the major part of the tumour cells. PNA binding is variable with both completely positive and negative areas. Neuraminidase digestion unmasks the Friedreich-Thomsen antigen thus rendering all tumour cells positive (E. Haneke, unpublished data). Differential diagnosis includes verrucae (even histologically) and keratoacanthoma which exhibits rapid growth and clinically aggressive behaviour.

Epithelioma cuniculatum should not be confused with squamous cell carcinoma as it is verrucous and histologically showing little anaplasia. Pseudoepitheliomatous hyperplasia shows very irregular, jagged, papillomatous downgrowths when compared to epithelioma cuniculatum (Coldiron *et al.* 1986).

Successful treatment requires Mohs micrographic surgery because of tissue-sparing capacity. Amputation is usually not necessary.

## References

Baran, R. & Haneke, E. (1990) Epithelioma cuniculatum. In: *XIth Congress of the International Society of Dermatological Surgery, Florence (Italy), Book of Abstracts*.

Coldiron, B.M., Brown, F.C. & Freeman, R.C. (1986) Epithelioma cuniculatum of the thumb: a case report and literature review. *Journal of Dermatologic Surgery and Oncology* 12, 1150–1154.

Haneke, E. & Baran, R. (1990) Epithelioma cuniculatum, histopathology, immuno and lectin histochemistry. In: *XIth Congress International Society of Dermatological Surgery, Florence (Italy), Book of Abstracts*.

Hitti, I.F., Sadowski, G., Statsinger, A.L. *et al.* (1987) Inverted variant of carcinoma cuniculatum of the toe. *Cutis* 39, 250–252.

McKee, R., Wilkinson, J.D., Black, M.M. *et al.* (1981) Carcinoma (epithelioma) cuniculatum: a clinico-pathological study of nineteen cases and review of the literature. *Histopathology* 5, 425–436.

Magnin, P.H., Label, M.G., Schroh, R. *et al.* (1986) Carcinoma cuniculatum localizado en el ledra subungual. *Revista Argentina de Dermatologia* 67, 68–72.

Schwartz, R.A. (1995) Verrucous carcinoma of the skin and mucosa. *Journal of the American Academy of Dermatology* 32, 1–21.

Tosti, A., Morelli, R., Fanti, P.A. *et al.* (1993) Carcinoma cuniculatum

origin. It has been reported in several patients with thumb involvement. Disto-lateral onycholysis and paronychia of the corresponding side was observed by McKee *et al.* (1981) in a 38-year-old woman; it had been present for at least 18 months. The second case started in an almost similar fashion. Progressively the inflammatory features were accompanied by subungual purulent material leading to disappearance of the nail plate. The nail bed was covered with multiple 'holes' extruding toothpaste like, foul smelling yellow-white material (Magnin *et al.* 1986). The patient of Coldiron *et al.* (1986) presented with a verrucous growth of the distal portion of the thumb. It was a friable mass erupting from the pulp. A biopsy revealed that the entire pulp was involved down to the bone. Subungual epithelioma cuniculatum was also seen in the racquet thumb of a retired internist where the role of possible repeated X-ray exposure cannot be excluded (Baran & Haneke 1990). Great toe (Hitti *et al.* 1987; Van Geertruyden *et al.* 1998) and 5th toe (Tosti *et al.* 1993) were involved with loss of the nail. Verrucous carcinoma does not metastasise except in some cases in which the tumours were treated with radiation (Schwartz 1995).

of the nail apparatus of two cases affecting the toenails. *Dermatology* **186**, 217–221.

Van Geertruyden, J.P., Olemans, C., Laporte, M. *et al.* (1998) Verrucous carcinoma of the nail bed. *Foot and Ankle International* **19**, 327–328.

## Malignant proliferating onycholemmal cyst (Fig. 11.47)

A 74-year-old woman was observed with a subungual lesion of her right thumb that had slowly enlarged. Curettage led to rapid recurrence. The nail bed showed a warty tumour that eventually destroyed most of her nail and was surrounded by swollen, livid red tissue. X-ray showed considerable bone resorption. After biopsy, the distal phalanx was amputated. Histopathology showed a malignant tumour invading the nail bed, proximal and lateral nail folds as well as the bone. The tumour showed many similarities with malignant proliferating trichilemmal cyst and was hence properly termed malignant proliferating onycholemmal cyst (Alessi *et al.* 1994). A similar case was also seen by Truchetet and Grosshans (personal communication).

### Reference

Alessi, E., Zorzi, F., Gianotti, R. & Parafiori, A. (1994) Malignant proliferating onycholemmal cyst. *Journal of Cutaneous Pathology* **21**, 183–188.

## Basal cell carcinoma (basalioma) (Fig. 11.48)

Although basal cell carcinoma is the most common malignant skin tumour, it is exceptionally rare in the subungual region. Only 15 cases have been reported since the first description by Eisenklam (1931).

The usual presentation is as a chronic paronychia or a periungual eczema often associated with ulceration, granulation tissue, and pain (Guana *et al.* 1994; Grine *et al.* 1997; Kim *et al.* 2000). Acquired longitudinal melanonychia in a white patient as the only manifestation of subungual basal cell carcinoma is unique (Rudolph 1987).

Basal cell carcinoma is usually present for many years before diagnosis.

In most of the cases, the lesions have occurred on the fingers, except for one lesion on a 5th toe (Mikhail 1985) and one on the great toe (Zaias 1990) developing into a large ulcerating mass (Waldman & Jacobs 1986).

The diagnosis can only be made by histological examination.

### References

Eisenklam, D. (1931) Über subunguale Tumoren. *Wiener Klinische Wochenschrift* **44**, 1192–1193.

Grine, R.C., Parlette, H.L. & Wilson, B.B. (1997) Nail unit basal cell carcinoma: a case report and literature review. *Journal of the American Academy of Dermatology* **37**, 790–793.

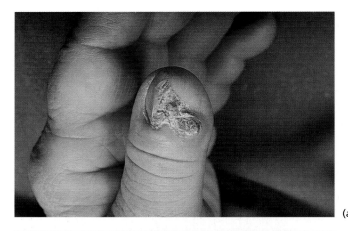

(a)

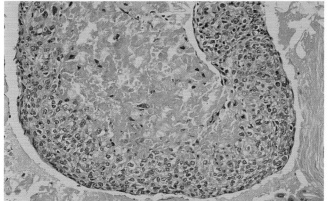

(b)

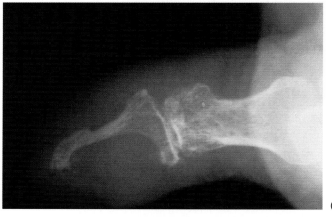

(c)

**Fig. 11.47** (a) Malignant proliferating onycholemmal cyst. (Courtesy of A. Alessi, Milan, Italy.) (b) Histology of the same lesion. (c) X-ray of the distal thumb tumour.

Guana, A.L., Kolbusz, R. & Goldberg, L.H. (1994) Basal cell carcinoma on the nailfold of the right thumb. *International Journal of Dermatology* **33**, 204–205.

Kim, H.J., Kim, Y.S., Suhr, K.B. *et al.* (2000) Basal cell carcinoma in the nail bed in a Korean woman. *International Journal of Dermatology* **39**, 397–398.

Mikhail, G.R. (1985) Subungual basal cell carcinoma. *Journal of Dermatologic Surgery and Oncology* **11**, 1222–1223.

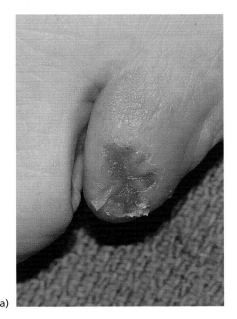

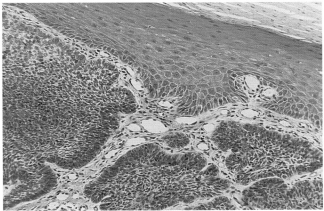

**Fig. 11.48** (a) Basal cell carcinoma of the 5th toe. (Courtesy of G. Mikhael, USA.) (b) Histology of the basal cell carcinoma seen in (a).

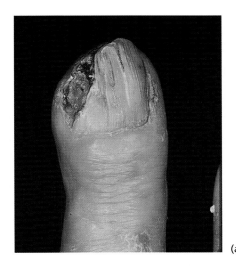

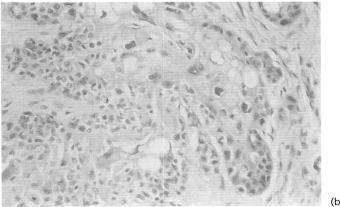

**Fig. 11.49** (a) Malignant eccrine poroma. (Courtesy of L. Requena, Spain.) (b) Histological changes of the same tumour.

Rudolph, R.I. (1987) Subungual basal cell carcinoma presenting as longitudinal melanonychia. *Journal of the American Academy of Dermatology* **16**, 229–233.

Waldman, M.H. & Jacobs, L.A. (1986) Malignant tumors of the foot. A report of 2 cases. *Journal of the American Podiatric Medical Association* **76**, 345.

Zaias, N. (1990) *The Nail in Health and Disease*, p. 225. Appleton & Lange. Norwalk, CT.

## Sweat gland carcinomas (Fig. 11.49)

Periungual porocarcinoma is very rare. Requena *et al.* (1990) reported a patient exposed to X-rays for many years which resulted in chronic radiodermatitis of several digits on both hands. He displayed an ulcer in the lateral nail fold of the right third digit which extended into the nail bed. Histology was consistent with malignant eccrine poroma. Another case was described by van Gorp and van der Putte (1993).

A mucinous adenocystic sweat gland carcinoma was seen on the distal aspect of the right great toe of a 30-year-old black woman. The tumour was located just plantar to the hyponychium measuring approximately 15 mm in diameter. The lesion was freely mobile and tender. Histopathology showed multiple lobules of either solid, papillary or trabecular tumour tissue with focally abundant mitoses. The diagnosis of adenocystic eccrine sweat gland carcinoma was made (Geraci *et al.* 1987).

Engel *et al.* (1991) reported a 21-year-old man who developed a nodule on the dorsolateral aspect of his right great toe at age 9. The lesion was cauterized on several occasions, locally excised at age 13 and histopathology then showed benign eccrine spiradenoma. The lesion rapidly recurred and grew very slowly until age 18 when it began to grow more rapidly. He eventually presented with a 40 mm bilobed painless fluctuant tumour involving the nail bed. Histological examination showed malignant degeneration in a benign eccrine spiradenoma.

A throbbing nodule of the left middle fingertip without bone involvement showed histologically an aggressive digital papillary adenocarcinoma (Inatoz *et al.* 2000). This tumour is indicative of potential metastasis and fatality in which aggressive surgical treatment by digit amputation is advocated.

A 77-year-old African-American man presented with a 9-month history of a non-tender, enlarging nodule on the right third fingernail bed. The patient stated that the lesion began as a pigmented streak 1–2 years previously and had been rapidly increasing in size for a few months before presentation. Physical examination showed an ulcerated, red, dome-shaped nodule involving the right third finger proximal nailfold and the proximal three-quarters of the nail bed with destruction and loss of the overlying nail plate. The remaining few millimetres of attached nail plate on either side of the tumour showed hyperpigmentation. No axillary or epitrochlear lymphadenopathy was found. Excisional biopsy down to bone was performed and showed a multilobular tumour extending from the epidermis. The tumour comprised polygonal-shaped epithelial cells with distinctly demarcated cytoplasmic borders and pale to clear cytoplasm. These cells displayed pleomorphism, hyperchromasia and nuclear atypia with numerous mitoses. Immunohistochemical stains revealed strong positivity with cytokeratin and rare scattered cells staining with S-100 and CEA. A diagnosis of hidradenocarcinoma was made (Nash *et al.* 2001).

## References

Engel, C.J., Meads, G.E., Joeph, N.G. & Stavraky, W. (1991) Eccrine spiradenoma: a report of malignant transformation. *Canadian Journal of Surgery* **34**, 477–480.

Geraci, T.L., Janis, L., Jenkinson, S. & Stewart, R. (1987) Mucinous (adenocystic) sweat gland carcinoma of the great toe. *Journal of Foot Surgery* **26**, 520–523.

van Gorp, J. & van der Putte, S.C.J. (1993) Periungual eccrine porocarcinoma. *Dermatology* **187**, 67–70.

Inatoz, H.S., Patel, G.K., Williamson, A.G. *et al.* (2000) Agressive digital papillary adenocarcinoma. In: *AAD 58th Annual Meeting.* 10–15 March. San Francisco. Poster abstract book no. 474.

Nash, J., Chaffins, M. & Krull, E. (2001) Hidradenocarcinoma. In: *AAD 59th Annual Meeting*, 2–7 March, Washington, DC. Poster abstract No. 376.

Requena, L., Sanchez, M., Aguilar, P. *et al.* (1990) Periungual porocarcinoma. *Dermatologica* **180**, 177–180.

## Sebaceous gland carcinoma

Kasdan *et al.* (1991) reported on a 46-year-old man with a six-month history of increasing swelling of the radial aspect of the distal phalanx of his right index finger. The swelling was neither painful nor tender. X-ray films did not reveal bone abnormalities and the presumptive diagnosis was epidermoid cyst. At operation a greyish white irregular mass was fixed to the skin well-circumscribed and pseudoencapsulated. It was composed of markedly malignant cells of epithelial origin,

organized in irregularly shaped islands with areas of focal necrosis. The cells exhibited a somewhat lobular pattern, with many mitotic nuclei showing hyperchromatism and pleomorphism. The cytoplasm was eosinophilic with vacuolation, suggesting sebaceous gland origin. The pathologic diagnosis was poorly differentiated pilosebaceous carcinoma.

A formal ray amputation of the finger was carried out.

## Reference

Kasdan, M.L., Stutts, J.T., Lassan, M.A. *et al.* (1991) Sebaceous gland carcinoma of the finger. *Journal of Hand Surgery* **16A**, 870–872.

## Soft tissue tumours

### Fibrous tumours

There are many different types of *fibroma* which may develop in the subungual and periungual area. They may represent separate entities, or be variants of the same pathology. These fibrous tumours comprise a large variety of clinical types ranging from fibrous dermatofibroma to digital fibrokeratoma. This contrasts markedly with the uniformity of the histology of some fibrous tumours. This is an argument for a continuum of a single pathological process including Koenen's tumour, acquired fibrokeratoma and dermatofibroma of the nail apparatus, though the location of the origin of the fibroblastic proliferation could offer a clue to the diagnosis (Baran *et al.* 1994). For all these reasons, fibrokeratoma, a fibroepithelial tumour, is described with the various fibrous tumours.

#### Benign

*Koenen's tumours* (Figs 11.50–11.52)

Koenen's periungual fibromas develop in about 50% of the cases of tuberous sclerosis (epiloia or Bourneville-Pringle disease) which is a dominantly inherited multisystem disease affecting

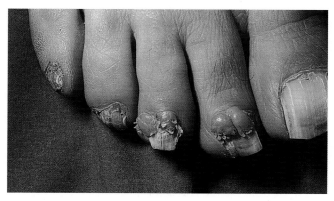

**Fig. 11.50** Koenen's tumours of tuberous sclerosis.

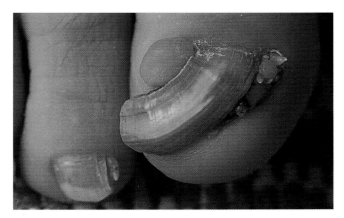

**Fig. 11.51** Koenen's tumours of tuberous sclerosis.

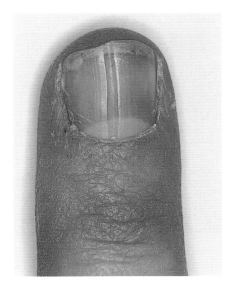

**Fig. 11.52** Koenen's tumours, small lesions under the proximal nail fold causing a groove in the nail plate.

the central nervous system, eyes, skin, cutaneous appendages, kidneys, heart, blood vessels, and bones. Two major gene loci have been identified where mutations can cause the tuberous sclerosis complex with apparently indistinguishable phenotypes: TSC1 at 9q34 and TSC2 at 16p13.3 (Sampson & Harris 1994). The periungual fibromas usually appear between the ages of 12 and 14 years and increase progressively in size and number with age. They are more frequent on toes than on fingers. Rarely are Koenen's tumours the only evidence of tuberous sclerosis (Webb *et al.* 1996) and we have seen a 47-year-old man who had multiple ungual fibromas on eight fingers whereas all toenails were unaffected and no further signs of tuberous sclerosis could be found. A 40-year-old man with familial retinoblastoma was seen to have typical multiple periungual fibrokeratomas without any other evidence of tuberous sclerosis. A germinal mutation of one allele of the RB gene (tumour suppressor gene) was found; since in some cases of tuberous sclerosis, a mutation of the tuberin gene, also a tumour suppressor gene, was demonstrated the authors speculated that multiple

periungual fibromas might indicate an anomaly of tumour suppressor genes (Dereure *et al.* 2000). Longitudinal erythronychia was associated with a subungual nodular tumour in the nail area.

Individual tumours are small, round, flesh-coloured, and asymptomatic, with a smooth surface (Figs 11.50 & 11.51). The tip of the tumour may be slightly hyperkeratotic, resembling fibrokeratoma. They grow out of the nail fold, eventually overgrowing the nail bed and destroying the nail plate. Depending on their location, they may cause longitudinal depressions in the nail plate. They sometimes also grow in the nail plate similar to a dissecting fibrokeratoma or onychomatricoma (Haneke 1998). Even a tiny hyperkeratotic lesion in the cuticle area may produce identical longitudinal nail grooves and have the same significance as Koenen's tumours (Colomb *et al.* 1976) (Fig. 11.52). However, a single ungual fibrokeratoma is apparently not a sign of a minor expression of tuberous sclerosis (Zeller *et al.* 1995). Excessively large tumours are often painful and should be excised at their base. Bone cysts may occur in tuberous sclerosis although those in the distal phalanx are excessively rare (Pontious & Labovitz 1997) and have to be differentiated from a number of other osseous lesions causing cystic defects in the distal phalanx (see aneurysmal bone cyst).

Histologically, no difference has been found between isolated ungual fibrokeratoma and Koenen's tumours (Zeller *et al.* 1995). In the Koenen's tumours we have examined (Kint & Baran 1988) two portions could be distinguished: a small distal segment with loose collagen and many blood vessels and a larger proximal part built up of dense collagen bundles and fewer capillaries. Neither neural or glial appearance (Nickel & Reed 1962) nor arteriovenous anastomoses (Knoth & Meyhöfer 1957) could be found. It thus appears that Koenen's tumour can be considered as a particular type of fibrokeratoma which can be subdivided according to its clinical appearance, its location, and its origin into the following groups:
1 Fibrokeratomas originating from the dermal connective tissue. These are post-traumatic or appear spontaneously and are usually located on the fingers (acquired digital fibrokeratoma).
2 Fibrokeratomas originating from the proximal nail fold or the surrounding connective tissue. They are located in the nail fold and can be hereditary (tuberous sclerosis) or acquired (for example, garlic-clove fibroma).

Koenen's tumours are cured by simple excision. Usually, no suture is necessary. Tumours growing out from under the proximal nail fold are removed after reflecting the proximal nail fold back by making lateral incisions down each margin in the axis of the lateral nail grooves. Subungual fibromas are removed after avulsion of the corresponding part of the nail plate.

## References

Baran, R., Perrin, C.H., Baudet, J. & Requena, L. (1994) Clinical and histological patterns of dermatofibromas (true fibromas) of the nail apparatus. *Clinical and Experimental Dermatology* **19**, 31–35.

Colomb, D., Racouchot, J. & Jeune, R. (1976) Les lésions des ongles dans la sclérose tubéreuse de Bourneville isolées ou associées aux tumeurs de Koenen. *Annales de Dermatologie et de Syphiligraphie* **103**, 431–437.

Dereure, O., Barnéon, G. & Guilhou, J.J. (2000) Multiple acral fibromas in a patient with familial retinoblastoma: a cutaneous marker of tumour and suppressor gene germline mutation? *British Journal of Dermatology* **143**, 856–859.

Haneke, E. (1998) Intraoperative differential diagnosis of onychomatricoma, Koenen's tumours, and hyperplastic Bowen's disease. 7th Cong Eur Acad Dermatol Venereol—Eur Nail Soc, Nice. *Journal of the European Academy of Dermatology and Venereology* **13** (Suppl.), S119.

Kint, A. & Baran, R. (1988) Histopathologic study of Koenen tumours. *Journal of the American Academy of Dermatology* **18**, 369–372.

Knoth, W. & Meyhöfer, W. (1957) Zur Nosologie des Adenoma sebaceum Typ Balzer, der Koenenschen Tumoren und des Morbus Bourneville-Pringle. *Hautarzt* **8**, 359–366.

Nickel, W.R. & Reed, J.R. (1962) Tuberous sclerosis. Special reference to the microscopic alterations in the cutaneous hamartomas. *Archives of Dermatology* **85**, 209–224.

Pontious, J. & Labovitz, J.M. (1997) Periungual fibromas associated with tuberous sclerosis. *Lower Extremity* **4**, 19–23.

Sampson, J.R. & Harris, P.C. (1994) The molecular genetics of tuberous sclerosis. *Human Molecular Genetics* **3**, 1477–1480.

Webb, D.W., Clarke, A., Fryer, A. & Osborne, J.P. (1996) The cutaneous features of tuberous sclerosis: a population study. *British Journal of Dermatology* **135**, 1–5.

Zeller, J., Friedmann, D., Clerici, T. & Revuz, J. (1995) The significance of a single periungual fibroma: report of seven cases. *Archives of Dermatology* **131**, 1465–1466.

### Acquired ungual fibrokeratoma

Acquired ungual fibrokeratoma is probably identical with acquired digital fibrokeratoma (Bart *et al.* 1968) (Fig. 11.53) and garlic clove fibroma (Steel 1965; LoBuono *et al.* 1979) (Fig. 11.54). They are acquired, benign, spontaneously developing, asymptomatic nodules with a hyperkeratotic tip and a narrow base which occur mostly in the periungual area (Fig. 11.55) or elsewhere on the fingers. They may be double and even triple and reach a considerable size (Tisa & Iurcotta

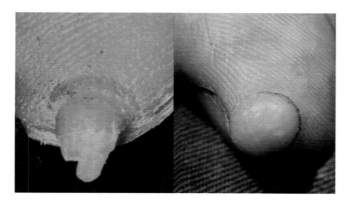

**Fig. 11.53** Acquired digital fibrokeratoma.

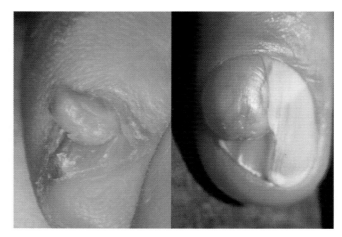

**Fig. 11.54** Garlic clove fibroma.

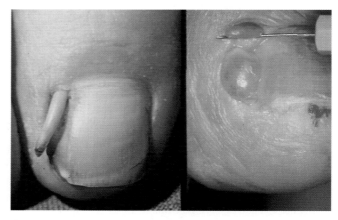

**Fig. 11.55** Acquired periungual fibrokeratoma.

1993). A giant fibrokeratoma of the nail bed was described by Hashiro *et al.* (1995). Takino and Mitoh (1983) reported a case in which the lesion was located beneath the nail and visible under the free margin of the great toe nail. Most ungual fibrokeratomas emerge from the most proximal part of the nail sulcus growing on the nail and causing a sharp longitudinal depression (Kikuchi *et al.* 1978) (Fig. 11.56). Some of these lesions originate from within the matrix and thus grow in the nail plate to eventually emerge in the middle of the nail; these intraungual fibrokeratomas are also called a 'dissecting ungual fibrokeratoma' because they divide the nail plate (Haneke 1998b). Subungual fibrokeratomas arise from the nail bed; they are rare.

*MRI accurately depicts the component emerging from the proximal nail fold in the split of the nail plate. Overall, MR images highlight the deep implantation close to the nail root (Fig. 11.57). The signal of the tumour depends on the different histologic types: very low signal on all sequences for the dense and numerous collagen bundle type, high signal on T2-weighted images in case of mucoid stroma. Intralesional septa and the acanthotic epidermal coverage show regular limits and*

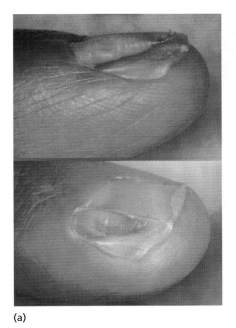

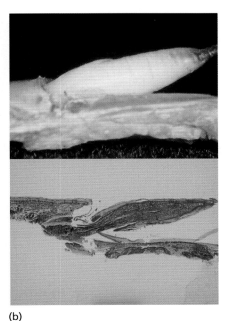

**Fig. 11.56** (a) Acquired periungual fibrokeratoma causing a longitudinal depression. (Courtesy of I. Kikuchi, Japan.) (b) Acquired periungual fibrokeratoma after operative removal (top); low-power histological changes (Masson stain) (bottom).

(a)

(b)

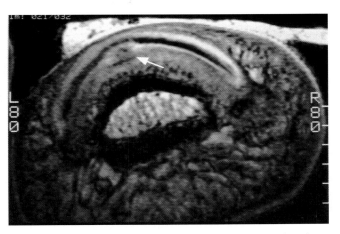

**Fig. 11.57** Acquired fibrokeratoma: deep implantation on the distal matrix (arrow). Axial gradient echo MR image.

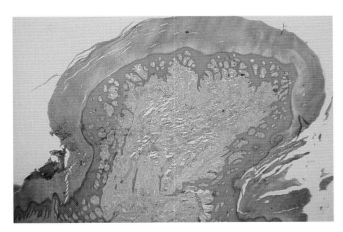

**Fig. 11.58** Acquired periungual fibrokeratoma (type I).

*a signal identical to that of normal epidermis. MRI is also able to depict a tumour involving the ventral aspect of the proximal nail fold with an epithelial invagination.*

Trauma is thought to be a major factor initiating acquired periungual fibrokeratoma. Biopsy is mandatory for the diagnosis of nail tumours: Haneke (1991) described a case of Bowen's disease simulating acquired ungual fibrokeratoma. Pseudo-fibrokertoma should be considered as a clue for Bowen's disease (Baran & Perrin 1994).

Histological examination of fifty cases of acquired digital fibrokeratoma (Kint *et al.* 1985) disclosed three histological variants of these lesions:

**I** a tumour composed of thick dense and closely packed collagen bundles, (Fig. 11.58).

**II** a variant with an increased number of fibroblasts in the cutis (Fig. 11.59).

**III** a type with an oedematous and poorly cellular structure (Fig. 11.60).

The acquired digital fibrokeratoma is considered to result from new collagen formation by fibroblasts. The acanthosis of the epidermis is probably secondary to the dermal alteration.

Immunohistochemistry shows that the fibroblasts are vimentin positive and many of them stain with HHF 35, a monoclonal antibody said to be specific for muscle actin. Surgical treatment is the same as for Koenen's tumours and will depend on the size and location of the fibroma. Usually the tumour is incised around its base and dissected from the bone. Superficial removal usually results in a recurrence (Haneke 2001).

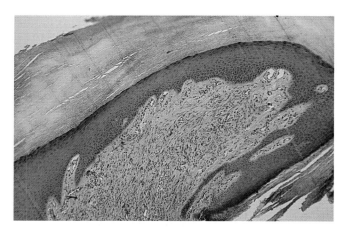

**Fig. 11.59** Acquired periungual fibrokeratoma (type II).

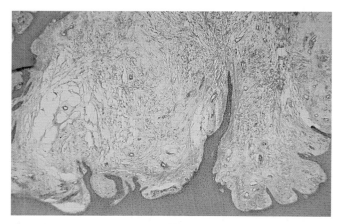

**Fig. 11.60** Acquired periungual fibrokeratoma (type III).

The differential diagnosis of acquired periungual fibroma includes fibroma, keloid, Koenen's tumour, recurring digital fibrous tumours of childhood, dermatofibrosarcoma, fibrosarcoma, cutaneous horn, eccrine poroma, pyogenic granuloma, verruca vulgaris and exostosis (Cahn 1977).

### *Invaginated fibrokeratoma* (Perrin & Baran 1994)

Three cases of a variant of a fibrokeratoma involving the ventral aspect of the proximal nail fold have been observed.

They have three characteristic features:

1 Proximal to the normal matrix, and in the same axis, there is epithelial invagination.

2 The floor of this infolding acts as an accessory matrix, without a granular layer, and gives rise to a 'pseudonail' made of keratin, similar to the normal nail plate.

3 This accessory nail apparatus, lying on a dermal fibrous nodule is sharply demarcated from the surrounding dermis, having a large base which narrows the tip, giving the typical appearance of an incipient fibrokeratoma of type I in Kint *et al.*'s classification.

### *Matrix fibroma*

Kinoshita *et al.* (1996) reported a case of dermatofibroma involving the matrix and noted bulging and thinning of the thumb nail plate. Two cases of 'unguioblastic fibroma' in the right middle finger of a 30-year-old man and the right thumb of a 45-year-old woman were recently described. The tumours were 1.5 and 2.4 cm in diameter, respectively, and involved the proximal nail fold. The lesions showed peripheral bands of benign appearing, basaloid epithelium forming a reticulated pattern of internal growth. Squamous differentiation mainly occurred were the epithelial retinacula merged. Mild papillomatous change was seen in some areas. The stroma was fibrocellular with a collagenous matrix and cells arranged in a parallel array. Mast cells were frequent. Stroma cells were positive for factor XIIIa and CD 34, squamoid epithelial cells stained for AE1–AE3 (Barr *et al.* 1996). We have seen two cases of matrix fibroma clinically producing transverse overcurvature. Histopathology showed a dense cellular stroma made up of very fine collagen fibres and thus resembling the stroma of onychomatricoma (Haneke 1998a).

### *Subungual filamentous tumour*

Subungual filamentous tumours are thread-like horny subungual lesions growing with the nail plate and emerging from under the free edge (Fig. 11.61). They are visible through the nail plate as a whitish, yellowish to brown streak of approximately 1 mm width, sometimes containing some clotted blood, but they are always wider than splinter haemorrhages. They may cause a longitudinal rim or a distal split in the nail. The diagnosis is confirmed by looking under the free edge of the nail plate where they appear as a horny pearl. It can be scraped off when cleaning the hyponchial space and pares down painlessly when the nail is cut. It was thought that this entity might be a narrow, extremely hyperkeratotic fibrokeratoma; however, in contrast to ungual fibrokeratoma, it never grows wider than 1–1.5 mm, is always located under the nail, and

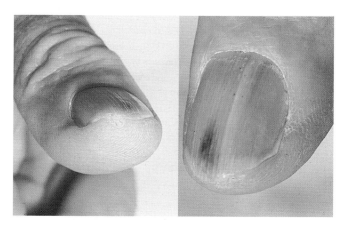

**Fig. 11.61** Subungual filamentous tumour.

**Table 11.3** Differential diagnostic features of fibrokeratoma and subungual filamentous tumour.

| Features | Ungual fibrokeratoma | Subungual filamentous tumour |
|---|---|---|
| Growth of lesion | Slow, insidious | Only keratin filament |
| Location | On, in or under nail | Always under nail plate |
| Differential diagnosis | Koenen's tumour, fibroma, wart, Bowen's disease | Onychopapilloma of the nail bed |

lacks a fibrotic core. It has therefore to be considered as another entity.

Differential diagnosis includes subungual onychopapilloma and subungual warty papilloma (page 528). (Table 11.3).

Radical treatment requires nail bed exposure and excision of the base of the lesion. Histology shows a subungual rim of keratinous substance in an irregular whorled arrangement. The nail bed may show a single slightly papillomatous projection with marked hypergranulosis.

## References

Baran, R. & Perrin, C. (1994) Pseudo-fibrokeratoma of the nail apparatus: a new clue for Bowen disease. *Acta Dermato-Venereologica* **74**, 449–450.

Barr, R., Headington, J.T., Molne, L. & Ternesten-Bratel, A. (1996) Unguioblastic fibroma—a histological and immunohistological study of a previously unrecognized neoplasm. *Journal of Cutaneous Pathology* **23**, 46.

Bart, R.S., Andrade, R., Kopf, A.W. & Leider, M. (1968) Acquired digital fibrokeratomas. *Archives of Dermatology* **97**, 120–129.

Cahn, R.L. (1977) Acquired periungual fibrokeratoma. *Archives of Dermatology* **113**, 1564–1568.

Haneke, E. (1991) Epidermoid carcinoma (Bowen's disease) of the nail simulating acquired ungual fibrokeratoma. *Skin Cancer* **6**, 217–221.

Haneke, E. (1998a) The spectrum of ungual fibromas. In: *Abstracts of Dermatology 2000, Singapore, May 1998.*

Haneke, E. (1998b) Intraoperative differential diagnosis of onychomatricoma, Koenen's tumours, and hyperplastic Bowen's disease. *Journal of the European Academy of Dermatology and Venereology* **11**, S 119.

Haneke, E. (2001) Differential diagnosis of ungual fibrokeratoma and subungual filamentous tumour (in preparation).

Hashiro, M., Fujio, Y., Tanaka, M. & Yamatodani, Y. (1995) Giant acquired fibrokeratoma of the nail. *Dermatology* **190**, 169–171.

Kikuchi, I., Ishii, Y. & Inoue, S. (1978) Acquired periungual fibroma. *Journal of Dermatology* **5**, 235–237.

Kinoshita, Y., Kojima, T. & Furusato, Y. (1996) Subungual dermatofibroma of the thumb. *Journal of Hand Surgery* **21B**, 408–409.

Kint, A., Baran, R. & De Keyser, H. (1985) Acquired (digital) fibrokeratoma. *Journal of the American Academy of Dermatology* **12**, 816–821.

LoBuono, P., Jothikumar, T. & Kornblee, L. (1979) Acquired digital fibrokeratoma. *Cutis* **24**, 50–51.

Perrin, C. & Baran, R. (1994) Invaginated fibrokeratoma of the nail apparatus. *British Journal of Dermatology* **130**, 654–657.

Steel, H.H. (1965) Garlic-clove fibroma. *Journal of the American Medical Association* **191**, 1082–1083.

Takino, C. & Mitoh, Y. (1983) A case of acquired ungual fibroma located beneath the nail. *Japanese Journal of Clinical Dermatology* **37**, 57–62.

Tisa, L.M. & Iurcotta, A. (1993) Solitary periungual angiofibroma. An unusual case report. *Journal of the American Podiatric Medical Association* **83**, 679–680.

### Fibrous dermatofibromas or 'true' fibromas

Fibromas usually develop as painless slow-growing nodular tumours. They may be spherical or oval in shape, and firm or elastic in consistency. They can develop in any epidermal structure of the nail apparatus and may be mobile or fixed (Butler *et al.* 1960).

Fibromas may become cherry-shaped or polypoid and lift the nail in the distal subungual area (Fig. 11.62). In addition to deformity of the nail, displacement of the finger pulp and erosion of the distal phalanx may lead to unnecessary amputation. The tumour is smooth on the dorsal aspect of the proximal fold, or on the nail bed. It is usually spherical, resembling a small pea, or alternatively may be ovoid (Fig. 11.63). On the lateral nail fold the fibroma may also be spherical but without the collar of slightly elevated skin seen in acquired periungual fibrokeratoma. Fibroma of the matrix results in nail dystrophy (Kinoshita *et al.* 1996) (Fig. 11.64). Therefore clinical features are variable according to the anatomical site, ranging from simple thinning of the nail plate to a longitudinal canal, which is sometimes partially covered by nail keratin to form a tunnel-like structure.

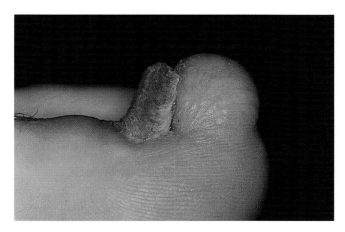

**Fig. 11.62** Fibroma lifting up the nail plate.

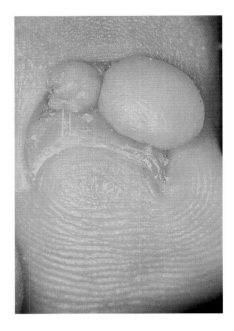

**Fig. 11.63** Spherical fibroma on the dorsum of the nail plate.

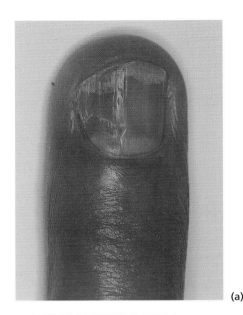

(a)

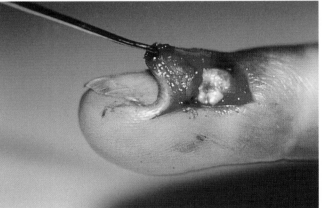

(b)

**Fig. 11.64** (a) Fibroma of the matrix resulting in nail dystrophy. (b) Fibroma at operation.

Lebouc (1889) described a plexiform fibroma of the nail bed which had developed after severe trauma. Heller (1902) described a sub and periungual fibroma, the size of a pigeon egg.

Histological features are a dermal hypocellular reticular nodule, composed of very dense connective tissue bundles with elastic fibres present with ill-defined demarcation and are similar in all our patients in spite of clinical variation (Baran *et al.* 1994). Factor XIIIa was negative on the core of the tumours but in one case, the papillary dermis above the tumour showed a slight increase of factor XIIIa cells surrounding the vessels.

Two types of dermatofibroma histology are classically described (Lever *et al.* 1983): fibroma (or fibrous dermatofibroma) (Fig. 11.66a.b) and histiocytoma. In the latter, uncommon in the nail apparatus, histiocytic proliferation is sometimes associated with an angiomatous component, most often referred to as sclerosing haemangioma. Rupp *et al.* (1957) reported a unique case with darkening of the right great toe nail, slight oedema, moderate erythema, and thickening of the nail, which proved to be a tumour mass within the distal phalanx. Focal erosion of the dorsal cortex with extension of the mass into the lower dermis was present. This was, histologically, a benign fibrous histiocytoma clinically mimicking a melanoma. Reed and Elmer (1971) in a review of 28 cases of solitary acral fibrous tumour distinguished three histological varieties: (a) acquired digital fibrokeratoma (ADFK); (b) irritation fibroma; and (c) fibroma molle. This classification is difficult to apply in the cases we have studied and should be discarded. Several authors (Yasuki 1985, Kojima *et al.* 1987) have assimilated periungual fibroma and periungual fibrokeratoma as interchangeable terms and have not used Reed's classification.

Several connective tissue tumours are easily ruled out (Table 11.4).

Three main histological clues distinguish isolated 'true' fibroma from ADFK and from other tumours of the nail apparatus:

1 the lesions are composed of areas of very thick, hypocellular, hyalinised collagen bundles, in a haphazard array;

2 there is an ill-defined nodule situated mostly in the reticular dermis;

3 the elastic fibres are most often absent or scarce.

*Radiographs may depict erosion of bone and a thickening of the soft tissues. There are no calcifications. MRI findings are suggestive with a mainly low signal nodule on all sequences and very dark irregular areas of extremely dense connective bundles (Fig. 11.65). These patterns and the lack of an obvious peripheral rim differentiate them from acquired fibrokeratomas. A faint and heterogeneous uptake of contrast media may be noted.*

**Table 11.4** Differential diagnosis of ungual true fibroma with other fibrous tumours of the nail apparatus.

*Sclerotic fibroma*
(Rapini & Golitz 1989; Tosti *et al.* 1999)
Well circumscribed
Overlying epidermis thin
Collagen bundle in a 'whorl-like' pattern

*Fibroma of tendon sheath*
Well circumscribed
Attachment to tendon or tendon sheath
Gradual transition between cellular and more hyalinized areas

*Pleomorphic fibroma*
Multinucleated cells with large hyperchromatic nuclei

*Keloid*
(Ackerman 1978; Lever & Schaumberg-Lever 1983; Mehregan 1986)
Well circumscribed
Papillary dermis normal
Hypocellular areas admixed with more cellular areas

*Leiomyoma*
(Requena & Baran 1994; Fitzpatrick *et al.* 1990)
Muscle stains red with Masson trichome (by contrast, fibroma stains blue)
Leiomyoma is labelled by smooth muscle action and desmin (Lever & Schaumberg-Lever 1983)

*Recurrent infantile digital fibromas*
First year of life
Characteristic inclusion bodies visualized with phosphotungstic acid haemotoxylin stain (Lever & Schaumberg-Lever 1983)

*Rudimentary supernumerary digits*
Present at birth
Involvement of the fifth digit
Multiple nerve bundles within the dermal core

*Dermatomyofibroma*
(Cheng & Nydorf 2001)
Uncommon cutaneous neoplasm of myofibroblastic origin)

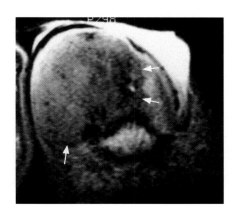

**Fig. 11.65** Subungual fibroma (arrows). Axial post-enhanced T1-weighted spin echo image.

A case of 'osteoid fibroma' of the tip of the right little finger in a 10-year-old girl was described by Stein (1959).

Subungual myxoid pleomorphic fibroma was seen in a 54-year-old man who had a 1-year history of a painless, slowly growing mass subungually in his right thumb. The nail was thickened with subungual hyperkeratosis and paronychia. Histopathology showed a hypocellular neoplasm with haphazard arrangement of thick collagen separated by myxoid stroma and dilated blood vessels. Among ordinary appearing fibroblasts were atypical cells with large pleomorphic and hyperchromatic nuclei, multinucleated cells some of which exhibited rosette arrangement. The cytoplasm was pale pink and scant. The cells were positive for vimentin, and many atypical large cells reacted strongly with anti-CD34 (Hassanein *et al.* 1998).

Tosti *et al.* (1999) described a case of storiform collagenoma (Fig. 11.66c), known as sclerotic fibroma (Rapini & Golitz

1989) and presenting as a 1 cm subungual nodule associated with onycholysis of the first left finger. This peculiar benign fibromatous tumour typically occurs in patients with Cowden's disease, which was not found in Tosti's case. The subungual fibrotic nodule reported by Sigel (1974) in a case of Cowden's disease was not explored histologically.

Dermatomyofibroma is a recently recognized, uncommon cutaneous neoplasm of myofibroblastic origin. Prior clinical reports of dermatomyofibroma show a predilection for the shoulder, axillae or upper arm. The authors have described a case of solitary dermatomyofibroma on the right 5th finger at the proximal nailfold that is thought to be the first reported case occurring at this location. The patient was a 58-year-old woman with an asymptomatic, slowly enlarging nodule. Pathology revealed interweaving fascicles of bland, uniform spindled cells within the reticular dermis. Adnexal structures were preserved within the lesion. The spindled cells demonstrated immunoreactivity for vimentin, muscle-specific actin and smooth muscle actin, consistent with a myofibroblastic origin. Together, these pathologic findings are those of a dermatomyofibroma.

## References

Ackerman, A.B. (1978) *Histologic Diagnosis of Inflammatory Skin Diseases.* Lea Febiger, Philadelphia.

Baran, R. & Perrin, C. (1995) Localised multinucleate distal subungual keratosis. *British Journal of Dermatology* **133**, 77–82.

Baran, R., Perrin, C., Baudet, J. & Requena, L. (1994) Clinical and histological patterns of dermatofibromas (true fibromas) of the nail apparatus. *Clinical and Experimental Dermatology* **19**, 31–35.

Butler, E.D., Hamill, J.P., Seipel, R.S. & de Lorimier, A.A. (1960) Tumours of the hand. *American Journal of Surgery* **100**, 293–302.

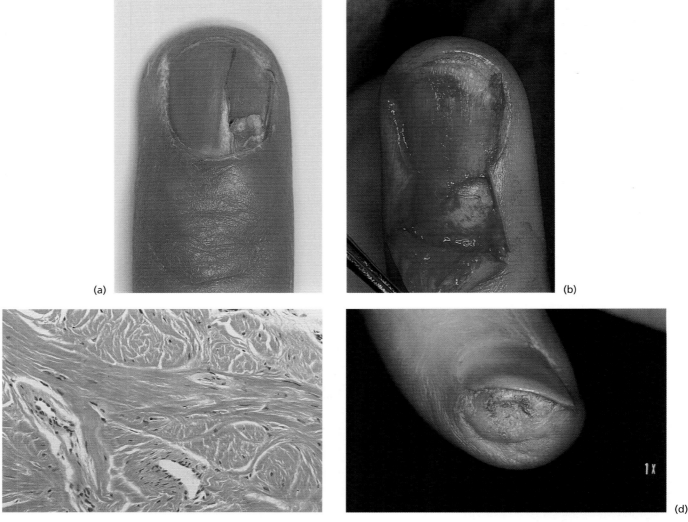

**Fig. 11.66** (a) Fibroma nail dystrophy. (b) Fibroma at operation showing the matrix location of the tumour. (c) Fibroma dermal microscopy, same patient. (d) Storiform colagenoma. (Courtesy of A-Tosti, Bologna, Italy.)

Cheng, A.M. & Nydorf, E.D. (2001) A case of dermatomyofibroma at the proximal nail fold. In: *AAD 59th Annual Meeting*, 2–7 March, Washington, DC. Poster abstract No. 462.

Fitzpatrick, J.E., Mellette, J.R., Hwang, R.J., *et al.* (1990) Cutaneous angiolipoleiomyoma. *Journal of the American Academy of Dermatology* **23**, 1093–1098.

Hassanein, A., Telang, G., Benedetto, E. & Speilvogel, R. (1998) Subungual myxoid pleomorphic fibroma. *American Journal of Dermatopathology* **20**, 502–505.

Heller, E. (1902) *Zur Kenntnis der Fibrome und Sarkome an Hand und Fingern*. Inaugural-Dissertation, Leipzig.

Kinoshita, Y., Kojima, T. & Furusato, Y. (1996) Subungual dermatofibroma of the thumb. *Journal of Hand Surgery* **21B**, 408–409.

Kojima, T., Nagano, T. & Uchida, M. (1987) Periungual fibroma. *Journal of Hand Surgery* **12A**, 465–470.

Lebouc, L. (1889) *Etude clinique et anatomique sur quelques cas de tumeurs sous-unguéales. Thèse pour le doctorat en médecine.* pp. 1–34. G. Steinheil, Paris.

Lever, W.F. & Schaumburg-Lever, G. (1983) *Histopathology of the Skin*, 7th edn. JB Lippincott, Philadelphia.

Mehregan, A.M. (1986) *Pinkus' Guide to Dermatohistopathology*, 4th edn. Appleton-Century-Crofts, Norwalk, CT.

Rapini, R.P. & Golitz, L.E. (1989) Sclerotic fibromas of the skin. *Journal of the American Academy of Dermatology* **20**, 266–271.

Reed, R.J. & Elmer, L.C. (1971) Multiple acral fibrokeratomas. Discussion of classification of acral fibrous nodules. *Archives of Dermatology* **103**, 286–297.

Requena, L. & Baran, R. (1994) Angioleiomyoma of the finger. *Journal of the American Academy of Dermatology* **110**, 476–477.

Rupp, M., Khalluf, E. & Toker, C. (1957) Subungual fibrous histiocytoma mimicking melanoma. *Journal of the American Podiatric Medical Association* **3**, 141–142.

Sawada, Y. (1988) Angioleiomyoma masquerading as a painful ganglion of the great toe. *European Journal of Plastic Surgery* **11**, 175–177.

Sigel, J.M. (1974) Tuberous sclerosis (forme fruste) vs. Cowden syndrome. *Archives of Dermatology* **110**, 476–477.

Stein, A.H. (1959) Benign neoplastic and nonneoplastic destructive lesions in the long bones of the hand. *Surgery, Gynecology and Obstetrics* **109**, 189–97.

Tosti, A., Cameli, N., Peluso, A.M. *et al.* (1999) Storiform collagenoma of the nail. *Cutis* **64**, 203–204.

Yasuki, Y. (1985) Acquired periungual fibrokeratoma. *Journal of Dermatology* **12**, 349–356.

### Keloid

Hypertrophic scars and keloids result from injuries to the nail fold or nail bed, but are rare in this location. They present as relatively large, smooth, firm nodules (Heller 1927) (Fig. 11.67). Large keloids were seen after electrosurgical resection of the hallux and second toenails because of recurrent ingrown nails in a 25-year-old man (E. Haneke, unpublished data).

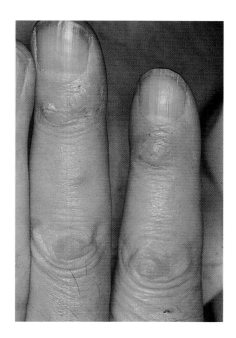

**Fig. 11.68** Knuckle pads.

Keloid exhibits hyalinised collagen bundles; the fibroblasts are contiguous with, and parallel to, the thick collagen bundles which are separated from the epidermis by nearly normal papillary dermis. Additionally, keloids are well-circumscribed and elastic fibres are not present.

### Reference

Heller, J. (1927) Die Krankheiten der Nägel. In: *Handbuch der Haut- und Geschlechtskrankheiten*, Bd VIII/2. *Spezielle Dermatologie* (ed. J. Jadassohn), pp. 150–172. Springer, Berlin.

### Knuckle pads

Knuckle pads are asymptomatic, persistent, flesh-coloured, keratotic, nodular plaques occurring on the dorsal surface of the interphalangeal joints (Fig. 11.68). Histology shows hyperkeratosis and an increase in the thickness of collagen bundles (Mulvaney *et al.* 1985). They rarely interfere with normal nail growth.

### Reference

Mulvaney, M.S., Salasche, S.J. & Hayes, T.J. (1985) Differential diagnosis of multiple acral nodules. *Journal of the Association of Military Dermatology* **11**, 24–27.

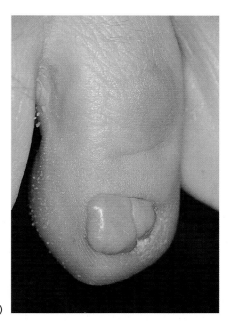

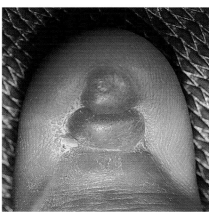

**Fig. 11.67** (a) Keloid of the nail bed. (b) Keloid following grafting of the nail bed. (Courtesy of S. Goettmann-Bonvallot, France.)

### Infantile digital fibromatosis (recurring digital fibrous tumours of childhood, benign juvenile digital fibromatosis) (Reye 1965)

Recurring digital fibrous tumours (RDFT) are round, smooth, dome-shaped, shiny (Oñate-Cuchet *et al.* 1989), firm to tense dermal nodules, with reddish or livid-red colour (Fig. 11.69).

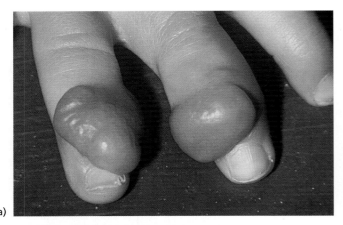

(a)

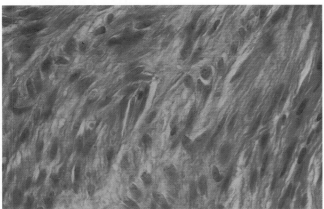

(b)

**Fig. 11.69** (a) Infantile digital fibromatosis. (b) Histology of infantile digital fibromatosis. (Courtesy of J.L. Verret, France.)

They are located on the dorsal and axial surfaces of the fingers and toes, characteristically sparing the thumbs and great toes. They may be present at birth or develop during infancy. Two cases were described in an adolescent and an adult, respectively (Demar 1975; Sarma & Hoffman 1980). Fingers are more often affected than toes. On reaching the nail unit, they may elevate the nail plate leading to dystrophy but not to destruction. The tumour may cause considerable distortion of the digits. Often the tumour is multicentric occurring on several digits.

Ryman and Bale (1985) reported thirty cases, seen over 36 years: 20 females and 10 males. Fingers and toes were equally affected. Multiple lesions occurred in 50% of patients, more often in the fingers, especially on adjacent fingers. Two patients had bilateral lesions. Dabney *et al.* (1986) and Piñol-Aguadé *et al.* (1971) observed firm plantar nodules in one of their three cases with infantile digital fibromatosis.

With recurrence occurring in 60% after excision, surgery should be attempted only if functional impairment occurs. Excessive growth has been treated by amputation of the involved digit in some cases (Poppen & Niebauer 1977). Surgery necessitates going down to the fascia and tendon to avoid recurrence. It can be mutilating. As this lesion is entirely benign and meta-

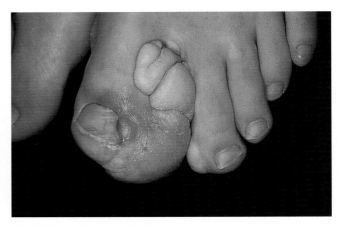

**Fig. 11.70** Cerebriform connective tissue naevus.

stasis has never been recorded, the amputations sometimes performed in the past (38 of 115 cases) can no longer be justified (Ryman & Bale 1985).

Conservative treatment is the best since the lesions have a natural course: a tumoral stage, followed by spontaneous resolution (Duran-McKinster *et al.* 1993; Kawaguchi *et al.* 1998). The lesions are not observed in adulthood (Sangüeza & Jove 1983). Cryosurgery may accelerate the natural involution.

Histologically (Fig. 11.69b), in about 2% of the fibroblasts, paranuclear inclusion bodies, 3–10 mm in diameter, can be seen in properly fixed specimens using stains such as iron haematoxylin, methyl green-pyronin, and phosphotungstic acid-haematoxylin (Mehregan 1981). They are also visible in haematoxylin and eosin stained sections as globules slightly smaller than erythrocytes (Haneke 1998). Zina *et al.* (1986) studied two cases of Reye's tumour by electron microscopy and immunohistochemistry, using rabbit anti-actin sera. The tumour cells were typical myofibroblasts, containing inclusion bodies and bundles of microfilaments. Immunohistochemistry has shown that the paranuclear inclusions consist of actin fibres.

Differential diagnosis includes pseudo-infantile digital fibromatosis with hypertrophic lateral lips of the great toe in early infancy (Chapter 3), fibrosarcoma and neurofibrosarcoma. Cerebriform connective tissue naevus (Bauer & Eisen 1985) (Fig. 11.70) and the multiple, soft dome-shaped tumours present in a patient with systemic sclerosis but histologically reminiscent of cutaneous focal mucinosis (Marzano *et al.* 1997) should also be ruled out. Progressive thickening of the soles of the feet was accompanied in a 10-year-old girl by fleshy, cerebriform elevations over the plantar surfaces with extension onto the sides and dorsal aspect of several toes. The most striking biochemical abnormality is the marked reduction in the production of collagenase. Similar patients have been reported (Cohen & Hayden 1979) also suffering multiple hamartomas including linear epidermal naevi. Histopathologically, Reye's fibrous tumour may be confused with dermatofibroma, fibroma and scar tissue.

## References

Bauer, E.A. & Eisen, A.Z. (1985) Biochemical changes in certain genodermatoses. *Clinics in Dermatology* **3**, 135–142.

Cohen, M.M. & Hayden, P.W. (1979) A newly recognized hamartomatous syndrome. *Birth Defects* **5B**, 291–296.

Dabney, K.W., MacEwen, G.D. & Davis, N.E. (1986) Recurring digital fibrous tumour of childhood. Case report with long-term follow-up and review of the literature. *Journal of Pediatric Orthopedics* **6**, 612–617.

Demar, L. (1975) Recurring digital fibrous tumor of childhood. *Archives of Dermatology* **111**, 1372–1373.

Duran-McKinster, C., Herrera, M., Reyes-Mugica, M. & Ruiz-Maldonado, R. (1993) Infantile digital fibromatosis: spontaneous regression in three cases. *European Journal of Dermatology* **3**, 192–194.

Haneke, E. (1998) Clinical and histopathological spectrum of ungual fibromas. In: *Clinical Dermatology 2000, Singapore, Book of Abstracts.*

Kawaguchi, M., Mitsuhashi, Y., Hozumi, Y. & Kondo, S. (1998) A case of infantile digital fibromatosis with spontaneous regression. *Journal of Dermatology* **25**, 523–526.

Marzano, A.V., Berti, E., Gasparini, G. *et al.* (1997) Unique digital skin lesions associated with systemic sclerosis. *British Journal of Dermatology* **136**, 598–600.

Mehregan, A. (1981) Superficial fibrous tumors in childhood. *Journal of Cutaneous Pathology* **8**, 321–334.

Oñate-Cuchet, M.J., Vargas Castrillon, J., Sanchez Gomez-Coronada, P. *et al.* (1989) Fibromatosis digital recurrente infantil. *Acta Dermato-Sifilitica* **80**, 15–18.

Piñol-Aguadé, J., Mascaro, J.M., Galy-Mascaro, C. *et al.* (1971) Etude clinique, histologique et ultrastructurale de la fibromatose juvénile bénigne des doigts. *Archives Medicals de l'Ouest (France)* **3**, 179–183.

Poppen, N.K. & Niebauer, J.J. (1977) Recurring digital fibrous tumour of childhood. *Journal of Hand Surgery* **2**, 253–255.

Reye, R.D.K. (1965) Recurring digital fibrous tumours of childhood. *Archives of Pathology* **80**, 228–231.

Ryman, W. & Bale, P. (1985) Recurring digital fibromas of infancy. *Australasian Journal of Dermatology* **26**, 113–117.

Sangüeza, P. & Jove, N. (1983) Fibromatosis digital infantil recidivante. *Medicina Cutanea Ibero-Latino-Americana* **11**, 307–310.

Sarma, D.P. & Hoffman, E.D. (1980) Infantile digital fibroma-like tumour in an adult. *Archives of Dermatology* **116**, 578.

Zina, A.M., Rampini, E., Fulcheri, E. *et al.* (1986) Recurrent digital fibromatosis of childhood. An ultrastructural and immunohistochemical study of 2 cases. *American Journal of Dermatopathology* **8**, 22–26.

### *Juvenile hyaline fibromatosis II* (Fig. 11.71)

Juvenile hyaline fibromatosis II is the name introduced by Kitano *et al.* (1972) to describe the condition previously reported as molluscum fibrosum, mesenchymal dysplasia (Puretic syndrome), systemic hyalinosis and fibromatosis. About 40 cases have been described in the world literature. It is characterized by skin lesions, muscle weakness, and flexion contractures of large joints. The skin lesions are multiple, large, subcutaneous,

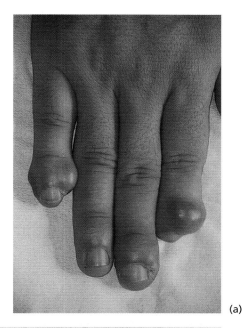

**Fig. 11.71** (a) Juvenile hyaline fibromatosis II. (b) Histology of the same lesion.

painless, hyaline tumours, or small, pink or pearly papules with a translucent appearance and gelatinous consistency. They are found in the head and neck region, on the trunk and at the tip of the digits where acroosteolysis may be seen. Distal osteolysis with destruction of the distal phalanx causes nail deformity (Puretic *et al.* 1962; Gutierrez *et al.* 1973) whereas no nail changes were described despite excessively large periungal hyaline fibromas in the case of Rimbaud *et al.* (1973) redescribed by Schaller *et al.* (1997).

The tumours exhibit a reduction of normal collagen and fibroblasts and show lake-like deposits of a hyaline substance. 'Chondroid' cells are seen in this eosinophilic substance. Electron microscopy showed the fibroblasts to contain a markedly dilated rough endoplasmic reticulum and Golgi apparatus filled with granular and fibrillar material (Finlay *et al.* 1983; Schaller *et al.* 1997). Excision of cutaneous lesions is almost always followed by local recurrences (Kan & Rogers 1989).

Juvenile hyaline fibromatosis is inherited as an autosomal recessive trait.

## References

Finlay, A.Y., Ferguson, S.D. & Holt, P.J.A. (1983) Juvenile hyaline fibromatosis. *British Journal of Dermatology* **108**, 609–616.

Gutierrez, G. *et al.* (1973) Fibromatosis hialinica multiple juvenile. *Medicina Cutanea Ibero-Latino-Americana* **7**, 283–286.

Kan, A.E. & Rogers, M. (1989) Juvenile hyaline fibromatosis: an expanded clinicopathologic spectrum. *Pediatric Dermatology* **6**, 68–75.

Kitano, Y., Horiki, M. & Aoki, T. (1972) Two cases of juvenile hyalin fibromatosis. Some histological, electron microscopy and tissue culture observations. *Archives of Dermatology* **106**, 877–883.

Puretic, S., Puretic, B., Fišer-Herman, M. *et al.* (1962) A unique form of mesenchymal dysplasia. *British Journal of Dermatology* **74**, 8–19.

Rimbaud, P., Jean, R., Meynadier, J., Rieu, D., Guilhou, J.J. & Barnéon, G. (1973) Fibro-hyalinose juvénile. *Bulletin de la Société Française de Dermatologie et de Syphiligraphie* **80**, 435–436.

Schaller, M., Stengel-Rutkowki, S. & Kind, P. (1997) Juvenile hyaline fibromatose. *Hautarzt* **48**, 253–257.

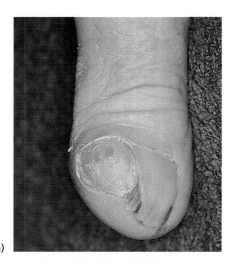

(a)

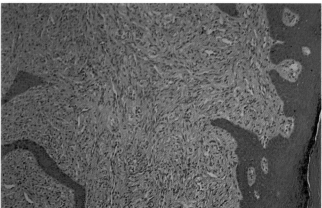

(b)

**Fig. 11.72** (a) Dermatofibrosarcoma protuberans. (Courtesy of A. Bories, France.) (b) Histology of the same lesion. (Courtesy of A. Claudy.)

## Malignant

### *Dermatofibrosarcoma protuberans*

A pink, firm, multilobulated, and painful mass involved the palmar aspect of the distal thumb of a 31-year-old black woman. The fibrous growth of rubbery consistence was surrounded by well-circumscribed skin (Coles *et al.* 1989).

A 55-year-old Japanese woman presented with a dark-brownish hyperkeratotic plaque on the dorsum of her first proximal to the posterior nail fold. The initial clinical diagnosis of wart prompted treatment with cryotherapy. After that, a glossy milky white tumour appeared (Hashiro *et al.* 1995).

Pigmented pachyonychia of the second toe was the clinical presentation of a subungual tumour in a 55-year-old caucasian woman (Fig. 11.72a). Histology revealed the characteristic histology of dermatofibrosarcoma (Dumas *et al.* 1998) (Fig. 11.72b).

## References

Coles, M., Smith, M. & Rankin, E.A. (1989) An unusual case of dermatofibrosarcoma protuberans. *Journal of Hand Surgery* **14A**, 135–138.

Dumas, V., Euvrard, S., Ligeron, C. *et al.* (1998) Dermatofibrosarcome de Darier–Ferrand sous-unguéal. *Annales de Dermatologie et de Vénéréologie* **125** (Suppl. 3), S93 (poster 37).

Hashiro, M., Fujio, Y., Shoda, Y. & Okumura, M. (1995) A case of dermatofibrosarcoma protuberans on the right first toe. *Cutis* **56**, 281–282.

## Vascular tumours

### Benign

#### *Haemangiomas*

Haemangiomas of the nail bed and tip of the digit are extremely rare. They exhibit the classic course with fast growth and slow spontaneous involution (Fig. 11.73).

#### *Capillary malformations (port-wine stains and telangiectases)*

Capillary malformations are developmental defects present from birth, and usually permanent. They may look violet through the nail (Fig. 11.74). Paradoxically, when the colour of the angioma is pronounced, true leuconychia can be observed (Fig. 11.75) (Enjolras & Riché 1990).

#### *Venous malformations*

Venous malformations of the nail apparatus are rare and should be left untreated. The shape of the nail may remain normal but the nail bed is blue (Enjolras & Riché 1990) (Fig. 11.76). It may blacken if thrombosed. Venous malformations

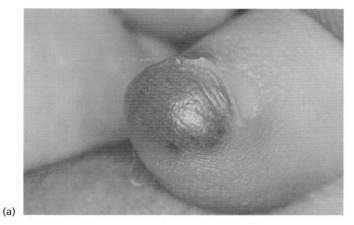

(a)

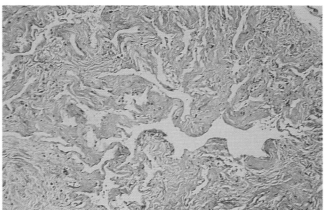

(b)

**Fig. 11.73** (a) Subungual haemangioma. (b) Subungual haemangioma—histological changes.

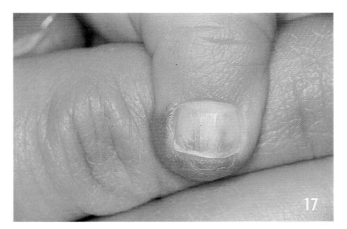

**Fig. 11.74** Port-wine stain.

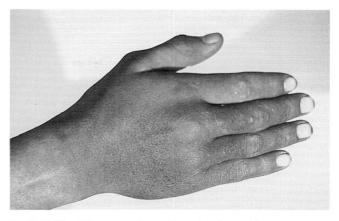

**Fig. 11.75** Klippel–Trenaunay syndrome with prominent leuconychia.

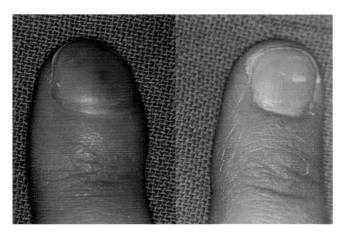

**Fig. 11.76** Venous malformation showing blue nail bed in an isolated finger. (Courtesy of P. Souteyrand, France.)

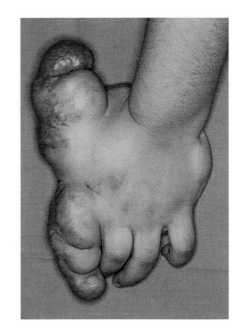

**Fig. 11.77** Klippel–Trenaunay syndrome—'venous' colour of the subungual area. (Courtesy of O. Enjolras, France.)

may arise in the bone or soft tissue (Fig. 11.77). When primary in the bone they have a characteristic radiological appearance of linear striations parallel to the shaft of the bone. Soft tissue venous malformations are more common lesions and may be radiographically manifested by local soft tissue masses,

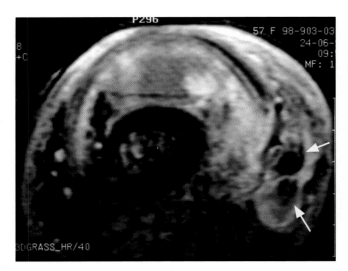

**Fig. 11.78** Venous malformation of the lateral nail fold and the nail bed. Axial post-enhanced gradient echo image. Note the flow void artifact in the lateral nail fold (arrows).

phleboliths in the soft tissue, and pressure erosion of the underlying bone (Monses & Murphy 1984).

Histopathology shows ectatic capillary or venous channels with normal-looking endothelial cells.

*MRI easily shows the vascular patterns of the malformation, but is not able to differentiate it from other vascular tumours. Images may be misleading without the injection of contrast media. Flow void artefacts, signal haemorrhage and a high enhancement after injection of gadolinium must be searched for. MRI also assesses the extension of the lesion in the soft tissues and the relations with the digital collateral vessels (Fig. 11.78). These relations may be better highlighted with angio-MRI sequences. The original location, soft tissues or bone, is easily depicted on MR images.*

Heller's case with 'angioelephantiasis' probably represented Klippel–Trenaunay's syndrome, i.e. a capillary and venous complex combined malformation, or a Parkes-Weber syndrome, i.e. a limb overgrowth syndrome due to arterio-venous fistula. The bed of the thumb was dark blue and four toenails were reduced to keratotic plugs (Heller 1927).

### References

Enjolras, O. & Riché, M.C. (1990) *Hémangiomes et malformations vasculaires superficielles.* Medsi/McGraw-Hill, New York.

Heller, J. (1927) Die Krankheiten der Nägel. In: *Handbuch der Haut- und Geschlechtskrankheiten*, Bd VIII/2. *Spezielle Dermatologie* (ed. J. Jadassohn), pp. 150–172. Springer, Berlin.

Monses, B. & Murphy, W.A. (1984) Distal phalangeal erosive lesions. *Arhritis and Rheumatism* **27**, 449–455.

### *Angiokeratoma circumscriptum* (Fig. 11.79)

Dolph *et al.* (1981) described a 12-year-old girl with a raised, firm, bluish-purple nodule over the dorsal aspect of the distal

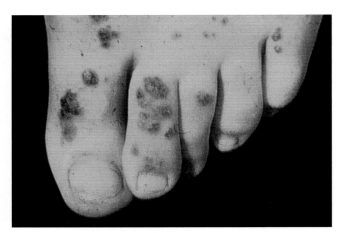

**Fig. 11.79** Angiokeratoma circumscriptum.

index finger. It enlarged with the concomitant appearance of several black dots at the periphery. Histology showed a typical angiokeratoma. The authors listed several tumours in the differential diagnosis, of which malignant melanoma was the most important.

### Reference

Dolph, J.L., Demuth, R.J. & Miller, S.H. (1981) Angiokeratoma circumscriptum of the index finger in a child. *Plastic and Reconstructive Surgery* **67**, 221–223.

### *Arteriovenous fistula (aneurysmal bone cyst)*

Arteriovenous fistulae may occur in the distal phalanx of young people. They are rapidly growing, painful lesions with marked, bulbous enlargement of the fingertip. Aneurysmal bone cyst is a distinct clinical entity separated from haemangiomas of bone and from other tumours in which giant cells are also a prominent feature. It has been named aneurysmal bone cyst because the contour of the affected bone suggests a blow-out type of distension which resembles the secular protrusion of the walls of an aneurysm and also because cystic blood-filled spaces are encountered at surgery. On X-ray, the phalanx may be excessively enlarged and almost completely occupied by osteolytic tissue simulating a malignant tumour (Schajowicz *et al.* 1970) (Fig. 11.80). Computed tomographic scans of aneurysmal bone cysts reveal fluid levels (Hudson 1984), but they are a non-specific finding (Kransdorf & Sweet 1995).

*MRI may be evocative of aneurysmal bone cyst with intraosseous cystic blood-filled spaces with horizontal levels (Schmutz et al. 1988). However, these findings are not pathognomonic.*

### References

Hudson, T.M. (1984) Fluid levels in aneurysmal bone cysts: a CT feature. *American Journal of Roentgenology* **141**, 1001–1004.

Kransdorf, M.J. & Sweet, D.E. (1995) Aneurysmal bone cyst: concept, controversy, clinical presentation and imaging. *American Journal of Roentgenology* **164**, 573–580.

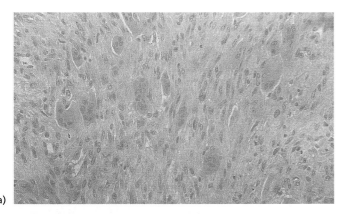

(a)

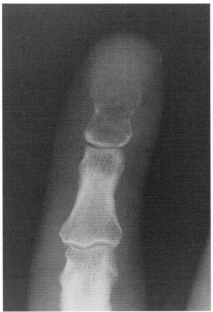

(b)

**Fig. 11.80** (a) Aneurysmal bone cyst—histiocytic, fibroblastic and multinucleate cells. (b) Aneurysmal bone cyst. (Courtesy of J.L. Schmutz, France.)

Schajowicz, F., Aiello, C. & Slullitel, I. (1970) Cystic and pseudocystic lesions of the terminal phalanx with special reference to epidermoid cysts. *Clinical Orthopedics and Related Research* **68**, 84–92.

Schmutz, J.L., Cuny, J.F., Duprez, A. *et al.* (1988) Kyste osseux anévrismal d'un orteil. *Recherche Dermatologique* **1**, 679–681.

### Subungual keratosis with longitudinal erythronychia (onychopapilloma of the nail bed)

This lesion was first described as 'acquired subungual superficial capillary malformation'.

### Intravascular papillary endothelial hyperplasia (pseudoangiosarcoma of Masson)

This rare reactive lesion usually occurs in dilated thrombosed veins. A 50-year-old male hair-dresser was observed who pre-

sented with a slightly tender, swollen, bluish-red tip of his right index finger suspicious of a metastasis to the terminal phalanx. The nail plate appeared enlarged, the radial nail wall had almost disappeared. The patient did not remember a specific traumatic event although repeated microtrauma was possible. X-ray examination did not reveal bony changes. An incision was made along the lateral aspect of the terminal phalanx and a dark-blue, segmented lesion became visible which upon further dissection turned out to be vascular. Histopathological examination revealed intravascular papillary endothelial hyperplasia in a thrombotic, thin-walled, very ectatic vein (Haneke *et al.* 1997).

### Reference

Haneke, E., Mainusch, O. & Hilker, O. (1997) Diaklinik der Hautklinik Wuppertal. *Zeitschrift für Dermatologie* **183**, 180–195.

### Periungual and subungual arteriovenous tumours (cirsoid angioma)

A firm, bluish, non-pulsatile vascular nodule has been reported in the lateral nail fold of the left little finger with histological findings consistent with cirsoid angioma (Burge *et al.* 1996).

In four cases an aequivid vascular tumour involved the subungual tissue. In another patient, a cirsoid angioma under the matrix of both thumbs caused transverse overcurvature and a distal split in the nails (E. Haneke, unpublished data). This sometimes painful lesion is distinguished from pyogenic granuloma by the prolonged history without enlargement or bleeding, while the absence of exquisite tenderness differentiates, clinically, from a glomus tumour. Cirsoid angioma should be considered in the differential diagnosis of causes of a longitudinal red line with distal fissuring in the nail. Some cases probably correspond to onychopapilloma of the nail bed.

### Reference

Burge, S.M., Baran, R., Dawber, R.P.R. & Verret, J.L. (1986) Periungual and subungual arteriovenous tumours. *British Journal of Dermatology* **115**, 361–366.

### Digital arteriovenous malformation

In digital arteriovenous malformations the digit and the nail bed have a purple hue with progressive resorption of the distal phalanx and shrinking of the nail plate presenting a slight transverse overcurvature (Fig. 11.81). In Kadono *et al.*'s (2000) patients, the lesions were acquired and occurred in young individuals with history of preceding trauma in some cases. Clinically the lesions consisted of collections of reddish dots. The colour faded on diascopy and returned immediately after decompression. Histologically, dilated venous and arterial vessels were present in the dermis. Pseudo-Kaposi syndrome can be seen (Enjolras & Riché 1990) (Fig. 11.82). Diagnosis is

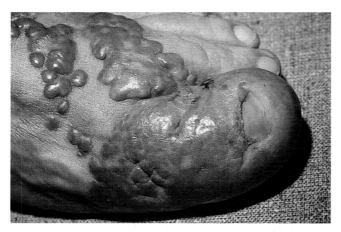

**Fig. 11.81** Arteriovenous fistula. (Courtesy of J.L. Schmutz, France.)

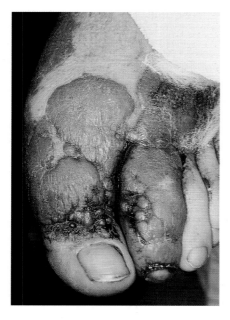

**Fig. 11.82** Pseudo-Kaposi syndrome.

easily made from Doppler ultrasound evaluation and digital arteriography. Heller's case with 'angioelephantiasis' (1927) probably represented Klippel–Trenaunay's syndrome or Parkes–Weber's syndrome.

## References

Enjolras, O. & Riché, M.C. (1990) *Hémangiomes et Malformations Vasculaires Superficielles.* Medsi/McGraw-Hill, New-York.

Heller, J. (1927) Die Krankheiten der Nägel. In: *Handbuch der Haut- und Geschlechtskrankheiten*, Bd VIII/2. *Spezielle Dermatologie* (ed. J. Jadassohn), pp. 150–172. Springer, Berlin.

Kadono, T., Kishi, A., Onishi, Y. *et al.* (2000) Acquired digital arteriovenous malformation: a report of six cases. *British Journal of Dermatology* 142, 362–365.

## Epithelioid haemangioma

Weiss and Enzinger (1982) proposed the term 'epithelioid haemangioendothelioma' to describe an unusual tumour of soft tissue having an epithelioid appearance. These tumours pursue a clinical course between that of a haemangioma and that of a conventional angiosarcoma. Similar neoplasms occur in other sites such as the lung, liver and bone.

Epithelioid haemangioma masquerading as a paronychia was described in a 42-year-old female who had a 6-month history of progressive swelling and some tenderness of the left great toe. The toe was diffusely swollen, the pulp was bluish-red and there was increased curvature of the nail of the left big toe. On X-ray a large lytic lesion of the distal phalanx was shown without any reactive new bone formation and with expansion of the proximal end of the phalanx and an associated large soft tissue mass. The typical multicentric morphology was recognized, on the basis of bone isotope scan. Multifocal epithelioid haemangioendothelioma of the sole of the foot and tip of the toes was observed in a 63-year-old female patient. The diagnosis was confirmed by the demonstration of the endothelial markers factor VIII, CD 31 and CD 34. MRI scan and digital subtraction angiography showed multifocal bone involvement. Treatment with interferon-alpha led to partial regression (Laskowski *et al.* 1999).

Histopathology of curetted tissue showed numerous vessels of varying size and development, many with large epithelioid endothelial cells. The associated inflammatory infiltrate contained foci of eosinophils (Kennedy *et al.* 1990).

Because of its rare occurrence, epithelioid haemangioma may be misdiagnosed as a metastatic carcinoma or other neoplasm (Tsuneyoshi *et al.* 1986).

## References

Kennedy, C.T.C., Burton, P.A. & Cook, P. (1990) Swollen toe due to epithelioid haemangioma of bone. *British Journal of Dermatology* 123 (Suppl. 37), 85–89.

Laskowski, J., Bamberg, C., Zimmermann, R. & Gross, G. (1999) Multifokales Hämangioendotheliom der unteren Extremität. *Hautarzt* 50 (Suppl. 1), S74.

Tsuneyoshi, M., Dorfman, H.D. & Bauer, T.W. (1986) Epithelioid hemangioendothelioma of bone. A clinicopathologic, ultrastructural, and immunohistochemical study. *American Journal of Surgery and Pathology* 10, 754–756.

Weiss, S.W. & Enzinger, F.M. (1982) Epithelioid haemangioendothelioma. A vascular tumor often mistaken for a carcinoma. *Cancer* 50, 970–981.

## Pseudo-pyogenic granuloma (histiocytoid haemangioma)

Avenel *et al.* (1982) described a 40-year-old woman with angiomatous nodules affecting the fingertip, lateral nail folds and nail bed (Fig. 11.83a). The histological and ultrastructural changes were consistent with a diagnosis of pseudo-pyogenic cytoplasmic vacuoles. The endothelial cells were positive for factor VIII and vimentin.

The collective term histiocytoid haemangioma (Rosai *et al.* 1979) encompasses a spectrum of diseases that share histological features characterized by distinctive histiocytoid endothelial cells. Several incompletely defined cutaneous and extracutaneous vascular tumours, including atypical pyogenic granuloma, pseudopyogenic granuloma, papular angioplasia, angiolymphoid hyperplasia with eosinophilia, Kimura's disease, and inflammatory arteriovenous haemangioma, have been included in this group.

## References

Avenel, M., Verret, J.L. & Fortier, P. (1982) Finger localisation of Wilson–Jones pseudo-pyogenic granuloma. In: *Case Presentations in XVI Congressus Int Dermatol Tokyo 1982*, p. 38. University of Tokyo Press, Japan.

Dannaker, C., Piacquadio, D., Willoughby, C.B. & Goltz, R.W. (1989) Histiocytoid hemangioma: a disease spectrum. *Journal of the American Academy of Dermatology* 21, 404–409.

Rosai, J., Gold, J. & Landy, R. (1979) Histiocytoid haemangiomas. *Human Pathology* 10, 707–729.

Tosti, A., Peluso, A.M., Fanti, P.A., Torresan, F., Solmi, L. & Bassi, F. (1994) Histiocytoid hemangioma with prominent fingernail involvement. *Dermatology* 189, 87–89.

Verret, J.L., Avenel, M., François, H., Baudoin, M. & Alain, P. (1983) Hémangiomes histiocytoïdes des pulpes digitales. *Annales de Dermatologie et de Vénéréologie* 110, 251–257.

Wilson-Jones, E. & Bleehen, S.S. (1969) Pseudo-pyogenic granuloma. *British Journal of Dermatology* 81, 804–816.

### Angiolymphoid hyperplasia with eosinophilia (ALHE)

Risitano *et al.* (1990) described a 23-year-old man with ALHE of the nail bed of his left ring finger and Imbing *et al.* (1996) reported on a 26-year-old black woman with slightly blue-black subungual discoloration in the right small fingernail together with more lesions on the palm. Ward *et al.* (1996) observed a 39-year-old man with a tender multinodular swelling of the left middle fingernail causing nail deformity and splitting.

Histology shows a benign vascular proliferation associated with a dense lymphocytic infiltrate with many eosinophils. The capillaries are lined with plump endothelial cells protruding into the lumen.

ALHE was considered to be identical with histiocytoid haemangioma (Ward *et al.* 1996) or epithelioid haemangioma (Imbing *et al.* 1996).

Pachydermoperiostosis was associated with ALHE involving the face and the palms in a patient of Kanekura *et al.* (1994).

## References

Imbing, F.D., Viegas, S.F. & Sánchez, R.L. (1996) Multiple angiolymphoid hyperplasia with eosinophilia of the hand: report of a case and review of the literature. *Cutis* 58, 345–348.

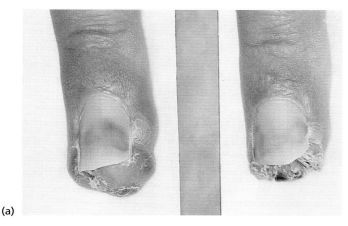

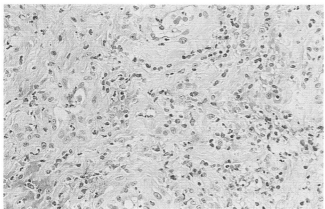

**Fig. 11.83** (a) Histiocytoid haemangioma. (Courtesy of J.L. Verret, Angers, France.) (b) Histology of histiocytoid haemangioma. (Courtesy of A. Tosti, Bologna, Italy.)

granuloma (Wilson-Jones & Bleehen 1969; Bosai *et al.* 1979; Verret *et al.* 1983); (Fig. 11.83b). Dannaker *et al.* (1989) reported a case with simultaneous cutaneous and bone involvement of histiocytoid haemangiomas. The patient, a 31-year-old Mexican-American man, presented with nail changes including onycholysis of the distal area, longitudinal splitting, subungual and periungual erythema, and paronychial swelling with purulent drainage. Biopsy specimens showed a proliferation of histiocytoid endothelial cells with intracytoplasmic vacuoles and associated vascular lumen formation. Radiation therapy resulted in significant clinical improvement. Tosti *et al.* (1994) observed a 47-year-old man with liver cirrhosis due to hepatitis C who had noted multiple painless lesions of the right middle finger and fingernail for 2 months. Apart from several 1–3-mm-large angiomatous papules, he had a 5-mm-large vegetating nodule that destroyed the nail plate, was bright red, smooth and superficially eroded. Biopsy revealed inflammatory cells, nests and cords of endothelial cells and abnormal vessels lined by large endothelial cells which had vesicular nuclei and prominent nucleoli. Small lumina were present within endothelial cell aggregates, and other lumina were formed by confluent

Kanekura, T., Mizumoto, J. & Kanzaki, T. (1994) Pachydermoperiostosis with angiolymphoid hyperplasia with easinophilia. *Journal of Dermatology* **21**, 133–134.

Risitano, C., Gupta, A. & Burke, F. (1990) Angiolymphoid hyperplasia with eosinophilia in the hand. *Journal of Hand Surgery* **15B**, 376–377.

Ward, K.A., Sheehan, A.L. & Kennedy, C.T.C. (1996) Angiolymphoid hyperplasia with eosinophilia (ALHE) of the digit. *British Journal of Dermatology* **135** (Suppl. 47), 43.

### Acral pseudolymphomatous angiokeratoma of children (APACHE)

Ramsay *et al.* (1983) described five children (four females, one male) who developed a unilateral eruption of multiple angiomatous papules on the extremities (in four patients on the feet and in one patient on the hand), between the ages of 2 and 13 years. The lesions were red-violaceous, discrete, irregularly shaped papules 1–4 mm in size with a hyperkeratotic collar occurring over acral sites (Fig. 11.84). The provisional diagnosis in three of the patients was angiokeratoma of Mibelli, but the lesions were more numerous and chilblains were not a feature. The lesions persisted, with some decrease in size, during follow-up periods of up to 16 years. Kaddu *et al.* (1994) reported a 16-year-old boy who had several deep-red, scaly papules and nodules on his left 1st and 5th toes with small papules also on the lateral nail wall.

Histological findings consist of hyperkeratosis, slight thinning of the overlying epidermis with elongated rete ridges at the margins and a well-circumscribed dense nodular lymphocytic infiltrate present throughout the dermis, extending from the subcutis to the dermoepidermal junction, but without involving the epidermis. There is an equal number of B and T cells and the T suppressor cells (CD8) outnumbered helper T cells (CD4) (Ramsay *et al.* 1990). In one patient the lesions were destroyed by curettage and did not recur.

Hara *et al.* (1991) reported on a 14-year-old Japanese girl presenting multiple lesions in a linear fashion on just one finger with involvement of the medial aspect of the nail as partial onycholysis. The histology corresponded to that of a pseudolymphoma but there was a lack of prominent thickened capillaries. There were epidermal changes including liquefaction degeneration of the basal cells with predominance of CD4 lymphocytes at the upper portion of the infiltrate and CD8 at the lower one.

### References

Hara, M., Matsunaga, J. & Tagami, H. (1991) Acral pseudolymphomatous angiokeratoma of children (APACHE). A case report and immunohistological study. *British Journal of Dermatology* **124**, 387–388.

Kaddu, S., Cerroni, L., Pilatti, A., Soyer, H.P. & Kerl, H. (1994) Acral pseudolymphomatous angiokeratoma. A variant of the cutaneous pseudolymphomas. *American Journal of Dermatopathology* **16**, 130–133.

Ramsay, B., Dahl, M.G.C., Malcolm, A.J., Soyer, H.P. & Wilson Jones, E. (1983) Acral pseudolymphomatous angiokeratoma of children (APACHE). *British Journal of Dermatology* **119** (Suppl. 33), 13.

Ramsay, B., Dahl, M.G.C., Malcolm, A.J. & Wilson-Jones, E. (1990) Acral pseudolymphomatous angiokeratoma of children. *Archives of Dermatology* **126**, 1524–1525.

### Pyogenic granuloma (granuloma telangiectaticum, botryomycoma)

Pyogenic granuloma is a benign eruptive haemangioma typically following a minor penetrating skin injury. It starts around the nail with a minute red papule which rapidly grows to the size of a pea or even a cherry. Its surface may become eroded by necrosis of the overlying epidermis. Crusting may mimic a malignant melanoma although the typical collarette can usually be seen. Pyogenic granuloma is commonly located at the proximal nail fold (Fig. 11.85), but may develop distally (Fig. 11.86) in the hyponychium region with onycholysis (Fig. 11.87a), in the nail bed or even the matrix after a penetrating wound of the nail plate. Prolonged frictional trauma may result in pyogenic granuloma in the toenail bed (Richert 2001). Tenderness and a ready tendency to bleed are characteristic features. Unilateral pyogenic granulomas associated with Beau's lines following hand trauma (Price *et al.* 1994) and with onychomadesis following cast immobilization (Tosti *et al.* 2001) have been reported. Extensive granulation tissue due to an ingrowing toenail may mimic a periungual pyogenic granuloma, and it has also been observed in patients treated with aromatic retinoids (Baran 1990) as well as with indinar (Bouscarat *et al.* 1998) and cyclosporin (Higgins *et al.* 1995). Differential diagnosis includes also cavernous angioma, pseudo-pyogenic granuloma, haemangiosarcoma and above all amelanotic melanoma.

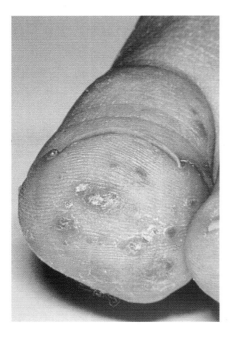

**Fig. 11.84** APACHE syndrome. (Courtesy of L. Dahl, Newcastle, UK.)

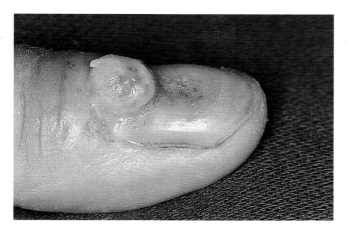

**Fig. 11.85** Pyogenic granuloma following pushing back of the cuticle (habit tic producing a nail depression).

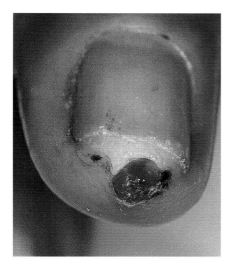

**Fig. 11.86** Pyogenic granuloma developed distally.

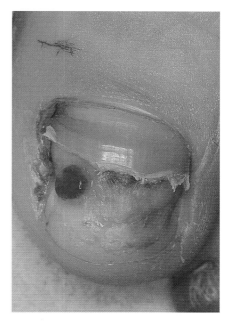

(a)

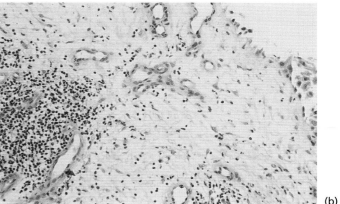

(b)

**Fig. 11.87** (a) Pyogenic granuloma of the nail bed resulting from frictional trauma. (b) Histological picture—patient in (a).

Histological investigation of the specimen is therefore essential (Fig. 11.87b). Therapy should be as simple as possible to avoid disfiguring scars or nail deformity. Pyogenic granuloma may be removed by excision at its base (Schulte *et al.* 1996) followed by electrodesiccation or application of Monsel's or aluminium chloride solution. The use of argon, $CO_2$ and 585 nm flashlamp-pumped pulsed dye lasers is also curative (Apfelberg *et al.* 1983; Modica 1988; González *et al.* 1996).

## References

Apfelberg, D.B., Maser, M.R., Lash, H. *et al.* (1983) Expanded role of the argon laser in plastic surgery. *Journal of Dermatologic Surgery and Oncology* **19**, 145–151.

Baran, R. (1990) Retinoids and the nails. *Journal of Dermatologic Treatment* **1**, 151–154.

Bouscarat, F., Bouchard, C. & Bachour, D. (1998) Paronychia and pyogenic granuloma of the great toes in patients treated with indinavir. *New England Journal of Medicine* **338**, 1776–1777.

González, S., Vibhagool, C., Falo, L.D., Jr, Momtaz, K.T., Grevelink, J. & González, E. (1996) Treatment of pyogenic granulomas with the 585 nm pulsed dye laser. *Journal of the American Academy of Dermatology* **35**, 428–431.

Higgins, E.M., Hughes, J.R., Snowdon, S. *et al.* (1995) Cyclosporin induced periungual granulation tissue. *British Journal of Dermatology* **132**, 829–830.

Modica, L.A. (1988) Pyogenic granuloma of the tongue treated by carbon dioxide laser. *Journal of the American Geriatric Society* **36**, 1036–1038.

Price, M.A., Bruce, S., Waidhofer, W. *et al.* (1994) Beau's lines and pyogenic granulomas following hand trauma. *Cutis* **54**, 248–249.

Richert, B. (2001) Frictional pyogenic granuloma in the nail bed. *Dermatology* **202**, 80–81.

Schulte, K.-W., Miller, A. & Neumann, N.J. (1996) Subunguale Tumoren. *Zeitschrift für Hautkrankheiten* **71**, 305.

Tosti, A., Piraccini, B.M. & Camacho-Martinez, F. (2001) Ony-chemadesis and pyogenic granuloma following cast immobilization. *Archives of Dermatology* **137**, 231–232.

### Coccal nail fold angiomatosis

A peculiar case of reactive vascular lesions growing out from under several nail folds was observed in a girl after her hand had been splinted for a wrist trauma. They were erosive, slightly oozing, asymptomatic tumours. The affected nails showed pronounced Beau's lines. Histopathology was reminiscent, but not identical with pyogenic granuloma with considerable vessel proliferation in an oedematous tissue rich in lymphocytes and plasma cells. Streptococci were grown in culture. Treatment with antibiotics led to complete cure (Davies 1995). Three patients have been seen with coccal nail fold angiomatosis, all after trauma of the hand or wrist, respectively (Haneke *et al.* 1997). Two identical cases were seen by Tosti and Camacho who speculate that this might be a peculiar type of sympathetic reflex dystrophy (personal communication). It is likely that the two cases described as Beau's lines and pyogenic granulomas following hand trauma were identical (Price *et al.* 1994).

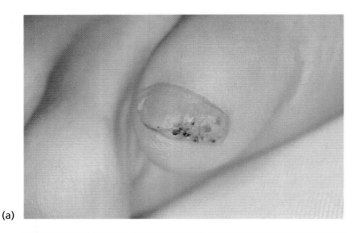

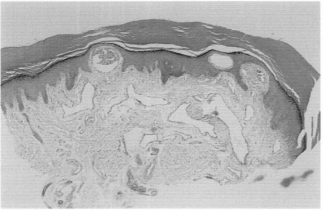

**Fig. 11.88** (a) Lymphangioma of the distal nail bed. (Courtesy of S. Goettmann-Bonvallot, France.) (b) Histology.

### References

Davies, M.G. (1995) Coccal nail fold angiomatosis. *British Journal of Dermatology* **132**, 162–163.

Haneke, E. Mainusch, O. & Hilker, O. (1997) Diaklinik der Hautklinik Wuppertal vom 10.9. 1997. *Zeitschrift für Dermatologie* **183**, 180–195.

Price, M.A., Bruce, S., Waidhofer, W. & Weaver, S.M. (1994) Beau's lines and pyogenic granulomas following hand trauma. *Cutis* **54**, 246–249.

### Lymphangioma circumscriptum (Fig. 11.88)

Appearing as a cluster of vesicles resembling frog spawn (some of the vesicles can be filled with fresh or altered blood) lymphangioma circumscriptum is rare on the distal digit.

Histopathology shows endothelium-lined spaces which may be so closely applied to the lower surface of the epidermis that they may simulate intraepidermal vesicles. They are in communication with large subcutaneous cisterns consisting of muscle coated lymphatic vessels and must be excised in order to effect cure. Therefore excision has to be wide and deep (Mehregan 1986).

### Reference

Mehregan, A. (1986) *Pinkus' Guide to Dermatopathology*, p. 558. Appleton, Norwalk, CT.

### Glomus tumour

The glomus tumour was first described by Wood (1812) as a painful subcutaneous 'tubercle'. Several cases were described as malignant angiosarcomas or colloid sarcomas until Barré and Masson (1924) published their investigations on two glomus tumours. Seventy-five per cent of glomus tumours occur in the hand, especially in the fingertips and particularly the subungual area. One to 2% of all hand tumours are glomus tumours (Rettig & Strickland 1977). The age of the patients at the time of diagnosis ranges from 30 to 50 years (Carroll & Berman 1972). Men are less frequently affected than women. Seven cases of subungual glomus tumours in von Recklinghausen's neurofibromatosis have been reported (Sawada *et al.* 1995).

The glomus tumour is characterized by intense, often pulsating pain that may be spontaneous or provoked by the slightest trauma. Even changes in temperature, especially from warm to cold, may trigger pain radiating up to the shoulder.

*Glomus tumours may be tested for by placing an ice cube on the nail to exacerbate the pain.*

Sometimes the pain is worse at night. A tourniquet placed at the base of the digit stops the pain, but also a blood pressure cuff inflated to 300 mmHg before or immediately after minor trauma abolishes the pain response (Hildreth 1970).

The tumour is seen through the nail plate as a small bluish to reddish-blue spot several millimetres in diameter, rarely ex-

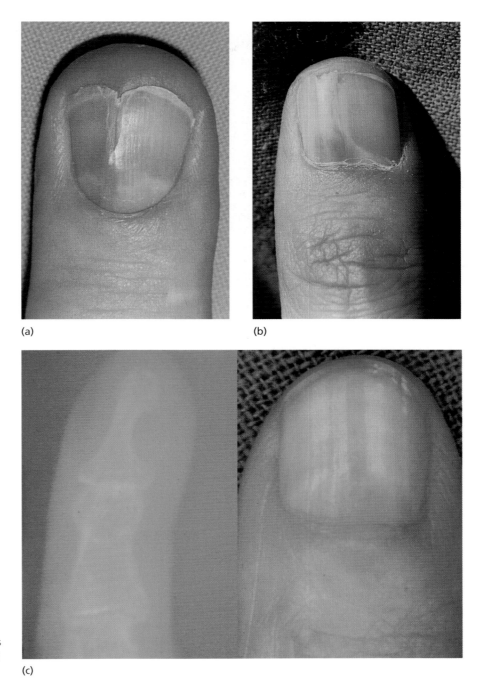

(a)

(b)

(c)

**Fig. 11.89** (a) Glomus tumour fissuring the nail plate. (b) Glomus tumour in the proximal nail bed presenting as a red spot. (c) Glomus tumour—depression on the dorsal surface of the distal phalanx.

ceeding 1 cm in diameter (Fig. 11.89). An erythematous focus that does not blanch totally with pressure and is associated with sharp pain probably represents a glomus tumour. Sometimes it causes a slight rise in surface temperature; this can be detected by thermography; dynamic telethermography shows the lesion about three times its actual size (Corrado *et al.* 1982). One-half of the tumours cause minor nail deformities, ridging and fissuring being the most common. Subungual hyperkeratosis with onycholysis is rare (Belanger & Weaver 1993). About 50% cause a depression on the dorsal aspect of the distal phalangeal

bone or even a cyst visible on X-ray (El Hachem *et al.* 1996; Van Geertruyden *et al.* 1996). Intraosseous location is unusual (Sugiura 1976; Johnson *et al.* 1993). Enlargement of the thickened nail and of the purple soft tissues with moderate pain of the 4th right finger was present for 20 years in a 95-year-old woman (Watelet *et al.* 1986). Probing and transillumination may help to localize the tumour if it is not clearly visible through the nail (Hidreth 1970; Love 1994). If the tumour cannot be localized clinically or on X-ray, arteriography may be performed; this will reveal a star-shaped telangiectatic zone

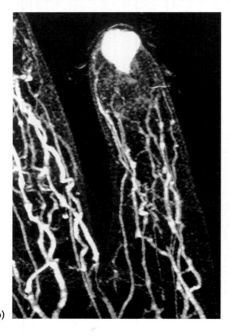

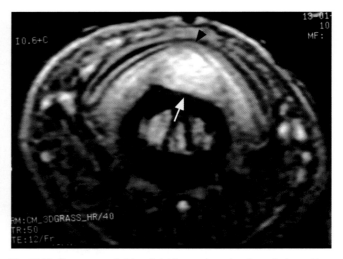

**Fig. 11.91** Glomus tumour (solid type). Axial post-enhanced gradient echo image. The tumour is faintly visible on the midline. Note the peripheral low-signal capsule and the bone erosion of the dorsal aspect of the phalanx (arrow). The nail matrix is lifted up (arrowhead).

**Fig. 11.90** Glomus tumour (vascular type). (a) Axial post-enhanced gradient echo image. Note the strong enhancement of the tumour and a thin peripheral capsule with low signal. (b) MR angiography with a strong and homogenous enhancement of the fingertip.

useful for diagnosis and localization of the tumour. (Natali *et al.* 1966; Camirand & Giroux 1970; Priollet *et al.* 1985). A painless nodular growth emerging from beneath the proximal nail fold of the left 4th toe of a 61-year-old man is a unique presentation. At surgery the stalk was followed down to its base and was seen to arise from the nail matrix (Lim *et al.* 1999).

*MRI may be preferable as it offers the highest sensitivity and a better assessment of the extent of the lesion.*

*High resolution MRI is able to depict normal glomus bodies with T2-weighted images and after injection of gadolinium. Three main findings are well highlighted by MRI: the signal, the location and the limits of the tumour.*

*MR findings can be equivocal and some studies in the literature report conflicting signal behaviour. Though most of the tumors presented a high signal on T2-weighted images, on the other hand on T1-weighted images the lesions could present a low signal (Kneeland* et al. *1987; Jablon* et al. *1990; Matloub*

et al. *1992), a high signal (haemorrhage or vascular component?) (Schneider & Bachow 1991), an intermediate (Holzberg 1992) or heterogeneous signal with a tumoral core (Hou* et al. *1993). In fact, the signal behaviour depends on histologic composition. Glomus tumours are the result of hyperplasia of one or several elements of the glomus bodies and may be considered hamartomas (Carroll & Berman 1972). Masson described different histological variants (Masson 1924). They are not routinely mentioned in pathological reports, as they have no prognostic significance. However, their knowledge is important to understand their involvement in the signal of tumour (Drapé* et al. *1995). The vascular type is composed of numerous vascular lumina. The enhancement is very high after injection of gadolinium and the signal is also elevated on T2-weighted images (Fig. 11.90). The cellular or solid type mainly represents a proliferation of epithelioid cells (glomus cells) and a relative poverty of vascular lumens. This type of tumour is quite difficult to detect with MRI. Its signal is close to that of the normal dermis of the nail bed on all sequences. The injection of gadolinium is of little use. In fact, thin 3-D contiguous gradient echo slices are the most helpful. They are the most appropriate to depict a peripheral capsule or a slight erosion of bone on the dorsal aspect of the distal phalanx (Fig. 11.91). The mucoid type with a mucoid degeneration of the stroma presents a faint enhancement, and on the other hand a very high signal on T2-weighted images due to the large amount of water in the stroma. Numerous tumours are a combination of these three features (Fig. 11.92).*

*Most often the tumour limits are well-defined with a peripheral pseudocapsule. This capsule is a reaction by the surrounding connective tissue. It presents a very low signal on all sequences, but is more visible on T2-weighted images or 3-D gradient echo images (Fig. 11.90). Its analysis is greatly facilit-*

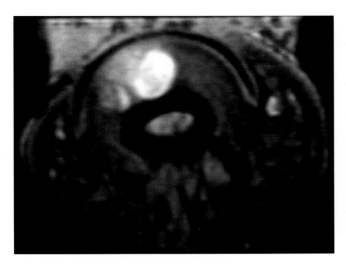

**Fig. 11.92** Glomus tumour (mixed types). Axial post-enhanced gradient echo image. The upper and the lateral parts of the tumour show a faint enhancement and ill-defined limits.

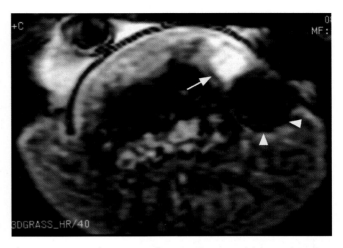

**Fig. 11.93** Recurrent glomus tumour after surgery 3 years ago. Axial post-enhanced gradient echo image. Note the 2-mm large tumour (arrow) deep to the dark artifact of the previous lateral surgical approach (arrowheads).

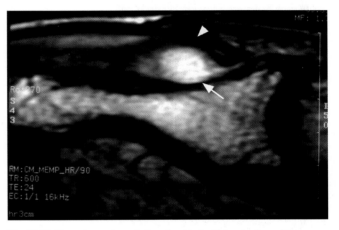

**Fig. 11.94** Glomus tumour beneath the nail matrix. Sagittal post-enhanced T1-weighted spin echo image. The nail matrix is lifted up (arrowhead). Note the high signal of the dermis tissue surrounding the tumour (arrow).

ated by high-resolution MRI (Drapé et al. 1996a). In our series, the capsule appears incomplete or absent in 23% of cases. Then the tumour limits are ill-defined and the injection of gadolinium may depict small foci of tumour extending in the nearby nail bed. Often in these cases, some adhesions with the nail bed are noted during surgery (Fig. 11.92). Local invasion of the capsule is debated and was reported on histological examinations in 1–2% of cases by Kohout and Stout (1961) and was not found by Carroll and Berman (1972). It is certain that the risk of recurrence is high if some tumoral tissue is left in situ during surgery of these ill-defined lesions. The recurrence rate varies from 12–24% in the literature (Carroll & Bermann 1972; Rettig & Strickland 1977; Varian & Cleak 1980; Davis et al. 1981). MRI appears particularly helpful in case of recurrent pain because it helps distinguish between postsurgical pain and pain due to residual or recurrent glomus tumour after surgery (Fig. 11.93). MRI is also able to depict multiple glomus tumours in the same fingertip. In these cases, the two tumours are usually close and may be located on each side of the median line. MRI is essential in these cases to plan the surgical approach.

In most cases, 66% in our series, the tumour is located in the subungual area, in the supporting tissue of the nail bed or the matrix. These locations are the most difficult to highlight with ultrasonography since the curvature of the nail plate disturbs the analysis of the lateral parts of the nail bed (Fornage 1988). Usually, the lesion is deep, close to the periosteum of the underlying phalanx. Often, a cortical erosion is depicted on the axial MR images (82% of our cases), although occult on radiographs. These axial slices are essential to distinguish the tumours on the median line from those of the lateral part of the nail bed, which sometimes extend into the pulp via the rima ungualum; an area delineated by the distal phalanx and Flint's

ligament. The surgical approach is planned according to the size and the location of the tumour. The lateral type may be excised by a lateral approach and lifting of the nail bed without disruption of the matrix. The median type may need a transungual approach, whose resection size will be adapted to the size of the tumour.

Sagittal slice MRI are essential to determine the relations between the tumour and the nail matrix. The lesions beneath the matrix are really difficult to detect. Clinically, they are often unsuspected, although they may lead to a nail fissure by a compression of the matrix. The supporting dermis of the matrix presents specific features with MRI, as an oval area with a high signal on T2-weighted images and a high enhancement after injection of gadolinium (Drapé et al. 1996b). These patterns decrease the contrast between healthy tissue and tumour on all sequences (Fig. 11.94). In addition, this oval area beneath the

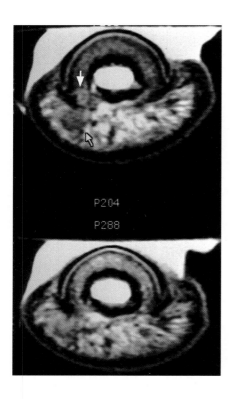

**Fig. 11.95** Glomus tumour. Axial T1-weighted spin echo image before (top) and after (bottom) injection of gadolinium. The bilobated tumour is implanted in the rima ungalum and extends toward the nail bed and the pulp (arrows).

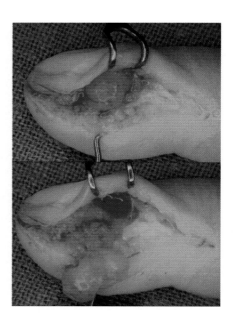

**Fig. 11.96** Glomus tumour—removal through a lateral incision.

*matrix may be particularly intense and must not be confused with a glomus tumour. Axial 3-D gradient echo images and the injection of gadolinium may help to highlight a faint cortical erosion and a peripheral capsule.*

*More seldom, the lesions may be located in the pulp or the posterior nail fold. In this case, the contrast of healthy tissue/tumour is completely different because of the fat tissue of the hypodermis surrounding the tumour. The low-signal tumour is spontaneously visible on T1-weighted images, surrounded by the high signal of fat. On the other hand, the injection of gadolinium blurs the tumour limits by levelling out the signals (Fig. 11.95). Fat-suppressed sequences or three-dimensional gradient echo images with the injection of gadolinium yield the best contrast between the low signal of the fat and the enhanced tumour.*

*Glomus tumours are easily distinguished from such other vascular lesions as angiomas, with their characteristic blood flow artifacts.*

Many patients give a history of trauma. The most common misdiagnoses are neuroma, causalgia, gout, and arthritis. These have resulted in disastrous therapeutic attempts such as posterior rhizotomy and amputation (Rettig & Strickland 1977). The differential diagnosis includes other painful lesions such as subungual warts, keratoacanthoma, subungual exostoses, enchondroma, leiomyoma, but also inflammatory processes like paronychia, osteitis and subungual whitlow.

Histology shows a highly differentiated, organoid tumour. It consists of an afferent arteriole, vascular channels lined with endothelium and surrounded by irregularly arranged cuboidal cells with round dark nuclei and pale cytoplasm. Primary collecting veins drain into the cutaneous veins. Myelinated and non-myelinated nerves are found and may account for the pain. The tumour is surrounded by a fibrous capsule. Mucinous stroma degeneration is not rare (Hisa *et al.* 1994). Since all the elements of the normal glomus are present, the glomus tumour may be considered a hamartoma rather than a true tumour.

A variant with transition from glomus cells to elongated mature smooth muscle cells was described under the term of glomangiomyoma. A single case of a painful subungual lesion was described by Quarterman *et al.* (1996).

Immunohistochemistry of glomus tumours showed the glomus cells positive for vimentin, a 42 kDa muscle actin (with HHF 35) and smooth muscle actin (CGA 7), and myosin (Daugaard *et al.* 1990), but negative for desmin, factor VIII-related antigen and several neural markers; however, nerve fibres contain protein S-100, Leu-7 antigen (HNK-I, 110kD), neuron-specific enolase and neurofilaments (Herbst *et al.* 1991). The endothelium clearly stains with factor VIII-related antigen, $\beta_2$-microglobulin and the lectin Ulex europaeus agglutinin (UEA) I, whereas only a few endothelial cells of the glomus tumour bind PNA in contrast to normal nail bed vessels the endothelial cells of which do not stain for PNA at all (E. Haneke, unpublished data). In a study of 20 glomus tumours, Daugaard *et al.* (1990) found that the cells were also negative for fibrillic acid protein and chromogranin.

The only treatment is surgical removal (Figs 11.96–11.98). Small tumours may be removed by punching a 6-mm hole into the nail plate, incising the nail bed longitudinally, or the distal matrix transversally and enucleating the lesion. The small nail disc is put back in its original position as a physiological dressing. Larger tumours may be treated after lifting of the proximal half of the nail plate; allowing access to the tumour. The matrix is carefully incised parallel to the lunula border and the lesion

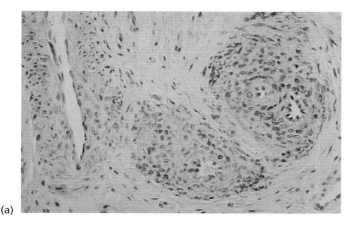

(a)

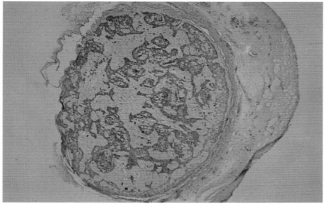

(b)

**Fig. 11.97** (a) Glomus body—normal aspect. (b) Glomus tumour—low power microscopy.

dissected. The lifted nail plate is laid back and sutured to the lateral nail sulcus. An H-shaped incision (Ekin *et al.* 1997) or cruciate incision (Rohrich *et al.* 1994) is only necessary in case of very large lesions. Glomus tumours in lateral positions are removed by an L-shaped incision parallel to and 4–6 mm on the volar side of the lateral nail fold. The nail bed is carefully

dissected from the bone until the tumour is reached and extirpated (Foucher *et al.* 1999). Extirpation is usually curative although the pain may take several weeks to disappear (Jepson & Harris 1970; Bao-guo *et al.* 1996). Recurrences occur in 10–20% of cases (Carroll & Berman 1972; Foucher *et al.* 1999) and may represent either incomplete excision, tumour overlooked at the initial operation or newly developed tumours (Cornell 1981; Ali Noor & Masbah 1997). More extensive surgery than is often carried out might achieve more first time cures (Varian & Cleak 1980). Amputation of the distal phalanx is an unnecessary mutilation (Watelet *et al.* 1986).

Only one case of malignant glomus tumour (glomangiosarcoma) on the radial aspect of the volar skin over the distal joint of the thumb has been described (Wetherington *et al.* 1997).

### References

Ali Noor, M. & Masbah, O. (1997) Synchronous glomus tumors in a distal digit: a case report. *Journal of Hand Surgery* **22A**, 508–510.
Bao-guo, S., Yun-tao, W. & Jia-zhen, L. (1996) Glomus tumours of the hand and foot. *International Orthopaedics (SICOT)* **20**, 339–341.
Barré, J.A. & Masson, P. (1924) Etude anatomo-clinique de certaines tumeurs sous-unguéales douloureuses (tumeurs du glomus neuro-myo-artériel des extrémités). *Bulletin de la Societé Française de Dermatologie et de Syphiligraphie* **31**, 149–159.
Belanger, S.M. & Weaver, T.D. (1993) Subungual glomus tumor of the hallux. *Cutis* **52**, 50–52.
Camirand, P. & Giroux, J.M. (1970) Subungual glomus tumour. *Archives of Dermatology* **102**, 677–679.
Carroll, R.E. & Berman, A.T. (1972) Glomus tumors of the hand: review of the literature and report of 28 cases. *Journal of Bone and Joint Surgery* **54A**, 691–703.
Cornell, S.J. (1981) Multiple glomus tumours in one digit. *Hand* **13**, 301–302.
Corrado, E.M., Passareti, U., Messore, L. & Lanza, F. (1982) Thermographic diagnosis of glomus tumour. *Hand* **14**, 21–24.
Daugaard, S., Jensen, M.E. & Fisher, S. (1990) Glomus tumours. An immunohistochemical study. *APMIS* **98**, 983–990.
Davis, T.S., Graham, W.P. III & Blomain, E.W. (1981) A ten-year experience with glomus tumors. *Annals of Plastic Surgery* **6**, 297–299.

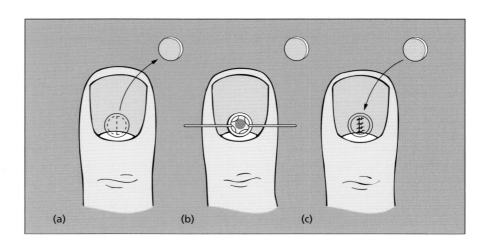

**Fig. 11.98** Sequence of events in the removal of a glomus tumour through the nail.

(a)    (b)    (c)

Drapé, J.L., Idy-Peretti, I., Goettmann, S. *et al.* (1995) MR imaging of subungual glomus tumors. *Radiology* **195**, 507–515.

Drapé, J.L., Idy-Peretti, I., Goettmann, S. *et al.* (1996a) Standard and high resolution magnetic resonance imaging of glomus tumors of toes and fingertips. *Journal of the American Academy of Dermatology* **35**, 550–555.

Drapé, J.L., Wolfram-Gabel, R., Idy-Peretti, I., Baran, R. *et al.* (1996b) The lunula: resonance imaging approach to the subnail matrix area. *Journal of Investigative Dermatology* **106**, 1081–1085.

Ekin, A., Özkan, M. & Kabaklioglu, T. (1997) Subungual glomus tumours: a different approach to diagnosis and treatment. *Journal of Hand Surgery* **22B**, 228–229.

El Hachem, M., Zicari, L. & Pastori, A. (1996) Osteolytic glomus tumor. A child case report. In: *Vth Congress of the European Society of Paediatric Dermatology, Rotterdam, Book of Abstracts*, p. 212.

Fornage, B.D. (1988) Glomus tumours in the fingers: diagnosis with ultrasound. *Radiology* **167**, 183–185.

Foucher, G., Le Viet, D., Dalliana, Z. *et al.* (1999) Les tumeurs glomiques de la région unguéale. A propos d'une série de 55 patients. *Revue de Chirurgie et Orthopédie* **85**, 362–366.

Herbst, W.M., Nakayama, K. & Hornstein, O.P. (1991) Glomus tumours of the skin: an immunohistochemical investigation of the expression of marker proteins. *British Journal of Dermatology* **124**, 172–176.

Hildreth, D.H. (1970) The ischemia test for glomus tumor: a new diagnostic test. *Reviews of Surgery* **27**, 147–148.

Hisa, T., Nakagawa, K. & Wakasa, K. (1994) Solitary glomus tumour with mucinous degeneration. *Clinical and Experimental Dermatology* **19**, 227–229

Holzberg, M. (1992) Glomus tumor of the nail. A 'red herring' clarified by magnetic resonance imaging. *Archives of Dermatology* **128**, 160–162.

Hou, S.M., Shih, T.T.F. & Lin, M.C. (1993) Magnetic resonance imaging of an obscure glomus tumour in the fingertip. *Journal of Hand Surgery* **18B**, 482–483.

Jablon, M., Horowith, A. & Bernstein, D.A. (1990) Magnetic resonance imaging of a glomus tumour of the fingertip. *Journal of Hand Surgery* **15A**, 507–509.

Jepson, R.P. & Harris, J.D. (1970) Glomus tumours. *Medical Journal of Australia* **2**, 452–454.

Johnson, D.L., Kuschner, S.H. & Lane, C.S. (1993) Intraosseous glomus tumor of the phalanx: a case report. *Journal of Hand Surgery* **18A**, 1026–1028.

Kneeland, J.B., Middelton, W.D., Matloub, H.S. *et al.* (1987) High resolution MR imaging of glomus tumor. *Journal of Computer Assisted Tomography* **11**, 351–352.

Kohout, E. & Stout, A.P. (1961) The glomus tumor in children. *Cancer* **14**, 555–556.

Lim, I.J., Pho, R.W.H. & Tock, E.P.C. (1999) Atypical extraungual manifestation of a subungual tumour. *British Journal of Plastic Surgery* **52**, 327–328.

Love, J.G. (1944) Glomus tumors: diagnosis and treatment. *Proceedings of the Mayo Clinics* **19**, 113–116.

Masson, P. (1924) Le glomus neuromyo-artériel des régions tactiles et ses tumeurs. *Lyon Chirurgical* **20**, 256–280.

Matloub, H.S., Muoneke, V.N., Prevel, C.D., Sanger, J.R. & Youssif, N.J. (1992) Glomus tumor imaging: use of MRI for localization of occult lesions. *Journal of Hand Surgery* **17A**, 472–475.

Natali, J., Ecarlat, B., Vinardi, G. *et al.* (1966) Artériographie d'une tumeur glomique. *Journal de Chirurgie* (*Paris*) **92**, 481–484.

Priollet, P., Pernes, J.M., Laurian, C. *et al.* (1985) Intérêt de l'artériographie dans l'exploration des tumeurs glomiques sous-unguéales. *Journal des Maladies Vasculaires* **10**, 363–365.

Quarterman, M.J., Lucas, J.G., Pellegrini, A.E. *et al.* (1996) Subungual glomangioleiomyoma: a case report. *Journal of Cutaneous Pathology* **23**, 90.

Rettig, A.C. & Strickland, J.W. (1977) Glomus tumor of the digits. *Journal of Hand Surgery* **2**, 261–265.

Rohrich, R.J., Hochstein, L.M. & Millwee, R.H. (1994) Subungual glomus tumors: an algorithmic approach. *Annals of Plastic Surgery* **33**, 300–304.

Sawada, S., Honda, M., Kamide, R. & Niimura, M. (1995) Three cases of subungual glomus tumors with von Recklinghausen neurofibromatosis. *Journal of the American Academy of Dermatology* **32**, 277–278.

Schneider, L.H. & Bachow, T.B. (1991) Magnetic resonance imaging of glomus tumor. *Orthopedic Reviews* **20**, 255–256.

Sugiura, I. (1976) Intra-osseous glomus tumour. *Journal of Bone and Joint Surgery* **58B**, 245–247.

Van Geertruyden, J., Lorea, P., Goldschmidt, D. *et al.* (1996) Glomus tumours of the hand. A retrospective study of 51 cases. *Journal of Hand Surgery* **21B**, 257–260.

Varian, J.P.W. & Cleak, D.K. (1980) Glomus tumors in the hands. *Hand* **12**, 293–299.

Watelet, F., Menez, D., Pageaut, G. *et al.* (1986) Tumeur glomique sous-unguéale. Un cas de forme inhabituelle. *Revue de Chirurgie et Orthopédie* **72**, 509–510.

Wetherington, R.W., Lyle, W.G. & Sangüeza, O.P. (1997) Malignant glomus tumor to the thumb: a case report. *Journal of Hand Surgery* **22A**, 1098–1102.

Wood, W. (1812) On painful subcutaneous tubercle. *Edinburgh Medical Journal* **8**, 283.

### Blue rubber bleb neavus

Blue rubber bleb naevus of the hand and fingers may be accompanied by leuconychia (Fig. 11.99).

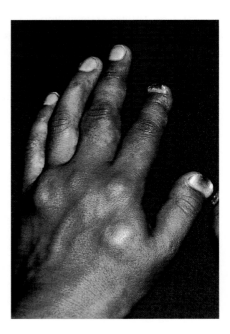

**Fig. 11.99** Blue rubber bleb naevus.

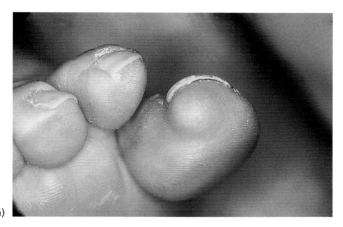

(a)

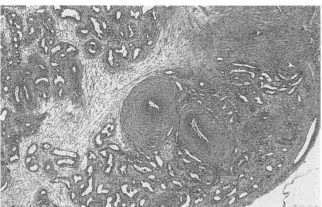

(b)

**Fig. 11.100** (a) Angioleiomyoma in the distal pulp. (b) Angioleiomyoma—histological changes with bundles of fibre interspersed with arterial and venous vessels.

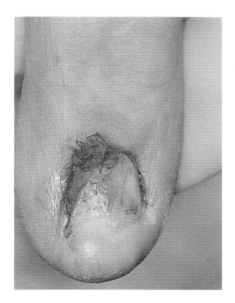

**Fig. 11.101** Angioleiomyoma in the matrix shelled out after transverse incision and resembling greyish grains of caviar-like substance.

### Angioleiomyoma

Lebouc (1889) described a case of subungual leiomyoma of the great toe. The pea-sized tumour consisted mainly of bundles of smooth muscle fibres intermingled with arterial and venous vessels. The muscular layer of the vessels was heavily hypertrophic, sometimes actually obliterating the lumen. Smooth muscle bundles were also found without vascular structures.

Conolly (1980) showed a clinical and radiological picture of a leiomyoma presenting as a slow growing tumour of the fingertip of a male aged 54 years. We have observed an apparently similar case in a young lady. The distal third of the nail plate was elevated and dystrophic. After avulsion of the nail plate, a small tumour was then seen directly distal to the lunula. Histology showed numerous blood vessels with a unique cushion-like hypertrophy of the smooth muscle which did not form a circular muscularis media layer. The patient had never experienced pain (E. Haneke, unpublished data).

We have seen (Requena & Baran 1993) a female presenting with a painless nodule disto-lateral to the distal groove with typical histology (Fig. 11.100). We have also observed a 70-year-old women with extensive onycholysis of her right index finger. The pain was paroxysmal and led to the diagnosis of glo-

mus tumour (Fig. 11.101). MRI located this tumour beneath the matrix and suggested the same diagnosis. An elliptical transverse incision enabled the lesion to be shelled out easily. It resembled greyish grains of caviar-like substance. Histology was typical of angioleiomyoma composed of muscle fibres with centrally located, thin, blunt-edged, 'eel-like' nuclei and eosinophilic vacuolated cytoplasm (Baran *et al.* 2000).

Clinically it is not possible to rule out cutaneous *angiolipoleiomyoma* (Fitzpatrick *et al.* 1990), a tumour histologically well circumscribed, and composed of smooth muscle, vascular spaces, connective tissue, and mature fat cells.

Sawada (1988) described a 53-year-old woman with a tender tumour of the tip of her right hallux. Upon surgery, it was a cystic round tumour of 20 mm in the subcutis. The nail was normal. Histopathology showed an angioleiomyoma with extensive myxoid degeneration.

There are neoplasms with gradual transition from glomus cells to elongated, mature smooth muscle cells. Even though, glomangioleiomyoma (Quaterman *et al.* 1996) is easily ruled out since there are no glomus cells in angioleiomyoma.

### References

Baran, R., Requena, L. & Drapé, J.L. (2000) Angioleiomyoma mimicking glomus tumour in the nail matrix. *British Journal of Dermatology* **142**, 1239–1241.

Conolly, W.B. (1980) *A Colour Atlas of Hand Conditions*, p. 167. Wolfe Medical Publications, London.

Fitzpatrick, J.E., Mellette, J.R., Hwang, R.J. *et al.* (1990) Cutaneous angiolipoleiomyoma. *Journal of the American Academy of Dermatology* **23**, 1093–1098.

Lebouc, L. (1889) *Etude clinique et anatomique sur quelques cas de tumeurs sous-unguéales. Thèse pour le doctorat en médecine*, pp. 1–34. G. Steinheil, Paris.

Quaterman, M.J., Lucas, J.G., Pellegrini, A.E. *et al.* (1996) Glomangioleiomyoma: a case report. *Journal of Cutaneous Pathology* **23**, 90.

Requena, L. & Baran, R. (1993) Digital angioleiomyoma: an uncommon neoplasm. *Journal of the American Academy of Dermatology* **29**, 1043–1044.

### Malignant

#### *Kaposi's sarcoma*

Kaposi's haemorrhagic sarcoma may involve the nail unit causing elevation or deformation of the nail plate (Zaias 1990). König (1899) described the case of a 61-year-old man with 'angiosarcoma multiplex' in the distal phalanges of three toes who later developed metastases in the calf.

Kaposi's sarcoma can involve the nail region in patients with AIDS (see p. 284). Most cases described before 1920 as subungual angiosarcoma (Kolaczeck 1878; Kraske 1887) were probably glomus tumours.

### References

Kolaczeck, J. (1878) Über das Angio-Sarkom. *Deutsche Zeitschrift für Chirurgie* **9**, 1–48.

Kraske, P. (1887) Über subunguale Geschwülste. *Münchene Medizinische Wochenschrift* **34**, 889–891.

Zaias, N. (1990) *The Nail in Health and Disease*, 2nd edn. Appleton and Lange, Norwalk, CT.

#### *Glomangiosarcoma*

(See page 573.)

#### *Malignant haemangioendothelioma (haemangiosarcoma, haemangioendothelioma)*

(See page 564.)

### Neuroendocrine tumour

#### Merkel cell tumour

Merkel cell carcinoma on a toe was reported in a teenage girl (Goldenhersh *et al.* 1992). The tumour clinically masqueraded as granulation tissue associated with an ingrown nail. On the medial aspect of the left great toe, at the junction of the lateral nail fold and the nail bed, there was a deep red, focally ulcerated, granular nodule. On cut section of the specimen, a poorly delineated tumour consisting of brown haemorrhagic tissue and measuring 0.7 cm in diameter was identified.

The tumour cells were present in dense sheets, and focally were arranged in a trabecular pattern at all levels of the dermis and in the superficial subcutaneous fat.

### Reference

Goldenhersh, M.A., Prus, D., Ron, N. *et al.* (1992) Merkel cell tumor masquerading as granulation tissue on a teenager's toe. *American Journal of Dermatopathology* **14**, 560–563.

## Tumours of peripheral nerves

Neurogenic tumours of the terminal phalanx are very rare.

### Neuroma

Post-traumatic neuromas are produced by the numerous nerve fibres in the nail bed and around the nail (Fig. 11.102). They may cause tenderness, elevation of the nail bed and nail dystrophy. Their treatment is by careful resection with preservation or reconstruction of the nail bed (Zook 1988) (Fig. 11.103).

*Ultrasonography and MRI can detect a well circumscribed nodule in the nail bed or the pulp. The signal of the lesion is low to intermediate on T1- and T2-weighted images. Usually there is no or a faint enhancement after injection of gadolinium (Fig. 11.103). This enhancement is increased by fat suppression.*

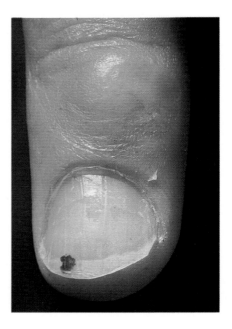

**Fig. 11.102** Post-traumatic neuroma.

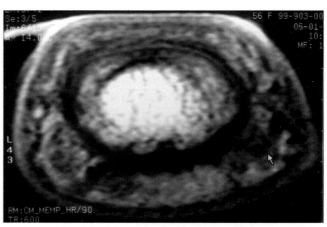

**Fig. 11.103** Post-traumatic neuroma (arrow). Axial post-enhanced T1-weighted spin echo image.

## So-called rudimentary supernumerary digits

The so-called rudimentary supernumerary digit is usually present at birth, often bilaterally symmetric and almost always located at the base of the metacarpophalangeal joint. The lesion is distinguished by the finding of multiple nerve bundles within the dermal core and especially at the proximal base of the nodule, and a large number of Meissner corpuscles in the dermal papillae. Meissner cells may be associated with the generation of cutaneous nerve plexus and nerve endings in the upper dermis, and possibly with the development of Meissner corpuscles, at the early stage of rudimentary polydactyly (Ban & Kitajima 2001).

## Neurofibroma

Neurofibromas in von Recklinghausen's neurofibromatosis (NF type I) are surprisingly rare in the nail region and most ungual neurofibromas are isolated. When located in the proximal nail fold they may produce a longitudinal depression (Zaias 1990), or even mimic Koenen's subungual tumours (Fröhlich 1939); a subungual location may cause onychodystrophy (Runne & Orfanos 1981; Fig. 11.104), or elevate the nail (Haneke *et al.* 1998). Surface ulceration with ready tendency to bleed made the latter look like a pyogenic granuloma (Haneke *et al.* 1998).

A solitary subungual neurofibroma on the right third finger of a 13-year-old female had deformed overall into a flattened dome shape and presented moderate tenderness from the ulnar half only. X-ray examination revealed mild compression atrophy of the ulnar side of the distal phalanx (Niizuma & Iijima 1991). Longitudinal ridging and increased convexity of the lateral half of the nail with associated subungual hyperkeratosis was reported in a 27-year-old female nurse (Bhushan *et al.* 1999). The nail dystrophy was accompanied by a diffuse painless non-confluent swelling beneath the proximal nail fold. Histology revealed a dermal tumour consisting of loosely

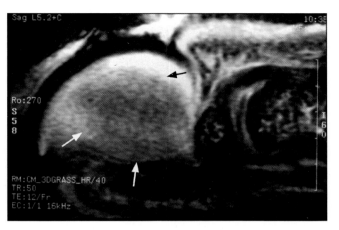

**Fig. 11.105** Neurofibroma of the nail bed (arrows). Sagittal post-enhanced gradient echo image.

arranged spindle cells with scanty, pale cytoplasm and elongated, wavy nuclei in a myxoid stroma. Chronic paronychia was the clinical presentation in a case of Fleeger and Zeinowicz (1990). MRI with injection of gadolinium shows a faintly to highly enhanced nodule of the nail bed lifting up the nail plate (Fig. 11.105).

Exploratory nail plate removal may be a diagnostic aid for treating this tumour which may be painful (Shelley & Shelley 1986). Diffuse neurofibroma of the distal phalanx of a thumb was shown to enlarge both the fingertip and the nail without causing gross nail deformity (Zaias 1990). We observed almost the same aspect on the distal phalanx of the thumb (Fig. 11.106a,b). Papules and associated nodules with intradermal naevi may resemble Recklinghausen's disease. They are ruled out by histopathology showing that ungual neurofibromas are virtually identical to those in other locations (Fig. 11.106c) (Baran & Haneke 2001).

## Systematized multiple fibrillar neuromas

These neuromas were observed by Altmeyer and Merkel (1981). Involvement of the tips of several fingers resulted in thickening of the periungual tissue without nail plate abnormalities.

## Plexiform 'Pacinian' neuroma

A plexiform 'Pacinian' neuroma was observed in the distal phalanx of an 11-year-old boy. The tumour was asymptomatic but hindered complete flexion of the distal interphalangeal joint. The nail plate was normal. Histology showed unusual connective tissue structures resembling Pacini's corpuscles (Altmeyer 1979). Runne (1977) described a case of multiple mucosal neuroma syndrome with marked thickening of the proximal nail folds which were shown to contain neuromas.

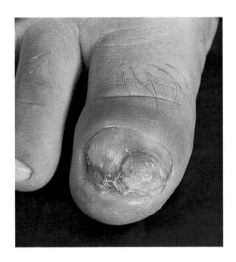

**Fig. 11.104** Neurofibroma of the nail bed. (Courtesy of U. Runne, Germany.)

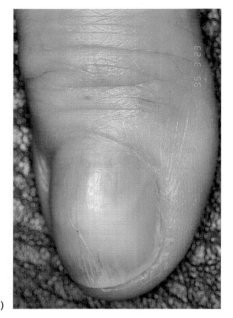

(a)

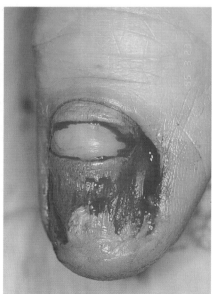

(b)

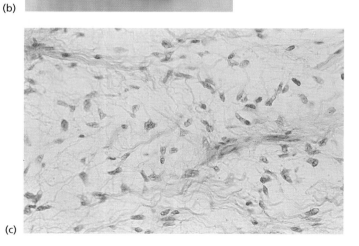

(c)

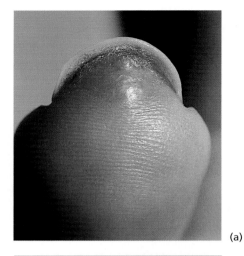

(a)

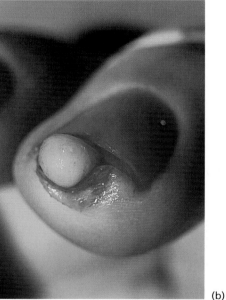

(b)

**Fig. 11.107** (a) Glioma. (Courtesy of J. Préaux, France.) (b) The distal subungual tumour is shelled out.

## Glioma, neurilemmoma, schwannoma

They rarely occur in a subungual position (Fig. 11.107) or in the proximal nail fold (Fig. 11.108).

A pigmented cutaneous lesion extending into the nailbed of the right index finger of a 71-year-old lady was the unique presentation of *malignant melanocytic schwannoma* (Elder *et al.* 1981). The superficial pigmented portion of the primary tumour consisted of epithelioid and somewhat spindle-shaped cells above the 'white' spindle cell portion demonstrating the biphasic nature of the lesion.

**Fig. 11.106** (right) (a) Neurofibroma—clubbed thumb. (b) Neurofibroma—transverse incision of the matrix showing the yellowish tumour. (c) Myxoid neurofibroma—histological changes.

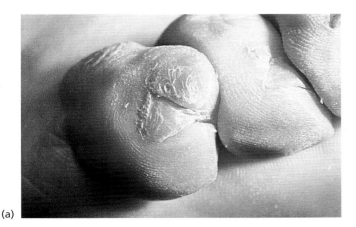

(a)

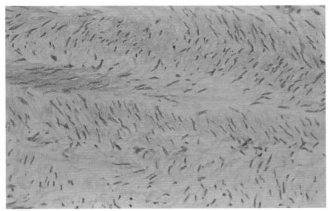

(b)

**Fig. 11.108** (a) Schwannoma in the proximal nail fold. (b) Histological changes.

*Schwannomas have sharp limits and show a strong enhancement of the whole or a part of the tumour on MR images. A cystic component is possible. The signal is high on T2-weighted images.*

### Granular cell tumour

Hasson *et al.* (1991) reported a tender verrucous periungual growth located deeply medially in the proximal nail fold of the great toe in a 35-year-old female producing a longitudinal groove in the nail plate (Fig. 11.109a). Peters and Crowe (1998) described a diffuse granular cell tumour in a 33-year-old woman causing enlargement of the left middle toe almost completely overgrowing the nail.

Histology showed a well-circumscribed cluster of tumour cells surrounded by strands of collagen fibres. The tumour cells were large with round or oval and centrally located nuclei and pale cytoplasm filled with faintly eosinophilic coarse granules (Fig. 11.109b). The lesion was excised.

### Malignant granular cell tumour (Urabe *et al.* 1991)

A reddish nodule that reached a size of 5 mm in diameter and destroyed the nail developed under the nail of the right index

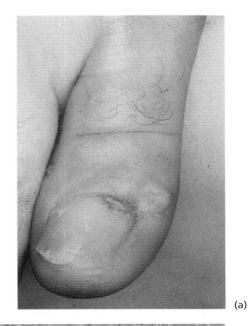

(a)

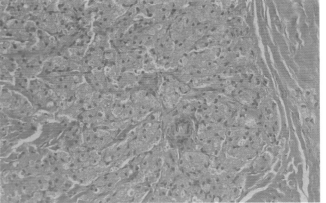

(b)

**Fig. 11.109** (a) Granular cell tumour. (Courtesy of L. Requena, Spain.) (b) Granular cell tumour—clusters of tumour cells surrounded by strands of collagen fibres.

finger of a 51-year-old Japanese woman (Fig. 11.110a). It recurred 2 years after resection and was firm, partly eroded and 25 mm in diameter when the finger was amputated. Multiple metastases appeared 6 months later and the patient eventually died. Histopathology of the primary and recurrent tumour (Fig. 11.110b) as well as a metastasis revealed polygonal eosinophilic granular cells with mitoses, some multinucleated giant cells and in the metastasis, anaplastic cells. Immunohistochemistry (protein S-100, Leu 7, vimentin) and electron-microscopy confirmed the diagnosis of malignant granular cell tumour.

### Perineurioma

Baran and Perrin (2001) have reported the first case of subungual perineurioma presenting as a monodactylous clubbing. Histological study showed a myxoid tumour but with, unexpectedly, a diffuse expression of CD34.

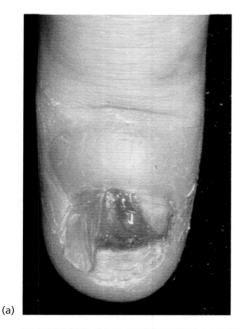

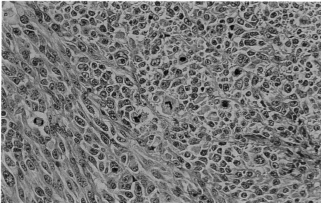

**Fig. 11.110** (a) Malignant granular cell tumour of the nail bed. (Courtesy of A. Urabe, Japan.) (b) Malignant granular cell tumour, histological changes.

## References

Altmeyer, H. (1979) Histologie eines Rankenneuroms mit Vater–Pacini–Lamellenkörper-ähnlichen Strukturen. *Hautarzt* **30**, 248–252.

Altmeyer, H. & Merkel, K.H. (1981) Multiple systematisierte Neurome der Haut und der Schleimhaut. *Hautarzt* **32**, 240–244.

Ban, M. & Kitajima, Y. (2001) The number and distribution of Merkel cells in rudimentary polydactyly. *Dermatology* **202**, 31–34.

Baran, R. & Haneke, E. (2001) Subungual myxoid neurofibroma on the thumb. *Acta Dermato-Venereologica* (in press).

Baran, R. & Perrin, C. (2001) Subungual perineurioma. *British Journal of Dermatology* (in press).

Bhushan, M., Telfer, N.R. & Chalmers, R.J.G. (1999) Subungual neurofibroma, an unusual cause of nail dystrophy. *British Journal of Dermatology* **140**, 777–778.

Elder, D.E., Ainsworth, M.A., Goldman, L.I. *et al.* (1981) Malignant melanocytic schwannoma. In: *Pathology of Malignant Melanoma* (ed. A.B. Ackerman), pp. 251–261. Masson Publishing, New York.

Fleegler, E.J. & Zeinowicz, R.J. (1990) Tumors of the perionychium. *Hand Clinics* **6**, 113–133.

Fröhlich, W. (1939) Fibromatosis subungualis. *Dermatologische Wochenschrift* **109**, 1211–1212.

Haneke, E., Mainusch, O. & Hilker, O. (1998) Subunguale Tumoren: Keratoakanthom, Neurofibrom, Nagelbett-Melanom. *Zeitschrift für Dermatologie* **184**, 86–102.

Hasson, A., Arias, M.C., Guttierez, A. *et al.* (1991) Periungual granular cell tumour. A light microscopic, immunohistochemical and ultrastructural study. *Skin Cancer* **6**, 41–46.

Niizuma, K. & Iijima, K.N. (1991) Solitary neurofibroma: a case of subungual neurofibroma on the right third finger. *Archives of Dermatological Research* **283**, 13–15.

Peters, J.S. & Crowe, M.A. (1998) Granular cell tumor of the toe. *Cutis* **62**, 147–148.

Runne, U. (1977) Syndrom der multiplen Neurome mit metastasierendem medullärem Schilddrüsenkarzinom ('Multiple mucosal neuroma-syndrome'). *Zeitschrift für Hautkrankheiten* **52**, 299–301.

Runne, U. & Orfanos, C.E. (1981) The human nail. *Current Problems in Dermatology* **9**, 102–149.

Shelley, E.D. & Shelley, W.B. (1986) Exploratory nail plate removal as a diagnostic aid in painful subungual tumours: glomus tumour, neurofibroma, and squamous cell carcinomas. *Cutis* **38**, 310–312.

Urabe, A., Imayama, S., Yasumoto, S. *et al.* (1991) Malignant cell tumor. *Journal of Dermatology* **18**, 161–166.

Zaias, N. (1990) *The Nail in Health and Disease*, 2nd edn. Appleton & Lange, Norwalk, CT.

Zook, E.G. (1988) Complications of the perionychium. *Hand Clinics* **2**, 407–427.

## Osteocartilaginous tumours

### Benign tumours

#### *Exostosis*

Subungual exostoses are not true tumours but rather outgrowths of normal bone or calcified cartilaginous remains. Whether or not subungual osteochondroma (Apfelberg *et al.* 1979) is a different entity is still not clear (de Palma *et al.* 1996). Norton (1980) listed differential features (see Table 11.2).

Subungual exostoses are rare; there were only 60 subungual exostoses in a series of 6034 benign osseous lesions (Dahlin & Unni 1986); however, they may be considerably underdiagnosed and underreported. A survey found more than 400 cases in the literature up to 1998. They are bony growths which are painful upon pressure and may elevate the nail (Fig. 11.111). They are particularly frequent in young people and mostly located in dorso-medial aspect of the tip of the great toe, though subungual exostoses may also occur in lesser toes (Stieler *et al.* 1989; Badawy Abdel-Naser *et al.* 1992; Davis & Cohen 1996; de Palma *et al.* 1996; Letts *et al.* 1998) or less commonly thumb or index fingers (Baran & Sayag 1978) (Fig. 11.112). Carroll *et al.* (1992) reported a series of 16 cases of subungual exostosis in the hand. Only 42 positively identified cases have been found in the literature to date (Iizuka *et al.* 1995; Davis & Cohen 1996; Guidetti *et al.* 1996; Fikry *et al.* 1998a; de Berker &

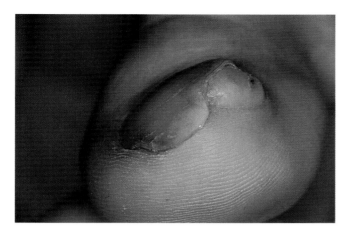

**Fig. 11.111** Subungual exostosis.

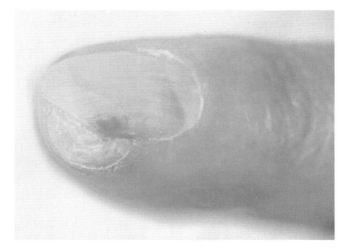

**Fig. 11.112** Finger exostosis.

Langtry 1999). Solitary subungual exostoses have never been observed to undergo malignant degeneration.

They start as small elevations of the dorsal aspect of the distal phalanx and may eventually emerge from under the nail edge or destroy the nail plate. If the nail is lost, the surface becomes eroded and secondarily infected, sometimes mimicking an ingrown toenail or even a melanoma (Velanovich 1994). Walking may be painful (Pambor & Neubert 1971).

James (1988) reported a case arising from the ventral aspect of the distal phalanx of the left index finger and causing enlargement of the fingertip. Proximal nail groove pain associated with bilateral exostoses on the proximal medial aspect of the base of the distal hallux phalanges is unusual (Chinn & Jenkin 1986). Trauma appears to be a major causative factor (Sebastian 1977; Davis & Cohen 1996; Fikry *et al.* 1998b) though some authors claim that a history of trauma is only occasionally found in subungual exostosis (Norton 1980) (see Table 11.2).

The triad of pain (the leading symptom), nail deformation and radiographic features is usually diagnostic. The exostosis is an ill-defined trabeculated osseous growth (Fig. 11.113) with an expanded distal portion covered with radiolucent fibrocartilage.

Lemont and Christman (1990) presented a new classification for subungual exostoses, in genetic and acquired type. This was based on the lesion's pathology, radiographic appearance, location, and age. They stated that the genetic subungual exostosis (type I) appears in the second and third decades of life, paronychia is frequent and only the medial aspect of the nail bed is hypertrophic. The acquired subungual exostosis (type II), in their study, is observed from the fourth through to the sixth decade of life with a blunt or sharp protuberance at the distal and dorsal aspect of the distal phalanx, without cartilage. The nail plate appears as an inverted U, with nail bed hypertrophy

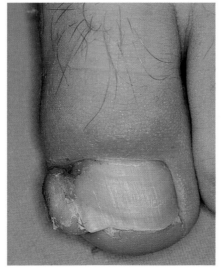

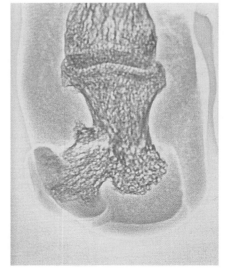

**Fig. 11.113** (a) Exostosis clearly visible on xeroradiography. (b) Xeroradiography.

(a)

(b)

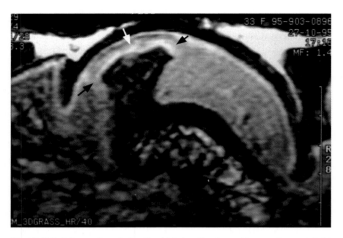

**Fig. 11.114** Subungual exostosis with a high signal hyaline cartilage cap (arrows). Axial gradient echo image.

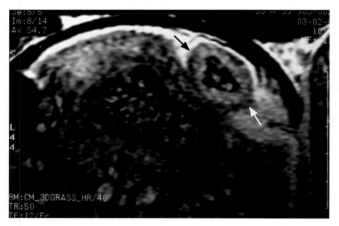

**Fig. 11.115** Subungual exostosis with a 1-mm thick fibrocartilage cap (arrows). Axial gradient echo image. Note the central core of trabecular bone.

being apparent. In fact this classification describes the osseous changes seen in pincer nails with type I being the inherited usually symmetrical type of overcurvature and type II characterizing the acquired type of pincer nails (Haneke 1992). This type of osteophyte formation is equivalent to what we call subungual hyperostosis. The type II hyperostosis may be due to an abnormal positional relationship between the first metatarsal and hallux, with secondary osteoarthritis.

*Most often, MRI is not necessary for the diagnosis but can easily depict a cartilaginous cap. The proton density-weighted images or the gradient echo images are the most accurate and can distinguish hyaline cartilage with high signal (Fig. 11.114) from fibrocartilage with lower signal (Fig. 11.115). These two components may be associated and the thickness of the cap can be accurately measured. The trabecular bone is nicely visible on gradient echo images, where the trabecular network is increased by the magnetic susceptibility artifacts. However, MRI is mainly indicated to highlight a purely radiolucent cartilaginous exostosis.*

Histology shows a proliferative fibrocartilaginous cap that merges into hyaline cartilage forming mature trabecular bone at its base by enchondral ossification. It appears probable that the cartilaginous cap is finally replaced by bone in mature lesions. Electron microscopy reveals that the tumour is composed of two types of cells, one, rich in cell organelles including rough endoplasmic reticulum, well developed Golgi apparatus, and glycogen granules; the other cell with few such cell organelles. The former cells seem to be osteoblasts actively engaged in bone formation, and the latter to be osteocytes related to those situated deeper in bone matrix of normal bone. However, ossification or calcification in subungual exostosis is rather casual, and osteocytes in this disorder may lack the capacity to elaborate compact bone.

### Osteochondroma

Osteochondroma, commonly evoking the same symptoms as subungual exostosis, is said to have a male predominance (Fig. 11.116). Its onset is usually between the ages of 10 to 25. There is also often a history of trauma (Apfelberg *et al.* 1979). Its growth rate is slow. X-ray shows a well-defined circumscribed pedunculated or sessile bone growth projecting from the dorsum of the distal phalanx near to the epiphyseal line. Therefore, nail dystrophy may be pronounced (Schulze & Hebert 1994; Kim *et al.* 1998). Histology shows a bony tumour with a hyaline cartilage cap (Fig. 11.117.) However, on the basis of the histopathological pattern, de Palma *et al.* (1996) claim that most subungual bone masses exhibit the features of conventional osteochondromas and not of subungual exostoses independent of their location at the distal phalanx. It must be differentiated from primary subungual calcification, particularly seen in elderly women, secondary subungual calcification due to trauma and psoriasis (Fischer 1982), and primary osteoma cutis (Burgdorf & Nasemann 1977).

The case of osteochondroma on the ulnar side of the distal phalanx of the small finger and penetrating the skin and the nail is unique (Ganzhorn *et al.* 1981).

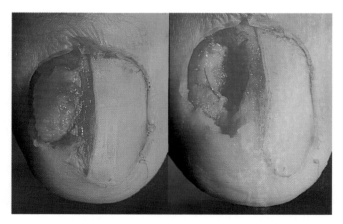

**Fig. 11.116** Osteochondroma.

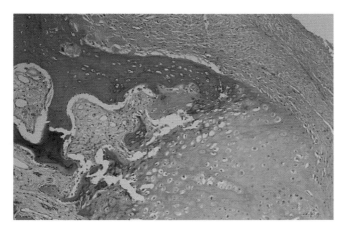

**Fig. 11.117** Subungual osteochondroma—histological changes clearly different from subungual calcification.

Differential diagnosis of subungual exostosis and osteochondroma rules out malignant melanoma, epithelioma, keratoacanthoma, glomus tumour, pyogenic granuloma, implantation cyst and wart (Tables 11.5 & 11.6) (Stieler *et al.* 1989).

Therapy of subungual exostosis and osteochondroma consists of local curettage (Senff *et al.* 1987) or excision of the excess bone under aseptic conditions. Conservative and thorough treatment of this pathology can be achieved using the appropriate tools in a dermatology day case setting (de Berker & Langtry 1999). If the tumour is located in the nail bed, the nail plate is partially removed and a longitudinal incision is made in the nail bed. Whenever possible, we prefer to remove the tumour by an L-shaped or a fish-mouth incision, in order to avoid avulsion of the nail plate. The osseous growth with its cartilaginous cap is carefully dissected using fine skin hooks to avoid damage to the fragile nail bed and the tumour is removed with a fine chisel. Most subungual exostoses are located in the medial aspect of the hyponychial area of the hallux elevating the distal margin of the plate. The overlying skin is usually extremely overstretched and has to be removed by a fusiform excision which also facilitates removal of the exostosis by a fine chisel or bone rongeur (Haneke 1991).

## References

Apfelberg, D.B., Druker, D., Maser, M. *et al.* (1979) Subungual osteochondroma. *Archives of Dermatology* **115**, 472–473.

Badawy Abdel-Naser, M., Zouboulis, C.C. & Anagnostopoulos, I. (1992) Subungual exostosis. *European Journal of Dermatology* **2**, 345–347.

Baran, R. & Sayag, J. (1978) Exostose sous-unguéale de l'index. *Annales de Dermatologie et de Vénéréologie* **105**, 1075–1076.

de Berker, D. & Langtry, J. (1999) Treatment of subungual exostoses by elective day case surgery. *British Journal of Dermatology* **140**, 915–918.

Burgdorf, W. & Nasemann, T. (1977) Cutaneous osteomas: a clinical and histopathologic review. *Archives of Dermatological Research* **260**, 121–135.

Carroll, R.E., Chance, J.T. & Inan, Y. (1992) Subungual exostosis in the hand. *Journal of Hand Surgery* **17B**, 569–574.

Chinn, S. & Jenkin, W. (1986) Proximal nail groove pain associated

**Table 11.5** Differential diagnosis of subungual exostosis and osteochondroma (Schulze & Hebert 1994; Davis & Cohen 1996).

| Feature | Subungal exostosis | Subungual osteochondroma |
|---|---|---|
| Aetiology | Trauma, repeated microtrauma, infection | Congenital or traumatic |
| Onset | Adolescence, young adults | 10–25 years |
| Male : female ratio | 1 : 2 | 2 : 1 |
| Location | Distal end of distal phalanx | Juxtaepiphyseal |
| Growth rate | Moderate | Slow |
| Radiology | Broad-based trabeculated bone with distal flare | Sessile bone with scalloped dome and radiolucent hyaline cartilage cap |
| Histopathology | Cancellous bone with fibrocartilaginous cap | Bone with hyaline cartilage cap |
| Malignant degeneration | None | Rare (1%) |
| Treatment | Complete removal | Complete removal |

**Table 11.6** Differential features of exostosis, osteochondroma, enchondroma and epidermoid cyst (Norton 1980).

| Tumour | Age (years) | Sex ratio | History of trauma | Rate of growth | X-ray |
|---|---|---|---|---|---|
| Exostosis | 20–40 | F : M, 2 : 1 | Occasionally | Moderate | Trabeculated osseous growth with expanded distal portion covered with radiolucent fibrocartilage |
| Osteochondroma | 10–25 | M : F, 2 : 1 | Often | Slow | Well-defined sessile bone growth with hyaline cartilage cap |
| Enchondroma | 20–40 | M + F | Often | Rapid | Lobulated bone cyst showing radiolucent defect, bone expansion and flecks of calcification |
| Epidermoid cyst | 8–83 | M : F, 2 : 1 | Almost always | Rapid | Radiolucent cyst: no calcification |

with an exostosis. *Journal of the American Podiatric Medical Association* **76**, 506–508.

Dahlin, D.C. & Unni, K.K. (1986) *Bone Tumors*, 4th edn. pp. 18–30. C.C. Thomas, Springfield.

Davis, D.A. & Cohen, P.R. (1996) Subungual exostosis. Case report and review of the literature. *Pediatric Dermatology* **13**, 212–218.

Fikry, T., Dkhiss, M., Harfaoui, A. *et al.* (1998a) Les exostoses sous-unguéales. Etude rétrospective d'une série de 28 cas. *Acta Orthopaedica Belgica* **64**, 35–40.

Fikry, T., Harfaoui, A., Zahid, M. *et al.* (1998b) Exostose sous-unguéale digitale. A propos d'un cas. *Main* **3**, 77–82.

Fischer, E. (1982) Subunguale Verkalkungen. *Fortschritte der Röntgenologie* **137**, 580–584.

Ganzhorn, R.W., Bahri, G. & Horowitz, M. (1981) Osteochondroma of the distal phalanx. *Journal of Hand Surgery* **6**, 625–626.

Guidetti, M.S., Stinchi, C., Vezzani, C. *et al.* (1996) Subungual exostosis of a finger resembling pterygium inversum unguis. *Dermatology* **193**, 354–355.

Haneke, E. (1991) Cirugía dermatológica de la región ungueal. *Monografias de Dermatologia* **4**, 408–423.

Haneke, E. (1992) Etiopathogénie de l'hypercourbure transversale de l'ongle du gros orteil. *Journal de Médecine Esthétique et Chirurgie Dermatologique* **29**, 123–127.

Iiszuka, T., Kinoshita, Y. & Fukumoto, K. (1995) Subungual exostosis of the finger. *Annals of Plastic Surgery* **35**, 330–332.

James, M.P. (1988) Digital exostosis causing enlargement of the fingertips. *Journal of the American Academy of Dermatology* **19**, 132.

Kim, S.W., Moon, S.E. & Kim, J.A. (1998) A case of subungual osteochondroma. *Journal of Dermatology* **25**, 60–62.

Lemont, H. & Christman, R.A. (1990) Subungual exostosis and nail disease and radiologic aspects. In: *Nails, Therapy, Diagnosis, Surgery* (ed. R. Scher & C.R. Daniel), pp. 250–257. W.B. Saunders, Philadelphia.

Letts, M., Davidson, D. & Nizalik, E. (1998) Subungual exostosis: diagnosis and treatment in children. *Journal of Trauma, Injury, Infection and Critical Care* **44**, 346–349.

Norton, L.A. (1980) Nail disorders. *Journal of the American Academy of Dermatology* **2**, 451–467.

de Palma, L., Gigante, A. & Specchia, N. (1996) Subungual exostosis of the foot. *Foot and Ankle International* **17**, 758–763.

Pambor, M. & Neubert, H. (1971) Tumorartige Begleitreaktionen der Haut bei Exostosen der Zehenendphalangen (Zur Differential-diagnose par-und subungualer Tumoren). *Dermatologische Monatsschrift* **157**, 532–537.

Schulze, K.E. & Hebert, A.A. (1994) Diagnostic features, differential diagnosis, and treatment of subungual osteochondroma. *Pediatric Dermatology* **11**, 39–41.

Sebastian, G. (1977) Subunguale Exostosen der Grosszehe, Berufsstigma bei Tänzern. *Dermatologische Monatsschrift* **163**, 998–1000.

Senff, H., Kuhlwein, A. & Janner, M. (1987) Subungual Exostose. *Zeitschrift für Hautkrankheiten* **62**, 1401–1404.

Stieler, W., Reinel, D., Jänner, M. & Haneke, E. (1989) Ungewöhnliche Lokalisation einer subungualen Exostose. *Aktuelle Dermatologie* **15**, 32–34.

Velanovich, V. (1994) Subungual pigmented lesion caused by a bone spur: a mimic of a subungual melanoma. *Military Medicine* **159**, 663.

Webber, J.M. & Miller, M.V. (1994) Subungual exostosis in a young women. *Pathology* **26**, 339–341.

## Multiple exostoses syndrome (diaphysial aclasis)

Multiple exostoses syndrome (MES) is a heritable disorder affecting enchondral skeleton during the period of growth in a variety of ways, but generally 'close to the knee and far from the elbow'. It is characterized by thickening and deformity of the growing bone with the formation of numerous cartilage-capped exostoses clustered around the areas of most active growth.

A 16-year-old boy presented with anonychia of his left index finger caused by a firm non-tender nodule affecting the proximal two thirds of the nail bed and the lunula with resultant slight elevation of the proximal nail fold (Fig. 11.118a). The outgrowth had started 2 years earlier. A lateral X-ray revealed an exostosis (Fig. 11.118b). His sister, aged 12, presented with multiple exostoses of the hands, clearly visible radiologically. They were located on the ventral aspect of the middle phalanx of the right index finger and the dorsal aspect of the distal phalanx of the right 5th digit and the 1st, 2nd and 3rd left digits where they slightly lifted up the nail plate (Baran & Bureau 1991).

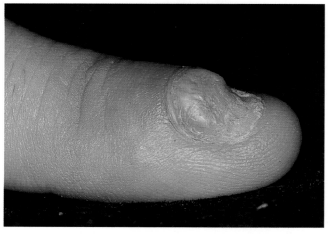

(a)

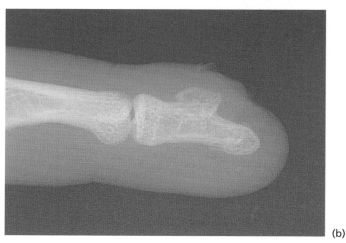

(b)

**Fig. 11.118** (a) Multiple exostoses syndrome—proximal bony swelling with anonychia. (b) Radiological appearance of (a).

Laugier *et al.* (1964) reported two cases in the French literature. In the first, exostosis of the base of the distal phalanx of the 4th finger of a 10-year-old boy resulted in a lateral deviation of the nail plate. Several fingers were affected in an 11-year-old girl presenting with various physical signs including a bump at the base of the right index nail, an overcurvature of the lateral aspect of the nail of the right middle finger, a red linear longitudinal line with a distal fissure on the right 5th finger nail, and distal fissures arranged in a fanwise manner on 2 other nails.

Hazen and Smith (1990) reported prominent elevation of the proximal portion of the nail and corresponding nail fold of several fingers by firm and non-tender nodules. Schmitt *et al.* (1997) reported 3 young children with lifting up of the nail plate which was fissured and covered with longitudinal ridges. In Del Rio *et al.*'s report (1992) nail plate deformity consisted of malalignment, longitudinal dystrophy and swelling of the proximal nail fold on several fingers that had developed slowly since birth.

When the disease involves the distal phalanx it seems to affect most often several digits simultaneously. Such a distribution should therefore alert the clinician to suspect MES with the possible risk of malignant changes to chondrosarcoma from 1 to 25% (Solomon 1974), despite the absence of malignancy reported in this location and in childhood (Smith 1988).

## References

Baran, R. & Bureau, H. (1991) Multiple exostoses syndrome presenting with anonychia on a single finger. *Journal of the American Academy of Dermatology* **25**, 333–335.

Del Rio, R., Navarra, E., Ferrando, J. *et al.* (1992) Multiple exostoses syndrome presenting as nail malalignment and longitudinal dystrophy of fingers. *Archives of Dermatology* **128**, 1655–1656.

Hazen, P.G. & Smith, D.E. (1990) Hereditary multiple exostoses, report of a case presenting with proximal nail fold and nail swelling. *Journal of the American Academy of Dermatology* **22**, 132–134.

Laugier, P., Gille, P., Gondy, B. *et al.* (1964) Maladie exostosante avec lésions unguéales (2 cas). *Bulletin de la Societé Française et de Syphiligraphie* **71**, 338.

Schmitt, A.M., Bories, A. & Baran, R. (1997) Exostoses sous-unguéale des doigts au cours de la maladie exostosante héréditaire. *Annales de Dermatologie et de Vénéréologie* **124**, 233–236.

Smith, D.W. (1988) *Recognizable Patterns of Human Malformation. Genetic, Embryologic and Clinical Aspects*, 4th edn. W.B. Saunders, Philadelphia.

Solomon, L. (1974) Chondrosarcoma in hereditary multiple exostosis. *South African Medical Journal* **48**, 671–676.

### Soft tissue chondroma

Swelling of the distal phalanx of the middle finger with progressive distortion of the nail was seen in a 37-year-old man. Magnetic resonance imaging revealed a $9 \times 11$ mm large, well-defined tumour in the nail bed and matrix. At operation, a bluish oval lesion was easily dissected from the surrounding tissue. Histology revealed fairly normal mature hyaline cartilage (Dumontier *et al.* 1997). Two more nail bed chondromas were described by Lichtenstein and Goldman (1964).

## References

Dumontier, C., Abimelec, P. & Drapé, J.-L. (1997) Soft-tissue chondroma of the nail bed. *Journal of Hand Surgery* **22B**, 474–475.

Lichtenstein, L. & Goldman, R.L. (1964) Cartilage tumors in soft tissue, particularly in the hand and foot. *Cancer* **17**, 1203–1208.

### Enchondroma

Solitary enchondroma accounts for 90% of all bone tumours of the hand but is rare in the distal phalanx. Though occurring in all age groups it is most frequently seen between 30 to 35 years of age. It is a painful tumour which expands the tip of the finger (Fig. 11.119a). Pathological fracture is frequently the presenting symptom, but up to 20% remain totally asymptomatic. It may present clinically as paronychia (Shelley & Ralston 1964; Pastinszky & Dévai 1968; Wawrosch & Rassner 1985), as clubbing with thickening, discoloration and longitudinal ridging of the nail (Yaffee 1965; Koff *et al.* 1996) or as a pearly-white tumour lifting the overlying nail plate (Carjaval *et al.* 1987). X-ray reveals a well-defined radiolucent defect with expansion of the distal phalanx and sometimes spotty calcifications (Schajowicz *et al.* 1970) (Fig. 11.119b). The enchondroma is typically located at the base or in the middle of the distal phalanx abutting the articular surface (Monsees & Murphy 1984). Pathological fractures may occur as a result of continuous thinning of the bone cortex.

Enchondroma involving the distal phalanx of the hand was monostotic in three cases and polyostotic in 30 cases after Takigawa's review (1971). Chondrosarcoma may arise in a pre-existing enchondroma (Bellinghausen *et al.* 1983; Nakajima *et al.* 1988). Histology shows hyaline cartilage proliferation with irregularly arranged cells (Fig. 11.119c).

Treatment is required to prevent further enlargement of the enchondroma and because of its symptoms. The tumour is usually enucleated under full aseptic conditions through a mid-lateral or dorsal incision (Shimizu *et al.* 1997). Curettage followed by autologous cancellous bone grafting usually yields the best results and the ilium can be recommended as a good donor site for such grafting. However, all lesions do not necessarily need such an operation as a certain degree of spontaneous healing may take place in some cases.

### Enchondromatosis (Ollier's chondrodysplasia)

Enchondromatosis results from cartilage failing to undergo normal ossification in an asymmetrical fashion (Fig. 11.120).

### Maffucci's syndrome (enchondromatosis, or chondrodysplasia with multiple soft tissue haemangiomas)

In Maffucci's syndrome multiple haemangiomas of the subcutis

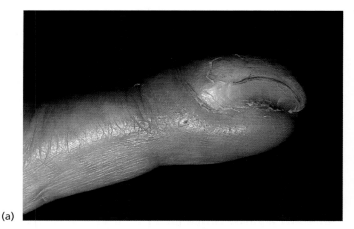

(a)

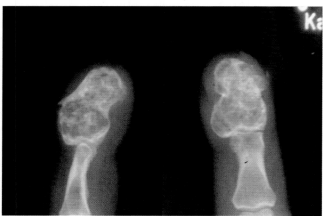

(b)

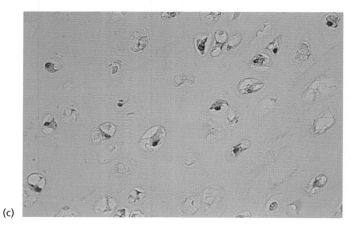

(c)

**Fig. 11.119** (a) Enchondroma. (b) X-ray showing expansion of the distal phalanx and irregular, spotty calcification (see a). (c) Enchondroma—hyaline cartilage proliferation with irregularly arranged cells (see a and b). (Courtesy of G. Rassner, Germany.)

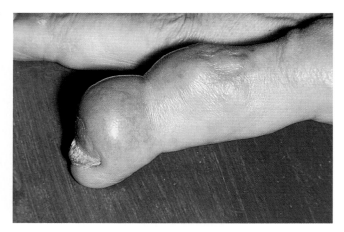

**Fig. 11.120** Enchondromatosis—Ollier's chondrodysplasia.

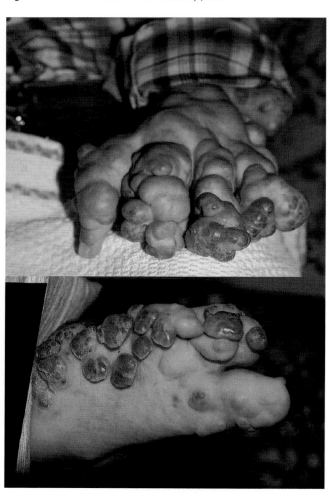

**Fig. 11.121** Maffucci's syndrome. (Courtesy of D. Tilsley, New Zealand.)

and internal organs as well as hard cartilaginous nodules near epiphyseal lines develop in childhood, with up to 25% being affected at birth or during infancy. The hands particularly develop vascular hamartomas often showing cauliflower-like growths. Gross skeletal deformities are due to masses and columns of uncalcified cartilage causing unequal growth of bones

and delayed healing of the easily sustained bone fractures. The hands and feet may be transformed into useless masses (Steudel 1892; Hackenbroch 1922).

Involvement of the terminal phalanx may result in gross deformity, dystrophy or loss of the nail (Fig. 11.121) (Tilsley

& Burden 1981; Yazidi *et al.* 1998). The most important complication is the high frequency of chondrosarcoma (Lewis & Ketcham 1973) or angiosarcoma, but other malignant neoplasms have also been observed (Yazidi *et al.* 1998).

The differential diagnosis of subungual chondroma (Ayala *et al.* 1983) includes most tumours occurring in a subungual location, such as subungual exostosis, pyogenic granuloma, common wart, glomus tumour, epidermoid cyst, keratoacanthoma, melanoma, neurofibroma and sarcoma, but the distinction between chondroma and low-grade chondrosarcoma is one of the most difficult to make histopathologically (Gottschalk & Smith 1963). A case of subungual melanoma with cartilaginous differentiation was recently described by Cachia and Kedziora (1999).

## References

Ayala, F., Lembo, G. & Montesano, M. (1983) A rare tumour. Subungual chondroma. *Dermatologica* **167**, 339–340.

Bellinghausen, H.W., Weeks, P.M., Young, L.V. & Gilula, L.A. (1983) Chondrosarcoma of distal phalanx. *Orthopedic Reviews* **12**, 97–100.

Cachia, A.R. & Kedziora, A.M. (1999) Subungual malignant melanoma with cartilaginous differentiation. *American Journal of Dermatopathology* **21**, 165–169.

Carvajal, L., Uraga, E., Garcia, I. *et al.* (1987) Tumours of the hallux, myxoma, osteochondroma and enchondroma. *Skin Cancer* **2**, 197–201.

Gottschalk, R.G. & Smith, R.T. (1963) Chondrosarcoma of the hand. *Journal of Bone and Joint Surgery* **45A**, 141–150.

Hackenbroch, M. (1922) Über Olliersche Waschstumsstörung und Chondromatose des Skeletts. *Fortschritte der Röntgenologie* **30**, 432–440.

Koff, A.B., Goldberg, L.H. & Ambergel D. (1996) Nail dystrophy in a 35-year-old man. *Archives of Dermatology* **132**, 223–228.

Lewis, R.J. & Ketcham, A.S. (1973) Maffucci's syndrome; functional and neoplastic significance. *Journal of Bone and Joint Surgery* **55A**, 1465.

Monsees, B. & Murphy, W.A. (1984) Distal phalangeal erosive lesions. *Arthritis and Rheumatism* **27**, 449–455.

Nakajima, H., Ushigome, S. & Fukuda, J. (1988) Case report 482: chondrosarcoma (grade 1) arising from the right second toe in patient with multiple enchondromas. *Skeletal Radiology* **17**, 289–292.

Pastinszky, I. & Dévai, J. (1968) Paronychia et onychodystrophia enchondromatosa. *Börgyógyászati és Venerelogiai Szemle* **44**, 176–178.

Schajowicz, F., Aiello, C. & Slullitel, I. (1970) Cystic and pseudocystic lesions of the terminal phalanx with special reference to epidermoid cysts. *Clinical Orthopedics and Related Research* **68**, 84–92.

Shelley, W.B. & Ralston, E.L. (1964) Paronychia due to enchondroma. *Archives of Dermatology* **90**, 412–413.

Shimizu, K., Kotoura, Y., Nishijima, N. & Nakamura, T. (1997) Enchondroma of the distal phalanx of the hand. *Journal of Bone and Joint Surgery* **79A**, 898–900.

Steudel, (1892) Multiple Endondrome der Knochen in Verbindung mit venösen Angiomen der Weichteile. *Beitrage zur Klinischen Chirurgie* **8**, 503–521.

Takigawa, K. (1971) Chondroma of the bones of the hand. *Journal of Bone and Joint Surgery* **53A**, 1591–1600.

Tilsley, D.A. & Burden, P.W. (1981) A case of Maffucci's syndrome. *British Journal of Dermatology* **105**, 331–336.

Wawrosch, W. & Rassner, G. (1985) Monströses Enchondrom des Zeigefingerendgliedes mit Nageldeformierung. *Hautarzt* **36**, 168–169.

Yaffee, H.W. (1965) Peculiar nail dystrophy caused by an enchondroma. *Archives of Dermatology* **91**, 361.

Yazidi, A., Benzekri, L., Senouci, K. *et al.* (1998) Syndrome de Maffucci avec carcinome épidermoïde du cavum. *Annales de Dermatologie et de Vénéréologie* **125**, 50–51.

## Osteoid osteoma

Osteoid osteoma (Jaffé 1935) is a distinct clinical and pathological entity (Rosborough 1966). About 8% of all osteoid osteomas occur in the phalanges, and 1 to 2% of hand tumours are osteoid osteomas; however, its location in the distal phalanx is quite rare (Aulicino *et al.* 1981) with index predominance. The usual incidence is two males to one female. They appear in young adults but Szabó and Smith (1985) reported one case which had probably existed since birth.

Osteoid osteoma causes swelling of the distal phalanx or even enlargement of the entire tip and clubbing. Thickening or enlargement of the nail may be associated (Fig. 11.122a). The

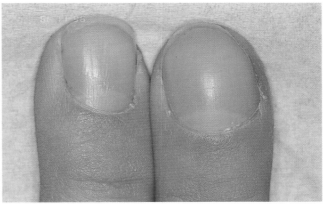

(a)

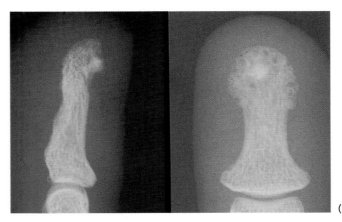

(b)

**Fig. 11.122** (a) Osteoid osteoma—pseudo-clubbed finger. (b) Osteoid osteoma—X-ray changes.

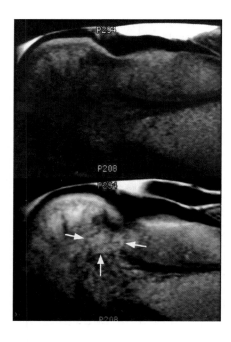

**Fig. 11.123** Osteoid osteoma of the tuft. Sagittal T1-weighted spin echo image before (top) and after injection of gadolinium (bottom). Note the enhanced nidus (arrows), and the oedema of the nail bed and the trabecular bone of the distal phalanx.

skin is either normal in colour or faintly violaceous. Increased sweating of the area has been described. Palpation with a blunt probe may help to localize the tender tumour on pressure. A nidus, characterized by a small area of rarefaction with surrounding sclerosis, is demonstrable radiologically in most cases and has been likened to a sleigh-bell (Foucher *et al.* 1987; Meng & Watt 1989) (Fig. 11.122b); it is located in the medulla, in the cortex, or subperiosteally with a very thin covering of bone over the nidus (Sullivan 1971). The hypervascularisation explaining the nail thickening, can be demonstrated by arteriography (Lindbom *et al.* 1960; Sullivan 1971), by thermography (O'Hara *et al.* 1975) or by scintigraphy (Braun *et al.* 1980).

*Computed tomography (CT) with thin contiguous slices is the best imaging technique to analyse and accurately locate the nidus previously guided by a bone scan. MRI is less sensitive than CT for the detection of a tiny intracortical nidus. The osteoid tissue is quite intense on gradient echo images and enhances. The large inflammatory reaction of the nail bed is very difficult to see with CT, although it is obvious with MRI, as the associated medullary oedema of the distal phalanx (Fig. 11.123). A synovitis of the distal interphalangeal joint may be associated.*

Young patients may have premature fusion of the adjacent epiphysis. Histologically, the nidus is a meshwork of osteoid trabeculae with varying degrees of mineralization in a background of vascular fibrous connective tissue. When they appear in the distal phalanx they present unusual diagnostic difficulties due to (a) atypical radiological appearance; (b) presence of soft tissue enlargement and nail deformity; (c) small size of the distal phalanx and consequent close approximation of lesions to the nail, growth plate and distal interphalangeal joint (Bowen *et al.* 1987).

Osteoid osteoma usually evokes a 'nagging' pain, accentuated at night, which is poorly localized and may extend proximal to the proximal joint of the affected digit. Local tenderness is present in about one-half of the cases. There is no evidence of inflammation. Relief of pain by salicylates is characteristic. However, symptoms may vary considerably. According to Saville (1980) naproxen given in low doses may prevent the pain of osteoid osteoma, offering useful non-surgical treatment and spontaneous regression leading even to complete cure is possible (Foucher *et al.* 1987).

Treatment is by en-bloc resection through a 'fish mouth' incision (Hamilos & Cervetti 1987). Curettage may fail to eradicate the lesion. Radiography does not seem to be helpful in deciding whether the whole lesion has been removed. After therapy the swelling regresses, a normal nail regrows and the pain gradually disappears. There are cases, however, where digital enlargement persisted after removal of the lesion. Therefore reducing the soft tissue and narrowing the nail at the same time the lesion is removed has been advocated (Giannikas 1977).

The differential diagnosis comprises glomus tumour, implantation epidermoid cyst, sclerosing osteitis of Garré, localized cortical bone abscess, syphilitic dactylitis, tuberculosis, chondroma and arteriovenous fistula. It is not possible to differentiate between osteoid osteoma and benign osteoblastoma (less painful, less sclerosis) on histological grounds alone (Table 11.7).

## References

Aulicino, P.L., DuPuy, T.E. & Moriarity, R.P. (1981) Osteoid osteoma of the terminal phalanx of finger. *Orthopedic Reviews* 10, 59–63.

Bowen, C.V.A., Dzus, A.K. & Hardy, D.A. (1987) Osteoid osteomata of the distal phalanx. *Journal of Hand Surgery* 12B, 387–390.

**Table 11.7** Differentiation between osteoid osteoma and benign osteoblastoma.

|  | Osteoid osteoma | Osteoblastoma |
| --- | --- | --- |
| Size | < 1 cm in diameter | Slow progressive enlargement |
| Symptoms | Painful | Less painful |
| X-ray | Considerable reactive bone and sclerosis | Less sclerosis |
| Location | Long bones | Flat bones |
| Histology |  | Indistinguishable |

Braun, S., Chevro, A., Tomeno, B. *et al.* (1980) Les ostéomes ostéoides phalangiens. *Médecine et Hygiène (Genève)* **38**, 1222–1229.

Foucher, G., Lemarechal, P., Citron, N. *et al.* (1987) Osteoid osteoma of the distal phalanx. A report of four cases and review of the literature. *Journal of Hand Surgery* **12B**, 382–386.

Giannikas, A., Papachristov, G., Tiniakos, G. *et al.* (1977) Osteoid osteoma of the terminal phalanges. *Hand* **9**, 295–300.

Hamilos, D.T. & Cervetti, R.G. (1987) Osteoid osteoma of the hallux. *Journal of Foot Surgery* **26**, 397–399.

Jaffé, H.L. (1935) Osteoid osteoma. A benign osteoblastic tumor composed of osteoid and atypical bone. *Archives of Surgery* **31**, 709–728.

Lindbom, A., Lindvall, N., Sodenberg, G. & Spujt, H. (1960) Angiography in osteoid osteoma. *Acta Radiologica Stockholm* **54**, 327–333.

Meng, Q. & Watt, I. (1989) Phalangeal osteoid osteoma. *British Journal Radiologica* **62**, 321–325.

O'Hara, J.P., Tegmeyer, C., Sweet, D.E. & MacCue, F.C. (1975) Angiography in the diagnosis of osteoid osteoma of the hand. *Journal of Bone and Joint Surgery* **57A**, 163–166.

Rosborough, D. (1966) Osteoid osteoma, report of a lesion in the terminal phalanx of a finger. *Journal of Bone and Joint Surgery* **48B**, 485–487.

Saville, P.D. (1980) A medical option for the treatment of osteoid osteoma. *Arthritis and Rheumatism* **23**, 1409–1411.

Sullivan, M. (1971) Osteoid osteoma of the fingers. *Hand* **3**, 175–178.

Szabó, R.M. & Smith, B. (1985) Possible congenital osteoid osteoma of a phalanx; case report. *Journal of Bone and Joint Surgery* **67A**, 815–816.

### Giant cell tumour of the bone

Giant-cell tumour may involve the distal bony phalanx of young adults. The most common complaint is pain that may be noted suddenly in the hand, following relatively mild trauma (Averill *et al.* 1980). A painful lesion is always tender to palpation with sometimes a palpable bony mass at the site of the lesion. Radiologically the lesions often show extensive destruction of the cortical and cancellous bone with one-third of the tumours expanding the cortex so that the bone widens to 2–3 times its normal diameter. Fracture of the cortex or complete destruction of the bone may be observed. Stippling or calcification within the tumour, has not been reported.

A 13-year-old child developed a lesion on her 3rd toe some months after cryotherapy for warts. This was curetted but recurred rapidly. It was then seen with a round, yellowish soft tumour in the distal nail bed which was tender on palpation. X-ray showed osteolysis and MRI revealed a phalangeal tumour invading the dermis. The lesion was removed with part of the terminal phalanx. Histology showed a tumour invading and fragmenting the underlying bone. The tumour had an eosinophilic cytoplasm and large nuclei with obvious nucleoli thus resembling histiocytes. There were many multinucleated giant cells, but neither atypical cells nor mitoses were seen (Goettmann *et al.* 1995).

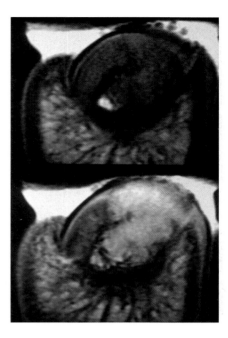

**Fig. 11.124** Giant cell tumour of the distal phalanx with invasion of the nail bed. Axial T1-weighted spin echo image before (top) and after (bottom) injection of gadolinium.

*On MR images, the signal behaviour of the tumour is identical to that of the surrounding soft tissues (Fig. 11.124). However, the lesion may have numerous cavities with high signal in case of an aneurysmal component.*

The tumour tissue is vascular, friable and reddish-brown. Since there is an 18% incidence of multicentric foci of giant-cell tumours of the hand, bone scan is advised when these tumours occur in the hand (Averill *et al.* 1980). Histological examination is necessary to confirm the diagnosis.

Curettage was found ineffective as a method of treatment. However, amputation is not necessary except for extreme cases.

### References

Averill, R.M., Smith, R.J. & Campbell, C.J. (1980) Giant-cell tumors of the bones of the hand. *Journal of Hand Surgery* **5**, 39–50.

Goettmann, S., Baran, R., Fraitag, S. *et al.* (1995) Tumeurs à cellules géantes osseuses avec atteinte unguéale. *Annales de Dermatologie et de Vénéréologie* **122** (Suppl. 1), S148–149.

### Solitary bone cyst

Solitary bone cyst of the distal phalanx is exceptional and may belong to the group of aneurysmal bone cysts. Goldsmith (1966) reported on clubbed nail deformity overlying a bulbous distal end of the left second toe which was tender. X-ray examination revealed an expanded distal phalanx with an ultra-thinned cortex and cystic-like loss of substance in the main body of bone.

### Reference

Goldsmith, E. (1966) Solitary bone cyst of the distal phalanx. A case report. *Journal of the American Podiatric Association* **5**, 69–70.

## Malignant tumours

### *Chondrosarcoma*

See page 594.

## Synovial tumours

### Giant cell tumour (benign synovioma, benign xanthomatous giant cell tumours, villo-nodular pigmented synovitis)

Giant cell tumour is a neoplasm derived from the tendon sheath or the joint synovialis. It is the second most common subcutaneous tumour of the hand. It is more frequent in females than in males. On the digits (Fig. 11.125a), it usually occurs on the dorsum of the distal interphalangeal joint and usually appears as a solitary, often lobulated, slow-growing, skin coloured and smooth surfaced nodule which tends to feel firm and rubbery. The tumour, which may present as multi-nodular (Schwartz & Southwick 1979) may enlarge to the size of a cherry and may cause pain on flexion by virtue of its dimen-

sions. Only rarely does the tumour interfere with the nail unit. In the region of the lateral nail fold, periodic inflammation and drainage may occur (Norton 1990). In contrast to malignant synovioma, no calcification is demonstrable on X-ray (Wright 1951).

A unique case of subungual giant cell tumour was published by Abimelec *et al.* (1996). They reported a 41-year-old man who had observed abnormal growth of his left ring finger nail. This was due to a firm non-inflammatory swelling of the matrix region.

A 24-year-old women presented with a cystic-appearing lesion adjacent to the nail of her right middle finger which caused a wide longitudinal groove in the nail plate (Batta *et al.* 1999). Another giant cell tumour involving the lateral nail fold and nail bed and interfering with nail growth was seen in a 37-year-old man (Richert & André 1999).

*MRI may suggest the diagnosis with a nodule close to the distal insertion of the flexor or extensor digitorum tendon or to the synovium of the distal interphalangeal joint. In typical cases, haemosiderin deposits lead to typical signal void artifacts on all MR images (Fig. 11.126). These deposits are less often visible in the fingers than in the knee. However, an intermediate to low signal of a part of the tumor is very frequent and must evoke the diagnosis. On the other hand, the signal enhancement after the injection of gadolinium is not specific.*

Histopathology (Fig. 11.125b) shows a cellular tumour composed of histiocytic and fibroblastic cells with a variable number of giant cells and some foam cells in a hyalin stroma. Siderophages may give the tumour a brown appearance.

Differential diagnosis includes a ganglion which tends to feel more cystic (aspiration or transillumination), fibroma of tendon sheath (Chung & Enzinger 1979; Humphreys *et al.* 1986), implantation epidermal cyst, fibrokeratoma, rheumatoid nodule, multicentric reticulohistiocytosis, metastatic tumour, tendinous xanthoma, chondro or osteo-sarcoma, reticulohistiocytoma whose histology may be indentical to giant cell

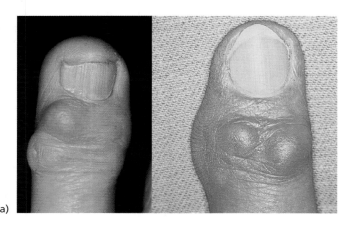

(a)

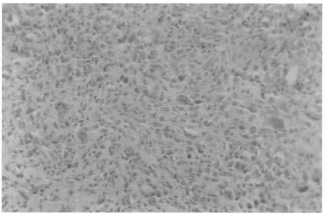

(b)

**Fig. 11.125** (a) Giant cell tumour—benign synovioma. (Courtesy of H.H. Wolff, Germany.) (b) Giant cell tumour—mainly histiocytic and fibroblastic cells, some giant cells and foam cells in a hyaline stroma.

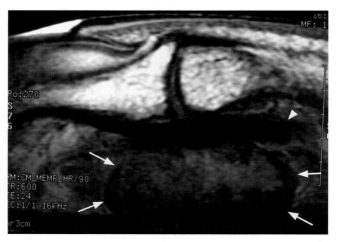

**Fig. 11.126** Giant cell tumour (arrows) of the sheath of the flexor digitorum profundus tendon (arrowhead). Sagittal gradient echo image.

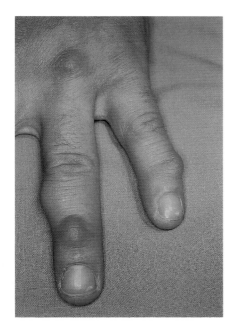

**Fig. 11.127** Granuloma annulare. (Courtesy of S. Salasche, USA.)

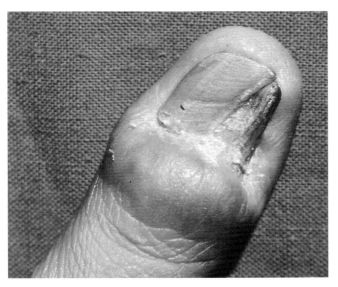

**Fig. 11.128** Erythema elevatum diutinum. (Courtesy of G. Moulin, France.)

tumour. Granuloma annulare (Fig. 11.127) and erythema elevatum diutinum (Fig. 11.128) should also be ruled out.

Treatment is by careful surgical removal. An oblique incision along the greatest axis of the tumour enables the multilobulated lesion to be exposed. It may penetrate the extensor tendon. Complete removal is necessary to prevent recurrences.

### References

Abimelec, P., Cambiaghi, S., Thioly, D., Moulonguet, I. & Dumontier, C. (1996) Subungual giant cell tumor of the tendon sheath. *Cutis* **58**, 273–275.

Batta, K., Tan, C.Y. & Colloby, P. (1999) Giant cell tumour of the tendon sheath producing a groove deformity of the nail plate and mimicking a myxoid cyst. *British Journal of Dermatology* **140**, 720–781.

Chung, E.B. & Enzinger, F.M. (1979) Fibroma of tendon sheath. *Cancer* **44**, 1945–1954.

Humphreys, S., McKee, P.H. & Fletcher, D.M. (1986) Fibroma of tendon sheath, a clinicopathologic study. *Journal of Cutaneous Pathology* **13**, 331–338.

Norton, L.A. (1990) Tumors. In: *Nails, Therapy, Diagnosis, Surgery* (eds R.K. Scher & C.R. Daniel), pp 202–213. Saunders Company, Philadelphia.

Richert, B. & André, J. (1999) Latero-subungual giant cell tumor of the tendon sheath: an unusual location *Journal of the American Academy of Dermatology* **41**, 347–348.

Schwartz, R.A. & Southwick, G.J. (1979) Solitary multinodular giant cell tumor of tendon sheath. *Journal of Surgery and Oncology* **12**, 191–197.

Wright, C.J.E. (1951) Benign giant-cell synovioma. An investigation of 85 cases. *British Journal of Surgery* **38**, 257–271.

## Lipomatous and myxomatous tumours

### Lipoma

Stein (1959) described a lipoma of the distal phalanx of the thumb causing a tender and painful swelling and destruction of the distal bony phalanx. We have seen a lipoma (Baran 1984) located in the lateral nail fold of a finger. The tumour underwent slow growth (Fig. 11.129). Histologically it resembled *naevus lipomatodes superficialis*. A subungual lipoma was seen in the right thumb of a 73-year-old women. Interestingly, there was a squamous cell carcinoma of the nail bed overlying this lipoma (Failla 1996).

A subungual lipoma of the ring finger (Higashi 1988) deformed the nail which became hemispherical with ridging and loss of lustre. The tumour mimicked a fibroma.

*Lipoma is easily recognized on MR images as a mass with a very intense signal on T1-weighted images. The signal is cancelled with a fat-suppression presaturation.*

### References

Baran, R. (1984) Periungual lipoma, an unusual site. *Journal of Dermatologic Surgery and Oncology* **10**, 32–33.

Failla, J.M. (1996) Subungual lipoma, squamous carcinoma of the nail bed, and secondary chronic infection. *Journal of Hand Surgery* **21A**, 512–514.

Higashi, N. (1988) Subungual lipoma. *Hifu* **30**, 447–448.

Stein, A.H. (1959) Benign neoplastic and nonneoplastic destructive lesions in the long bones of the hand. *Surgery, Gynecology and Obstetrics* **109**, 189–197.

### Myxoma

Eisenklam (1931) described a pea-sized subungual myxoma elevating the nail of the great toe of a 65-year-old woman.

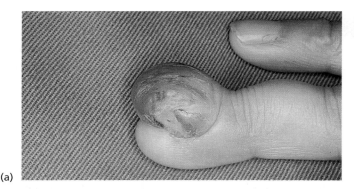

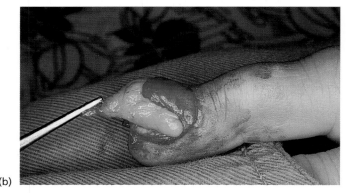

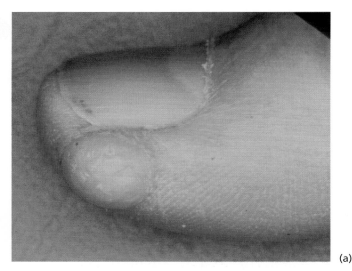

(a)

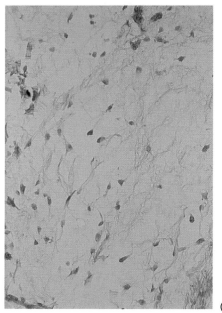

(a)

(b)

**Fig. 11.129** (a) Lipoma. (Courtesy of N. Higashi, Japan.) (b) Appearance of the tumour at operation.

**Fig. 11.130** (a) Myxoma of the lateral nail fold. (Courtesy of J. Martel, France.) (b) Myxoma—histological appearance.

Subsequently Sanusi (1982) reported a case presenting with a growth at the tip of his right thumb; this gradually increased in size raising and distorting the nail. X-ray examination showed an osteolytic lesion surrounded by sclerotic edges. Myxoma in a subungual position differs from the exceptional myxoma affecting the distal bony phalanx, which has only been described in the toe. A cylindrical deformity of the nail plate was secondary to nail matrix myxoma in Gourdin and Lang's case (1996). Another subungual myxoma of the left thumb was seen in a 59-year-old woman that had expanded and rounded the nail and fingertip. Magnetic resonance imaging showed a 15 mm oval subungual homogeneous, expansile lesion which was removed by a radial incision leaving a normal nail after 8 months (Rozmaryn & Schwartz 1998). A firm pea-sized tumour involving the distal portion of the lateral nail wall of the right thumb was observed by Donzel and Martel (1991) in a 58-year-old male with a normal bony phalanx (Fig. 11.130).

Carvajal *et al.* (1987) reported the case of a 43-year-old woman presenting with a slow growing subungual tumour of the left hallux lifting the nail and occupying all the subungual surface with mild pain on pressure. Biopsy of this greyish white myxoid tumour showed a small amount of spindle shaped cells and stellate cells in the dermis (Fig. 11.130b).

Armijo (1981) reported a case of a large myxoma of the dorsal aspect of the terminal segment of the middle finger allegedly developing 2 years after an injury. The patient presented with a pinkish-violet, somewhat translucent, firm tumour. It was widely excised and the defect covered with a full-thickness skin graft. Injection of methylene blue solution did not demonstrate a cystic space or communication with the joint.

Armijo (1981) listed the salient differences between cutaneous myxoma and myxoid cyst. The differential diagnosis includes a group of neoplasms in which myxomatous change is a prominent secondary feature and a variety of conditions characterized by mucinous degeneration of the skin or soft tissues (Sanusi 1982).

Marzano *et al.* (1997) observed large, cystic appearing tumours over the interphalangeal joints of both hands of a 40-year-old man with systemic sclerosis. A yellowish mucinous material could be aspirated but the lesions reappeared quickly.

# References

Armijo, M. (1981) Mucoid cysts of the fingers. *Journal of Dermatologic Surgery and Oncology* **7**, 317–322.

Carvajal, L., Uraga, E., Garcia, I. *et al.* (1987) Tumours of the hallux, myxoma, osteochondroma and enchondroma. *Skin Cancer* **2**, 197–201.

Donzel, J.P. & Martel, J. (1991) Myxome digital du pouce droit. *Nouvelle Dermatologie* **10**, 706–707.

Eisenklam, D. (1931) Über subunguale Tumoren. *Wiener Klinische Wochenschrift* **44**, 1192–1193.

Gourdin, I.W. & Lang, P.G. (1996) Cylindrical deformity of the nail plate secondary to subungual myxoma. *Journal of the American Academy of Dermatology* **35**, 846–848.

Marzano, A.V., Berti, E., Gasparini, G. *et al.* (1997) Unique digital skin lesions associated with systemic sclerosis. *British Journal of Dermatology* **136**, 598–600.

Rozmaryn, L.M. & Schwartz, M.A. (1998) Treatment of subungual myxoma preserving the nail matrix: a case report. *Journal of Hand Surgery* **23A**, 178–180.

Sanusi, D. (1982) Subungual myxoma. *Archives of Dermatology* **118**, 612–614.

# Sarcomas

Sarcomas arising in the finger tip are very rare. The disease has usually been present long before the diagnosis is made and the lesion treated; a very painful oozing growth sheds the nail plate or grows out from under the nail.

## Phalangeal sarcoma

Phalangeal sarcoma with osteolytic lesions may enlarge the distal phalanx to three times its normal size and present with a warm and extremely painful clinical appearance, similar to a paronychia (Marcove & Charosky 1972). A case of osteogenic sarcoma arising in the distal phalanx of the thumb of a dentist after chronic intermittent exposure to X-ray irradiation is unique (Carroll & Godwin 1956). Keratotic material progressed and gradually replaced two thirds of the nail bed.

Metastases to regional lymph nodes occurred very early. Therefore, excisional biopsy of the entire ulcerating lesion is the only effective treatment.

Due to its rarity, osteogenic sarcoma is not often considered in the differential diagnosis of phalangeal tumours. 'Florid reactive periostitis of the tubular bones of the hands and feet' (Spjut & Dorfman 1981), also called 'fibro-osseous pseudotumour of the digits' (Dupree & Enziger 1986; Chan *et al.* 1993), is a benign lesion which may simulate osteosarcoma. This reactive lesion of the digits occurs in the soft tissue of young adults, also in the distal phalanx and subungually (Chan *et al.* 1993). Enlargement of the distal phalanx and onycholysis may result from its insidious growth. Magnetic resonance imaging reveals a benign appearing mass with calcification (Moon *et al.* 1997). It may, microscopically, resemble myositis ossificans (Dupree & Enziger 1986). It is not clear whether 'bizarre parosteal

osteochondromatous proliferations of the tubular bones of hands and feet' are different from fibro-osseous pseudotumours. One case presenting as paronychia of the right thumb was described by Derrick *et al.* (1994).

## Epithelioid sarcoma

This sarcoma usually occurs in the soft tissues of young adults. It may arise from the synovia of the distal interphalangeal joint and cause 'diffuse swelling' (Zanolli *et al.* 1992) whereas others mimic hard ganglion cysts. This spreads to affect the dorsal aspect of the tip of the digit (Fig. 11.131a). A case was reported in a 12-year-old girl involving the distal left index finger as a tumoral lesion, which was ulcerated and painful (Tsoitis *et al.* 1996). Diagnosis is difficult and often delayed. Although the majority of the patients are otherwise asymptomatic, pain and tenderness is a complaint of some. An ulcerated tumour of the dorsum of the digit or its ventral aspect (Carloz *et al.* 1991) may recur in the stump and eventually metastasise to lymph nodes and lungs.

Histologically the individual cells usually display a marked eosinophilia and grow as nodular proliferations of plump, epithelial appearing cells blending with fusiform cells (Chase & Enzinger 1985) (Fig. 11.131b,c). The tumour usually has a strikingly granulomatous appearance with central necrosis. Immunohistochemistry is positive for vimentin and focally positive for cytokeratin and epithelial membrane antigen.

Differential diagnosis includes necrobiotic granuloma, giant cell tumour, malignant fibrous histiocytoma, squamous cell carcinoma, malignant melanoma, synovial sarcoma and epithelioid haemangioendothelioma.

## Xanthomatous giant cell sarcoma

Hartert (1913) described a case of xanthomatous giant cell sarcoma of the foot secondarily involving the fifth toe and its terminal phalanx.

## Glomangiosarcoma

See page 573.

## Epithelioid leiomyosarcoma

A 63-year-old man had a non traumatic avulsion of this right great toenail after a 3-week history of pain. Histopathological examination showed a neoplasm composed mainly of interlacing bundles of spindle cells with indistinct cell borders, eosinophilic cytoplasm and pleomorphic nuclei. Immunohistological stains were positive for desmin and muscle-specific actin, but negative for S-100, HMB 45, cytokeratin, carcinoembryonic and factor VIII-related antigens. The diagnosis was epitheloid leiomyosarcoma (Bryant 1992).

Microscopic differential diagnosis includes fibrosarcoma, malignant fibrous histiocytoma and leiomyosarcoma.

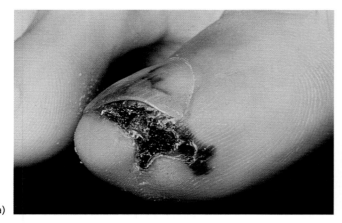

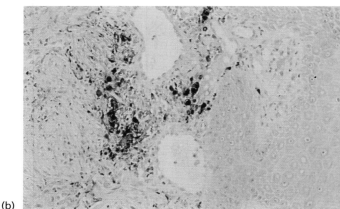

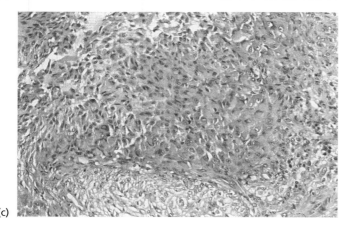

**Fig. 11.131** (a) Epithelioid sarcoma. (Courtesy of J. Revuz, Paris.) (b,c) Histological changes showing many eosinophilic cells of plump epithelial cells blending with fusiform cells.

## Fibrosarcoma

Fibrosarcoma usually arises superficially as a hard, fixed, painful tumour, but may present as a deep swelling, often reaching a large size with a tendency to invade the skin and neighbouring tissues. The tumour may grow slowly over a period of many years and then demonstrate rapid growth, or may be rapidly invasive from the start. Metastases to the lung and, less com-

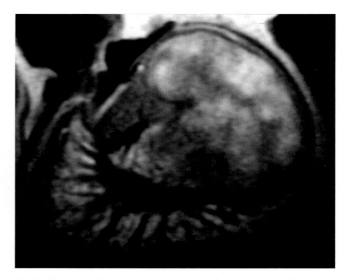

**Fig. 11.132** Grade 2 chondrosarcoma of the distal phalanx with invasion of the nail bed. Axial post-enhanced TI-weighted spin echo image.

monly, to regional nodes occur early. Amputation offers the best chance for cure (Butler *et al*. 1960).

## Chondrosarcoma

In chondrosarcoma, pain and swelling are common symptoms (Gargan *et al*. 1984). In contrast, patients with benign cartilaginous tumours of these bones rarely have pain unless pathologic fracture has occurred (Dahlin & Salvador 1974).

Radiologically a chondrosarcoma is a large and well-defined lesion with expanded bone contours and endosteal scalloping. Cortical destruction and extraosseous extension with tiny calcifications in clusters are indicative of active and more aggressive lesions (Bellinghausen *et al*. 1983).

*On early radiographs, these patterns may be subtle and the diagnosis is difficult. MRI is helpful and shows abnormal patterns for a simple enchondroma. The extension to the nail bed may be large with lifting of the nail plate. Some areas show a typical signal behaviour of hyaline cartilage, but other areas present an unusual mottled enhancement (Fig. 11.132).*

Although the incidence of malignant transformation of a solitary enchondroma is less than 1%, it may be as high at 50% in Ollier's disease and 18% in Maffucci's syndrome. The risk of malignant changes in the multiple exostoses syndrome varies from 1 to 25% but there is no report of malignancy in the distal phalanx.

A combination of squamous cell carcinoma and chondrosarcoma, the *carcinosarcoma*, has been reported as a painful exophytic mass on the tip of the middle finger of the right hand, involving the distal part of the nail bed (Lee *et al*. 1998).

## Haemangiosarcoma (haemangioendothelioma)

This malignant tumour of blood vessels is quite rare. The size of the tumour ranges from that of a pea to that of a plum. It is dark or bluish red, moderately soft and non tender. Davies *et al.* (1990) reported on a cutaneous haemangioendothelioma developed on a toe nail bed of a patient who had worked with polyvinyl chloride (Fig. 11.133a). Histology showed plump cells in a loose connective tissue stroma (Fig. 11.133b,c). Some were clumped; others formed capillary-sized channels with open lumina. Cellular pleomorphism and bizarre mitotic figures were marked and reticulin fibers were frequent.

### Epithelioid angiosarcoma

Epithelioid angiosarcoma developed in an arterio-venous fistula of a 61-year-old man who had undergone haemodialysis and eventually received a kidney transplant and was treated with azathioprine, cyclosporin and prednisolone. Apart from small nodules on other finger tips, violaceous red swelling appeared under and around his right thumb that necrotized within 15 days. Histopathology revealed a proliferation of epithelioid tumour cells with large nuclei, obvious nucleoli and abundant eosinophilic cytoplasm. The tumour showed multiple vascular spaces lined with a proliferating endothelium. Despite amputation of the arm, he finally died from lung metastasis (Bessis *et al.* 1995).

### Ewing's sarcoma

When the bone is primarily involved, it is designated as Ewing's sarcoma (Dick *et al.* 1971). This presents with a painless swelling with ulceration of the tip of the digit. Radiographs reveal a lytic lesion of the distal phalanx. Biopsy is the key of the diagnosis. Radical resection is the treatment of choice.

### References

Bellinghausen, H.W., Weeks, P.M., Young, L.V. *et al.* (1983) Roentgen Rounds 64. Chondrosarcoma. *Orthopedic Reviews* **XII**, 97–100.

Bessis, D., Sotto, A., Chabrier, P.-E. *et al.* (1995) Angiosarcome épithélioïde survenant sur fistule artério-veineuse chez un hémodialysé: implication de l'endothéline. *Annales de Dermatologie et de Vénéréologie* **122** (Suppl. 1), S144–S145.

Bryant, J. (1992) Subungual epithelioid leiomyosarcoma. *Southern Medical Journal* **85**, 560–561.

Butler, E.D., Hamil, J.P., Seipel, R.S. *et al.* (1960) Tumors of the hand. A ten-year survey and report of 437 cases. *American Journal of Surgery* **100**, 293–302.

Carloz, B., Bioulac, P., Gavard, J. *et al.* (1991) Recidives multiples d'un sarcome épithélioïde. *Annales de Dermatologie et de Vénéréologie* **118**, 623–628.

Carroll, R.E. & Godwin, J.T. (1956) Osteogenic sarcoma of phalanx after chronic Roentgen-ray irradiation. *Cancer* **9**, 753–755.

Chan, K.W., Khoo, U.S. & Ho, C.M. (1993) Fibro-osseous pseudotumor of the digits: report of a case with immunohistochemical and ultrastructural studies. *Pathology* **25**, 193–196.

Chase, D.R. & Enzinger, F.M. (1985) Epithelioid sarcoma. *American Journal of Surgery and Pathology* **9**, 241–263.

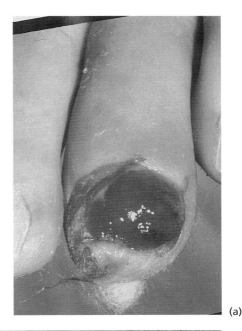
(a)

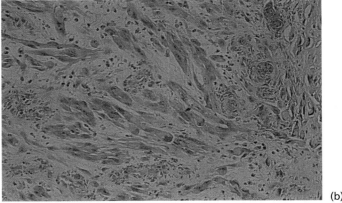
(b)

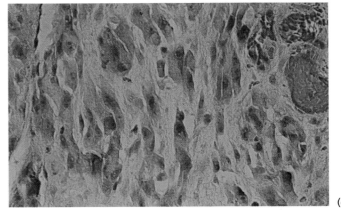
(c)

**Fig. 11.133** (a) Haemangioendothelioma. (b,c) Histological changes of (a).

Dahlin, D.C. & Salvador, A.H. (1974) Chondrosarcomas of the bones of the hands and feet. A study of 30 cases. *Cancer* **34**, 755–760.

Davies, M.F.P., Curtis, M. & Howat, J.M.T. (1990) Cutaneous haemangioendothelioma, possible link with chronic exposure to vinyl chloride. *British Journal of Industrial Medicine* **47**, 65–67.

Derrick, E.K., Darley, C.R. & Tanner, B. (1994) Bizarre parosteal osteochondromatous proliferations of the tubular bones of the hands and feet. *Clinical and Experimental Dermatology* **19**, 53–55.

Dick, H.M., Francis, K.C. & Johnston, A.D. (1971) Ewing's sarcoma of the hand. *Journal of Bone and Joint Surgery* **53A**, 345–348.

Dupree, W.B. & Enziger, F.M. (1986) Fibro-osseous pseudotumour of the digits. *Cancer* **58**, 2103–2109.

Gargan, T.J., Kanter, W. & Wolfort, F.G. (1984) Multiple chondrosarcomas of the hand. *Annals of Plastic Surgery* **12**, 542–546.

Hartert, W. (1913) Zur Kenntnis der pigmentierten riesenzellenhaltigen Xanthosarcome an Hand und Fuss. *Beiträge der Klinische Chirurgie* **84**, 546–562.

Lee, E.K., Yoon, D.H., Tim, T.Y. *et al.* (1998) Carcinosarcoma of the skin. A new combination of squamous cell carcinoma and chondrosarcoma. *Annals of Dermatology* **10**, 81–85.

Marcove, R.C. & Charosky, C.B. (1972) Phalangeal sarcomas simulating infections of the digits. *Clinical Orthopedics and Related Research* **83**, 224–231.

Moon, S.E., Kim, J.A. & Park, B.S. (1997) Subungual fibro-osseous pseudotumor. *Acta Dermato-Venereologica* **77**, 247–248.

Spjut, J.H. & Dorfman, H.D. (1981) Florid reactive periostitis of the tubular bones of the hands and feet. *American Journal of Surgery Pathology* **5**, 423–433.

Tsoitis, G., Asvesti, Z., Papadimitriou, C. *et al.* (1996) Epithelioid sarcoma. Abstract 86. In: *European Society of Pediatric Dermatology, Rotterdam, Book of Abstracts*, p. 133.

Zanolli, M.D., Wilmoth, G., Show, J.A. *et al.* (1992) Epithelioid sarcoma, clinical and histologic characteristics. *Journal of the American Academy of Dermatology* **26**, 302–305.

## Pseudotumours

### Myxoid pseudocysts of the digits

*This common deformity of the nail bed is due to distal interphalangeal joint ganglions, which have been called clear cysts, mucus cysts, myxoid cysts and other names (Moss et al. 1985; Zaias 1990) Kleinert et al. (1972) reported a communication between these cysts and the joint and proposed that they were ganglions rather than a local soft tissue degeneration. He found that most occurred at an osteoarthritic spur on the DIP joint, which allowed egress of joint fluids filling and expanding the cystic structure.*

*Pressure on the germinal matrix may cause a deformed nail. When the cystic expansion of the ganglion is between the dorsal skin and nail fold the pressure causes a groove in the nail. If the cyst forms between the periosteum and the germinal matrix it will cause disruption of the nail (Fig. 11.134). The treatment is debridement of the joint to remove the connection between the cyst and the osteophyte (Brown et al. 1991). It is not necessary*

*to remove the cyst, but only puncture and drain it. Ninety per cent of nails return to normal with this treatment and without recurrence (Gingrass et al. 1995).*

*Ganglions sometimes rupture and drain via the nail fold. I recommend no operative procedure until the drainage has stopped and the ganglion sealed. Proximal migration of bacteria through the cyst and into the joint may cause joint contamination and infection.*

Whereas some authors regard it as a synovial cyst, some others believe it to be a degenerative lesion. Quite often, true myxomatous areas are seen in the vicinity of cystic appearing cavities so that the different aspects may be manifest as the lesion ages (de Berker 1995): fresh lesions are myxomatous, mature lesions cystic.

Myxoid pseudocysts occur more often in women. They are typically found in the proximal nail fold of the fingers and rarely on toes; middle, index fingers and thumb are most frequently affected. Location of the tumour at the corner of the cul-de-sac following subungual haematoma (Higashi 1992) is exceptional. Subungual myxoid cysts result in increased transverse curvature of the nail. This takes the form of a pincer nail if the cyst is central, or lateral ingrowing if the cyst lies eccentrically (de Berker & Baran 1999). The colour of the lunula is red or blue, and only rarely is it normal. Those occurring above the matrix are usually asymptomatic varying from soft to firm, cystic to fluctuant, and may be dimpled, dome-shaped or smooth-surfaced (Figs 11.135a & 11.136). Transillumination confirms their cystic nature. They are always located to one side of the midline and rarely exceed 10 to 15 mm in diameter. The skin over the lesion is often thinned and may be verrucous or may even ulcerate. Rarely a paronychial fistula may develop beneath the proximal nail fold (Fig. 11.137) and exceptionally under the nail plate. Longitudinal grooving, which is often very marked, results from pressure on the matrix (Fig. 11.135b). Manipulation with a needle will release a thick, clear, gelatinous fluid (Fig. 11.138). This decompresses the matrix and nail growth is normal until the cyst refills. Purulent drainage due to infection and development of septic arthritis of the distal interphalangeal joint has been reported (Rangarathnam & Linscheid 1984).

Spontaneous rupture and release of the content into the cul-de sac beneath the proximal nail fold is frequent and can be seen as dried material emerging in the longitudinal groove from under the cuticle. Irregular wash-board grooving is the result of multiple ruptures with release of pressure from the matrix. Subungual digital mucinous pseudocyst may produce a nail dystrophy (Fig. 11.139) and livid-blue discoloration without abnormalities of the periungual skin (Westrom & Finlay 1986); often there is a marked acquired overcurvature of the affected nail (Goettmann *et al.* 1996; Karte *et al.* 1996). Degenerative, 'wear and tear' osteoarthritis, frequently with Herberden's nodes, is present in almost all cases (Götz & Koch 1956; Brown *et al.* 1991; Kasdan *et al.* 1994; Gingrass *et al.* 1995; Fritz *et al.* 1997).

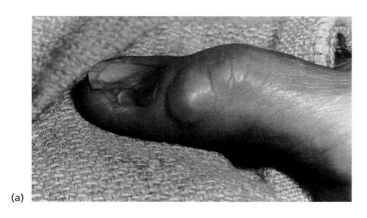

(a)

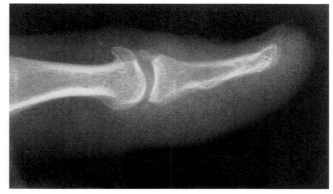

(b)

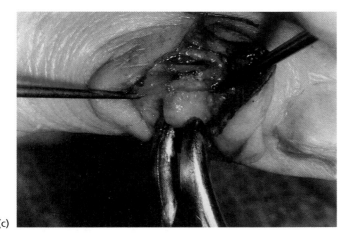

(c)

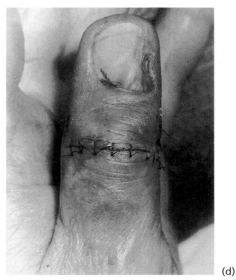

(d)

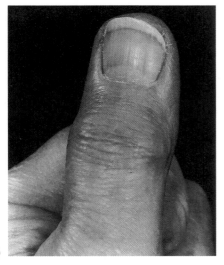

(e)

**Fig. 11.134** (a) A ganglion of the DIP joint causing significant nail deformity. (b) X-ray of the joint showing osteophyte formation. (c) Debridement of the osteophyte through a dorsal incision. (d) The incision closed and the ganglion drained. (e) The patient's nail 1 year later. © E. Zook.

*MR imaging is not necessary for the diagnosis in most cases. Our MR findings are based on a review of 23 MRI of mucoid cysts (Drapé et al. 1996). Most of the cysts are solitary and located on the proximal nail fold. Their appearance is specific* *with thin regular walls, a low signal on T1-weighted images, very high signal on T2-weighted images. Intracystic septa are best seen on T2-weighted images in 39% of cases (Fig. 11.140). The injection of gadolinium shows an early faint peripheral enhancement. With time, the enhancement moves toward the center of the cyst. MRI is able to highlight satellite cysts or sagging multiloculated cysts. These later forms may be difficult to detect clinically, unless a typical story of swelling and discharge of a thick fluid from the proximal nail fold is found. In these infrequent forms (22%) we could not detect a connection with the distal interphalangeal joint. These cysts may develop independently from the underlying joint and result from in situ metaplasia. This process may be compared to the cutaneous myxomas with a focal storage of mucoid material in the dermis.*

*A peduncle connecting the cyst and the distal interphalangeal joint is visible in most cases with MRI (82% of cases). In all cases, the peduncle is lateral, beneath the insertion of the extensor digitorum tendon on the base of the distal phalanx (Fig. 11.141). The cysts may be compared to synovial cysts. When the surgical decision is made, the peduncle must be detected and tied up or removed in order to avoid the frequent recurrences.*

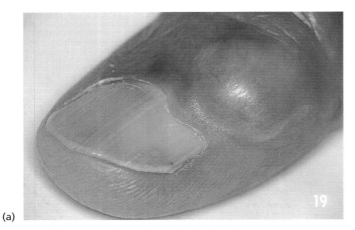

(a)

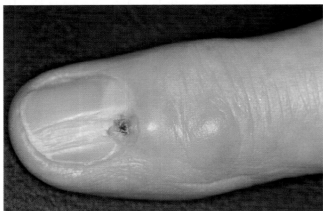

(b)

**Fig. 11.135** (a) Myxoid pseudocyst with large depression. (b) Double myxoid pseudocyst—nail plate gutter sign.

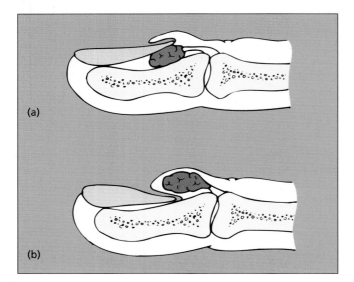

(a)

(b)

**Fig. 11.136** Myxoid pseudocyst, showing types of attachment to the distal interphalangeal joint. (After E. Zook.)

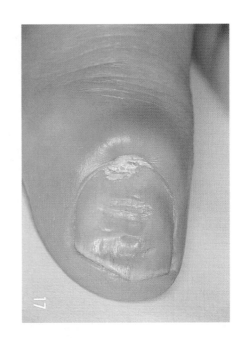

**Fig. 11.137** Myxoid pseudocyst—mimicking chronic paronychia.

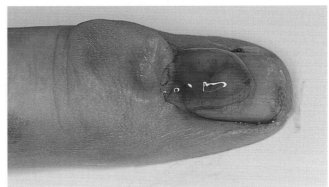

**Fig. 11.138** Myxoid pseudocyst—gelatinous contents exuded after pricking the lesion.

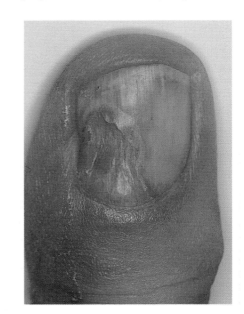

**Fig. 11.139** Myxoid pseudocyst located beneath the nail matrix producing onychodystrophy.

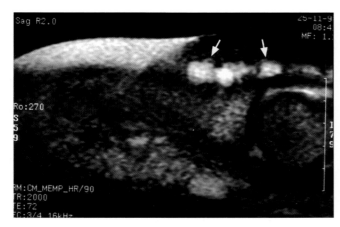

**Fig. 11.140** Myxoid pseudocyst of the posterior nail fold (arrows). Sagittal T2-weighted spin echo image.

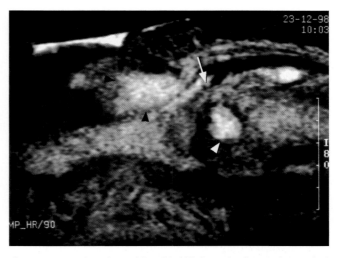

**Fig. 11.142** Myxoid pseudocyst of the nail bed (black arrowhead). Sagittal T2-weighted spin echo image. Note the dorsal osteophyte (arrow) at the insertion of the extensor tendon. Severe osteoarthritis of the distal interphalangeal joint with a bone cyst of the head of the middle phalanx (white arrowhead).

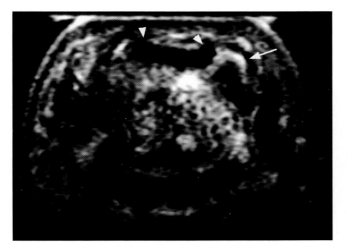

**Fig. 11.141** Myxoid pseudocyst of the posterior nail fold. Axial T2-weighted spin echo image. Note the peduncle (arrow) beneath the distal insertion of the extensor tendon (arrowhead).

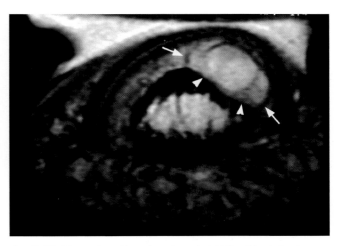

**Fig. 11.143** Subungual myxoid pseudocyst (arrows). Axial T2-weighted spin echo image. Note the bone erosion of the cortex of the distal phalanx (arrowheads) and the intracystic septa.

*An osteoarthritis of the distal interphalangeal joint is noted in 70% of cases on radiographs (Drapé et al. 1996). A dorsal osteophytosis of the head of the middle phalanx may injure the insertion of the extensor digitorum tendon (Fig. 11.142). All these cases present a mucoid cyst with a peduncle. The dorsal osteophyte must be removed at the same time as the cyst and the peduncle in order to avoid a recurrence. A thickening and an enhancement of the synovium of the distal interphalangeal joint is depicted in half of cases. This hyperplasia of the synovium associated with the osteophytes may contribute to the Heberden's nodes (Sonnex 1986).*

*Mucoid cysts extend into in the nail bed in 30% of cases (Drapé et al. 1996). This location is poorly known, and rarely mentioned in the literature. High-resolution MR imaging alone is able to detect this type of cyst. Symptoms may mislead to the diagnosis of a glomus tumour when the cyst is painful. When the cyst is large, an erosion of the cortex of the underlying*

*phalanx may occur in the confined space of the nail bed. The cyst is in the dermis beneath the nail matrix, close to the distal interphalangeal joint (Fig. 11.143). The matrix compression may induce a fissure of the nail plate with a claw deformity (Fig. 11.144). Most often, the cyst is bilobed with a component in the proximal nail fold and more rarely in the pulp, associated with the nail bed component. The submatrical extension may be clinically occult and responsible for recurrence. The detection of a peduncle is crucial, since its resection may be enough to collapse the cyst and avoid a direct access to the matrix.*

Histopathology reveals the pseudocystic character (Fig. 11.145). The structure is essentially myxomatous with inter-

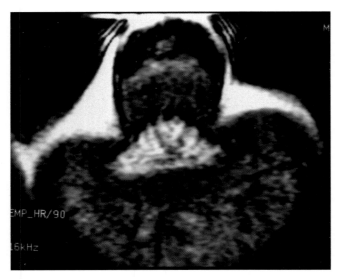

**Fig. 11.144** Subungual myxoid pseudocyst with a claw deformity of the nail plate. Axial T1-weighted spin echo image.

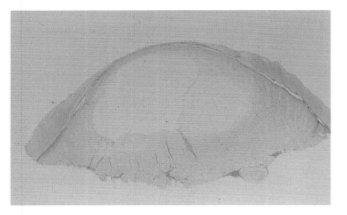

**Fig. 11.145** Myxoid pseudocyst—showing the gross microscopic appearance.

spersed fibroblasts. Areas of myxomatous degeneration may merge to form a multilocular pseudocyst. In the cavities, a jelly-like substance is found which stains positively for hyaluronic acid. Cavities without synovial lining are located in an ill-defined fibrous capsule. Goldman *et al.* (1977) found a mesothelial-like lining only in the stalk connecting the pseudocyst with the distal interphalangeal joint. Electron microscopy does not show a synovial lining of the pseudocyst but myofibroblasts which are also abundant in the mucopolysaccharide-like stroma. Immuno-histochemically, these cells mainly stain for vimentin, but some are faintly desmin positive (Haneke 1986).

A multitude of treatments have been recommended, including repeated incision and drainage, simple excision, multiple needlings and expression of contents (Epstein 1979), electro-cautery, chemical cautery with nitric acid, trichloracetic acid or phenol, massages or injection of proteolytic substances,

hyaluronidase, steroids (flurandrenolone tape) (Ronchese 1974) or injections, freezing with liquid nitrogen, carbon dioxide laser vaporization (Huerter *et al.* 1987; Karrer *et al.* 1999), infra-red coagulation (Kemmert & Colvert 1994) radical excision and even amputation (cit. Kleinert *et al.* 1972). X-ray treatment is obsolete. Tomoda *et al.* (1982) reported a case that had had more than 20 recurrences each treated by incision, the cyst eventually moving from the characteristic dorsal to a sub-ungual position, producing a defect in the nail plate.

Sonnex *et al.* (1982) used liquid nitrogen cryosurgery with an 86% cure rate. The field treated included the cyst and the adjacent proximal area to the transverse skin creases overlying the terminal joint. Two freeze/thaw cycles were carried out, each freeze time being 30 s after the ice field had formed, the intervening thaw times being at least 4 min; if this method is adopted then longer freeze times must be avoided or permanent matrix damage may occur. Böhler-Sommeregger and Kutschera-Hienert reported a success rate of 89%. Salasche (1984) suggested nail fold excision for distal lesions of the posterior nail fold. The injection of a sclerosing agent, such as 1% sodium tetradecyl sulphate (Sotradecol*) into mucoid pseudocysts may well have superseded the previous treatments (Audebert 1989). After the cyst has been pierced and its jelly-like material expressed 0.10–0.20 mL is injected, painlessly. One single proced-ure may be enough. A second or a third one can be performed at 1 month interval.

Kleinert *et al.* (1972) recommend the careful extirpation of the lesion. A tiny drop of methylene blue solution, mixed with fresh hydrogen peroxide, is injected into the distal inter-phalangeal joint at the volar joint crease. The joint will accept only 0.1–0.2 mL of dye (Newmeyer *et al.* 1974). This clearly identifies the pedicle connecting the joint to the cyst and the cyst itself which may look like a subcutaneous teno-arthro-synovial 'hernia' (Armijo 1981). This procedure sometimes also reveals occult satellite cysts. The incision line is drawn on the finger including a portion of the skin directly over the cyst and continu-ing proximally in a gentle curve to end dorsally over the joint (Fig. 11.146). The lesion is meticulously dissected from the sur-rounding soft tissue and the pedicle traced to the joint capsule and resected. Dumb-bell extension of cysts to each side of the extensor tendon is easily dissected by hyperextending the joint. Osteophytic spurs adjacent to the joint must be removed with a fine chisel or bone rongeur. We have treated more than 50 cases using this technique, and have only seen one recurrence (Haneke 1988). More recently, the importance of removing the osteophytes was stressed (Brown *et al.* 1991; Kasdan *et al.* 1994; Gingrass *et al.* 1995), identical success rates were found with osteophytectomy with and without removal of the cystic lesion. Nail deformities resolved in more than two thirds of the cases. Complications following resection of myxoid pseudo-cysts are mainly joint stiffness, loss of residual motion, persist-ent swelling, pain, deviation of the distal interphalangeal joint, and infection (Fritz *et al.* 1997).

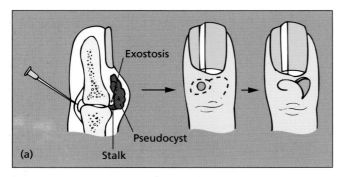

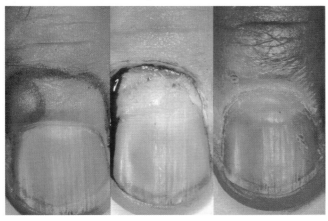

**Fig. 11.146** (a) Myxoid pseudocyst—one method of removal. (b) Crescent removal of pseudocyst located in the distal portion of the proximal nail fold.

## References

Armijo, M. (1981) Mucoid cysts of the fingers. *Journal of Dermatologic Surgery and Oncology* 7, 317–322.

Audebert, C. (1989) Treatment of mucoid cysts of fingers and toes by injection of sclerosant. *Dermatologic Clinics* 7, 179–182.

Brown, R.E., Zook, E.G., Russell, R.C. *et al.* (1991) Fingernail deformities secondary to ganglions of the distal interphalangeal joint (mucous cysts). *Plastic and Reconstructive Surgery* 87, 718–725.

de Berker, D. (1995) Treatment of myxoid cysts. *Journal of Dermatologic Treatment* 6, 55–57.

de Berker, D.A.R. & Baran, R. (1999) Clinical features of subungual myxoid cysts. *British Journal of Dermatology* 141 (Suppl. 55), 111–112.

Drapé, J.L., Idy-Peretti, I., Goettmann, S. *et al.* (1996) MR imaging of digital mucoid cysts. *Radiology* 200, 531–536.

Epstein, E. (1979) A simple technique for managing digital mucous cysts. *Archives of Dermatology* 115, 1315–1316.

Fritz, R.G., Stern, P.J. & Dickey, M. (1997) Complications following mucous cyst excision. *Journal of Hand Surgery* 22B, 222–225.

Gingrass, M.K., Brown, R.E. & Zook, E.G. (1995) Treatment of fingernail deformities secondary to ganglions of the distal interphalangeal joint. *Journal of Hand Surgery* 20A, 502–505.

Goettmann, S., Drapé, J.L. & Bélaïch, S. (1996) Pseudo-kystes mucoïdes sous-ungéaux. Intérêt diagnostic de l'IRM. *Annales de Dermatologie et de Vénéréologie* 123 (Suppl. 1), S165.

Goldman, J.A., Goldman, L., Jaffe, M.S. & Richfield, D.F. (1977) Digital mucinous pseudocysts. *Arthritis and Rheumarism* 20, 997–1002.

Götz, H. & Koch, R. (1956) Zur Klinik, Pathogenese und Therapie der sogenannten 'Dorsalzysten'. *Hautarzt* 7, 533–537.

Haneke, E. (1986) Dorsal finger cyst. In: *Society of Cutaneous Ultrastructure Research and European Society of Comparative Skin Biology (Joint meeting) Paris, May 28–31, Book of Abstracts*, p. 43.

Haneke, E. (1988) Operative Therapie der myxoiden Pseudozyste. In: *Fortschritte des operativen Dermatologie*. Vol. 4. *Gegenwärtiger Stand der operativen Dermatologie* (ed E. Haneke). Springer Verlag, Berlin.

Higashi, N. (1992) A case of myxoid cyst. *Hifu* 34, 315–319.

Huerter, C.J., Wheeland, R.G., Bailin, P. *et al.* (1987) Treatment of digital myxoid cysts with carbon dioxide laser vaporisation. *Journal of Dermatologic Surgery and Oncology* 13, 723–727.

Karrer, S., Hohenleutner, U., Szeimies, R.M. *et al.* (1999) Treatment of digital mucous cysts with a carbon dioxide laser. *Acta Dermato-Venereologica* 79, 224–225.

Karte, K., Bocker, T. & Wollina, U. (1996) Acquired clubbing of the great toenail. *Archives of Dermatology* 132, 223–228.

Kasdan, M.L., Stallings, S.P., Leis, V.M. & Wolens, D. (1994) Outcome of surgically treated mucous cysts of the hand. *Journal of Hand Surgery* 19A, 504–507.

Kemmert, D. & Colver, G.B. (1994) Myxoid cysts treated by infrared coagulation. *Clinical and Experimental Dermatology* 19, 118–120.

Kleinert, H.E., Kutz, J.E., Fishman, J.H. & McCraw, L.H. (1972) Etiology and treatment of the so-called mucous cyst of the finger. *Journal of Bone and Joint Surgery* 54A, 1455–1458.

Moss, S.H., Schwartz, K.S., von Drasek-Ascher, G. *et al.* (1985) Digital venous anatomy. *Journal of Hand Surgery* 10A, 473–482.

Newmeyer, W.L., Kilgore, E.S. & Graham, W.P. (1974) Mucous cyst, the dorsal distal interphalangeal joint ganglion. *Plastic and Reconstructive Surgery* 53, 313–315.

Rangarathnam, C.S. & Linscheid, R.L. (1984) Infected mucous cyst of the finger. *Journal of Hand Surgery* 9a, 245–246.

Ronchese, F. (1974) Treatment of myxoid cyst with flurandrenolone tape. *Rhode Island Medical Journal* 57, 154–155.

Salasche, S.J. (1984) Myxoid cyst of the proximal nail fold, a surgical approach. *Journal of Dermatologic Surgery and Oncology* 10, 35–39.

Sonnex, T.S. (1986) Digital myxoid cysts: a review. *Cutis* 37, 89–94.

Sonnex, T.S., Leonard, J., Ralfs, I. & Dawber, R.P.R. (1982) Myxoid cysts of the finger, treatment by liquid nitrogen spray cryosurgery. *British Journal of Dermatology* 107 (Suppl.), 21.

Tan, C.Y., Marks, R. & Payne, P. (1981) Comparison of xeroradiographic and ultrasound detection of corticosteroid induced dermal thinning. *Journal of Investigative Dermatology* 76, 126–128.

Tomoda, T., Ono, T., Ohyama, K. & Kojo, Y. (1982) Subungual myxoid cysts producing an ulcer in the nail plate. *Japanese (Rinsho) Dermatology* 9, 451.

Westrom, D.R. & Findlay, R.F. (1986) Subungual mucinous pseudocyst. *Journal of Dermatologic Surgery and Oncology* 12, 558–559.

Zook, E.G., Van Beek, A.L., Russell, R.C. *et al.* (1980) Anatomy and physiology of the perionychium: a review of the literature and anatomic study. *Journal of Hand Surgery* 5, 528–536.

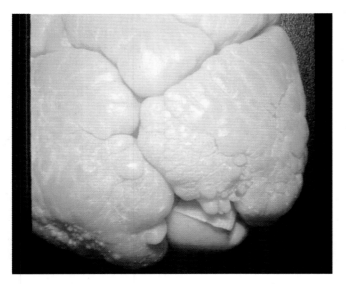

**Fig. 11.147** Severe 'pretibial myxoedema' hiding the nails. (Courtesy of P. Lazar, USA.)

## Pretibial myxoedema

The pink or fleshed coloured mucinous plaques may involve the dorsal aspect of the foot and exceptionally the toes partially hiding the nails (Fig. 11.147).

## Primary osteoma cutis

The following three types of calcinosis cutis are usually recognized: (i) idiopathic calcinosis cutis, which is a primary calcinosis, occurs in apparently normal cutaneous tissue when normal calcium and phosphorus serum levels are present; (ii) metastatic calcinosis cutis, a secondary calcinosis that occurs in the presence of abnormalities in the calcium/phosphorus metabolism or serum levels; and (iii) dystrophic calcinosis cutis, a secondary calcinosis that occurs in damaged cutaneous tissues in the absence of abnormalities in the calcium/phosphorus metabolism or serum levels. Cambiaghi *et al.* (2000) reported a case of a baby showing periodic transepidermal elimination of calcified nodules from her fingertips.

Burgdorf and Nasemann (1977) used the term 'primary osteoma' of the distal extremities to identify osteomas in six patients presenting with firm nail bed tumours in five toes and one finger. Bone alone was found in four cases and ossifying cartilage in two.

Blatière *et al.* (1999) reported on a 16-year-old girl presenting with a longitudinal haemorrhagic streak associated with distal splitting of her left 3rd finger nail (Fig. 11.148a). Histology of the tiny tumour found within the nail matrix revealed an osteoma cutis (Fig. 11.148b).

## References

Blatière, V., Baran, R. & Barneon, G. (1999) An osteoma cutis of the

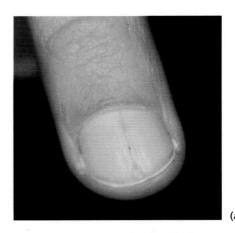

(a)

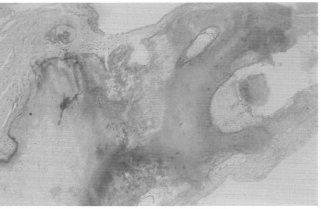

(b)

**Fig. 11.148** (a) Primary osteoma cutis in the nail matrix. (b) Histological changes of case shown in (a).

nail matrix. *Journal of the European Academy of Dermatology and Venereology* **12** (Suppl. 2 S), 126.

Burgdorf, W. & Nasemann, T. (1977) Cutaneous osteomas. A clinical and histopathologic review. *Archives of Dermatological Research* **260**, 121–135.

Cambiaghi, S., Imondi, D., Gangi, S. *et al.* (2000) Fingertip calcinosis cutis. *Cutis* **66**, 465–467.

## Subungual calcifications

Primary subungual calcifications in the normal nail bed of the digits are occasionally seen in the elderly, especially women (Fischer 1982) (Fig. 11.149). The frequency decreases from the 2nd to the 5th digit. In about 10% of cases the subungual calcifications of the fingers are combined with subungual calcifications of the toes (Fischer 1983a). Soft tissue calcification at the margin of the distal phalanges of the fingers occurs in 7% of normal adults (Fischer 1983b). In the normal toenail bed they begin in women during their thirties and reach an incidence of 47% in their eighties. These calcifications appear in men two decades later and obtain an incidence of only 4% in old age. The 1st toe is involved three times as often as the 5th toe (Fischer 1984). Secondary subungual calcification occurs

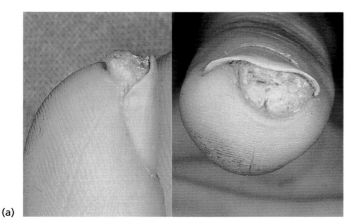

(a)

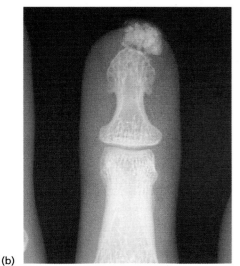

(b)

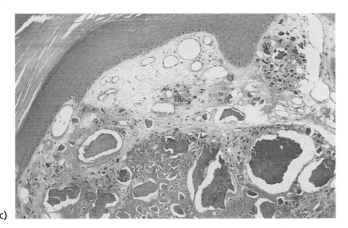

(c)

**Fig. 11.149** (a) Subungual calcification of the distal nail bed and the hyponychium. (Courtesy of C. Beylot, France.) (b) X-ray revealing calcifications in case shown in (a). (c) Calcification involving sequelae of haemangioma case shown in (a). (Courtesy of C. Perrin, France.)

occasionally after trauma and in psoriasis (Fischer 1982). The soft tissue calcification at the margin of the tuberosity of the distal phalanx of fingers results from mechanical injury of the collagen fibres close to their insertion into the bone (Fischer 1983).

## References

Fischer, E. (1982) Subunguale Verkalkungen. *Fortschritte der Röntgentherapie* 137, 580–584.

Fischer, E. (1983a) Subunguale Verkalkungen im normalen Nagelbett der Finger. *Hautarzt* 34, 625–627.

Fischer, E. (1983b) Weichteilverkalkungen am Rand der Tuberositas phalangis distalis der Finger. *Fortschritte der Röntgentherapie* 139, 150–157.

Fischer, E. (1984) Subunguale Verkalkungen im normalen Nagelbett der Zehen. *Radiologie* 24, 31–34.

## Cutaneous calculi

Winer (1952) first recognized 'solitary congenital nodular calcification of the skin' as a distinct entity. This rare condition presents from birth as slowly enlarging hard yellowish-white warty nodules at the side of a finger or a toenail (Fig. 11.150). In fact they are not always solitary and frequently not congenital (Woods and Kellaway 1963). The distal aspect of the involved digit may appear erythematous, with a solid chalky white, well circumscribed lesion, not tender to palpation. Radiographs demonstrate a radiopaque mass, consisting of multiple calcified fragments located adjacent to the distal phalanx (Mendoza *et al.* 1990) in a subepidermal location. Cutaneous calculi may be difficult to separate from calcinosis circumscripta.

## References

Mendoza, L.E., Lavery, L.A. & Adam, R.C. (1990). Calcinosis cutis circumscripta. A literature review and case report. *Journal of the American Podiatric Medical Association* 80, 97–99.

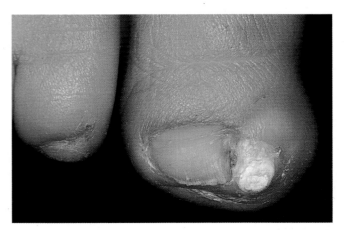

**Fig. 11.150** Congenital calcification involving lateral nail fold of the toe. (Courtesy of P. Souteyrand, France.)

Winer, L.H. (1952) Solitary congenital nodular calcification of the skin. *Archives of Dermatology and Syphilis* **66**, 204–211.

Woods, B. & Kellaway, T.B. (1963) Cutaneous calculi. *British Journal of Dermatology* **75**, 1–11.

## Oxalate granuloma

Several pink, lightly keratotic, tender subungual nodules affecting two digits combined with multiple tiny tender, yellow-tan papules on several fingertips were reported in a 46-year-old white man with chronic renal failure treated by haemodialysis for 20 years (Fig. 11.151a). Biopsy specimen of a subungual nodule showed a corymbus arrangement of calcium oxalate crystals surrounded by foreign body granulomas in the dermis (Sina & Lutz 1990) (Fig. 11.151b,c).

### Reference

Sina, B. & Lutz, L.L. (1990) Cutaneous oxalate granuloma. *Journal of the American Academy of Dermatology* **22**, 316–317.

## Foreign body granuloma

See Chapter 10.

## Gout

See Chapter 6.

---

# Histiocytic, lymphomatous and metastatic processes

## Histiocytic process

### Xanthoma

Keller (1960) reported a case of hypercholesterolaemic xanthomatosis in a 61-year-old woman exhibiting pseudo-Koenen's tumours periungually in the second and third toes.

### Reference

Keller, P.H. (1960) Hypercholesterinämische Xanthomatose. *Dermatologische Wochenschrift* **14**, 336–337.

### Verruciform xanthoma

Verruciform xanthoma is a rare skin condition characterized histologically by uniform epithelial acanthosis without atypia and foam cells within elongated dermal papillae. Verruciform xanthoma also occurs, rarely, as a secondary reaction in lesions with marked epidermal hyperplasia, such as epidermal naevus and ILVEN. Chyu *et al.* (1987) reported a 36-year-old black woman with verruciform xanthoma on the toes of a lymphoe-

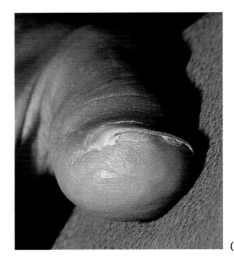

(a)

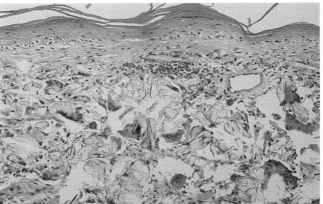

(b)

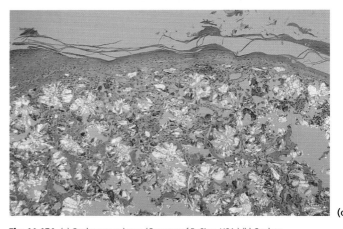

(c)

**Fig. 11.151** (a) Oxalate granuloma. (Courtesy of B. Sina, USA.) (b) Oxalate granuloma—many crystals surrounded by granuloma cells (from a). (c) Oxalate granuloma—micrograph showing the crystals within the dermis (from a).

dematous leg. This was a reccurent yellow-tan tumour on the right first toe present for 18 months, slowly increasing in size, as 2 cm yellowish, fungating, verrucous nodule involving the proximal nail fold. It was asymptomatic until its size interfered with the fit of her shoe.

Multiple verruciform xanthomas (Mountcastle & Lupton 1989) presented with a fingernail which was severely dystrophic and for the most part absent. The remaining part of the lesion measured 1 × 1.5 cm and appeared verrucous, with some crusted exudate that encompassed the nail bed.

## References

Chyu, J., Medenica, M. & Whitney, D.H. (1987) Verruciform xanthoma of the lower extremity—report of a case and review of literature. *Journal of the American Academy of Dermatology* **17**, 695–697.

Mountcastle, E.A. & Lupton, G.P. (1989) Verruciform xanthomas of the digits. *Journal of the American Academy of Dermatology* **20**, 313–317.

### Juvenile xanthogranuloma (see Fig. 6.63)

Juvenile xanthogranuloma is a benign self-limited histiocytic proliferative disorder most frequently seen in children. In Frumkim's case (1987) a progressive deformity of the second toenail developed after a trauma leading to a brown, opaque nail lifted from the nail bed resembling onychogryphosis. After nail avulsion, the whole nail bed and the matrix were seen to be occupied by a round, yellow, soft tumour 6 mm in diameter. Histology revealed lipidized macrophages intermingled with lymphocytes, eosinophils, foam cells and giant cells of the foreign body and Touton types. These latter exhibited the characteristic 'wreath' of nuclei. Another subungual juvenile xanthogranuloma was seen under the right index finger nail of a 2½-year-old boy. The lesion lifted up the nail plate, partially destroyed by the tumour on its ulnar portion. After nail avulsion, a yellow firm nodule appeared with ill-defined border, not tender under pressure. Histopathology showed a well-circumscribed histiocytic lesion with multiple multinucleated cells with a wreath arrangement of nuclei (Chang *et al.* 1996).

## References

Chang, P., Baran, R., Villanueva, C. *et al.* (1996) Juvenile xanthogranuloma beneath a finger nail. *Cutis* **58**, 173–174.

Frumkin, A., Roytan, M. & Johnson, S. (1987) Juvenile xanthogranuloma underneath a toenail. *Cutis* **40**, 244–245.

### Multicentric reticulohistiocytosis

See Chapter 6.

### Lymphoma

See Chapter 6.

### Metastases

Metastases to the fingertip or nail region (Fig. 11.152) are quite

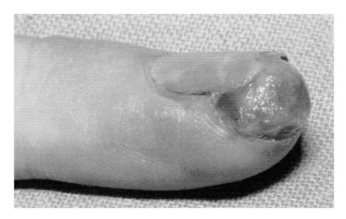

**Fig. 11.152** Metastasis of a chondrosarcoma. (Courtesy of D. Lambert, France.)

rare (about 150 cases reported, Baran & Tosti 1994) and are often initially misdiagnosed as acute infection in and around the nail apparatus and treated as such by incisions. These lesions may be the first manifestation of an internal neoplasm (Camiel *et al.* 1969). Most metastatic tumours primarily affect the bone with subsequent spread to soft tissues. Primary soft tissue metastases of the distal digit may secondarily involve the underlying bone.

The symptoms and signs of metastases are very variable and include dusky red painful or painless swelling (Fig. 11.153a), expansile pulsation, pseudo-clubbing (Hödl 1980) (Fig. 11.154), nail dystrophy, and changes simulating acute or chronic paronychia, a finger infection such as whitlow or osteomyelitis (Marmor & Horner 1959), and even benign lesions such as glomus tumour (Wu & Guise 1978) and early rheumatoid arthritis (Karten & Bartfeld 1962). A clinical picture of necrotizing vasculitis involving the nail area was mimicked by metastatic hypopharyngeal carcinoma (Nigro *et al.* 1992). Whatever symptoms occur, the signs increase out of proportion to the pain, and in the absence of injury or infection this suggests the possibility of metastases (Baran & Tosti 1992). With time, a reddish-purple nodule in the distal nail bed, hyponychial region may become ulcerated.

X-rays usually show an osteolytic focus (Fig. 11.153b) which may resemble spina ventosa or osteitis. Distal phalangeal metastases usually do not cross the articular surface. In fact they characteristically preserve a thin margin of subchondral cortical bone and sometimes, a blown-out cortical shell (Monsees & Murphy 1984) Aspiration or incision biopsy is necessary to classify the tumour and exclude a primary bone growth but even this may fail to reveal the true nature of the primary lesion.

Bronchial carcinoma represents 50% of phalangeal metastases (Fig. 11.153c). The other primary tumours include breast (15% in female), kidney, colon, rectal and parotid gland carcinoma (Falkinburg & Fagan 1956), seminoma (Gartmann 1958), melanoma (Kolmsee & Schultka 1972; Retsas & Samman 1983; Zaun & Dill-Müler 1997), neuroblastoma, plasmocytoma, chondrosarcoma; also skin, and adrenal gland.

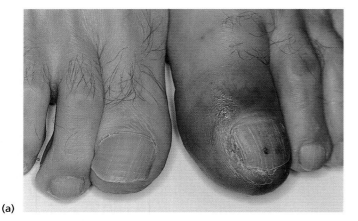

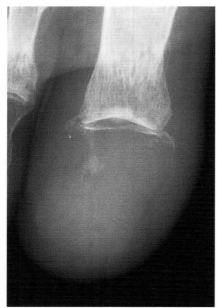

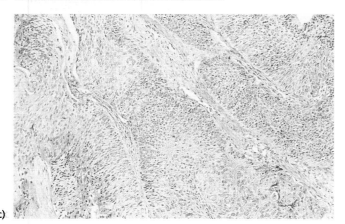

**Fig. 11.153** (a) Metastasis—lung carcinoma. (b) Metastasis—distal phalanx bronchial carcinoma (from a). (c) Metastasis—from bronchial carcinoma.

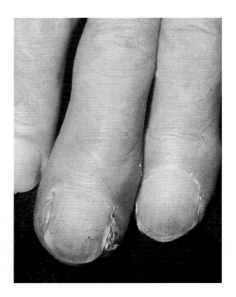

**Fig. 11.154**
Metastasis—pseudo-clubbing: bronchial carcinoma. (Courtesy of S. Hödl, Austria.)

## References

Baran, R. & Tosti, A. (1994) Metastatic bronchogenic carcinoma to the terminal phalanx of the toe. Report of 2 cases and review of the literature. *Journal of the American Academy of Dermatology* **31**, 259–263.

Barnett, L.S. & Morris, J.M. (1969) Metastases of renal-cell carcinoma simultaneously to a finger and a toe. *Journal of Bone and Joint Surgery* **51A**, 773–774.

Camiel, M.R., Aron, B.S., Alexander, L.L., Benninghoff, D.L. & Minkowitz, S. (1969) Metastases to palm, sole, nailbed, nose, face, and scalp from unsuspected carcinoma of the lung. *Cancer* **23**, 214–220.

Falkinburg, L.W. & Fagan, J.H. (1956) Malignant mixed tumor of the parotid gland with a rare metastasis. *American Journal of Surgery* **91**, 279–282.

Gartmann, H. (1958) Seminommetastasen der Haut. *Dermatologische Wochenschrift* **138**, 828–829.

Hödl, S.T. (1980) Fingermetastasen bei Bronchuscarcinom. *Aktuelle Dermatologie* **6**, 249–254.

Karten, I. & Bartfeld, H. (1962) Bronchogenic carcinoma simulating early rheumatoid arthritis. *Journal of the American Medical Association* **179**, 162–164.

Kolmsee, I. & Schultka, O. (1972) Keratoma palmare et plantare dissipatum hereditarium, Pachyonychia congenita und Hypotrichosis lanuginosa, malignes Melanom, Möller-Huntersche Glossitis, Vasculitis allergica superficialis (Bildberichte). *Hautarzt* **23**, 459–460.

Marmor, C. & Horner, R. (1959) Metastasis to a phalanx simulating infection in a finger. *American Journal of Surgery* **97**, 236–237.

Monsees, B. & Murphy, W.A. (1984) Distal phalangeal erosive lesions. *Arthritis and Rheumatism* **27**, 449–455.

Nigro, M.A., Chieregato, G. & Castellani, L. (1992) Metastatic hypopharyngeal carcinoma mimicking necrotizing vasculitis of the skin. *Cutis* **49**, 187–188.

Retsas, S. & Samman, P.D. (1983) Pigment streaks in the nail plate due to secondary malignant melanoma. *British Journal of Dermatology* **108**, 367–370.

Wu, K.K. & Guise, E.R. (1978) Metastatic tumours of the hand, a report of six cases. *Journal of Hand Surgery* 3, 271.

Zaun, H. & Dill-Müler, D. (1997) *Krankhafte Veränderungen des Nagels*, 7th edn. p. 74. Spitta Verlag, Balingen.

# Melanocytic lesions

## Subungual melanocytic lesions

Melanocytes are present in the nail matrix and nail bed although they usually remain functionally inactive in Caucasians. When they become active and produce melanin in amounts that can no longer be degraded by the keratinocytes of the matrix, melanin will continuously be enclosed in the growing nail plate to give rise to a longitudinal light brown to black band (Figs 11.155 & 11.156). A rapid enlargement of a sub-ungual pigmented lesion may be seen as a stripe that is wider in its proximal part; estimation of the nail growth rate and measurement of the difference in width proximally and distally allows an exact calculation of the growth of the pigment-producing lesion. Except for 'subungual linear keratotic melanonychia' (Baran & Perrin 1999) (see p. 528), pigmented lesions in the nail bed *usually* do not cause a longitudinal melanonychia but shine through the nail as a greyish to brown or black spot.

## Longitudinal melanonychia

Longitudinal melanonychia (LM) is characterized by a tan, brown, or black longitudinal streak within the nail plate (Fig. 11.157). LM results from increased melanin deposition in the nail plate. This deposition may result from greater melanin synthesis by normally nonfunctional matrix melanocytes (Figs 11.158 & 11.159) or from an increase in the total number

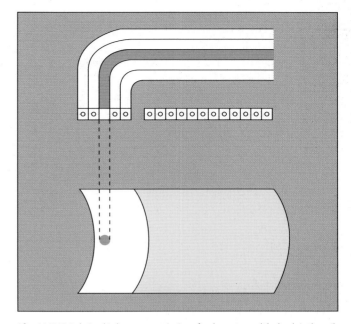

**Fig. 11.156** Relationship between matrix sites of melanocytes and the levels in the nail plate that their pigment will reside in.

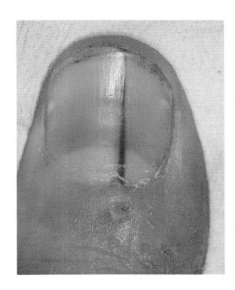

**Fig. 11.157** Longitudinal melanonychia. Proximal widening of the band should make the clinician suspicious.

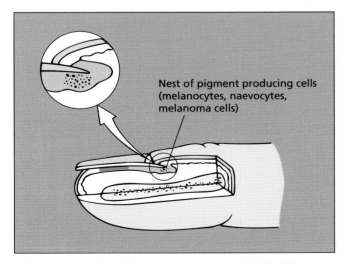

Nest of pigment producing cells (melanocytes, naevocytes, melanoma cells)

**Fig. 11.155** The main site of functionally active melanocytes in health and disease.

of matrix melanocytes that synthetize melanin; in either instance, melanocytes may be normal or abnormal. Perrin *et al.* (1997) have demonstrated that proximal nail melanocytes contain premelanosomes and melanosomes I and II, but not the 'mature' melanosomal compartment; therefore the dormant melanocytes are predominant. In the distal matrix, the same authors observed an active melanin synthesis compartment, i.e. functionally differentiated, associated with a dormant melanocyte compartment. In contrast to common belief, LM originates more often in the distal matrix not secondary to the larger melanocyte density, but because only the distal matrix contains melanocytes with active melanin synthesis. This is a

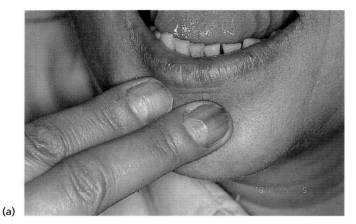

(a)

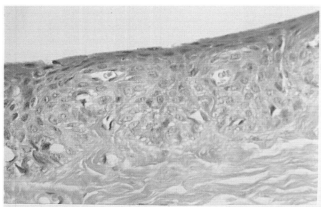

(b)

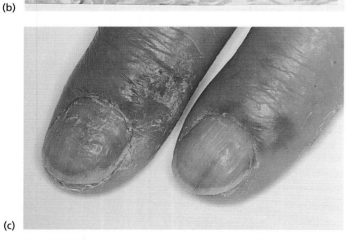

(c)

**Fig. 11.158** (a) Laugier syndrome—nail and lip pigmentation. (b) Laugier syndrome showing normal-looking melanocytes. (c) Laugier syndrome—longitudinal melanonychia and periungual pigmentation with pseudo-Hutchinson's signs.

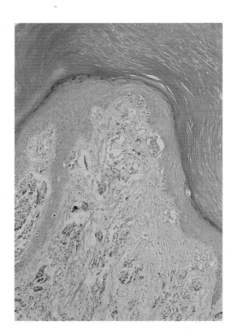

**Fig. 11.159** Junctional lentiginous naevus.

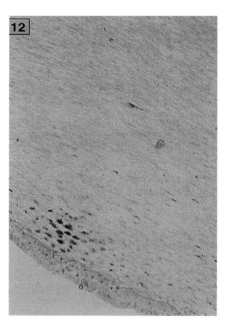

**Fig. 11.160** Pigment within the deep layer of the distal nail plate (Fontana stain).

fortunate circumstance because permanent nail plate deformity is less common when surgery is performed in the distal rather than in the proximal matrix. The more proximal the origin, the more superficial is the melanin within the nail plate (Fig. 11.156). It is possible to identify the site of origin of pigmentation in LM within the matrix by staining a nail plate clipping with Fontana-Masson's argentaffin reaction (Fig. 11.160).

When distal matrix origin seems likely, the cuticle can sometimes be retracted proximally to confirm the distal origin of LM without incision of the proximal nail fold.

LM is common in darkly pigmented persons. LM occurs in 77% of African-Americans over 20 years of age and in almost 100% who are older than 50 years; the thumbs and index fingers are most frequently involved. LM occurs in 10% to 20% of Japanese people; the thumbs, index and middle fingers are most frequently involved in this group. LM is also common in Hispanics and other dark-skinned groups. Among white people, LM is unusual.

The distribution of LM between digits coincides with relative digital use; LM is most common in frequently used fingers. The thumb, always used in grasping, is the digit that most often demonstrates LM. The index, middle, 4th, and 5th fingers are employed with diminishing frequency for grasping objects and demonstrate a correspondingly lower incidence of LM. More frequently used digits are also subject to greater trauma. Several authors have implicated trauma in the pathogenesis of subungual melanoma (SM) (Roberts 1984; Saccone & Rayan 1993; O'Toole *et al.* 1995; Pearce 1995).

The distribution of LM and SM is remarkably similar. SM develops slightly more often on the hand than on the foot. Forty-five per cent to 60% of SM arise on the hand; 40% to 55% arise on the foot. On the foot, SM usually occurs in the great toe. Is the incidence of SM higher in the thumb and great toe because each digit is subject to greater trauma; because LM, which commonly occurs on the thumb (and presumably the great toe), is a precursor of SM; or because the thumb and great toe occupy relatively large surface areas and afford greater opportunity for SM to develop?

To distinguish the small number of patients with subungual melanoma from, by far, the larger group of patients with non-malignant LM is difficult. Both are alike in several ways. In the hand, each arises most often in the thumb, index fingers or both. LM has been reported to precede the onset of SM and may be an early sign of SM. Both are more common in dark-skinned persons.

In a Japanese study, 31% of SM started as LM and became ulcerated or painful several years later (Takematsu *et al.* 1985). In a Belgian study, six of 10 white patients with SM described as their first sign a longitudinal pigmented band of their nail (Nogaret *et al.* 1986). Other authors have reported similar findings.

Approximately 1–3% of malignant melanomas in white persons are SM (Finley *et al.* 1994; Banfield *et al.* 1999). In Japanese persons, the proportion of SM was similar to that in white persons in two studies (Obata *et al.* 1979; Takahashi & Seiji 1983), but higher, 10%, in a third one (Miura & Jimbow 1985), and 30% in that of Saida and Oshima (1989). In African-Americans, the proportion of SM was higher and varied from 15% to 20% (Collins 1984). A study from Cape Town, RSA, of 20 subungual melanomas revealed 7 white and 13 black patients (Krige *et al.* 1995). The proportion among Chinese people, 17%, was similar to that in African-Americans. The highest proportion of 33% was seen in a small study of American Indians (Black & Wiggino 1985). In general, when melanoma occurs in dark-skinned persons, a higher percentage of melanomas are likely to arise in the nail apparatus (Shah & Goldsmith 1971), palm or sole whereas melanoma in light-skinned persons a lower percentage are likely to arise in the nail apparatus (Fig. 11.161).

A thorough history and physical examination should enable the various exogenous causes of a single band of LM to be distinguished. The most common pigmented lesion is subungual

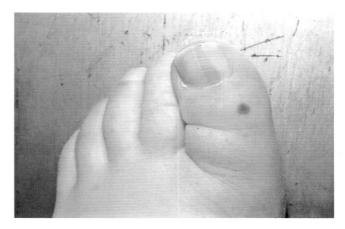

**Fig. 11.161** Melanoma, very pale longitudinal band.

haematoma and it is easily distinguished from LM. It usually migrates distally and its proximal margin is gently curved in one transverse axis. If the nail plate is notched with a scalpel at the proximal margin of the spot, distal migration of the haematoma can be accurately measured as the nail plate grows (Fig. 11.162). Non-migratory haematomas and foreign bodies, however, do not follow this rule and require more extensive evaluation. Silver nitrate staining may sometimes be linear. It also grows out. Histopathology shows jet-black granules in the superficial layers of the nail plate (Haneke 1998).

Periungual spread of pigmentation to the proximal and lateral nail folds as well as to the tip of a single digit is called Hutchinson's sign and corresponds to the radial growth phase of subungual melanoma. It is, therefore, the most important indicator of SM. When this sign is present, SM is the presumptive diagnosis (Fig. 11.163). This sign, however, particularly when subtle, is not absolutely pathognomonic for SM.

'Benign' 'non-melanoma' and 'illusory' variants of pseudo-Hutchinson's sign occur in the absence of subungual melanoma (Baran & Kechijian 1996). Each is characterized by periungual hyperpigmentation occurring in association with LM. Each represents a potentially misleading clue to the diagnosis of SM. The variants do not negate the importance of Hutchinson's sign. Rather, they oblige the clinician to consider the diagnostic possibilities other than SM. Likewise, the absence of periungual pigmentation does not preclude the diagnosis of SM. The clinician must carefully evaluate the individual patient for clues to the diagnosis of SM.

In addition to a detailed history of the present illness, careful clinical examination of the lesion, general physical examination, the history of the patient including drug ingestion, past treatments, hobbies and illnesses, family history, racial origin, and general appearance must be evaluated. If the diagnosis of SM seems likely, an adequate biopsy of involved nail unit is performed. In this manner, the pathologist is able to examine the tissue sufficiently to confirm or rule out SM. The relevance of Hutchinson's sign to the diagnosis of SM has withstood the

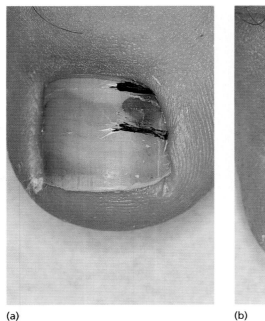
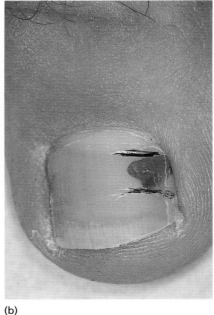
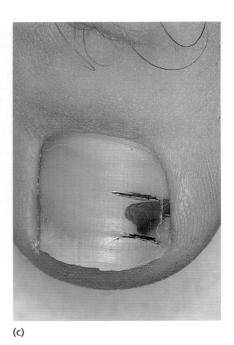

(a)                                    (b)                                    (c)

**Fig. 11.162** (a) Subungual haematoma. (b, c) Subungual haematoma notching the proximal and the distal margin of the lesion confirms its distal movement.

test of time. If the possibility of pseudo-Hutchinson's variants is kept in mind, the clinician is less likely to overdiagnose this important malignancy and more likely to address the problem with confidence and precision (Table 11.8).

1 Peri-ungual spread of pigmentation without SM may occur in the Laugier–Hunziker–Baran syndrome (Fig. 11.158) (Baran & Barrière 1986; Branco Ferreira *et al*. 1999), a disorder recognizable by the association of LM with macular pigmentation of the lips and mouth, (Dupré & Viraben 1990; Haneke 1991; Engelmann & Kunze 1992) as well as the genital (Vazquez *et al*. 1993) and esophagal mucosa (Yamamoto *et al*. 1999). This condition may also demonstrate isolated nail involvement (Haneke 1991; Stenier *et al*. 1992).

2 Periungual pigmentation of a congenital naevus of the nail region (Asahina *et al*. 1993) (Fig. 11.63e) and periungual recurrence of pigmentation after nail surgery for a naevus (Kopf & Waldo 1980).

3 LM and periungual hyperpigmentation after X-ray therapy for a finger dermatitis (Shelley *et al*. 1964).

4 Pigmented bands and periungual hyperpigmentation resulting from malnutrition (Bisht & Singh 1962) and some drugs.

5 LM and periungual hyperpigmentation have been described in association with minocycline therapy.

6 The theoretical association of LM with acral pigmentation in Peutz–Jeghers syndrome.

7 LM and pigmentation of the distal pulp have been reported in patients with AIDS even before the institution of systemic treatment (Gallais *et al*. 1992).

8 Naevoid nail area melanosis and nail matrix naevus in children may represent spontaneous regression (Kikuchi *et al*. 1993).

9 Sometimes LM that is dark brown simulates pigmentation of the overlying cuticle and proximal nail fold. The pigmentation is visible because of the relative transparency of the cuticle and proximal nail fold and not because of melanin deposition within these tissues. This can be identified by careful inspection. In good lighting, it is usually possible to establish whether pigment is present within the periungual tissues or beneath them in the underlying nail plate.

10 Also, previous silver nitrate treatment of granulation tissue may give a black halo which is easily distinguished from Hutchinson's melanotic whitlow (Haneke *et al*. 1998).

Besides Hutchinson's sign, other clues to the diagnosis of SM can be important. The clinician should be suspicious when LM:

1 begins in a single digit of a person during the fourth to sixth decade of life or later, however, melanonychia due to subungual melanoma has even been observed in children (see p. 621);

2 develops abruptly in a previously normal nail plate;

3 becomes suddenly darker or wider (Fig. 11.157);

4 occurs in either the thumb, index finger, or great toe;

5 occurs in a person who gives a history of digital trauma;

6 occurs singly in the digit of a dark-skinned patient, particularly if the thumb or great toe is affected;

7 demonstrates blurred, rather than sharp, lateral borders;

8 occurs in a person who gives a history of malignant melanoma;

9 occurs in a person in whom the risk for melanoma is increased (e.g. dysplastic naevus syndrome (Kechijian 1991) (Fig. 11.164);

10 is accompanied by nail dystrophy, such as partial nail destruction or disappearance.

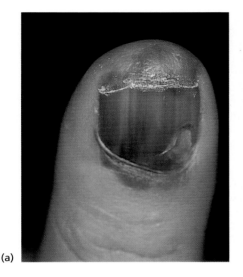

(a)

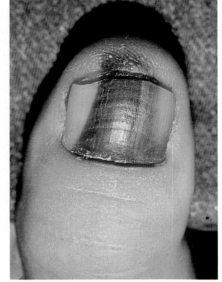

(b)

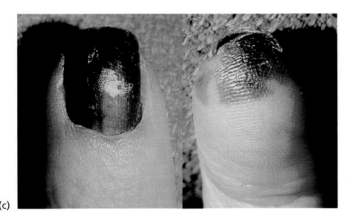

(c)

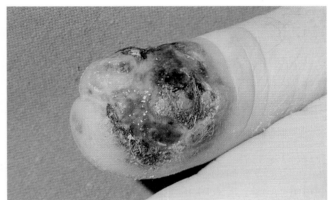

(d)

Other signs are noteworthy, but not necessarily helpful, in establishing the likelihood of malignancy:

1 Although amelanotic SM has been reported (Fig. 11.165), lightly pigmented bands of LM rarely represent SM, but do exist (Fig. 11.161); the pathologist may have difficulty even visualizing the melanin and melanocytes that constitute light-banded LM. We have seen two patients with pigmented nail bed melanoma without nail plate pigmentation.

2 Darker shades of brown do not necessarily represent SM because naevi and melanoma may manifest identical shades of brown. In white persons, black bands may be an important clue to SM; in African-Americans, however, 'jet-black' bands are not unusual. Theoretically, colour variegation suggests SM; however, variegation is common in persons with multiple 'benign' LM.

3 Theoretically, wide bands suggest SM; however, the critical width that signifies SM has yet to be established although a width of > 5 mm is usually critical.

4 Bands that do not extend distally to the free edge of the nail are unlikely to represent SM because they do not take their

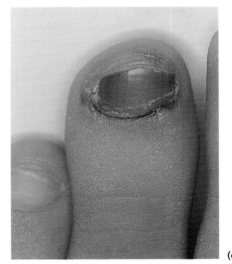

(e)

**Fig. 11.163** (a–c) Melanoma—Hutchinson's sign. (d) Melanoma—Hutchinson's sign. Nail disappearance. (e) Pseudo-Hutchinson's sign in congenital naevus.

**Table 11.8** Conditions accompanied by pseudo-Hutchinson's sign (after Baran & Kechijian 1996).

| Condition | Clinical features |
|---|---|
| *Benign* | |
| Illusory pigmentation (Baran & Kechijian 1996) | Dark colour transverses the transparent cuticle and thin nail fold |
| Ethnic pigmentation | Pigmentation of proximal nailfold in dark-skinned persons; lateral nailfolds not involved; longitudinal melanonychia not always present; often exaggerated in thumbs |
| Laugier syndrome (Baran & Barrière 1986) | Macular pigmentation of lips, mouth, and genitalia; one or several fingers involved |
| Peutz–Jeghers syndrome | Hyperpigmentation of fingers and toes; macular pigmentation of buccal mucosa and lips |
| Radiation therapy (Shelley *et al.* 1964) | Reported after treatment of finger dermatitis, psoriasis and chronic paronychia |
| Malnutrition (Bisht & Singh 1962) | Polydactylous involvement |
| Minocycline (Mooney & Bennet 1988) | Polydactylous involvement |
| Patients with AIDS (Gallais *et al.* 1992) | Polydactylous involvement; zidovudine produces similar pigmentation |
| Trauma induced (Baran 1987, 1990; Bayerl & Moll 1993) | Friction, nail biting and picking, and boxing |
| Congenital naevus (Asahina *et al.* 1993) | |
| Congenital naevus after biopsy (Kopf & Waldo 1980) | Pigment recurrence after biopsy of longitudinal melanonychia in acquired and congenital melanocytic naevi, often striking cytological atypia |
| Regressing nevoid melanosis in childhood (Kikuchi *et al.* 1993) | Monodactylic; initial increase in dyschromia followed by subsequent pigment regression; perplexing disorder |
| Subungual haematoma | Exceptionally, blood spreads to nail folds and hyponychial areas |
| Silver nitrate | For treatment of granulation tissue, may produce a black halo |
| *Malignant* | |
| Bowen's disease | Monodactylic with longitudinal melanonychia (Sau *et al.* 1994) |
| | Polydactylic (Dominguez-Cherit, unpublished data) |

origin from the nail matrix. However, they may represent metastatic melanoma or LM arising from the nail bed (see see p. 620). The management of black patients with pigmented bands can be difficult. Although multiple nails demonstrate LM, there may be substantial variability in the colour and width of bands within a single nail plate and among different nails in the same patient. Whether LM in a thumb or great toe represents SM or racial variation is not necessarily easily determined by history and inspection alone. Change in the morphology of LM, in particular widening and darkening, is the most important clue to the possibility of SM in these patients. A streak that is wider proximally than distally represents growth of the lesion in the matrix.

Multiple bands of LM are usually not neoplastic in origin although bilateral SM of the great toes has been observed once (Leppard *et al.* 1974). A drug history and complete general review to rule out relevant systemic disorders and a thorough examination of the skin and nails to exclude nail infection and associated cutaneous disorders may reveal the underlying cause of multiple LM.

However, despite meticulous evaluation, the aetiology of LM remains obscure, and biopsy becomes necessary to avoid pitfalls. The biopsy of a solitary longitudinal melanonychia revealed a subungual melanoma in a patient receiving phototherapy and this was followed by a new pigmented nail streak on an other finger where histological findings showed benign melanocytic hyperplasia (Beltrani & Scher 1991). There is no consensus among dermatopathologists regarding the melanocytic causes of LM. Therefore, the following histopathological classification represents an attempt to organize the causes into a practicable list.

## Benign melanocytic hyperplasia–focal melanocyte activation (Fig. 11.158)

Benign melanocytic hyperplasia is due to an increase in melanocyte activity and/or number causing a circumscribed pigmented macule in the matrix. When melanocyte hyperplasia indicates the presence of an increased number, there are more than 6.5 cells per mm of basal membrane length of melanin-containing melanocytes within the basal and suprabasal layers of the nail matrix (Tosti *et al.* 1998). Melanocytic hyperplasia in the matrix may also be induced by repeated trauma such as friction and X-irradiation. A circumscribed increased number of normal looking melanocytes is found in the matrix in the Laugier–Hunziker–Baran syndrome (Haneke 1991).

## Lentigo simplex and melanocytic naevus

Lentigo simplex is characterized by a considerable increase in highly active melanocytes accompanied by epidermal hyperplasia. There is a basal proliferation of melanocytes arranged as single cells, rather in nests. Typically, but not always, lentigo is associated with elongation of the rete ridges (lentiginous

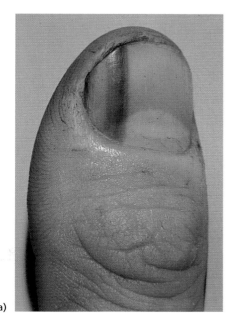

(a)

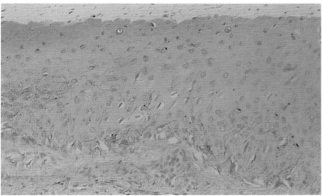

(b)

**Fig. 11.164** (a) Melanoma *in situ*. (Courtesy of P. Kechijian, USA.) (b) Melanoma *in situ*.

epithelial hyperplasia). The nature of the underlying melanotic lesion responsible for the pigmented band cannot be determined by clinical examination alone. The same holds true for subungual melanocytic naevi corresponding to a benign melanocytic hyperplasia with, at least, one nest (Fig. 11.159).

In a series of 22 naevi reported by Tosti *et al.* (1996) periungual pigmentation was present in one third of the cases. According to Leauté–Lebrèze *et al.* (1996), since LM can occur at the age when other naevi appear, surgical excision should not be undertaken on different grounds than with other congenital or acquired naevi in children. In a clinical and histopathological study of 40 cases of LM in children below 16 years, Goettmann-Bonvallot *et al.* (1999) found a lentigo in 12 cases, a naevus in 19 cases and functional LM in nine children. Ohtsuka *et al.* (1978) reported a case of congenital naevocytic naevus of the tip of the little finger in a Japanese female infant. This caused discoloration, overcurvature and subungual hyperkeratosis giving rise to an appearance similar to the nail of a

monkey. An unusual case of extremely large junctional naevus of the nail bed with histological atypia in a 6-year-old Japanese child was described by Pomerance *et al.* (1994).

Congenital subungual naevi are usually excised to prevent exceptional secondary malignant melanoma (Coskey *et al.* 1983; Wong *et al.* 1991; Libow *et al.* 1995) and the management of 'naevoid nail area melanosis' in Japanese children (Kikuchi *et al.* 1993) is still debatable. There is therefore a great deal of controversy about: (a) the malignant potential of small congenital naevi; (b) the malignant potential of subungual naevi; and (c) the relationship of childhood lentigines to the evolution of naevi and to the development of melanomas (Wong *et al.* 1991). DNA ploidy analysis is likely to provide information for evaluating the biological behaviour of subungual melanocytic lesions (Asahina *et al.* 1993).

Kawabata *et al.* (1999) consider that dermatoscopic features of melanoma *in situ* can be distinguished from pigmental naevi.

## Atypical melanocytic hyperplasia and nail melanoma

Atypical melanocytic hyperplasia shows an increased number of melanocytes with larger, hyperchromatic, pleomorphic nuclei, more prominent nucleoli, increased mitoses, and long branching dendrites. Thus, atypical melanocytic hyperplasia (Fig. 11.166a) may be considered to be incipient malignant melanoma *in situ* (Kopf & Waldo 1980; Kamino & Ackerman 1981).

Melanomas of the nail region are now better understood since the identification and analysis of acrolentiginous melanoma (ALM), the most frequent type (Clark *et al.* 1979; Feibleman *et al.* 1980). Superficial spreading melanoma (SSM) is unfrequent and nodular melanoma is very rare in subungual area despite Milton's *et al.* (1985) findings in Australia (7 cases out of 30 individuals), and Miura and Jimbow's (1985) questionnaire survey of 108 cases of subungual melanomas in Japan, indicating that ALM was present in 80% of cases, nodular melanoma in 15% and SSM in 5%. Some cases are unclassifiable for two main reasons:
1 there may be an histological transition between SSM and ALM (Sondergaard 1983) indicating a close biologic relationship between the two types;
2 poor quality of the biopsy specimen (Blessing *et al.* 1991).

Approximately 1% to 3% of melanomas in Caucasians (Paul *et al.* 1992; Finley *et al.* 1994; Banfield *et al.* 1999), and 15% to 20% in blacks are located in the nail apparatus (Oropeza 1976). However, since malignant melanoma is rare in black people, the absolute number of ungual melanoma in Caucasians and black people does not significantly differ. In Caucasians, most patients with SM have a fair complexion, light hair, and blue or hazel eyes. There is no sex predominance. The mean age is 60 years. Most tumours are located on the thumbs and great toes—22 lesions out of 24 subungual melanomas—(Rigby & Briggs 1992), but develop more commonly on the foot than on the hand.

Melanomas are often asymptomatic, pain and bleeding being rare. The clinical appeareance of the tumour varies (Patterson

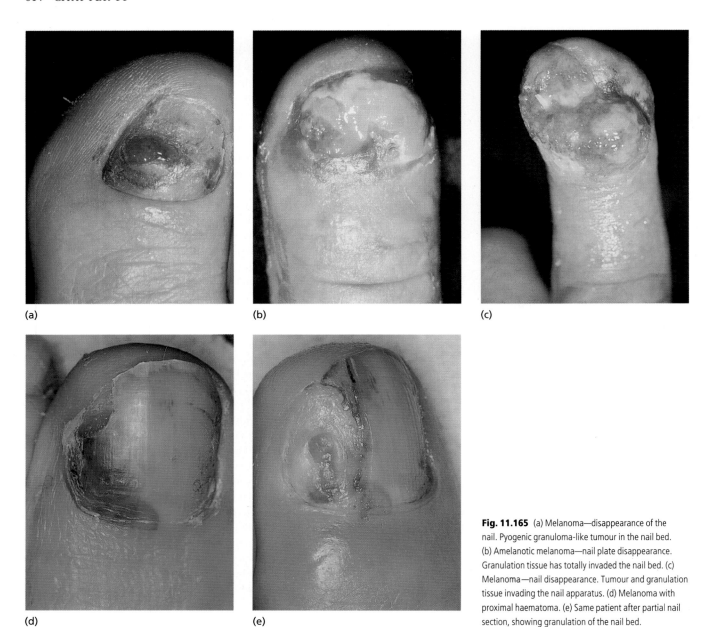

(a)

(b)

(c)

(d)

(e)

**Fig. 11.165** (a) Melanoma—disappearance of the nail. Pyogenic granuloma-like tumour in the nail bed. (b) Amelanotic melanoma—nail plate disappearance. Granulation tissue has totally invaded the nail bed. (c) Melanoma—nail disappearance. Tumour and granulation tissue invading the nail apparatus. (d) Melanoma with proximal haematoma. (e) Same patient after partial nail section, showing granulation of the nail bed.

& Helwig 1980), but half the patients note a mass below the nail, usually associated with partial destruction of the nail, or total loss (Figs 11.165 & 11.167).

Periungual infection, ulceration of the nail bed, and granulation tissue occur in about one-third of the patients (Zanone *et al.* 1993). In another third, discoloration of the nail area is the presenting sign:

1 Some lesions begin as a longitudinal melanonychia. This pigmented (brown to black) linear streak of variable width runs through the whole length of the visible nail. It was the first feature in 6 out of 10 patients with malignant melanoma (Nogaret *et al.* 1986). After some months or years, the borders of the band widen, become blurred and ulceration appears. It must be stressed that neither the width nor the intensity of the brown pigmentation are proof of, or exclude, subungual melanoma.

2 A spot can appear in the matrix or nail bed. This may vary in colour from brown to black and may be homogeneous or irregular. It is seldom painful.

3 Less frequent is Hutchinson's sign (1886) (Fig. 11.163), an irregular brown black pigmentation of the matrix, nail bed, nail plate, and surrounding tissues. It represents the radial growth phase of subungual melanoma and has proved to be a valuable clue to the clinical diagnosis of malignancy (Kopf 1981) after pseudo-Hutchinson's signs have been ruled out (see p. 613). Its presence means that the entire nail apparatus must be removed (without prior incisional biopsy).

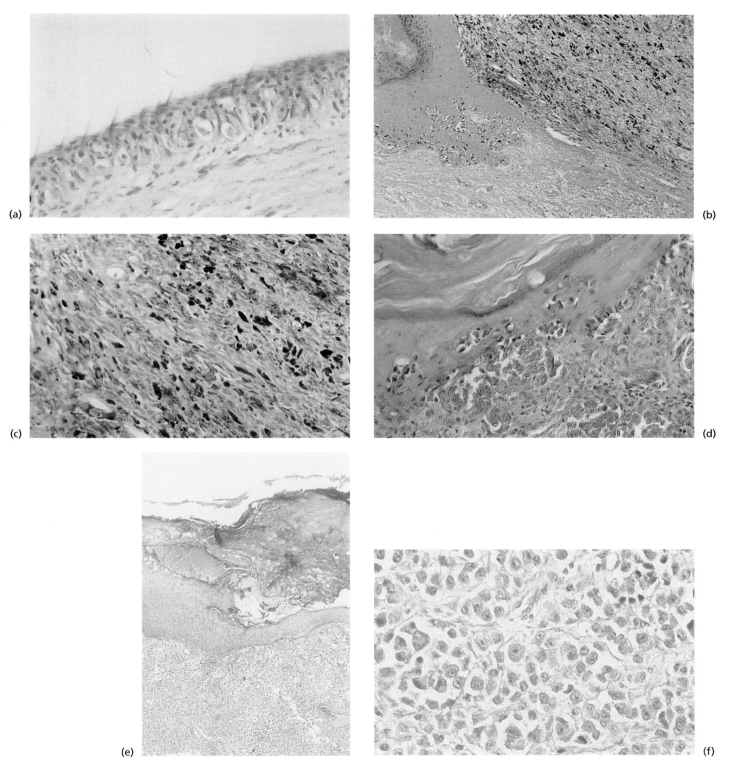

**Fig. 11.166** (a) Melanoma *in situ* (×20). (Courtesy of J.P. Varini, France.) (b) Invasive subungual melanoma (×20). (Courtesy of J. Graham, USA.) (c) Same patient (×40). (Courtesy of J. Graham, USA.) (d) Invasive melanoma (×40). (Courtesy of J.P. Varini, France.) (e) Amelanotic melanoma (×20). (Courtesy of J.P. Varini, France.) (f) Same patient (×100). (Courtesy of J.P. Varini, France.)

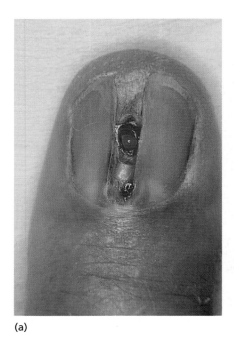

(a)

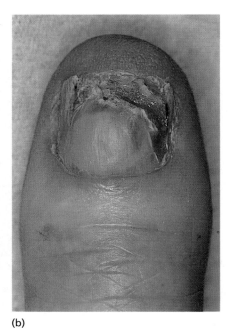

(b)

**Fig. 11.167** (a) Amelanotic melanoma—large central fissure of the nail plate showing granulation tissue in the nail bed. (b) Amelanotic melanoma with ulceration of the distal and lateral nail bed.

This technique enables serial sections to be examined which is particularly important in acral lentiginous melanoma in which histology may be difficult to interpret. The radial growth phase of malignant melanoma in the subungual region is easily confused histologically with junctional naevus and the clinician must be wary of a benign histological report in any subungual lesion showing Hutchinson's sign. The vertical phase with its abrupt onset when compared temporally with the slowly evolving radial growth phase is manifested by the focal appearance of a discrete blue, black or pink nodule in tumours of subungual site causing partial or total permanent destruction of the nail plate (Clark *et al.* 1979).

Approximately 25% of melanomas are amelanotic (Fig. 11.167) and may present as pyogenic granuloma, granulation tissue (Fig. 11.165), ingrowing nail and mycobacterial infections with nail dystrophy. The risk of misdiagnosis is therefore particularly high in these cases.

Nail melanoma must be considered in the differential diagnosis (Shukla & Hughes 1989) in all patients affected by unexplained chronic paronychia, whether painful or not, torpid granulomatous ulceration of the proximal nail fold, pyogenic granuloma (Rathi *et al.* 1995), pseudo-verrucous keratotic alterations of the nail bed and lateral nail groove, and persistence of a lesion following trauma of the nail. Pathologic fracture secondary to subungual melanoma may be the presenting sign (Gregorcyk *et al.* 1996).

Subungual melanoma may be mimicked by subungual haematoma which is not rare and may even be present without a history of severe trauma (Fig. 11.162). It may follow repeated minor trauma which escapes the patient's attention such as in tennis toe or following trauma from hard ski boots or windsurf board. Haematoma following isolated trauma usually grows out in one piece rather than as longitudinal streak due to continuous production of pigment but subungual melanoma following a single injury to the digit was observed in several cases after an interval of between nine months and seven years (Roberts 1984; Saccone & Rayan 1993; O'Toole *et al.* 1995; Pearce 1995). Repeated trauma may cause difficulties in differential diagnosis and a non-migrating haematoma should be ruled out. Alkiewicz and Pfister (1976) suggest that the lesion should be examined with a loup, after it has been covered by a drop of oil. Epi-illumination microscopy is now used successfully (see p. 623). The pigmented nail should be clipped and tested with the argentaffin reaction in order to rule out melanin pigmentation. Subungual haemoglobin is not degraded to haemosiderin and remains therefore Prussian blue negative. Scrapings or small pieces of the nail boiled with water in a test tube gives a positive benzidine reaction with conventional haemostix. However, it has to be stressed that any erosive bleeding tumour will also give a positive benzidine reaction. Therefore a diagnostic nail biopsy should be performed for the investigation of any persistent, clinically suspicious, pigmented nail lesion (Banfield & Dawber 1999). The difference between blood and melanotic pigment, sometimes rather difficult to discern by routine histological methods, is easily seen by ultra-structural techniques—since haem pigment is intercellular while melanin is mainly intracellular (Achten 1982).

### Blue naevus

Soyer and Kerl (1984) found a slightly infiltrated black area well-demarcated with a small periungual nodule (Fig. 11.168a) on the dorsum of the left big toe of a 4-year-old girl. In the

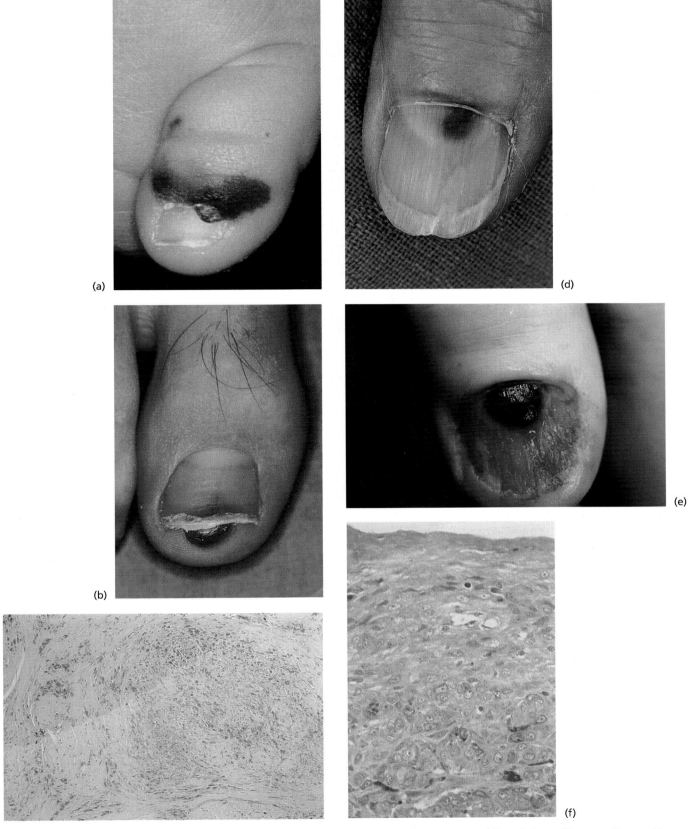

**Fig. 11.168** (a) Blue naevus of the proximal nail fold with satellites of the proximal phalanx. (Courtesy of H.P. Soyer & H. Kerl, Austria.) (b) Distal subungual blue naevus. (Courtesy of L. Requena, Spain.) (c) Histology—case shown in (b). (d,e) Atypical blue naevus involving the nail matrix. (f) Histology—case shown in (d). (Courtesy of E. Duhard, France.)

neighbouring skin several pinhead-sized satellite nodules were found with enlarged lymph nodes of the left groin. Epithelioid, dendritic and spindle-shaped melanocytes were found in the capsule and in some parts of certain lymph nodes. The case was interpreted as an example of periungual combined naevus with benign lymph node metastasis (metastasing pseudomelanoma) from the blue naevus component.

Vidal *et al.* (1997) reported on distal subungual blue naevus (Fig. 11.168b,c) as an asymptomatic nodule, present since birth, and growing slowly on the right great toe. Histology of the 9 mm diameter nodule demonstrated elongated, slightly spindly cells with long branching dendritic processes. These cells were arranged in fascicles and were dispersed as solitary units among collagen bundles. Dermal melanocytes were mostly orientated with their long axes parallel to the epidermis and many were filled with fine granules of melanin.

Atypical blue naevus is an exceptional tumour (Tran *et al.* 1998) which may involve the nail matrix (E. Duhard, unpublished data) (Fig. 11.168d–f).

## Pseudo-Recklinghausen intradermal naevi (Fig. 11.169)

Abnormal naevoblast migration may mimic neurofibromatosis (Lycka *et al.* 1991), where hundreds of papules and nodules on both feet and toes have been reported as intradermal naevi. A similar clinical presentation was shown in a black male (Cavelier-Balloy *et al.* 1992).

The main difference was in the presence of only blue naevi in the latter case. Leu 7 and myelin basic protein were negative which also ruled out neurofibromatosis (Gray *et al.* 1990).

However, is the case of nail melanoma of the great toe of a neurofibromatosis patient reported by Karakayali *et al.* (1999) just a coincidence or an association?

## Histopathology of subungal melanoma (Fig. 11.166)

Subungual melanoma is a particular form of acrolentiginous melanoma. This type of melanoma is defined by its location on palms, soles and under the nails rather than by a specific microscopic morphology; however, some authors distinguish subungual nodular melanoma and subungual superficial spreading melanoma from acrolentiginous melanoma (Miura & Jimbow 1985; Takematsu *et al.* 1985; Diepgen *et al.* 1991).

It is also very important to stress that a major proportion of patients suffering from subungual melanoma have undergone some minor form of surgery before the diagnosis of subungual melanoma has been made. This is not only the consequence of patients' neglect but also of physicians' misdiagnoses, false biopsy techniques and insufficient histopathological techniques and knowledge. Thus the importance of proper biopsy and histopathology for the prognosis cannot be overestimated (Baran & Haneke 1984; Baran & Kechijian 1989). Recent series as well as our own experience has shown that ML in young people is mostly due to lentigines or junctional naevi (Leauté–Labrèze

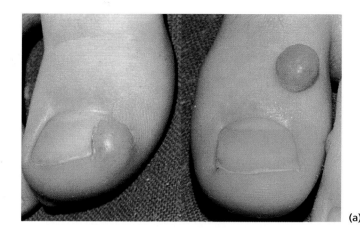

(a)

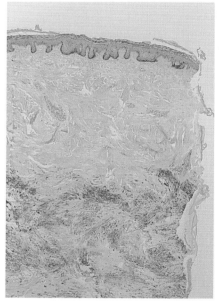

**Fig. 11.169** (a) Pseudo-Recklinghausen intradermal naevus. (b) Intradermal blue naevus (same patient). (Courtesy of Cl. Beylot, France.)

(b)

*et al.* 1996; Tosti *et al.* 1996). Histopathology thus shows melanocytes and naevus cells mainly in the basal zone of the matrix epithelium. Subungual melanoma may arise from suprabasal melanocytes (Tomizawa 2000). Therefore, a biopsy technique was developed that ensures almost scarless healing and gives excellent tissue specimens for histopathological work-up (Haneke 1999b). This is essentially a superficial, tangential excision of the pigmented lesion of the matrix performed after lifting the nail plate at its proximal third (Haneke 1999, 2001).

Migration of melanoma cells into suprabasal epidermal layers is a characteristic feature also seen in acral lentiginous melanoma. These cells and cell clusters eventually reach the horny layer or nail plate, respectively. Therefore, clippings of subungual melanoma nail plates sometimes contain pycnotic tumour cells (Kerl *et al.* 1984) which retain their protein S-100 positivity (Haneke & Binder 1978).

There is usually no difficulty making the histopathological diagnosis of advanced invasive subungual melanoma. Most subungual acrolentiginous melanomas exhibit a lentiginous pattern with pleomorphic, often dendritic atypical melanocytes being arranged singly or in irregular clusters in the basal and suprabasal epithelial layers. Sheets of melanoma cells either spindle, epithelioid, polygonal, small, dendritic, or bizarre and pleomorphic, extend from the epithelium into the dermis. Large round melanoma cells are dispersed throughout the entire epidermis in a pagetoid (SSM-like) pattern. The nodular pattern is rare and shows subepidermal tumour cells usually with little junctional cell complexes and at least part of the overlying epithelium is necrotic; to our experience, subungual nodular melanoma appears to be primarily located rather in the nail bed than the matrix. Mixed features of lentiginous and pagetoid patterns are not rare. Especially the lentiginous type of subungual melanoma may exhibit a dense population of atypical melanocytes in the basal epithelial layers which may give rise to artificial bulla formation due to lack of cohesion between melanoma cells and nail bed and matrix epithelium upon sectioning and is also one cause of nail atrophy in subungual melanoma (Haneke 1986). Melanoma cells migrating up to the superficial matrix layers may be included in the nail plate and can be seen microscopically (Haneke & Binder 1978), sometimes even in nail clippings (Kerl *et al*. 1984). Subungual nodular melanoma with no junctional component may be difficult to distinguish from lymphoma, anaplastic and small cell carcinoma as well as other malignant tumours including metastases all of which are rare in this location. Several cases of desmoplastic subungual melanoma have been reported (Patterson & Helwig 1980; Pearce 1995; Rongioletti *et al*. 1995) (Fig. 11.170) some with perineural extension. Characteristic intraneural invasion and extension along the median nerve has been demonstrated in a case of acral lentiginous melanoma of the right thumb nail bed (Iyadomi *et al*. 1998). SM may even extend along the ulnar, median and musculocutaneous nerves for a distance of 30 cm (Ogose *et al*. 1998). They may also masquerade as fibrous histcytic tumours (Hara *et al*. 1993) and have even been observed to produce cartilage (Cachia & Kedziora 1999). Immunohistochemical demonstration of S-100 protein or another melanoma marker such as HMB 45 aids in making the correct diagnosis.

The most difficult problem in subungual pigmented lesions is to differentiate benign melanocytic hyperplasia that may eventually develop into a benign junctional or compound naevus, from the earliest changes of subungual melanoma (Table 11.9). One has always to keep in mind that there are many well-documented cases with histories longer than 20 or 30 years. These cases often started with a light-brown longitudinal stripe in the nail. We have seen three cases of subungual melanoma *in situ* with only a very light longitudinal melanonychia; however, the pigmented bands were wider than 5 mm.

In the case of a pigmented spot in the matrix or nail bed the lesion should be completely excised and serial and step sections are a must. It is common to see only few melanocytes which tend to be variable in size but some of which have enlarged

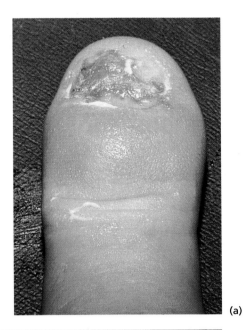
(a)

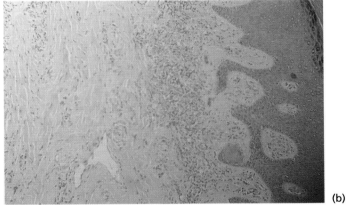
(b)

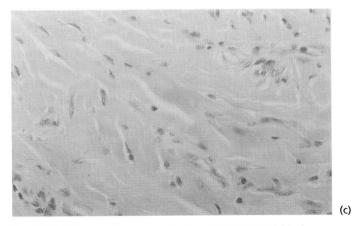
(c)

**Fig. 11.170** (a) Desmoplastic melanoma. (Courtesy of F. Rongioletti, Italy.) (b, c) Histology—case shown in (a). (Courtesy F. Rongioletti.)

**Table 11.9** Differential diagnosis of melanocytic naevi from malignant melanoma of the nail solely by signs in the cornified layer/nail plate. (Adapted from Kerl *et al.* 1984.)

| Junctional and compound melanocytic naevi | Subungual melanoma |
| --- | --- |
| Modest numbers of melanocytes and melanin granules | Abundant melanocytes and melanin granules |
| No or few, mostly small clumps of melanocytes with uniform shape | Large clumps of melanocytes with marked variation in size and shape |
| Usually no atypical melanocytes | Usually atypical melanocytes |
| Melanin granules distributed focally and in vertical or oblique columns | Melanin in diffuse distribution |
| More melanin than melanocytes | Melanin as prominent as melanocytes |
| No S-100 positive cells in nail plate | S-100 and HMB45 positive cells in nail plate |

hyperchromatic nuclei. Serial sections increase the likelihood of detecting limited areas with more pronounced hyperplasia of atypical melanocytes that may be seen in suprabasal layers and exhibit large, hyperchromatic, pleomorphic nuclei. Mitoses are very rare. There may be a sparse mononuclear infiltrate beneath the lesion but it is often inconspicuous. Although macrosopically, visible, the melanin is frequently less conspicuous in histological sections, even when Fontana-stained. Clear-cut *in situ* subungual melanoma usually shows junctional nests of melanoma cells.

Histopathology of Hutchinson's melanotic whitlow is virtually identical with the lentiginous pattern of acrolentiginous melanoma *in situ* of palms and soles (Kerl *et al.* 1984). Atypical melanocytes, often polygonal or even dendritic, are dispersed mainly in the basal layer of the periungual epidermis with relatively few cells being localized suprabasally.

Histopathology is compulsory for the diagnosis of any melanin-induced pigmentation in, under, and around the nail. Both the biopsy techniques (Baran & Haneke 1984; Baran & Kechijian 1989; Haneke 2000) and histological techniques, numbers of serial and step sections as well as the expertise of the investigating dermatopathologist are crucial for the correct diagnosis. However, the clinician is probably the most important person, because he or she has to decide on whether to biopsy or not, how to do it, to whom to send the specimen and to carefully or properly mark the tissue so that orientation will be possible in the laboratory. Neither gender, nor localization, nor age must influence the decision for biopsy since subungual melanomas do occur on fingers with aesthetic importance as well as in children (Kato *et al.* 1989).

In conclusion, the pathologist must know the details of the clinical picture, and the clinician must be wary of benign histological report in any subungual lesion showing Hutchinson's sign (Clark *et al.* 1979).

## Metastasis (Fig. 11.171)

Ungual melanomas are generally assumed to have a poor prognosis. This is due to the delay in diagnosis which in turn, is the cause for the presentation of very thick melanomas in many patients. The appearance of pigmented streaks in the nail plates is an unusual metastatic manifestation of malignant melanoma (Retsas & Samman 1983). In a cohort of 40 patients with subungual melanoma, 31 were in clinical stage I, and nine in stage

II. 35 patients were treated with amputation and 33 of them also underwent regional lymph node dissection. Only one patient in clinical stage I already had lymph node metastases whereas all stage II patients had positive lymph nodes. Elective lymph node dissection was therefore not supported for clinical stage I (Rodriguez-Cuevas & Luna-Perez 1993). We have therefore adopted the sentinel lymph node dissection for invasive subungual melanoma (Haneke *et al.* 1999).

*The necessity for lymph node dissection and its timing is controversial (Fortner* et al. *1964; Goldsmith 1979; Glat et al. 1996). Recently the use of 'sentinel node' intraoperative biopsy has shown promising results to determine whether lymph node dissection should be carried out (Jigalin & Mainusch 1999).*

Adjuvant therapies including isolated regional perfusion with cytotoxic drugs (Baas *et al.* 1989) did not improve the survival rate.

## Prognosis of subungual melanoma

The diagnosis of ungual melanomas is commonly delayed by 18 to 30 months, fingernail and pigmented tumours are usually treated earlier. Hence it follows that the prognosis of toenail melanomas is worse than that of fingernails.

Recently reported series of ungual melanomas (Table 11.10) have shown many patients with advanced invasive tumours and that many of these had been inadequately biopsied prior to definitive therapy. Two independent series reporting 124 British nail melanoma patients had a mean Breslow depth of 4.7 mm giving evidence of an apalling neglect by patients and physicians of nail lesions. These studies also demonstrated that tumour thickness is the single most important prognostic factor on which further significant factors such as ulceration, mitotic activity and vascular invasion depend. At the time of treatment, the melanoma subtype itself, whether acral lentiginous, superficial spreading, or nodular melanoma is not significantly associated with prognosis although acral lentiginous melanomas often have a history of many years or even decades and the development of nodular ungual melanomas is frequently very rapid.

The experience from recently published series of thick (sub)ungual melanomas is in contrast to our own experience with more than 20 *in situ* and early subungual melanomas.

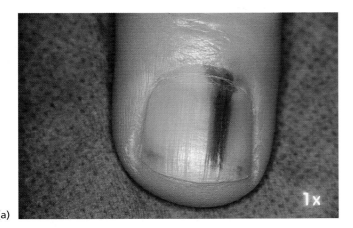

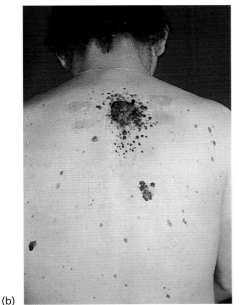

(a)

(b)

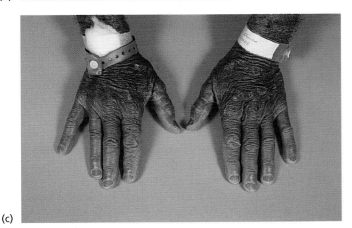

(c)

**Fig. 11.171** Metastatic melanoma—longitudinal bluish melanonychia which does not reach the free edge. (b) Melanoma of the back with satellites—case shown in (a). (c) Metastatic melanoma—diffuse pigmentation of the skin. (Courtesy of R. Sinclair, Australia.)

**Table 11.10** Survival rates of ungual melanomas.

| Reference | Period | % Survival |
|---|---|---|
| Das Gupta & Brasfield 1965 | 5 years | 38 |
| Graham 1973 | 5 years | 50 |
| Panizzon & Krebs 1980 | 5 years | 25 |
| Patterson & Helwig 1980 | 5 years | 16 |
| Krementz et al. 1982 | 5 years | 63 |
| Takematsu et al. 1985 | 5 years | 40 |
| Blessing et al. 1991 | 5 years | 41 |
| Rigby et al. 1992 | 10 months | 29 |
| Paul et al. 1992 | 5 years | 51 (fingers 57) (toes 48) |
| | 10 years | 28 (fingers 41) (toes 22) |
| Glat et al. 1995 | 5 years | 66 |
| Banfield et al. 1999 | 5 years | 51 |
| Metzger et al. 1998 | 5 years | 68.5 |

**Table 11.11** Correspondence between clinical warning signs of subungual and cutaneous melanoma (after de Berker).

| Subungual melanoma | Cutaneous melanoma |
|---|---|
| *Anatomical criteria* | *ABCD/Glasgow* |
| • Hutchinson's sign | B/D |
| • Nail dystrophy | E |
| • Pigment full lenth | Beware |
| | |
| *Melanocytic criteria* | |
| • >6 mm diameter | D |
| • Variegated colour | C |
| • Blurred edges | A/B |
| • Change or abrupt onset | Glasgow 1–3 |

ABCD/Glasgow differs from ABC rule for clinical detection of subungual melanoma (Levit et al. 2000).

However, any acquired longitudinal melanonychia as well as any periungual pigmentation no matter how light they might have been were totally removed and examined histopathologically using a large number of serial sections. Early treatment of lesions suggestive of melanoma is mandatory to improve the cure rate and to successfully use a more conservative surgical approach in order to avoid amputation. (Tables 11.11 & 11.12).

## Nail melanoma in childhood (Fig. 11.172)

Malignant melanoma is certainly exceptional in childhood. Lyall (1967) reported on a pigmented spot of the tip of the right middle fingernail of a 12 month male, not preceded by LM. Pensler *et al.* (1993) observed a case affecting a caucasian child (but not documented). Ruiz-Maldonado *et al.* (2001) observed a melanoma associated with a black toe nail in a hispanic 9-year-old child (Fig. 11.172). Goettmann-Bonvallot *et al.* (unpublished date) have seen the appearance of a melanoma in

| Treatment | Reference |
|---|---|
| *Surgery* | |
| Proximal amputation | Pack & Oropeza 1967; Papachristou & Fortner 1982 |
| Distal amputation | Finley *et al.* 1994; Glat *et al.* 1996; Quinn *et al.* 1996 |
| Local amputation | Saida & Oshima 1989; Banfield *et al.* 1998 |
| Nail ablation | Haneke & Binder 1978 |
| Mohs | Banfield *et al.* 1999 |
| Elective lymph node dissection | Kato *et al.* 1996; Quinn *et al.* 1996 |
| Sentinel node biopsy | Jigalin & Mainusch 1999 |
| | |
| *Adjuvant therapy* | |
| Chemotherapy | Kato *et al.* 1996 |
| • Dacarbazine | |
| • Ac. nitrosourea | |
| • Vincristine | |
| Limb perfusion therapy | Lingham *et al.* 1995 |
| Radiotherapy | Krige *et al.* 1995 |
| Other modalities | No reported experience in subungual melanoma |
| • Interferon | |
| • Interleukin | |
| • Vaccination therapy | |

**Table 11.12** Modalities of treatment of subungual melanoma. (After de Berker.)

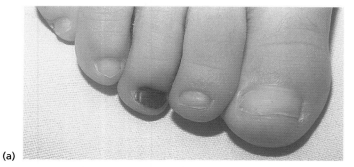

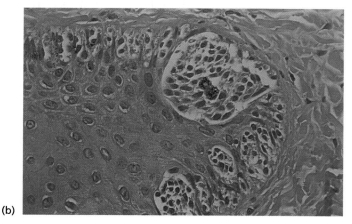

**Fig. 11.172** Nail melanoma in childhood. (Courtesy of R. Ruiz-Maldonado, Mexico DF.)

an 18-year-old girl presenting with a longitudinal melanonychia for several years.

By contrast, there are some reports of malignant melanoma in oriental children. Ohno *et al.* (1988) presented the case of

a 7-year-old girl with a LM and seen at age 27 with a deformed nail and Hutchinson's sign. Histology revealed malignant melanoma and lymph node metastases. Mori and Fukui (1993) reported a case of LM starting at age nine, following an injury at age four, which developed into malignant melanoma at age 32. Uchiyama and Minemura (1979) observed a sudden increase in pigmentation at the base of the right middle fingernail, which appeared one month after birth. It then developed into melanoma with lymph node metastasis following a minor injury at the age of seven years. All except three cases of melanoma *in situ* of the nail apparatus which have been reported in Japan developed from pigmented bands in the nail after the age of 20 (Saida and Oshima 1988). Kato *et al.* (1989) described a 2-year-old child with melanoma *in situ* as did Hori *et al.* (1988) a 3-year-old girl, and Kiriyu (1998) in the finger nail of another 3-year-old girl.

## Nail melanoma in deeply pigmented races

LM is found in 90–100% of individuals in deeply pigmented races. The common presenting sign of subungual melanoma is an alteration in colour intensity or width of LM.

However, the pigmented band shows an indistinct border, sometimes widens rapidly, and the longitudinal streak becomes jet black rather than the normal brown. The diagnosis may be aided by comparing them with the brown streaks in other nails or by occurrence of Hutchinson's sign.

## Nail melanoma in transplant recipients

Of clinical importance is the development of malignant melanomas in transplant recipients. Merkle *et al.* (1991) reported a slowly enlarging tumour on the tip of the middle finger in a 59-year-old man. This verrucous and erosive nonpigmented tumour involving the distal nail bed was a nodular malignant melanoma in a patient treated with corticosteroids and azathioprine and who had undergone kidney transplantation 7 years earlier.

The diagnosis of malignant melanoma may be made only by maintaining a high index of suspicion with any persistent nail bed lesion, irrespective of the presence of pigmentation. Incisional biopsy should be performed in all suspected cases, followed by definitive treatment (Winslet and Tejan 1990).

Recent advances in the management of malignant melanoma have been made through knowledge of determinants such as primary depth of invasion, thickness, presence of ulceration and status of regional lymph nodes (Daly *et al.* 1987).

## Incident light microscopy of pigmented nail disorders (J.F. Kreusch, Luebeck, Germany)

Incident light microscopy (ILM) permits reliable atraumatic differentiation of pigmented disorders of the nail (Kreusch & Rassner 1991a, 1992). However, features of subungual melanoma differ from the ones encountered in tumours on regular skin, e.g. asymmetry and diameter are not applicable to subungual tumours. Criteria for identifying lesions of melanocytic origin are simple and help to differentiate non-melanocytic tumours from being suspected as melanoma.

The instrument used should magnify 40-fold at least. Stereoscopic view is particularly helpful as it allows identification of the pigment bearing stratum of the nail plate rendering valuable diagnostic information. A portable stereomicroscope with magnifications to be varied between 20–60-fold is shown in Fig. 11.173a. Operation microscopes may be used as well. However, they are very expensive and cannot be handled easily. Subungual haemorrhage invariably shows colours of fresh or clotted blood, varying between bright red and violet to black (Fig. 11.173b,c). Centrally the pigment is homogenous. Round droplets are present near the edges or splinters of blood are included in the nail plate.

Pigmentation in secondary fungal infection varies between a reddish brown for trichophyton infections and greenish-yellowish black for *Candida* and *Pseudomonas*. In onychomycosis almost invariably the nail plate shows whitish streaks at the edge of the lesion corresponding to destruction of keratin caused by the fungi (Fig. 11.173d,e).

As in cutaneous melanocytic tumours subungual naevi and melanoma display the typical colours of melanin; e.g. brown to grey to black (Kreusch & Rassner 1991b). Particles resembling pepper-grains are visible if the nail is viewed at sufficient magnification (at least 30-fold), their diameter is approx. 20 μm. With a stereomicroscope the location of the corpuscles within the nail plate can be determined easily by adjusting the focal plane up and down through the nail. This helps to define the site for taking a biopsy of the nail matrix. If the granules are encountered in the upper or lower strata of the nail plate, the biopsy has to be taken from the proximal or distal nail matrix, respectively.

It is most important that even in clinically 'amelanotic' melanoma corpuscles containing melanin can be found microscopically (Fig. 11.173f,g).

As naevi and melanoma are mostly located within the nail matrix corpuscles with colours of melanin in the nail just give the clue to the cell type responsible for the pigmentation. It is not possible to differentiate subungual melanocytic naevi and early subungual melanoma. However, microscopy of the nail helps to exclude many other sources of pigment. Thus, unnecessary biopsies and destruction of the growth area of the nail can be avoided.

## References

Kreusch, J. & Rassner, G. (1991a) *Auflichtmikroskopie pigmentierter Hauttumoren. Ein Bildatlas.* G. Thieme Verlag, Stuttgart.
Kreusch, J. & Rassner, G. (1991b) Standardisierte auflichtmikroskopische Unterscheidung melanozytischer und nichtmelanozytischer Pigmentmale. *Hautarzt* **42**, 77–83.
Kreusch, J. & Rassner, G. (1992) Auflichtmikroskopische Beurteilung pigmentierter Nagel veränderungen. *Deutsche Dermatologie* **40**, 1–6.

## Spontaneous regression of melanocytic lesions

### Longitudinal melanonychia

Longitudinal melanonychia, as a sign of the 'naevoid nail area melanosis' observed in Japanese children may demonstrate spontaneous regression and even disappearance (Kikuchi *et al.* 1992) (Fig. 11.174). The histological features of these pigmented lesions are lacking. LM from a matrix naevus was also observed to fade with time (Tosti *et al.* 1994) (Fig. 11.175). Complete disappearance of LM occurring in a 4-year-old Caucasian has been observed after 16 years in a patient of Grosshans (1994) (Fig. 11.176).

### Melanoma of the nail apparatus

The pathologists now more readily recognize the subtle features of histological regression since step sections through the entire block are more often being done. Regression was found in 27.1% of SSM and 17.4% of lentigo maligna melanomas and was not identified in nodular melanomas (Trau *et al.* 1983). Histological regression, however, played only a marginal role as a prognostic factor in SSM, deriving its significance mainly from its close relationship to the thickness of the melanoma.

Clinical examples of spontaneous regression of malignant melanomas of the nail apparatus are exceptional (Fig. 11.177) and have not been histologically documented.

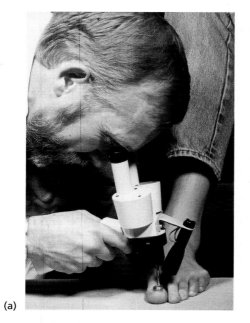
(a)

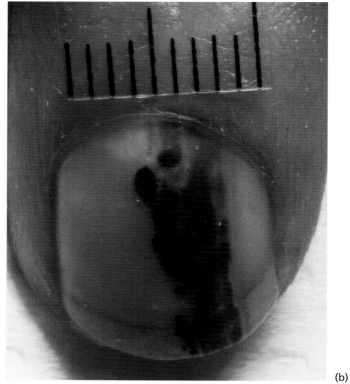
(b)

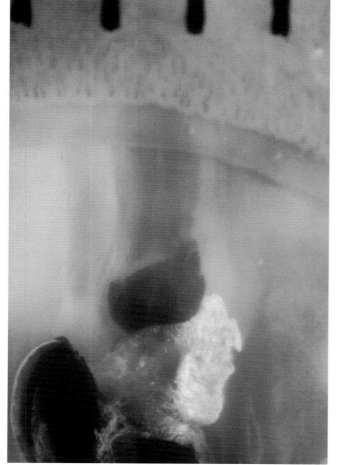
(c)

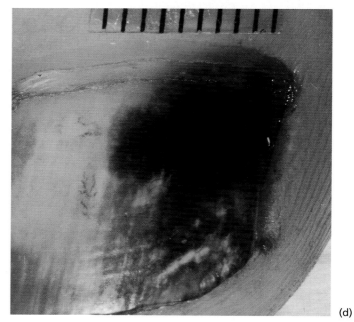
(d)

**Fig. 11.173**  (a) Dermoscopy—inspection of toenail with a portable stereomicroscope according to Kreusch. (b) Subungual haemorrhage of a fingernail—clinical view. (c) Dermoscopy—incident light microscopy of haemorrhage: colours vary between red and black. No granular structure can be seen (bars at 1 mm intervals). (d) Pigmented onychomycosis of toenail (*T. rubrum*). (From Georg Thieme Verlag, Stuttgart.) (*cont'd*)

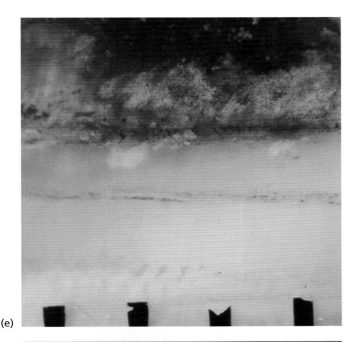

(e)

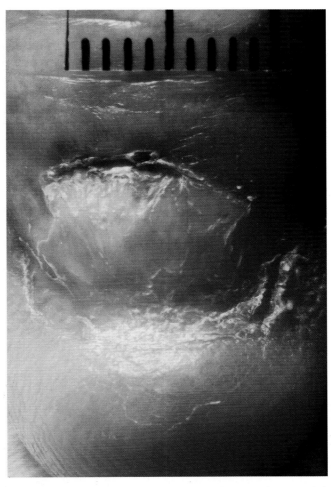

(f)

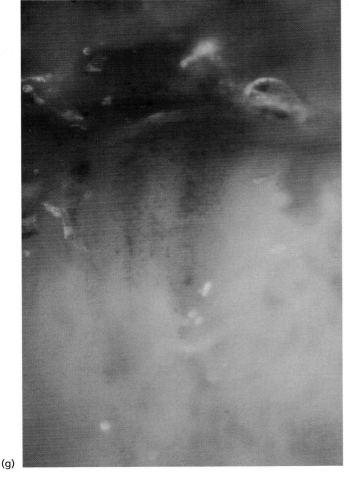

(g)

**Fig. 11.173** (cont'd) (e) Dermoscopy—microscopic view of (d). Brownish pigment which cannot be resolved into single corpuscles (bars at 1 mm intervals). Note the whitish streaks within the nail keratin. They do not extend under the cuticle. (f) Loss of the nail plate due to subungual melanoma. Clinically, barely any pigment is visible. (g) Dermoscopy—high-power microscopic view of (f) (×60). Short streaks of granular pigmentation at the edge of the cuticle. The colour is typical for melanin. This was the clue for the melanocytic origin of the process. (a–g courtesy of J. Kreusch, Germany.)

## References

Achten, G. (1982) What's new about normal and pathologic nail. In: *XVI International Congress of Dermatology Abstracts Tokyo*, pp. 17–18.

Alkiewicz, J. & Pfister, R. (1976) *Atlas der Nagelkrankheiten.* Schattauer Verlag, Stuttgart.

Asahina, A., Matsuyama, T., Tsuchida, T. *et al.* (1993) Two cases of infantile subungual pigmented nevi with Hutchinson's sign. *Japanese Journal of Dermatology* **99**, 899–906.

Banfield, C.C. & Dawber, R.P.R. (1999) Nail melanoma: a review of the literature with recommendations to improve patient management. *British Journal of Dermatology* **141**, 628–632.

Banfield, C.C., Redburn, J.C. & Dawber, R.P.R. (1998) The incidence and prognosis of nail apparatus melanoma. A retrospective study of

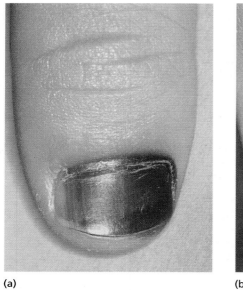

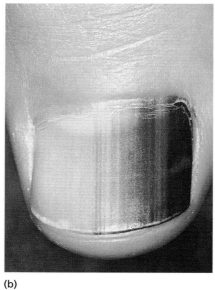

(a)                                    (b)

**Fig. 11.174** (a) Congenital melanonychia with pseudo-Hutchinson's sign. (b) Same patient several years later. (Courtesy of I. Kikuchi, Japan.)

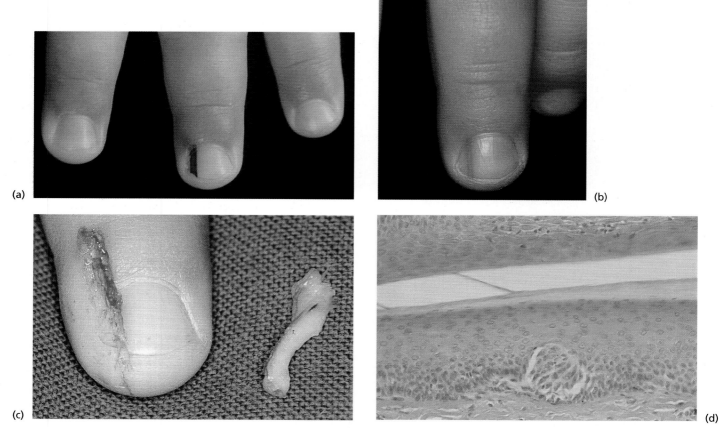

(a)                                                                    (b)

(c)                                                                    (d)

**Fig. 11.175** (a) Longitudinal melanonychia in a 9-month-old baby. (b) Finger shown in (a) 4 months afterwards. Note the fading of the band. (c) Lateral–longitudinal excisional biopsy. (d) Histology showing a typical naevus—case shown in (a). (Courtesy of A. Tosti, Bologna, Italy.)

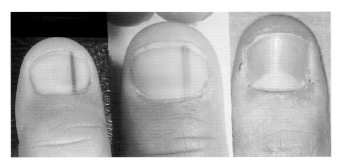

**Fig. 11.176** Young child presenting with longitudinal melanonychia—progressive fading disappearance at age 19. (Courtesy of E. Grosshans, Strasbourg, France.)

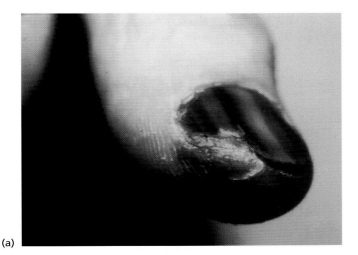

(a)

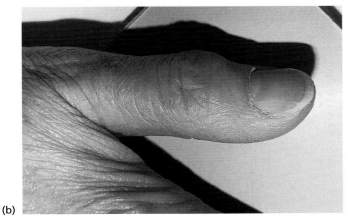

(b)

**Fig. 11.177** (a) Clinical presentation of subungual melanoma with Hutchinson's sign. (b) Spontaneous resolution five years afterwards. (Courtesy Charpentier, France.)

105 patients in four English regions. *British Journal of Dermatology* **139**, 276–279.

Banfield, C.C., Dawber, R.P., Walker, N.P. *et al.* (1999) Mohs micrographic surgery for the treatment of *in situ* nail apparatus melanoma: a case report. *Journal of the American Academy of Dermatology* **40**, 98–99.

Baas, P.C., Hoekstra, H.J., Koops, S.H. *et al.* (1989) Isolated regional perfusion in the treatment of subungual melanoma. *Archives of Surgery* **124**, 373–376.

Baran, R. (1987) Frictional longitudinal melanonychia: a new entity. *Dermatologica* **174**, 280–284.

Baran, R. (1990) Nail biting and picking as a possible cause of longitudinal melanonychia. *Dermatologica* **181**, 126–128.

Baran, R. & Barrière, H. (1986) Longitudinal melanonychia with spreading pigmentation in Laugier–Hunziker syndrome, a report of two cases. *British Journal of Dermatology* **115**, 707–710.

Baran, R. & Haneke, E. (1984) Diagnostik und Therapie der streifenförmigen Nagelpigmentierung. *Hautarzt* **35**, 359–365.

Baran, R. & Kechijian, P. (1989) Longitudinal melanonychia (melanonychia striata): diagnosis and management. *Journal of the American Academy of Dermatology* **21**, 1165–1175.

Baran, R. & Kechijian, P. (1996) Hutchinson's sign: a reappraisal. *Journal of the American Academy of Dermatology* **34**, 87–90.

Bayerl, C. & Moll, I. (1993) Longitudinal melanonychia with Hutchinson sign in a boxer. *Hautarzt* **44**, 476–479.

Beltrani, V.P. & Scher, R.K. (1991) Evaluation and management of melanonychia striata in a patient receiving phototherapy. *Archives of Dermatology* **127**, 319–332.

de Berker, D. (1999) Treatment of the black nail. In: *Proceedings of the European Nail Society*, Amsterdam.

Bisht, D.B. & Singh, S.S. (1962) Pigmented bands on nails, a new sign in malnutrition. *Lancet* **1**, 1175–1181.

Black, W.C. & Wiggino, C. (1985) Melanoma among Southwestern Indians. *Cancer* **55**, 2899–2902.

Blessing, K., Kernohan, N.M. & Park, K.G.M. (1991) Subungual malignant melanoma. Clinicopathological features of 100 cases. *Histopathology* **19**, 425–429.

Branco Ferreira, M.J., Macedo Ferreira, A., Pinto Soares, A. *et al.* (1999) Laugier–Hunziker syndrome: case report and treatment with the Q-switched Nd–YAG laser. *Journal of the European Academy of Dermatology and Venereology* **12**, 171–173.

Cachia, A.R. & Kedziora, A.M. (1999) Subungual malignant melanoma with cartilaginous differentiation. *American Journal of Dermatopathology* **21**, 165–169.

Cavelier-Balloy, B., Aractingi, S., Verola, O. *et al.* (1992) Naevus géant congénital avec naevi bleus multiples disséminés [poster]. *Journées Dermatologiques de Paris* **115**, 18–21.

Ceballos, P.I. & Barnhill, R.L. (1993) Spontaneous regression of cutaneous tumors. In: *Advances in Dermatology*, Vol. 8 (eds Callen, Dahl, Golitz, Greenway, Schachner). Mosby, St Louis.

Clark, W.H., Bernardino, E.A., Reed, R.J. & Kopf, A.W. (1979) Acral lentiginous melanomas. In: *Human Malignant Melanoma* (eds W.H. Clark & L.I. Goldman, Mastrangero), pp. 109–124. Grune & Stratton, New York.

Collins, R.J. (1984) Melanomas in the Chinese of Hong Kong. *Cancer* **54**, 1482–1483.

Coskey, R.J., Magnel, T.D. & Bernarcki, E.G. (1983) Congenital subungual naevus. *Journal of the American Academy of Dermatology* **9**, 747–751.

Daly, J.M., Berlin, R. & Urmacher, C. (1987) Subungual melanoma, a 25-year review of cases. *Journal of Surgery and Oncology* **35**, 107–112.

Das Gupta, T. & Brasfield, R. (1965) Subungual melanoma. *Annals of Surgery* **161**, 545–552.

Diepgen, T.L, Schell, H., Müller, A. *et al.* (1991) Maligne Melanome an den Akren-Häufigkeit, Klinik und Prognose. *Zeitschrift für Hautkrankheiten* **66**, 631–636.

Dupré, A. & Viraben, R. (1990) Laugier's disease. *Dermatologica* **181**, 183–186.

Engelmann, L. & Kunze, J. (1992) Laugier–Hunziker–Baran Syndrom mit ungewöhnlichem Verteilungsmuster. *Zentralblatt für Haut- und Geschlechtskrankheiten* **161**, 22.

Feibleman, C.E., Stoll, H. & Maize, J.C. (1980) Melanomas of the palm, sole, and nailbed, a clinicopathologic study. *Cancer* **46**, 2492–2504.

Finley, R.K. III, Driscoll, D.L., Blumenson, L.E. & Karakousis, C.P. (1994) Subungual melanoma: an eighteen-year review. *Surgery* **116**, 96–100.

Fortner, J.G., Booher, R.J. & Pack, G.T. (1964) Results of groin dissection for malignant melanoma in 220 patients. *Surgery* **55**, 485–494.

Gallais, V., Lacour, J.P.H., Perrin, C. *et al.* (1992) Acral hyperpigmentated macules and longitudinal melanonychia in AIDS patients. *British Journal of Dermatology* **126**, 387–391.

Glat, P.M., Shapiro, R.L., Roses, D.F., Harris, M.N. & Grossman, J.A.I. (1995) Management considerations for melanonychia striata and melanoma of the hand. *Hand Clinics* **11**, 183–189.

Glat, P.M., Spector, J.A., Roses, D.F. *et al.* (1996) The management of pigmented lesions of the nail bed. *Annals of Plastic Surgery* **37**, 125–134.

Goettmann-Bonvallot, S., André, J. & Bélaich, S. (1999) Longitudinal melanonychia in children: A clinical and histopathological study of 40 cases. *Journal of the American Academy of Dermatology* **41**, 17–22.

Goldsmith, H.S. (1979) Melanoma: an overview. *CA Cancer Journal for Clinicians* **29**, 194–215.

Graham, W.P. (1973) Subungual melanoma. *Pennsylvania Medicine* **76**, 56.

Gray, M.H., Smoller, B.R., McNult, N.S. *et al.* (1990) Neurofibromas and neurotized melanocytic nevi are immunohistochemically distinct neoplasm. *American Journal of Dermatopathology* **12**, 234–241.

Gregorcyk, S., Shelton, R.M., Ladaga, L.E. *et al.* (1996) Pathologic fracture secondary to subungual melanoma. *Journal of Surgery and Oncology* **61**, 230–233.

Grosshans, E. (1994) Mélanines, mélanomes. *Nouvelle Dermatologie* **13**, 497–498.

Haneke, E. (1986) Pathogenese der Nageldystrophie beim subungualen Melanom. *Verhandlungen der Deutschen Gesellschaft für Pathologie* **70**, 484.

Haneke, E. (1991) Laugier-Hunziker-Baran-Syndrom. *Hautarzt* **42**, 512–515.

Haneke, E. (1998) Silver nitrate staining of the nail. *Collegium Dermato-Pathologicum*, Turin.

Haneke, E. (1999) Operative Therapie akraler und subungualer Melanome. *Fortschritte der operativen und onkologischen Dermatologie* **15** (Suppl.), 210–214.

Haneke, E. (2000) Clinical judgement. A lesson derived from a subungual melanoma. *Dermatopathology Practical and Conceptual* **6**, 73–76.

Haneke, E. (2001) Tangential matrix excision for longitudinal melanonychia (submitted).

Haneke, E. & Binder, D. (1978) Subunguales Melanom mit streifiger Nagelpigmentierung. *Hautarzt* **29**, 389–391.

Haneke, E., Mainusch, O. & Hilker, O. (1998) Subunguale Tumoren: Keratoakanthom, Neurofibrom, Nagelbett-Melanom. *Zeitschrift für Dermatologie* **184**, 86–102.

Hara, M., Kato, T. & Tagami, H. (1993) Amelanotic acral melanoma masquerading as fibrous histiocytic tumours. *Acta Dermato-Venereologica* **73**, 283–285.

Hori, Y., Yamada, A., Tanizaki, T. *et al.* (1988) Pigmented small tumors. *Japanese Journal of Pediatric Dermatology* **7**, 117–120.

Hutchinson, J. (1886) Melanosis often not black, melanotic whitlow. *British Medical Journal* **1**, 149.

Iyadomi, M., Ohtsubo, H., Gotoh, Y. *et al.* (1998) Neurotropic melanoma invading the median nerve. *Journal of Dermatology* **25**, 379–383.

Jigalin, A. & Mainusch, O. (1999) Selektive Schildwächter-Lymphknoten dissektion. *Zeitschrift für Dermatologie* **185**, 27–30.

Kamino, H. & Ackerman, A.B. (1981) Malignant melanoma *in situ*. In: *Pathology of Malignant Melanoma* (ed. A.B. Ackerman). Masson, New York.

Karakayali, G., Güngör, E., Lenk, N. *et al.* (1999) Neurofibromatosis and cutaneous melanoma—coincidence or association? *Journal of the European Academy of Dermatology and Venereology* **12**, 190–192.

Kato, I., Usuba, Y., Takematsu, H. *et al.* (1989) A rapidly growing pigmented nail streak resulting in diffuse melanosis of the nail. *Cancer* **64**, 2191–2197.

Kato, I., Suetake, T., Sugiyma, Y. *et al.* (1996) Epidemiology and prognosis of subungual melanoma in 34 Japanese patients. *British Journal of Dermatology* **134**, 383–387.

Kawabata, Y., Ohara, K., Hino, H. *et al.* (1999) Dermatoscopic features of malignant melanoma of the nail apparatus *in situ* distinguish it from pigmented naevi of the nail apparatus. *Japanese Journal of Dermatology* **109**, 1323–1332.

Kechijian, P. (1991) Subungual melanoma *in situ* presenting as longitudinal melanonychia in a patient with familial dysplastic nevi. *Journal of the American Academy of Dermatology* **24**, 283.

Kerl, H., Trau, H. & Ackerman, A.B. (1984) Differentiation of melanocytic nevi from malignant melanomas in palms, soles, and nail solely by signs in the cornified layer of the epidermis. *American Journal of Dermatopathology* **6** (Suppl. 1), 159–161.

Kikuchi, I., Inoue, S., Sakaguchi, E. *et al.* (1993) Regressing nevoid nail area melanosis in childhood. *Dermatology* **186**, 88–93.

Kiryu, H. (1998) Malignant melanoma *in situ* arising in the nail unit of a child. *Journal of Dermatology* **25**, 41–44.

Kopf, A.W. (1981) Hutchinson's sign of subungual malignant melanoma. *American Journal of Dermatopathology* **3**, 201–202.

Kopf, A.W. & Waldo, E. (1980) Melanonychia striata. *Australasian Journal of Dermatology* **21**, 59–70.

Krementz, E.T., Reed, R.J., Coleman, W.P. *et al.* (1982) Acral lentiginous melanoma: a clinico-pathologic entity. *Annals of Surgery* **195**, 632.

Krige, J.E.J., Hudson, D.A., Johnson, C.A. *et al.* (1995) Subungual melanoma. *South African Journal of Surgery* **33**, 10–15.

Leauté-Labrèze, C., Bioulac-Sage, P. & Taïeb, A. (1996) Longitudinal melanonychia in children. A study of eight cases. *Archives of Dermatology* **132**, 167–169.

Leppard, B., Sanderson, K.V., Behan, F. (1974) Subungual malignant melanoma. Difficulty in diagnosis. *British Medical Journal* **1**, 310–312.

Levit, E.K., Kagen, M.H., Scher, R.K. *et al.* (2000) The ABC rule for clinical detection of subungual melanoma. *Journal of the American Academy of Dermatology* **42**, 269–274.

Libow, L.F., Casey, T.J. & Varela, C.D. (1995) Congenital subungual nevus in a black infant. *Cutis* **56**, 154–156.

Lingam, M.K., McKay, A.J., Mackie, R.M. *et al.* (1995) Single-centre prospective study of isolated limb perfusion with melphalan in the treatment of subungual malignant melanoma. *British Journal of Surgery* **82**, 1343–1345.

Lyall, D. (1967) Malignant melanoma in infancy. *Journal of the American Medical Association* **202**, 1153.

Lycka, B., Krywonis, N. & Hordinsky, M. (1991) Abnormal nevoblast migration mimicking neurofibromatosis. *Archives of Dermatology* **127**, 1702–1704.

Merkle, T., Landthaler, M., Eckert, F. *et al.* (1991) Acral verrucous malignant melanoma in an immunosuppressed patient after kidney transplantation. *Journal of the American Academy of Dermatology* **24**, 505–506.

Metzger, S., Ellwanger, U., Stroebel, W. *et al.* (1998) Extent and consequences of physician delay in the diagnosis of acral melanoma. *Melanoma Research* **8**, 181–186.

Milton, G.W., Shaw, H.M. & McCarthy, W.H. (1985) Subungual malignant melanoma. A disease entity separate from other forms of cutaneous melanoma. *Australasian Journal of Dermatology* **26**, 61–64.

Miura, S. & Jimbow, K. (1985) Clinical characteristics of subungual melanoma in Japan, case report and questionnaire survey of 108 cases. *Journal of Dermatology (Tokyo)* **12**, 393–402.

Mooney, E. & Bennet, R.G. (1988) Periungual hyperpigmentation mimicking Hutchinson's sign associated with minocycline administration. *Journal of Dermatologic Surgery and Oncology* **14**, 1011–1013.

Mori, T. & Fukui, V. (1993) A case of malignant melanoma originating from subungual pigmented lines which has existed since childhood. *Japanese (Rinsho) Dermatology* **35**, 808–809.

Nogaret, J.M., André, J., Parent, D. *et al.* (1986) Le mélanome des extrémités, diagnostic méconnu et traitement délicat. Revue des 20 observations. *Acta Chirurgica Belgica* **86**, 238–244.

Obata, M., Kato, T. & Seiji, M. (1979) Eight cases of subungual melanoma. *Japanese Journal of Clinical Dermatology* **33**, 515–521.

Ogose, A., Emura, I., Iwabuchi, Y. *et al.* (1998) Malignant melanoma extending along the ulnar, median, and musculocutaneous nerves: a case report. *Journal of Hand Surgery* **23A**, 875–878.

Ohno, M., Veda, M. & Mishima, Y. (1988) Subungual malignant melanoma. Especially on precursor lesions of ALM and nodular melanoma. *Hifu Rinsko* **30**, 1041–1048.

Ohtsuka, H., Hori, Y. & Ando, M. (1978) Naevus of the little finger with a remarkable nail deformity. *Plastic and Reconstructive Surgery* **61**, 108–111.

Oropeza, R. (1976) Melanomas of special sites. In: *Cancer of the Skin*, Vol. 2 (eds R. Andrade, S.L. Gumpert, G.L. Popkin & T.D. Rees), pp. 974–987. Saunders, Philadelphia.

O'Toole, E.A., Stephens, R., Young, M. *et al.* (1995) Subungual melanoma: a relation to direct injury? *Journal of the American Academy of Dermatology* **33**, 525–528.

Pack, G.T. & Oropeza, R. (1967) Subungual melanoma. *Surgery, Gynecology and Obstetrics* **124**, 571–582.

Panizzon, R. & Krebs, A. (1980) Das subunguale maligne Melanom. *Hautarzt* **31**, 132–140.

Papachristou, D.N. & Fortner, J.G. (1982) Melanoma arising under the nail. *Journal of Surgery and Oncology* **21**, 219–222.

Patterson, R. & Helwig, E.B. (1980) Subungual melanoma, a clinical pathological study. *Cancer* **46**, 2074–2087.

Paul, E., Kleiner, H. & Bodeker, R.H. (1992) Epidemiologie und Prognose subungualer Melanome. *Hautarzt* **43**, 286–290.

Pearce, R.L. (1995) Subungual desmoplastic melanoma in an Aboriginal woman. *Medical Journal of Australia* **162**, 611–612.

Pensler, J.M., Hijjawi, J. & Palle, A.S. (1993) Melanoma in prepubertal children. *International Surgery* **78**, 247–249.

Perrin, C.H., Michiels, J.F., Pisani, A. *et al.* (1997) Anatomic distribution of melanocytes in normal nail unit. An immunohistochemical investigation. *American Journal of Dermatopathology* **19**, 462–467.

Pomerance, J., Kopf, A.W., Ramos, L. *et al.* (1994) A large pigmented nail bed lesion in a child. *Annals of Plastic Surgery* **33**, 80–82.

Quinn, N.J., Thompson, J.E., Crotty, K. *et al.* (1996) Subungual melanoma of the hand. *Journal of Hand Surgery* **21A**, 506–511.

Rathi, S., Dogra, D. & Khanna, N. (1995) Subungual malignant melanoma clinically resembling granuloma pyogenicum. *Indian Journal of Dermatology, Venereology and Leprosy* **61**, 373–374.

Retsas, S. & Samman, P.D. (1983) Pigment streaks in the nail plate due to secondary malignant melanoma. *British Journal of Dermatology* **108**, 367–370.

Rigby, H.S. & Briggs, J.C. (1992) Subungual melanoma, a clinicopathological study of 24 cases. *British Journal of Plastic Surgery* **45**, 275–278.

Roberts, A.H.N. (1984) Subungual melanoma following a single injury. *Journal of Hand Surgery* **9B**, 328–330.

Rodriguez-Cuevas, S. & Luna-Perez, P. (1993) Subungual melanoma. Is elective regional lymph node dissection mandatory? *Journal of Experimental Clinical Cancer Research* **12**, 173–178.

Rongioletti, F., Gambini, C., Semino, M. *et al.* (1995) Mélanome sous-unguéal, desmoplastique et neurotrope. *Annales de Dermatologie et de Vénéréologie* **122**, 707–710.

Ruiz-Maldonado, R. *et al.* (2001) Subungual melanoma in a 3-year-old boy (in press).

Saccone, P.G. & Rayan, G.M. (1993) Subungual malignant degeneration following chronic perionychial infection. *Orthopedic Reviews* **22**, 623–626.

Saida, T. & Oshima, Y. (1988) Clinical and histopathological characteristics of the early lesions of subungual melanoma. *Cancer* **63**, 556–560.

Sau, P., McMarlin, S.L., Sperling, L.C. *et al.* (1994) Bowen's disease of the nail bed and periungual area: a clinicopathological analysis of seven cases. *Archives of Dermatology* **130**, 204–209.

Shah, M.P. & Goldsmith, H.S. (1971) Malignant melanoma in the North American Negro. *Surgery, Gynecology and Obstetrics* **133**, 437–439.

Shelley, W.B., Rawnsley, H.M. & Pillsbury, D.M. (1964) Post-irradiation melanonychia. *Archives of Dermatology* **90**, 174–176.

Shukla, V.K. & Hughes, L.E. (1989) Differential diagnosis of subungual melanoma from a surgical point of view. *British Journal of Surgery* **76**, 1156–1160.

Sondergaard, K. (1983) Histological type and biological behavior of primary cutaneous malignant melanoma. 2. An analysis of 86 cases located on so-called acral regions as plantar, palmar, and subparungual areas. *Virchows Archiv. A, Pathological Anatomy and Histopathology* **401**, 333–343.

Soyer, H.P. & Kerl, H. (1984) Congenital blue naevus with lymph node metastases and Klippel–Trenaunay syndrome. In: *European Society of Pediatric Dermatology Clinical Case Reports. Dia-Klinik*, pp. 28–29.

Stenier, C., de Beer, P., Creusy, C., Wiart, T. & Driba, M. (1992) Maladie de Laugier isolée de l'ongle. *Nouvelle Dermatologie* 11, 24–26.

Takahashi, M. & Seiji, M. (1983) Acral melanoma in Japan. *Pigment Cell* 6, 150–166.

Takematsu, H., Obata, M., Tomita, Y. *et al.* (1985) Subungual melanoma. A clinicopathologic study of 16 Japanese cases. *Cancer* 55, 2725.

Tomizawa, K. (2000) Early malignant melanoma manifested as longitudinal melanonychia: subungual melanoma may arise from suprabasal melanocytes. *British Journal of Dermatology* 143, 431–434.

Tosti, A., Baran, R., Morelli, R. *et al.* (1994) Progressive fading of longitudinal melanonychia due to a nail matrix melanocytic nevus in a child. *Archives of Dermatology* 130, 1076–1077.

Tosti, A., Baran, R., Piraccini, B.M. *et al.* (1996) Nail matrix nevi: a clinical and histopathological study of twenty-two patients. *Journal of the American Academy of Dermatology* 34, 765–767.

Tosti, A., Piraccini, B.M. & Baran, R. (1998) The melanocyte system of the nails and its disorders. In: *The Pigmentary System* (eds J.J. Nordlund, R.E. Boissy, V.J. Hearing, R. King & J.P. Ortonne), pp. 937–943. Oxford University Press, New York.

Trau, H., Kopf, A.W., Rigel, D.S. *et al.* (1983) Regression in malignant melanoma. *Journal of the American Academy of Dermatology* 8, 363–368.

Tran, A.T., Carlson, J.A., Basaca, P.C. *et al.* (1998) Cellular blue nevus with atypia (atypical cellular blue nevus): a clinicopathologic study of nine cases. *Journal of Cutaneous Pathology* 25, 252–258.

Uchiyama & Minemura (1979) Two cases of malignant melanoma in young persons. *Nippon Hifuka Gakkai Zasshi* 89, 668.

Vazquez, J., Peteiro, C. & Toribio, J. (1993) Enfermedad de Laugier-Hunziker. *Acta Dermato-Sifilitica* 84, 454–457.

Vidal, S., Sanz, A., Hernandez, B. *et al.* (1997) Subungual blue naevus. *British Journal of Dermatology* 137, 1023–1025.

Winslet, M. & Tejan, J. (1990) Subungual amelanotic melanoma: a diagnostic pitfall. *Postgraduate Medical Journal* 66, 200–202.

Wong, D.E., Brodkin, R., Rickert, R. & McFalls, S.G. (1991) Congenital melanonychia. *International Journal of Dermatology* 30, 278–280.

Yamamoto, O., Yoshinaga, K., Asahi, M. *et al.* (1999) A Laugier-Hunziker syndrome associated with esophageal melanocytosis. *Dermatology* 199, 162–164.

Zanone, M., Macchi, R., Sard, A. & Linri, A. (1993) Il melanoma maligno subunguale. *Minerva Ortopedica e Traumatologica* 44, 449–453.

# Index

Note: page numbers in *italic* refer to figures or tables.